Options for the Control of Influenza IV

Options for the Control
of Influenza IV

Proceedings of the World Congress on Options for the Control of Influenza IV
held in Crete, Greece 23rd – 28th September 2000

Editors:

Albert D.M.E. Osterhaus
Institute of Virology
Erasmus University Rotterdam
Dr. Molewaterplein 50
Rotterdam
The Netherlands

Nancy Cox
Influenza Branch
Centers for Disease Control and Prevention
Atlanta, Georgia
USA

Alan W. Hampson
WHO Collaborating Centre for Reference
and Research on Influenza
Melbourne
Australia

 2001

EXCERPTA MEDICA
Amsterdam – London – New York – Oxford – Paris – Shannon – Singapore – Tokyo

ELSEVIER SCIENCE B.V.
Sara Burgerhartstraat 25
P.O. Box 211, 1000 AE Amsterdam, The Netherlands

First edition 2001

Library of Congress Cataloging-in-Publication Data

World Congress on Options for the Control of Influenza (4th : 2000 : Crete, Greece)
  Options for the control of influenza IV : proceedings of the World Congress on Options for
the Control of Influenza IV, held in Crete, Greece, 23rd–28th September 2000. / editors, Albert
D.M.E. Osterhaus, Alan W. Hampson, Nancy Cox.
    p. ; cm. -- (International congress series, ISSN 0531-5131 ; no. 1219)
  Includes bibliographical references and index
  ISBN 0-444-50575-X (HC : alk. paper)
  1. Influenza--Congresses.   I. Osterhaus, Albert. II. Hampson, Alan W. III. Cox, Nancy
(Nancy J.) IV. Title. V. Series.
  [DNLM: 1. Influenza--prevention & control--Congresses. 2. Influenza--virology
--Congresses. 3. Influenza Vaccine--Congresses.   WC 515 W927o 2001]
  RC150. W585 2000
  614.5'18--dc21

                                                                2001050144

International Congress Series No. 1219
ISBN: 0444 50575 X

Preface

The fourth "Options for the Control of Influenza" meeting, held in Hersonissos, Crete, Greece from 23rd–28th September 2000 was attended by more than 850 participants representing virtually all the fields of current influenza research. It was organised by the European Scientific Working Group on Influenza (ESWI) with the help of the organising committee, the international program committee, advisors and sponsors. It followed the tradition established at the first "Options" meeting in 1985, aiming to provide a scientific program bringing together experts involved with all aspects of influenza, in order to advance our understanding and control of this important disease. The splendid venue, the hospitality of the hosts and the social events all contributed to the pleasant and informal atmosphere, which facilitated the stimulating scientific discussions, which took place during and between the sessions. As expected, the data presented clearly illustrated that the field of influenza research has changed and advanced rapidly during the last decade. The awareness of the public health impact of influenza has increased considerably in many countries, and both fundamental and applied research efforts have increased our understanding of the influenza virus and of its clinical and economical impact. New generations of vaccines, antiviral agents and diagnostics have become available, which has extended the options for prevention and treatment. This has encouraged health policy makers and authorities in many countries to endorse effective prevention programs for the control of influenza. The scientific program has clearly highlighted all these developments and pointed at new avenues to be explored. It also showed that although considerable achievements have been made in many of these areas, still little is known about the disease and its impact in large parts of the world with a limited public health infrastructure and insufficient financial means for studying influenza.

Like the previous "Options" meetings, the fourth "Options" meeting brought together influenza scientists from all over the world, who shared their latest information and ideas. In this way it contributed to the establishment of new international collaborations in all fields of influenza research.

Since the third "Options" meeting in 1996 a number of major events have occurred, which have all been addressed extensively by the fourth "Options" meeting: the H5N1 chicken flu pandemic warning in Hong Kong, the further characterization of the 1918 "Spanish flu" virus, advances in reverse genetics techniques and the advent of a new generation of antiviral agents which have now been registered for human us, just to name a few. Also the role of the WHO in the worldwide combat of influenza was addressed extensively at the meeting. Not only the world-wide surveillance network for influenza, which has now successfully operated for more than 50 years and has contributed in an unprecedented way to the annual identification of vaccine strains, but also the recent recommendations about pandemic preparedness and interpandemic prevention of influenza, were highlighted. Possibilities to further extend the influenza surveillance network both into new geographical areas and into the animal world were discussed, as were the possibilities to form new platforms and collaborations with all stakeholders in the field. In the light of the continuing pandemic threat of influenza in the 21st century and the continuing burden of the disease between pandemics, such collaborations are essential to allow an even better focussing of research efforts and the future applications of the scientific data in all the relevant fields, to minimize the impact of the disease in the new millennium. We feel that the meeting has indeed been successful in providing a platform for all the participants, to establish such collaboration.

Looking back at the fourth "Options" meeting we would like to thank all those who made the meeting to the success it was, the sponsors for their generous financial contributions without which the meeting could not have been organised. Biomedia, the agency that took care of the logistics of the organisation and ESWI for accepting the overall responsibility. Last but not least, all the participants, who by their contributions and discussions created the platform for the exchange of ideas.

The co-ordinators of the Scientific Committee

Contents

Epidemiology and surveillance: human influenza viruses

Insights into the host defence mechanisms

Insights into the structure and replication of the virus
Surface glycoproteins

M gene products

Viral genome structure and replication

Virus-host interaction: at the cellular level

Current strategies for improved control by vaccination
Opportunities for improved use of existing vaccines

Current strategies for improved control by antivirals
Neuraminidase inhibitors: effectiveness

Influenza:
the scope of the problem

International Congress Series 1219 (2001) 3–7

Striking the balance

Walter R. Dowdle

Task Force for Child Survival and Development, One Copenhill, Atlanta, GA 30307, USA

Keywords: Influenza virus; Influenza pandemics; Influenza epidemiology

Last year, about this same time, at the height of the Y2K scare, I was returning to Atlanta from London. My seatmate turned out to be a young lady who was the Y2K coordinator for a large hotel chain. I was delighted to have the opportunity to ask her whether elevators were really going to fall out of the sky and whether my reservations for London next year would be made for 1900 in Timbuktu. Her answer was no. The elevators do not care what day it is, let alone what year it is. Furthermore, for years, their hotels had been making reservations well into the 2000s. Then, I asked, why did they need a Y2K coordinator? Why the company did not just say there was no problem and be done with it?

The obvious answer, she said, was self-interest. She would be out of a job. But that was not the real answer. The real answer was that the public was so sensitized to Y2K fears by enterprising authors, pundits and the news media that the company had no choice except to go through the Y2K exercise. It was out of their control. If they announced too early there was no problem, then customers would not believe they had looked. They, like most other large corporations, would go through the exercise and announce in December that all Y2K problems had been resolved.

Incredible. It is even more incredible now that January 1, 2000 is behind us. The real potential for Y2K problems in a few special areas had been extrapolated to the computerized universe. The response to theY2K fears in the US was estimated to have cost a staggering US$365 for every man, woman and child.

Where is the balance? Once started, these extrapolated fears take on a life of their own.

Balancing fears, of course, are hardly limited to the electronic field. In our own field of infectious diseases, our inability to prove the negative has led to story after story about impending biological warfare and bioterrorism. Anthrax, plague, smallpox, ebola and even genetic hybrids containing the most horrible features of smallpox and ebola, whatever that is, have become household words. I am surprised that designer influenza viruses have not yet been added to the list.

Not heard much in all this is a rational discussion of the technical obstacles and a careful analysis of the real risks of biological warfare and bioterrorism. Where is the balance? How do we put all of this into perspective? There are those who maintain the world should have never eradicated smallpox.

In fact, at a recent presentation on polio eradication, a rather hostile member of the audience asked me how could I, in good consciousness, participate in a program that by eradicating polio was creating the most potent weapon yet for bioterrorism.

This is not, by the way, an isolated comment.

I personally doubt that polio would give the dramatic effect that a terrorist might like. But who can say? There is no answer. Everyone can play this game. We are only limited by our imagination.

But have we reached the point in this world where our extrapolated fears are given priority over the real fear of death or paralysis of a real child from polio?

Are we really to allow over 350,000 cases of real polio annually in the developing world just to prevent the theoretical use of the virus as a terrorist weapon in the developed world?

There is no doubt in my mind that Y2K was an important concern for a few special sectors. There is also no doubt in my mind that we need to be prepared to respond to bioterrorist acts. But how do we keep that balance between observation and extrapolation?

That question of balance really struck home just a few months ago. I had given a brief talk to a group of clinical and public health folks about pandemic planning. I pointed out how difficult it was to plan, because influenza pandemics, as defined by antigenic shifts, have ranged in modern history all the way from a disastrous 1918 to a relatively mild 1968, and technically speaking, to an even milder 1977. Afterward, a very respected, knowledgeable academic physician came up to me and said he had not been aware that the consequences of an antigenic shift could be similar to a large epidemic.

In our pandemic planning exercise, are we headed down the same path of extrapolation?

As we should have learned by now, in influenza as has been said about other fields [1], there can be two diseases: influenza and influenza extrapolitis. Both influenza and influenza extrapolitis are contagious, and both can have very serious consequences.

How many of you in the audience have made the statement to the effect that "We cannot be certain when there will be another pandemic, but we can be certain there will be one".

Now, before you begin to look around at your neighbor, I will confess, I have. In fact, I have made that statement on more than one occasion. It is great. It is very quotable, very dramatic, and very, very safe. Impossible to prove you wrong. And there is just an outside chance you may be right.

But, in truth, we cannot be certain. We cannot be certain there will be an influenza pandemic in our lifetime, and if there is, we cannot be certain how severe it may be. Our track record over the years for predicting influenza events leaves much to be desired.

Given the prevailing thought in 1968, who among us would have believed that 32 years later the same virus would be with us, happily evolving, circulating the globe, and accomplishing its purpose in life and, wonder of wonders, sharing its ecological niche with an H1 virus. To know anything at all about the natural history of influenza is to know we have a lot yet to learn.

We cannot predict the future. On the other hand, our cumulative experience with influenza continues to grow. Surely, that counts for something.

The distant past may not be all that helpful. We cannot be certain that the influenza-like pandemics that occurred about 40–60 years apart over the past few centuries were [2], in fact, results of antigenic shifts, or even type A. Nor can we be certain that during the intervening years, there were no additional antigenic shifts that failed to register on the crude mortality scale of the day.

Furthermore, the world has changed over the past 300 years; so likely has the epidemiology of influenza. Global population at the time of the assumed 1729–1733 pandemic was less than a billion. Today, it is 6 billion. Intercontinental travel is measured in hours rather than weeks or months, and travelers in many millions circle the globe each day. Just as modern day transportation must affect influenza epidemiology, so must have the explosion in the number of sailing ships in the 18th century and the steamships of the 19th century, with navies, armies, colonialist, merchants, immigrants and missionaries crossing the seas.

In short, our modern knowledge of influenza really begins only in the later part of the 19th century, with the pandemic of 1889–1891. This was the first pandemic to be described as truly global. It is also the first pandemic to which we can attach a probable etiology.

So that leaves us with four pandemic models over the last 110 years: H3 in 1890, H1 in 1918, H2 in 1957, and H3 again in 1968, in addition to whatever you would like to call H1 in 1977 [3]. And even then, influenza epidemiology must have undergone major changes between the pandemics of 1890 and 1957.

"Populations of influenza naive" are likely to have been major factors in the 1890 and 1918 pandemics. Many communities and populations are likely not to have had influenza for many years, and many individuals not at all. We all know the stories of 1918 wherein entire remote villages were wiped out. Even in the period shortly after the emergence of the 1957 H2 virus, stories abound of the devastating effect on remote island communities that had not had flu for many years. Hardest hit were the influenza naive older children and young adults. The proportion of influenza naive in the 18th and 19th century may have contributed as much to the devastating morbidity and mortality of pandemics as any other factor.

Little or no influenza had been recorded anywhere in the world between 1847 and the big pandemic of 1890 [4]. There were also limited reports of influenza outbreaks between 1893 and the possible herald waves beginning in 1916. The swine virus appears to be the original antigenic sin for most of the population who were under 25–30 years old at the time of the 1918 pandemic. The unprecedented movement of people during World War I and a high number of immunologically naive young adults surely must have exerted some influence on the unusual course of the pandemic, consistent with the increased pneumonia and influenza deaths in the 20–30-year age group.

Today, populations of influenza naive are highly unlikely, given the speed and thoroughness in which influenza viruses are now transported around the world. Influenza A has virtually become endemic, resulting in wide spread immunological experience. Excess mortality per 100,000 population associated with individual influenza events since 1918 has dramatically decreased or stabilized.

Opportunities for virus spread, immunological experience with influenza, better general health, better health care all make the epidemics of the past poor models for the future.

Perhaps even more importantly, repeated frequent exposure to influenza viruses may help maintain heterosubtypic memory, providing population protection against the most severe form of the disease.

The second factor in our cumulative experience that must be considered is the remarkable protection provided by infection with the same or similar viruses many years earlier. Excess mortality in the 1968–1972 H3N2 pandemic was virtually nonexistent among those who had been born before 1899 [5]. They were presumably protected by immunity acquired in the 1890 H3N8 pandemic and the following decade or so of continued H3 virus circulation.

In 1977, the absence of disease among those born before1957, the end of the H1N1 era, was equally striking. These observations raise the question that if the swine flu H1N1 virus really had emerged in the human population in 1976, would the picture have been any different than that of the H1N1 of 1977? Infection with the swine flu virus in Fort Dix, NJ in 1976 was restricted to several hundred military recruits. I am not aware that anyone born before 1956 was infected. Furthermore, if an H2 virus were to return tomorrow, could we not expect a similar reduction in severe disease among those born before 1968, the previous H2N2 era? These observations, plus the current cocirculation of the H1N1 and H3N2 viruses, suggest that a disastrous pandemic caused by any known human subtype within the next few years is highly unlikely.

So which is our model? Is it 1918 with 20 million deaths worldwide? Is it 1957 with one-tenth the mortality rate of 1918 and one-fifth that of 1890? Or, is it 1968 with a rate half that again? In truth, all the available data point us away from the 1918, and even the 1890, model.

Some might argue that the Hong Kong H5 experience raises the spectra of a killer pandemic with a novel animal influenza virus. An incredible 30% of those infected in Hong Kong died. Extrapolate that to the whole world. Those were a scary few months. Very scary. No one knows that better than the Hong Kong health department and the international team. They did a remarkable job.

On the other hand, in retrospect, we have no evidence that the Hong Kong H5N1 virus was or ever would be a candidate for human-to-human transmission. It was a zoonotic disease. Humans were accidental hosts. Furthermore, if an H5N1/H1N1 or H3N2 reassortant had emerged in the human population, the Hong Kong experience may not have been a model at all.

So the question is, if all the cumulative experience points us away from the 1890 and 1918 models, what does that say about the next pandemic? And the answer is, we do not know. The potential virulence of a pandemic strain of animal origin is completely unknown, which is exactly why pandemic planning is so important. John Maynard Keynes noted that: "As living and moving beings, we are forced to act, even when our existing knowledge does not provide a sufficient basis for a calculated mathematical expectation". Not to do pandemic planning would be derelict indeed.

We must plan for an antigenic shift in the influenza type A virus. With that shift comes a wide range of epidemiologic possibilities, including a pandemic of unknown severity. But we cannot let our extrapolations of a severe pandemic overshadow the equally real possibility of a far lesser, but still bad enough, event. All of you in this room are aware of that. We must make certain that the policy makers and the public are also aware of the wide range of possibilities that an antigenic shift may bring.

You might say that, to this point, pandemic planning has been less threatened by extrapolated fears than by public inertia. True, national authorities do not like to appropriate funds on the basis of "It might happen and it might not, and if it does happen it might be severe, and it might not". But this can change overnight with reports of an outbreak with a new subtype somewhere.

The architects of the WHO Pandemic Plan are to be commended. The document goes a long way in striking the balance between planning for an antigenic shift and recognizing the critical need to reduce extrapolated fears. All of you in this audience have an important responsibility to provide that balance, no matter what country you represent or what job you have. You are the influenza experts.

The agenda for Options IV reflect that vital mix between basic research and public health action that has been a hallmark of the influenza field. Options IV also exemplifies the extraordinary progress that has been made over the past few decades in understanding the virus and addressing the public health needs. Influenza awareness is up. Vaccination rates are up. Influenza is a much more mature field.

But if an antigenic shift were to occur tomorrow, regardless of how mild or how severe it may be, are we ready? Hardly. Only some in the developed world and virtually none in the developing world would have access to vaccines, antivirals, or any other effective means of prevention.

As we begin this conference, remember how far we still have yet to go.

References

[1] R. Coker, Extrapolitis, A disease more threatening than TB in Russia? European Journal of Public Health 10 (2000) 148–155.

[2] C.W. Potter, Chapter 1: Chronicle of influenza pandemics, in: K.G. Nicholson, R.G. Webster, A.J. Hay (Eds.), Textbook of Influenza, Blackwell, Malden, MA, 1998, pp. 3–18.

[3] W.R. Dowdle, Influenza A virus recycling revisited, Bulletin of the World Health Organization 77 (1999) 820–828.

[4] G.R. Noble, Chapter 2: Epidemiological and clinical aspects of influenza, in: A.S. Beare (Ed.), Basic and Applied Influenza Research, CRC Press, Boca Raton, FL, 1982, pp. 11–50.

[5] W.J. Houseworth, M.M. Spoon, The age distribution of excess mortality during A2 Hong Kong epidemics compared with earlier A2 outbreaks, American Journal of Epidemiology 94 (1971) 348–350.

International Congress Series 1219 (2001) 9–11

The importance of global influenza surveillance for the assessment of the impact of influenza

Daniel Lavanchy*, Pilar Gavinio

Department of Communicable Disease Surveillance and Response, World Health Organization, Geneva, Switzerland

Keywords: Surveillance; Epidemic; Pandemic; Epidemiology; Morbidity; Mortality

Morbidity and mortality associated with influenza have been recognized for years. However, the true burden of disease has been difficult to determine. Precise quantification of morbidity and mortality therefore underlines the need for vigilant surveillance, and a greater need for virological confirmation of cases that do not exhibit typical clinical manifestations of influenza. Delayed identification of a new virus variant that may cause another pandemic may be even more devastating than the 1918 pandemic.

1. The global surveillance network

For more than 50 years, the main objectives of the WHO global influenza surveillance have remained the same. These objectives are to measure the impact of the disease by collection and analysis of epidemiological information on morbidity and mortality, and to anticipate future epidemics, and pandemics, by the collection and analysis of influenza viruses [1]. Influenza activity is currently monitored both globally through the four WHO Collaborating Centres for Reference and Research for Influenza, Centers for Disease Control and Prevention (CDC), Atlanta, USA; WHO Collaborating Centre for Reference and Research for Influenza, National Institute for Medical Research (NIMR), London, United Kingdom; WHO Collaborating Centre for Reference and Research for Influenza, Melbourne, Australia; and the WHO Collaborating Centre for Reference and Research for Influenza, National Institute of Infectious Diseases, Tokyo, Japan; and nationally through a network of 110 National Influenza

---

* Corresponding author.

Centres located in 82 countries. Together, these form the WHO global influenza surveillance system.

The system ensures the collection of epidemiological data and viral isolates for early detection of epidemics and rapid identification of virus variants which serve as the basis for the recommended vaccine composition in February intended for the Northern Hemisphere, and in September intended for the Southern Hemisphere. The system also facilitates the standardization of epidemiological information entered by the 110 national centres to the web-based database (http://oms2b3e.jussieu.fr/flunet), the WHO electronic global influenza surveillance system (FluNet) [2], which was developed in collaboration with the Institut National de la Santé et de la Recherche Médicale (INSERM), to provide international and national authorities, the public and the media with an early-alert information system for the global monitoring of influenza activity. The quality of epidemiological data submitted to WHO is controlled by the laboratory diagnosis of influenza through the standardized reagent kit developed by the WHO collaborating centre at the CDC. These kits are distributed to all national influenza centres before the start of the season.

Currently, of the 110 WHO National Influenza Centres, 23 have their own network within the country, which allows a standardised system of reporting. However, globally the network does not cover all regions uniformly. There are gaps in Eastern Europe, Asia and most especially Africa, and therefore, there is a need to expand and improve surveillance for a better worldwide coverage. The proper monitoring of outbreaks and prevention of the spread of infection, and an exchange of information between geographically distributed public health institutions must be facilitated. With the existing gaps in the regions worldwide, new virus variants may not be detected, which would mean failure in prevention and control measures.

Although the impact of influenza on morbidity and mortality causing substantial health resource utilization and cost have been estimated in temperate countries [3,4], this is not reflective of the true burden of disease globally. Assessment tools in most countries, particularly those in the tropics, do not exist. In many countries, national morbidity and mortality figures are simply not available. In those countries where such statistics are available, the procedures adapted for their collection, analysis, and dissemination vary according to the type of information and the source. In countries where no statistics are gathered, other means of obtaining a measure of morbidity and mortality must be investigated. The toll of deaths during the 1918 pandemic [5] underlines the periodic cause of great morbidity and mortality by influenza and the importance of constant and vigilant surveillance. Of particular importance for surveillance are those countries/areas where animal hosts and humans live in close proximity and which are the most likely places where new influenza variants may appear. Constant surveillance is therefore needed both in humans and in animals [6]. In addition, this will allow WHO and national public health authorities to monitor a pandemic that may emerge through an antigenic shift in an influenza virus.

2. The role of WHO

The most important role for WHO is to help national health services obtain early and accurate information on changes in the strains of influenza viruses, therefore enabling them to develop and apply appropriate control measures. Based on the global surveillance system, recommendations are made for the composition of influenza vaccines for the northern and southern hemisphere, respectively, in February and September each year. It is vital to have a more effective vaccine, rapid isolation of influenza viruses, early recognition of new virus variants and rapid transport of these strains for immediate identification, accompanied by epidemiological data. However, the existing surveillance system needs to be strengthened by:

- improving geographical and community coverage;
- ensuring rapid isolation and characterization of viral isolates and providing logistic support to National Influenza Centres to ensure quick and safe shipment of isolates to the WHO Collaborating Centres;
- ensuring rapid, more detailed, widespread and free exchange of information about the epidemiology globally.

The threat of another pandemic is always there. Unless the global surveillance system is able to rapidly detect the appearance of a new influenza virus which could behave as the 1918 virus, unparalleled tolls of illness and death would be expected. Early detection, reporting and investigation of potential pandemic strains are essential. The Pandemic plan by WHO has been prepared to assist medical and public health leaders to better respond to such an event [7].

Evaluating epidemiological information on influenza is fraught with difficulties. Influenza-related deaths or notifications do not capture the true impact of the disease and are probably prone to underreporting. Sentinel systems based on less specific information drawn either from mortality or morbidity data are efficient early-alert tools for outbreak detection at a local or national level. However, these systems do not exist in all countries and are not linked to each other using harmonized data formulas. Therefore, the global impact of influenza is not well understood as yet. This is also true for many countries that have not assessed the specific impact of influenza within their borders. Particularly alarming is the lack of data related to subtropical and tropical countries. WHO strongly advocates the design and implementation of studies to assess the impact in these areas.

National and regional decisions are required to set priorities and objectives in guidance on resource allocation for the prevention and control of influenza within the context of national public health.

References

[1] M. Pereira, F.A. Assaad, P.J. Delon, Influenza surveillance, Bull. W. H. O. 56 (2) (1978) 193–203.

[2] A. Flahault, V. Dias-Ferrao, P. Chaberty, K. Esteves, A.D. Valleron, D. Lavanchy, FluNet as a tool for global monitoring of influenza on the Web, JAMA 280 (15) (1998) 1330–1332 (Oct. 21).

[3] L. Simonsen, The global impact of influenza on morbidity and mortality, Vaccine 17 (1999) S3–S10.

[4] A. Klimov, L. Simonsen, K. Fukuda, N. Cox, Surveillance and impact of influenza in the United States, Vaccine 17 (1999) S42–S46.

[5] W. Beveridge, Influenza: The Last Great Plague, Heinman, London, 1977.

[6] R. Webster, W. Bean Jr., Evolution and ecology of human influenza viruses: interspecies transmission, Textb. Influenza (1998) 109.

[7] Influenza Pandemic Preparedness Plan, The Role of WHO and Guidelines for National and Regional Planning, 1999, WHO/CDS/EDC/99.1.

International Congress Series 1219 (2001) 13–19

Influenza-related morbidity and mortality among children in developed and developing countries

Lone Simonsen*

National Institute of Allergy and Infectious Diseases, National Institutes of Health, 6700B Rockledge Drive, Bethesda, MD 20892-7630, USA

Abstract

More than 20% of all childhood deaths are thought to be acute respiratory (ARI) deaths; most of these occur in developing countries. Bacterial pathogens are implied in 70–90% of pediatric ARI deaths, while 10–30% are attributed to respiratory syncytial viruses (RSV). This implies that influenza is not an important cause of severe pediatric ARI. Influenza A,B virus infections may nevertheless cause ARI deaths by triggering bacterial superinfections. The mechanism of triggering is still poorly understood, as well as the consequences in terms of disease burden. However, recent studies have shed additional light on the triggering mechanism and provided an example of an influenza-triggered outbreak of severe pediatric pneumococcal disease. Further, new studies have quantified the impact of influenza on pediatric hospitalizations in the US — and argued that they may be similar in magnitude to that of RSV. In the tropics, the year-round circulation of influenza viruses prohibits the use of traditional tools to observe and quantify the attributable burden as the increase in severe ARI outcomes during influenza periods. Also, several studies of pathogens isolated from ARI-hospitalized children suggest a minor role of influenza viruses. However, since influenza may trigger bacterial super infections it is likely that undiagnosed influenza infections cause a significant subset of ARI deaths in developing countries. The void of data demonstrating the impact on ARI hospitalizations and deaths in the tropics has put influenza viruses at a disadvantage in terms of being recognized as serious pathogens. With the availability of new mucosal live-attenuated influenza vaccine formulations, it may be prudent to re-examine this issue for children living in tropical developing countries. Vaccine probe studies are needed to assess the true influenza-related disease burden. © 2001 Elsevier Science B.V. All rights reserved.

Keywords: Influenza; ARI; Pneumonia; Children; Hospitalizations; Mortality; Global

* Tel.: +1-301-402-8487; fax: +1-301-402-3255.
E-mail address: Lsimonsen@niaid.nih.gov (L. Simonsen).

0531-5131/01/$ – see front matter © 2001 Elsevier Science B.V. All rights reserved.
PII: S 0 5 3 1 - 5 1 3 1 (0 1) 0 0 3 2 2 - 3

1. Introduction

Children under 5 years of age account for a large proportion of all deaths in the world each year; the majority of which occur among children born in developing countries. More than 20% of all childhood deaths are thought to be attributable to acute respiratory infections (ARI), corresponding to a figure of at least 4 million annual ARI deaths in this age group [1]. In terms of mild morbidity, ARI is considered a global leading cause of lost disability-adjusted life-years (DALYs) [2].

The bacterial pathogen *Streptococcus pneumoniae* is widely regarded as the leading cause of childhood ARI deaths, followed by *Haemophilus influenza*. Overall, about 70% to 90% of all childhood ARI deaths are attributed to bacterial pathogens while 10–30% are attributed to Respiratory Syncytial Virus (RSV) [3].

This implies that influenza infections are not important in terms of severe outcomes of childhood ARI. Unfortunately, the void of disease burden estimates has put influenza viruses at a disadvantage in terms of being regarded as a serious pathogen. In this paper, the question of a possible burden of influenza will be re-examined. With the availability of new antiviral drugs and near-future availability of a mucosal live-attenuated vaccine, it is imperative to better assess the influenza-related disease burden, in order to make better public health decisions regarding the use of influenza vaccines in pediatric populations world wide.

2. The likely role of influenza as a trigger of secondary bacterial ARI

2.1. Influenza epidemiology: temperate versus tropical climates

Each year, influenza A and/or B viruses circulate during winter months in the temperate climates of the Northern and Southern hemisphere, causing extensive epidemics of ARI with 5–15% of the total population infected. A recent study found even higher attack rates among infants with several siblings (50% during the first year of life) [4]. In terms of disease burden, the 1918 A(H1N1) pandemic was associated with some 20 million deaths globally [5]. Each of the three influenza pandemics of this century: 1918 A(H1N1), 1957 A(H2N2) and 1968 A(H3N2), was associated with many-fold increased risk of influenza-related mortality among younger persons [6]. Of the currently circulating strains, most seasons dominated by A(H3N2) viruses are associated with a sharp increase in ARI mortality among the elderly, while A(H1N1) and influenza B seasons are rarely associated with excess mortality. The cumulative number of deaths associated with inter-pandemic influenza far exceeds the number of deaths associated with the two most recent pandemics [6,7].

In contrast, influenza in the tropics has received little attention, despite surveillance data documenting influenza A(H1N1), A(H3N2) and influenza B virus activity each year. As influenza occurs year-round or biannually with no distinct pattern in the tropics, the impact of influenza cannot be visualized as spikes and seasonality in ARI mortality data. As a consequence, very little is known about influenza attack rates and the attributable burden on morbidity and mortality in the tropics where a large proportion of the world's population resides.

2.2. The triggering hypothesis

Consider the possibility that influenza viruses cause a considerable proportion of childhood ARI disease, and that a couple of weeks following this primary infection, a subset of the affected children develop complications such as bacterial pneumonia and death (Fig. 1). In such cases, influenza infection as a triggering event is highly likely to be missed at the time of diagnosis of bacterial pneumonia: firstly, the virus is not easily cultured, and secondly, the influenza virus infection may have already been cleared by the immune system. It follows that some proportion of ARI deaths currently attributed to bacterial pathogens may indeed be preventable by influenza vaccine—and that influenza is currently underrepresented as an underlying cause of childhood ARI deaths.

Influenza infections have long been known to trigger secondary bacterial infections and other serious complications. For example, during the influenza A(H3N2) pandemic of 1968 in the US, a three-fold increase in the incidence of pneumonia due to *S. aureus* was observed [8]. The triggering effect has been attributed to influenza viruses damaging the cells in the respiratory tract and thereby facilitating secondary bacterial infections [9,10].

Most recently, a study based on a mouse model demonstrated a synergistic lethal effect of influenza infection and certain bacterial pathogens including *S. pneumoniae* and *H. influenzae* [11]. Mice that were infected with influenza virus and then 3–7 days later were challenged with a bacterial pathogen had 100% lethal outcome (control mice infected with influenza or a bacterial pathogen alone, or both simultaneously, survived). This study proposes the mechanism of triggering to be an influenza-mediated change in the cell surface receptors in the respiratory tract that facilitates secondary bacterial infections such as *S. pneumonia* and *H. influenzae*.

Additional support for the importance of influenza infection as a trigger of severe pediatric ARI was a recent outbreak investigation of severe pneumococcal childhood pneumonia in the US during the winter 1995–1996, which provided direct and

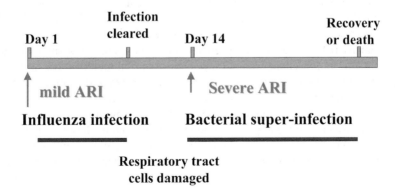

Fig. 1. The triggering hypothesis. A primary influenza virus infection triggers a secondary bacterial pulmonary infection. Cultures at the time of hospitalizations may only yield the bacterial pathogen.

indirect evidence that a preceding influenza A(H1N1) infection led to severe pneumococcal pneumonia. The authors concluded that prevention of pneumococcal disease
among children should be considered among the potential benefits of influenza
vaccination [12].

3. The impact of influenza on morbidity and mortality: classical tools

3.1. The impact of influenza on ARI hospitalizations and mortality in the US: an example of a developed country with a temperate climate

The 1918–1919 A(H1N1) pandemic was associated with a dramatic increase in
childhood infectious disease mortality [13]. A recent study of pneumonia and influenza
(P&I) mortality during 1939–1996 demonstrated a strong downward trend, which is
probably attributable to the introduction of antibiotics around 1950 and the general
improved access to health care in the US during the 1960s and 1970s [14]. The impact
of the most severe influenza seasons could be visualized as an increase in the annual
rate of P&I deaths: visible increases in childhood P&I deaths associated with the
1957–1958 A(H2N2) pandemic as well as the 1943–1944 A(H1N1) epidemic are
consistent with an excess in influenza-related mortality. In contrast, in recent years
(including the 1968–1969 pandemic), influenza-related deaths did not visibly increase
the total yearly number of childhood pneumonia deaths compared to surrounding years.
In summary, in recent years children in developed countries have a far greater chance
than they did pre-WW2 of surviving severe ARI disease, including influenza-related
events—due to prompt and effective medical treatment and the availability of
appropriate antibiotics.

The traditional method for assessing influenza-related pneumonia mortality is to
estimate the excess in pneumonia (P&I) deaths above a baseline during influenza-
epidemic periods. The monthly numbers of P&I deaths and the timing of influenza
epidemic periods for the years 1968 through 1976 show definite winter peaks
coinciding with influenza (Fig. 1; original data). Considerable seasonality and excess
in P&I mortality attributable to influenza occurred during the last season of A(H2N2)
virus circulation (1967–1968), the 1968–1969 pandemic season and during two of the
first four inter-pandemic A(H3N2) seasons (Fig. 2). Over the next decades, this
seasonal pattern largely disappeared and pneumonia mortality rates continued to
decline; a pattern consistent with little or no influenza-related childhood deaths after
1976 (data not shown).

This excess methodology for assessment depends on influenza seasonality in the
data and may not be appropriate for studying childhood pneumonia deaths due to
concurrent RSV epidemics. A recent study teased out the effects of influenza and RSV
on ARI hospitalizations during two recent influenza seasons in the US. Using virus
surveillance data to define the RSV and influenza-epidemic periods, combined with a
variant of the excess mortality methodology, the seasonal impact of influenza on ARI
hospitalizations was found to be similar to that of RSV, both for children <24 months
of age (∼100–150 per 100,000 infants per season), for children 2–4 years of age

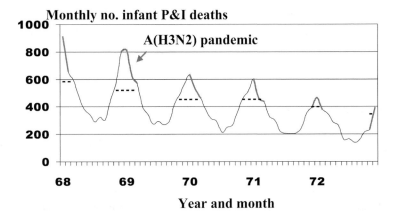

Fig. 2. The impact of influenza on P&I infant mortality in the US. During 1968–1972, there was a steep downward secular trend in all infant pneumonia deaths. The influenza-attributable proportion of P&I deaths can be visualized as the increases/spikes during periods with epidemic influenza activity (thicker solid lines). (Original data; Source: NCHS, multiple-cause-of-death tapes; monthly numbers of deaths with a P&I diagnosis as the underlying cause of death).

($\sim 15–26$ per 100,000) as well as for older children (0–5 per 100,000) [15]. In addition, another recent US-based study found that infants < 12 months of age had considerable excess cardio-pulmonary hospitalization rates during influenza periods ($\sim 500–1000$ per 100,000) than in the surrounding months, placing infants at a risk similar to that of high-risk adults [16].

In summary, recent studies have revealed a considerable influenza-related disease burden in the US, leading to a proposal by CDC to consider routine influenza vaccination in healthy infants and young children in the US [15].

3.2. The burden of influenza in the tropics

Due to the lack of a definite epidemic pattern in the tropics, the burden of influenza cannot be visualized as a single peak in ARI mortality—and, consequently, the traditional methodology of estimating excess in mortality is difficult to apply.

Several reports studied the distribution of pathogens isolated from throat culture in cohorts of hospitalized children. A viral pathogen was identified in 21–45% of cultures; RSV was always the dominant viral pathogen while influenza A and B viruses accounted for 3–15% of all viral isolates [17].

Two recent studies set in Cuba and Singapore found a strong age-related pattern of RSV versus influenza in the tropics [18,19]. RSV was the dominant viral pathogen isolated from ARI-hospitalized infants, but during early childhood influenza became equally important and for older children influenza was dominant (Fig. 3).

In developing countries, the disease burden of influenza is likely to be similar or greater than in the US pre-antibiotic era: children have limited access to care and antibiotics, while

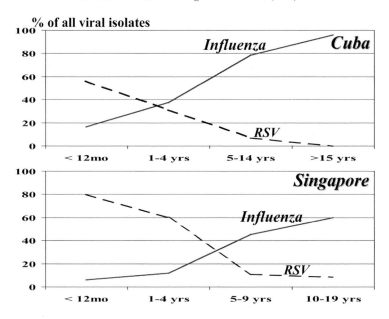

Fig. 3. Relative impact of influenza A,B and RSV. The graphs depict the percentage of all viral isolates that were influenza or RSV, among age groups of children hospitalized with ARI in two tropical settings. (Based on analysis of data from Cuba [18] and Singapore [19]).

commonplace malnutrition, immunosuppression and parasitic diseases may further increase the risk of severe complications of influenza infection [9]. In summary, there are many a priori reasons to believe that influenza is associated with a significant childhood disease burden in the tropics—and that this disease burden cannot be assessed using traditional tools.

4. New assessment tools needed: vaccine probe studies

An alternative method to estimate the burden of influenza among children in developing tropical countries is to probe with an influenza vaccine of known high efficacy. Such a vaccine probe study recently demonstrated a 20–30% reduction in outcomes such as febrile illnesses and otitis media during winter months among infants vaccinated with a live attenuated mucosal vaccine in the US [20]. With a vaccine efficacy of 85%, the differences in disease rates among vaccinees and placebo recipients in this study represent a low estimate of the total influenza-attributable burden of febrile illness and otitis media during winter months.

Similar vaccine probe studies set in developing tropical regions of the world would be the best method to document the disease burden of influenza. In a sufficiently large study cohort it would be possible to assess the burden of influenza on severe ARI morbidity and mortality in the developing world.

References

[1] M. Garenne, C. Ronsmans, H. Campbell, The magnitude of mortality from acute respiratory infections in children under 5 years in developing countries, Rapp. Trimmest. Stat. Sanit. Mond. 45 (1992) 180–191.

[2] C.J. Murray, A.D. Lopez, Global mortality, disability, and the contribution of risk factors: global burden of disease study, Lancet 349 (9063) (1997) 1436–1442.

[3] J. Leowski, Mortality from acute respiratory infections in children under 5 years of age: global estimates, World Health Stat. Q. 39 (2) (1986) 138–144.

[4] W.P. Glezen, L.H. Taber, A.L. Frank, et al., Influenza virus infections in infants, PID 16 (1997) 1065–1068.

[5] G.R. Noble, Epidemiological and clinical aspects of influenza, in: A.S. Geare (Ed.), Basic and Applied Influenza Research, CRC Press, Boca Raton, FL, 1982, pp. 1–50.

[6] L. Simonsen, M.J. Clarke, L.B. Schonberger, et al., Pandemic versus epidemic influenza mortality: a pattern of changing age distribution, JID 178 (1998) 53–60.

[7] L. Simonsen, M.J. Clarke, G.D. Williamson, et al., The impact of influenza epidemics on mortality: introducing a severity index, Am. J. Public Health 87 (1997) 1944–1950.

[8] S. Schwarzmann, J. Adler, R. Sullivan, et al., Bacterial pneumonia during the Hong-Kong influenza epidemic of 1968–69, Arch. Intern. Med. 127 (1971) 1037–1041.

[9] M.W. Leigh, J.L. Carson, F.W. Denny Jr., Pathogenesis of respiratory infections due to influenza virus: implications for developing countries, Rev. Inf. Dis. 13 (Suppl. 6) (1991) S501–S508.

[10] J.-M. Hament, J.L.L. Kimpen, A. Fleer, et al., Respiratory viral infection predisposing for bacterial disease: a concise review, FEMS Immunol. Med. Microbiol. 26 (1999) 189–195.

[11] J.A. McCullers, E.I. Tuomanen, R.G. Webster, Lethal synergism of influenza A virus and *streptococcus pneumoniae* in a mouse model, These proceedings.

[12] K.L. O'Brien, M.I. Walters, J. Sellman, et al., Severe pneumocuccal pneumonia in previously healthy children: the role of preceeding influenza infection, CID 30 (2000) 784–789.

[13] G.L. Armstrong, L.A. Conn, R.W. Pinner, Trends in infectious disease mortality in the United States during the 20th Century, J. Am. Med. Assoc. 281 (1999) 61–66.

[14] S. Dowell, B.A. Kupronis, E.R. Zell, et al., Mortality from pneumonia in children in the United States, 1939 through 1996, NEJM 342 (2000) 1399–1407.

[15] H.S. Izurieta, W.W. Thompson, P. Kramarz, et al., Influenza and the rates of hospitalization for respiratory disease among infants and young children, NEJM, (2000) 232–239.

[16] K.M. Neuzil, B.G. Mellen, P.F. Wright, et al., The effect of influenza on hospitalizations, outpatient visits and courses of antibiotics in children, NEJM 342 (2000) 225–231.

[17] M.W. Weber, E.K. Mulholland, B.M. Greenwood, Respiratory syncytial virus infection in tropical and developing countries, Trop. Med. Int. Health 3 (4) (1998) 268–280.

[18] R. Cancio, C. Savon, I. Abreu, et al., Diagnostico rapido de los principales virus respiratorios en Ciudad de la Habana, 1995–1997, Rev. Argent. Microbiol. 32 (2000) 21–26.

[19] F.T. Chew, S. Doraisingham, A.E. Ling, et al., Seasonal trends of viral respiratory tract infections in the tropics, Epidemiol. Infect. 121 (1) (1998) 121–128.

[20] R.B. Belshe, W.C. Gruber, Prevention of otitis media in children with live attenuated influenza vaccine given intranasally, PID 19 (2000) S66–S71.

International Congress Series 1219 (2001) 21–23

Influenza present: the impact of the 1999/2000 epidemic on morbidity and mortality in the UK

John M. Watson[a,*], Nichola Goddard[a], Carol Joseph[a],
Maria Zambon[b]

[a]Epidemiology Division, PHLS Communicable Disease Surveillance Centre, London NW9 5EQ, UK
[b]Respiratory Virus Unit, PHLS Central Public Health Laboratory, London NW9 5HT, UK

Keywords: Influenza; Morbidity; Mortality

The aim of this paper is to summarise the activity of influenza in the United Kingdom (UK) in the winter of 1999/2000 using surveillance indices, and to provide an overview of the impact that resulted in the disruption of hospital services and considerable political controversy.

Isolates of the "Sydney" strain of influenza A subtype H3N2 were first reported in week 41 of 1999 and began to increase rapidly from week 46. The strain had first circulated in the UK in the winter of 1997/1998 when it had been associated with only limited influenza activity, and again in 1998/1999 when it was associated with "higher than expected seasonal activity" (Fig. 1), based on consultation rates with general practitioners in the sentinel surveillance scheme of the Royal College of General Practitioners in England [1]. Attack rates for influenza-like illness in the 1998/1999 season had been particularly high in the elderly and associated with considerable mortality.

Clinical indices of influenza activity began to rise above "baseline" levels in week 50 of 1999. This coincided with the annual rise in respiratory syncytial virus (RSV) infections which peaked at the turn of the year. In addition to a rise in influenza-like illness, consultations for acute bronchitis in the RCGP scheme also rose sharply. Attack rates for both influenza-like illness and acute bronchitis were highest in older adults (45–64 years) and the elderly (65 years and older).

A similar pattern of activity was seen in the north, central and southern parts of England, and also in Wales (based on data from a general practice sentinel surveillance scheme coordinated by the Communicable Disease Surveillance Centre, Wales) and in

---

* Corresponding author.

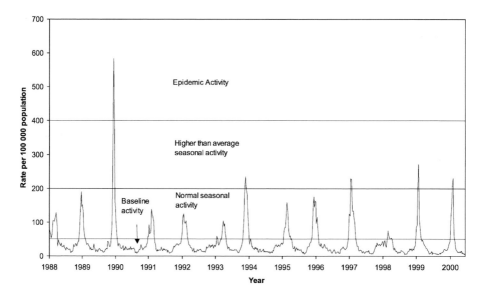

Fig. 1. RCGP weekly consultation rate for influenza and influenza-like illness.

Scotland (based on a similar scheme coordinated by the Scottish Centre for Infection and Environmental Health).

Although the activity peak, based on consultations with general practitioners, occurred in week 2 of 2000, the true peak may have been a little earlier at the turn of the year. This coincided not only with the annual holiday for the Christmas festivities but also with the extended holiday associated with the beginning of the new millennium. Access to general practitioner services was reduced during this period.

The peak level of activity, based on consultation rates reported in England, Scotland and Wales, reached the level described as "higher than expected seasonal activity", which was similar to that seen in 1998/1999 but considerably less then the "epidemic" level seen in the 1989/1990 winter.

The high attack rates of acute respiratory illness in the elderly resulted in a substantial increase in pressure for hospital admissions for complications of the initial infections. Mortality also rose, reaching a weekly peak of 20,772 deaths due to all causes in the first week of 2000. Excess mortality (Table 1) during the 1999/2000 influenza season (weeks 1999/40 to 2000/20 inclusive) was calculated at 15,706 deaths, compared with 14,071 in the previous year and 21,133 in the winter of 1989/1990 (PHLS unpublished data).

In conclusion, although influenza activity was substantial in the United Kingdom in the winter of 1999/2000, it was not very high, based on consultation rates with general practitioners. However, the peak of activity coincided with the peak of RSV infections in the population and the extended Christmas and Millennium holiday period. The high attack rates of both influenza-like illness and acute bronchitis in the elderly lead to increased hospitalisations and substantial mortality. The resulting extra pressure on hospital services caused considerable disruption. It also led to political debate as the

Table 1
Excess mortality due to influenza in England and Wales

Year	Number of excess deaths
1989/1990	21,133
1990/1991	1324
1991/1992	1787
1992/1993	0
1993/1994	19,584
1994/1995	0
1995/1996	8111
1996/1997	23,729
1997/1998	0
1998/1999	14,071
1999/2000	15,706

PHLS unpublished data.

government was asked to explain the apparent inability of the National Health Service to cope with "expected" annual winter pressures.

Reference

[1] Commun. Dis. Public Health 2 (1999) 273–279.

International Congress Series 1219 (2001) 25–27

Surveillance and assessment of influenza activity in the UK and Europe

John M. Watson

Epidemiology Division, PHLS Communicable Disease Surveillance Centre, London NW9 5EQ, UK

Keywords: Surveillance; Influenza; Europe

This paper outlines the range of measures of influenza activity in European countries, discusses problems with standardisation and interpretation, and considers some future options.

Clinical indices of influenza activity together with virological surveillance form the basis of surveillance in most European countries. Sentinel general practitioner surveillance schemes recording consultations for influenza-like illness (ILI) or other acute respiratory illness (ARI) have become the single most important element of clinical surveillance in many European countries. A number of factors make it difficult to compare results from the different schemes. These include the definition and ascertainment method for a case for surveillance (the numerator), the denominator used (sometimes based on the total number of consultations and sometimes on the population served by the reporting practitioners), and the overall system of health care in the country in question. In the United Kingdom, for example, baseline and peak levels of consultations for ILI over a number of seasons vary considerably between England, Wales and Scotland (Fig. 1), which share a similar health service.

Other clinical indices of activity employed in some countries include sickness absence statistics, school attendance, pharmacy sales and admissions to hospital. Issues of specificity for influenza, population representativeness and timeliness of data availability all limit the usefulness of these indices.

Both qualitative and quantitative virological surveillance for influenza is carried out in most European countries. Viruses are obtained for characterisation and included in reports, through National Influenza Centres, to WHO FluNet [1]. Weekly numbers of laboratory diagnosed influenza infections are also collated in some countries. In recent years, virological sampling for influenza has been linked to general practitioner sentinel

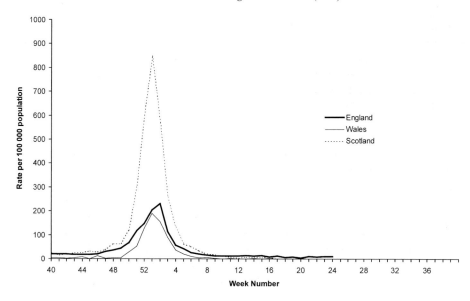

Fig. 1. GP consultation rates for influenza and influenza like illness for England, Wales and Scotland, 1999–2000.

surveillance schemes so as to obtain isolates, which are representative of these occurring in the community.

The development, by WHO, of the network of National Influenza Centres in 1947 led to considerable improvements in the quality and comparability of the results of culture of isolates of influenza virus. Nevertheless, considerable variation remains between countries in the methods used for the diagnosis of influenza infection as well as differences in the approach to the ascertainment of cases, sampling, storage and transport methods. In a review of the methods used in different European countries, Hannoun and Tumova concluded that although there was considerable consensus on the general approach to the collection and use of clinical specimens, and the diagnostic techniques involved, the details of the techniques are heterogeneous, and the results are therefore not really comparable [2].

An influenza surveillance network has been formed between clinical, virological and epidemiology/public health experts in European countries to exchange information on influenza activity, provide early warning to national administrations and collate a database for research on the impact of influenza in Europe [3]. Members of the network, the European Influenza Surveillance Scheme (EISS), submit weekly rates of consultations fir ILI or ARI from regional or national sentinel surveillance schemes combined with the results of virology conducted on a sample of the reported cases. The weekly data is available on the EISS web site www.eiss.org). The network, which currently includes twelve countries, also aims to standardise surveillance methods so as to facilitate comparison of surveillance data.

More limited information is available on the impact of influenza in European countries and much of the data that are available cannot be directly compared between countries.

The burden of influenza in general practice has been compared between England and the Netherlands [4]. The overall proportion of the population consulting with ILI is almost double in the Netherlands compared with England over comparable influenza seasons.

Admissions to hospital relating to influenza are also difficult to assess and are substantially affected by the health system of the country concerned. Between one and two admissions per 1000 inhabitants are estimated to occur each year on average in the Netherlands [5] compared with 0.18 per 1000 inhabitants in England during influenza periods [6].

Estimates of excess mortality, which are produced in a number of European countries, are also plagued with problems of comparability. Neither influenza deaths alone, nor influenza and pneumonia deaths, provide a realistic assessment of the mortality associated with influenza as a result of the large number of deaths due to other conditions such as chronic heart disease, which are exacerbated by influenza. In addition, estimation of the baseline of mortality in the absence of influenza, and subsequent estimation of the excess above this baseline, are highly dependent on the statistical methodology employed. Excess mortality due to all causes in England and Wales, using unpublished Public Health Laboratory Service data, varies from 0 to 2000 in the quietest influenza seasons to 20,000–25,000 in epidemic winters such as 1989/1990.

In conclusion, many European countries adopt a broadly similar approach to clinical and virological surveillance of influenza, although methodological differences make direct comparisons difficult. There is currently only limited information on the impact of influenza on European countries. Collaborative European surveillance offers not only the opportunity to provide early warning of influenza activity but also to promote standardisation of methods to assess influenza activity. New developments, such as national telephone-based health advice services (e.g. NHS Direct in England and Wales (www.nhsdirect.nhs.uk)) and near-patient tests, provide opportunities to improve further the usefulness of influenza surveillance information in Europe.

References

[1] http://oms2.63e.jussieu.fr/flu net/.

[2] C. Hannoun, Tumove Band European Scientific Working Group Influenza (ESWI), Survey of influenza laboratory diagnostic and surveillance methods in Europe, Eur. J. Epidemiol. 16 (2000) 217–222.

[3] J.C. Manuguerra, A. Mosnieu, Surveillance of influenza in Europe from October 1999 to February 2000, Eurosurveillance 5 (2000) 63–68.

[4] D.M. Fleming, M. Zambon, A.I.M. Bartelds, Populated estimates of pressure rpesenting to general practitioners with influenza-like illness, 1987–96: a study of the demography of influenza-like illness in sentinel practice networks in England and Wales, and in the Netherlands, Epidemiol. Infect. 124 (2000) 245–253.

[5] M.J.W. Sprenger, The Impact of Influenza, An Epidemiological Study of Morbidity, Direct Mortality and Related Mortality, Erasmus University, Rotterdam, 1990.

[6] D.M. Fleming, The contribution of influenza to combined acute respiratory infections, hospital admissions and deaths, in winter, Comm. Dis. Public Health 3 (2000) 32–38.

International Congress Series 1219 (2001) 29–32

Recent progress in national policy against influenza in Japan

Masato Tashiro

Department of Viral Diseases and Vaccine Control, National Institute of Infectious Diseases, Gakuen 4-7-1, Musashi-Murayama, Tokyo, 208-0011, Japan

Abstract

Fundamental policies against influenza in Japan have been severely cut back since the obligatory annual immunization program to all school children was withdrawn in 1994. After that, the number of vaccines was extremely reduced in Japan and the manufacturing facilities were also cut down accordingly. In 1997, the Ministry of Health recognized the impact of influenza pandemics as a matter of crisis management and decided to reconstruct comprehensive national influenza politics. National Influenza Pandemics Committee was organized to discuss influenza issues from many aspects. The document of the committee concluded that pandemic planning should be based on year-to-year measures against annual influenza epidemics. The committee made a blueprint of influenza planning and guidelines to carry out the measures. In 1999, the Law of Infectious Diseases Control and Prevention was amended drastically, in which influenza is underlined as a specifically important infectious disease that requires extensive national measures. Vaccinations to elderly persons are strongly recommended by the government, and the Preventive Immunization Law will be amended again to facilitate the new policy. Many plans have been put into practice gradually and the general attitude to influenza in Japan has been improved greatly. © 2001 Elsevier Science B.V. All rights reserved.

Keywords: National policies of Japan; Vaccination program; Vaccine efficacy; Influenza measures

Fundamental policies against influenza in Japan have been severely collapsed since the annual immunization program to all school children was withdrawn in 1994 (Table 1). Before that time, a mass immunization program had been carried out according to the Preventive Immunization Law for more than 20 years, in which all school children between six and 15 years of age received influenza vaccines obligatorily. This was based on a hypothesis that children, who are most susceptible to influenza virus infections, spend most day time in schools in a close contact with one another. By that, influenza should be amplified in schools and children bring back influenza to their homes and spread to the

Table 1
History of influenza vaccination in Japan

1957	Introduction of influenza vaccines (inactivated whole virion vaccines)
1962	Voluntary immunization to school children recommended
1972	Introduction of ether-split vaccines
1976	Obligatory mass immunization program to all school children based on the Preventive Immunization Law
1985	Actions against the immunization program
1987	Parent's consent required
1994	Withdrawal of the mass immunization program
1994	Influenza policies collapsed
2000	Amendment of the Preventive Immunization Law, Immunization to the elderly recommended and supported by the government

community. It was, therefore, considered reasonable that immunization of all school children with influenza vaccines could control influenza epidemics in the community and protect the high-risk groups, including elderly persons from infection with the viruses.

Although the annual mass immunization had been done to all school children, little evidence was obtained that influenza epidemic was controlled efficiently. On the other hand, rare adverse events associated with the vaccination had been exaggerated by mass media. Action groups against immunizations performed big campaigns to stop the immunization program, claiming that influenza vaccines are useless and the obligatory mass-immunization program violates the children's right.

Due to the pressures, the Ministry of Health abolished the immunization program by changing the Preventive Immunization Law in 1994. In the meantime, the Ministry said that influenza vaccines are effective to prevent vaccines from developing severe complications and recommended being vaccinated at one's own expense. However, these messages were not transmitted to the public adequately because of prejudice of mass media influenced by the action groups. Moreover, the government neither recommended vaccination to the high-risk groups, including the elderly, nor proposed any alternate preventive measures against influenza. Most people believed that the government authorized the uselessness of the vaccines and, therefore, withdrew the vaccination program. After that, the number of vaccines was extremely reduced in Japan, resulting in 80 times declines of vaccine production from 40 to only 0.5 million shots, and the manufacturing facilities were also cut down accordingly.

In 1997, upon arguments about possible pandemic influenza, the Ministry of Health recognized the impact of influenza pandemics as a matter of crisis management and decided to reconstruct the comprehensive influenza politics in Japan. Outbreak of H5N1 avian influenza in Hong Kong facilitated the change of policies. The National Pandemic Influenza Committee was organized to discuss influenza issues from scientific, medical, public health and political aspects. The document of the committee concluded that pandemic planning should be based on year-to-year measures against annual influenza epidemics. Cumulative health damages and social impact due to annual influenza epidemics should exceed those of a pandemic influenza. The committee has drawn a blueprint of the influenza planning and guidelines to carry out the measures.

In 1999, the Law of Infectious Diseases Control and Prevention was amended drastically in which Influenza, as well as tuberculosis and AIDS, is underlined as a specifically important infectious disease that requires extensive national measures. Vaccinations to elderly persons are strongly recommended by the government, and the Preventive Immunization Law will be amended again to facilitate the new policy. Many plans have been put into practice gradually and general attitude to influenza in Japan has been improved greatly.

One of our progresses was a change in the vaccination policy. We have an increasing number of elderly persons in Japan, and many of them are in institutions. Recently, the media has reported sensationally have severe outbreaks of influenza in nursing homes. Under these circumstances, the government has concluded that the priority target of vaccination is the elderly group. Although many people now understand the impact and importance of influenza in the elderly group, most people and also many doctors in Japan still doubt the efficacy and safety of influenza vaccines. Therefore, convincing scientific evidence for the efficacy and safety of influenza vaccines to the elderly should have been made before new vaccination program is introduced by the government (Table 2). Otherwise, action groups and mass media must oppose the new policy again.

A research group was organized by the Ministry of Health and performed a prospective study for 3 years in 21 nursing homes and hospitals in four different regions. A total of 2166 inhabitants older than 65 years of age were involved. Vaccination to the elderly in institutions was shown to reduce significantly relative risk of high fevers, complications requiring hospitalization to 0.3–0.5, and death to 0.18. Based on these results, the Government of Japan decided to introduce a new vaccination policy to elderly persons.

Table 2
Efficacy of influenza vaccination to elderly persons in nursing homes (1998/1999)

Event	Region	Relative risk	(95% confidential)
Fever (>38 °C)	A	0.62	(0.40–0.96)*
	B	0.61	(0.41–0.89)*
	C	0.72	(0.54–0.94)*
	D	0.74	(0.67–0.82)*
	Total	0.62	(0.52–0.74)*
Fever (>39 °C)	A	0.38	(0.16–0.86)*
	B	0.49	(0.26–0.90)*
	C	0.57	(0.33–0.96)*
	D	0.50	(0.40–0.63)*
	Total	0.45	(0.34–0.60)*
Hospitalization	A	0.48	(0.12–1.45)
	C	0.51	(0.36–1.18)
	D	0.30	(0.14–0.59)*
Death	A	0.20	(0.02–2.19)
	B	0.00	(0.00–0.88)*
	C	0.13	(0.01–1.13)
	D	0.13	(0.32–0.77)*
	Total	0.18	(0.13–0.24)*

* $P < 0.01$.

Recent progresses in the national influenza politics in Japan include the following.

(1) Fundamental national policies of influenza measures were changed. The government settled three acts for influenza prevention and control:

(a) National Pandemic Influenza Planning, 1997;
(b) The New Law of Infectious Disease Control and Prevention, 1999;
(c) National Planning for Interpandemic Influenza Control, 1999.

(2) National surveillance system of influenza has been improved and enhanced:

(a) The Law of Infectious Diseases Control and Prevention was amended to enhance surveillance systems, 1998;
(b) Infectious Disease Surveillance Center was established in National Institute of Infectious Diseases, 1997;
(c) Sentinel stations for influenza surveillance were potentiated from 2400 pediatric clinics to total 5000 stations, including 3000 pediatric and 2000 internal medicine clinics and hospitals, 1999;
(d) 74 public health institutes of local governments isolate and characterize about 10000 influenza viruses a year.

(3) Vaccination to the elderly has been strongly recommended by the Ministry of Health and Welfare since 1998. The Preventive Immunization Law is scheduled to be amended to support the immunization cost to the elderly and to compensate for possible adverse events.
(4) Production of influenza vaccines has been facilitated:

(a) Structures and facilities of vaccine manufactures for influenza vaccines are reconstructed to facilitate vaccine production under the BSL3 safety condition, by the financial support by the government;
(b) Single radial immunodiffusion test has been introduced to quality control process of influenza vaccines instead of mouse immunization/egg neutralizing test.

(5) Introduction of anti-influenza drugs: Amantadine and neuraminidase inhibitors have been licensed and the costs are/will be covered by the health insurance systems.
(6) Several rapid diagnostic test kits for influenza viruses were launched and the cost of clinical diagnostic test is covered by the health insurance systems.
(7) National collections of animal influenza virus strains: For rapid development of new vaccines and diagnostic test kits in case of new influenza pandemics, systematic collection and storage of animal influenza viruses have been prepared.
(8) International collaboration, including global surveillance activities, has been enhanced.

Acknowledgements

The data of field study of vaccine efficacy was kindly provided by Dr. H. Kamiya, National Mie Hospital, Japan.

International Congress Series 1219 (2001) 33–36

Alternative models for estimating influenza-attributable P&I deaths in the US

W. Thompson*, L. Brammer, D. Shay, E. Weintraub, N. Cox, K. Fukuda

Influenza Branch, A-32, Division of Viral and Rickettsial Diseases, National Center for Infectious Diseases, Centers for Disease Control and Prevention, 1600 Clifton Road, N.E., Atlanta, GA 30333, USA

Abstract

Introduction: This study examined alternative models for estimating influenza-attributable pneumonia and influenza (P&I) deaths in the United States which included influenza specific measures of viral activity as well as measures of RSV activity. *Materials and methods*: P&I deaths in the United States were modeled from 1976 to 1997. Predictors in the models included influenza subtypes A(H1N1), A(H3N2), and B and RSV. We analyzed data from 1976 to 1997. RSV data was available from 1990 through 1997 and therefore separate models were fit that included and excluded RSV measures. *Results*: Influenza accounted for an average of 4773 P&I deaths per year from 1976 to 1997. The results were highly correlated with previous estimates of P&I deaths in the United States ($r = 0.74$, $p < 0.001$). From 1990 to 1997, after controlling for RSV, influenza accounted for an average of 7900 P&I deaths per year. RSV was associated with 563 P&I deaths per year during this time period. *Discussion*: The models in this paper provide strain specific estimates of the association between influenza and P&I deaths in the United States. The models are well suited for providing more precise measurements of the association between influenza and deaths. Published by Elsevier Science B.V.

Keywords: Excess deaths; Mortality; Cyclical regression

1. Introduction

Several alternative statistical methods have been used to estimate annual numbers of influenza-attributable deaths in the United States [1–4]. Methods that include

---

* Corresponding author. Tel.: +1-404-639-4656; fax: +1-404-639-3866.
E-mail address: wct2@cdc.gov (W. Thompson).

0531-5131/01/$ – see front matter. Published by Elsevier Science B.V.
PII: S 0 5 3 1 - 5 1 3 1 (0 1) 0 0 3 2 3 - 5

measures of influenza virus activity [5–7] have been proposed but not implemented widely because reliable measures of influenza virus activity have not been available until recently.

Models that exclude measures of influenza viral activity have been criticized because they have not been validated to ensure that wintertime baselines are free of influenza activity [8]. These models tend to label epidemic periods with B influenza as non-epidemic and bias the non-epidemic baselines higher than expected [8]. The models also require several additional assumptions. Specifically, the models assume that all deviations from non-epidemic baselines represent influenza-attributable deaths. However, influenza is not the only cause of hospitalizations and deaths during the winter period when influenza is circulating. Several recent papers suggest that respiratory syncytial virus (RSV) contributes to a significant number of hospitalizations and deaths during the winter period in the United States in both young children and the elderly [9–11].

Our objective was to estimate both influenza-attributable and RSV-attributable P&I deaths in the United States using models that include measures of viral activity for both influenza and RSV. The models provide more precise estimates of the independent contributions of influenza and RSV on mortality in the United States.

2. Material and methods

Data for deaths in the United States were obtained through the National Center for Health Statistics (NCHS) [12]. Deaths were classified based on the International Classification of Diseases, eighth revision, adapted (ICD-8) or ninth revision (ICD-9) [13–15]. For ICD-8, the pneumonia and influenza (P&I) deaths were coded as 480 through 486 (bacterial and viral pneumonia) and 470–474 (influenza). For ICD-9, pneumonia deaths were coded as 480–486 and influenza deaths were coded 487.

Weekly influenza virus isolation data were obtained from the U.S. World Health Organization (WHO) Collaborating Laboratory Reports from the 1976 to 1977 season through 1996 to 1997 season. Over this 21-year period, 50–75 WHO collaborating virology laboratories in the United States reported the total number of respiratory specimens tested and the number of positive tests for influenza by type and subtype each week [16].

Weekly RSV data were obtained from the National Respiratory and Enteric Virus Surveillance System (NREVSS) from 1990 through 1997. A total of 100 clinical and public health laboratories in 47 states have reported to NREVSS the number of specimen tested for RSV by the antigen detection and virus isolation method, and the number of positive results [17].

Annual influenza-attributable P&I deaths were estimated using a previously described regression model [5,6]. The regression models used in this paper included seasonal variables that controlled for unmeasured effects such as temperature. The models also included a linear term to account for the secular trend in deaths over time, three separate terms for each of the influenza subtypes (A(H3N2), A(H1N1), and B), and a term for RSV virus circulation.

3. Results

3.1. Descriptive statistics

From 1976 to 1996, the average number of P&I deaths in the United States was 67,727 (range 47,094–87,660). The number of P&I deaths increased an average of 1500 deaths per year during this time period. WHO collaborating laboratories in the United States tested an average of 23,512 specimens per year. The number of specimens tested increased during this time period an average of 1200 tests per year.

3.2. Influenza-attributable P&I deaths

For the model fit to data from 1976 to 1997, RSV data were not included as a covariate in the model. From 1976 to 1997, the average number of influenza-attributable P&I deaths was 4773 (range 49–10,191). A(H3N2) viruses were associated with an average of 4014 P&I deaths (range 0–9089). Similarly, influenza B viruses were associated with an average of 759 P&I deaths (range 1–1878). During this time period, A(H1N1) viruses were not statistically associated with P&I deaths.

For the model fit to data from 1990 to 1997, RSV data were included as a covariate in the model. From 1990 to 1997, the average number of influenza-attributable P&I deaths was 7900 (range 4195–11,634). A(H3N2) viruses were associated with an average of 6121 P&I deaths (range 1214–9791), influenza B viruses were associated with an average of 1398 P&I deaths (range 62–2755) and A(H1N1) viruses were associated with 381 P&I deaths. RSV was associated with an average of 563 P&I deaths (range 25–1155).

4. Discussion

Estimates of the annual numbers of influenza-attributable P&I deaths from 1976 to 1997 were positively correlated ($r = 0.74$, $p < 0.01$) with previous estimates published by the CDC [3,4]. On average, the estimates of influenza-attributable P&I deaths were 16% lower than previous CDC estimates (4773 versus 5675). After accounting for RSV circulation, influenza viruses were associated with an average of 7900 P&I deaths annually from the 1990 to 1991 season through the 1996 to 1997 season. Overall, 77% of influenza-attributable deaths were associated with A(H3N2) viruses, 18% with B viruses and 5% with A(H1N1) viruses. RSV was associated with approximately 563 P&I deaths annually, a finding consistent with previously published estimates [9,18].

There are several reasons why our results represent a step forward in the understanding of influenza-attributable deaths in the United States. First, these models provide influenza subtype-specific estimates of the association between influenza activity and deaths in the United States. Second, the models address several previous criticisms of influenza excess death models. For example, we did not label B influenza seasons as non-epidemic and a substantial number of deaths were attributed to influenza B viruses. Third, the effect of influenza viruses varies throughout the influenza season; these models allow the influenza measure to vary week-by-week. When the percentage of influenza-positive isolates was high for a particular week, the model predicted that a greater number of deaths were associated with influenza. Fourth, the models do not impute epidemic periods. Fifth, the models allow for the inclusion of the effects of another respiratory virus associated with wintertime mortality, RSV. Finally, the models can be adapted to include other important confounders such as temperature.

References

[1] R.E. Serfling, Methods for the current statistical analysis of excess pneumonia–influenza deaths, Public Health Rep. 78 (1963) 494–506.

[2] K.J. Lui, A.P. Kendal, Impact of influenza epidemics on mortality in the United States from October 1972 to May 1985, Am. J. Public Health 77 (1987) 712–716.

[3] L. Simonsen, M. Clarke, G.D. Williamson, et al., The impact of influenza epidemics on mortality: introducing a severity index, Am. J. Public Health 87 (1997) 1944–1950.

[4] L. Simonsen, M.J. Clarke, D.F. Stroup, et al., A method for timely assessment of influenza-associated mortality in the United States, Epidemiol. 8 (1997) 390–395.

[5] R.E. Clifford, J.W.G. Smith, H.E. Tillett, P.J. Wherry, Excess mortality associated with influenza in England and Wales, Int. J. Epidemiol. 6 (1977) 115–128.

[6] D.W. Alling, W.C. Blackwelder, C.H. Stuart-Harris, A study of excess mortality during influenza epidemics in the United States, 1968–1976, Am. J. Epidemiol. 113 (1981) 30–43.

[7] P.W. Glezen, Serious morbidity and mortality associated with influenza epidemics, Epidemiol. Rev. 4 (1982) 25–44.

[8] P.W. Glezen, Emerging infections: pandemic influenza, Epidemiol. Rev. 18 (1996) 64–76.

[9] Han, Alexander, Anderson, Respiratory syncytial virus pneumonia among the elderly: an assessment of the disease burden, J. Infect. Dis. 179 (1999) 25–30.

[10] H.S. Izurieta, W.W. Thompson, P. Kramarz, et al., Influenza and the rates of hospitalization for respiratory disease among infants and young children, N. Engl. J. Med. 342 (2000) 232–239.

[11] D.K. Shay, R.C. Holman, R.D. Newman, L.L. Liu, J.W. Stout, L.J. Anderson, Bronchiolitis associated hospitalizations among US children, 1980–1996, JAMA 282 (1999) 1440–1446.

[12] Vital Statistics Mortality Data, Multiple Cause Detail, 1972–1997. Public use data tapes contents and documentation package. National Center for Health Statistics, Hyattsville, MD, 1992.

[13] World Health Organization, International Classification of Diseases, Eight Revision, Adapted for Use in the United States, US Government Printing Office, Washington, DC, 1975.

[14] Manual of the International Statistical Classification of Diseases, Injuries, and Causes of Death. Based on Recommendations of the Ninth Revision Conference, 1975, and adopted by the Twenty-Ninth World Health Assembly. World Health Organization, Geneva, Switzerland, 1997.

[15] W.H. Barker, J.P. Mullooly, Impact of epidemic type A influenza in a defined adult population, Am. J. Epidemiol. 112 (1980) 798–811.

[16] L.T. Brammer, H.S. Izurieta, K. Fukuda, et al., Surveillance for influenza—United States, 1994–95, 1995–96 and 1996–97 seasons, MMWR 49 (SS-3) (2000) 13–28.

[17] CDC, Update: Respiratory Syncytial Virus Activity–United States, 1998–1999 Season, MMWR 48 (1999) 1104.

[18] D. Shay, R.C. Holman, G.E. Roosevelt, M.J. Clarke, L.J. Anderson, Bronchiolitis associated mortality and estimates of repiratory syncytial virus associated deaths among U.S. children, 1979–1997, J. Infect. Dis., in press.

International Congress Series 1219 (2001) 37–42

Influenza present: the impact of the 1999–2000 epidemic on morbidity and mortality in the USA

N.J. Cox*, T.L. Brammer, A. Postema, A.I. Klimov, W. Thompson, K. Fukuda

Influenza Branch, G-16, Centers for Disease Control and Prevention, 1600 Clifton Road, N.E. Atlanta, GA 30333, USA

Abstract

Background: During the 1999–2000 influenza season, influenza A (H3N2) viruses predominated in the United States and worldwide. Typically, influenza seasons in which influenza A (H3N2) viruses predominate are more severe than seasons in which influenza A (H1N1) and influenza B viruses are the primary circulating viruses. Three of the four indices used to monitor the impact of influenza in the US indicated that the 1999–2000 season was a typical H3N2 season; however, the P and I mortality reporting system and many media reports indicated that it was particularly severe. *Methods*: During the seasons covered (1996–1997 through 1999–2000), CDC received weekly reports from October through May from (1) collaborating laboratories that report on the total number of respiratory specimens tested and those that are influenza positive; (2) State and Territorial Epidemiologists who report on estimates of influenza activity in their state or territory; (3) sentinel physicians who report on the total number of patient visits and the number of cases of influenza-like illness (ILI); and (4) vital statistics offices in major US cities that report on the number of deaths related to pneumonia and influenza (P and I). *Results*: During the 1999–2000 influenza season, the percentage of respiratory specimens testing positive for influenza peaked at 33%; the state and territorial epidemiologists reports peaked at 44 states reporting either regional or widespread influenza activity; the percentage of patient visits for ILI peaked at 6%; and the proportion of deaths attributed to pneumonia and influenza peaked at 11.2%. *Conclusions*: Influenza activity during the 1999–2000 influenza season was similar to the three previous influenza seasons as indicated by reports from state and territorial epidemiologists, the percentage of respiratory specimens positive for influenza, and the proportion of visits for ILI. The percentage of deaths attributed to P and I reported by 122 US cities was higher than the peaks of the previous three seasons; however, part of the observed increase is apparently due to changes in reporting. Published by Elsevier Science B.V.

Keywords: Influenza surveillance; Influenza variation; Morbidity; Mortality

* Corresponding author. Tel: +1-404-639-3591; fax: +1-404-639-2334.
E-mail address: ncox@cdc.gov (N.J. Cox).

0531-5131/01/$ – see front matter. Published by Elsevier Science B.V.
PII: S0531-5131(01)00404-6

1. Introduction

Epidemics of influenza occur nearly every year during the winter months in the United States and are responsible for substantial morbidity and mortality [1,2]. It has been estimated that in recent decades an annual average of over 110,000 hospitalizations and over 20,000 deaths can be attributed to influenza [3–5]. The Influenza Branch conducts surveillance for influenza in the United States each year from October through mid-May. Through voluntary reporting of influenza data by the states, CDC determines when influenza viruses are circulating, identifies circulating strains, detects antigenic and genetic changes in the viruses, monitors influenza-related illnesses and measures the impact of influenza on deaths. During the 1999–2000 influenza season, media reports indicated that the influenza season was particularly severe. We compared the morbidity and mortality observed for the past four seasons in order to determine if the 1999–2000 influenza season was more severe than other recent years.

2. Methods

CDC's influenza surveillance system is comprised of the following four components.

(1) World Health Organization (WHO) Collaborating Laboratories and National Respiratory and Enteric Virus Surveillance System (NREVSS) Laboratories. Approximately 75 WHO collaborating laboratories and approximately 50 NREVSS laboratories located throughout the United States report the total number of respiratory specimens tested and the number positive for influenza by type and subtype each week. A subset of the influenza viruses isolated is sent to CDC for antigenic and genetic characterization.

(2) State and Territorial Epidemiologist Reports. The level of state- or territory-wide influenza activity, as assessed by the state or territorial epidemiologist, is reported to CDC weekly from October through May. When activity occurs, it is reported as sporadic (cases of ILI or lab-confirmed influenza reported), regional (outbreaks of ILI or laboratory-confirmed influenza occurring in geographic areas containing less than 50% of the state's population), or widespread (outbreaks of ILI or laboratory-confirmed influenza occurring in geographic areas representing more than 50% of the state's population). Methods for assessing activity levels vary from state to state.

(3) US Influenza Sentinel Physicians Surveillance Network. Each week from October through May, approximately 450 (out of a total of approximately 900) sentinel physicians report the number of patients seen each week and the number of these patients seen for ILI by age group. Baseline levels of total patient visits for ILI ranged from 0% to 3%.

(4) 122 Cities Mortality Reporting System (MRS). Each week during the years 1996–1998, the vital statistics offices in 122 cities report the total number of death certificates filed and the number of death certificates in which either pneumonia was identified as the underlying cause of death or influenza was identified anywhere on the death certificate. CDC modified the 122 cities case definition for reporting deaths for the 1999–2000 season. Cities were asked to report total deaths and the number of deaths when either pneumonia or influenza was listed anywhere on the death certificate [3]. These data are used to calculate the proportion of all deaths attributed to pneumonia and influenza (P and

I), as well as a P and I mortality curve. A periodic regression model that incorporates a robust regression procedure is applied to produce a seasonal baseline of P and I deaths and to calculate "excess" deaths above the baseline. An increase of 1.645 standard deviations above the seasonal baseline of P and I deaths was considered the epidemic threshold (i.e., the point at which the observed proportion of deaths attributed to pneumonia or influenza was significantly higher than would be expected at that time of the year in the absence of influenza).

3. Results

During the 1999–2000 influenza season, influenza type A (H3N2) viruses were the predominant viruses circulating in the United States. The national percentage of respiratory specimens positive for influenza peaked at 33% during mid-December. During the previous three influenza seasons (1996–1997, 1997–1998, and 1998–1999), the peak percentages of specimens testing positive for influenza viruses ranged from 28% to 34% (Fig. 1).

State and Territorial Epidemiologists reports peaked during mid-January when 44 states reported either regional or widespread influenza activity. This figure compares with 39, 46, and 42 states reporting regional or widespread influenza activity for the 1996–1997, 1997–1998, and 1998–1999 seasons, respectively (Fig. 1).

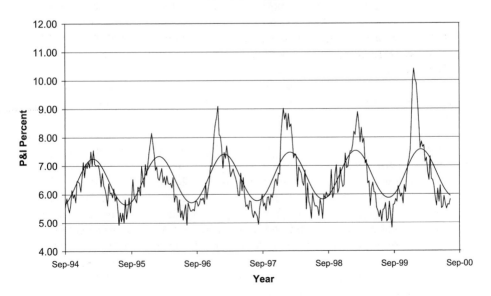

Fig. 1. Results of three influenza surveillance systems by week and year: United States, 1996–2000.

Influenza Surveillance, United States
1996-97 through 1999-2000

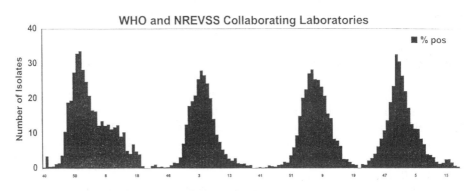

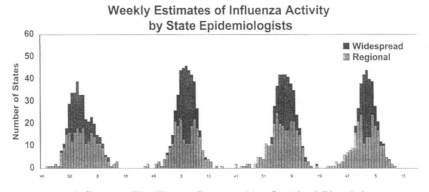

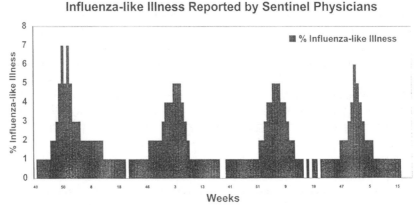

Fig. 2. Adjusted percentage of mortality attributable to pneumonia and influenza (P and I) in 122 cities, by week of report: United States 1994–2000.

The percentage of patient visits for ILI peaked at 6% during late December, 1999. During the previous 3 years, the peak percentages for such visits ranged between 5% and 7% (Fig. 1).

The percentage of deaths attributed to P and I peaked at 11.2% during the week ending January 22 (week 33). During the previous three influenza seasons, peak percentages of deaths attributed to P and I was 9.2%, 9.0%, and 8.8% for the 1996–1997, 1997–1998, and 1998–1999 influenza seasons, respectively. Analysis of P and I data from the previous four seasons compared to the 1999–2000 season indicated that there had been a shift upward of approximately 0.8% in the baseline, coincident with the change in reporting definition. Using this analysis to adjust the baseline, we found that the percentage of deaths peaked at approximately 10.4% during the 1999–2000 influenza season (Fig. 2).

4. Discussion

During the 1999–2000 season, influenza A/Sydney/05/97-like (H3N2) viruses predominated with peak activity occurring during late December (weeks 51 and 52). Peak activity for this season occurred approximately 4–6 weeks earlier than peak activity during the 1997–1998 and 1998–1999 influenza seasons, but at approximately the same time as the 1996–1997 season. The percentage of respiratory specimens testing positive for influenza viruses was 33% for 1999–2000, as compared with 28% to 34% for the previous three seasons. During the 1999–2000 season, the highest combined number of reports of either widespread or regional influenza activity by state and territorial epidemiologists was 44 for the week ending January 15 (week 2). During the previous three influenza seasons, the highest total numbers of widespread or regional reports ranged from 39 to 46. The percentage of patient visits for ILI peaked at 6% in the 1999–2000 influenza season. During the three previous seasons, the peak percentages of visits for ILI ranged from 5% to 7%. Thus, using these three influenza surveillance components, the 1999–2000 influenza season appears to be fairly typical compared to the previous three seasons. However, the peak percentage of deaths attributed to P and I in the 122 cities MRS was higher than levels seen during the previous three influenza seasons. Before the 1999–2000 season, vital statistics offices participating in the 122 cities MRS were asked to report a death as a P and I death when pneumonia was listed in part 1 of the death certificate or when influenza was listed anywhere on the death certificate (part I or part II). However, this case definition did not allow P and I mortality cases to be identified easily in computerized mortality systems, and an evaluation of the 122 cities MRS conducted in 1999 showed that the case definition was not used consistently by all cities (CDC, unpublished data, 1999). Some large cities reported P and I deaths on the basis of underlying causes of death. In addition, in January 1999, CDC's National Center for Health Statistics implemented the International Statistical Classification of Diseases and Related Public Health Problems, 10th Revision (ICD-10) [6]. Coding rules for the underlying causes of death for pneumonia in ICD-10 substantially differ from those in International Classification of Diseases, Ninth Revision (ICD-9). In response to inconsistent use of the old case definition and the impact of the change from ICD-9 to ICD-10 on reporting to the 122 cities MRS, CDC modified the 122 cities case definition for reporting P and I deaths for the 1999–2000 season. Cities were asked to report a death as a P and I death when either pneumonia or influenza was listed anywhere on the death certificate. This new case definition is simpler and more compatible with computerized mortality systems. The effect of the change in the case definition and concurrent ICD-9 to ICD-10 change is not yet completely resolved. However, it appears that reporting changes resulted in an upward change of approximately 0.8% in the seasonal baseline. Even after taking this baseline change into account, it appears that the 1999–2000 influenza season resulted in substantial influenza-related mortality.

References

[1] G.R. Noble, Epidemiological and clinical aspects of influenza, in: A.S. Beare (Ed.), Basic and Applied Influenza Research, CRC Press, Boca Raton, FL, 1982, pp. 11–50.
[2] N.J. Cox, K. Subbarao, Global epidemiology of influenza: past and present, Annu. Rev. Med. 51 (2000) 407–421.
[3] L. Simonsen, L.B. Schonberger, D.F. Stroup, N.H. Arden, N.J. Cox, The impact of influenza on mortality in the USA, in: L.E. Brown, A.W. Hampson, R.G. Webster (Eds.), Options for the Control of Influenza III, Elsevier, Amsterdam, 1996, pp. 26–33.
[4] K.J. Lui, A.P. Kendal, Impact of influenza epidemics on mortality in the United States from October 1972 to May 1885, Am. J. Public Health 77 (1987) 712–716.
[5] L. Simonsen, K. Fukuda, L.B. Schonberger, N.J. Cox, The impact of influenza epidemics on hospitalizations, J. Infect. Dis. 181 (2000) 831–837.
[6] World Health Organization, International Statistical Classification of Diseases and Related Public Health Problems, 19th revision, World Health Organization, Geneva, Switzerland, 1993.

International Congress Series 1219 (2001) 43–51

The impact of pandemic influenza, with special reference to 1918

Stephen C. Schoenbaum*

The Commonwealth Fund, One East 75th Street, New York, NY 10021 USA

Abstract

Pandemic influenza, by definition, affects the overwhelming majority of countries and population subgroups in the world in a very short period of time. The impact of pandemics is not merely a matter of the biology of the particular virus in individuals. Pandemics are a social phenomenon affected by prevailing social circumstances, e.g., war, economic conditions, crowding, and food supply. In turn, pandemics affect social organization and events, e.g., governance and famine. Much of the study of pandemic influenza has been in industrialized countries in temperate zones; the occurrence of excess morbidity and mortality, and the strain on health care and other services in these countries are well known. A conference in 1998 brought together an increasingly large body of historical research about the pandemic of "Spanish influenza" in 1918–1919. It included interesting contributions about the impact of the pandemic in areas such as sub-Saharan Africa, India (where mortality is estimated at 17 million, or about half the world total), and the Pacific Islands. There are important lessons for contemporary society from the impact of the pandemic of 1918–1919 and other pandemics. One can make a compelling case for pandemic preparedness, including developing and executing strategies both to prevent and to ameliorate pandemic spread. © 2001 Elsevier Science B.V. All rights reserved.

Keywords: Pandemic influenza; Impact; History; Pandemic preparedness; "Spanish influenza"

1. Introduction

In a short period of time, weeks to months, influenza pandemics wreak destruction throughout the world, causing enormous numbers of illnesses and staggering numbers of deaths. In a few months of 1918 and 1919, approximately 30 million people died. In India

* Corresponding author. Tel.: +1-212-606-3505; fax: +1-212-606-3515.
 E-mail address: SCS@cmwf.org (S.C. Schoenbaum).

alone, the influenza pandemic of 1918, interacting with famine, is now believed to have taken the lives of 17 million persons [1]. Gina Kolata, in her recent book, "Flu", makes the following observations on the worldwide impact of the 1918 pandemic: "In comparison, AIDS had killed 11.7 million people through 1997. World War I was responsible for 9.2 million combat deaths...World War II for 15.9 million combat deaths. Historian (Alfred) Crosby remarks that whatever the exact number felled by the 1918 flu, one thing is indisputable: the virus 'killed more humans than any other disease in a period of similar duration in the history of the world' [2]."

It is easy to characterize the pandemic of 1918 as an extremely unusual event and believe that nothing like it will ever occur again. It is much more appropriate, however, to consider pandemic influenza in relation to large storms, such as hurricanes, or earthquakes, or volcanic eruptions. In short, pandemic influenza, even of the magnitude of 1918, is an event that is likely to occur again. We just do not know when.

In this paper, we shall examine some of the attributes of pandemic influenza, its effect on individuals and on societies, and why these effects make a compelling case for pandemic preparedness, particularly planning to prevent or ameliorate pandemic spread.

2. Definition of pandemic influenza

There has not been a constant definition of the terms "pandemic influenza" or "influenza pandemics" over time. One type of definition is strictly epidemiologic: some use the term simply to refer to apparent worldwide spread of influenza epidemics. With this use of the term, it is possible to have "pandemics" of influenza every few years and to speak of the degree to which they are associated with severe illnesses or deaths. Others use the term to refer to worldwide spread of severe epidemics, ones associated with high rates of illness, complications such as pneumonia, and death. Even with this use of the term, it is possible to have "pandemics" of influenza every few years. More recently, the term has been used to refer to a combination of an epidemiologic and a virologic event. Thus, some use the term to refer to worldwide spread of severe epidemics in association with an antigenic shift in at least the hemagglutinin of the prevailing influenza A viruses. Finally, when there is an antigenic shift, it has been common for multiple waves of illness and deaths in the same "influenza season" to occur in at least some geographic locations. It also is common to see multiple epidemics in a couple of years period before there is significant antigenic drift in the newly shifted virus. Some use the term "influenza pandemic" to refer to the first major occurrence of the newly shifted virus (e.g., the Asian influenza pandemic of 1957), or to the first season of the newly shifted virus (e.g., the Asian influenza pandemic of 1957–1958), or to the period before there was significant antigenic drift (e.g., the Asian influenza pandemic of 1957–1959).

For the purposes of this paper, I shall use the term "influenza pandemic" to refer to unusually extensive and severe epidemics of influenza A, compared to recent experience with influenza, with the epidemics occurring throughout the world, in association with a major antigenic shift in at least the hemagglutinin. I shall generally confine the use of the term to either the first major occurrence of the newly shifted virus or to the first influenza season in which it appeared. In my use of the term, by definition, "pandemic influenza" must have a large impact on populations. Also, my use of the term leaves some question of how to characterize the "herald wave" that occurred in some places in the early months of 1918 and likely resulted in seeding the virus throughout much, though not all, of the world. This wave of illness, unnoticed in many areas, was significant enough in Spain to lead to the name "Spanish influenza" that then stuck to the pandemic when global illness began to occur in the later months of 1918.

With the definition I am using, there were three influenza pandemics in the 20th century: 1918–1919, 1957–1958, and 1968–1969. Deaths were greatest in 1918–1919, and least in 1968–1969. The first two were associated with a major shift in both the prevailing influenza A hemagglutinin and neuraminidase, whereas, only the hemagglutinin shifted in 1968. The last pandemic prior to 1918 was in 1890, and it, too, had enormous impact. The hemagglutinin of the virus responsible for the 1890 pandemic appears to have been related to the H3 hemagglutinin that appeared in 1968 [3]. Elderly persons in 1968 had pre-existing antibody against this hemagglutinin and appeared to be relatively protected [3]. That, and the fact that there was no shift in the neuraminidase in 1968, may have been related to the relatively lesser impact of the pandemic of 1968–1969 compared to 1957–1958. Interestingly, in 1977, another major shift in the influenza A virus appeared. The H1N1 strains that began to circulate then were virtually identical to strains that had circulated in the 1950s and much of the adult population had been exposed to and had antibody to similar strains. Though worldwide epidemics of the new H1N1 strains occurred (the so-called "Russian flu"), the severity of these epidemics was not great, even among younger persons; and by the definition I am using, we will not consider the appearance of these H1N1 strains to have been associated with an influenza pandemic.

3. What is special about influenza pandemics?

Influenza pandemics occur irregularly. When they occur, most of the population is susceptible to the newly shifted influenza A strain, so that attack rates can range as high as 40–50% of the population. Further, the infections tend to be associated with viral pneumonia, which can be fatal, and to predispose other infected persons to secondary bacterial pneumonias, which also can be fatal. In 1918, it was common for persons to go from being perfectly healthy to dying of primary viral pneumonia in a matter of a couple of days. Although some infected persons are asymptomatic and although many, indeed most, of the illnesses associated with an influenza pandemic are mild (symptoms occur but the person remains ambulatory) or moderate (require the ill person to go to bed), pandemics are nonetheless associated with large epidemics of emergency room visits, hospitalizations for pneumonia, and deaths, in most affected geographic areas. In just one hospital in Atlanta, GA, in the pandemic of 1968–1969, medical emergency clinic visits doubled, pneumonia admissions and deaths attributable to pneumonia and influenza increased about seven-fold [4]. This puts an enormous strain on the healthcare system; and the 1968–1969 pandemic had relatively low impact compared to 1957–1958 and 1918–1919. Furthermore, when so many persons become ill in such a short period of time, there are significant economic and social effects, which we shall discuss below.

3.1. The impact of influenza pandemics in the United States

First, however, it is worth noting that pandemics, as defined above, have somewhat different patterns of morbidity and mortality than interpandemic epidemics of influenza A, even very large interpandemic epidemics. Recently, Simonsen et al. [5] have shown that with the pandemics of 1918, 1957, and 1968, mortality in the United States was relatively higher for younger persons (< 65) than with subsequent epidemics of influenza A viruses carrying the same hemagglutinin. In 1918, with the emergence of H1N1 influenza, there were approximately 550,000 excess pneumonia and influenza deaths in the United States, and almost half of all excess deaths occurred among persons aged 20–40 [6]. That, however, is only part of the story. In 1918, virtually 100% of excess deaths were in persons < 65; whereas, by 1936–37, only about 60% of excess deaths were in persons < 65; and, by 1943–44, only 30% of excess deaths were in persons < 65. In the Asian influenza (H2N2) era, a similar pattern was observed, at a lesser order of magnitude. In 1957–1958, there were two waves of illness and excess deaths. Overall, total excess mortality for the season was about 65,000, and 36% of the excess deaths were in persons < 65. By 1967–1968, with the last appearance of Asian influenza in the United States, there were an estimated 22,000 excess deaths; and only 4% were in persons < 65. Finally, in the Hong Kong (H3N2) era, the first appearance in 1968–1969 was associated with total excess mortality of approximately 28,000 and pneumonia and influenza excess mortality of approximately 16,000, of which over 40% were in persons < 65. Since 1982, the H3N2 epidemics in the United States have been accompanied by less than 10,000 excess deaths per year and less than 10% of those have been in persons < 65.

What are the implications of these patterns of mortality? First, we have become used to the notion that the principal impact of influenza is on the elderly. Not only is that not necessarily true; but Simonsen's analyses suggest that in pandemics, even if the principal impact happens to be among older individuals, younger ones are disproportionately affected. In any pandemic, it is likely that the effect on younger persons will be noticeable; and, should there be a large total impact of the pandemic, which is quite possible, this could lead to a significant social effect. In short, the next major pandemic should affect disproportionately countries with younger populations; and, throughout the world, there will be epidemics of children plunged precipitously into single-parent families or orphaned!

Simonsen et al. [7] have also looked at the impact of influenza epidemics on hospitalizations by studying the years 1970–1995. Not surprisingly, patterns in hospitalization tend to be similar to patterns in excess mortality. This includes the fact that the greatest proportional hospitalization for persons < 65 tends to occur in the earliest years after emergence of a pandemic strain and decline over the years. Thus, again, one would predict that a next pandemic would lead to a noticeable increase in hospitalizations for pneumonia and influenza among younger persons, not just the elderly.

It is easy to think that, at least in Western countries, our medical capability for treating pneumonia and influenza is much greater today than during the pandemics of the 20th century. We have more antibiotics and better intensive care units. But, such thinking does not take into account a couple of important facts. (1) A pandemic of 1918 proportions, occurring in the United States today, would potentially cause 1.5 million deaths and several times that number of hospitalizations. The United States, with its emphasis on efficiency in hospital care, is unlikely to have a fraction of the intensive care capacity necessary to bring state-of-the art treatment to most of the persons who would need it. (2) Secondary bacterial pneumonias in patients with influenza are not necessarily curable with current therapy. The most common cause of secondary pneumonia has been pneumococcal; but higher case-fatality has been associated with pneumonias caused by *Staphylococcus aureus*, Group A beta hemolytic streptococci, and *Hemophilus influenzae*. Even when these organisms are exquisitely sensitive to available antibiotics, the infections can be fatal. In 1918, of course, there were no available antibiotics; but in 1957, penicillin-resistant staphylococci proved to be particularly problematic. Now, there is increasing resistance of pneumococci to penicillin, and staphylococci are increasing resistant to methicillin. In the next pandemic of influenza, secondary bacterial pneumonias could prove to be very difficult to treat with existing antibiotics.

Meltzer et al. [8] have evaluated the potential economic impact of a moderately large pandemic of influenza in the United States, with 89,000–207,000 deaths, 314,000–734,000 hospitalizations, and 18–42 million outpatient visits. Such an occurrence would have an economic impact of US$71–166 billion, "excluding disruptions to commerce and society". The latter, of course, would be enormous.

3.2. The worldwide impact of influenza pandemics

It is common to focus on the impact of influenza in Western countries, particularly those, such as the United States, where systematic information on mortality has been available for many years. Pandemics, by definition, have global impact, and it is important to consider some of the features of this impact, to the extent it can be estimated. Although, regrettably, there is very little information about the impact of the Asian and Hong Kong influenza pandemics throughout the world, over the years, historians have paid increasing attention to the 1918 pandemic.

Patterson and Pyle [1], the source of the modern estimate of 30 million deaths around the world in this pandemic, have tried to compile mortality figures by region and country. Despite what was mentioned above about the enormous impact of the pandemic in the United States, in Patterson and Pyle's estimates, "the highest death rates are generally from Africa and Asia, and the lowest from North America, Australia, and Europe. Not surprisingly, poor populations suffered more than wealthier ones with better food and shelter. Differential access to health care probably also had some impact; there was no specific therapy for influenza or its complications, but supportive care was useful." In their estimates, mortality ranged from about 5 per 1000 in Europe and North America, to about 9 per 1000 in Latin America, to about 15 per 1000 in Africa, to 20–34 per 1000 in Asia. As mentioned before, India appears to have had the highest mortality.

In 1998, Professor Howard Phillips, in the Department of History at the University of Cape Town, and Professor David Killingray organized a conference, entitled, "Reflections on the Spanish Flu Pandemic after 80 years: causes, course and consequences" (see http://www.uct.ac.za/depts/history/conf.htm). Papers presented at this conference painted a picture of the social impact of influenza that is seldom as vivid in the epidemiologic literature. For example, Ramanna [9] chronicled some of the measures taken to cope with the pandemic in and around Bombay, including setting up special hospitals, organizing volunteer medical support and charitable collections, and providing ways for cremating the huge number who died. Wakimura [10] recorded the inter-relationship between famine and influenza in India. On the one hand, failure of the monsoon led to reduced crops and very high prices for food, with attendant increases in malnutrition, which increased the impact of influenza infection. On the other hand, after influenza began to occur, the high mortality disrupted agricultural activities and increased the impact of the famine.

Sub-Saharan Africa appears not to have been affected by the "herald wave" in the early months of 1918 [1]. Influenza arrived in the region by ship in about August, 1918, and spread largely by ship, river boat, and railway [11,12]. Although case-fatality was much less than it had been for plague in Senegal, overall mortality was considerably greater [11]. In Tanzania, owing to the very large number of deaths, many chiefs suspended the traditional funerals, a step not taken lightly. In a number of areas, as in India, there was again an interaction between influenza and famine. Social disruption was significant. As Musambachime pointed out, "Mining areas in Northern Rhodesia (Zambia), Katanga, Southern Rhodesia (Zimbabwe) and South Africa were closed and labor recruitment for these and other employment centers was suspended for 4 months between October 1918 and February 1919... Both missionaries and administrative officers were unable to tour outlying areas to collect taxes" [13].

Western Polynesia was also affected, for the most part severely, by the 1918 pandemic [14]. Many of the islands there adopted quarantine policies, as did other island nations such as Mauritius and Australia. These policies mostly delayed outbreaks, but occasionally avoided them. As Herda [14] points out, "Western Samoa, which did not close off its port suffered one of the world's worst death rates from the pandemic, while American Samoa, about 50 km away, avoided the pandemic entirely due to a full and effective quarantine. Western Samoan anger and bitterness over the pandemic—both the circumstances of its entry as well as its management by the colonial administration—was deep and fueled the formation of a proto-independence movement, known as the Mau, in the 1920s". The administrator, from New Zealand, was removed from his post.

Overall, despite the fragmentary history available to us from around the world of the impact of the pandemic of 1918, and despite the fact that there was much less impact of the pandemics of 1957 and 1968, it seems clear that these events can cause enormous demands on medical services and enormous costs. Key individuals may become incapacitated or die, literally changing the course of history (for example, Crosby [15] documents the possible effects that influenza had on the European peace process in late 1918 and 1919). Social disruption can occur from interrupted services, owing to massive illness among workers and from sudden deaths of parents. There are likely to be unpredictable consequences such as loss of confidence in a government's ability to handle the situation.

4. What would be different now?

Overall, as one reviews the history of the 1918 pandemic, it is striking that the occurrence of disease, although global, affecting almost all countries and almost all sub-populations within a country, most severely affected persons who were poor, lived in crowded conditions, or were affected by hunger, pregnancy, or other concurrent illnesses. These situations persist today, and it does not take much imagination to realize that the effect of an influenza pandemic today in some of the poorer parts of the world could be enormous. A predictable tragedy would occur in countries in which there are large numbers of HIV infected persons. Furthermore, we have already reviewed the fact that even in first-world countries, medical facilities and resources would probably not be adequate to blunt the impact of a newly shifted influenza A virus infecting a population.

By 1889–1890, transportation by steamships and railroads was sufficiently well developed to support "a truly worldwide pandemic" [16]. In the 21st century, there should be no transportation barrier to spreading a potential pandemic strain of influenza A throughout the world in a very short period of time.

Thus, the only difference between then and now is our growing understanding of influenza virology and our ability to consider preventing or ameliorating pandemic spread. There seem to be several possibilities for doing this. (1) First, there can and should be global surveillance for novel strains infecting humans. It requires global organization and financial support to have a tight and effective surveillance network. Nonetheless, it is possible that the identification of the H5N1 infections in Hong Kong and the eradication of the avian reservoir (chickens and ducks) that appeared to be related to those infections, was an example of prevention of the emergence of a pandemic strain. (2) There is evidence that persons who have had natural exposure to similar strains exhibit some protection later in life when a pandemic strain emerges [3]. An important question is whether some similar sort of protection might occur with prior immunization to prototypes of the influenza A hemagglutinins? In other words, could prior immunization ameliorate illness during a subsequent pandemic? Furthermore, if it could, what would be the optimal time to begin giving the vaccine (for example, in early childhood, so as possibly to induce the phenomenon of "original antigenic sin" that occurs with natural infection in childhood [17]) and should the vaccine be live or inactivated? This set of questions merits thought since there are only 14 influenza A hemagglutinin types, and it should be possible with current technology to develop polyvalent vaccines and give them periodically through life. (3) A related strategy would be developing vaccines for prototype strains of influenza A viruses carrying the various hemagglutinin types and stockpiling them for use when a potential pandemic emerged. Although this approach would avoid "unnecessary" immunization, it raises practical issues about manufacturing and maintaining stockpiles. (4) Since pandemics often consist of more than one wave in an influenza season, or lead to recurrent epidemics in the next year or two, with the emergence of a potential pandemic strain, countries should consider immediate production of a vaccine, even if it appears that it cannot be produced in time to prevent the first epidemic wave. (5) There are now several antivirals that are effective at preventing influenza infection or modifying illness when given early enough. A next pandemic could be ameliorated if it were possible to have sufficient supplies of one or more of these antivirals available. (6) Although secondary pneumococcal pneumonia is less lethal than some of the other secondary bacterial pneumonias, it is the most common type of secondary bacterial pneumonia. Pneumococcal vaccination at the time of emergence of a potential pandemic influenza strain might ameliorate the impact of the pandemic.

All of the above merit serious consideration and form an agenda for pandemic planning and for research. I find it troublesome that with the currently available knowledge and technology, most of the above options are unlikely to make much of a difference for all but the most affluent nations. The impact of the next major pandemic, although great in affluent nations, is likely to be even greater in the poorest nations. The first option, increasing global surveillance, is within our technical grasp and is clearly a critical part of developing a global strategy for thwarting emerging pandemic strains. A second consideration of great importance is focusing on methods for rapid development and production of inexpensive influenza vaccines that might be used for the general population of the world.

References

[1] K.D. Patterson, G.F. Pyle, The geography and mortality of the 1918 influenza pandemic, Bull. Hist. Med. 65 (1991) 4–21.

[2] G. Kolata, Flu: The Story of the Great Influenza Pandemic of 1918 and the Search for the Virus that Caused it, Farrar, Straus and Giroux, New York, 1999, p. 330 (p. 7).

[3] S.C. Schoenbaum, M.T. Coleman, W.R. Dowdle, S.R. Mostow, Epidemiology of influenza in the elderly: evidence of virus recycling, Am. J. Epidemiol. 103 (1976) 166–173.

[4] S.W. Schwarzmann, J.L. Adler, R.J. Sullivan Jr., W.M. Marine, Bacterial pneumonia during the Hong Kong influenza epidemic of 1968–1969, Arch. Intern. Med. 127 (1971) 1037–1041.

[5] L. Simonsen, M.J. Clarke, L.B. Schonberger, N.H. Arden, N.J. Cox, K. Fukuda, Pandemic versus epidemic influenza mortality: a pattern of changing age distribution, J. Infect. Dis. 178 (1998) 53–60.

[6] S.D. Collins, Age and sex incidence of influenza and pneumonia morbidity and mortality in the epidemic of 1928–29 with comparative data for the epidemic of 1918–19, Public Health Rep. 33 (1931) 1909–1937.

[7] L. Simonsen, K. Fukuda, L.B. Schonberger, N.J. Cox, The impact of influenza epidemics on hospitalizations, J. Infect. Dis. 181 (2000) 831–837.

[8] M.I. Meltzer, N.J. Cox, K. Fukuda, The economic impact of pandemic influenza in the United States: priorities for intervention, Emerging Infect. Dis. 5 (1999) 659–671.

[9] M. Ramanna, Coping with the influenza pandemic, 1918–1919: the Bombay experience, in: S. Phillip, D. Killingray (Eds.), The Spanish Influenza Pandemic of 1918–19: New Perspectives, Routledge, London (in press).

[10] K. Wakimura, The Indian experience of influenza pandemic 1918–19: why the mortality was so huge?, in: S. Phillip, D. Killingray (Eds.), The Spanish Influenza Pandemic of 1918–19: New Perspectives, Routledge, London (in press).

[11] M. Echenberg, The dog that did not bark: evidence for the 1918 influenza pandemic in Senegal, in: S. Phillip, D. Killingray (Eds.), The Spanish Influenza Pandemic of 1918–19: New Perspectives, Routledge, London (in press).

[12] J.G. Ellison, A fierce hunger: tracing the impacts of the 1918–1919 influenza pandemic in southwest Tanzania, in: S. Phillip, D. Killingray (Eds.), The Spanish Influenza Pandemic of 1918–19: New Perspectives, Routledge, London (in press).

[13] M.C. Musambachime, A great catastrophe: the blood of the dead soldiers is killing us: African reactions to the influenza pandemic of 1918/1919 in Northern Rhodesia (Zambia) and Nyasaland (Malawi), in: S. Phillip, D. Killingray (Eds.), The Spanish Influenza Pandemic of 1918–19: New Perspectives, Routledge, London (in press).

[14] P.S. Herda, Disease and colonialism in the Pacific: the 1918 pandemic in Western Polynesia, in: S. Phillip,

D. Killingray (Eds.), The Spanish Influenza Pandemic of 1918–19: New Perspectives, Routledge, London (in press).

[15]　A.W. Crosby Jr., Epidemic and Peace, 1918, Greenwood Press, Westport, CT, 1976, p. 337.

[16]　K.D. Patterson, Pandemic Influenza 1700–1900: A Study in Historical Epidemiology, Rowman and Little-field, Totawa, NJ, 1986, p. 118 (p. 3).

[17]　T. Francis Jr., F.M. Davenport, A.V. Hennessy, A serologic recapitulation of human infection with different strains of influenza virus, Trans. Assoc. Am. Physicians 66 (1953) 231–239.

International Congress Series 1219 (2001) 53–59

Influenza future: the impact of new vaccines and antivirals

Arnold S. Monto*

*Department of Epidemiology, School of Public Health, The University of Michigan,
109 Observatory Street, Ann Arbor, MI 48109-2029, USA*

Abstract

The new vaccines and antivirals may change the way influenza is controlled, but we need first to remember that the current inactivated vaccines are effective and underutilized. A trivalent live-attenuated vaccine has recently been demonstrated to be 93% efficacious in preventing isolation-confirmed influenza and to be 86% efficacious when a drifted strain was circulating. The antivirals zanamivir and oseltamivir shorten the duration of illnesses from 1 to 3 days and prevent complications requiring antibiotics. Both are efficacious in prophylaxis, including postexposure in the family. We can expect to see, in the future, expanded prevention and control of influenza, not only in the traditional groups, but in additional segments of the population, such as working adults and children. © 2001 Elsevier Science B.V. All rights reserved.

In this paper, I will attempt to predict how the impact of influenza will evolve into the future. I do not intend to predict how the virus itself will evolve; we all know the dangers of that sort of prognostication. Rather, I would like to look at the exciting new interventions that have either been approved for use or appear to be in final stages of development, and to speculate how they will affect influenza morbidity and even influenza mortality. These interventions are new vaccines, particularly the live attenuated ones, as well as the new antivirals, the neuraminidase inhibitors. In this discussion, given the limitation of time, I will be very selective. Omitting an approach does not mean it will not play an important role.

To begin, I want to remind you of the continued under-utilization of the current inactivated vaccines, especially in many countries and regions of the world. Let us look at the new horizons that open to us with the live vaccines. I recognize that there are concerns about their safety on a population rather than on an individual basis, and I would suggest

---

* Tel.: +1-734-764-5453; fax: +1-313-764-3192.
E-mail address: asmonto@umich.edu (A.S. Monto).

0531-5131/01/$ – see front matter © 2001 Elsevier Science B.V. All rights reserved.
PII: S0531-5131(01)00325-9

that this might be addressed, as are concerns about population resistance to antivirals, that is by systematic global monitoring. The live vaccines will give us a unique opportunity to address influenza morbidity. I do not want to get into a debate on whether they are more or less efficacious than the inactivated vaccines. Given the vagaries of influenza attack rates and other variables encountered in clinical trials, only a head-to-head comparison can answer this question. It is sufficient to say that they are highly efficacious. This efficacy was most clearly demonstrated in a population that has been little evaluated with inactivated vaccine, young children between 15 months and 6 years of age. The pivotal trial, lead by Belshe [1] (see Fig. 1), demonstrated a clinical efficacy of 93% in preventing isolation-confirmed influenza caused by types $A(H_3N_2)$ and type B. No cases of type $A(H_1N_1)$ were observed. Vaccine was given in 1996–1997 in two doses to most of the children (82%). The remainder received a single dose, but it seemed to be equally protective at both dose levels. This was probably because the major concern in immunogenicity was type $A(H_1N_1)$, which did not occur in that year. Another important observation was the prevention of febrile otitis media; this, as in the situation with the antivirals, confirms the role of influenza (and certainly other respiratory viruses) as the primary cause of this condition. Even without doing virology, the impact of the vaccine might have been noticed, with overall reduction by 21% in febrile respiratory illness [1].

The ideal influenza vaccine would not only be highly efficacious, but it would also protect well in years with antigenic drift, and for that matter would not have to be given annually, the major problem in sustaining programs and demonstrating cost effectiveness. Concerning the second point, protecting in spite of antigenic drift, the live vaccine seems to have performed well in a year when the inactivated vaccine did not. In a follow-up to the 1996–1997 year, the investigators mainly revaccinated the previous participants (85%). The vaccine used was similar to that in the inactivated vaccine, but the drifted strain, A/Sydney, caused most of the illness in the United States that year (1997–1998). In spite of that, the protective efficacy was 86% against A/Sydney in this population [2]

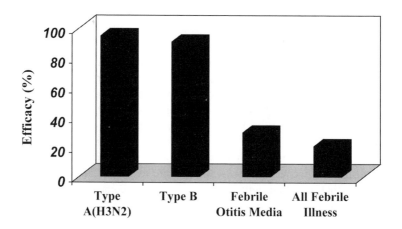

Fig. 1. Efficacy of cold-adapted (US) influenza vaccine in preventing influenza and complications in 15–71-month-old children, 1996–1997.

(see Fig. 2). In the same year, only low efficacy was demonstrated in those given inactivated vaccine. The good efficacy with the live vaccine might partially be a result of most individuals being serially vaccinated, but it still suggests strongly that these vaccines, which protect by infection, may well have the hope for advantage of inducing a broadened immunity. That conclusion is reinforced by the study of this vaccine in the same year by Nichol et al. [3] in working adults vaccinated once, which also demonstrated significant protection against febrile respiratory illness.

Let us move to the new neuraminidase inhibitors. They will be considered as a class, with illustrations being drawn from trials with either zanamivir or oseltamivir. Starting with prophylaxis, again in the A/Sydney year, both were shown to be as effective historically as a well-matched vaccine. In Fig. 3, results of two seasonal prophylaxis studies are shown. Zanamivir was given over a 4-week period, and oseltamivir over a 6-week period, both once per day [4,5]. Two laboratory-confirmed illness endpoints were used in the zanamivir study, the first, not requiring fever. The second requiring fever gave 84% protection and is probably a better reflection of efficacy since it is a more specific measure. Of interest is that there was even significant protection against all febrile illnesses during the season (43%), with or without laboratory confirmation. This is similar to the result observed with the live vaccines. With oseltamivir, only febrile illnesses were evaluated. In the zanamivir study, two sites were used and they had similar attack rates. That was not true with oseltamivir. The Virginia site had an attack rate similar to that seen in the zanamivir study, and the protective efficacy was 84%, identical to that observed with zanamivir. Their South Central US site had a lower attack rate, so that the average efficacy in the study was 76%.

Seasonal antiviral prophylaxis is more proof of principle than a way drug would be extensively used. Both drugs have been demonstrated to be effective when used for shorter post-exposure in the household setting. They have also been demonstrated to be highly protective in nursing home elderly populations, most of whom have received inactivated

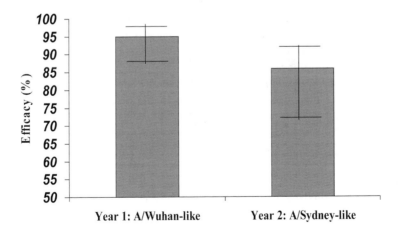

Fig. 2. Efficacy of cold-adapted (US) vaccine against isolation confirmed clinical influenza cause by the circulating type A(H₃N₂) virus.

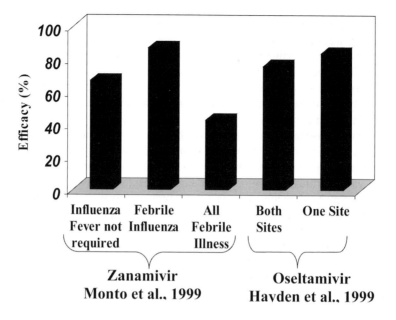

Fig. 3. Prevention of influenza by zanamivir and oseltamivir in seasonal prophylaxis.

vaccine. In this setting, there has not yet been any evidence of antiviral resistance, sometimes a problem with the M2 inhibitors, amantadine and rimantadine [6].

I shall only briefly review the treatment studies with the neuraminidase inhibitors. The ones currently available for scrutiny are mainly in healthy adults. Both oseltamivir and zanamivir have been given twice daily for 5 days. An alleviation endpoint has been used for both drugs, which is an artificial point when certain symptoms required at entry have been significantly reduced or are absent. Results have been fairly similar for both drugs, even though the alleviation endpoint is defined somewhat differently. On average, there is a reduction in time to this alleviation endpoint of 1 1/2 days. However, this does not tell the whole story. Significant reductions in reported symptoms start within one day of start of therapy, so benefit begins long before the alleviation endpoint is reached [7]. Also, the longer the duration of illness would have been in the placebo group, the greater the reduction in duration in the treated group. This has been analyzed in the zanamivir trials by identifying those who were classified as more severely ill at the start of treatment. The reduction in duration here is 3 or more days, with similar reduction seen in other severity categories [8].

The trials so far reported are mainly in healthy adults, individuals not thought to develop frequent complications. However, with both drugs, there have been significant reductions in complications, mainly in illnesses requiring antibiotics [9,10]. This reinforces the observation that such complications do occur in this group. Results in children, the elderly and high-risk groups will soon become available, which will help in demonstrating the economic benefit of using these drugs. Prevention of complications adds an important element to factors such as earlier return to work and use of less symptomatic relief medications.

The impact of use of new vaccines and antivirals is likely to be very large, but also gradual. It will also be different in different parts of the world. As their availability spreads and as knowledge of them increases, we are likely to see an increased awareness of the impact of influenza in population groups that have not traditionally been thought of as targets of influenza prevention and treatment. One such group will be children. We have known for many years that there is serious morbidity and even mortality in young children. The classic pandemic mortality curves show it, hospitalization rates show it and recent studies have teased out the impact of influenza in the under 5-year olds and especially in the under 1-year olds [11,12] (see Fig. 4). It is clear from the work of several groups that it is not just high-risk children who have severe morbidity but previously healthy children, as well. The attraction of the live attenuated vaccine is not only its demonstrated efficacy, but also its delivery system. This would be of particular merit for use in young children, especially given the need to vaccinate annually. However, if the strategy is to prevent severe disease in the under 1-year-old population, we have a problem. The pivotal study excluded children under age 15 months and the median age in this study was 43 months, so further evaluation would be needed before the vaccine is used in the very young [1]. So, the major target might be prevention of illness in those who are most likely to develop it: children under 5 years of age.

Not all previously healthy children would be vaccinated each year, even in those countries that move to that approach. There are cost-effective issues, as well as logistic problems of vaccinating every year in this large group. Prevention is always better than treatment, but if use of antivirals, particularly the neuraminidase inhibitors, reduces duration of illness, and most importantly prevents complications, then it could be a reasonable alternative. It is likely that many pathways will be taken to control influenza in children, and this will be one.

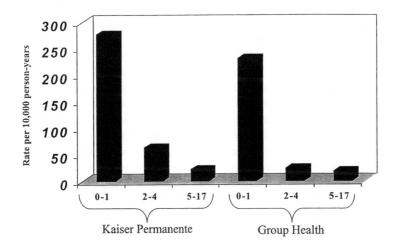

Fig. 4. Rate of hospitalizations during predominate influenza seasons in non-high-risk children.

Before leaving the issue of children, I shall touch on the use of the live vaccine in preventing community spread by vaccinating school-age children [13]. There are theoretic approaches to interruption in transmission, mainly with vaccine preventable infections in children [13]. In general, high transmissibility of an agent is demonstrated by early age of infection. Before vaccine availability, most children were already infected by measles at an early age, but not by rubella. Influenza is even less transmissible, and interruption should occur at a lower level of antibody prevalence. We demonstrated that this was possible originally during the $A(H_3N_2)$ pandemic, using a single dose of inactivated vaccine [14]. In a somewhat different experiment, our Russian colleagues reduced illness in unvaccinated schoolmates and in unvaccinated teachers by vaccinating a large portion of school children in Novgorod with their live attenuated vaccine [15]. This experience is being readdressed using managed health care approaches in Texas.

Healthy adults do not experience high hospitalization rates, but they are economically the most productive part of society. We also know that the inactivated vaccine is highly efficacious in this population. Some studies have also demonstrated high levels of cost effectiveness [16]. It is in this population that we are likely to see a great deal of healthy competition between strategies for prevention and treatment. We also need to have further independent comparative studies of cost effectiveness, if not using actual experimental interventions then using simulations. Since health economics varies from country to country, national as well as international studies are needed. One thing, though, that I cannot accept is that in countries with mature health care systems, a febrile ill individual with influenza should be denied treatment with an effective antiviral and told to take symptomatic therapy, given our state of knowledge of the various benefits that accrue.

I shall only mention use of inactivated vaccines in at-risk populations. To reduce mortality, we obviously need more use of vaccine in those industrialized countries where it is underused. There may be a role for vaccines of improved immunogenicity for older individuals since we know that such improvement is desirable [17]. However, demonstration of significantly increased protection will be required for widespread adoption of such a vaccine for this highly vulnerable population.

Discussion up to now has focused on a small proportion of the population of the world: those in industrialized countries. Not only does most of the world's population live in other countries, but that population is aging. The new global recommendations urge recognition of the impact of influenza in these countries and addressing it in a sequential manner, mainly with inactivated vaccines [18]. This may have the greatest impact on global mortality of anything that we do in prevention and treatment.

In summary, the new studies with vaccine and antivirals confirm that we have underestimated the impact of influenza, especially in terms of complications produced, so there is a greater job to be done. As the new interventions are introduced, they will also further result in increased recognition of the importance of influenza and make influenza more visible as a specific entity. The existing interventions are underutilized. This particularly applies to inactivated influenza vaccine, the one product that is globally available. The old and new interventions should be compared for their relative advantages in different population groups and the results may be different. With many new interventions available or about to become available, there is an unprecedented opportunity to achieve better control of influenza. All of us, whatever our particular interests, should work together to achieve this goal since it all starts from achieving greater recognition of the importance of the impact of influenza and of its control.

References

[1] R.B. Belshe, P.M. Mendelman, J. Treanor, J. King, W.C. Gruber, P. Piedra, et al., The efficacy of live attenuated, cold-adapted, trivalent, intranasal influenzavirus vaccine in children, N. Engl. J. Med. 338 (1998) 1405–1412.

[2] R.B. Belshe, W.C. Gruber, P.M. Mendelman, I. Cho, K. Reisinger, S.L. Block, J. Wittes, et al., J. Pediatr. 136 (2000) 168–175.

[3] K.L. Nichol, P.M. Mendelman, K.P. Mallon, L.A. Jackson, G.J. Gorse, R.B. Belshe, et al., Effectiveness of live, attenuated intranasal influenza virus vaccine in healthy, working adults: a randomized controlled trial, JAMA 282 (1999) 137–144.

[4] A.S. Monto, D.P. Robinson, M.L. Herlocher, J.M. Hinson Jr., M.J. Elliott, A. Crisp, Zanamivir in the prevention of influenza among healthy adults, JAMA 282 (1999) 31–35.

[5] F.G. Hayden, R.L. Atmar, M. Schilling, C. Johnson, D. Poretz, D. Paar, et al., Use of the selective oral neuraminidase inhibitor oseltamivir to prevent influenza, N. Engl. J. Med. 341 (1999) 1336–1343.

[6] A.S. Monto, N.H. Arden, Implications of viral resistance to amantadine in control of influenza A, Clin. Infect. Dis. 15 (1992) 362–367.

[7] A.S. Monto, A. Webster, O. Keene, Randomized, placebo-controlled studies of inhaled zanamivir in the treatment of influenza A and B: pooled efficacy analysis, JAC 44 (1999) 23–29.

[8] A.S. Monto, A.B. Moult, S.J. Sharp, Effect of zanamivir on duration and resolution of influenza symptoms, Clin. Ther., in press.

[9] J.J. Treanor, F.G. Hayden, P.S. Vrooman, R. Barbarash, R. Bettis, D. Riff, et al., Efficacy and safety of the oral neuraminidase inhibitor oseltamivir in treating acute influenza, JAMA 283 (2000) 1016–1024.

[10] K.G. Nicholson, F.Y. Aoki, A.D. Osterhaus, S. Trottier, O. Carewicz, C.H. Mercier, et al., Lancet 355 (2000) 1845–1850.

[11] H.S. Izurieta, W.W. Thompson, P. Kramarz, D.K. Shay, R.L. Davis, F. DeStefano, et al., Influenza and the rates of hospitalization for respiratory disease among infants and young children, N. Engl. J. Med. 342 (2000) 232–239.

[12] K.M. Neuzil, B.G. Mellen, P.F. Wright, E.F. Mitchel, M.R. Griffin, The effect of influenza on hospitalizations, outpatient visits, and courses of antibiotics in children, N. Engl. J. Med. 342 (2000) 225–231.

[13] A.S. Monto, Interrupting the transmission of respiratory tract infections: theory and practice, Clin. Infect. Dis. 28 (1999) 200–204.

[14] A.S. Monto, F.M. Davenport, J.A. Napier, T. Francis Jr., Modification of an influenza outbreak in Tecumseh, Michigan by vaccination of school children, J. Infect. Dis. 22 (1970) 16–25.

[15] L.G. Rudenko, A.N. Slepushkin, A.P. Kendal, A.S. Monto, A.L. Beljaev, E.I. Burtseva, et al., Comparative studies of live and inactivated vaccines in Novgorod: description of study design and results of reactogenicity and immunogenicity of vaccines, in: C. Hannoun, et al. (Eds.), Options for the Control of Influenza II, Elsevier, Amsterdam, Netherlands, 1993, pp. 91–96.

[16] K.L. Nichol, A. Lind, K.L. Margolis, et al., The effectiveness of vaccination against influenza in healthy, working adults, N. Engl. J. Med. 333 (1995) 889–893.

[17] S.E. Ohmit, M.N. Arden, A.S. Monto, Effectiveness of inactivated influenza vaccine among nursing home residents during an influenza type A (H3N2) epidemic, JAGS 47 (1999) 165–171.

[18] Influenza vaccines: recommendations for the use of inactivated influenza vaccines and other preventive measures, Wkly. Epidemiol. Rec. 75 (35) (2000) 281–288.

International Congress Series 1219 (2001) 61–66

Quantifying the burden of influenza: a prospective household contact study in France[☆]

Fabrice Carrat [a,*], Camille Sahler[a], Marianne Leruez[b],
Christine Rouzioux[b], Sylvie Rogez[c], François Freymuth[d],
Bruno Housset[e], Abdelkader El-Hasnaoui[f], Marlène Nicolas[f]

[a]Institut National de la Santé Et de la Recherche Médicale INSERM Unit 444,
Hôpital Saint-Antoine, Paris, France
[b]Laboratoire de virologie, CHU Necker Enfants-Malades, Paris, France
[c]Laboratoire de bactériologie, virologie et hygiène, CHU Dupuytren, Limoges, France
[d]Laboratoire de virologie humaine et moléculaire, CHU Côte de Nâcre, Caen, France
[e]Service de pneumologie, Centre Hospitalier Inter-Communal, Créteil, France
[f]Glaxo-Wellcome, Marly-le-roi, France

Abstract

Background: The actual impact of influenza epidemics cannot be accurately estimated from medical practice-based surveillance data. A prospective household contact study was performed in order to quantify the burden of influenza. *Methods*: The study took place in France between January and March 2000. A total of 947 households were recruited by 161 general practitioners (GP), from an "index-case" who consulted the GP for influenza-like illness. Virological specimens were collected for diagnosis of influenza and other respiratory pathogen infections. All household members were asked to complete a questionnaire, which included a 15-day follow-up, with details of clinical events, healthcare resources and work–sick leave. *Results*: Identified among household contacts were 395 influenza type A-positive index cases and 313 secondary cases. The median time to alleviation of major influenza symptoms was 8 days in index cases and 6 days in secondary cases. Forty-two percent of secondary cases did not consult while 15% consulted more than once. The mean number of treatments taken was respectively 3.7 and 2.2 in index and secondary cases. Work–sick leave was mainly associated with the severity of the illness.

☆ On behalf of the EPIGRIPPE group: M. Bungener (Paris), F. Carrat (Paris), F. Denis (Limoges), A. Flahault (Paris), F. Freymuth (Caen), A. El Hasnaoui (Marly le Roi), I. Goderel (Paris), M. Guiguet (Paris), B. Housset (Créteil), C. Le Gales (Le Kremlin Bicêtre), M. Leruez (Paris), M. Nicolas (Marly le Roi), G. Pannetier (Paris), S. Rogez (Limoges), C. Rouzioux (Paris), C. Sahler (Paris), M. Schwarzinger (Paris) and 161 GPs involved in recruitment of households.
* Corresponding author. Tel.: +33-144-738-458; fax: +33-144-738-453.
E-mail address: carrat@u444.jussieu.fr (F. Carrat).

Conclusion: These results could help for quantifying the burden of influenza epidemics. © 2001 Elsevier Science B.V. All rights reserved.

Keywords: Influenza; Household contact study; Morbidity

1. Introduction

Quantifying the actual burden of influenza is difficult to achieve for several reasons. First, based on clinical grounds only, it is not easy to distinguish illnesses due to influenza infection from illnesses caused by other respiratory pathogens [1]. Second, illnesses due to influenza infection are highly variable in terms of severity, and the clinical consequences of influenza range from asymptomatic infection to severe disease and sometimes death [2]. Third, usual estimates obtained from medical practice-based influenza surveillance systems, either associated with a virological collection of specimens or not, give an incomplete picture of the influenza societal burden. It has been shown in retrospective studies that 30% of subjects suffering from influenza-like illness do not consult a practitioner [3]. On the other hand, the number of consultations in medical practice per individual has never been described in observational studies.

A prospective household contact study has been performed during the 1999/2000 influenza epidemic, in order to describe the clinical outcomes of illnesses caused by influenza infection and their consequences in terms of healthcare use or work–sick leave. The main objective of the study was to achieve precise quantification of the influenza burden in ambulatory care.

2. Material and methods

The study took place in France, between January and March 2000, during an influenza epidemic. One hundred sixty one general practitioners (GPs) involved in influenza-like illness surveillance [4] included households from the consultation of an 'index-case'—a household member suffering from influenza-like illness who consulted for the first time and who was presumed to be the first influenza-like illness case within the household. Virological samples were collected in the index case for the diagnosis of influenza A and B infection by an immunofluorescent method, culture (on MDCK cells) and PCR. Also, the diagnoses of RSV, adenoviruses and parainfluenza viruses infections were systematically performed (immunofluorescent method). During the consultation, the GP completed an inclusion form describing symptoms, treatments taken before the consultation or prescribed at the end of the consultation, and composition of the household. The GP also delivered to the index-patient a questionnaire to be completed by all household members (the index-case and the contacts). The questionnaire included detailed description of baseline and sociodemographic characteristics as well as daily records for all household members regarding symptoms, healthcare use, treatments that were taken and absence from work (in working adults). The length of the follow-up was 15 days.

Telephone interviews were performed successfully at days 3 and 15 of the follow-up, in 92% of the households.

A daily symptom score was computed by dividing the number of reported symptoms with the maximum number of possible symptoms (13 in the diary cards). A work–sick leave index was calculated in working adults, by applying the following rule: for working days only, a complete absence from work was quoted 1, an absence from work less than 1 day was quoted 0.5 and a disruption in professional activity but no absence from work was quoted 0.25.

A secondary case was defined as a contact subject presenting at least two of the following: cough, sore throat, myalgia, fatigue, headache, rhinorrhea or sneezing or fever (>37.7 °C), feverishness occurring within the first 5 days of follow-up. Note that virological samples were not collected in secondary cases.

Statistical analyses used Chi-square or Fisher's exact test for qualitative variables, Student's t-test or Anova for quantitative variables, or Kaplan–Meier estimates and Log-rank test for survival variables. Anova for repeated measurements was used for comparison of quantitative variables in time. All statistical analyses were performed with SAS v 6.12 (SAS Institute, North Carolina, USA).

3. Results

Nine hundred fifty six households were included, 503 (53%) of which were associated with an influenza type A-positive index case; 714 households (75%) returned the questionnaire, of which 395 corresponded to influenza positive index cases. According to the GP inclusion form, there was no difference between households lost to follow-up and those with the questionnaire returned in terms of severity of the illness in the index case, rate of influenza positive samples or household composition. The number of contact subjects for influenza-positive index cases was 891. For 74 contacts, daily registration of symptoms was incomplete and did not allow classification as a secondary case. For the remainder, 313 (38%) contact subjects were classified as secondary cases.

3.1. Clinical outcomes and healthcare use

Table 1 presents the clinical outcomes and healthcare use results in both index and secondary cases. Overall, the mean age was equal to 33.9 (±21) years, which was consistent with the mean age described for patients consulting with influenza-like illness during the epidemic observed by the French Sentinelles system (unpublished data). The time between the inclusion and onset of disease in the secondary cases was 1.4 days (±1.5). The index cases were, on average, more severely ill than the secondary cases. This result was mainly explained by the difference in case-definitions used for inclusion of index case and classification of secondary cases. This is illustrated by a longer course of disease—a median of 8 days in index cases and 6 days in secondary cases, ($p<0.001$), and a greater mean symptom score in index than in secondary cases at days 1, 5 and 10 of the disease ($p<0.001$—Anova with repeated measurements). Forty

Table 1

Clinical outcomes and healthcare use in influenza type A-positive index cases and secondary cases; Epigrippe Study, January to March 2000, France

	Index cases	Secondary cases
Age, year	36.7 ± 19	30.4 ± 20
Male sex, n (%)	186 (51)	150 (49)
Influenza vaccination, n (%)	38 (10)	21 (7)
Chronic disease, n (%)	88 (24)	39 (14)
Smoker, n (%)	77 (19)	53 (17)
Time, days		
inclusion → onset of disease	–	1.4 ± 1.5
onset of disease → consultation	1.0 ± 1.5	1.1 ± 2.0
Time to alleviation of major influenza symptoms, days (median 95% CI)	8 (7–8)	6 (6–7)
Symptoms score		
day 1	0.69 ± 0.18	0.39 ± 0.21
day 5	0.29 ± 0.20	0.23 ± 0.21
day 10	0.11 ± 0.13	0.07 ± 0.13
Number of consultations, n (%)		
0	–	126 (42)
1	285 (72)	129 (43)
2	86 (22)	37 (12)
3+	24 (6)	10 (3)

Plus–minus values are means $\pm$ SD.

two percent of secondary cases did not consult while 15% had consulted more than once. Seeking advice from a practitioner was mainly associated with the symptom score at day 1 of the disease ($p < 0.001$), age — U shape with higher rates in the young and the elderly ($p < 0.001$), and individual habits in terms of consultation for influenza-like illness ($p = 0.02$).

At day 1 of the disease, the mean number of treatments taken was 3.7 (± 1.5) and 2.2 (± 1.6), respectively, in index and secondary cases. Almost all cases had taken antipyretics or analgesics and 82% of index cases and 68% of secondary cases had used medications for cough. Fifty three percent of index cases and 44% of secondary cases had taken antibiotics for a median duration of 6 days (95% CI: 6–7). Few patients, 5% of those who had consulted, had taken neuraminidase inhibitor. Finally, the median time of treatment of any type was 8 days in index cases and 6 days in secondary cases.

3.2. Work–sick leave

One hundred ninety one index cases and 126 secondary cases were working adults. Among the index cases, 10% did not stop working; this rate equaled 29% in secondary cases. Fig. 1 shows the mean work–sick leave index as a function of the day of the disease. The mean cumulative work–sick leave was 4.0 (± 3), 2.9 (± 3) and 0.2 (± 0.1) days in index cases, secondary cases that consulted and secondary cases that did not consult, respectively. Work–sick leave was mainly associated with the severity of the

Work sick-leave index (per working day)

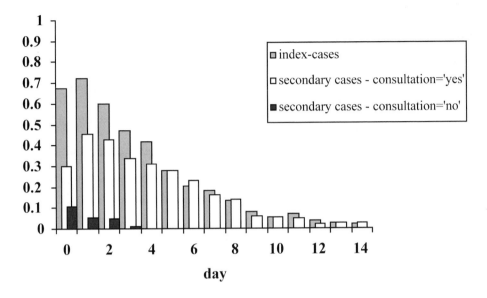

Fig. 1. Impact of influenza type A illness on work sick–leave, as a function of the day of the illness. Epigrippe Study, January to March 2000, France. The values ranged between 0 (normal working day) and 1 (complete absence from work).

illness ($r = 0.21$, $p = 0.004$ in index cases; $r = 0.35$, $p = 0.03$ in secondary cases) itself linked with consultations.

4. Discussion

From our results, it appears that the influenza disease burden could be much greater than the estimates derived from a medical practice-based influenza surveillance system. In fact, 42% of persons presenting with illness attributable to influenza will not seek advice from a practitioner, thus will not be registered on any influenza surveillance system. A precise quantification is however important if one wishes to evaluate strategies for controlling influenza, such as vaccination or treatment with neuraminidase inhibitors.

The other major result, while expected, was that the individual burden was highly correlated with the severity of illness exhibited by the subject, even if the study was restricted to ambulatory care.

We used a prospective household contact study design. Compared with the traditional cohort approach, the prospective household contact study offered advantages of decreasing the length of the follow-up period, while increasing the chance of observing influenza illnesses among contacts. However, this design implies that persons living alone cannot be included. We do not believe that excluding persons living alone would dramatically bias the results obtained from contacts of an index case. The variable that was the most correlated with healthcare use was the severity of the illness, and there is no reason to believe that severity could correlate with living alone or not. Moreover, no relationship between healthcare use and socio-demographic characteristics of the case was found (results not shown). A second potential source of bias is linked with the possible change of behavior of household members enrolled in the study, regarding healthcare use for influenza illness. This sort of bias is difficult to avoid in observational prospective studies of any type, though much lower than in clinical trials. No recommendation was given either to the GP, or to the household members as exemplified by the high rate of first-line antibiotic consumption or the high rate of secondary cases who did not consult. Again, we do not believe that our estimates are biased by participation.

The next step in this study will be to translate all outcomes into monetary units, in order to assess the economic burden of influenza epidemic.

References

[1] F. Carrat, A. Tachet, C. Rouzioux, B. Housset, A.-J. Valleron, Evaluating clinical case-definitions of influenza: a detailed investigation of patients during the 1995–96 epidemic, Clin. Infect. Dis. 28 (1999) 290–293.
[2] T.R. Cate, Clinical manifestations and consequences of Influenza, Am. J. Med. 82 (1987) 15–19 (Suppl. 6A).
[3] A.G. Elder, B. O'Donnell, E.A.B. McCruden, I.S. Symington, W.F. Carman, Incidence and recall of influenza in a cohort of Glasgow healthcare workers during the 1993–4 epidemic: results of serum testing and questionnaire, Br. Med. J. 313 (1996) 1241–1242.
[4] F. Carrat, A. Flahault, E. Boussard, N. Farran, L. Dangoumeau, A.-J. Valleron, Surveillance of Influenza-like illness in France: the example of the 1995/1996 epidemic, J. Epidemiol. Community Health 52 (1998) 32S–38S (Suppl. 1).

International Congress Series 1219 (2001) 67–71

How much are patients willing to pay for an earlier alleviation of influenza?[☆]

Fabrice Carrat[a,*], Camille Sahler[a], Catherine Le Galès[b],
Michael Schwarzinger[b], Marlène Nicolas[c], Martine Bungener[d]

[a]Institut National de la Santé Et de la Recherche Médicale INSERM Unit 444, Hôpital Saint-Antoine,
27 rue Chaligny, 75012 Paris, France
[b]Institut National de la Santé Et de la Recherche Médicale INSERM Unit 537, Le Kremlin Bicêtre, France
[c]Glaxo-Wellcome, Marly-le-roi, France
[d]Institut National de la Santé Et de la Recherche Médicale INSERM Unit 502, Paris, France

Abstract

Background: The willingness-to-pay (WTP) method, i.e. the maximum amount of money an individual is willing to pay for a health intervention, is increasingly used for measuring health benefits. We studied how much individuals were willing to pay for an earlier alleviation of influenza symptoms. *Methods*: 527 household members were interviewed by telephone as a part of a prospective household contact study in January 2000 in France. Scenarios describing drug treatment and influenza alleviation varied with the respondent, depending on the age of the first household (index) case of influenza-like illness (child or adult) and the status of the respondent (index-case or not). A double-bounded dichotomous choice method was used for valuation, with health benefits (1 or 3 days without influenza) and bids selected randomly. *Results*: Median WTP was FF 209 (95%CI: 180–241) for 1 day and FF 340 (95%CI: 293–389) for 3 days without influenza in adults, with no difference whether the respondent was the index-case or not. Median WTP was FF 334 (95% CI: 237–499) for 1 day and FF 548 (95% CI: 389–805) for 3 days without influenza in children. *Conclusions*: These results could be used in a cost-benefit analysis

☆ On behalf of the EPIGRIPPE group: M. BUNGENER (Paris), F. CARRAT (Paris), F. DENIS (Limoges), A. FLAHAULT (Paris), F. FREYMUTH (Caen), A. EL HASNAOUI (Marly le Roi), I. GODEREL (Paris), M. GUIGUET (Paris), B. HOUSSET (Créteil), C. LE GALES (Le Kremlin Bicêtre), M. LERUEZ (Paris), M. NICOLAS (Marly le Roi), G. PANNETIER (Paris), S ROGEZ (Limoges), C ROUZIOUX (Paris), C.SAHLER (Paris), M. SCHWARZINGER (Paris) and 161 GPs involved in recruitment of households.

* Correspondence author. Tel.: +33-144-738-458; fax: +33-144-738-453.
E-mail address: carrat@u444.jussieu.fr (F. Carrat).

as valuation of health benefits linked with earlier alleviation of influenza symptoms. © 2001 Elsevier Science B.V. All rights reserved.

Keywords: Influenza; Willingness-to-pay; Cost-benefit studies

1. Introduction

Clinical effectiveness of neuraminidase inhibitors for treating influenza has been demonstrated in randomized trials [1], but little is known about their societal economic impact. Focusing on healthy individuals, for whom influenza infection is associated with uncomplicated acute illness of short duration, a fundamental question for the public health decision maker is whether the treatment could save money by reducing the length of the disease.

In cost-benefit analysis, costs of the intervention are put in balance with benefits, and the usual decision rule is that the intervention should be undertaken if benefits exceed costs. In health economics two methods are used for valuing benefits of health interventions in monetary terms. The first one is the 'cost-of-illness' (COI) method, where benefits are directly calculated by the difference between the evaluated costs of illness with the intervention and the costs of illness without the intervention. Costs are generally derived from observations of market values or their proxies. The second method, which has been widely used in environmental economics, is the 'willingness-to-pay' (WTP) method—i.e., the maximum amounts of money individuals are willing to pay in order to have access to the intervention. WTP translates into monetary terms the perceived usefulness of the intervention—thus, providing valuation of perceived health benefits, including intangible benefits. Both COI and WTP methods have their advantages and limits—that discussion is beyond the scope of this paper. To our knowledge, no WTP study has been performed on interventions targeting influenza. It has been recently suggested that WTP could be used for measuring the impact of healthcare program for the prevention and control of influenza [2]. Our objective was to quantify the benefit of an earlier alleviation of influenza symptoms using the WTP method.

2. Material and methods

The study was nested into a prospective household contact study described elsewhere [3], which took place in France between January and March 2000. Households were recruited from the general practice of an index-case — a household member suffering from influenza-like illness who consulted for the first time and who was presumed to be the first influenza-like illness case within the household. The first 527 households were included in the WTP nested study. The WTP questionnaire was delivered during a telephone interview of household members at day 3 of the follow-up. Three scenarios describing drug treatment and influenza alleviation were used accordingly with the age of the index-case (child or adult) and the status of the respondent when the index-case was

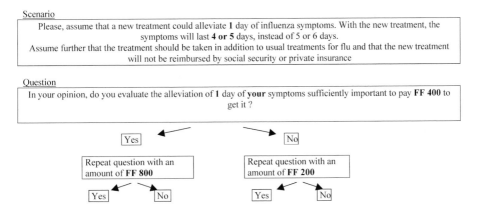

Scenario

| Please, assume that a new treatment could alleviate **1** day of influenza symptoms. With the new treatment, the symptoms will last **4 or 5** days, instead of 5 or 6 days. Assume further that the treatment should be taken in addition to usual treatments for flu and that the new treatment will not be reimbursed by social security or private insurance |

Question

| In your opinion, do you evaluate the alleviation of **1** day of **your** symptoms sufficiently important to pay **FF 400** to get it ? |

Fig. 1. Example of WTP questions. The respondent was the index case, the health outcome was equal to 1-day earlier alleviation and the initial bid was FF 400. All values indicated in bold varied with the respondent.

an adult (index-case or contact subject). Thus, from a health economics point of view, the WTP study evaluated the benefit of an earlier alleviation from a patient perspective (Strata 1, the respondent was the index-case), and from an 'altruistic' perspective (Strata 2, the respondent was a contact subject and the index-case was another adult; Strata 3, the respondent was a contact subject and the index-case was a child). Whatever the scenario, respondents were randomized either to answer for 1- or 3-day earlier alleviation of influenza symptoms. We have used the recommended strategy for asking individuals how much they were willing to pay, by using double-bounded dichotomous choice responses [4] with initial bids selected randomly between FF 25 (approximately US$ 4; FF 1 = US$ 0.153—01/01/2000) and FF 800 (US$ 120). Fig. 1 described an example of questionnaire, where the respondent was the index-case; the health outcome was equal to 1-day earlier alleviation and the initial bid was FF 400.

Analysis was stratified according to the respondent status. The medians WTP were estimated by logistic regression model designed for this type of data [5]. A parametric bootstrap method was used for the computation of confidence intervals.

3. Results

Of 507 households included in the WTP study, 11 refused to participate. Fig. 2 shows an example of WTP results for 1-day earlier alleviation of influenza symptoms, when the respondent was the index-case ($n = 172$). The figure represents the decreasing cumulative rate of subjects as a function of the maximum amount of money they were willing to pay for an earlier alleviation. For example, it was estimated that 13% subjects would not pay (whatever the amount). The median WTP was FF 198 (95% CI: 168–235) (US$ 30; 95% CI: 26–36); 12% of subjects were willing to pay a maximum amount of FF 400 (US$ 61).

The analysis was repeated across the various strata for 1- or 3-day earlier alleviation of influenza symptoms : when the index-case was an adult, medians WTP were, respectively, FF 198 (US$ 30) and FF 247 (US$ 38) for 1-day alleviation, and FF 347 (US$ 53) and FF

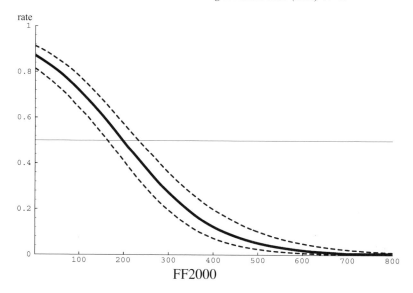

Fig. 2. The WTP function corresponding to scenario described in Fig. 1: the index case was the respondent, valuation of 1-day earlier alleviation of influenza symptoms.

308 (US$ 47) for 3-day alleviation, with no difference regarding the status of the respondent. On the other hand, medians WTP were higher when the index-case was a child, either for 1 day (FF 334—US$ 51) or 3-day earlier alleviation of influenza symptoms (FF 548—US$ 84) ($p < 0.05$).

4. Discussion

Our study shows that the median WTP was around FF 209 (US$ 32) for 1-day earlier alleviation of influenza symptoms, and FF 340 (US$ 52) for 3-day earlier alleviation in adults, irrespective of whether or not the respondent was the index-case. Median WTP estimates were 1.6 times greater for children. It is important to note that these values compared favorably with the cost of neuramidase inhibitors in France (FF 150, US$ 23 — prescribed for adult only and not reimbursed by the social security). Since the clinical effectiveness of neuraminidase inhibitors—in intent-to-treat analysis—is ranging from 1- to 2.5-day earlier alleviation of influenza symptoms [6], it is likely that treatment is cost-savings from the individual's perspective.

A possible limitation was that our study was not conducted from a societal perspective—the recommended perspective in health economics studies. For the societal perspective, we would need to evaluate the maximum amount of money that individuals would be willing to pay for general access to the treatment, with uncertainties about the risk of having influenza (e.g. 5% risk per year)—thus regardless of who incurs the costs and who obtains the effects. Since influenza is a very common disease that has been experienced by almost all adults in the population, it is likely that a study performed from the societal perspective on a random sample would have led to even greater benefit. In fact, a median WTP above FF 10.5 ($=$ FF 209 $\times$ 5% risk) for 1-day earlier alleviation of influenza would provide the same net benefit observed in our study.

The analysis is not finished yet. We will explore how WTP depends on sociodemographic factors or severity of the disease. Finally, we believe that the method could be used for valuing benefits linked with other interventions for controlling influenza, for example, focusing on more severe outcomes such as hospitalizations or death.

References

[1] A.S. Monto, D.M. Fleming, D. Henry, et al., Efficacy and safety of the neuraminidase inhibitor zanamivir in the treatment of influenza A and B virus infections, J. Infect. Dis. 180 (1999) 254–261.

[2] S. Birch, A. Gafni, B. O'Brien, Willingness to pay and the valuation of programmes for the prevention and control of influenza, Pharmacoeconomics 16 (Suppl. 1) (1999) 55–61.

[3] F. Carrat, C. Sahler, M. Leruez, et al., Quantifying the burden of influenza: a prospective household contact study in France, in: A. Osterhaus, et al. (Eds.), Options for the Control of Influenza IV, Excerpta Medica International Congress Series, Elsevier, Amsterdam, 2001, 52–57.

[4] R.D. Smith, The discrete-choice willingness-to-pay question format in health economics: should we adopt environmental guidelines?, Med. Decis. Making 20 (2000) 194–206.

[5] M. Hannemann, J. Loomis, B. Kanninen, Statistical efficiency of double-bounded dichotomous choice contingent valuation, Am. J. Agric. Econ. 73 (1991) 1255–1263.

[6] A.S. Monto, A. Webster, O. Keene, Randomized, placebo-controlled studies of inhaled zanamivir in the treatment of influenza A and B: pooled efficacy analysis, J. Antimicrob. Chemother. 44 (Suppl. B) (1999) 23–29.

International Congress Series 1219 (2001) 73–79

Rapid flu test and neuraminidase inhibitors in healthy adults: a cost-benefit analysis

Michael Schwarzinger[a], Bruno Housset[b], Fabrice Carrat [a,*]

[a]*Institut National de la Santé Et de la Recherche Médicale INSERM Unit 444, Hôpital Saint-Antoine,*
27 rue Chaligny, 75012 Paris, France
[b]*Centre Hospitalier Inter-Communal, Créteil, France*

Abstract

Background: Neuraminidase inhibitors (NI) reduce the number of days of symptomatic illness in influenza-positive patients. New rapid flu tests (RFT) should increase the number of influenza-positive patients who receive NI appropriately. *Objective*: The objective is to estimate the economic effects of implementing RFT and NI among healthy working adults, considering varying proportions of influenza infections among patients with influenza-like illness (ILI). *Methods*: By the means of a decision tree, the number of flu days averted and societal costs were compared for three strategies: RFT with a conditional NI prescription, systematic NI prescription, and no NI. *Results*: During flu epidemics, systematic NI prescription provided the best health outcome (0.4 flu days averted) and minimized societal costs (reduced by US$41.20 per person, in 1999 dollars, from the US$280.80 associated with no NI). RFT with conditional NI averted 0.32 flu days and saved US$33.10 per person. When the proportion of influenza-positive patients exceeded 56%, the systematic NI strategy was dominant, regardless of any other variations. For lower proportions, RFT with conditional NI could be preferred depending on RFT characteristics (sensitivity exceeding 94% with 80% specificity or RFT cost lesser than US$6.60). *Conclusions*: Systematic NI prescription without RFT for unvaccinated healthy working adults consulting within 2 days of the onset of ILI symptoms was a dominant strategy during flu epidemics. © 2001 Elsevier Science B.V. All rights reserved.

Keywords: Influenza; Decision trees; Predictive value of tests; Immunologic tests; Reagent kits; diagnostic; Outpatients

* Corresponding author. Tel.: +33-144-738-458; fax: +33-144-738-453.
E-mail address: carrat@u444.jussieu.fr (F. Carrat).

0531-5131/01/$ – see front matter © 2001 Elsevier Science B.V. All rights reserved.
PII: S0531-5131(01)00328-4

1. Introduction

In 1999, the US Food and Drug Administration approved two antiviral drugs, zanamivir and oseltamivir, for the treatment of uncomplicated influenza infection. The efficacy of both these neuraminidase inhibitors (NI) was similar when they were administered within 2 days of the onset of influenza-like illness (ILI) symptoms; they reduced the median duration of symptomatic illness by 1 day [1] In addition to annual vaccination, NI could alleviate much of the influenza burden in healthy workers.

NI prescription will be effective when the clinical case definition of influenza infection has a high positive predictive value. Rapid flu tests (RFT) suitable for point-of-care use in physicians' offices will soon be available for both A and B viruses. Using a decision analysis model, we estimated the costs related to implementation of RFT and NI and compared them with the savings from the secondary infectious complications averted and the societal benefits of productivity gains. Our primary objective was to compare three strategies for management of healthy unvaccinated working adults younger than 65 years, consulting within 2 days of the onset of ILI symptoms during flu epidemics: (A) RFT with a conditional NI prescription, (B) a systematic NI prescription without RFT, and (C) neither RFT nor NI.

2. Methods

2.1. Decision analysis model

The RFT with NI strategy aims to maximize the proportion of influenza-positive patients receiving NI (Fig. 1). We assumed that NI is prescribed only after a positive test. In the systematic NI strategy, all patients with ILI receive NI, and RFT is accordingly irrelevant. The reference option is the no NI strategy, when physicians prescribe neither NI nor RFT. Secondary infectious complications (implying follow-up visits and antibiotic use) and over-the-counter (OTC) medication were assumed to depend on both influenza infection and NI prescription. Our model did not include the adverse effects of NI.

Cost-benefit analysis was performed from the societal perspective and included the costs of productivity loss [2]. We also performed sensitivity analyses to assess the uncertainty among plausible ranges for all variables. We used Data software to program the decision tree (Data (version 3.0), TreeAge Software, Williamstown, MA, USA).

2.2. Outcome estimates

We used the duration of ILI symptoms from NI clinical trials as the primary health outcome (Table 1). We considered conservatively that during flu epidemics, 40% of unvaccinated patients with ILI are infected with influenza [3], even if this proportion was substantially higher during NI clinical trials.

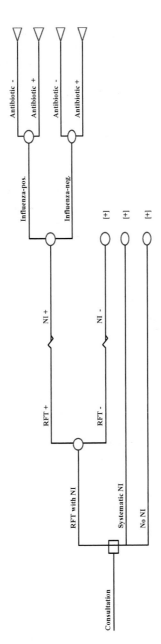

Fig. 1. Three clinical strategies for management of healthy working adults consulting within 2 days of the onset of influenza-like illness symptoms.

Table 1
Health outcomes, probabilities of health outcomes, and resource use for the model

	Base case	Sensitivity analysis	Sources
Influenza infections among patients with ILI	40%	30–80%	[3]
Median duration of ILI symptoms			[1]
NI-treated influenza-positive patients	5 days	–	
Untreated influenza-positive patients	6 days	–	
Other ILI patients	6 days	–	
Rapid flu test characteristics			
Sensitivity	80%	50–100%	Assumption
Specificity	80%	50–100%	Assumption
Baseline values of antibiotic and OTC consumption			
Antibiotics	15%	15–30%	[10,11]
OTC relief medications	80%	50–100%	[10,11]
NI-related reduction in medical consumption			
Antibiotics and follow-up visits	50%	0–100%	[10]
OTC relief medications	25%	0–50%	[11]
Mean number of lost work days	1.2 days	0.5–3 days	[7]
NI-related reduction in lost work days	1 day	–	

2.3. Medical and societal cost estimates

The cost of NI was fixed at US$28 by assumption, and of RFT at US$10 [4]. Secondary infectious complications added the cost of a follow-up visit (US$60 by assumption) and antibiotic costs, which we estimated as the product of the published average wholesale price (AWP) of amoxicillin at US$8.00 [5] and an average 5-day use. OTC treatment costs were also estimated at US$12.50, the mean AWP for antipyretics, cough mixtures, and decongestants. Productivity losses were measured by the human capital approach: a lost work day was valued at the daily earnings lost. The mean number of lost work days in the reference (no NI) group was derived from the placebo arm of influenza vaccination trials in US populations of full-time worker [6,7]. We assumed that the reduction of lost work days attributable to NI was identical to the median reduction of ILI symptomatic days. The US Census Bureau estimated the mean annual earnings of full-time, year-round workers, male and female, at least 15 years old, at US$39,156 in 1998 [8]. Assuming that such employees worked 240 days/year, mean lost earnings for 1 day equaled US$163.20. All costs are presented in 1999 US dollars with use of the Consumer Price Index.

3. Results

During flu epidemics, systematic NI prescription for healthy working adults consulting within 2 days of the onset of ILI symptoms provided the best health outcome (0.4 flu days averted) and minimized societal costs (reducing the US$280.80 per person associated with no NI by US$41.20, i.e., a decrease of 15%) (Table 2). The RFT with NI strategy averted 0.32 flu days, saving US$33.10 per person (i.e., a decrease of 12%)

Table 2
Economic benefits associated with RFT with NI and systematic NI strategies compared with no NI

Outcome variables	Average costs (savings) per person (1999 US$)	
	RFT with NI	Systematic NI
Medical costs		
RFT	10	0
NI	12.30	28
Antibiotic and follow-up visit	(2.40)	(3)
OTC	(0.80)	(1)
Total medical costs	19.10	24
Productivity losses	(52.20)	(65.20)
Total costs	(33.10)	(41.20)

compared with the societal costs of no NI. The medical costs associated with no NI were US$85 per person and went up 28% with systematic NI and 22% with RFT and conditional NI.

In sensitivity analyses, RFT with NI resulted in greater savings when RFT cost less than US$1.80 or when RFT sensitivity exceeded 94% with 80% specificity (the sensitivity threshold ranged from 87% to 100% when the proportion of influenza infections among ILI patients varied from 30% to 55%; it ranged from 88% to 100% when RFT specificity varied between 100% and 60%, respectively). Finally, the most cost-saving strategy changed when daily earnings changed: systematic NI saved the most when they were greater than US$61, RFT with NI when they were between US$61 and US$59.80, and no NI at below US$59.80. The most cost-saving strategy also depended on the proportion of influenza infections among ILI patients. Under the standard model, no NI yielded the greatest societal savings when this proportion was less than 13%, RFT with NI at between 13% and 24%, and systematic NI at higher levels.

4. Discussion

4.1. Major findings

During flu epidemics, defined by a proportion of influenza infections among patients with ILI of 40% or higher, systematic NI prescription without RFT was a dominant strategy for healthy working adults consulting within 2 days of the onset of ILI symptoms since it provided the best health outcome (0.4 flu days averted) and minimized societal costs (saved US$41.20 per person). When the rate of influenza infections exceeded 56%, systematic NI was always dominant in every sensitivity analysis through all plausible ranges for every variable.

Systematic NI during flu epidemics prevented secondary infectious complications and thus reduced antibiotic use and follow-up visits with savings of US$3 per person. We did not consider the unnecessary antibiotics prescribed to meet the expectations of patients with ILI.

4.2. Limitations

We adopted a societal approach as recommended by the Panel on Cost-Effectiveness in Health and Medicine [2]. The measurement of productivity gains (or losses) remains controversial, however, and involved three decisions related to ILI particularities: the cost method, the measurement of daily earnings lost, and the reduction of absenteeism related to NI. Our cost method, justified by the current full employment situation in the US, was based on the human capital approach and approximated productivity gains by multiplying additional work days by their related mean earnings. The friction cost method might also apply since the short duration of influenza-related absenteeism might either be compensated for locally in up to 60% of cases [9] or permit patients to make up their missed work on their return. Using the friction cost method would have minimized the productivity gains associated with NI. The results did not change, however, when we decreased the mean number of lost work days from 1.2 to 0.5 in the sensitivity analysis. On the other hand, the mean number of lost work days relied solely on the lack of physical presence and thus did not take into account the productivity losses that occur when a worker with ILI symptoms nonetheless comes to work. In NI controlled trials, patients in the NI group returned to normal activities a median of 2 days earlier than untreated patients [10].

The second decision was our choice to measure earnings lost based on the mean annual earnings from wages and salary of full-time, year-round workers, who represented 73.7% and 56.3 %, respectively, of the 77.3 million men and 68.8 million women at least 15 years old who worked in 1998 [8]. Full-time, year-round workers were included in influenza vaccination trials [7]. Using mean annual earnings from wages and salary, non-farm self-employment, and farm self-employment (US$30,387 in 1998) [8] would not have changed the results.

Thirdly, because the NI controlled trials did not directly study the reduction of lost work days attributable to NI, a societal rather than strictly medical outcome, we assumed that it was identical to the median reduction of ILI symptomatic days—1 day. The greater efficacy of NI in the more symptomatic patients, in particular those with fever, supported this assumption; fever was the most common reason for absence from work [9]. It was also the main symptom that induced patients with ILI to visit physicians, accounting for half the visits [9].

References

[1] Centers for Disease Control and Prevention, Prevention and control of influenza: recommendations of the Advisory Committee on Immunization Practices (ACIP), MMWR Morb. Mortal. Wkly. Rep. 49 (2000) 1–38.

[2] M.R. Gold, J.E. Siegel, L.B. Russell, et al., Cost-effectiveness in Health and Medicine, Oxford Univ. Press, New York, 1996.

[3] F. Carrat, A. Tachet, C. Rouzioux, et al., Evaluation of clinical case definitions of influenza: detailed investigation of patients during the 1995–1996 epidemic in France, Clin. Infect. Dis. 28 (1999) 283–290.

[4] S.J. Todd, L. Minnich, J.L. Waner, Comparison of rapid immunofluorescence procedure with TestPack RSV and Directigen FLU-A for diagnosis of respiratory syncytial virus and influenza A virus, J. Clin. Microbiol. 33 (1995) 1650–1651.

[5] 1995 Drug Topics Red Book, Medical Economics, Montvale, NJ, 1995.

[6] K.L. Nichol, P.M. Mendelman, K.P. Mallon, et al., Effectiveness of live, attenuated intranasal influenza virus vaccine in healthy, working adults: a randomized controlled trial, JAMA 282 (1999) 137–144.

[7] K.L. Nichol, A. Lind, K.L. Margolis, et al., The effectiveness of vaccination against influenza in healthy, working adults, N. Engl. J. Med. 333 (1995) 889–893.

[8] U.S. Census Bureau, Current Population Reports, P60-206. Money Income in the United States: 1998. U.S. Government Printing Office, Washington (DC), 1999.

[9] M. Keech, A.J. Scott, P.J. Ryan, The impact of influenza and influenza-like illness on productivity and healthcare resource utilization in a working population, Occup. Med. 48 (1998) 85–90.

[10] J.J. Treanor, F.G. Hayden, P.S. Vrooman, et al., Efficacy and safety of the oral neuraminidase inhibitor oseltamivir in treating acute influenza: a randomized controlled trial. US oral neuraminidase study group, JAMA 283 (2000) 1016–1024.

[11] A.S. Monto, D.M. Fleming, D. Henry, et al., Efficacy and safety of the neuraminidase inhibitor zanamivir in the treatment of influenza A and B virus infections, J. Infect. Dis. 180 (1999) 254–261.

International Congress Series 1219 (2001) 81–85

Health economics in decision making for influenza management

Paul A. Scuffham*, John W. Posnett, Peter A. West

York Health Economics Consortium, University of York, Heslington, York, England YO10 5DD, UK

Abstract

Background: The aim of this study was to compare the cost-effectiveness of vaccination programmes with antiviral prophylaxis and antiviral treatment programmes. We estimated the cost-effectiveness of these various strategies for the high risk and elderly populations in UK, France and Germany. *Methods*: This was a decision analysis approach with Country-specific data collected from national sources. The effectiveness of interventions reported in meta-analyses was applied to the risk groups. *Results*: The cost per death averted ranged from €3643 to €21,031 with vaccination strategies, from €243,061 to €770,227 with antiviral prophylaxis strategies, and from €1962 to €22,305 with antiviral treatment programmes. Antiviral prophylaxis strategies with either neuraminidase inhibitors (NIs) or ion channel inhibitors (ICIs) were expensive compared with all other strategies. Sensitivity analyses indicated prophylactic strategies remained the most expensive strategy under all realistic scenarios modelled. The antiviral treatment strategies were based on an optimal set of assumptions and were highly sensitive to small changes in these assumptions; reducing the effectiveness in averting complications by 50%, increased the cost per death averted sevenfold. Antiviral treatment was also sensitive to the number seeking GP treatment and the timing of that treatment. Vaccination strategies were relatively robust to changes in effectiveness and rate of side effects. The greatest number of cases, hospitalizations and deaths could be averted from vaccination compared with other strategies. *Conclusions*: Vaccination programmes represent the most feasible option for the management of influenza in Europe. © 2001 Elsevier Science B.V. All rights reserved.

Keywords: Vaccine; Antiviral prophylaxis; Antiviral treatment; Cost-effectiveness; Health policy

* Corresponding author. Tel.: +44-1940-433-620; fax: +44-1940-433-628.
  E-mail address: pas8@york.ac.uk (P.A. Scuffham).

0531-5131/01/$ – see front matter © 2001 Elsevier Science B.V. All rights reserved.
PII: S 0 5 3 1 - 5 1 3 1 (0 1) 0 0 3 2 9 - 6

1. Introduction

Several choices are available to health policy decision makers for the management of influenza in the population. Vaccination programmes may be opportunistic (i.e. individuals consulting a GP may be offered vaccination) or comprehensive (i.e. a targeted programme with identification of individuals at risk, a register of who has had a vaccination, and active recruitment and recall of patients). The targeted risk group may also vary.

The ion channel inhibitors (ICIs) are active against influenza A but not influenza B. The neuraminidase inhibitors (NIs) may be active against both influenza A and B viruses. Antiviral prophylaxis may be given as a short course (e.g. 1 week) or an extended course lasting 4–6 weeks. When antivirals are used for treatment of influenza, the treatment must be initiated within the first 2 days following infection to gain the full benefit. Six independent potential strategies for the control of influenza are available from these vaccination and antiviral options (Table 1).

Policy decisions about public health choices should be based not only on the information about effectiveness but also on cost-effectiveness, resources available and the impact on the health care funders' budget. Previous studies indicate that vaccination is a cost-effective approach to prevent and control of influenza [1,2]. However, the cost-effectiveness of antiviral strategies is unknown. In addition, NIs are more expensive and more effective than ICIs, and the cost-effectiveness of the two classes is open to economic appraisal. Furthermore, the cost-effectiveness and optimal strategy may differ between countries and risk groups as the propensity to consult a GP for treatment, admission in the hospital, and definition of population risk groups varies between countries.

2. Objective

The aim of this project was to estimate the costs, consequences and cost-effectiveness of six independent potential strategies for the control of influenza in UK, France and Germany. We estimated the cost-effectiveness of each strategy for the high risk groups and the elderly from the perspective of a third-party health care funder.

3. Methods

A decision analysis approach was used to model the costs and consequences for each strategy and country. The incremental costs, consequences and cost-effectiveness are estimated by comparing each intervention to a "no intervention" base-case scenario (i.e. no vaccination, no prophylactic antivirals, and no treatment with antivirals).

Country-specific baseline data included current vaccination rates, attack rates of influenza-like illness (ILI), excess GP consultations, excess hospitalizations for influenza (including pneumonia and other respiratory illness) and excess deaths associated with influenza. The "excess" morbidity associated with ILI is the number of incidents over and above those that occur in the absence of influenza epidemics after accounting for seasonal effects and trends.

Current vaccination rates are used for modelling opportunistic vaccination programmes. For a comprehensive programme, we assumed that coverage rates would increase to 65% for all groups except for the French elderly, where we assumed coverage could be increased to 90% (79% of the elderly are currently vaccinated). In addition, we assumed that 0.1% would consult a GP with side effects of the vaccine.

We assumed coverage rates for chemoprophylaxis equal to current (opportunistic) vaccination rates. A medical doctor must prescribe chemoprophylaxis. We assumed most would obtain chemoprophylaxis on an opportunistic basis but 10% would consult a GP specifically to obtain chemoprophylaxis. We assumed a non-compliance dropout rate of 5% per week based on observational studies of prophylaxis compliance [3]. ICIs may produce severe side effects. Based on Myint et al. [4], we assumed that of the 5% who dropout from ICI prophylaxis, 24% consult a GP and 15% of these are admitted to hospital. We also assumed antivirals would be effective for the proportion of the influenza season they are used and that the risk of infection returns to baseline for the remaining period.

For early treatment, we assumed that current rates of GP consultations for ILI would double and 50% would commence treatment within 2 days of the onset of symptoms (85% in France). We assume that 90% of those presenting within 2 days of symptoms would be prescribed antivirals.

The effectiveness of each intervention (reduction in relative risks) was obtained from published meta-analyses [5]. The effects of NIs in the elderly and high risk groups are unknown at this time but we assumed that the effectiveness for healthy adults (a 74% reduction in ILI cases [6]) would be attained in these groups and for all levels of illness severity. This is a clear overestimate but is a conservative assumption with a bias in favour of NIs. Likewise, we assumed the effectiveness of ICIs in healthy adults, a 23% reduction in ILI cases [6], would apply to the elderly and high risk populations and all levels of illness severity. Early treatment with antivirals may reduce antibiotic prescribing and complications by 7% and 13%, respectively [7]. We assumed this reduction in complications from early treatment would apply to excess hospitalizations and deaths and for both NIs and ICIs. We also assume there are no adverse events and only those with ILI symptoms get treatment. These effectiveness parameters and assumptions were uniformly applied to each country and are all biased in favour of antivirals.

Country-specific data were used to estimate the resource use and costs for each population group in each country. Cost-effectiveness outcomes reported here are the incremental costs per case and per death averted. We also performed sensitivity analyses to identify influential factors in the models.

4. Results

Incremental consequences and costs are those in addition to the base case. Incremental cost-effectiveness ratios are obtained from incremental consequences and costs (Table 1).

Comprehensive vaccination programmes can prevent more cases and deaths but cost more in administration. The additional costs are most noticeable for Germany where the cost of comprehensive vaccination is 40% more than an opportunistic programme.

Table 1
Incremental cost-effectiveness ratios for the high risk and elderly populations

	Prophylaxis strategies				Treatment strategies	
	Opportunistic vaccination	Comprehensive vaccination	ICIs	NIs	ICIs[a]	NIs
High risk groups[b]						
UK						
Cost per case averted	479	668	23,608	30,657	–	–
Cost per death averted	9351	13,053	559,883	727,051	1732	7589
France						
Cost per case averted	200	344	13,945	13,589	–	–
Cost per death averted	5199	8956	440,966	429,703	3610	11,179
Germany						
Cost per case averted	253	557	18,886	32,003	–	–
Cost per death averted	3643	8030	243,061	411,001	6336	8810
Elderly groups[b]						
UK						
Cost per case averted	439	629	23,400	41,287	–	–
Cost per death averted	9063	12,978	431,402	761,178	1962	2591
France						
Cost per case averted	259	393	18,403	13,947	–	–
Cost per death averted	7113	10,797	342,529	451,954	4164	10,043
Germany						
Cost per case averted	481	786	18,923	32,225	–	–
Cost per death averted	12,884	21,031	452,300	770,227	17,709	22,305

All units are in Euro (€).

[a] Only for influenza A.

[b] The high risk and elderly groups represent 22%, 23% and 33% of the UK, French and German adult populations, respectively.

Similarly, vaccination in high risk groups is more cost-effective compared with the elderly. All chemoprophylaxis strategies are relatively expensive in all countries. The cost-effectiveness ratios of the relatively expensive but effective NIs were similar to the low cost and weakly effective ICIs. The most realistic comparison is between vaccination and early treatment. Opportunistic vaccination is the most cost-effective strategy in Germany but early treatment with ICIs is more cost-effective in UK and France.

Our sensitivity analyses indicate that the cost-effectiveness of chemoprophylaxis strategies remains relatively high even when the effectiveness is doubled (cost per case averted is 20–30 times more than vaccination). Early treatment with either ICIs or NIs is extremely sensitive to the assumptions used. When more patients attend the GP, early treatment is less viable, but when the proportion that commences treatment within 2 days increases, early treatment becomes more viable. These two factors (number consulting and the proportion that consult within 2 days) act in opposite directions. The cost per death averted increases sevenfold when the effectiveness of early treatment is halved. Vaccination strategies were relatively robust to changes in effectiveness and the rate of side effects. Prevention strategies become considerably more and early treatment becomes less cost-effective when large epidemics were modelled.

5. Discussion

The economic outcomes of the strategies for the control of influenza presented in Table 1 were based on assumptions favourable to antiviral treatment. We expect that if an early treatment policy was implemented, then the number of GP consultations could increase substantially more than current levels, and it is likely that antivirals would be given to those without true influenza. Furthermore, serious concerns have been raised regarding the safety of influenza treatment with antivirals [8]. Vaccination programmes prevent between 3.2 and 7.0 times the numbers of deaths that could be prevented in early treatment strategies and without the increased demand on GP resources required from early treatment. Given these results, the lack of evidence that antivirals reduce complications and the sensitivity of the estimates of early treatment strategies, vaccination programmes appear to represent the most feasible influenza management option.

Acknowledgements

We are thankful to MAPI Values, France, and the Institute of Empirical Health Economics, Germany for their comments and assistance in obtaining the necessary data. We are grateful for the educational grants received from five pharmaceutical companies.

References

[1] D.S. Fedson, Evaluating the impact of influenza vaccination a North American perspective, Pharmaco-Economics 9 (Suppl. 3) (1996) 54–61.
[2] K.L. Nichol, M. Goodman, The health and economic benefits of influenza vaccination for healthy and at-risk persons aged 65–74 years, PharmacoEconomics 16 (Suppl. 1) (1999) 63–71.
[3] H. Kastrissios, T.F. Blaschke, Medication compliance as a feature in drug development, Annu. Rev. Pharmacol. Toxicol. 37 (1997) 451–475.
[4] M.W.W. Myint, C. Kng, C.P. Wong, C. Mak, Use of amantadine as prophylaxis for influenza A in a subvented care and attention home in Hong Kong, Hong Kong Pract. 20 (10) (1998) 534–543.
[5] P.A. Gross, A.W. Hermogenes, H.S. Sacks, J. Lau, R.A. Levandowski, The efficacy of influenza vaccine in elderly persons, Ann. Intern. Med. 123 (7) (1995) 518–527.
[6] V. Demicheli, T. Jefferson, D. Rivetti, J. Deeks, Prevention and early treatment of influenza in healthy adults, Vaccine 18 (11–12) (2000) 957–1030.
[7] NICE, Fast Track Appraisal of Zanamivir (Relenza): Summary of Evidence, National Institute for Clinical Excellence, London, 2000.
[8] FDA, Important Drug Warning: Zanamivir for Inhalation. U.S. Food and Drug Administration, Washington.

A global pattern for influenza activity

T.A. Reichert[a,b,*], A. Sharma[a], S. Pardo[a]

[a]*Becton Dickinson and Company, New Jersey, USA*
[b]*Entropy Limited, Upper Saddle River, NJ, USA*

Abstract

In two papers at this conference, we showed influenza to be the cause of $\sim 70\%$ of seasonal variation in human mortality. Seasonal mortality, therefore, is a surrogate for the force of influenza infection. We asked whether there might be a geographical pattern. *Methods*: Monthly all-cause mortality data were collected for 37 countries for 1962–1965, 1968–1971 and 1978–1981. Deaths above baseline of summer (DABS) were determined for three winters in each period, and the ratio to the summer baseline (SB) was calculated. The average of this ratio for each period was plotted against geographical factors. Spline fits were made of each plot. *Results*: Plots of average DABS/SB ratio versus latitude reveal an asymmetric bell shape. The outliers are instructive. Plots of DABS/SB against midwinter temperature are bell-shaped, also with instructive outliers. The height of both "bells" diminishes from 1960s to 1980s. Mortality curves of outlier countries, in the plot against temperature, exhibit a broadened winter peak. The peak of the curve lies between 5 and 9 °C and at 38–44° degrees latitude. *Conclusions*: A surrogate for force of influenza infection, seasonal mortality, varies smoothly with latitude and mid-winter temperature. The large variation argues that influenza control programs should be tailored locally. © 2001 Elsevier Science B.V. All rights reserved.

Keywords: Seasonal mortality

1. Introduction

Sakamoto-Momiyama [1] demonstrated that, as countries attain economic development, plots of monthly all-cause mortality change universally, from one which exhibits both a large summer peak and a broad and lower winter elevation, to one with a summer trough

* Corresponding author. 262 W. Saddle River Rd, Upper Saddle River, NJ 07458, USA. Tel.: +1-201-934-9365; fax: +1-201-934-1467.
E-mail address: doctom_us@yahoo.com (T.A. Reichert).

0531-5131/01/$ – see front matter © 2001 Elsevier Science B.V. All rights reserved.
PII: S 0 5 3 1 - 5 1 3 1 (0 1) 0 0 3 8 2 - X

and a sharp peak occurring in mid-winter. The summer peak likely represents gastro-intestinal/diarrheal disease, which is eliminated by effective sanitation and water supply; and the winter peak is thought to result from an association with malnutrition and/or failures in food preservation late in winter. The former is usually resolved before the latter.

Countries with developed economies have monthly mortality curves which are sharply peaked in a mid-winter month. This is true for both all-cause mortality and for disease-specific mortality. In the paper by Reichert and Sharma [2] in these proceedings, such data are presented, and it is demonstrated that

- the winter-seasonal component of the mortality curve for each disease is the same, for all diseases, in each of three widely separated countries,
- seasonal variation differs by a factor of about two between the US and Japan, with Australia intermediate,
- seasonal mortality is most variable in the height of the mid-winter peak, and that variability is highly correspondent with country–local influenza activity,
- inhibition of local influenza activity (by comprehensive vaccination) dramatically reduced the seasonal component of mortality, and
- cessation of inhibition restored the pre-intervention level of seasonal variability.

We infer, then, that seasonal variation of disease-specific or all-cause monthly mortality is a good surrogate for influenza activity within a healthcare system. We asked whether the

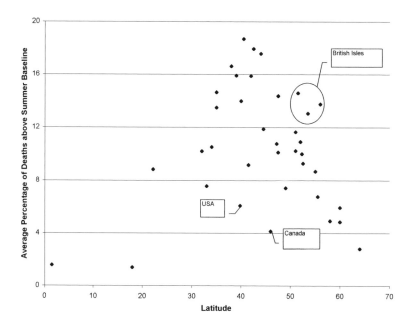

Fig. 1a. The distribution of seasonal mortality as a percentage of total annual mortality for 37 countries versus latitude, for the time period 1962–1965. Three instructive outliers are called out.

variability seen in the three countries might be a part of a global pattern for influenza activity.

2. Methods

Monthly mortality data were obtained for approximately 50 countries for the periods 1962–1965 [3], 1968–1971 [4] and 1978–1981 [5]. Countries for which a plot of monthly mortality exhibited a summer peak or multiple, irregular peaks, were eliminated from the database; and countries for which data were not available for all periods were not considered. Thirty-seven countries in all three hemispheres met these criteria.

The Summer Baseline for any winter period was defined as the average of the mortality for the preceding and following summer months (June–September, in the northern hemisphere, and December–March, in the southern hemisphere). Deaths above the baseline of summer (DABS) were defined as the sum of the non-negative differences between the monthly mortality and the summer baseline, for each non-summer month. The ratio of DABS to the total annual all-cause mortality is the fraction of deaths that occur in the winter season (DABSFrac). This fraction compensates, after a fashion, for differences among countries in population number and age distribution.

The population centrum was defined, for each country, as a point placed at the approximate population-weighted center of gravity for that country. DABSFrac was

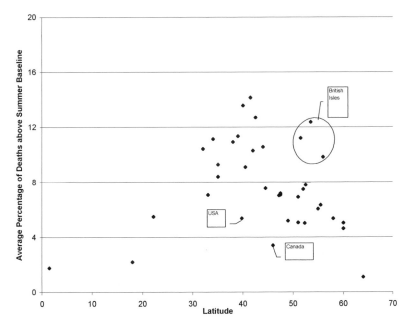

Fig. 1b. The distribution of seasonal mortality as a percentage of total annual mortality for 37 countries for the period 1978–1981. The same outliers appear.

plotted for each country versus the latitude of the population centrum. The mean mid-winter temperature (in January for countries in the northern hemisphere, July in the southern hemisphere) was obtained for capitol cities in each country [6]. These were also plotted against DABSFrac. The resulting scatter plots were fitted using the locally weighted regression (Lowess) [7].

3. Results

Fig. 1a displays the distribution of DABSFrac with latitude for the earliest time period (∼1965), and Fig. 1b, the latest period (∼1980). There is significant scatter, but there is also an obvious bell-shaped relationship, which is somewhat lower in the later period. There are also obvious outliers, which appear consistently in all three periods and are noted in the figure. The USA, Canada and the British Isles all have in common the fact that their winter temperatures are atypical for their latitude. The first two are much colder, the last much warmer. Eliminating these outliers, Lowess fits for all periods are

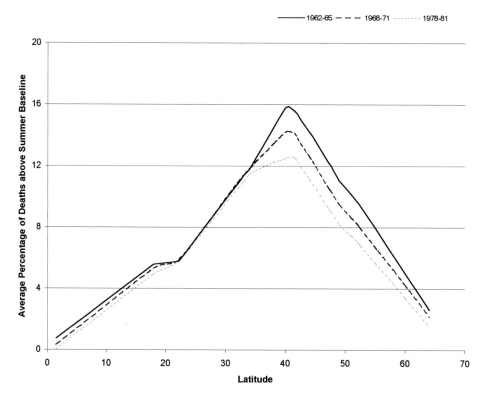

Fig. 2. Locally weighted regression fits to the distribution of winter seasonal mortality as a percentage of total mortality versus latitude for 37 countries, for three time periods.

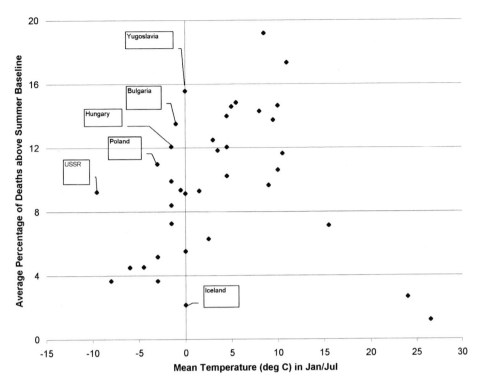

Fig. 3. The seasonality of mortality as a percentage of annual mortality for 37 countries versus the mean temperature in a mid-winter month in the capitol city, averaged for the time period 1968–1971.

shown in Fig. 2. The result is a bell-shaped curve, which has a broad maximum spanning latitudes, 38–43, for each period and a general lowering of the maximum with advancing time.

DABSFrac was also plotted against mean, mid-winter month temperature. Fig. 3 displays this relationship, for the middle period (∼ 1970). Again, a bell-shaped trend is obvious, with outliers, which are now different. Fig. 4 displays the Lowess fits for all three time periods.

4. Discussion

The distribution among economically developed countries of the fraction of all-cause deaths, which occur as a winter excess above the summer baseline, varies smoothly and consistently in all three hemispheres, in both latitude and in mean temperature of a central mid-winter month. A locally weighted regression fit to these distributions makes the underlying pattern manifest as bell-shaped curves, with maxima between 38° and 44° latitude and at 5–9 °C. The bells are relatively symmetric, at least near the peak, dropping

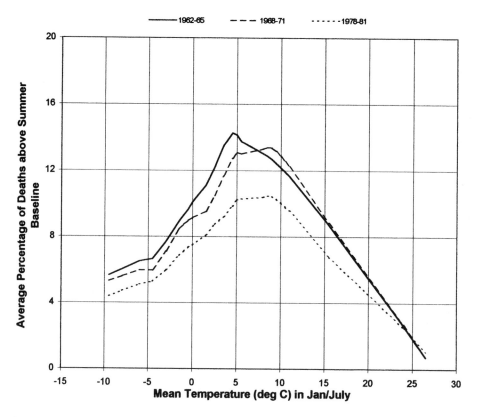

Fig. 4. Locally weighted regression fits to the distribution of winter seasonal mortality as a percentage of total annual mortality, versus the mean mid-winter temperature in the capitol city, for 37 countries, for three time periods.

to half of peak values at ±12° of latitude and 10 °C. Data is relatively scant in low latitudes (<30 degrees) and high winter temperatures (>12 °C). Therefore, our ability to draw conclusions relative to tropical regions is limited.

In latitude, the global pattern of seasonal mortality decreased with about equal amounts between each pair of the three time periods; about 25% in toto, in peak magnitude. This is consistent with the general worldwide reduction in the activity of influenza over the same time. Relative to mid-winter average temperature, the global pattern also declined, about 1/3 in magnitude, with less distinction between the two earlier periods.

We are not the first to suggest a relationship between mid-winter temperature, seasonal mortality and influenza. Curwen [8], reviewing some of the same data, demonstrated that winter quarter mortality was strongly associated with both mean temperature and deaths attributed to influenza. Unfortunately, this author considered only monotonic relationships and, therefore, found data from the period around and after 1980 troubling to his hypothesis.

The presently proposed pattern of influenza activity versus mid-winter mean temperature exhibits outliers not noted by previous authors. All such outlier countries (except Iceland, for which seasonal mortality is lower than trend) were members of the so-called Soviet bloc at the index time. The USSR and Bulgaria are consistently outliers in each time period. There are at least two plausible explanations. Either the temperature assigned is lower than a more appropriate average, or some consistent element acted to elevate the apparent seasonality. The additional outliers, in Fig. 3, suggest that one such element might be a broadening of the winter mortality peak. Each of the "outlier" countries, for that period, has a relatively broad winter peak, spanning 3 or 4 months, rather than 1 or 2. Many factors might conspire to produce such a broadening. However, Sakamoto-Momiyama [1] noted that the sharpening of the winter peak occurs relatively later in economic development than does the loss of the summer peak. Factors such as failure of food storage facilities, food scarcity, and in particular, lack of availability of vitamin-rich foodstuffs may produce both malnutrition and an increased susceptibility to an array of diseases. The above are plausible, but remain to be speculative bases for the noted departure from the apparent pattern.

Seasonal variation in all-cause mortality is relatively easy to measure in any healthcare system, and these data appear to be reliable at low levels of sophistication in data collection. For this reason, the surrogate association of the winter excess of mortality with influenza activity is a powerful tool for both global assessment and pandemic planning. Figs. 2 and 4 readily demonstrate that influenza activity in severely affected regions may be large integer factors greater than that in other countries of similar levels of economic development. We note that countries located near the peak of activity are those which are often cited as the plausible origin of historical influenza pandemics, and cities with peak characteristics are overwhelmingly represented in the list of viral isolates used in vaccines in the modern era.

The above model does not include factors plausibly important in the rise and propagation of influenza epidemics, such as complex temperature patterns, population density, wind and transportation patterns, and humidity. We suggest, however, that even the crude nature of the global pattern thus far elucidated is sufficiently compelling that it should be considered for use in global pandemic planning. It is obvious, for example, that new viral variants are most likely to arise where the largest number of susceptibles are exposed to the highest level of viral activity. It would follow, then, that the placement of an efficient array of surveillance centers should be guided by the global distribution of viral activity. It is equally obvious that vaccination strategies appropriate for one level of activity may be less optimal for lower or higher levels of force of infection of the viral agent. Longini et al. [9] demonstrate that the level of coverage needed to produce community protection varies strongly with the local force of viral infection, and earlier models [10,11] demonstrated that factors such as national policy and resource availability interact with the force of infection to determine the locally optimal tactical implementation of influenza control. Every developed country has steadily increased the level of influenza vaccination within its citizenry over time [12], and many are now approaching coverage levels at which discernible effects might be seen. Integration of the global pattern of influenza activity would significantly increase the effectiveness of most of these programs, even at present resource levels and presently enunciated policy provisions.

References

[1] M. Sakamoto-Momiyama, Seasonality in Human Mortality, Univ. Tokyo Press, Tokyo, 1972.

[2] T.A. Reichert, A. Sharma, The seasonality of human mortality: the role of influenza, in: A.D.M.E. Oster-haus, et al. (Eds.), Options for the Control of Influenza IV, Elsevier, Amsterdam, 2001(in press).

[3] Table 19, 1966 Demographic Yearbook, United Nations, New York, 1968, pp. 361–378.

[4] Table 32, 1974 Demographic Yearbook, United Nations, New York, 1976, pp. 982–999.

[5] Table 30, 1985 Demographic Yearbook, United Nations, New York, 1987, pp. 732–748.

[6] National Geographic Atlas of the World, National Geographic, Washington, 1999, p. 136.

[7] W.S. Cleveland, Robust locally weighted regression and smoothing scatterplots, J. Am. Stat. Assoc. 74 (1979) 829–836.

[8] M. Curwen, Excess winter mortality: a British phenomenon? Health Trends 22 (1990/1991) 169–175.

[9] I.M. Longini Jr., M.E. Halloran, A. Nizam, et al., Estimation of the efficacy of live, attenuated influenza vaccine from a two-year, multi-center vaccine trial: implications for influenza epidemic control, Vaccine 18 (2000) 1902–1909.

[10] I.M. Longini, E. Ackerman, L.R. Elveback, An optimization model for influenza A epidemics, Math. Biosci. 38 (1978) 141–157.

[11] I.M. Longini Jr., J.S. Koopman, M. Haber, G.A. Cotsonis, Statistical inference for infectious diseases: risk-specific household and community transmission parameters, Am. J. Epidemiol. 128 (1988) 845–859.

[12] F. Ambrosch, D.S. Fedson, Influenza vaccination in 29 countries: an update to 1997, Pharmacoeconomics 16 (Suppl. 1) (1999) 47–54.

International Congress Series 1219 (2001) 95–101

The seasonality of human mortality: the role of influenza

T.A. Reichert[a,*], A. Sharma[b]

[a]Becton Dickinson and Company/Entropy Limited, Upper Saddle River, NJ, USA
[b]Becton Dickinson and Company, Franklin Lakes, NJ, USA

Abstract

Background: In economically developed countries, the pattern of mortality attributable to major disease classes appears similar in shape to the excess mortality attributed to pneumonia and influenza. We asked to what extent influenza activity is correlated with seasonality of all mortality. *Methods*: Monthly mortality, for all-causes and five disease classes plus influenza, was assembled for 50 years for the US, Japan and Australia. A transformation, z-scaling, was performed on the time trace of each mortality class; and the time-local coefficient of variation (moving CV) was calculated. An epidemiological version of the Henle–Koch postulates was defined. *Results*: All mortality classes z-scaled to a single curve for each country, the most variable feature of which correlated well with influenza activity. The moving CV of all vascular diseases is similar in each country and the variability in pulmonary disease was everywhere two to three times greater. Overall, variability in Japan was $2 \times$ the US and $1.5 \times$ Australia. A "notch", in the z-scale and moving CV, for all Japanese mortality classes, coincided with the national program of schoolchildren vaccination. *Conclusions*: In developed countries, there is a common cause for all seasonal mortality due to disease. Influenza is the dominant element in this set of causes. © 2001 Elsevier Science B.V. All rights reserved.

Keywords: Seasonality of mortality; z-scale; Moving CV; Koch's postulates; Schoolchildren vaccination

1. Introduction

The temporal pattern of death in undeveloped countries is bimodal, with peaks in late winter and mid-summer associated with infectious disease [1]. With economic development, this pattern yields to a unimodal curve with a peak in one of the winter months; and

* Corresponding author. 262 W. Saddle River Road, Upper Saddle River, NJ 07458, USA. Tel.: +1-201-934-9365; fax: +1-201-934-1467.
E-mail address: doctom_us@yahoo.com (T.A. Reichert).

for which both the level and the variability are reduced. Sakamoto-Momiyama [1] also observed that the unimodal curve was further flattened, "deseasonalized", in certain countries, most especially the US, Canada, and countries in northern Europe. She and others suggested that the basis of deseasonalization lay in advances in environmental support infrastructure, especially home heating [2,3]. Keatinge et al. [4] examined the home heating issue in England and Wales and found no discernible reduction in excess winter mortality attributable to cardiovascular or cerebrovascular disease, but excess mortality attributable to respiratory causes dropped about 70%.

A number of authors have shown that deaths due to cardiovascular disease, cerebro-vascular disease, and pneumonia occur with a frequency inversely related to temperature [1,5,6,7]. Countries in more temperate climes have steeper slopes, and while the slopes of the temperature relationship of cardio- and cerebrovascular disease about equal one another in nearly every country, that for respiratory disease is inevitably two to three times greater.

Correlates of seasonal mortality, such as arterial blood pressure and blood chemistry and hematological parameters have been sought by many authors, but the magnitude of the seasonal change in these elements appears sufficient to account for at most one-half the observed winter excess of mortality. At least one author [8] noted that concomitants of infection vary directly with the observed changes in the hemostatic factors; and suggested that respiratory infections may be predisposing factors for acute vascular events. Spodick et al. [9] noted an increased prevalence of symptoms of respiratory infection in acute myocardial infarction patients; and Bainton et al. [10] observed a direct relationship between influenza activity and the number of cases of pulmonary embolism and acute myocardial infarction.

Several population-based, retrospective studies have demonstrated that influenza vaccination is effective in reducing not only hospitalization and reports of illness, but also, all-cause mortality during winter influenza epidemic periods [11–13]. Nichol et al. [14] directly demonstrated, in an elderly population with chronic obstructive pulmonary disease, that seasonal variation in both hospitalizations and death was all but eliminated by influenza vaccination. The estimated reduction in risk of death was 70%. In Japan, from 1977 to 1994, $\sim 80\%$ of schoolchildren were vaccinated against influenza [15]. During this period, all-cause excess mortality rates dropped by 2/3 [16].

Reductions in all-cause mortality and that attributable to pneumonia are clearly related to the temporal occurrence of influenza. However, it is not known whether the seasonal variation in other diseases is idiosyncratic to the particular disease, whether a case for a common cause can be advanced; and whether it is likely and to what extent, that causation may be laid to influenza. To this end, we reviewed 50 years of mortality data on the major causes of death due to disease, from three countries, each in a different hemisphere, for signs of commonality.

2. Methods

Monthly mortality data were obtained for the US, Japan and Australia, from 1949 to the latest year available (1997 or 1998) for all-cause mortality, ischemic heart disease (IHD), cerebrovascular disease (stroke), diabetes mellitus, malignant disease, pneumonia, influenza, and chronic pulmonary disease (CPD) [17–19]. The labeling of these categories of disease was neither constant nor consistent over the 48-year period. Each country made slightly different coding choices within the version of the International Coding of Disease, then current.

The number of monthly deaths was adjusted to a standard, 30.4-day, month. Each adjusted monthly mortality was "detrended" by subtracting the 13-month moving average from the adjusted deaths for the index month. The overall standard deviation of each detrended mortality was calculated. For each month, the detrended number of deaths was divided by this overall standard deviation. The result is a set of scaled values, with mean, zero, and standard deviation, one. The above-described process is called z-scaling in analogy to the calculation of the z-score, a commonly used statistical tool for comparing different kinds of measurements.

The ratio of the standard deviation to the average is called the coefficient of variation or CV. It provides a measure of relative variability useful in comparing effects with different average values. The CV was computed as both an overall quantity, and locally, in time. In concert with each 13-month moving average, we calculated the moving standard deviation and the ratio of the two, the moving CV.

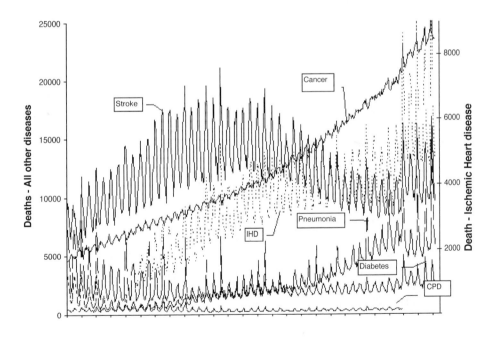

Fig. 1. Disease-specific monthly mortality in Japan for 50 years. Six diseases are plotted. Deaths due to malignant disease (cancer), diabetes, cerebrovascular disease (stroke), pneumonia and chronic respiratory disease (CRD) are plotted against the left-hand axis. Ischemic heart disease (IHD) mortality is plotted against the right-hand axis. Statistics for IHD were not published for years earlier than 1958.

3. Results

The time course of every mortality class listed, in all three countries, consists of a secular trend, plus a variable, annual cycle, with sharp peaks in a winter month. Fig. 1 displays the monthly mortality for six disease classes for Japan. Peak excursions in the annual peak mortality are invariably synchronized, for every class of mortality.

For each of the three countries, the z-scaling process produces essentially the same curve, regardless of mortality class. Fig. 2 displays the z-score curve for the above five disease classes for Japan and the US for a representative 12-year segment from 1967 to 1979. The z-score curves for malignant disease and for all-cause mortality would also fall directly atop each collective z-score displayed. The former is a bit noisy, due to the small variation. Fig. 2 also includes the number of deaths attributed to influenza. The z-score curve, for all three countries, is most variable, year-to-year, in the winter peak height. Excursions in the annual z-score peak unfailingly coincide with epidemic influenza activity within the country.

The overall CV for each disease class is very similar, for the three vascular diseases (diabetes, IHD, and stroke; data not shown), within each country. The CV for malignant disease is the same, and very low, in all countries. The CV for respiratory disease is, in each case, between two and three times that for vascular disease, and acute respiratory disease is more variable (between 30% and 50%) than chronic disease. Over all, for mortality classes, the variability is about twice as great in Japan as the US, with Australia lying about halfway between.

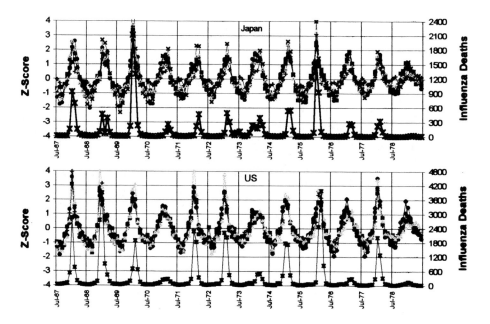

Fig. 2. The z-scale curve for five diseases for Japan (upper panel) and the US, for a representative 12-year period. The overlap is virtually complete. Monthly deaths attributed to influenza are plotted against the right-hand axis.

4. Discussion

The specific disease classes selected here accounted for about 60% of all deaths in 1995. Non-disease causes of death (suicide, homicide, accidents, etc.) have a very different seasonality. The overlap of the z-score curves for all individual diseases, for the US and Australia is very tight. In the US, only chronic respiratory disease shows a departure from the common seasonal z-score curve, and this only for the period earlier than 1958, for which period the coding used was not representative of the class. The fact that the z-score curves for very different diseases, which account for the majority of all deaths in three countries, in all hemispheres, completely overlap for decades argues that the driving force of seasonal variation in all these diseases must be a common one.

Fig. 3 is a plot of the moving CV of vascular disease in Japan. The most striking feature is the notch, which occurs beginning in 1971 and ends abruptly in 1995. Seasonal variability in mortality due to vascular and respiratory disease and all-causes plummeted, and peak excursions were attenuated for this 24-year period [16]. There is a further drop in level beginning in 1977. These effects correspond to the timing of the Japanese School-children Vaccination Program. During this period, death rates dropped by a factor of three to four; and at least 37,000 deaths per year were averted.

Like the inverse relationship in disease-specific mortality, the moving CV data also demonstrate similar values for cardiovascular and cerebrovascular disease and values two to three times greater for respiratory disease, with increased levels in countries with more temperate climates. This body of evidence leads to a conclusion that the single, root cause of seasonal variation in mortality produces an effect that is very similar for all forms of

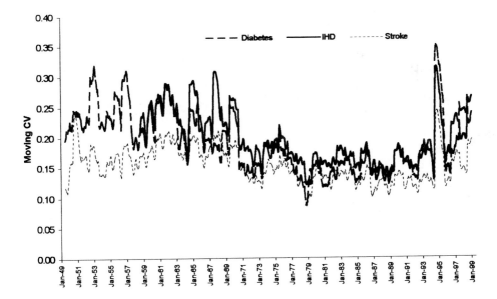

Fig. 3. The moving coefficient of variation (CV) for vascular disease in Japan over 50 years. The "notch" in values between 1972 and 1995 occurs in precise timing with the Japanese Schoolchildren Vaccination Program.

vascular disease, and greater for respiratory disease. The level of seasonal variation varies from country to country, both overall, and in the relative magnitude seen in respiratory disease compared to vascular disease. This ratio may depend on microclimate control infrastructure.

The most variable feature of seasonal mortality is excursions in the mid-winter peak height and these excursions inexorably follow the course of influenza activity, which is different in each country. This evidence is strongly suggestive of, but does not establish a causal relationship between influenza and the seasonality of mortality phenomenon. Rather, in epidemiological analogy to the molecular form of Koch's postulates [20], we suggest that this evidence satisfies the equivalent of the first postulate.

(1) The seasonality of mortality is singular in cause and significantly associated with the occurrence and non-occurrence of epidemic influenza.

We suggest, further, that the data from Japan [16] satisfy the epidemiological equivalent of the latter two postulates given below.

(2) Specific and substantive inhibition of the activity of the influenza virus leads to a measurable decrease in seasonality mortality.

(3) Restoration of full pathogenicity leads to recrudescence in the seasonality phenomenon.

We assert this to be proof of a causal relation between influenza and seasonal mortality in economically developed human populations.

The question remaining is whether the seasonality of mortality phenomenon is wholly derived from influenza or whether other agents, acting contemporaneously, form an equivalence set. The consensus of the seasonality of mortality literature is that the development of microclimate control has reduced measures of this phenomenon, but only in respiratory disease. There is no evidence that microclimate control has reduced seasonality in mortality due to vascular disease. The Japanese schoolchildren vaccination program reduced all-cause and pneumonia and influenza (P&I) excess mortality rates by two-thirds, by indirect effect. Nichol et al. [14] showed that direct vaccination of the population at risk against influenza can reduce all-cause mortality by 70%. These observations suggest that influenza plays a very large role in the putative equivalence set. Since these two strategies could be overlapping, additive or synergistic, it is not clear how to synthesize further. These lines of evidence do combine, however, to argue that influenza is at least 70% of the cause of seasonal mortality. We conclude that the equivalence set must consist of either influenza alone, or must include entities which have a temporal distribution strongly associated with that of influenza.

References

[1] M. Sakamoto-Momiyama, Seasonality in Human Mortality, Univ. Tokyo Press, Tokyo, 1972.
[2] M. Curwen, Excess winter mortality: a British phenomenon? Health Trends 22 (1990/1991) 169–175.
[3] D. Seretakis, L. Pagona, L. Lipworth, L.B. Signorello, K.J. Rothman, D. Trichopoulos, Changing seasonality of mortality from coronary heart disease, JAMA, J. Am. Med. Assoc. 278 (1997) 1012–1014.
[4] W.R. Keatinge, S.R.K. Coleshaw, J. Holmes, Changes in seasonal mortalities with improvement in home heating in England and Wales from 1964 to 1984, Int. J. Biometeorol. 33 (1989) 71–76.
[5] T.W. Anderson, W.H. Le Riche, Cold weather and myocardial infarction, Lancet 7 (1970) 291–296 (February).

[6] G.M. Bull, Meteorological correlates with myocardial and cerebral infarction and respiratory disease, Brit. J. Prev. Soc. Med. 27 (1973) 108–113.

[7] G.M. Bull, J. Morton, Environment, temperature and death rates, Age Ageing 7 (1978) 210–224.

[8] P.R. Woodhouse, K.T. Khaw, M. Plummer, A. Foley, T.W. Meade, Seasonal variations of plasma fibrinogen and Factor VII activity in the elderly: winter infections and death from cardiovascular disease, Lancet 343 (1994) 435–439.

[9] D.H. Spodick, A.P. Fleiss, M.M. Johnson, Association of acute respiratory symptoms with onset of acute myocardial infarction: prospective investigation of 150 consecutive patients and matched control patients, Am. J. Cardiol. 53 (1984) 481–482.

[10] D. Bainton, G.R. Jones, D. Hole, Influenza and ischaemic heart disease—a possible trigger for acute myocardial infarction? Int. J. Epidemiol. 7 (1978) 231–239.

[11] D.S. Fedson, A. Wajda, J.P. Nicol, G.W. Hammond, D.A. Kaiser, L.L. Roos, Clinical effectiveness of influenza vaccination in Manitoba, JAMA, J. Am. Med. Assoc. 270 (1993) 1956–1961.

[12] K.L. Nichol, K.L. Margolis, J. Wuorenma, et al., The efficacy and cost effectiveness of vaccination against influenza among elderly persons living in the community, N. Engl. J. Med. 331 (1994) 778–784.

[13] K.L. Nichol, J. Wuorenma, T. von Sternberg, Benefits of influenza vaccination for low-, intermediate-, and high-risk senior citizens, Arch. Intern. Med. 158 (1998) 1769–1776.

[14] K.L. Nichol, L. Baken, A. Nelson, Relation between influenza vaccination and outpatient visits, hospitalization, and mortality in elderly persons with chronic lung disease, Ann. Intern. Med. 130 (1999) 397–403.

[15] W.R. Dowdle, J.D. Millar, L.B. Schonberger, F.A. Ennis, J.R. LaMontagne, Influenza immunization policies and practices in Japan, J. Infect. Dis. 141 (1980) 258–264.

[16] T.A. Reichert, N. Sugaya, D.S. Fedson, W.P. Glezen, L. Simonsen, M. Tashiro, The Japanese experience with vaccinating schoolchildren against influenza, N. Engl. J. Med. 344 (2001) 889–896.

[17] National Center for Health Statistics, Vital Statistics of the United States, 1949–1992, vol. II, mortality, part A. Washington: Public Health Service, 1951–1994, Advance report of final mortality statistics, 1993–1998, Monthly Vital Statistics Report, Hyattsville, Maryland: National Center for Health Statistics, 1994–1998. US: 1949–1992.

[18] Vital Statistics of Japan, Statistics and Information Department, Minister's Secretariat, Ministry of Health and Welfare, Tokyo, 1949–1998.

[19] Vital Statistics of Australia, Australian Institute of Health and Welfare, Melbourne, 1949–1998.

[20] S. Falkow, Molecular Koch's postulates applied to microbial pathogenicity, Rev. Infect. Dis. 157 (1988) 1124–1133.

International Congress Series 1219 (2001) 103–106

The value of a database in surveillance and vaccine selection

C. Macken*, H. Lu, J. Goodman, L. Boykin

Theoretical Division, T-10 Mail Stop K710, Los Alamos National Laboratory, Los Alamos, NM 87545, USA

Abstract

The Influenza Sequence Database (ISD) is a curated, specialized database of influenza genomic and protein sequences, and influenza-specific sequence analysis tools that have a web interface available to the public http://www.flu.lanl.gov). Contents are primarily those influenza sequences that have been deposited in GenBank. A growing number of sequences are deposited directly into the ISD by WHO surveillance sites around the world. The core function of the interface is a database search. Analysis tools are a combination of developments by ISD staff and adaptation of existing, freely available software. Future developments of the database and its web site will be driven by user needs and by output from our in-house research. Projects underway include a layered, secure interface with the database to allow variable access privileges to sensitive data, and clickable mapping of a homology model if Influenza B hemagglutinin. Published by Elsevier Science B.V.

Keywords: Influenza; Sequence; Database

1. Introduction: the Influenza Sequence Database today

The Influenza Sequence Database (ISD) is a curated, specialized database of influenza genomic and protein sequences, and influenza-specific sequence analysis tools that have a web interface available to the public http://www.flu.lanl.gov). Contents are primarily those influenza sequences that have been deposited in GenBank. A growing number of sequences are deposited directly into the ISD by WHO surveillance sites around the world. These unpublished sequences are identified by accession numbers beginning with "ISD" and are credited with authorship and ownership according to the

---

* Corresponding author. Tel.: +1-505-665-6464; fax: +1-505-665-3493.
E-mail address: cmacken@lanl.gov (C. Macken).

0531-5131/01/$ – see front matter. Published by Elsevier Science B.V.
PII: S 0 5 3 1 - 5 1 3 1 (0 1) 0 0 3 3 0 - 2

depositor's directions. The web interface provides simple, menu-driven access to data and tools for analysis.

The core function of the web interface is a database search. Searching can be done in one of three modes: (a) search only; (b) search nucleotide or protein sequences, align, and clip sequences to a region of interest (such as the cleavage region); and (c) search protein sequences, align and highlight a pattern of interest (such as glycosylation site). Sequences can be downloaded in a variety of formats. Since all sequences in the database are prealigned by type of influenza (across serotype, for Influenza A), alignments also can be downloaded using the Region Search function.

Analysis tools are a combination of developments by ISD staff and adaptation of existing, freely available software. Currently available analytical tools allow the user to: BLAST, a nucleotide or protein sequence against the influenza sequence database; analyze prealigned protein sequences by chemical alphabet or hydrophobicity code; plot sites of interest on a 3-D graphic of A (H3N2) hemagglutinin subunit one (HA1) molecule; translate accession numbers to strain names on phylogenetic trees.

2. Why a specialized database?

Knowledge of an organism can lead to improved curation, beyond that possible in an all-purpose database, such as GenBank. One of the first actions that we carry out when adding sequences to the ISD is a check for redundancy of sequences at the nucleotide level. We distinguish duplication (same strain, same sequence) from identity (different strain, same sequence) and multiplicity (same strain, different sequence). Duplicates are removed from the database; multiple sequences are triggers to contact the authors for clarification. In addition, we attempt to fill all relevant fields of information associated with a sequence, by searching the literature and/or contacting authors. Curation leads to efficient data analysis and refined data selection.

The database is designed and developed largely in response to interaction with users and hence are tailored to their needs. For example, vaccine selection pages were designed to answer a need by the CDC to disseminate sequences of current vaccine strains, possibly before their publication in GenBank. The Region Search tool was developed in response to users' requests for alignments, and for the simplicity of viewing only those regions of a sequence that are of interest. Users can similarly define future developments of the database.

3. The value of the ISD in surveillance and vaccine selection

The initial impetus for the database was to collect, in a central location, the many unpublished sequences that reside in disparate databases around the world. Communications with various influenza surveillance laboratories have led to fledgling efforts to deposit sequences from current and/or past season's influenza surveillance into the ISD directly. We have a very simple protocol for sequence deposition, and attempt to obtain all basic epidemiological and laboratory information that is important for sequence analysis.

When large amounts of data are to be deposited, we develop individualized protocols tailored to the needs of the depositing author. We have an agreement with GenBank to send sequences directly to them from the ISD, thus, circumventing the need for authors to resubmit sequences upon their eventual publication.

Our procedure for accepting unpublished sequences into the ISD is an element of a larger plan that is currently under development. Our goal is to develop an interface with our database that allows different levels of access to its contents, with appropriate security maintained on sensitive data not intended for public use. Experts on distributed database design in the Advanced Computing Laboratory at Los Alamos National Laboratory (LANL) are advising us on the design of this multilevel access and security schema. Ultimately, we foresee the ISD as a common site for securely sharing information among specified groups of users, as well as a site for analyzing private data within the context of public data, using analytical tools available at the ISD site. Such a centralized function of the ISD may be particularly useful for laboratories whose collection is localized rather than global.

In addition to the above plans for sequence collection, there are two new tools under development that are designed for use in surveillance and vaccine selection. A prototype for the first can be viewed at http://www.flu.lanl.gov/FluTool.htm. It is intended for mapping seasonal genetic drift of influenza hemagglutinin sequences. (It could easily be expanded to map the drift of other gene segments, or to map antigenic drift.) As this tool is developed, it will interface with the database to extract sequences collected within a specified time period and plot the location of collection of these sequences on a map of the world. The map will color code countries by the frequency of isolation per time period, and give a pie-chart summary of the representation of isolates by phylogenetic lineage. With these two data summaries, it is easy to visualize the worldwide time course of genetic drift.

The second new tool that will help to assess the potential impact of genetic change on influenza evolution derives from our research into structural modeling of influenza proteins. Currently, we are developing a model for the Influenza B hemagglutinin HA1 subunit, suing homology. We have calculated a well-supported model by using information from the crystal structures of the Influenza A HA1 and Influenza C hemagglutinin-esterase function subunit 1(HEF1) molecules. We use our model as a mechanism for gaining insight into the basis for continuing evolution, and divergence, of sublineages of Influenza B HA1. Once published, the model structure will be presented at the web site for clickable mapping of residues of interest, in a tool that matches the currently available clickable 3-D map of the crystal structure of Influenza A HA1.

4. How might the ISD be of further value?

In the course of our activities in influenza sequence analysis and database development, we have gained considerable understanding of the evolutionary behavior of influenza, in particular with respect to its impact on phylogenetic analysis. We also have access to supercomputers at LANL that allow us, in a timely fashion, to build trees for large data sets using maximum likelihood estimation, and to calculate bootstrap support for the trees.

These capabilities could be utilized to provide reference trees to the influenza research community. To date, we have received expressions of interest in such reference trees, but no consensus on the appropriate reference data sets. Our goal is to ascertain a basic collection of preferred reference data sets, and then develop web tools for quickly placing user, or database, sequences on a user-selected tree.

As users familiarize themselves with the capabilities of the ISD, we shall continue to respond to their needs for further data collection and expanded analysis, thereby supporting the community in their efforts to provide timely surveillance and accurate decisions on vaccine selection.

Acknowledgements

The Influenza Sequence Database is supported by an interagency agreement with the Influenza Branch of the Centers for Disease Control and Prevention, USA, and by various grants from the USA Department of Energy, and the University of California.

International Congress Series 1219 (2001) 107–118

Seven integrated influenza surveillance systems in Taiwan

Chwan-Chuen King[a,b,*], Chuan-Liang Kao[c], Ding-Ping Liu[d],
Min-Chu Cheng[e], Hui-Lin Yen[a,b], Min-Shiuh Lee[f],
Ching-Ping Tsai[g], Shin-Ru Shih[h], Happy K. Shieh[f],
Jen-Pang Hsiu[d], Shu-Fang Li[d], Hour-Young Chen[d], Hsu-Mei Hsu[d],
Shing-Jer Twu[d], Nancy J. Cox[i], Robert G. Webster[j,k]

[a]*Institute of Epidemiology, College of Public Health, National Taiwan University (NTU), Taipei, Taiwan*
[b]*Takemi Program in International Health, School of Public Health, Harvard University, Boston, MA 02115, USA*
[c]*School of Medical Technology, College of Medicine, NTU and Division of Virology,*
Department of Laboratory Medicine, NTU Hospital, Taipei, Taiwan
[d]*Centers for Disease Control, Taipei, Taiwan*
[e]*Council of Agriculture, Animal Health Research Institute, Taipei, Taiwan*
[f]*National Chung Hsing University, Taichung, Taiwan*
[g]*Pig Research Institute in Taiwan, Taiwan*
[h]*Department of Medical Technology, Chang-Gung University, Taoyuan, Taiwan*
[i]*Influenza Branch, Centers for Disease Control and Prevention, Atlanta, USA*
[j]*Department of Virology and Molecular Biology, St. Jude Children's Research Hospital, Memphis, TN, USA*
[k]*WHO Collaborating Center for Studies on the Ecology of Influenza in Animals and Birds, USA*

Abstract

Background: Influenza surveillance in recent decades in Taiwan showed that the major virus isolates were A/Hong Kong/68-like (H3N2), A/England/42/72-like (H3N2), A/Taiwan/1/86 (H1N1), A/Texas/36/91-like (H1N1), A/Taiwan/112/96 (H1N1), and A/Taiwan/118/96 (H1N1) based on passive virologic surveillance before 1999. *Materials and methods*: To prevent the potential public health threat of a newly emerged influenza A strain like H5N1 in Hong Kong, seven surveillance systems have been established in Taiwan since 1999, including severe case reporting, sentinel physician, contract-laboratory, poultry market, domestic avian, wild bird and pig surveillance. Scientific exchanges and possible public health actions are discussed in regular meetings during the winter season. *Results*: The isolation rates of influenza A virus were higher among ducks than

* Corresponding author. Institute of Epidemiology, College of Public Health, National Taiwan University, 1 Jen-Ai Road Section 1, Taipei, Taiwan. Tel.: +886-2-2341-4347; fax: +886-2-2351-1955.
E-mail address: a1234567@ccms.ntu.edu.tw (C.C. King).

chickens in both domestic avian and market surveillance systems. Ten subtypes of influenza A virus can be found in migrating wild birds, which may serve as a reservoir for the genetic and antigenic changes of the virus. The H6 subtype was isolated from both wild birds and market surveillance systems. Pig surveillance found that H3 occurred more in the winter, whereas H1 appeared predominantly in the summer. Human virologic surveillance also demonstrated summer and winter peaks. Market surveillance in Taipei showed H6, H4, and H3 subtypes isolated from ducks only. Sentinel physician surveillance experience has taught us the importance of involving local clinics, particularly in farm areas. The traditional passive physician reporting surveillance provided limited information and it was replaced by severe case reporting. Most elderly physicians in Taiwan did not like to report influenza even after implementation of direct electronic reporting through a worldwide web system. More modern technology will be applied to increase the timeliness and representativeness of influenza surveillance in preparing for future pandemics. *Conclusion*: Integration of animal and human influenza surveillance systems in the high population density in Taiwan serves as a model in the efforts of global influenza surveillance to detect newly emerged influenza virus strains via several channels, particularly useful in detecting severity of cases and inter-species transmission. © 2001 Elsevier Science B.V. All rights reserved.

Keywords: Surveillance; Influenza A; Taiwan; Interspecies transmission

1. Introduction

Pandemic influenza is caused by new human influenza A virus which arises due to genetic reassortment of animal influenza viruses or direct intra-species transmission and has global public health significance [1]. In addition, epidemic influenza is responsible for respiratory morbidity, hospitalization and mortality worldwide [2–4]. The impact of the next influenza A pandemic on the USA has been estimated as 89,000–207,000 deaths, 314,000–734,000 hospitalized cases, 18–42 million clinical visits, 20–47 million additional people ill and 71–166 billion American dollars in social disruption [5]. Surveillance is the most effective public health prevention and control strategy by providing early detection of an epidemic, defining high risk populations in a given year, investigating the extent and distribution of severe cases, identifying the current circulating subtypes of the virus, monitoring for antigenic shift, tracing the origin of the newly emergent/re-emergent virus, and developing vaccines for immunization programs [6–9].

Surveillance involves the systematic collection, consolidation, and evaluation of morbidity and mortality reports and other relevant data such as risk or preventive factors [10]. Public health surveillance has a responsibility for disease control activities, which is distinct from epidemiologic surveillance, that focuses mainly on epidemiologic research. In general, public health professionals at local, state/provincial, national and international levels regularly analyze surveillance data and use this information for taking appropriate action [11–14]. Effective disease control and prevention programs depend primarily on sensitive and representative surveillance systems to detect infectious disease problems early enough to take an immediate action [15]. In particular, influenza surveillance requires close collaboration both at the various levels of the health system within a country and between countries in order to take immediate global efforts to prevent pandemic. Since it was established in 1947, the WHO global surveillance for influenza has grown to 110 designated National Influenza Centers in 80 countries [16]. There are many different national influenza surveillance systems, however, most of these are directed primarily at the detection of human cases and few of them are integrated with animal influenza surveillance systems in order to fully understand the ecology, evolution and mechanisms contributing to the emergence of virulent influenza A viruses.

Taiwan is located in a subtropical area of Southeast Asia with an extremely high population density in most urban areas, particularly the capital City of Taipei. Therefore, respiratory infections including influenza have a public health priority. The incentive to improve infectious disease surveillance systems in this area has attracted more attention since a large-scale epidemic of enterovirus 71 occurred in Taiwan in 1998. In addition, frequent travel by Taiwanese to Hong Kong, mainland China and other Southeast Asian countries, where the origin of several pandemics of flu had been documented in the past, have also provided an impetus to monitor influenza A virus activity by establishing sensitive, representative and integrated surveillance systems. Furthermore, the epidemic of influenza A (H5N1) in Hong Kong in 1997 [17] and the finding of human H9N2 isolates in China and Hong Kong in 1999 [18,19] imply that influenza A viruses are widespread in Asian poultry. Under these circumstances of potential public health threats, we became the first country to integrate all seven influenza surveillance systems, including both human and animal surveillance, prior to the epidemic season 1999–2000. This report describes the strengths and weaknesses of each influenza surveillance system with more emphasis on our valuable experience with respect to successes, failures and future efforts.

2. Materials and methods

2.1. Influenza surveillance systems in Taiwan before 1998

Three major influenza surveillance systems had been operating from 1970s until 1998, including human virologic surveillance at the national level, domestic avian surveillance in central Taiwan and swine flu surveillance in the Institute of Pig Research in Miaoli. Unfortunately, similar to most other countries, there was little exchange of influenza A virus of activity and data analysis between animal and human influenza surveillance systems on a regular basis. In addition, prior to 1998 while influenza-reporting data were passively collected on a weekly and monthly basis, summary data was compiled annually and published in Chinese Epidemiology Bulletin. However, most Chinese physicians did not like to report influenza and only two to three sentinels located in Taipei sent regular respiratory specimens each month for virologic identification [20]. On the other hand, local Health Centers and Bureaus obtained infectious disease morbidity and mortality data passively and three different organizations (Bureau of Communicable Disease, National Institute of Preventive Medicine and National Quarantine Service) were responsible for the final infectious disease surveillance report before the large-scale epidemic of enterovirus 71 throughout Taiwan in the summer of 1998. Following this epidemic the Center for Disease Control was initiated to combine all of the above three organizations in order to increase the efficiency of infectious disease surveillance and health policy. Therefore, several improved surveillance systems, including severe case reporting, sentinel physician reporting and virologic laboratory reporting systems for human influenza were evaluated since then.

In animal influenza A surveillance, both pig and avian influenza surveillance systems were mainly seroepidemiologically oriented although strains of influenza A were sometimes isolated [21,22]. The pig surveillance collected nasal swabs from collaborating pig farms, whereas the avian flu surveillance, a passive system, regularly diagnosed infections such as Newcastle disease, etc., among sick chickens and ducks. In addition, influenza A viruses were occasionally isolated from organs of wild birds. However, there was no selective monitoring of migrating birds.

2.2. Systematic changes in influenza surveillance process

Because the elderly are at greater risk for influenza-related complications and the numbers of elderly persons have been increasing rapidly in recent years, systematic approaches to improve current human flu surveillance have become necessary in Taiwan. The transmission of H5N1 influenza viruses to humans, which resulted in six fatal cases of 18 infected persons, highlighted the role of chickens as a potential intermediate host for human infection [17,19]. Furthermore, the isolation of H9N1 influenza viruses from humans in mainland China and Hong Kong again illustrates that the most effective surveillance systems should involve animal reservoirs or intermediate hosts together with human surveillance systems [27,28]. Taiwan has more than 100,000 businessmen and travelers who visit Hong Kong and China each year. There has been little information regarding the gene pools of influenza A viruses among migrating birds and domestic avian species in Asia, therefore, seven different surveillance systems of influenza A have been integrated since 1998–1999.

2.2.1. Wild bird virologic surveillance

Feces of wild birds including residential and migratory birds were collected monthly from several bird roosting areas distributed all over Taiwan main island (the south, central, east, west, and north) and Kinmen isolated islet, during seasonal months when birds (wild water fowls) were flying into Taiwan. Systematic stratified sampling of 30 ducks per group and 1–2 groups were collected at each surveillance site [23]. In addition, cloacal swabs of banded birds were also obtained. These samples were inoculated directly into 10-day-old embryonated chicken eggs for the isolation of influenza virus. Subtyping of hemaglutinin (H antigen) was undertaken using reference serum samples obtained from Dr. Hiroshi Kida, Hokkaido University, Japan and Dr. D.J. Alexander in NCVL, England. Sequence analysis of H5 and H7 subtypes were undertaken to determine the presence of basic amino acid sequences, which contribute to virulence of the virus.

2.2.2. Domestic avian influenza surveillance

Sick domestic birds were sent to Dr. Happy Shieh's laboratory at the Department of Veterinary Medicine at the National Chung-Hsing University, Taichung, Taiwan. Viruses were isolated, identified and sequenced using the primer sets designed based on the local Taiwan avian sequence data bank [24].

2.2.3. Market avian virologic surveillance

With the consultation and technical guidance from Dr. R. Webster, we initiated a market avian virologic surveillance system at the College of Public Health, National Taiwan University and selected a large wholesale market located in Taipei selling live chickens, ducks, and geese from different parts of Taiwan. Faeces of white chickens, brown chickens, black-bone chickens, and ducks were collected early in the morning once each week from November 1999 to June 2000 [25].

2.2.4. Swine influenza surveillance

Both serologic and virologic surveillance systems were employed to monitor the virus activity at the Pig Research Institute in MiaoLi, Taiwan. Tracheal samples were collected from pigs manifesting respiratory symptoms/signs. The six sentinel sites included two pig farms with about 4000–5000 pigs each in Northern (TaoYuan, MiaoLi), Central (Taichung, Changhwa) and Southern Taiwan (Kaohsiung, Pingtung). Specimens were inoculated into 10-day-old specific pathogen free embryonated chicken eggs. Human and pig flu A subtypes were compared frequently [26].

2.2.5. Sentinel physician surveillance

Since 1990 sentinel physician surveillance in Taiwan has been in place established to monitor chickenpox, measles, mumps, rubella and neonatal tetanus. Upper respiratory disease sentinel surveillance system was initiated in the 39th week of 1995 and sentinel physicians were selected according to their past reporting records and enthusiasm. The influenza-like illness (ILI) sentinel surveillance was initiated in January 1999 to predict trends and provide early warning of epidemics. The case definition of ILI includes patients with fever (ear temperature over 38 °C), respiratory symptoms/signs and muscle pain/headache/exhaustion. Patients with rhinitis, tonsillitis and bronchiolits were excluded [27].

2.2.6. Human virologic surveillance

Nationwide human influenza virologic surveillance linking the sentinel physician and laboratory surveillance systems was initiated in March 1999. Specimens were inoculated in MDCK cells, immunofluorescence and hemaglutination inhibition tests were used to identify subtypes and selected strains were sent to WHO collaborating laboratories or Centers for Disease Control and Prevention in Atlanta, USA, for antigenic studies and confirmation. This system involves virology laboratories distributed in southern (Kaohsiung Medical College in Kaohsiung, ChengKung University in Tainan), central (ChangHwa Christian Hospital in Changhwa) and eastern (TzeChi Hospital in HwaLien) and northern (National Taiwan University Hospital and ChangGun Memorial Hospital in Taipei) Taiwan in July 1999 [28].

2.2.7. Severe case surveillance

Since many infections may have similar symptoms/signs to influenza, most physicians in Taiwan do not like to report these. The passive physician-based surveillance system had very limited values in timeliness and specificity and was replaced by a hospital based severe case surveillance in January 2000.

3. Results

3.1. Use and strengths of animal influenza surveillance systems

Because influenza A is a zoonotic disease which may contribute new virulent human strains, information obtained from animal virologic surveillance is crucial [29].

3.1.1. Wild bird flu surveillance

Wild bird surveillance system provides monthly data of flu virus activity, geographic and host species distribution of different subtypes of influenza A viruses, and prevailing environmental conditions. Influenza A virus activity was strongly associated with the seasonal movement of migrating wild water ducks. Ten different H and N subtypes, including H4N2, H4N6, H3N8, H4N8, H10N7, H2N3, H7N1, H1N3, H4N7 and H1N1 were all isolated [23]. Tests indicated that none of these viruses were virulent for chickens.

One area located in northeastern Taiwan close to a duck raising farm was further investigated and monitored for their virus activity. H subtypes of newly isolates from domestic ducks and market surveillance have been communicated and compared frequently. Because the peaking months of bird flu virus appeared before human flu peaking months, the director of the Center for Disease Control in Taiwan in charge of human influenza prevention and control activities was immediately notified about updated bird flu surveillance data.

3.1.2. Domestic avian flu surveillance

The isolation rates varied in different geographic areas. Ducks in areas with potential contact of migrating birds and open farming had the higher flu A virus isolation rate. Health education and changing the farming style were then implemented by educating poultry farmers how to avoid contact with wild birds. The isolation rates of influenza A virus decreased since the widespread introduction of closed farming methods. Because sequence data currently in gene bank consists mostly of influenza A viruses isolated from European and American birds, Asian avian flu A sequences are urgently required to optimise primer design for the reverse-transcriptase polymerase chain reaction (RT-PCR) and to monitor genetic changes and their possible role in viral pathogenesis [24].

3.1.3. Market flu surveillance

Chinese markets selling live chickens or ducks provide the best opportunity for contact between domestic avians and the human population and potential exchange of viruses. Phylogenetic studies on all eight segments of the influenza A viruses isolated from markets provide information useful in evaluating both the possible pandemic potential of viruses, due to reassortment, and also their possible sources by sequence homology. Until to now, no influenza A virus have been isolated from chickens in Taiwan, whereas ducks had the highest influenza A virus isolation rate. Nine subtypes were isolated, including H3N1, H3N2, H3N6, H3N8, H4N1, H4N2, H4N4, H4N6 and H6N1 [25]. Sequence data for the eight gene segments were determined in Dr. Robert Webster's laboratory.

Because of public health concerns, seroepidemiologic study on the extent of infection due to these isolates was investigated among veterinarians, poultry workers and market salesmen. A study of 195 poultry workers and 146 veterinarians distributed throughout Taiwan were found seronegative to the H4 and H6 subtypes. Questionnaire data analysis showed that weather, altitude, number of animals raised or species were not the major influential factors of interspecies transmission.

3.1.4. Swine flu surveillance

Swine flu surveillance has the highest priority because Taiwan has the largest swine population in Asia. Monthly and geographic distributions of swine influenza A viruses have been monitored. For hygiene reasons contacts between humans and pigs have now been minimized by industrialization of pig farms in most areas, however, swine influenza viruses were frequently isolated. Both H1 and H3 subtypes were isolated with different subtypes predominating in different years. The monthly pattern of H subtypes in swine flu was consistent with those found in human influenza A in the same year in 1998–2000, even the shift from H3 to H1 subtype. There was no striking geographic variation of swine flu viruses and sequence data for H and N genes indicated the possibility of human flu A genes existed in pigs. Both the representativeness and specificity of this surveillance will be further improved in coming years.

3.2. Improvement of human flu surveillance

Several human influenza surveillance systems were compared. ILI reported by sentinel physicians and laboratory surveillance showed an increase in activity in the same month. The laboratory surveillance detected the virus activity one month earlier than previous years due to the improved sampling through the sentinels and increased numbers of sentinels.

3.2.1. Direct computer reporting from physicians

Due to the unwillingness of physicians to report influenza, a program for direct computer reporting was initiated in December 1999. Unfortunately, older physicians do not adapt to the computer system. Further improvement is in process.

3.2.2. Representative of sentinel physician surveillance system

The proportion of sentinel physicians was planned to cover 1.5% of the total Taiwan population with an aim of approximately one sentinel physician per 750 people. Sampling was based on 63 medical care network districts. The greatest number of surveillance sites was located in areas of high population density, Taipei City and County, particularly pediatricians whose patients are living or working close to market or farm areas. On the other hand, rural areas with avian or pig farms or wild birds roosting areas were considered as potential sites for the sources of newly emerging influenza viruses and surveillance sites were, therefore, recruited based not only on total population but also considering the potential sources of influenza viruses.

3.2.3. Initiating contract laboratory virologic surveillance system

Virology laboratories in Taiwan are mostly found in teaching hospitals. Four contract virology laboratories commenced operation in March 1999 to collect clinical specimens for isolation of influenza viruses and to extend geographic sampling to the east and central part of Taiwan, two more contract laboratories with fewer well-trained technical laboratory personnel were added and supervised in July 1999. A further five laboratories, including the largest military hospital in Taipei and two more hospitals in central and southern Taiwan, catering for patients from rural areas, have been invited to increase the sensitivity of virologic surveillance. Data were collected each week for rapid feedback data analysis. The highest isolation rates of influenza viruses were found in the core laboratory, which collected more clinical samples from several local clinics and had pediatricians with virologic training, than the other virologic sentinel sites. The reasons include better communication with the local physicians and trained enthusiastic pediatricians who pay much greater attention to viral diseases. Analysis indicated that most district and community hospitals where patients have more potential exposure to farm animals might not be detected by the current human virologic surveillance. More comprehensive surveillance will assist in selecting virus strains for immunization program. In 1999–2000 in Taiwan, there was a decrease in A(H3N2) A/Sydney/5/97-like strains and the appearance of A/Moscow/10/99-like isolates, A(H1N1) A/New Caledonia/20/99-like strains and B/Beijing/184/93-like strains.

3.2.4. Clinical severe case surveillance

To avoid the possible chaos associated with the emergence of pandemic strains, a clinical severe case surveillance system was established in January 2000. Epidemiologic investigations will be initiated if a clustering of cases in place or time occurs or unusual epidemiological characteristics are seen.

3.3. Integration of animal and human flu surveillance systems

3.3.1. Regular scientific exchanges

Following consultation with Dr. Nancy Cox at the Centers of Disease Control and Prevention at Atlanta, GA, USA, regular monthly scientific exchange meetings were instituted during influenza seasonal months commencing with a meeting at the Institute of Epidemiology, National Taiwan University in December 1999. Data from each surveillance system is presented and discussed for public health actions and future research. Suggestions and future collaborative efforts were discussed with consensus.

3.3.2. Integrated study design

Collaborative research projects were initiated in December 1999 with more integration of study sites, selection of study populations and data analysis of different surveillance systems. In addition, both virologic isolation and seroepidemiologic investigation are complementary in determining the magnitude of infection and spread of a new subtype of influenza A virus.

3.4. Epidemiologic trends of human flu virologic surveillance at the National Taiwan University Hospital

The virological surveillance data at NTU Hospital showed that the predominant influenza season was winter to spring, although influenza isolates were found in late

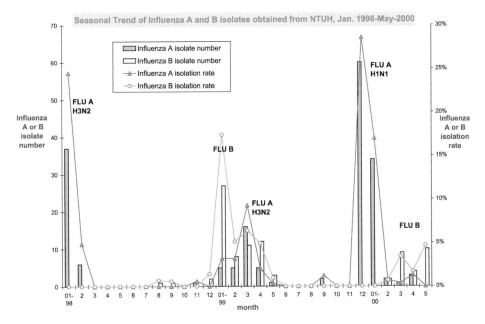

Fig. 1. Seasonal trend of influenza A and B isolates obtained from National Taiwan University Hospital, January 1998 – May 2000.

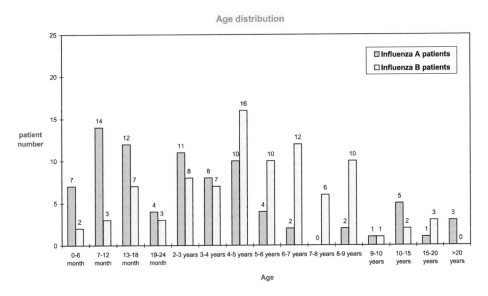

Fig. 2. Age distribution of influenza A and B patients at National Taiwan University Hospital, January 1998 – May 2000.

summer or autumn. Both NTU Hospital and the national virologic surveillance systems can detect influenza virus activity even during the summer time (Fig. 1). Although H3N2 and H1N1 were co-circulating in recent years in Taiwan, different serotypes of the virus were dominant in different years. Comparing the age distribution of influenza A and B patients under 10 years old, we found that influenza A patients were significantly younger than influenza B patients ($p < 0.01$). Age distribution of different serotypes also varies indicating that different selective pressure may exist among H3N2 versus H1N1 (Fig. 2).

4. Discussion

Influenza A viruses continue to evolve by antigenic drift and shift in humans, pigs and horses. Both pigs and aquatic birds may contribute to the emergence of pandemic influenza viruses for humans [29]. Therefore, a network of surveillance, which integrates both human and animal surveillance systems considering sources of new emergent influenza virus strains, intermediate hosts, inter-species transmission and mild and severe human cases, is important to public health. Such surveillance systems mean that prevention strategies for future pandemics of influenza A in humans become feasible [30,31]. The timeliness of reporting, representative, sensitivity, specificity, flexibility, simplicity, feed-back responses, effectiveness of coordination and the ability to detect unusual events and outbreaks in each surveillance system for etiologic agents with pandemic potential require ongoing evaluation each year.

Routine operation of surveillance must consider: (1) number and type of reporting channels and sources, (2) efficient method(s) of transmitting reporting data and relevant information, and (3) amount and type of information necessary to establish clinical and laboratory diagnosis. While active surveillance provides more timely data than passive surveillance it is time consuming. Simple surveillance systems gain the greatest compliance in data collection, efficient operation, and rapid distribution of key messages for effective prevention and control. Continuous evaluation of the process of surveillance is necessary and we have found that biweekly meetings are very helpful to facilitate changes. In addition, other surveillance systems such as emergency room surveillance, ICU surveillance, school students' absenteeism, work absenteeism and drug usage may also help to increase the sensitivity of the current surveillance systems in Taiwan.

Future efforts to improve our influenza surveillance will include: (1) application of rapid viral diagnosis tests to surveillance, particularly for rural, suburban and isolated areas where more animal–human contacts are possible [32], (2) examining the molecular evolution of H3 and H1 viruses in both humans and animals by phylogenetic analysis of all eight viral gene segments [33], (3) establishing gene pool data base in different parts of Taiwan by linking epidemiologic findings and public health policy for better decision-making, and (4) integrating our surveillance from study design, selection of sentinels, study sites and populations to data analysis. For those areas where more virulent or diverse subtypes of influenza A virus are isolated from wild waterfowl, chickens, ducks and pigs, more pediatric sentinel physicians will be added to monitor the subsequent virus activities in both humans, domestic avians and pigs. We believe international collaboration on flu surveillance among Asian countries and areas, particularly Hong Kong, Taiwan and China, will contribute more understanding to avoid future pandemics [31].

References

[1] R.G. Webster, Influenza: an emerging microbial pathogen, in: R.M. Krause (Ed.), Emerging Infections, Academic Press, New York, 1998, pp. 275–300.

[2] T.D. Szucs, Influenza: the roles of burden-of-illness research, PharmacoEconomics 16 (Suppl. 1) (1999) 27–32.

[3] K.M. Sullivan, Health impact of influenza in the United States, PharmacoEconomics 9 (Suppl. 3) (1996) 26–33.

[4] D.M. Fleming, The impact of three influenza epidemics on primary care in England and Wales, PharmacoEconomics 9 (Suppl. 3) (1996) 38–45.

[5] S. Klimov, Global influenza surveillance and vaccine strain selection, "International Conference on Emerging Infectious Diseases", July 16–19, Atlanta, Georgia, USA.

[6] Y.P. Lin, M. Shaw, V. Gregory, K. Cameron, W. Lim, A. Klimov, K. Subbarao, Y. Guan, S. Krauss, K. Shortridge, R. Webster, N. Cox, A. Hay, Avian-to-human transmission of H9N2 subtype influenza A viruses: relationship between H9N2 and H5N1 human isolates, Proc. Natl. Acad. Sci. U. S. A. 97 (17) (2000) 9654–9658.

[7] A.I. Karasin, M.M. Schutten, L.A. Cooper, C.B. Smith, K. Subbarao, G.A. Anderson, S. Carman, C.W. Olsen, Genetic characterization of H3N2 influenza viruses isolated from pigs in North America, 1977–1999: evidence of wholly human and reassortant virus genotypes, Virus Res. 68 (1) (2000) 71–85.

[8] Centers for Disease Control and Prevention, Delayed supply of influenza vaccine and adjunct ACIP influenza vaccine recommendations for the 2000–2001 influenza season, Advisory Committee on Immunization Practices, JAMA 284 (6) (2000) 687–688.

[9] A.H. Reid, T.G. Fanning, T.A. Janczewski, J.K. Taubenberger, Characterization of the 1918 "Spanish" influenza virus neuraminidase gene, Proc. Natl. Acad. Sci. U. S. A. 97 (12) (2000) 6785–6790.

[10] A.D. Langmuir, The surveillance of communicable diseases of national importance, N. Engl. J. Med. 268 (1963) 182–192.

[11] R.M. Zweighaft, D.W. Fraser, M.A.W. Hattwick, W.G. Winkler, W.C. Jordan, M. Alter, M. Wolfe, H. Wulff, K.M. Johnson, Lassa fever: response to an imported case, N. Engl. J. Med. 297 (1977) 803–807.

[12] S.B. Thacker, R.L. Berkelman, Public health surveillance in the United States, Epidemiol. Rev. 10 (1988) 164–190.

[13] M.S. Gottlieb, R. Schroff, H.M. Schanker, et al., *Pneumocystis carinii* pneumonia and mucosal candidiasis in previous healthy homosexual men: evidence of a new acquired cellular immunodeficiency, N. Engl. J. Med. 305 (1981) 1425.

[14] C.C. King, Infectious disease surveillance, in: C.H. Chiou (Ed.), Public Health Textbook, HwaHsin Publisher, Taipei, Taiwan, 1999, pp. 222–250 (in Chinese).

[15] G. Pugliese, M.S. Favero, Surveillance of unexplained illness and death, Inf. Control Hosp. Epidemiol. 19 (1998) 285–286.

[16] A.W. Hampson, N.J. Cox, Global surveillance for pandemic influenza: are we prepared?, in: L.E. Brown, A.W. Hampson, R.G. Webster (Eds.), Options for the Control of Influenza III, Elsevier, Amsterdam, 1996.

[17] E.C.J. Classs, OsterhausR.V. Beek, J.C. Jong, G.F. Rimmelzwaan, D.A. Senne, S. Krauss, K.F. Shortridge, R.G. Webster, Human influenza A H5N1 virus related to a highly pathogenic avian influenza virus, Lancet 351 (1998) 472–477.

[18] Y.J. Guo, S. Kraus, D.A. Senne, I.P. Mo, K.S. Lo, X.P. Xiong, M. Norwood, K.F. Shortridge, R.G. Webster, Characterization of the pathogenicity of members of the newly established H9N2 influenza virus lineage in Asia, Virology 267 (2000) 279–288.

[19] Y. Guan, K.F. Shortridge, S. Krauss, R.G. Webster, Molecular characterization of H9N2 influenza viruses: were they the donors of the "internal" genes of H5N1 viruses in Hong Kong?, Proc. Natl. Acad. Sci. U. S. A. 96 (1999) 9363–9367.

[20] R.K. Tseng, H.Y. Chen, C.B. Horng, Influenza virus infections in Taiwan from 1979–1994, J. Formosan Med. Assoc. 94 (1995) S126–S136.

[21] H.K. Shieh, W.J. Huang, J.H. Shien, S.Y. Chiu, L.F. Lee, Y.S. Lu, Studies on avian influenza in Taiwan, R.O.C. (III): isolation, identification and pathogenicity tests of the virus isolated from breeding chickens, Taiwan J. Vet. Med. Anim. Husb. 59 (1992) 45–55.

[22] C.P. Chang, A.E. New, G.S. Irving, H.S. Chiang, J.F. Taylor, A surveillance of human influenza virus in swine in southern Taiwan, Int. J. Zoonoses 4 (1977) 25–30.

[23] M.C. Cheng, Wild bird influenza A virologic surveillance in Taiwan, Sept. 1998–Dec. 1999, Options for the Control; of Influenza IV Conference, Abstract #p2-84, Crete, Greece, p. 152.

[24] M.S. Lee, Typing and subtyping of avian influenza viruses by reverse transcriptase polymerase chain reaction (RT-PCR), Master Degree Thesis, 1999, National Chung-Hsing University, Taichung, Taiwan, R.O.C.

[25] H.L. Yen, Epidemiological study of interspecies transmission of avian influenza viruses in Taiwan, Master Degree Thesis 2000, Institute of Epidemiology, College of Public Health, National Taiwan University, Taipei, Taiwan, R.O.C.

[26] C.P. Tsai, M.C. Cheng, D.T. Lin, C.M. Chen, The prevalence of hemaglutination–inhibition (HI) antibodies to influenza viruses A/swine/Iowa/15/30 (H1N1) and A/Swine/Obihiro/10/85 (H3N2) in Taiwan Pigs, July 1993–Mar. 2000, Proc. 16th IPVS Congress Melbourne, Australia, 257.

[27] J.P. Hsu, Sentinel Physician Surveillance System Plan, Government Report 1999, Center for Disease Control, Department of Health, Taipei, Taiwan.

[28] D.P. Liu, Influenza Laboratory Surveillance., Government Report 2000, Center for Disease Control, Department of Health, Taipei, Taiwan.

[29] G. Webster Robert, Antigenic variation in influenza viruses, in: E. Domingo, R. Webster, J. Holland (Eds.), Origin and Evolution of Viruses, Academic Press, San Diego, 1999, pp. 377–390 (Chap. 14).

[30] T. Ito, Interspecies transmission and receptor recognition of influenza A viruses, Microbiol. Immunol. 44 (6) (2000) 423–430.

[31] E. Hoffmann, J. Stech, I. Leneva, S. Krauss, C. Scholtissek, P.S. Chin, M. Peris, K.F. Shortridge, R.G. Webster, Characterization of the influenza A virus gene pool in avian species in southern China: was H6N1 a derivative or a precursor of H5N1?, J. Virol. 74 (14) (2000) 6309–6315.

[32] D.P. Offringa, V. Tyson-Medlock, Z. Ye, R.A. Levandowski, A comprehensive systematic approach to identification of influenza A virus genotype using RT-PCR and RFLP, J. Virol. Methods 88 (1) (2000) 15–24.

[33] A.I. Karasin, M.M. Schutten, L.A. Cooper, C.B. Smith, K. Subbarao, G.A. Anderson, S. Carman, C.W. Olsen, Protein, Nucleotide Genetic characterization of H3N2 influenza viruses isolated from pigs in North America, 1977–1999: evidence for wholly human and reassortant virus genotypes, Virus Res. 68 (1) (2000) 71–85 (Jun).

International Congress Series 1219 (2001) 119–122

Further development of influenza surveillance in China and global impact on influenza control

Hitoshi Oshitani*

*World Health Organization, Western Pacific Regional Office, P.O. Box 2932,
UN Avenue, 1000 Manila, Philippines*

Abstract

Influenza surveillance is important both on a local and a global basis for several reasons. Information obtained from surveillance is critical for the development and support of control and prevention strategies in China. Influenza surveillance in China also has serious global implications. It is known that China has been a source of new influenza strains, which include both "antigenic drifted" and "antigenic shifted" strains. Over the past 10 years, many of the vaccine strains recommended by WHO originated in China. Some of the pandemic strains are also thought to have originated from China. WHO, in collaboration with Centres for Disease Control and Prevention, the US and National Institute of Infectious Diseases, Japan has provided technical and financial support to the Ministry of Health (MOH), China. Currently, provincial and municipal laboratories in 10 provinces are actively monitoring influenza viruses under the National Influenza Centre in Beijing. MOH, with technical assistance from WHO, is finalizing a National Influenza Surveillance Plan. Over the next 5 years, we can expect the number of surveillance laboratories to increase to as many as 20. An influenza disease surveillance system will also be established. © 2001 Elsevier Science B.V. All rights reserved.

Keywords: Influenza; Surveillance; China; World Health Organization

Influenza causes significant outbreaks generally every winter in northern China. In southern China, influenza circulates year round. Influenza is considered to be a significant cause of morbidity and mortality in China. However, the health and economic impact of influenza has not been well documented. The adverse impact of influenza is expected to increase due to the rapidly aging population and the anticipated increase in

---

* Tel.: +63-2-528-9730; fax: +63-2-521-1036.

the number of those with chronic medical conditions. Development of a national surveillance system is a vital step toward establishing a sound policy for controlling and preventing influenza in China.

Influenza surveillance in China also has serious global implications. China is known to have been a source of new variants of influenza viruses. In the past decade, more than half of vaccine strains recommended by World Health Organization (WHO) were first isolated in China (Fig. 1) [1]. Historical evidence suggests that some of the past pandemic strains also originated in China. In the 20th century, there were four pandemics. Three of these pandemics, A/H3N2 in 1957 (known as the "Asian flu"), A/H2N2 in 1968 (known as the "Russian flu") and A/H3N2 in 1977 (known as the "Hong Kong flu") were probably caused by strains originating from China. The geographical origin of strain of A/H1N1 in 1918 (known as the "Spanish flu"), which caused the most severe pandemic in the 20th century is uncertain. However, this A/H1N1 may also have originated in China [2]. Recent outbreaks of A(H5N1) and A(H9N2) in Hong Kong (China) give strong support to the importance of this area for early detection of potential pandemic strains.

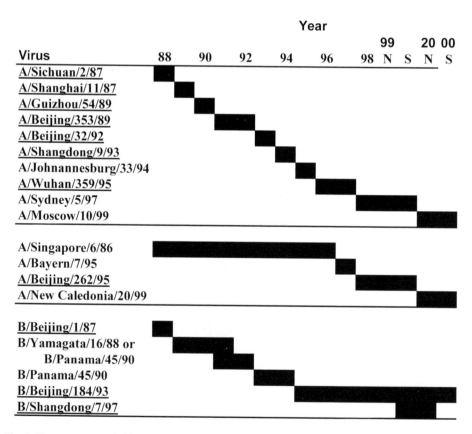

Fig. 1. Viruses recommended by the World Health Organization for inclusion in the influenza virus vaccines, 1988–2000 [1]. Strains originating from China are underlined.

The National Influenza Center (NIC) was established in 1957 in the Institute of Virology, Chinese Academy of Preventive Medicine, Beijing, to conduct national influenza surveillance and to provide guidance for influenza control and prevention activities. The NIC has been actively participating in the WHO global influenza surveillance network [3]. Influenza surveillance has improved significantly in recent years. WHO, in collaboration with WHO Collaborating Centres, particularly National Institute of Infectious Diseases (NIID) in Tokyo, and the Centers for Disease Control and Prevention (CDC) in Atlanta has provided considerable support in strengthening influenza surveillance. This has resulted in many provincial and municipal laboratories upgrading their abilities to conduct influenza surveillance.

Currently, Beijing, Shanghai, Harbin, Wuhan, Shenzhen, Guangxi, Guangdong, Henan, Yunan, Hubei and Hunan provinces (or cities) are actively monitoring influenza activity. Over the past few years, over 300 strains annually have been sent to WHO Collaborating Centres for further analysis and consideration in WHO recommended vaccine composition. These achievements have contributed to both national and global efforts in the fight against influenza. However, both the Ministry of Health (MOH), China, and WHO acknowledge that further improvement in influenza surveillance is necessary. Development of a coordinated national surveillance system is a vital step toward establishing a sound and effective policy for control and prevention of influenza in China. Improved influenza surveillance in China also supports the strengthening of global surveillance efforts. It is therefore proposed that MOH, China with technical support from WHO,

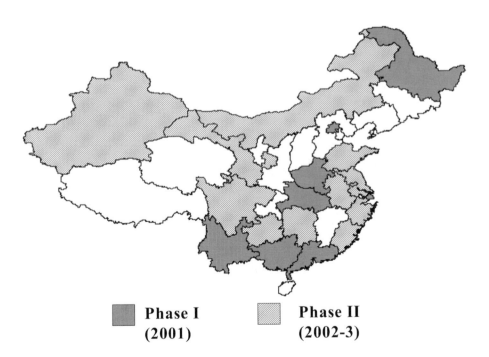

Phase I (2001)   **Phase II (2002-3)**

Fig. 2. Strengthening of influenza surveillance in China in a 5-year national plan.

establish a National Influenza Surveillance Plan. The objective of this plan is to develop a more coordinated and effective surveillance system over the next 5 years (2001–2005).

In the first phase (2001), capacities in the currently participating eight provinces will be strengthened. In the second phase (2002–2003), an additional 12 provinces will be targeted for surveillance capacity strengthening (Fig. 2). In addition to virological surveillance, more systematic influenza disease surveillance will also be established. This comprehensive influenza surveillance system will greatly assist both China and the world in efforts to reduce the impact of the disease.

References

[1] WHO, WHO Report on Global Surveillance of Epidemic Prone Infectious Diseases, Geneva: World Health Organization (WHO/CDS/CSR/ISR/2000.1), 2000.
[2] A.W. Hampson, Surveillance for pandemic influenza, J. Infect. Dis. 176 (Suppl. 1) (1997) S8–S13.
[3] D. Lavanchy, The importance of global surveillance of influenza, Vaccine 17 (Suppl. 1) (1997) S24–S25.

International Congress Series 1219 (2001) 123–129

Surveillance of influenza viruses in Guangdong Province, China in 1998: a preliminary report

Weishi Chen*, Hanzhong Ni, Ping Huang, Huiqiong Zhou, Shaomei Liu

Institute of Epidemic Control and Research of Guangdong Province, 176 Xin Gang Xi Road, Guangzhou 510300, China

Abstract

Background: Since cases of humans infected with avian influenza A(H5N1) virus were reported in Hong Kong, the world has been surprised. Guangdong Province has a similar climate and geographic environment to Hong Kong, and a prosperous poultry market gives rise to the potentiality of an epidemic or outbreak of human infection with A(H5N1) virus. Therefore, a strengthened surveillance of influenza viruses was carried out in eight cities of Guangdong Province during March–October 1998. *Methods*: Samples of throat swabs were taken from outpatients with influenza-like illness and inpatients with bronchitis, pneumonia or other infections in the lungs, and of pharynx fluid from chickens in farming markets, and then inoculated into embryonated chicken eggs for isolation of influenza viruses. The hemagglutination (HA)-positive fluid derived from the embryonated eggs was then identified by the hemagglutination inhibition (HAI) test. Sera of the occupational group of raising, selling and slaughtering chickens and the general group were taken and tested for antibody to influenza viruses by HAI. *Results*: A total of 8563 specimens of human throat swabs were collected and 242 isolates were identified as flu viruses. Of 242 isolates, 193 were A(H3N2), 4 were A(H1N1), 36 were type B and 9 were A(H9N2). A(H5N1) virus was not found. The predominant strain was A(H3N2), making up 79.8% of the all isolates, followed by type B (14.8%). Of 9 A(H9N2) viruses, 4 were isolated in Shaoguan City and 5 in Shantou City, respectively. The time distribution of influenza viruses isolated was 10 isolates in March, 52 in April, 45 in May, 52 in June, 34 in July, 28 in August, 17 in September and 4 in October. Of 9 A(H9N2) viruses, 2 strains were isolated in July, 6 in August and 1 in September, respectively. HAI titers of H9 antibody were 1:160 in one of nine suspected cases from whom A(H9N2) were isolated.

---

* Corresponding author.

Antibodies to A(H5N1) were not detectable in 1512 sera of occupational group and 885 sera of general individuals. *Conclusions*: In the surveillance of influenza, 242 influenza viruses were isolated from 8563 specimens of human throat swabs viruses in Guangdong Province, China 1998. The predominant strain was A(H3N2). Nine strains of A(H9N2) were isolated from human throat swabs. © 2001 Elsevier Science B.V. All rights reserved.

Keywords: Surveillance; Influenza virus

Since cases of humans infected with avian influenza A(H5N1) virus were reported in Hong Kong [1,2], the whole world has been surprised. Adjoining Hong Kong, Guangdong Province has similar climate and geographic environment to Hong Kong, and a prosperous poultry market gives rise to the potentiality of an epidemic or outbreak of human infection with A(H5N1) virus. Therefore, a strengthened surveillance of influenza viruses was carried out in eight cities of Guangdong Province during March–October 1998.

1. Material and methods

1.1. Surveillance sites

Eight cities of Guangzhou, Shenzhen, Zhuhai, Shaoguan, Shantou, Zhanjiang, Foshan and Yunfu were selected as surveillance sites. Eleven hospitals were chosen as surveillance hospitals from the cities above.

1.2. Surveillance subjects

1. Outpatients with influenza-like illness. The clinical features included fever for 3 days, 38 °C or more of body temperature, accompanied by two or more other influenza-like symptoms as described by WHO.
2. Inpatients with bronchitis, pneumonia or other infections in lungs.
3. Occupational group of raising, selling and slaughtering chickens.
4. General group (individuals that were exclusive from the groups given above).
5. Chickens in farming markets or chicken farms.

1.3. Surveillance contents

1.3.1. Epidemiological surveillance

1. Total numbers of outpatients and cases with respiratory infection in departments of internal medicine and pediatrics, inpatients and deceased patients with respiratory infection were counted in surveillance hospitals.
2. When outbreak of influenza occur, surveillance sites should conduct epidemiological investigation and epidemic control.

1.3.2. Pathogenic surveillance

Samples of throat swabs (25 samples per hospital per week) were collected mostly from outpatients and partly from inpatients to isolate influenza A(H5N1), A(H3N2), A(H1N1), A(H9N2) and B viruses. Samples of pharynx fluid were collected from chickens to isolate influenza A(H5N1), A(H7) and A(H9N2) viruses.

1.3.3. Serological surveillance

Antibodies to influenza A(H5N1) viruses were tested in samples of sera from occupational groups. Antibodies to A(H9N2) were tested in sera from where A(H9N2) was isolated from.

1.4. Sampling methods

Throat swabs of human: a dry cotton swab was used to vigorously swab the posterior pharynx and tonsil. The tip of the swab was put into a vial containing 2–3 ml of transport medium and the applicator stick was broken off. For patients less than 5 years old, the cotton swab should be soaked in Hank's fluid (pH 7.4), pressed against the wall of the tube, and then swabbed as described above.

Pharynx fluid of chickens: a dry cotton swab was used to collect the pharynx fluid of the chicken, and then placed into a vial as described above.

The samples collected were kept at 4–8 °C and are transported to the sentinel health and epidemic prevention stations (HEPSs) within 24 h for isolation of influenza virus.

1.5. Testing methods

1.5.1. Isolation of influenza virus

Each sample of throat swab from human or pharynx fluid from chickens was inoculated into amniotic and allantoic cavities of 9–10-day-old embryonated chicken eggs. Three eggs were inoculated per specimen. After inoculation at 33–34 °C for 48 h, amniotic and allantoic fluids were harvested from one to two eggs. The left egg was harvested in 72 h. The amniotic and allantoic fluids were tested by hemagglutination (HA) test. The HA-positive fluid was divided into two vials, one was sent to the provincial influenza laboratory for identification, another to the Chinese National Influenza Center (CNIC) at 4 °C. MDCK also could be used for influenza virus isolation in laboratories if the condition allowed.

1.5.2. Identification of influenza isolates

Hemagglutination inhibition (HAI) test was adopted for identification of influenza isolates. The amniotic and allantoic fluids, with HA-positive, isolated from human throat swabs were initially identified by using reference antisera of influenza A(H1N1), A(H3N2) and B viruses. The HA-positive fluid which was not able to react with antisera of influenza viruses above would then be identified with reference antisera of influenza A(H5N1, H7 and H9N2) viruses.

The amniotic and allantoic fluids, HA-positive, isolated from pharynx fluid of chickens were identified by using reference antisera of influenza A(H5N1, H7, and

H9N2) viruses. Antisera of influenza A/Beijing/53/97(H1N1), A/Wuhan/359/95(H3N2) and B/Beijing/12/97 were offered by CDC from WHO and CNIC, and reference antisera of influenza A(H5N1, H7 and H9N2), by Harbin Veterinary Institute, Agricultural Academy, China.

1.5.3. Test of antibody to influenza A(H5N1) virus in sera

Hemagglutination-inhibition (HI) tests were performed to analyze antibody to influenza A(H5N1). The inactivated strain of influenza A(H5N1) virus was offered by CDC from WHO. A titer of 1:20 or more was diagnosed to be positive.

All sera were treated with red blood cells (RBC) of chicken before analysis and 20% of RBC was used to absorb non-specific inhibitors and hemagglutinin.

2. Results

A total of 1,291,980 outpatients were recorded from out-departments of internal medicine and pediatrics in 11 surveillance hospitals. Of them, 490,503 cases suffered from respiratory infection. There were 6763 inpatients, 53 of whom died of respiratory infection.

A total of 8563 samples of throat swabs were collected from patients and 242 strains of influenza viruses were isolated. The average positive rate of isolation was 2.8%.

Of 242 isolates, 193 were identified as A(H3N2), 4 as A(H1N1), 36 as B and 9 as A(H9N2), respectively. No H5N1 virus was found. The predominant strain was A(H3N2), making up 79.8% of the all isolates, followed by type B (14.8%). The geographical distribution was shown as 182 isolates in Guangzhou, 38 in Shenzhen, 11 in Shantou, 7 in Shaoguan and 2 in Foshan cities. Of 9 A(H9N2) viruses isolated from human throat swabs, 4 were isolated in Shaoguan City and 5 in Shantou City, respectively.

The time distribution of influenza viruses isolated was 10 isolates in March, 52 in April, 45 in May, 52 in June, 34 in July, 28 in August, 17 in September and 4 in October. The isolates were mainly distributed during April–July. Of 9 A(H9N2) viruses, 2 strains were isolated in July, 6 in August and 1 in September, respectively.

The relationship between cases with respiratory infection and isolation rates of influenza virus is shown in Fig. 1.

From Fig. 1, it can be seen that the isolation rate of influenza virus was higher than the number of cases with respiratory infection among the 3 months of May, June and July, while lower than the cases in April, August, September and October, especially in October. It was a reverse relationship between the isolation rate of influenza virus and number of cases with respiratory infection during the 3 months of August, September and October.

The HI antibody to A(H9N2) were tested in eight of nine suspected cases, since one suspected case was missing. HI titers of H9 antibody were 1:120 to 1:160 in only one suspected case from Shaoguan City, while the others were less than 1:20 (details will be published elsewhere).

Antibodies to A(H5N1) were not detectable in 1512 sera of occupational group and 885 sera of general individuals.

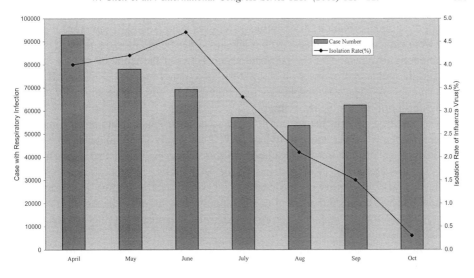

Fig. 1. Relationship between cases with respiratory infection and isolation rates of influenza virus in Guangdong, China 1998.

A total of 436 specimens of pharynx fluid were collected from chickens and 73 isolates of influenza A(H9N2) were isolated and identified, with a 16.7% positive rate of isolation. There was no H5N1 virus isolated from chickens.

It was reported that 724 cases suffered from influenza-like illness clinically in 10 outbreak sites of influenza in Guangzhou City in March. A total of 32 specimens of throat swabs were collected from suspected cases with influenza and 6 were isolated and identified as influenza A(H3N2) viruses, with 18.8% of positive rate. Influenza A(H5N1) and A(H9N2) viruses were not found.

3. Discussion

Since the cases with infection of influenza A(H5N1) were reported in Hong Kong in 1997 [1,2], there have not been any new cases reported over the world. In the past, it was considered that influenza viruses had strict specific hosts among human and animals, and avian influenza viruses could not cross the species barrier into humans. However, recent findings indicated that the A(H5N1) virus was responsible for the severe human disease that occurred in Hong Kong in 1997 and are reassortants that obtained their internal genes from avian H9N2 virus [3], and studies of these viruses indicated that genetic reassortment between avian and human influenza viruses has not occurred [1,4]. It implies that avian influenza viruses can infect humans directly.

Among the types of influenza viruses isolated in this surveillance, type A(H3N2) made up 79.8% (193/242) of the all viruses isolated. It indicated that the predominant strain was still type A(H3N2), followed by type B in Guangdong Province in 1998.

From the time distribution, more influenza viruses were isolated from April to August, which were coincident with the period (spring and summer) of epidemic peak of influenza in Guangdong Province. The reverse relationship between the isolation rate of influenza virus and the number of cases with respiratory infection were not coincident. It implied that the number of cases with respiratory infection might not be a good index for revealing the relationship to the influenza virus.

It was the first time influenza A(H9N2) was isolated from a human in Guangdong Province, China. However, the infectivity of H9N2 to human is still not clear. The fact that the influenza A(H9N2) virus was isolated from a human indicated that avian influenza A(H9N1) virus could also infect humans besides A(H5N1).

Influenza A(H9N2) virus is considered to be widespread in poultry [5]. However, it does not appear to cause high rates of death in poultry as did influenza A(H5N1) in Hong Kong [6]. Therefore, it was not surprising to isolate so many A(H9N2) viruses from chickens in the study.

According to the serological test, HAI antibody of A(H9N2) was found to be positive only in one case, while the others were not detectable. The blood collection time was in intervals of about 2–3 months after their onset of diseases and the ages of the cases were distributed widely. After they were infected by A(H9N2) virus, generally speaking, the HAI antibody of A(H9N2) should be produced and could not have disappeared completely in the serum. This remains to be followed up and studied further.

Certainly, a neutralization assay should be performed for further confirmation of the HAI result. Professor Shortridge, et al. at the University of Hong Kong have found that an HI titer of 1:40 corresponds generally with detectable virus infectivity neutralizing (VN) activity. Thus, VN titrations in cell culture need to be done to make the finding credible. The reason for this is unclear. The impact of cross-reacting of H9 with H3, H2 and H4 must be fully considered when detecting HI antibodies [7].

Acknowledgements

The authors thank the cooperation of the sentinel hospitals and health and the epidemic prevention stations of eight cities, the support from the Health Department of Guangdong Province, the offer of reference antisera of influenza by the CDC in the USA, the Chinese National Influenza Center and the Harbin Veterinary Institute, Agricultural Academy, China.

References

[1] CDC, Isolation of avian influenza A(H5N1) viruses from humans—Hong Kong, May–December 1997, MMWR 46 (1997) 1204–1207.

[2] CDC, Prevention and control of influenza: recommendations of the Advisory Committee on Immunization Practices (ACIP), MMWR 46 (1997), no. RR-9.

[3] Y. Guan, K.F. Shortridge, S. Krauss, R.G. Webster, Molecular characterisation of H9N2 viruses: were they the donors of the internal genes of H5N1 viruses in Hong Kong?, Proc. Natl. Acad. Sci. U. S. A. 96 (1999) 9363–9369.

[4] C. Bender, H. Hall, J. Huang, A. Klimov, N. Cox, A. Hay, V. Gregory, K. Cameron, W. Lim, K. Subbarao, Characterization of the surface proteins of influenza A (H5N1) viruses isolated from humans in 1997–1998, Virology 254 (1) (1999) 115–123.

[5] D.J. Alexander, A review of avian influenza, Symposium on Animal Influenza Viruses, University of Ghent, Ghent, Belgium, 1999, pp. 42–43.

[6] CDC, Influenza A(H9N2) infections in Hong Kong, Media Relations Division (404) 639–3286.

[7] M. Peiris, W.C. Yam, K.H. Chan, P. Ghose, K.F. Shortridge, Influenza A H9N2: aspects of laboratory diagnosis, J. Clin. Microbiol. 37 (1999) 3426–3427.

International Congress Series 1219 (2001) 131–137

Surveillance of influenza: a pan European perspective

J.-C. Manuguerra*,[1]

National Influenza Centre (France-North), Institut Pasteur, 25 rue du Docteur Roux, 75724 Paris cedex 15, France

Abstract

Although influenza is essentially an international disease, its surveillance, however, must be performed at a very local level, both in terms of morbidity data and of virological collections. Throughout Europe, surveillance is scattered among a number of national systems, making it difficult to picture influenza activity at the continental level. Gradually, the need to centralise the follow up of influenza activity was felt and EuroGROG was created in the early 1990s by C. Hannoun. The aim of this new system was to systematically gather morbidity and virological reports from a variety of institutions throughout Europe. EuroGROG is an extensive system since it covers 24 countries. Data is collected each week mainly by fax and e-mail. Data management is a core activity of EuroGROG. In the EuroGROG Bulletin, the situation in each country is summarised in a maximum of two lines. The level of influenza activity is reported and, when necessary, regional details are added. When available, qualitative virological data is given. The EuroGROG Bulletin is sent by e-mail, post and is also available on the Internet. This paper describes the EuroGROG system and the type of data collected over five influenza seasons (1995–2000). The European Influenza Surveillance Scheme (EISS), in operation since 1996 in its current form, is a more formal system, comprising 11 countries that are also part of EuroGROG. Whereas any contributor can join EuroGROG, EISS accepts only new members filling strict inclusion criteria. EISS is EuroGROG's future when both systems will eventually be geographically superimposed. © 2001 Elsevier Science B.V. All rights reserved.

Keywords: Influenza; Surveillance; Europe; Network

---

* Tel.: +33-1-4061-3354; fax: +33-1-4061-3241.
  E-mail address: jmanugu@pasteur.fr (J.-C. Manuguerra).
[1] On behalf of the EuroGROG contributors.

Table 1
Example showing the fifth issue of the EuroGROG bulletin of the 1999–2000 season

Weeks 2000/02 to 2000/04   **EUROGROG Bulletin No. 5**
New information received from 19 European countries.
Influenza activity is still high but has reached a plateau or is declining (sometime sharply) in many western European countries such as Great Britain, France, the Netherlands, Belgium, Germany, Spain and Switzerland. It seems that influenza activity is now increasing in eastern Europe, including Russia. A(H3N2) is by far the predominant sub-type. Sporadic laboratory confirmed cases of influenza A(H1N1) and B are still reported.

AUSTRIA **	Widespread influenza activity due to type A.	24/01/2000
BELGIUM **	ARI and influenza at epidemic levels but the epidemic is now receding. Activity mainly due to A(H3N2) viruses although sporadic A(H1N1) and B viruses have been reported week 2000/02.	Week 2000/02 16/01/2000
BULGARIA	No sign of influenza activity	09/12/1999
CROATIA **	Influenza A(H3N2) isolates are reported.	31/01/2000
CZECH REPUBLIC **	Widespread influenza activity due to A(H3N2) viruses.	Week 2000/04 28/01/2000
DENMARK **	Local outbreaks of influenza activity, due to A(H3N2) viruses.	Week 2000/03 26/01/2000
FINLAND **	Influenza activity after reaching regional to widespread levels is now decreasing. Activity mainly due to type A viruses.	Week 2000/03 25/01/2000
FRANCE **	Widespread influenza activity due to A(H3N2) viruses. Globally the peak is behind although activity is high everywhere, still increasing in some regions whereas decreasing in others.	Week 2000/03 26/01/2000
GERMANY **	Influenza activity still at widespread epidemic levels. Activity due to A(H3N2) viruses.	Week 2000/03 26/01/2000
GREECE	Three isol./detections of influenza A are reported. ILI levels are increasing in Southern Greece.	
HUNGARY	Increasing ILI levels. So far seven influenza A(H3N2) and two influenza B cases have been reported.	Week 99/52 12/01/2000
ITALY **	A(H3N2) isolates from northern and central Italy.	Week 2000/03 25/01/2000
LITHUANIA **	Influenza activity reached epidemic levels, mainly due to type A viruses.	Weeks 2000/02 to 2000/04 28/01/2000

Country	Description	Date
THE NETHERLANDS **	Influenza activity still at widespread epidemic levels. Activity due to A(H3N2) viruses.	Week 2000/03
NORWAY **	Decreasing ILI levels. Influenza activity due to type A viruses.	Week 2000/03 25/01/2000
POLAND **	Increasing ILI levels in association with isolations/detections of influenza A viruses.	Week 2000/03 25/01/2000
PORTUGAL **	Influenza activity due to type A(H3N2) viruses.	Week 2000/03
ROMANIA **	The levels of ARI and influenza activity are increasing, reaching epidemic levels in some regions (North and North-East). Influenza A(H3N2) isolates are reported.	31/01/2000
SLOVAK REPUBLIC	ARI levels increasing slightly. No virus detections/isolation so far.	30/12/1999
SPAIN **	Influenza activity decreasing and now at regional epidemic levels. Activity due to A viruses.	Week 2000/03
SWEDEN	No report so far.	
SWITZERLAND **	Receding influenza activity due to A(H3N2) viruses. Globally, ILI are still at widespread epidemic levels.	Week 2000/03
RUSSIA and CIS c. **	Increasing influenza activity reaching the epidemic threshold in 5 out 42 Russian cities. Influenza A(H3N2), A(H1N1) and B viruses are reported.	Week 2000/02 20/01/2000
GREAT BRITAIN **	Sharp decline of influenza activity across England, Wales and Scotland. Influenza activity is due to A(H3N2) viruses.	Weeks 2000/02 and 2000/03 27/01/2000 (Update 14)

The names of the countries represented in EISS are underlined. The general layout of the Bulletin presented here was slightly modified to adapt to the type of publication. Elsewhere in the World: USA: (Week 2000/02 15/01/2000): Influenza activity at regional levels in 12 states and at widespread levels in 30 states. Influenza activity due to A(H3N2) which is by far the predominant sub-type since week 99/40. The proportion of deaths attributed to pneumonia and influenza is 'above the epidemic threshold and is unusually high'.

1. Introduction

Throughout Europe, surveillance is scattered among a number of national systems, making it difficult to picture influenza activity at the continental level. Gradually, the need to centralise the follow up of influenza activity was felt and EuroGROG was created in the early 1990s by C. Hannoun. The main goal of this new system was to systematically gather morbidity and virological reports from a variety of institutions throughout Europe. EuroGROG is an extensive and informal system covering 24 countries, which is focused on Europe and does not require the responsibility of an international organisation. The same need to improve communication between European networks gave birth to other European schemes as EuroGROG started to function. The Eurosentinel project, which lasted from 1987 to 1991 [1], was followed by the ENS-CARE Influenza system which operated from 1992 to 1995 [2], under the initiative of the World Health Organisation (WHO) regional office for Europe, and the help of the Directorate General (DG) XIII of the European Union. In 1995, following these two initiatives, the early warning influenza system called "European Influenza Surveillance Scheme" (EISS) was created [3]. EISS, in operation since 1996 in its current form, is a more structured system, comprising 11 countries that are also part of EuroGROG. Whereas any contributor can join EuroGROG, EISS accepts only new members filling strict inclusion criteria. EISS and EuroGROG fully cooperate and convergence is a primary objective for EuroGROG. This paper describes the EuroGROG system and data collected through it over five influenza seasons (1995–2000).

2. Material and methods

2.1. Geographical area covered by the EuroGROG system

Until the 1999–2000 season, the following 24 countries were represented in the EuroGROG network as shown in Table 1: Austria, Belgium, Bulgaria, Croatia, Czech Republic, Denmark, Finland, France, Germany, Great Britain, Greece, Hungary, Italy, Lithuania, The Netherlands, Norway, Poland, Portugal, Romania, Russia and the Community of Independent States, Slovak Republic, Spain, Sweden, and Switzerland. As shown in Table 1, half of them were, at that time, members of EISS. For the 2000–2001 season, two more EuroGROG countries will be part of EISS. For this season, EuroGROG will welcome two new contributing countries: Iceland and Latvia.

2.2. Time unit of data collection and transmission

Seventeen countries adopted the calendar week as the basic time unit and reported regularly on this basis. Until the 1999–2000 season, one country collected data on a fortnightly basis. The other countries released summary reports at regular intervals.

2.3. Type and nature of data

As previously mentioned, institutions throughout Europe contributed to the 24 country data for influenza surveillance. It is noteworthy that each country may have a number of reporting organisations, which contributed to the overall EuroGROG reports. Data is collated and then assessments made, based on an 'overall' perspective. All national networks contributing to EuroGROG provided, in one way or another, both virological and clinical data. Clinical data varied from weekly attack rates in the population, broken into age groups, calculated on population based denominator, to a simple or already formatted "expert" assessment about the overall situation. Virological data were either weekly figures or cumulated values. To a certain extent, all networks were able to give the numbers of positive samples by antigen or nucleic acid detection or by viral isolation. Some systems provided EuroGROG with information on the type, sub-type and variants on a regular basis, others simply reported the type of influenza viruses detected. A minority of national correspondent gave serological data.

2.4. Data transmission (input)

Data was collected each week mainly by fax and e-mail. Data management is a core activity of EuroGROG as data formats are extremely variable as are the collected items.

2.5. Data management and data output

In the EuroGROG Bulletin, the situation in each country was summarised in a maximum of two lines. The level of influenza activity was reported and, when necessary, regional details were added. When available, qualitative virological data were given, such as the first detection or isolation for each influenza type and sub-type, the nature of the main circulating virus in the case of co-circulation and the antigenic characteristics of the isolates. The current bulletin was produced in standard 'Word' format and then exported to a web page ready for the Internet.

Table 2
Structure of the table containing the 24 countries reporting information, where ** indicates new information since the previous bulletin

Country	Activity	Period	Report Date
Finland **	Influenza activity after reaching regional to widespread levels is now decreasing. Activity mainly due to type A viruses.	Wk 2000/03	25/01/2000
France **	Widespread influenza activity due to A(H3N2) viruses. Globally, the peak is behind although activity is high everywhere, still increasing in some regions while decreasing in others.	Wk 2000/03	26/01/2000

The names of the countries represented in EISS are underlined. Examples were taken from the 1999–2000 season Bulletin number five, shown in Table 1.

The structure of the bulletin was made up of a header paragraph. This paragraph was a basic overview of the above-mentioned data. The next table contained the 24 countries reporting information. This was structured as shown in Table 2. Finally a section entitled 'Elsewhere in the World' was a basic inclusion of influenza activity in areas outside Europe. The information was produced in a timely and easy to read format.

Once complete, the bulletin was sent out via email and a paper copy via postal mail or fax. The EuroGROG Bulletin was also available on the Internet.

3. Results

During the past five seasons, from 1995–1996 to 1999–2000, a minimum of 5 (1999–2000 season) and a maximum of 13 (1996–1997 season) issues had been released each season. The first bulletin of the season was released between the 14th of November (1996–1997 season) and the 1st of December (1998–1999 season) and the last issue was released between the 31st of January (1999–2000 season) and 14th of April (1996–1997 season). The number of issues and the length of EuroGROG reporting depended on the timing and intensity of influenza epidemics. The earlier the epidemic, the lesser number of EuroGROG bulletin issues and vice versa. The rate of weekly participation of each country was consistently good and varied from 50% to 92%. The rate of participation during the overall seasons varied from 59% (1996–1997 season) to 78% (1998/1999 season). An example of EuroGROG bulletin is shown in Table 1.

4. Discussion

EuroGROG has found its place in the complex systems of networks involved in influenza surveillance. Its modest goals were reached as the EuroGROG system created informal bonds among the European contributors to influenza surveillance at large. Its dedication to a large Europe spanning from Ireland in the west, to Eastern Russia at the Far East, was a main feature of the bulletins. Its focus on Europe meant that EuroGROG was not redundant, with more global information systems such as the World Health Organisation more ambitious in their scope. The emergence of EISS has not yet modified the need for a pan European system. EuroGROG contributors and other readers of the bulletin, express their wish for more bulletins, mainly because of its European focus and concise/easy to read format. EuroGROG needs to be more regular and not limit its bulletin to release during the influenza epidemic period. The current operating procedure poses operational difficulties. (1) Reporting institutions currently have no structure to the reports that are filed. These reports are sent through by fax or email and can be as brief as one sentence, or as long as a full A4 sheet. While these 'Text' reports can provide vital information on local or regional outbreaks, detailed information can sometimes be omitted or simply not included. (2) The data collection method used to assess information from these manual reports can take a large amount of time, and can only be completed by a qualified influenza specialist. Because of this, the reported information can sometimes be outdated by the time the bulletin is produced and circulated. One of the drawbacks of these difficulties is that the bulletin is not issued as often and as regularly as it should be. To try to overcome these problems, it is planned that the EuroGROG system be made available on the Internet in the way of a fully interactive service. This would provide the data contributors with a means to send through their reports to EuroGROG via the Internet. The European Influenza Surveillance Scheme (EISS) is a more formal system, comprising 11 countries that are also part of EuroGROG. Whereas any contributor can join EuroGROG, EISS accepts only new members filling strict inclusion criteria. EISS is EuroGROG's future when both systems will eventually be geographically superimposed.

Acknowledgements

The author wants to thank all EuroGROG contributors for their data and dedication to provide the system with regular input.

References

[1] R. Snacken, J. Lion, V. Van Casteren, et al., Five years of sentinel surveillance of acute respiratory infections (1985–1990): the benefits of an influenza early warning system, European Journal of Epidemiology 8 (1992) 485–490.

[2] R. Snacken, M. Bensadon, A. Strauss, The CARE telematics network for the surveillance of influenza in Europe, Methods of Information in Medicine 34 (1995) 518–522.

[3] R. Snacken, J.-C. Manuguerra, P. Taylor, European influenza surveillance scheme on the internet, Methods of Information in Medicine 37 (1998) 266–270.

International Congress Series 1219 (2001) 139–145

Phylogenetic studies of South African influenza A viruses: 1997–1999

Terry G. Besselaar*, Barry D. Schoub, Jo M. McAnerney

National Institute for Virology, Private Bag X4, Sandringham, 2131, Johannesburg, South Africa

Abstract

Background: The National Institute for Virology (NIV) in Johannesburg has an active surveillance programme to monitor influenza activity and to obtain viral isolates for characterisation at both the antigenic and the molecular level. These data also provide a clearer understanding of the genetic relationships of the South African viruses with those circulating in other countries. *Methods*: Influenza A H3N2 and H1N1 viruses isolated from 1997 to 1999 were analysed by sequence analysis of the viral haemagglutinin gene, and phylogenetic relationships were determined. *Results*: Most influenza activity was due H3N2 viruses, while H1N1 activity was generally low. The H3N2 viruses responsible for the major epidemic in 1998 were found to be due to the introduction of the antigenically distinct A/Sydney/5/97-like strains into the country in April. The 1999 H3N2 isolates exhibited drift from the A/Sydney/5/97 virus at the genetic level and shared a close homology with some recent Australian and New Zealand virus isolates. Phylogenetic analysis revealed that several 1997 H1N1 isolates were similar to the A/Wuhan/371/95-like variants. These were the first H1N1 viruses of this lineage to be isolated in the Southern Hemisphere. The 1998 and 1999 H1N1 isolates were genetically more related to the previous A/Jhb/82/96 vaccine strain than to the 1999 A/Beijing/262/95 vaccine strain. *Conclusions*: These studies have shown that the viruses present in South Africa during a specific year are not always closely related to those in other Southern Hemisphere countries and thus provide a valuable contribution to the Southern Hemisphere vaccine formulation decision. © 2001 Elsevier Science B.V. All rights reserved.

Keywords: Molecular epidemiology; Haemagglutinin; Vaccine; Surveillance

* Corresponding author. Tel.: +27-11-321-4200; fax: +27-11-321-4212.
E-mail address: terryb@niv.ac.za (T.G. Besselaar).

0531-5131/01/$ – see front matter © 2001 Elsevier Science B.V. All rights reserved.
PII: S 0 5 3 1 - 5 1 3 1 (0 1) 0 0 6 4 8 - 3

1. Introduction

Surveillance and monitoring of the antigenicity of influenza viruses in circulation each year is necessary to identify any new variant strains so that vaccines can be updated annually. Many countries in Africa do not have the financial and human resources to carry out influenza surveillance. In South Africa, however, an active influenza surveillance programme has been operating since 1984 at the National Institute for Virology (NIV) in Johannesburg, to obtain virus isolates and to monitor influenza epidemics [1]. The influenza laboratories at NIV serve as one of the National Influenza Centres of the WHO and provide data annually to the Collaborating Centres for Reference and Research on Influenza.

In recent years, the molecular epidemiology of influenza viruses has helped elucidate what occurs during antigenic drift. These studies rely primarily on sequencing the HA1 subunit of the HA (haemagglutinin) genes coupled with phylogenetic analysis of the sequencing data. Molecular characterisation of South African influenza virus isolates by sequence analysis of the viral HA1 subunit has been carried out since 1993 to detect any new mutations relative to previous strains [2,3]. In this study, we examined the phylogenetic relationships of the HA genes of South African H1N1 and H3N2 viruses isolated between 1997 and 1999 and compared these with viruses isolated from other countries, particularly those in the Southern Hemisphere.

2. Methods

2.1. Patients and sources of specimens

The active surveillance programme of the South African National Institute for Virology consists of some 15 centres servicing a cross-section of the population residing mainly in the densely populated Gauteng province. These centres include general medical practitioners, paediatric out-patient departments at hospitals, a paediatrician, primary health care centres at several mines, a university clinic and the staff clinic at NIV. In addition to the active surveillance programme, influenza isolates were also obtained from routine diagnostic specimens sent for analysis for the presence of respiratory viruses, as well as specimens collected from infants hospitalized with severe acute respiratory infection at the Chris Hani/Baragwanath Hospital. This hospital is the largest in the world, servicing the population (estimated to be over 2 million) of Soweto, close to Johannesburg. A further source of influenza specimens was recruited from a baseline study for an antiviral clinical trial. Individuals of all age groups presenting with acute respiratory disease were sampled.

2.2. Virus detection, isolation and subtyping

Viruses were detected using the shell vial method described by Besselaar et al. [3]. Influenza-positive specimens were processed and inoculated intra-amniotically into 12-day-old embryonated eggs as described by Schoub et al. [4]. Specimens were also inoculated into 24-well MDCK cell cultures in serum-free DMEM supplemented with

2.5 µg/ml trypsin and incubated for 3–5 days at 33 °C. Chorioallantoic or cell culture supernatants were tested for haemagglutination (HI) as outlined by Schoub et al. [4], but using turkey red blood cells rather than fowl cells. Virus isolates in chorioallantoic or tissue culture fluid were typed by haemagglutination inhibition (HAI) with reference antisera supplied by the WHO Collaborating Centre for Influenza, CSL, Melbourne.

2.3. Molecular characterisation

Influenza A H3N2 and H1N1 viruses isolated during 1997–1999 in South Africa were analysed by nucleotide sequencing of the HA1 subunit of the HA gene. The strains selected for genetic analysis were chosen to represent isolates obtained at the beginning, middle and end of the seasons each year.

RNA was extracted from 140 µl of infectious tissue culture supernatant or allantoic fluid using the QIAamp Viral RNA extraction kit (Qiagen, Hilden, Germany). The amplification

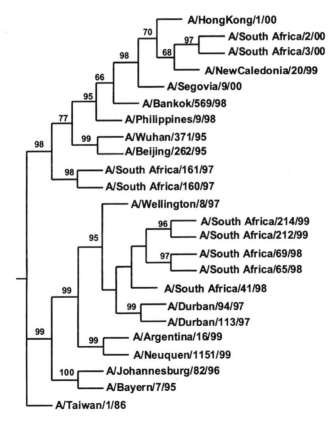

Fig. 1. Phylogenetic tree of influenza A (H1N1) virus HA1 gene nucleotide sequences (979 bp). The tree was generated using neighbor-joining analysis by PHYLIP and 1000 × bootstrap resampling. The number at each branch point indicates percentage probability that the resultant topology is correct.

of the HA1 coding region by PCR was carried out under the conditions described previously [3]. The H3 PCR products were 1073 base pairs (bp) in size while the H1 amplicons were 1112-bp long.

Sequencing of the 1997 and 1998 PCR products was done manually as described by Besselaar et al. [3]. In 1999, sequencing was performed using the Big Dye Terminator Cycle sequencing kit (PE Biosystems, CA, USA) and the reaction products separated on 4.25% polyacrylamide urea gels using an ABI Prism 377 Genetic Analyser (PE Biosystems). The data were analysed using the HIBIO DNASIS programme (Hitachi Software Engineering, Brisbane, CA, USA).

BLAST-searches of the Los Alamos National Laboratory (LANL) database [5] were performed using version 2.0 of BLAST to find sequences related to the South African nucleotide data. Additional nucleotide sequence data were obtained from the WHO Centre for Reference and Research on Influenza in London. Phylogenetic analysis of the

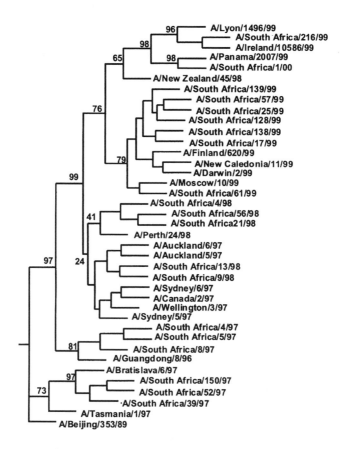

Fig. 2. Phylogenetic tree of influenza A (H3N2) virus HA1 gene nucleotide sequences (921 bp). The tree was generated using neighbor-joining analysis by PHYLIP and 1000 × bootstrap resampling. The number at each branch point indicates percentage probability that the resultant topology is correct.

sequencing data was carried out using the PHYLIP neighbor-joining programme, followed by 1000 replications of bootstrap resampling. The trees were generated using the Drawgram programme.

3. Results

Eighty three of the respiratory specimens received at NIV during 1997 were positive for influenza A, 366 specimens for influenza A in 1988, while in 1999, 115 influenza A isolates were made.

During the study period, the number of H3N2 viruses isolated each winter season were far greater than the subtype H1N1 viruses. In 1997, the percentage of H3N2 isolates was 79.4%; in 1998, it was 92.4%, and in 1999, it increased to 97.4%. The only H1N1 viruses, which were isolated during the 1997 winter season, came from Durban in the KwaZulu/Natal province. Three H1N1 isolates were made in November that year from the Gauteng province.

The results of the phylogenetic analysis of the HA1 sequence data generated from representative South African H1N1 viruses are shown in Fig. 1. The majority of the H1N1 viruses isolated during 1997–1999 grouped with the A/Bayern/7/95-like viruses. The South African isolates were related to the New Zealand strain A/Wellington/8/97. Several of the 1997 viruses, however, clustered with the A/Wuhan/371/95-like variant viruses.

Fig. 2 shows the phylogenetic tree constructed for the H3N2 South African isolates. The 1997 viruses grouped into two distinct clusters. The viruses isolated in 1998 were unrelated to the 1997 viruses, and were more similar to the A/Sydney/5/97-like strains. The 1999 H3N2 isolates exhibited genetic drift from the A/Sydney/5/97-like viruses and were more closely related to the reference A/Finland/620/99 strain. The A/South Africa/216/99 virus, which was isolated in December, exhibited further drift and clustered with the reference A/Panama/2007/99 strain.

4. Discussion

In the past decade, phylogenetic studies of human influenza viral nucleotide sequences have helped to determine the extent of drift of circulating viruses from vaccine strains [6] and provide a better understanding of the intercontinental spread of the virus [7]. Bush et al. [8] have also recently developed a method for predicting the evolution of human A H3N2 virus using phylogenetic trees.

The phylogenetic tree generated for the H1N1 sequences clearly revealed that two separate lineages of H1N1 viruses circulated in South Africa in 1997. The viruses that were isolated during the winter had evolved from the A/Bayern/7/95 and A/Johannesburg/82/96 lineage, while the H1N1 viruses isolated later in the year were derived from the A/Wuhan/371/95 lineage. This finding was of some significance as this was the first time that viruses of the latter lineage had been isolated in the Southern Hemisphere. These viruses did not continue to circulate in South Africa the following year, however, as all the 1998 and 1999 isolates fell into the A/Bayern/7/95 lineage. The South African viruses grouped together with the New Zealand A/Wellington/8/97 strain in the same sub-lineage. In terms of matching vaccine strains, they were genetically more related to the previous A/ Johannesburg/82/86 vaccine virus than to the 1999 A/Beijing 262/95 vaccine strain.

With regard to the H3N2 South African viruses, two different sub-lineages of the strains isolated in 1997 were identified. The isolates made earlier in the season were similar to the A/Guandong/8/96 strain, while the later isolates were in the same sub-lineage as the A/ Bratislava/6/97 and A/Tasmania/1/97 strain. None of the South African 1997 strains clustered in the same lineage as the A/Sydney/5/97-like variant viruses.

The 1998 H3N2 South African viruses, on the other hand, were genetically distinct from the viruses which had been circulating in the country in 1997 and grouped with the A/Sydney/5/97-like viruses. The introduction of these new viruses into South Africa in 1998 caused the unusually early and severe epidemic previously documented [3]. Genetic drift of the South African 1999 viruses from the A/Sydney/5/97 vaccine strain was evident from the fact that they were on the same sub-lineage as the A/Finland/620/99 reference strain and the Australian A/Darwin/2/99 isolate. The H3N2 virus A/South Africa/216/99 showed even greater drift from the vaccine strain and was more related to the A/Panama/ 2007/99 reference strain. This South African virus was isolated in December when H3N2 viruses were circulating in Europe and North America [9].

These phylogenetic studies on the influenza A H1N1 and H3N2 viruses have provided a clearer understanding of the genetic relationships of the South African viruses with those circulating in other countries. They have shown that the viruses present in South Africa during a specific year are not always closely related to those in other Southern Hemisphere countries and thus make an important contribution to the Southern Hemisphere vaccine formulation decision.

Acknowledgements

We wish to thank Vicky Gregory at the WHO Centre for Reference and Research on Influenza, London, for sending sequences from recent virus isolates. This work was supported by a grant from the Polio Research Foundation.

References

[1] B.D. Schoub, S. Johnson, J.M. McAnerney, E. Martin, I.L. Dos Santos, Laboratory studies of the 1984 influenza epidemic on the Witwatersrand, S. Afr. Med. J. 70 (1986) 815–818.
[2] T.G. Besselaar, N.K. Blackburn, B.D. Schoub, The molecular characterization of influenza virus strains isolated in South Africa during 1993 and 1994, Res. Virol. 147 (1996) 239–245.
[3] T.G. Besselaar, B.D. Schoub, N.K. Blackburn, Impact of the introduction of A/Sydney/5/97 H3N2 influenza virus into South Africa, J. Med. Virol. 59 (1999) 561–568.
[4] B.D. Schoub, S. Johnson, J.M. McAnerney, N.K. Blackburn, Benefits and limitations of the Witwatersrand influenza and acute respiratory infections surveillance programme, S. Afr. Med. J. 84 (1994) 674–678.
[5] Web site: http://www.flu.lanl.gov.
[6] N.J. Cox, H.L. Regnery, Global influenza surveillance: tracking a moving target in a rapidly changing world, in: L.E. Brown, A.W. Hampson, R.G. Webster (Eds.), Options for the Control of Influenza III, Elsevier, Amsterdam, 1996, pp. 591–598.

[7] W.M. Fitch, R.M. Bush, C.A. Bender, N.J. Cox, Long term trends in the evolution of H(3) HA1 human influenza type A, Proc. Natl. Acad. Sci. U. S. A. 94 (1997) 7712–7718.

[8] R.M. Bush, C.A. Bender, K. Subbarao, N.J. Cox, W.M. Fitch, Predicting the evolution of human influenza A, Science 286 (5446) (1999) 1921–1925.

[9] FluNet web site: http://oms.b3e.jussieu.fr/flunet/flunet.html.

International Congress Series 1219 (2001) 147–153

Predicting influenza evolution:
the impact of terminal and egg-adapted mutations

Robin M. Bush[a,*], Walter M. Fitch[a], Catherine B. Smith[b],
Nancy J. Cox[b]

[a]Department of Ecology and Evolutionary Biology, 321 Steinhaus, University of California,
Irvine, CA 92697, USA
[b]Influenza Branch, Centers for Disease Control and Prevention, Atlanta, GA 30333, USA

Abstract

Background: The hemagglutinins (HA) of human influenza viruses adapt during growth in chicken eggs. Amino acid replacements in HAs of egg-grown viruses generally appear on the terminal branches of phylogenetic trees. Our method for predicting human influenza HA evolution, which tracks replacements at positively selected codons across trees, is more accurate with terminal mutations excluded. *Methods*: We extracted the sequence data that contain the majority of egg-adapted replacements from our original data set, and replicated our prediction tests analyzing both internal and terminal mutations. We contrasted these results with those obtained analyzing (1) only internal mutations and (2) analyzing all mutations in our full data set. *Results*: Excluding egg-adapted replacements did not increase the accuracy of our predictions when other terminal mutations remained in the analysis. Deleting all terminal mutations produced the best prediction of success of viral lineages. *Conclusions*: Amino acid replacements on terminal branches interfered with our ability to identify which codons were under positive selection. Therefore, we recommend limiting such analyses to the internal branches of phylogenetic trees. The effects of terminal mutations may be caused by the criteria used for selecting viruses for HA sequencing. © 2001 Elsevier Science B.V. All rights reserved.

Keywords: H3N2; Hemagglutinin; Phylogeny; Molecular evolution; Host-mediated

1. Introduction

The hemagglutinin (HA) gene of human influenza viruses adapts in response to propagation in embryonated chicken eggs in the laboratory [1]. The egg-adapted amino

---

* Corresponding author. Tel.: +1-949-824-2243; fax: +1-949-824-2181.
E-mail address: rmbush@uci.edu (R.M. Bush).

0531-5131/01/$ – see front matter © 2001 Elsevier Science B.V. All rights reserved.
PII: S0531-5131(01)00643-4

acids, which are often located around the receptor binding pocket of the HA1 domain, represent residues that either were not present or were at very low frequency in the human host. Egg-adapted changes in sequence data resulting from laboratory culture will generally appear on the terminal branches of phylogenetic trees ([4], Fig. 1). These artifacts should be extracted from studies that examine evolution of the virus during replication in humans.

We recently developed a method for predicting human influenza A evolution using phylogenetic analysis of H3 HA1 hemagglutinin sequence data. Our prediction method identifies codons at which amino acid replacements have provided a selective advantage in the past, as indicated by an excess of non-synonymous relative to synonymous nucleotide substitutions [2]. We tested our prediction method retrospectively for 11 recent influenza seasons [3]. In 9 of 11 seasons, the method successfully identified the ancestor of future lineages as the isolate with the greatest number of amino acid replacements at positively selected codons (Fig. 1).

To exclude egg-adapted replacements from our analyses, we eliminated all "terminal mutations" (nucleotide substitutions on terminal branches) from our trees [2]. This reduced the mutations available for determining positive selection by 70%, but gave more accurate evolutionary predictions than analyses including terminal mutations ([3],

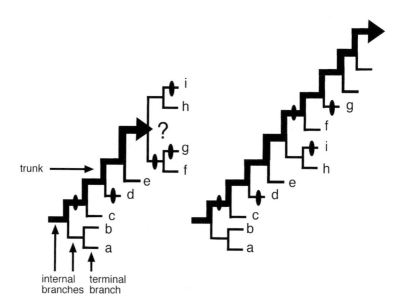

Fig. 1. Retrospective prediction of H3 influenza A evolution. The tree on the left depicts HA1 sequence evolution during a period of time in the past, with the root in the lower left corner. A single evolutionarily successful lineage, or "trunk lineage," characteristic of H3 evolution, is shown as a bold line. The question mark indicates the point where we can no longer discern the course of the trunk near the top of the tree. The lineage undergoing the greatest number of amino acid replacements at positively selected codons (ovals) terminates at the sequence from isolate g. An accurate prediction test is illustrated; isolate g is more closely related to subsequent lineages than are isolates a–f.

Table 2). However, this increase in accuracy did not necessarily result solely from excluding egg-adapted replacements. It could have resulted from excluding terminal mutations irrespective of whether they were egg-adapted.

In this paper, we compare our original prediction results with results from two alternative tests designed to determine the effects of egg-adapted replacements and terminal mutations on our analyses. Our results suggest that terminal mutations confound studies of positive selection regardless of whether they were egg-adapted. We propose that terminal mutations confound the analysis because of the way in which viral isolates are chosen for HA sequencing during influenza surveillance.

2. Materials and methods

Laboratory studies comparing sequences from isolates passaged in eggs with sequences from cell-passaged isolates or from direct PCR of the original clinical specimen suggest that at least 22 of the 329 codons in the HA1 domain may undergo egg-adapted replacements (reviewed in Ref. [2], Table 1). Some codons, such as 145, 156 and 186, are particularly well known to change during growth of influenza viruses in eggs [1]. Others, such as 111, have been reported to adapt to eggs but do not vary in our data set. Little is known about differences in the frequency of egg-adapted replacements among codons, thus we considered all 22 codons equivalently susceptible to adaptation to eggs in this study.

A prediction test has two steps. In the first step, we identify codons that show evidence for having been under positive selection. These are codons having a significant excess of non-synonymous versus synonymous substitutions [2]. An excess of non-synonymous substitutions results when selection had, in the past, favored amino acid replacement at a site in the hemagglutinin. In the second step, we identify the currently circulating viral strain carrying the greatest number of additional replacements at the positively selected codons. We predict that this strain should be the ancestor of future lineages [3]. A successful prediction test is illustrated in Fig. 1.

2.1. Internal-Branches test

In our original study of 357 HA1 sequences, we estimated positive selection using only substitutions on internal tree branches to avoid introducing error due to egg-mediated changes into our analyses [2]. Here, we compare our previous results with three new tests.

2.2. All-Branches test

We estimated positive selection using mutations on both the internal and terminal branches of our original phylogenetic trees [2,3]. All-Branches prediction tests could be less accurate than our original prediction tests for three reasons: egg-adapted replacements could introduce error into the estimation of positive selection; egg-adapted replacements could cause errors in phylogenetic reconstruction; and deleterious or neutral mutations on terminal branches could obscure evidence for positive selection.

Table 1

Ratios of non-synonymous to synonymous nucleotide substitutions at codons in the HA1 domain of human influenza A subtype H3

Codon	Internal-Branches	All-Branches	All-Egg-Excluded
2	1/0	4/0	4/0
50	4/1	9/3	9/3*
53	0/0	6/1	6/1*
78	3/0	6/0*	6/0*
80	2/0	7/0*	7/0*
111[E]	0/0	0/0	0/0
121	5/0*	10/1*	10/1*
124	5/0*	6/2	6/2
126[E]	0/0	2/0	0/0
128	0/0	8/0*	8/0*
133	8/0*	12/0*	12/0*
135	5/0*	12/1*	12/1*
137[E]	0/0	12/1*	3/0
138[E]	6/0*	22/0*	17/0*
142	4/0*	8/1*	8/1*
144[E]	3/0	6/1	4/0
145[E]	8/0*	19/0*	14/0*
155[E]	1/2	3/4	2/3
156[E]	9/1*	24/2*	13/2*
157	2/0	6/3	6/3
158[E]	5/0*	8/0*	7/0*
159[E]	3/1	14/3*	4/2
172	3/0	9/1*	9/1*
174	2/0	5/0*	5/0*
182	0/0	7/1*	7/1*
185[E]	0/1	0/3	0/3
186[E]	9/1*	23/5*	14/4*
189	2/0	3/0	3/0
190	4/0*	13/0*	13/0*
193[E]	4/0*	24/1*	7/1*
194[E]	4/0*	13/2*	7/2
196	3/1	12/1*	12/1*
197	4/0*	5/3	5/3
198	2/0	7/1*	7/1*
199[E]	0/0	0/0	0/0
201	4/0*	6/1	6/1*
216	2/0	6/1	6/1*
219[E]	5/3	13/3*	9/3*
220	0/0	5/0*	5/0*
226[E]	20/1*	38/3*	30/3*
229[E]	3/1	10/4	9/3*
246[E]	3/2	16/4*	8/3
248[E]	0/3	10/6	5/5
260	1/0	6/1	6/1*
262	4/0*	7/2	7/2
275	6/0*	10/0*	10/0*
276[E]	2/0	11/0*	5/0*
290[E]	0/0	0/0	0/0

Table 1 (continued)

Codon	Internal-Branches	All-Branches	All-Egg-Excluded
310	2/2	9/2*	9/2*
312	1/0	8/0*	8/0*
322	1/0	4/0	4/0

These codons either show evidence for positive selection (* = a significant ($p < 0.05$) excess of non-synonymous substitutions) or are known to undergo egg-adapted replacements (E). Positive selection was estimated using mutations on Internal Branches, on All Branches, or in the All-Egg-Excluded test, on all branches excluding egg-adapted replacements. Statistical significance differs among some tests having identical ratios because expectations depend on the proportion of non-synonymous substitutions in each data set.

2.3. All-Egg-Excluded test

In this test, we excluded mutations from our analyses if they were in one of the 22 codons known to undergo egg-adapted change and they occurred on a branch attaching an egg-grown isolate to the tree. These 22 codons show an excess of non-synonymous substitutions, but not of synonymous substitutions, on such branches. We had previously estimated, by comparing mutation rates on branches attaching cell-cultured and egg-cultured isolates to the tree, that about 59 non-synonymous substitutions in our data set were egg-adapted [4]. For this test, we excluded 8 synonymous and 110 non-synonymous substitutions. The remaining data set consisted of 595 synonymous substitutions and 635 non-synonymous substitutions. With the egg-adapted replacements excluded, we estimated positive selection using all internal and terminal mutations.

2.4. Alternative Egg-Exclusion test

In the All-Egg-Excluded test, we removed egg-adapted replacements after phylogenetic reconstruction. In this test, we excluded egg-adapted replacements before building

Table 2
Accurate (x) retrospective prediction tests for 11 recent influenza seasons

	Internal-Branches	All-Branches	All-Egg-Excluded
1987	x		
1988			
1989		x	
1990	x	x	x
1991	x	x	x
1992	x	x	
1993	x	x	x
1994	x		
1995	x	x	
1996	x	x	x
1997	x		

See Table 1 for descriptions of data sets.

the tree. Results were very similar, so only the test done excluding the replacements after tree construction, the All-Egg-Excluded test, is reported here.

3. Results

Our original (Internal-Branches) analysis identified 18 positively selected codons ([2], Table 2). All-Branches, the test using all mutations, identified 30 positively selected codons. The test with potentially egg-adapted replacements excluded, All-Egg-Excluded, identified 32 positively selected codons (Table 1).

Retrospective prediction tests, which track change at the positively selected codons as illustrated in Fig. 1, were accurate in 9 of 11 influenza seasons for the Internal test, in 7 seasons for the All-Branches test, and in 4 seasons for All-Egg-Excluded test (Table 2).

4. Discussion

Our results suggest that excluding all terminal mutations improves accuracy of prediction more than excluding only the egg-adapted replacements. The way in which viral isolates are selected for sequencing may explain this result. Sequence analysis of influenza viruses has been purposefully biased toward sequencing strains that are antigenically dissimilar from the established reference strains. This bias inflates the frequency of amino acid replacements on terminal branches, and may cause us to mistakenly identify codons as positively selected when replacements are neutral or deleterious.

Amino acid replacements on internal branches more accurately reflect changes in the influenza population than replacements on terminal branches. Replacements in the HA1 domain that are retained in the H3 viral population over time (that is, on internal branches) are generally in residues on the surface of the hemagglutinin trimer [5]. These surface-exposed residues are susceptible to attack by antibodies. Most of the 18 positively selected codons from our original analysis were also surface exposed, and 78% of them were associated with antibody combining sites A and B and/or the receptor binding pocket. By contrast, few of the additional codons found to be positively selected when terminal mutations were included in our analyses were associated with these functionally important sites [2]. Thus, internal amino acid replacements provide important information about viral evolution, whereas terminal replacements may be influenced by sampling bias.

Acknowledgements

This work was supported by NIH grant 1R01AI44474-01 and also by funds provided by the University of California for the conduct of discretionary research by Los Alamos National Laboratory, conducted under the auspices of the US Department of Energy. We gratefully acknowledge the technical expertise of Huang Jing and the helpful advice of Steve Frank.

References

[1] J.S. Robertson, Clinical influenza virus and the embryonated hen's egg, Rev. Med. Virol. 3 (1993) 97–106.

[2] R.M. Bush, W.M. Fitch, C.A. Bender, N.J. Cox, Positive selection on the H3 hemagglutinin gene of human influenza virus A, Mol. Biol. Evol. 16 (1999) 1457–1465.

[3] R.M. Bush, C.A. Bender, K. Subbarao, N.J. Cox, W.M. Fitch, Predicting the evolution of human influenza A, Science 286 (1999) 1921–1925.

[4] R.M. Bush, C.B. Smith, N.J. Cox, W.M. Fitch, Effects of passage history and sampling bias on phylogenetic reconstruction of human influenza A evolution, PNAS 97 (2000) 6974–6980.

[5] J.J. Skehel, B. Barrere, S.A. Wharton, R. Bizebard, D. Fleury, M. Eisen, D.C. Wiley, Antibody recognition of influenza hemagglutinin, in: F. Brown, D. Burton, P. Doherty, J. Mekalanos, E. Norrby (Eds.), Vaccines 97: Molecular Approaches to the Control of Infectious Diseases, Cold Spring Harbor Laboratory Press, Plainview, NY, 1997, pp. 1–7.

International Congress Series 1219 (2001) 155–161

Early herald wave outbreaks of influenza in 1916 prior to the pandemic of 1918

J.S. Oxford[a,*], A. Sefton[a], R. Jackson[a], W. Innes[a], R.S. Daniels[b], N.P.A.S. Johnson[c]

[a]*Department of Medical Microbiology and Retroscreen Ltd. (http://www.retroscreen.com) Virology, St. Bartholomew's and The Royal London School of Medicine and Dentistry, Queen Mary and Westfield College, London E1 4NS, UK*
[b]*Virology Division, NIMR, London NW7 1AA, UK*
[c]*Department of Geography, University of Cambridge, Cambridge CB2 3EN, UK*

Abstract

The 1918 outbreak dwarfed the immediately preceding pandemic of 1889 and the subsequent 1957 and 1968 pandemics in mortality and morbidity. In retrospect, much can be learnt about the source, the possibly subterranean spread of virus and the genetic basis of virulence. In the recent pandemics of 1957 and 1968, there were so-called 'herald waves' either in the summer months, or in particular countries up to 6 months before more worldwide outbreaks. These localised outbreaks would lengthen the time available for preparation of new vaccines and stockpiling of antiviral compounds. We present new epidemiological and mortality evidence of early outbreaks of influenza in France, UK, Norway, Germany and USA in the years 1915 to 1917. Certain of these focal outbreaks which had a very high mortality in the young occurred during the winter months, and were respiratory with a heliotrope cyanosis so prominent in the clinical diagnosis in the world outbreak of 1918. Thus, the upturn of influenza activity in Norway in 1916 was associated with an unusual level of mortality in young adults. Similarly, the outbreak at Etaples in France and Aldershot barracks in the UK in 1916–1917 caused mortality in 25–35 year olds. We deduce from an analysis of these outbreaks that early focal outbreaks occurred mainly in Europe and on the balance of probability the Great Pandemic was not initiated in Spain in 1918 but possibly in another European country, either France or England, in 1915, 1916 or 1917. © 2001 Elsevier Science B.V. All rights reserved.

Keywords: Pandemic; Heliotrope cyanosis; 'Epidemic' catarrh

---

* Corresponding author.

0531-5131/01/$ – see front matter © 2001 Elsevier Science B.V. All rights reserved.
PII: S 0 5 3 1 - 5 1 3 1 (0 1) 0 0 3 3 6 - 3

1. Introduction

The so-called Great Spanish Pandemic of 1918–1919 appeared at first sight to emerge very rapidly and spread around the entire world in a 2–3 month period. Thus, the short period from late September 1918 to November 1918 saw the death of the US Army private, Private Vaughan, in South Carolina [1] and the deaths of another soldier at Camp Upton in the USA; of 'Lucy' at Brevig Mission, Alaska [2]; and of six Norwegian coal miners in Spitsbergen [3]. Reports of influenza deaths in countries as widely spread as Norway, Sweden, Finland, Canada, Spain, Britain, France, Germany, Senegal, Tanzania, Nigeria, Ghana, Zimbabwe, South Africa, India and Indonesia were recorded [4]. The very wide geographical spread of these deaths in such a short period, in the absence of air travel at that time, suggests that the disease had spread around the globe prior to this time and that 'seeding' had occurred.

We have searched the early medical literature and also historical medical records at the Wellcome Museum, The British Library and The Army records at Kew for early herald waves of influenza. The term influenza now used to describe the respiratory disease with acute onset, headache and generalised pains (Stuart-Harris et al. [5]) was not commonly used between its first mention in the medieval period in Florence until the end of the 19th Century. Alternative names were epidemic bronchitis or epidemic catarrh [6]. We therefore investigated explosive outbreaks of respiratory disease, affecting young persons, in the winter periods prior to 1918 with high mortality and with the characteristic heliotrope cyanosis. All these features characterised the 1918–1919 pandemic.

2. Results and discussion

2.1. Outbreaks in the army

Hammond et al. [7] described an outbreak of respiratory infection termed purulent bronchitis in a huge British army base at Etaples in Northern France in the winter of 1916 (Fig. 1). The soldiers were admitted to the base hospital, suffering from an acute respiratory infection, high temperature and cough at a time when recognised influenza was present. Etaples was a large camp, with 100,000 soldier inhabitants at any time and 24 hospitals. This outbreak was further characterised by cyanosis and extremely high mortality. Clinical examination showed, in most cases, signs of bronchopneumonia, and histology showed an acute purulent bronchitis. Our clinical microbiological review of the paper now ranks the description as classic influenza being essentially similar to the extensive literature of deaths in 1918–1919 [8].

An almost identical epidemic of purulent bronchitis with bronchopneumonia, with cases showing the peculiar dusky heliotype cyanosis and mortality rates of 25–50%, was described in Aldershot barracks in March 1917 [9].

At present, no clinical samples have been located from the above two outbreaks in France and the UK, which could be analysed for influenza genes by RT PCR. Therefore, the question remains as to whether these earlier outbreaks were caused not by influenza

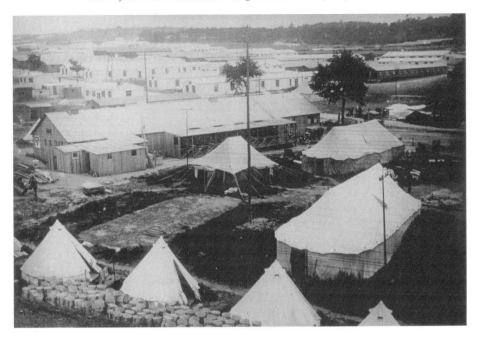

Fig. 1. The British Army Base Camp at Etaples, France showing a hospital section.

but for example, by pneumococcus or mycoplasma. Undoubtedly, pneumococcal super-infection contributed to the high mortality in soldiers hospitalised and nursed together in open wards [8]. However, it is unlikely that this organism alone could have caused explosive outbreaks of pneumonia in young persons. Bacteriological analysis of the two outbreaks [7,9] detected a range of bacteria. Similarly, a wide range of gram-positive and gram-negative bacteria were recovered from sputum and lung samples during the main pandemic of 1918–1919 [8].

Corroborative evidence that these early outbreaks could be herald waves from the autumn pandemic of 1918 comes from Eyre and Malloch [9] who with recent and up to date experience of the Spanish pandemic reiterated that the morbid anatomy and histology of the lungs of 1917 epidemic bronchitis cases were very similar to influenza cases of 1918 [10]. Furthermore, in an independent report, Abercrombie [11] recorded: "Early in 1917, I had under my care in France a large number of (young) soldiers suffering from a grave form of purulent bronchitis proceeding in some cases to bronchopneumonia The cases exhibited dysponea, a heliotrope cyanosis, pyrexia and a high mortality".

2.2. Outbreaks in civilian populations

When influenza and/or pneumonia mortality for many locations is plotted (Fig. 2a, b and c), it is apparent that 1915–1916 saw an increase in influenza activity in many locations, including England and Wales [12], Scotland [13], Ireland [14], USA [15,16], Denmark [17], Norway [18] and Sweden [19].

Additional indirect evidence of seeding comes from Norwegian data where the age distribution of mortality suggests that the upturn in influenza activity in 1915

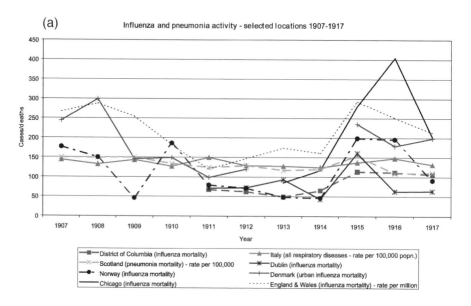

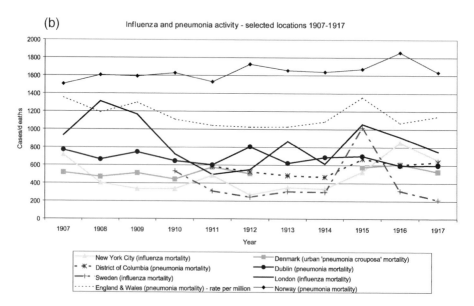

Fig. 2. (a) Influenza deaths and cases—selected locations (b) Influenza deaths and cases—selected locations. (c) Influenza deaths and cases—selected locations.

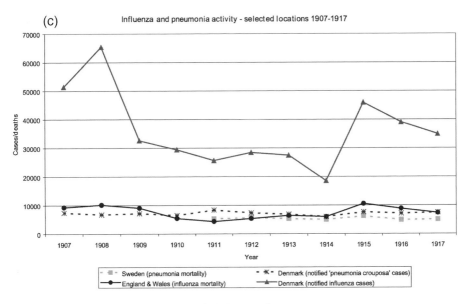

Fig. 2 (*continued*).

and 1916 was associated with an unusual level of mortality among young adults—a feature that was to be so characteristic of the later 1918–1919 pandemic itself [20].

3. Conclusions

In anticipation of the first influenza pandemic of the 21st century, WHO has published a template pandemic plan as have many National Authorities [21]. A recent analysis [21] of the changing factors which could increase the rate of spread of a new pandemic virus such as air travel, global tourism, increased population has been balanced against the potential effectiveness of the new anti-NA drugs and the greatly increased capacity to produce influenza vaccine, which globally now exceeds 200 million doses per year.

The term 'herald wave' has been used previously to describe a late outbreak of influenza in a season that, with virus isolation and analysis, can be used as a predictor of virus strains in the following seasons [22]. We use the term here for the first time to analyse the early steps in the emergence of a pandemic virus. It is noteworthy that in the well-documented influenza A (H2N2) pandemic of 1957, the first virus was isolated in China in February. Subsequently, the virus spread to Australia, South East Asia by June reaching the rest of Europe and South America by July–September. By December 1957, every continent of the world had been infected. Therefore, a period of 10 months was required for global spread. In the influenza A (H3N2) pandemic of 1968, the virus spread from China in July but although the virus was introduced in the rest of Asia by August, the explosive outbreak was delayed by 6 months. Similarly in the UK and Europe, seeding occurred early but explosive outbreaks were delayed for 12–14 months. Early detection of these events would prolong the lead-time necessary for vaccine production distribution and initiation of general strategies with the new anti-neuraminidase drugs.

The protracted period that we postulate for the emergence of the Great Pandemic of 1918, almost 2 years, could be explained by the absence of air travel and the distortion and restriction of travel during the Great War itself. Conversely, demobilisation in the autumn of 1918 would have provided an ideal set of circumstances for intimate person-to-person spread and wide dispersion as young soldiers returned home by sea and rail to countries around the entire globe.

References

[1] J.K. Taubenberger, A.H. Reid, A.E. Krafft, K.E. Bijwaard, T.G. Fanning, "Spanish" influenza virus, Science 275 (1997) 1793–1796.

[2] A.H. Reid, T.G. Fanning, J.V. Hultin, J.K. Taubenberger, Origin and evolution of the 1918 "Spanish" influenza hemagglutin gene, Proc. Natl. Acad. Sci. 96 (1999) 1651–1656.

[3] J.L. Davis, et al., Application of ground penetrating radar in permafrost to locate the bodies of seven victims of the 1918 "Spanish Flu", J. Forensic Sci. 20 (2000) 68–76.

[4] The Spanish influenza pandemic of 1918–1919: new perspectives, in: H. Phillips, D. Killingray (Eds.), Social history of medicine series, Routledge, 2001, in press.

[5] C.H. Stuart-Harris, G.C. Schild, J.S. Oxford, Influenza, the Virus and the Disease, Edward Arnold, London, 1984.

[6] T. Thompson, Annals of Influenza or Epidemic Catarrhal Fever in Great Britain from 1510 to 1837, Sydenham Society, London, 1852.

[7] J.A.R. Hammond, W. Rolland, T.H.G. Shore, Purulent bronchitis: a study of cases occurring amongst the British troops at a base in France, Lancet ii (1917) 41–45.

[8] E.L. Opie, F.G. Blake, J.C. Small, T.M. Rivers, in: H. Kimpton (Ed.), Epidemic Respiratory Disease: The Pneumonias and Other Infections of the Respiratory Tract Accompanying Influenza and Measles, 1921, pp. 402, London.

[9] A. Abrahams, N.F. Hallows, J.W.H. Eyre, H. French, Purulent bronchitis: its influenza and pneumococcal bacteriology, Lancet ii (1917) 377–380; J. Eyre, T.H. Malloch, Influenza, a Discussion, Royal Society of Medicine, (1918) 97–102 Nov.

[10] W.G. Macpherson, W.P. Herringham, T.R. Elliott, A. Balfour, in: W.G. Macpherson, W.P. Herringham, T.R. Elliott, A. Balfour (Eds.), History of the Great War 174, HMSO, London, 1920, pp. 211–214.

[11] 83rd Annual Report of Registrar General, England and Wales, and London, 1922, p. 21.

[12] 66th Annual Report of the Registrar General for Scotland, Scotland, 1922, p. cxxiii.

[13] Yearly Summary of the Weekly Returns of Births and Deaths in the Dublin Registration Area, Dublin, 1910 and 1921.

[14] New York City, Chicago and Washington D.C. Ministry of Health, Report on the pandemic of influenza 1918–1919. London, 1920, pp. 306, 309-310 and 315-316.

[15] J.S.N. Van Tam, Epidemiology of Influenza, in: Textbook of Influenza. Edited by K. Nicholson, A. Hay, W.R.G. Webster.

[16] Statistik Aarborg, 1910, 1914, 1919 and 1921. Denmark.

[17] Statistical yearbooks of Norway, 1900–1921. Norway.

[18] Statistisk Årsbok for Sverige, 1919 and 1923. Sweden.

[19] Statistical yearbooks of Norway, 1914–1917. Norway.

[20] Influenza Pandemic Plan, in: The Role of WHO and guidelines for National and Regional Planning. World Health Organization, Geneva, Switzerland 1999.

[21] J.S. Oxford, Influenza A pandemics of the 20th century with special reference to 1918: virology, pathology and epidemiology, Rev. Med. Virol. 10 (2000) 119–133.

[22] W.P. Glezen, R.B. Couch, H.R. Six, The influenza herald wave, Am. J. Epidemiol. 116 (1982) 589–598.

International Congress Series 1219 (2001) 163–168

The 1918 Spanish flu epidemic in Geneva, Switzerland

Catherine E. Ammon*

Louis Jeantet Institute for the History of Medicine, University of Geneva, Geneva, Switzerland

Abstract

Methods: This historical research was accomplished by reviewing the city archives, medical publications and the daily press of 1918–1919. Data relating to the Spanish flu epidemic in Geneva were collected. *Results*: More than 50% of the population was hit by the infection during three consecutive waves in 1918. Mortality was highest for the age group 21–40 years. Mortality and morbidity rates were much higher in males. In Geneva, the flu first appeared in July 1918 among soldiers back from the border posts. It was then followed by a rapid spread within the civilian population. The second wave, which occurred in October–November was the deadliest. The third outbreak was observed at the end of 1918. The Geneva authorities (Conseil d'Etat) held two emergency meetings in October and made immediate decisions to temporarily close all public and private schools, and to prohibit any meeting and public gathering (religious service, funeral, leisure, theatres, balls, sport events, etc.). They opened an emergency hospital and authorised burials within 48 h of death. To avoid the spread of contagion through dust, it was made compulsory to spray streets, staircases and flats with a powerful disinfectant. The epidemics caused havoc in the private and public sectors. Some companies reported that as many as 80% of their staff were sick. Postal and phone services were disrupted, as well as public transportation. Medical doctors were difficult to reach and the hospital refused new admissions. Doubts and misinformation were common in the press (medical and mass media) regarding the disease, its prevention, its cure, and personal or public hygiene measures. Nearly every article or letter published in the press was denied, refuted or followed by counter-information, which added insecurity in an already difficult war-time period. *Conclusions*: The analysis of this historical case-study can be of some help in the understanding of present-day and future flu epidemics and pandemics, in particular, with respect to the biological history of

* Present affiliation: Swiss Federal Office of Public Health, Epidemiology and Infectious Diseases, P.O. Box 3003 Bern, Switzerland. Tel.: +41-31-323-13-39; fax: +41-31-323-87-95.
  E-mail address: catherine.ammon@bag.admin.ch (C.E. Ammon).

viruses and hosts, and public concerns about the disease. © 2001 Elsevier Science B.V. All rights reserved.

Keywords: Spanish flu epidemic; Mortality; Morbidity

This historical research is based on various documents dating from the 1918 epidemic of Spanish flu such as Government and State archives, medical publications, daily and weekly newspapers, enhanced with oral testimonies. It is mainly focused on the city of Geneva, but some data relate to the whole of Switzerland.

In 1918, the context is that of war: able-bodied men mobilised in the army, rationed food, scarcity of fuel; the population is deprived and conditions are hard.

The flu epidemic hit Switzerland in three major waves. The first occurred in July 1918, the deadliest in October–November that year, followed by the third peak at the end of 1918. The latter peak declined sharply but with residual cases occurring until January–February 1919. A smaller peak recurred at the beginning of 1920. The first cases appeared among soldiers based at the border posts [1] and in the foreign soldiers' camps situated in several villages in Central Switzerland [2]. The epidemic rapidly spread to civilians. More than 50% of the total population was hit by the infection during 1918, and 58% during the 2 years of the epidemic [3] (Figs. 1 and 2).

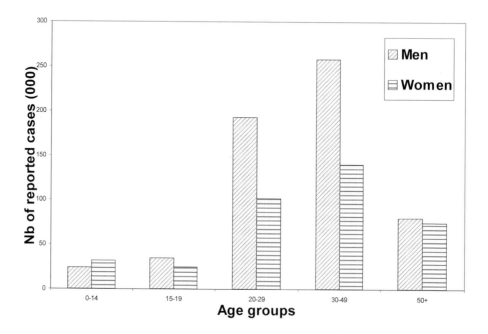

Fig. 1. Flu morbidity per sex and age group, Switzerland (1918).

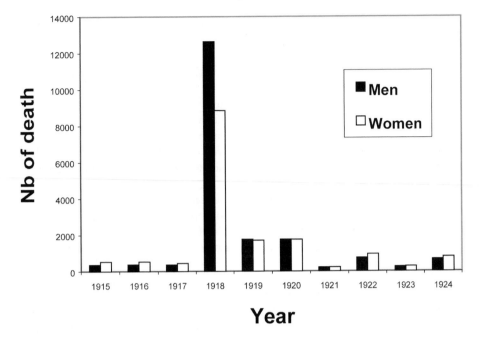

Fig. 2. Flu mortality per sex, Switzerland (1915–1924).

The flu symptoms were the same as seen today, but the peak that occurred in autumn brought fulminant clinical forms with deadly complications, typically characterised by cyanosed extremities followed by death within 24 h. It seems that people infected during the early waves were subsequently protected.

Mortality and morbidity rates were highest among the adult population, especially in the age group 21–40 years, and were higher in males. It is hypothesised that the cramped conditions within the soldiers' living quarters facilitated the spread of the virus among the troops, while women and civilians were slightly less at risk. A possible immunity from the previous epidemic of 1889–1891 might still have had protective effects for the elderly in 1918.

The Swiss health authorities immediately (18 July 1918) delegated the power to act to the Cantons [4]. In Geneva, the Conseil d'Etat held two emergency meetings (5 and 30 October 1918) in addition to the regular scheduled sessions of the Grand Conseil. The main decisions taken were as follows:

- Closure of private and public schools (at various times)
- Prohibition of all meetings and public gatherings (church services, masses and funerals; theatres and movies; public balls and dancing parties; sports and leisure events; etc.)
- Prohibition of visits to hospitals
- Mandatory spraying of disinfectant on the streets

- Prohibition of dry wiping of floors, staircases and court yards (i.e. mandatory use of water for cleaning)
- Setting up of an emergency hospital
- Authorisation of burials within 48 h of death (i.e. without the usual legal delay).

Disruption in the private and public sectors was widespread. Some companies reported as many as 80% of their staff sick [5]. The administration was badly affected by the epidemic. Postal services were disrupted, and many post offices were simply closed. Telephone and telegraph services functioned with reduced opening hours [6]. Public transportation was less frequent and irregular, facilitating the spread of the disease with overcrowded vehicles.

The sanitary and medical sectors also experienced a high degree of disruption. Medical doctors were difficult to reach due to the phone restrictions imposed by the phone companies [7], and also because they had to visit their patients [8]. Some physicians were sick and many young doctors died. Taxi companies were ordered to refuse to transport patients to the hospitals, as only disinfected special ambulances were authorised to carry patients [9]. At the major peak of the epidemic in October–November 1918, the Geneva hospital accepted no new admissions [10]. In the army, 50–80% of the troops as well as 50% of the staff from the sanitary services fell sick within 2 days [11], emergency hospitals were set up (see Fig. 3). There were requests in newspapers for volunteers to help

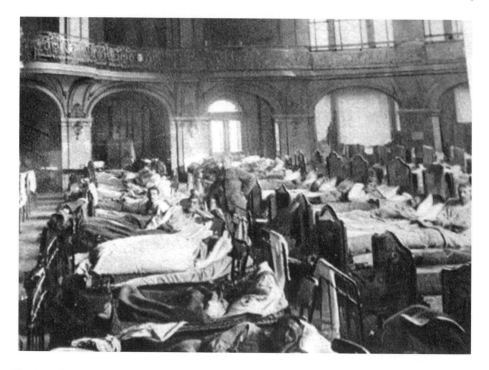

Fig. 3. Tonhalle converted in a military hospital for soldiers with flu, Zurich (1918) (Source: La Patrie Suisse, 1918 (858), p. 293 — Foto W. Schneider Zurich).

at the hospital [12]. A doctor from Geneva was fined by the national sanitary authorities court for having failed to notify cases [13].

The climate was one of the fears. Doubts and misinformation were common in the press (both medical and mass media) regarding the disease, its origin, its transmission, its treatment, and the personal or public hygiene measures required to prevent it. Virus transmission was thought to originate from the army dirty laundry [14], washed by civilians and Red Cross volunteers, or through mail received from soldiers [15].

The measures taken were severe. No leisure events regrouping individuals were allowed. In some Cantons, access to restaurants and cafés was restricted and opening hours reduced. Theatres, cinemas and night clubs were closed.

Churches could give no direct spiritual relief as services were prohibited. In Lausanne, religious services were held outdoors (see Fig. 4). In Valais, the church bells no longer rang to announce death [16]. In Geneva, two ministers were fined for having conducted a mass in church [17] despite the prohibition. Funerals were perfunctory and processions were prohibited.

A lack of continuity and the instability was demonstrated by schools closing, opening, and closing again, increasing the feeling of insecurity. Also, there was no specific reassurance from authorities, leading to doubts among the population as to the real control of the situation.

In the press, death announcements filled pages after pages, lowering morale and reinforcing fear of the plague. Statistics from hospitals were published daily throughout the epidemic, stating the number of admissions, discharges, deaths and patients refused. Medical doctors disagreed among themselves, for example some suggested the con-

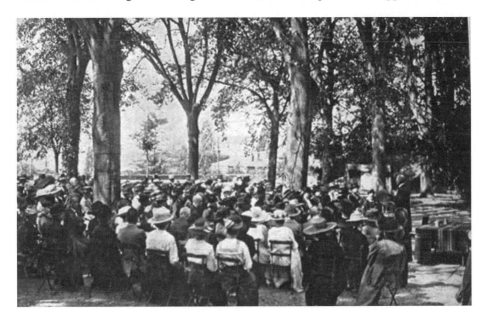

Fig. 4. Religious service held outdoors, Lausanne (1918) (Source: La Patrie Suisse, 1918 (650), p. 204 — Foto E. Würgler, Lausanne).

sumption of alcohol, while others strongly rejected it [18]. Although there was no specific treatment for the flu, advertisements for medical products and "miracle" cures appeared frequently in newspapers. In the daily press, letters from readers were controversial regarding the measures taken. Nearly every article or letter published was denied, refuted or followed by counter-information, which added insecurity in an already difficult wartime period.

The importance of the lack of consistent information and comprehensible messages has to be stressed. The analysis of this historical case-study can be of some help in the understanding of present-day and future flu epidemics, in particular, with respect of the biological history of viruses and hosts, the public concerns about the disease, and the reaction of authorities and population. There are lessons that can still be learned from the Spanish epidemic of 1918.

References

[1] La Suisse, 5 July 1918.

[2] La Suisse, 7 July 1918.

[3] L'influenza en Suisse en 1918/1919, Hygiène pratique. Prophylaxie. Statistique médicale, etc. Rapport du Service d'Hygiène publique, Rapport du Conseil Fédéral, 1919.

[4] Letter from the President of the Confederation Gallandé and the Vice-Chancelier David, Department of Public Economy, Service of Public Hygiene to the Conseil d'Etat, Canton of Geneva, dated 18 July 1918.

[5] La Tribune de Genève, 28 August 1918.

[6] La Suisse, 15 October 1918; La Feuille, 23 October 1918; La Tribune de Genève, 26 October 1918.

[7] Journal de Genève, 26 and 31 October 1918.

[8] La Suisse, 25 October 1918.

[9] La Suisse, 20 October 1918; Journal de Genève, 30 October 1918; La Tribune de Genève, 1 November 1918.

[10] La Tribune de Genève, 23 August 1918.

[11] La Tribune de Genève, 19 July 1918.

[12] La Tribune de Genève, 20 August 1918.

[13] Jugement de la Cour de Justice du Canton de Genève (notification par les médecins des cas de grippe soignés par eux), Jugements et recours, 31 May 1919.

[14] La Tribune de Genève, 4–5 August 1919; La Suisse, 5 August 1918.

[15] La Tribune de Genève, 19 July 1918; La Suisse, 10 July 1918.

[16] Personal communication, Mrs Anne Gaillard, Valais.

[17] La Tribune de Genève, 4–5 and 23 August 1918.

[18] E. Cottin, P. Gautier, C. Saloz, La Grippe de 1918 — Ses formes cliniques, Revue Suisse de Médecine 25 (1919) 504–522, 10 December; A. Thélin, Département de l'Intérieur, Service Sanitaire, A propos de la grippe, lettre circulaire à Messieurs les Préfets, et par eux aux Municipalités et aux médecins de canton, Gazette d'Hygiène, de Médecine et de Sciences sociales de la Suisse Romande 13 (1918) 1–2, 9 July.

International Congress Series 1219 (2001) 169–171

Global surveillance of animal influenza for the control of future pandemics

H. Kida[a,*], K. Okazaki[a], A. Takada[a], H. Ozaki[a], M. Tashiro[b],
D.K. Lvov[c], K.F. Shortridge[d], R.G. Webster[e]

[a]*Department of Disease Control, Hokkaido University Graduate School of Veterinary Medicine,*
Sapporo 060-0818, Japan
[b]*National Institute of Infectious Diseases, Tokyo, Japan*
[c]*Ivanovsky Institute of Virology, Moscow, Russia*
[d]*University of Hong Kong, Hong Kong, China*
[e]*St. Jude Children's Research Hospital, Memphis, USA*

Abstract

Influenza viruses of different subtypes were isolated from fecal samples of ducks in their nesting areas in Siberia in summer from 1996 to 1999. Phylogenetic analysis of the NP genes of the isolates in Siberia and Japan on their flyway of migration to the south indicate that influenza viruses perpetuated in ducks nesting in Siberia should have contributed genes in the emergence of the H5N1 virus in Hong Kong. Inactivated vaccine prepared from an avirulent H5N4 virus isolated from a migratory duck in Japan showed enough potency to induce protective immunity against the pathogenic H5N1 virus in mice. To expand surveillance for influenza viruses in migratory and domestic ducks and geese, chickens, quail, and pigs of the world and be informed about what influenza viruses are dominant in the animal reservoirs, we have started the "Programme of Excellence in Influenza". Influenza virus strains isolated from animal species in the surveillance should be thoroughly characterized, stored, and be provided for the use of diagnosis and vaccine preparation for the control of future pandemics. © 2001 Elsevier Science B.V. All rights reserved.

Keywords: Avian influenza; Surveillance; Vaccine strain

All of the known subtypes of influenza A viruses are circulating in ducks. The 1957 Asian H2N2 and A/Hong Kong/68 (H3N2) strains obtained their HA, PB1, and NA genes, and HA and PB1 genes from avian viruses and the remaining genes were from the preceding human strains, respectively. Since avian viruses of any subtype can contribute

* Corresponding author. Tel.: +81-11-706-5207; fax: +81-11-706-5273.
E-mail address: kida@vetmed.hokudai.ac.jp (H. Kida).

genes in the generation of reassortants in pigs [1], none of the 15 HA and 9 NA subtypes can be ruled out as potential candidates for future pandemics.

To provide information on the distribution of influenza viruses in the natural reservoir, virological surveillance of duck influenza was carried out in Alaska during their breeding season in summer. Influenza viruses of different subtypes were isolated from fecal samples of ducks and water samples of the lakes where they nest in Alaska. Viruses were isolated from the lake water still in autumn after the ducks had left for migration to the south. The results support the notion that influenza viruses are maintained in duck population by water-borne transmission and revealed the mechanism of year-by-year perpetuation of the viruses in the frozen lake water while ducks are absent. Phylogenetic analysis of the NP genes of the isolates showed that they belonged to the North American lineage of avian influenza viruses, suggesting that the host ducks nesting in the lakes on Yukon Flat and reservoiring influenza viruses migrate to North America and not to southern China, an influenza epicenter [2].

The transmission of H5N1 influenza viruses from domestic poultry to humans in Hong Kong in 1997 further emphasized the need to have information on influenza viruses circulating in avian species in the world. It is, therefore, essential to expand surveillance for influenza viruses in migratory and domestic ducks and geese, chickens, quail, and pigs of the world and be informed about what influenza viruses are circulating in the animal reservoirs. Influenza virus strains isolated from avian species in the surveillance should be characterized, stored, and be provided for the use of diagnosis and vaccine preparation for the prevention and control of pandemic influenza.

1. Results and discussion

To provide information on the precursor gene of future pandemic influenza viruses, virological surveillance of avian influenza was carried out in Siberia where ducks nest in summer and in Hokkaido, Japan where ducks congregate on their flyway of migration from Siberia to the South in autumn. Influenza A viruses of different subtypes were isolated from fecal samples of ducks in their nesting areas in Siberia in summer from 1996 to 1999. Phylogenetic analysis of the NP genes of the isolates in Siberia and those in Hokkaido revealed that they belong to the Eurasian lineage of avian influenza viruses. It is noted that the genes of the isolates in Siberia are closely related to those of H5N1 influenza virus strains isolated from chickens and humans in Hong Kong in 1997 as well as to those of isolates from domestic birds in southern China. The results indicate that influenza viruses have been perpetuated in ducks nesting in Siberia and that these viruses should have contributed genes in the emergence of the H5N1 virus in Hong Kong [3].

In the H5N1 influenza virus incident in Hong Kong in 1997 signaled the possibility of an incipient pandemic. However, it was not possible to prepare a vaccine against the virus in the conventional embryonated egg system because of the lethality of the virus for chicken embryos, and the high level of biosafety therefore required for vaccine production. Alternative approaches, including an avirulent A/duck/Hokkaido/67/96 (H5N4) influenza virus isolated from a duck in Hokkaido, Japan as a surrogate virus and H5N1 virus as a reassortant with avian virus H3N1 were explored. Both vaccines were formalin-inactivated. Intraperitoneal immunization of mice with each of vaccines elicited the production of hemagglutination-inhibiting and virus-neutralizing antibodies.

Then we tested whether these vaccines induce mucosal immune response. Each vaccine was dropped three times into the nostrils of 15 mice. Samples were taken from five mice for each group. The remaining 10 mice of each group were challenged with the highly pathogenic H5N1 virus. Intranasal vaccination without adjuvant induced both mucosal and systemic antibody responses that protected the mice from lethal H5N1 virus challenge [4]. Thus, intensive surveillance study of aquatic birds worldwide is stressed to provide information on the future pandemic influenza virus strains and for vaccine preparation.

Influenza surveillance in Taiwan and Siberia is being continued. In Taiwan, more than 200 influenza viruses have been isolated mainly from migratory ducks. Confirmed hemagglutinin subtypes of these viruses are so far H3, H4, and H7. Virological surveillance of avian influenza including that in live poultry markets is now under way in Taiwan, Thailand, Korea, and China.

References

[1] H. Kida, T. Ito, J. Yasuda, Y. Shimizu, C. Itakura, K.F. Shortridge, Y. Kawaoka, R.G. Webster, Potential for transmission of avian influenza viruses to pigs, J. Gen. Virol. 75 (1994) 2183–2188.

[2] T. Ito, K. Okazaki, Y. Kawaoka, A. Takada, R.G. Webster, H. Kida, Perpetuation of influenza A viruses in Alaskan waterfowl reservoirs, Arch. Virol. 140 (1995) 1163–1172.

[3] K. Okazaki, A. Takada, T. Ito, M. Imai, H. Takakuwa, M. Hatta, H. Ozaki, T. Tanizaki, T. Nagano, A. Ninomiya, V.A. Demenev, M.M. Tyaptirganov, T.D. Karatayeva, S.S. Yamnikova, D.K. Lvov, H. Kida, Precursor genes of future pandemic influenza viruses are perpetuated in ducks nesting in Siberia, Arch. Virol. 145 (2000) 885–893.

[4] A. Takada, N. Kuboki, K. Okazaki, A. Ninomiya, H. Tanaka, H. Ozaki, S. Itamura, H. Nishimura, M. Enami, M. Tashiro, K.F. Shortridge, H. Kida, Avirulent avian influenza virus as a vaccine strain against a potential human pandemic, J. Virol. 73 (1999) 8303–8307.

International Congress Series 1219 (2001) 173–178

The pig as an intermediate host for influenza A viruses between birds and humans

Ian H. Brown*

Virology Department, Veterinary Laboratories Agency-Weybridge, Addlestone, Weybridge, UK

Abstract

Swine influenza (SI) was first observed at the time of the pandemic in humans in 1918, and since that time, subtypes H1N1 and H3N2 have been widely reported in pigs, frequently associated with respiratory disease. These include classical swine H1N1, avian-like H1N1 and human- and avian-like H3N2 viruses. Swine husbandry practices influence directly the evolution of SI viruses through reduced immune pressure and constant availability of susceptible hosts. The pig has been the leading contender for the role of intermediate host for reassortment of influenza A viruses, since they are the only mammalian species which are susceptible to, and allow productive replication of avian and human influenza viruses due to the presence of receptors for both virus types ($\alpha2,3$ and $\alpha2,6$, respectively), and this can result in modification of the receptor binding specificities of avian influenza viruses from $\alpha2,3$ to $\alpha2,6$ linkage, thereby providing a potential link from birds to humans. Several independent introductions of avian viruses to pigs have occurred, primarily involving H1N1 that has led to the establishment of stable lineages, but more recently with H4N6 and H9N2 viruses. Although H3N2 viruses related closely to early human strains continue to circulate long after their disappearance from the human population, there have also been frequent transmissions of the prevailing human strains and these may also be able to persist. In addition, reassortant viruses of H3N2 and H1N2 subtype derived from mixed lineages and usually containing genes encoding surface glycoproteins from human viruses have been reported widely in pigs. Numerous transmissions of virus from pigs to humans have occurred but without apparent secondary spread. Pigs may be important in the generation of 'new' strains, some of which may have the potential to transmit to other species including humans. Crown Copyright © 2001 Published by Elsevier Science B.V. All rights reserved.

Keywords: Swine; Reassortment; Transmission

---

* Tel.: +44-1932-357-339; fax: +44-1932-357-239.
E-mail address: ibrown.vla@gtnet.gov.uk (I.H. Brown).

1. The potential role of the pig

Given the worldwide interaction between humans, pigs, birds and other mammalian species, there is a high potential for cross-species transmission of influenza viruses in nature. Pigs are an important host in influenza virus ecology since they are susceptible to infection with both avian and human influenza A viruses, often being involved in interspecies transmission, facilitated by regular close contact with humans or birds. Pigs serve as major reservoirs of H1N1 and H3N2 influenza viruses, and the maintenance of these viruses in pigs and the frequent introduction of viruses from other species may be important in the generation of 'new' strains of influenza, some of which may have the potential to transmit to other species including humans.

The pig has been the leading contender for the role of intermediate host for influenza A viruses. Pigs are the only mammalian species, which are domesticated, reared in abundance and are susceptible to, and allow productive replication of avian influenza viruses. This susceptibility is due to the presence of both $\alpha 2,3$- and $\alpha 2,6$-galactose sialic acid linkages in cells lining the pig trachea which can result in modification of the receptor binding specificities of avian influenza viruses from $\alpha 2,3$ to $\alpha 2,6$ linkage [1], which is the native linkage in humans, thereby providing a potential link from birds to humans.

It has been shown that humans occasionally contract influenza viruses from pigs. The internal protein genes of human influenza viruses share a common ancestor with the genes of some swine influenza viruses. A number of authors have proposed the nucleoprotein (NP) gene as a determinant of host range which can restrict or attenuate virus replication [2–4], thereby controlling the successful transmission of virus to a 'new' host. These observations support the potential role of the pig as a mixing vessel of influenza viruses from avian and human sources. The pig appears to have a broader host range in the compatibility of the NP gene in reassortant viruses [2] than both humans and birds. Studies by Kida et al. [5], investigating experimentally the growth potential of a wide diversity of avian influenza viruses in pigs, indicate that these viruses (including representatives of subtypes H1 to H13), with or without HA types known to infect humans, can be transmitted to pigs. Therefore, the possibility for the introduction of avian influenza virus genes to humans via pigs could occur. Furthermore, these studies showed that avian viruses, which do not replicate in pigs, can contribute genes in the generation of reassortants when coinfecting pigs with a swine influenza virus.

2. Pigs in the 'influenza epicentre'

The majority of pandemic strains has apparently originated in China raising the possibility that this region is an influenza epicentre. In China, influenza viruses of all subtypes are prevalent in ducks and in water frequented by ducks. This region accounts for over 60% of the world pig population, and agricultural practices provide that there is close contact between wild aquatic birds, domestic ducks, pigs and humans, thereby presenting the opportunity for interspecies transmission and genetic exchange among influenza viruses, with the pig acting as an intermediary between domestic ducks and humans. However, the interface between pigs and other species, particularly humans, is also significant in many other parts of the world (see pig to human transmission).

3. Transmission of avian influenza viruses to pigs

In Eurasia, there have been several introductions of avian H1N1 viruses to pigs that have led to the establishment of stable lineages. These viruses have spread widely in pigs in this region and are often associated with disease epizootics [6,7]. Recently, H9N2 viruses have apparently been introduced to pigs in South-East Asia, possibly from poultry, although the potential of these viruses to spread and persist in pigs remain unknown. In 1999, an avian H4N6 virus was isolated from pigs in Canada with respiratory symptoms. There was local spread on the farm, which was located next to an area of open water where waterfowl congregate. The genotype of the virus was entirely avian, although there were some modifications in the receptor binding pocket on the HA gene which may have facilitated binding to receptors with $\alpha 2,6$ linkage [8].

4. Genetic reassortment in the pig

4.1. Eurasia

Evidence for the pig as a mixing vessel of influenza viruses of non-swine origin has been demonstrated in Europe by Castrucci et al. [9], who detected reassortment of human and avian viruses in Italian pigs. Phylogenetic analyses of human H3N2 viruses circulating in Italian pigs revealed that genetic reassortment had been occurring between avian and 'human-like' viruses since 1983 [9]. The unique co-circulation of influenza A viruses within European swine may lead to pigs serving as a mixing vessel for reassortment between influenza viruses from mammalian and avian hosts with unknown implications for both humans and pigs. It would appear that human H1 viruses are able to perpetuate in pigs following genetic reassortment. Furthermore, these viruses may be maintained in pigs long after one or both of the progenitor viruses have disappeared from their natural hosts. Reassortant viruses of H1N2 subtype derived from human and avian viruses [10] or H1N7 subtype derived from human and equine viruses [11] have been isolated from pigs in Great Britain. The H1N2 viruses derived from a multiple reassortant event, spreading widely within pigs in Great Britain and subsequently to other parts of Europe. Viruses of H1N2 subtype have also been derived from genetic reassortment of strains endemic in pigs, and have been established in pigs in Japan since 1978 [12,13]. Similar viruses were detected in France but apparently failed to become established [14].

4.2. North America

Since 1998, H3N2 viruses isolated from pigs in the USA have contained combinations of human, swine and avian genes. Furthermore, the HA gene of these viruses was derived from a human virus circulating in the human population in 1995 [15]. These newly emerged H3N2 viruses appear to be established in pigs in North America and are able to reassort with classical H1N1 viruses producing another unique genotype of H1N2 virus [16].

5. Transmission between pigs and humans

Transmission of influenza A viruses from pigs to humans occurs on a regular basis, however, subsequent transmission of these viruses within the human population is very rare. Serological studies of people having occupational contact with pigs support frequent transmissions through the detection of antibodies to swine influenza viruses. Pigs were implicated as the source of infection when an H1N1 virus was isolated from a soldier who had died of influenza at Fort Dix, NJ, USA. The virus was identical to viruses isolated from pigs in the USA. Furthermore, five other servicemen were shown to be infected by virus isolation, and serological evidence suggested that some 500 personnel at Fort Dix were, or had been, infected with the same virus [17]. Subsequently, there have been several reports of classical swine H1N1 influenza virus being isolated from humans with respiratory illness, occasionally with fatal consequences. All cases examined followed contact with sick pigs. Perhaps of greater significance for humans is a report of two distinct cases of infection of children in the Netherlands during 1993 with H3N2 viruses whose genes encoding internal proteins were of avian origin [18]. Genetically and antigenically related viruses had been detected in European pigs [9], raising the possibility of potential transmission of avian influenza virus genes to humans following genetic reassortment in pigs. These concerns were substantiated further by the results of serological studies in Italy, which indicated that these 'swine' H3N2 viruses had apparently been transmitted to young, immunologically naive persons [19].

The prevailing strains in the human population transmit to pigs frequently but it would appear that only H3N2 viruses can establish stable lineages without genetic reassortment. Human H3N2 viruses are endemic in most pig populations worldwide, where they persist many years after their antigenic counterparts have disappeared from humans, and therefore, present a reservoir of virus which may in the future infect a susceptible human population. However, there is no apparent evidence of pigs being infected with this subtype prior to the pandemic in humans in 1968.

6. Adaptation of 'new' influenza viruses to pigs

Following interspecies transmission and/or genetic reassortment, an influenza virus may undergo many pig-to-pig transmissions because of the continual availability of susceptible pigs. The mechanisms whereby an avian virus is able to establish a new lineage in pigs remain unclear, although following the introduction of an avian virus into European pigs in 1979, the virus was relatively unstable for approximately 10 years [20], but the mutation rate of this virus did not subsequently increase [21]. Furthermore, adaptation of this virus to pigs resulted in the virus acquiring altered receptor specificity, preferentially recognizing receptors with $\alpha 2,6$ linkage [1], the native linkage in humans (see Role of the pig). It would appear that the adaptive processes can take many years as occurred, following transmission of both avian H1N1 and human H3N2 viruses to pigs. Following new introductions of influenza A virus to pigs, close monitoring of the epizootiology of SI in a population is essential to determine the rate of change, which, if elevated, may facilitate further transmissions across the species barrier with potential implications for disease control in a range of other species including humans.

References

[1] T. Ito, J. Nelson, S.S. Couceiro, S. Kelm, L.G. Baum, S. Krauss, M.R. Castrucci, I. Donatelli, H. Kida, J.C. Paulson, R.G. Webster, Y. Kawaoka, Molecular basis for the generation in pigs of influenza A viruses with pandemic potential, J. Virol. 72 (1998) 7367–7373.

[2] C. Scholtissek, H. Burger, O. Kistner, K.F. Shortridge, The nucleoprotein as a possible major factor in determining host specificity of influenza H3N2 viruses, Virology 147 (1985) 287–294.

[3] S.F. Tian, A.J. Buckler-White, W.J. London, L.J. Recle, R.M. Channock, B.R. Murphy, Nucleoprotein and membrane protein genes are associated with restriction of influenza A/mallard/NY/78 virus and its reassortants in squirrel monkey respiratory tract, J. Virol. 53 (1985) 771–775.

[4] M.H. Snyder, A.J. Buckler-White, W.T. London, E.L. Tierney, B.R. Murphy, The avian influenza virus nucleoprotein gene and a specific constellation of avian and human virus polymerase genes each specify attenuation of avian human influenza A/Pintail/79 reassortant viruses for monkeys, J. Virol. 61 (1987) 2857–2863.

[5] H. Kida, T. Ito, J. Yasuda, Y. Shimizu, C. Itakura, K.F. Shortridge, Y. Kawaoka, R.G. Webster, Potential for transmission of avian influenza viruses to pigs, J. Gen. Virol. 75 (1994) 2183–2188.

[6] M. Pensaert, K. Ottis, J. Vandeputte, M.M. Kaplan, P.A. Bachmann, Evidence for the natural transmission of influenza A virus from wild ducks to swine and its potential importance for man, Bull. W.H.O. 59 (1981) 75–78.

[7] Y. Guan, K.F. Shortridge, S. Krauss, P.H. Li, Y. Kawaoka, R.G. Webster, Emergence of avian H1N1 influenza viruses in pigs in China, J. Virol. 70 (1996) 8041–8046.

[8] A.I. Karasin, I.H. Brown, S. Carmen, C.W. Olsen, Isolation and characterization of H4N6 avian influenza viruses from pigs with pneumonia in Canada, J. Virol., in press.

[9] M.R. Castrucci, I. Donatelli, L. Sidoli, G. Barigazzi, Y. Kawaoka, R.G. Webster, Genetic reassortment between avian and human influenza A viruses in Italian pigs, Virology 193 (1993) 503–506.

[10] I.H. Brown, P.A. Harris, J.W. McCauley, D.J. Alexander, Multiple genetic reassortment of avian and human influenza A viruses in European pigs, resulting in the emergence of an H1N2 virus of novel genotype, J. Gen. Virol. 79 (1998) 2947–2955.

[11] I.H. Brown, D.J. Alexander, P. Chakraverty, P.A. Harris, R.J. Manvell, Isolation of an influenza A virus of unusual subtype (H1N7) from pigs in England, and the subsequent experimental transmission from pig to pig, Vet. Microbiol. 39 (1994) 125–134.

[12] T. Sugimura, H. Yonemochi, T. Ogawa, Y. Tanaka, T. Kumagai, Isolation of a recombinant influenza virus (Hsw1N2) from swine in Japan, Arch. Virol. 66 (1980) 271–274.

[13] A. Ouchi, K. Nerome, Y. Kanegae, M. Ishida, R. Nerome, K. Hayashi, T. Hashimoto, M. Kaji, Y. Kaji, Y. Inaba, Large outbreak of swine influenza in southern Japan caused by reassortant (H1N2) influenza viruses: its epizootic background and characterisation of the causative viruses, J. Gen. Virol. 77 (1996) 1751–1759.

[14] J.M. Gourreau, C. Kaiser, M. Valette, A.R. Douglas, J. Labie, M. Aymard, Isolation of two H1N2 influenza viruses from swine in France, Arch. Virol. 135 (1994) 365–382.

[15] N.N. Zhou, D.A. Senne, J.S. Landgraf, S.L. Swenson, G. Erickson, K. Rossow, L. Liu, K.J. Yoon, S. Krauss, R.G. Webster, Genetic reassortment of avian, swine and human influenza A viruses in American pigs, J. Virol. 73 (1999) 8851–8856.

[16] A.I. Karasin, C.W. Olsen, G.A. Anderson, Genetic characterization of an H1N2 influenza virus isolated from a pig in Indiana, J. Clin. Microbiol. 38 (2000) 2453–2456.

[17] R.A. Hodder, J.C. Gaydos, R.G. Allen, F.H. Top, T. Nowosiwsky, P.K. Russell, Swine influenza A at Fort-Dix New Jersey January–February 1976. Extent of spread and duration of outbreak, J. Infect. Dis. 136 (1977) S369–S375.

[18] E.C.J. Claas, Y. Kawaoka, J.C. DeJong, N. Masurel, R.G. Webster, Infection of children with avian–human reassortant influenza virus from pigs in Europe, Virology 204 (1994) 453–457.

[19] L. Campitelli, I. Donatelli, E. Foni, M.R. Castrucci, C. Fabiani, Y. Kawaoka, S. Krauss, R.G. Webster, Continued evolution of H1N1 and H3N2 influenza viruses in pigs in Italy, Virology 232 (1997) 310–318.

[20] S. Ludwig, L. Stitz, O. Planz, H. Van, W.M. Fitch, C. Scholtissek, European swine virus as a possible source for the next influenza pandemic? Virology 212 (1995) 555–561.

[21] J. Stech, X. Xiong, C. Scholtissek, R.G. Webster, Independence of evolutionary and mutational rates after transmission of avian influenza viruses to swine, J. Virol. 73 (1999) 1878–1884.

International Congress Series 1219 (2001) 179–185

Recent examples of human infection by animal and avian influenza A viruses in Hong Kong

Y.P. Lin[a,*], W. Lim[b], V. Gregory[a], K. Cameron[a],
M. Bennett[a], A. Hay[a]

[a]National Institute for Medical Research, The Ridgeway, Mill Hill, London, NW7 1AA, UK
[b]Queen Mary Hospital, Hong Kong SAR, China

Abstract

Recent intensive surveillance in Hong Kong resulted in the detection of two novel viruses in children during 1999—two cases of infection by an H9N2 avian virus in March and a single case of infection by an H3N2 swine virus in September. The two human H9N2 isolates are similar in antigenic and genetic characteristics to an H9N2 virus isolated from a quail in late 1997, but are antigenically distinct from other lineages of H9N2 viruses circulating in other species of birds as well as those isolated from pigs during 1998. It is likely, therefore, that as for the H5N1 viruses in 1997, these infections are the result of direct avian-to-human transmission. A striking similarity between the six internal genes of the H9N2 and H5N1 human isolates indicates that they are related by reassortment. The H3N2 virus A/HK/1774/99 is distinct from contemporary human H3N2 viruses and is similar in antigenic and genetic properties to H3N2 viruses recently circulating in pigs in Europe. Although the source of infection was not traced, the likely presence of similar viruses in pigs in Hong Kong has subsequently been confirmed. These two instances provide further evidence for the direct transfer of avian and swine viruses in causing human disease and highlights the potential for emergence, either by adaptation or genetic reassortment with a circulating human strain, of a novel human pathogen. © 2001 Elsevier Science B.V. All rights reserved.

Keywords: H9N2; Surveillance; Transmission; Swine; Human; Hong Kong

1. Introduction

One of the principal objectives of the WHO Global Surveillance Network is the early detection and characterization of novel influenza A viruses which enter the human

---

* Corresponding author. Tel.: +44-20-8959-3666x2152; fax: +44-20-8906-4477.
E-mail address: lyipu@nimr.mrc.ac.uk (Y.P. Lin).

0531-5131/01/$ – see front matter © 2001 Elsevier Science B.V. All rights reserved.
PII: S0531-5131(01)00379-X

population and may have the potential to cause a pandemic. Influenza A viruses comprise a diverse array of antigenically distinguishable subtypes, which include various combinations of 15 HA subtypes and 9 NA subtypes [1]. The natural host is aquatic birds in which the viruses replicate mainly asymptomatically in the intestinal tract. Only a few subtypes have become established for significant periods of time in mammalian species, e.g. two (H7N7 and H3N8) in horses, three (H1N1, H3N2 and H1N2) in pigs and three (H1N1, H2N2 and H3N2) in the human population. That the strict species barrier can be breached with potentially devastating consequences was starkly demonstrated by the Hong Kong 'bird flu' incident in which 18 cases of human infection by an H5N1 virus resulted in six deaths [2,3]. In this instance domestic chickens, the source of most infections, appeared to act as an intermediate host in avian-to-human transmission. Pigs, which are readily infected by avian and human viruses, may act as an intermediate host both for transmission and in facilitating genetic reassortment between avian and human viruses, as may have occurred prior to the emergence of the 1957 H2N2 and 1968 H3N2 pandemic viruses [4].

In this paper, we consider further recent examples in Hong Kong of avian-to-human transmission of novel H9N2 viruses and swine-to-human transmission of an H3N2 virus similar to H3N2 viruses circulating in pigs in Europe.

2. Avian-to-human transmission of H9N2 viruses

In late 1997 during the H5 outbreak, several subtypes were identified in domestic poultry in addition to H5N1, of which H9N2 was the most prevalent [5]. The isolation of H9N2 viruses from pigs in Hong Kong in mid-1998 (D. Markwell and K. Shortridge, personal communication) raised concerns about their possible transmission to the human population, which was confirmed by reports in early 1999 of human isolates in Southern China [6]. In March 1999, A/HK/1073/99 and A/HK/1074/99 were isolated in Hong Kong from two patients with mild influenza, a 4-year-old girl and a 13-month-old girl, respectively [7].

Haemagglutination inhibition (HI) tests using post-infection ferret antisera showed that the HAs of these two human viruses were antigenically indistinguishable and were closely related to the HA of a quail H9N2 virus isolated in late 1997, A/quail/Hong Kong/G1/97 (Qa/HK/G1/97) and that these three viruses were clearly distinguishable from the closely related chicken and swine H9N2 viruses, A/chicken/Hong Kong/G9/97 (Ck/HK/G9/97) and A/swine/Hong Kong/9/98 (Sw/HK/9/98). The antigenic relationships were confirmed by sequence analyses which showed that the HA genes of the human and quail isolates shared 99% sequence homology and were distantly related to the HA genes of other H9N2 viruses which fall into phylogenetically distinguishable lineages.

Comparisons of the nucleotide sequences of all eight genes of the two human isolates with those of H9N2 viruses isolated from different species of birds in Hong Kong in 1997 emphasized the striking similarity between the human and quail/G1 isolates (99% or greater homology; Table 1). This contrasts with the differences (85–96% homology) between the genes of the human viruses and those of, e.g. A/duck/Hong Kong/Y280/97 (Dk/HK/Y280/97) and A/chicken/Hong Kong/Y439/97 (Dk/HK/Y439/97), which are representative of different phylogenetic lineages (Ref. [5]; Table 1). The similarity to

Table 1
Genetic relationships between H9N2 and H5N1 viruses

Gene	(% Homology to A/HK/1073/99)					
	A/HK/97 (H5N1)	Qa/HK/G1/97	Ck/PK/2/99	Ck/SA/[a]224/98	Dk/HK/Y280/97	Dk/HK/Y439/97
PB2	98	99	98	90	85	87
PB1	99	99	98	89	90	91
PA	98	99	98	90	90	90
H9	–	99	97	95	91	85
NP	99	99	99	94	90	94
N2	–	99	97	98	94	89
M	98	99	99	98	96	91
NS	98	100	98	90	93	91

[a] Based on partial sequences.

Qa/HK/G1/97 indicates that the two human viruses did not acquire, by genetic reassortment, any genes from another source including contemporary human viruses and that the human infections were most likely due to direct transmission of virus from infected birds, although the actual source is not known. Furthermore, it is evident that a swine virus similar to Sw/HK/9/98 was not an intermediate in transmission.

A particularly notable feature is the similarity between the internal genes (encoding PB2, PB1, PA, NP, M and NS proteins) of the two human H9N2 viruses and Qa/HK/G1/97 and those of the H5N1 viruses which cocirculated in poultry in late 1997 and caused fatal human infections. Thus, on the one hand, one or other or both of the virus subtypes may have arisen by genetic reassortment; the progenitor virus remains to be identified [8]. On the other hand, this common feature suggests that some (or all) of these genes may facilitate avian-to-human transmission; however the factors important for interspecies transmission are poorly understood.

A feature of the HA which is important in determining host range is its receptor specificity and changes in preference for sialic acid (SA) linked to the penultimate

Table 2
Comparisons of the genes of A/HK/1774/99 with the genes of recent human H3N2 viruses, European swine viruses and viruses circulating recently in pigs and avian species in Hong Kong

Gene	Homology (%)				
	European swine[a]	A/HK/1073/99	DK/HK/Y280/97	Sw/HK/168/93[b]	Human (H3N2)[c]
PB2	96	86	88	90	83
PB1	95	88	88	90	86
PA	95	87	86	86	85
H3	95	–	–	–	83
NP	97	89	90	91	81
N2	95	81	81	–	87
M	97	90	91	91	87
NS	97	90	89	89	85

[a] Indicates the highest homology with genes of H3N2 or H1N1 viruses.
[b] Data based on partial nucleotide sequences of PB1, PB2 and PA genes.
[c] Representative recent human viruses.

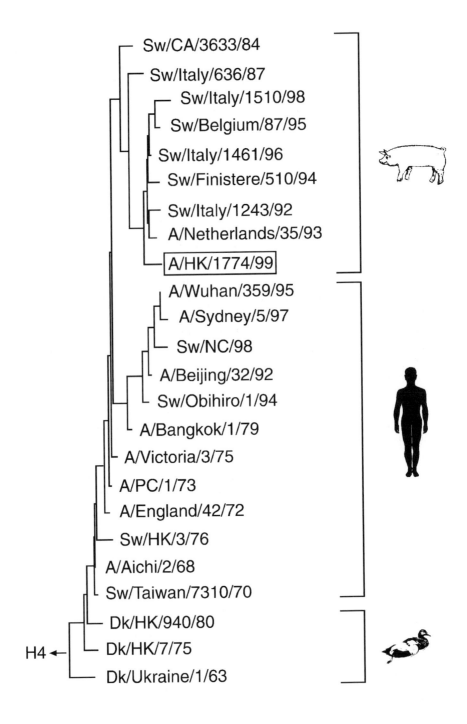

galactose (gal) of the receptor by an α2,3 bond (SA α2,3 gal) to one linked by an α2,6 bond (SA α2,6 gal) has been observed to accompany establishment of avian viruses (or their HAs) in human and swine hosts [9]. Differences in "conserved" amino acids in the receptor binding site [10] which distinguish the human and quail G1 viruses from other H9N2 viruses is the combination of histidine 183, glutamic acid 190 and leucine 226 (numbered according to H3) which was present in early human H3N2 viruses [7]. Whether these amino acids have a role in increasing affinity for SA α2,6 gal receptors and increasing the probability of human infection has yet to be determined. In this context, however, the H5N1 viruses, which caused human infections, were shown like other avian viruses to have a preference for SA α2,3 gal receptors [11].

3. H9N2 viruses in Pakistan

H9N2 viruses are widespread and have recently been responsible for outbreaks of disease in poultry in various parts of the world, notably Middle Eastern countries such as Iran, Pakistan and Saudi Arabia. Comparison of partial HA sequences showed that the H9s of viruses isolated during 1998 and 1999 in Germany, Iran, Pakistan and Saudi Arabia were closely related to the H9s of the human and quail G1 viruses isolated in Hong Kong and distinct from other phylogenetic lineages of H9 [12,13]. Comparison of the genes of one of the more closely related viruses (in terms of HA) A/chicken/Pakistan/2/99 (Ck/Pk/2/99) showed that it was closely related (97–99% sequence homology) in all 8 genes to the human and quail G1 viruses (Table 1). Thus, H9N2 viruses closely related to those which infected the two children in Hong Kong SAR are circulating more widely in other parts of Asia. Whether these viruses do in fact possess a similar capacity for interspecies transmission to humans is unknown. Although Ck/Pk/2/99 is typical of other viruses isolated in Pakistan, further analyses of the viruses isolated in Germany, Iran and Saudi Arabia showed that they represent reassortants, deriving genes from other previously characterized lineages of H9N2 viruses ([5]; Y. Lin, K. Cameron, V. Gregory and J. Banks, unpublished results). For example, whereas the NA and M genes of A/chicken/Saudi Arabia/224/98 (Ck/SA/224/98), in addition to the HA, correspond to the quail G1 lineage, the other five genes are more closely related to those of the lineages represented by Dk/HK/Y439/97 or A/chicken/Korea/6/96 (Table 1).

4. Swine-to-human transmission

In September 1999, an H3N2 virus A/HK/1774/99 was isolated in Hong Kong SAR from a 10-month-old girl with mild influenza symptoms [14]. It was antigenically distinct from A/Sydney/5/97-like (H3N2) viruses recently circulating in the human population and was closely related to early human and swine H3N2 viruses such as A/Port Chalmers/1/73

Fig. 1. Phylogenetic comparisons of nucleotide sequences encoding H3 HAs (nucleotides 1–994). Sequences were obtained as in Ref. [14] or from Genbank. Dk, duck; Sw, swine; CA, Cotes d'Armor; HK, Hong Kong; NC, North Carolina; PC, Port Chalmers.

(A/PC/1/73) and A/swine/Cotes d'Armor/3633/84 (Sw/CA/3633/84), respectively. Comparisons of the nucleotide sequences of the eight genes of A/HK/1774/99 with available sequence data demonstrated a close relationship to H3N2 viruses recently circulating in European pigs (Table 2). For example, phylogenetic analyses showed that the HA (Fig. 1) and NA genes of A/HK/1774/99 were most closely related (95% homology) to the Italian isolate A/swine/Italy/1461/96. Analyses of amino acid sequences showed that the HA of A/HK/1774/99 contains several residues which are typical of the H3 s of swine viruses isolated in Europe during the 1990s when compared with similar H3N2 viruses circulating prior to 1987. Although a number of variants have been distinguished among recent H3N2 viruses none was particularly closely related to A/HK/1774/99.

A/HK/1774/99 is thus similar in antigenic and genetic characteristics to H3N2 viruses recently prevalent in European pigs and had not acquired by reassortment any genes from other genetically distinguishable viruses circulating recently in human, pig (e.g., A/swine/HK/163/93, Table 2) or domestic poultry (e.g., A/HK/1073/97 and Dk/HK/Y280/97, H9N2) populations in South East Asia. There were no reports of isolation of similar viruses from pigs in Hong Kong prior to isolation of A/HK/1774/99. The more recent identification of related viruses in pigs in Hong Kong (K. Shortridge, personal communication) is consistent with local pigs as the source of infection, although it is not clear how the child contracted the infection. A serological study of family members confirmed infection of the child but failed to demonstrate conclusively whether or not other family members may also have been infected; no family member had recent contact with pigs. Of particular interest is the antigenic and genetic similarity between A/HK/1774/99 and two viruses, A/Netherlands/5/93 and A/Netherlands/35/93, which infected two children in the Netherlands in 1993 [15]. This incident in Hong Kong therefore represents another example of sporadic human infection by a swine influenza virus with little evidence of human-to-human transmission. An important property of these viruses, like other viruses circulating in European pigs since about 1987 [16], is their resistance to the anti-influenza A drugs, amantadine and rimantadine. Their wider geographical distribution in pigs, which have been implicated in the emergence, by genetic reassortment, of novel pandemic subtypes [4], thus increases the potential for the emergence of drug-resistant human viruses.

Acknowledgements

We acknowledge the contributions of many scientists (some cited in original papers, Refs. [7,13,14]) in various laboratories who collaborated on global surveillance and characterization of human, animal and avian viruses to the work reviewed in this article.

References

[1] R.G. Webster, W.J. Bean, O.T. Gorman, T.M. Chambers, Y. Kawaoka, Microbiol. Rev. 56 (1992) 152–179.
[2] E. Claas, A. Osterhaus, R. van Beek, J. De Jong, G. Rimmelzwaan, D. Senne, S. Krauss, K. Shortridge, R.G. Webster, Lancet 351 (1998) 447–472.

[3] K. Subbarao, A. Klimov, J. Katz, H. Regnery, W. Lim, H. Hall, M. Perdue, D. Swayne, C. Bender, H. Jing, et al., Science 279 (1998) 393–396.

[4] C. Scholtissek, H. Burger, O. Kistner, K.F. Shortridge, Virology 147 (1985) 287–294.

[5] Y. Guan, K.F. Shortridge, S. Krauss, R.G. Webster, Proc. Natl. Acad. Sci. U. S. A. 96 (1999) 9363–9367.

[6] Y. Guo, J. Li, X. Cheng, M. Wang, Y. Zhou, X.H. Li, F. Cai, H.L. Miao, H. Zhang, F. Guo, et al., Chin. J. Exp. Clin. Virol. 13 (1999) 105–108.

[7] Y.P. Lin, M. Shaw, V. Gregory, K. Cameron, W. Lim, A. Klimov, K. Subbarao, Y. Guan, S. Krauss, K. Shortridge, R. Webster, N. Cox, A. Hay, Proc. Natl. Acad. Sci. U. S. A. 97 (2000) 9654–9658.

[8] E. Hoffman, J. Stech, I. Leneva, S. Krauss, C. Scholtissek, P.S. Chin, M. Peiris, K.F. Shortridge, R.G. Webster, J. Virol. 74 (2000) 6309–6315.

[9] R.J. Connor, Y. Kawaoka, R.G. Webser, J.C. Paulson, Virology 205 (1994) 17–23.

[10] W. Weis, J.H. Brown, S. Cusack, J.C. Paulson, J.J. Skehel, D.C. Wiley, Nature (London) 333 (1988) 426–431.

[11] M. Matrosovich, N. Zhou, Y. Kawaoka, R. Webster, J. Virol. 73 (1999) 1146–1155.

[12] J. Banks, E.C. Speidel, P.A. Harris, D.J. Alexander, Avian Pathol. 29 (2000) 353–360.

[13] K.R. Cameron, V. Gregory, J. Banks, I.H. Brown, D.J. Alexander, A.J. Hay, Y.P. Lin, Virology 278 (2000) 36–41.

[14] V. Gregory, W. Lim, K. Cameron, M. Bennett, A. Klimov, N. Cox, A.J. Hay, Y.P. Lin, (2000) submitted for publication.

[15] E.C.J. Claas, Y. Kawaoka, J.C. De Jong, N. Masurel, R.G. Webster, Virology 204 (1994) 453–457.

[16] M. Bennett, S. Grambas, K. Cameron, Y. Lin, A. Hay, (2001) submitted for publication.

International Congress Series 1219 (2001) 187–193

Two lineages of H9N2 influenza viruses continue to circulate in land-based poultry in southeastern China

Y. Guan[a,b,*], K.F. Shortridge[a], S. Krauss[b], P.S. Chin[a], K.C. Dyrting[c], T.M. Ellis[c], R.G. Webster[a,b], M. Peiris[a]

[a]Department of Microbiology, The University of Hong Kong, University Pathology Building,
Queen Mary Hospital, Hong Kong SAR, China
[b]Department of Virology and Molecular Biology, St. Jude Children's Research Hospital,
Memphis, TN 38105, USA
[c]Department of Agriculture Fisheries and Conservation, Hong Kong SAR, China

Abstract

Background: The transmission of H9N2 influenza viruses to humans and the realization that the A/Hong Kong/156/97-like (H5N1/97-like) internal genome complex is still present in southeastern China necessitated a study of the distribution and characterization of H9N2 viruses in poultry in the Hong Kong SAR in 1999. *Methods*: Virus isolation, serological identification and genetic analysis. *Results*: Two lineages of H9N2 influenza viruses were isolated in the live poultry markets and are represented by A/Quail/Hong Kong/G1/97 (Qa/HK/G1/97) and A/Duck/Hong Kong/Y280/97 (Dk/HK/Y280/97). No reassortment between the two H9N2 virus lineages was detected despite their co-circulation in the poultry markets. The Qa/HK/G1/97-like viruses were isolated most frequently from quail and Dk/HK/Y280/97-like viruses from chicken. *Conclusion*: The high prevalence of quail infected with Qa/HK/G1/97-like virus that contains six gene segments genetically highly related to H5N1/97-like virus emphasizes the need for continued surveillance of mammals including humans for the H9N2 virus. © 2001 Elsevier Science B.V. All rights reserved.

Keywords: H9; H9N2; Poultry; Evolution

1. Introduction

The "bird flu" H5N1 incident in Hong Kong in 1997 caused global concern because of its high case fatality rate in humans and potential for a pandemic. Surveillance in the

---

* Corresponding author. Department of Microbiology, The University of Hong Kong, University Pathology Building, Queen Mary Hospital, Hong Kong SAR, China. Tel.: +852-2855-4892; fax: +852-2855-1241.
E-mail address: yguan@hkucc.hku.hk (Y. Guan).

poultry markets in December 1997 revealed that H9N2 influenza viruses co-circulated with H5N1 viruses in the markets. Subsequent studies suggested that H9N2 (Qa/HK/G1/ 97-like) and H6N1 (Teal/HK/W312/97-like) influenza viruses were the possible precursors providing all of the internal genes for the H5N1/97 virus [1,2].

Even though H5N1/97-like viruses have not been isolated since the poultry were depopulated across the SAR in late December 1997, isolation studies indicate that H9N2 viruses are still present in poultry in southern China [3]. The transmission to humans of H9N2 viruses that contain the H5N1/97-like internal genes [4,5] emphasizes the need for better understanding of the occurrence and evolution of these viruses in the poultry markets of Hong Kong.

2. Materials and methods

2.1. Sampling and virus isolation

Different types of poultry presenting in 35 live retail poultry markets of Hong Kong were sampled. Samples were inoculated into 9- to 10-day-old chicken embryos and virus isolates were identified as previously described [6,7]. In the current study, only land-based birds were sampled, as live aquatic birds are no longer present in these markets.

2.2. Gene sequencing and analysis

Viruses used in the present study are given in Table 1 and Fig. 1. Viral gene sequencing and analysis were carried out as previously described [1]. Sequence data were edited and analyzed using the Wisconsin Sequence Analysis Package, Version 10.0 (GCG, Madison, WI). The nucleotide sequences are available from GenBank under accession numbers AF222606 through AF222681.

3. Results

3.1. Isolation of H9N2 influenza viruses from poultry in the Hong Kong SAR in 1999

Of the 35 markets tested from April–November 1999, 27 contained H9N2 influenza viruses and overall 5.2% of faecal samples from cages of domestic poultry contained H9N2 viruses. These viruses were found in the faeces of most types of poultry examined. The majority of H9N2 influenza virus isolates were from chicken (62%) quail (17%), silky chicken (7%) and the remainder from pheasant, Guinea fowl, and pigeon.

3.2. Characterization of H9N2 viruses isolated in the poultry markets in Hong Kong

3.2.1. Antigenic analysis
Ferret or chicken antisera to the reference strain of the lineages found previously in the SAR [1] were included in the analysis. The H9N2 influenza viruses isolated in 1999 belong

Table 1
Antigenic analysis of H9N2 influenza viruses

Virus[a]	HI titers with chicken antisera to	HI titers with ferret antisera to		
	Dk/HK/Y280/97	Qa/HK/G1/97	Ck/HK/G9/97	HK/1073/99
Qa/HK/G1/97	80	320	<	80
Qa/HK/A17/99[b]	80	160	<	1280
Pg/HK/FY6/99	80	40	<	640
Ck/HK/NT16/99	160	160	<	1280
Qa/HK/SSP10/99	80	160	<	1280
Ph/HK/SSP11/99	80	40	<	640
Dk/HK/Y280/97	640	<	320	<
Ck/HK/SF2/99[b]	2560	40	1280	80
Ck/HK/FY20/99	2560	<	1280	80
Qa/HK/NT28/99	640	<	160	<
Ck/HK/KC12/99	1280	<	640	80
SCk/HK/SF44/99	2560	<	1280	80
Dk/HK/Y439/97	80	<	<	<
Ck/Kor/006/96	160	<	<	<

[a] Virus abbreviation: Poultry — quail, Qa; chicken, Ck; pigeon, Pg; pheasant, Ph; duck, Dk; silky chicken, SCk. Place — Hong Kong, HK; Korea, Kor.

[b] Viruses shown in bold are strains isolated as part of this study. Starting dilution of antisera 1:40.

to either the Qa/HK/G1/97-like or the Dk/HK/Y280/97-like virus lineages (Table 1). It is noteworthy that most of the H9N2 viruses similar to Qa/HK/G1/97 were from quail, while viruses represented by Dk/HK/Y280/97 were mainly from chicken with fewer isolates from

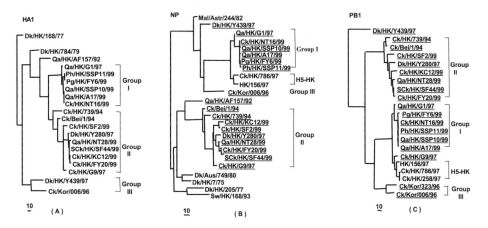

Fig. 1. Phylogenetic trees for the H9 HA1 (A), NP (B) and PB1(C) genes of influenza A viruses. The nucleotide sequences of the HA1, NP and PB1 genes were analyzed with PAUP by using a maximum-parsimony algorithm. Nucleotides 55–1014 (960 bp) of H9 HA1, nucleotides 48–1398 (1351 bp) of NP gene and nucleotides 67–1428 (1362 bp) of PB1 gene were used for the phylogenetic analysis. The HA1 phylogenetic tree is rooted to A/Duck/Alberta/60/76 (H12N5). The NP phylogenetic tree is rooted to A/Equine/Prague/1/56 (H7N7), and the PB1 tree is rooted to B/Lee/40. All viruses underlined in the NP and PB1 gene trees are H9N2 influenza viruses. Groups I, II and III designations are based on phylogenetic relationships of the HA1 gene.

silky chicken. No virus belonging to the Ck/Korea/006/96 lineage was isolated in 1999 from poultry in Hong Kong.

3.2.2. Molecular analysis

To provide complete genotyping of H9N2 influenza viruses isolated five representative isolates of the Qa/HK/G1/97-like and Dk/HK/Y280/97-like viruses were analyzed (Table 2). Each of the gene segments was partially sequenced and their homologies compared with representative strains from 1997. A/Quail/Hong Kong/A17/99 (A17) is representative of all the viruses in its group and closely related to Qa/HK/G1/97 in all eight gene segments. These viruses also have their six gene segments highly related to H5N1/97. A17 was distinguishable in all gene segments from Dk/HK/Y280/97. Conversely, A/Chicken/Hong Kong/FY20/99 (FY20) had all eight gene segments closely related to Dk/HK/Y280/97 and six of which were also closely related to Ck/HK/G9/97. It is noteworthy that no virus containing the full gene complement of Ck/HK/G9/97 has been found since 1997.

3.2.3. Phylogenetic analysis

To further understand the evolutionary relationship between these viruses phylogenetic analysis of the HA1, NP and PB1 of representative H9N2 influenza viruses isolated from 1999 were carried out (Fig. 1). In the HA1 tree, the quail, pigeon and pheasant isolates represented by A17 are phylogenetically (Fig. 1A) similar to Qa/HK/G1/97 (Group 1). The

Table 2
Homology of the gene segments of 1999 H9N2 influenza viruses with reference strain

Viruses (represented by)	Gene segments	Homology[a], % with the following influenza viruses			
		Qa/HK/G1/97	Dk/HK/Y280/97	Ck/HK/G9/97	HK/156/97(H5N1)
Qa/HK/A17/99	PB2	**98.8** (98.9)[b]	85.6 (85.7)	**97.4** (97.5)	**97.8** (97.9)
	PB1	**99.2** (99.2)	91.0 (90.8)	**98.2** (98.1)	**98.3** (98.3)
	PA	**98.7** (98.7)	88.9 (88.9)	88.4 (88.3)	**97.4** (97.4)
	HA	**98.9** (98.7)	90.1 (90.1)	90.7 (90.7)	–[c]
	NP	**99.1** (99.2)	88.7 (88.7)	89.0 (89.1)	**97.7** (97.8)
	NA	**99.2** (99.2)	93.5 (93.4)	93.1 (93.0)	–
	M	**99.3** (99.2)	96.7 (96.6)	96.5 (96.4)	**99.2** (99.1)
	NS	**99.9** (99.9)	93.7 (93.7)	93.3 (93.3)	**98.6** (98.6)
Ck/HK/FY20/99	PB2	86.4 (86.0)	**99.0** (98.5)	86.3 (85.8)	86.3 (86.0)
	PB1	90.6 (90.7)	**97.9** (97.8)	90.8 (90.8)	90.4 (90.4)
	PA	89.1 (89.1)	**98.9** (98.3)	**96.5** (96.7)	88.7 (88.8)
	HA	89.4 (90.0)	**98.5** (98.5)	**96.5** (97.0)	–
	NP	89.2 (88.9)	**98.5** (98.3)	**98.2** (98.1)	89.4 (89.1)
	NA	93.5 (93.2)	**99.6** (98.8)	**94.5** (94.2)	–
	M	95.9 (96.2)	**99.0** (99.1)	**98.5** (98.6)	96.0 (96.3)
	NS	93.0 (93.1)	**98.1** (97.8)	**97.9** (97.6)	93.5 (93.7)

[a] Homologies were calculated based on the nucleotide sequences of PB1 (988–2289), PB1 (67–1428), PA (19–1677), HA (88–1077), NP (34–1398), NA (20–1421), M (50–982), and NS (41–879).

[b] Mean homologies for the 5 viruses shown in bold type in each group in Table 1 which were isolated in 1999.

[c] Different HA or NA subtypes.

chicken and silky chicken isolates represented by FY20 are phylogenetically highly related to Dk/HK/Y280/97 (Group II). Similar topologies are also observed in the NP and PB1 gene trees (Fig. 1B,C). All H9N2 viruses isolated in 1999 clustered either into Qa/HK/G1/97 lineage or Dk/HK/Y280/97 lineage. No virus related to Ck/HK/G9/97 or Ck/Korea/006/96 viruses was isolated in 1999.

In addition to the 10 strains of H9N2 isolates from 1999 shown in Fig. 1, 34 other H9N2 isolates were genotyped by partial sequencing of the HA1 gene. Overall these 44 strains were from chicken ($n=18$), silky chicken ($n=5$), chukka ($n=1$), quail ($n=12$), pigeon ($n=2$), pheasant ($n=3$), Guinea fowl ($n=1$) and from cages with mixed birds ($n=2$). Seventeen (94%) chicken isolates, 1 quail, 1 pigeon, 1 pheasant, 1 chukka and all 5 silky chicken isolates were of the Dk/HK/Y280/97 lineage. In contrast, 11 of 12 (92%) quail, 1 chicken, 1 pigeon, 2 pheasant and 1 Guinea fowl isolates belonged to the Qa/HK/G1/97 lineage. The apparent specificity of the two lineages for chicken and quail is maintained even within the same market on any given occasion.

4. Discussion

The present studies establish that two phylogenetic lineages of H9N2 influenza viruses continue to circulate in the poultry of southeastern China. One lineage is circulating predominantly in quail and is represented by Qa/HK/G1/97; members of this lineage carry six internal gene segments highly related to those found in H5N1/97 that transmitted directly to humans from chicken causing lethal infection in 6 of 18 persons in 1997 [8,9]. Viruses almost identical in all gene segments with Qa/HK/G1/97 transmitted to two children in Hong Kong in 1992 [4,5].

Antigenic and genetic analyses confirmed that the two lineages of H9N2 viruses circulating in southeastern China in 1999 are distinguishable and are clearly separated phylogenetically. This applies to each of the eight gene segments of the viruses in each lineage. It is noteworthy that we failed to detect reassortants between the Qa/HK/G1/97-like and the Dk/HK/Y280/97-like viruses even though both viruses were isolated in the same market on the same day. Earlier studies demonstrated that reassortants between these lineages were present in 1997 [1]. The Ck/HK/G9/97 virus was a reassortant possessing PB1 and PB2 genes similar to Qa/HK/G1/97 and the remainder being most homologous with Dk/HK/Y280/97-like virus (Table 2). The Ck/HK/G9/97-like viruses were widespread in the poultry markets in 1997 together with H5N1/97 strains. Neither has been detected since their depopulation and cleaning in December 1997. The possibility exists that both the H5N1/97-like and the Ck/HK/G9/97-like viruses are reassortants [1,10,11] that arose in the poultry markets of the SAR. While the failure to detect reassortants between the two co-circulating H9N2 lineages in 1999 may reflect the relatively small number of viruses that have been completely genotyped, it is apparent that no reassortants between the H9N2 lineages have become dominant in the poultry markets in 1999.

The present studies establish that viruses with internal genes closely related to H5N1/97 and Qa/HK/G1/97 are still circulating in poultry in southeastern China. The transmission of H9N2 influenza viruses to humans was confirmed in two children in Hong Kong [4,5]. The viruses that transmitted to humans in Hong Kong belonged to the Qa/HK/G1/97-like lineage. In the H9N2 envelope, the virus seemingly has a lower propensity to spread to humans than in the H5N1 envelope. The absence of basic amino acids at the cleavage site in the H9 HA [3] may be one factor that modulates the pathogenicity of the H9N2 viruses. The fact that H9N2 viruses of the Qa/HK/G1/97-like genotype can transmit to and cause respiratory disease in humans [4] confirms that the surface glycoproteins can fulfill their primary functions in mammals. The presence of the H5N1 internal genome complex probably contributes significantly to the ability of these viruses to transfer to and replicate in humans.

The present studies on H9N2 influenza viruses from poultry markets confirm that viruses belonging to two lineages represented by Qa/HK/G1/97 and Dk/HK/Y280/97 viruses are wide spread in poultry in southeastern China and that the Qa/HK/G1/97-like viruses are prevalent in quail in the live poultry markets. The continued circulation of Qa/HK/G1/97-like viruses in poultry, especially in quail, alerts us to the need for continuing surveillance for these viruses in humans and pigs in this region.

Acknowledgements

These studies were supported by Public Health Research Grant AI29680 and AI95357 from the National Institute of Allergy and Infectious Diseases, Wellcome Trust Grant 057476/Z/99/Z, Cancer Center Support CORE Grant CA-21765, and the American Lebanese Syrian Associated Charities.

References

[1] Y. Guan, K.F. Shortridge, K. Krauss, R.G. Webster, Molecular characterisation of H9N2 influenza viruses; were they the donors of the "internal" genes of H5N1 viruses in Hong Kong? Proc. Natl. Acad. Sci. U. S. A. 96 (1999) 9363–9367.

[2] E. Hoffmann, J. Stech, I. Leneva, S. Krauss, C. Scholtissek, P.S. Chin, M. Peiris, K.F. Shortridge, R.G. Webster, Characterization of the influenza A gene pool in avian species in Asia: was H6N1 a derivative or a precursor of H5N1? J. Virol. 74 (2000) 6309–6315.

[3] Y.J. Guo, S. Krauss, D.A. Senne, I.P. Mo, K.S. Lo, X.P. Xiong, M. Norwood, K.F. Shortridge, R.G. Webster, Y. Guan, Characterization of the pathogenicity of members of the newly established H9N2 influenza virus lineages in Asia, Virology 267 (2000) 279–288.

[4] M. Peiris, K.Y. Yuen, C.W. Leung, K.H. Chan, K.F. Shortridge, P.L.S. Ip, R.W.M. Lu, W.K. On, Human infection with influenza H9N2, Lancet 354 (1999) 916–917.

[5] Y.P. Lin, M. Shaw, V. Gregory, K. Cameron, W. Lim, A. Klimov, K. Subbarao, Y. Guan, S. Krauss, K. Shortridge, R. Webster, N. Cox, A. Hay, Avian-to-human transmission of H9N2 subtype influenza A viruses: relationship between H9N2 and H5N1 human isolates, Proc. Natl. Acad. Sci. U. S. A. 97 (2000) 9654–9658.

[6] K.F. Shortridge, W.K. Butterfield, R.G. Webster, C.H. Campbell, Isolation and characterization of influenza A viruses from avian species in Hong Kong, Bull. W. H. O. 55 (1977) 15–19.

[7] K.F. Shortridge, N.N. Zhou, Y. Guan, P. Gao, T. Ito, Y. Kawaoka, S. Kodihalli, S. Krauss, D. Markwell, K.G. Murti, M. Norwood, D. Senne, L. Sims, A. Takada, R.G. Webster, Virology 252 (1998) 331–342.

[8] K. Subbarao, A. Kilmov, J. Katz, H. Regenery, W. Lim, H. Hall, M. Perdue, D. Swayne, C. Bender, J. Huang, M. Hemphill, T. Rowe, M. Shaw, X. Xu, K. Fukuda, N. Cox, Characterization of an avian influenza A (H5N1) virus isolated from a child with a fatal respiratory illness, Science 279 (1998) 393–396.

[9] K.Y. Yuen, P.K.S. Chan, M. Peiris, D.N.C. Tsang, T.L. Que, K.F. Shortridge, P.T. Cheung, W.K. To, E.T.F. Ho, R. Sung, A.F.B. Cheng, Members of the H5N1 Study Group, Clinical features and rapid diagnosis of human disease associated with avian influenza A H5N1 virus, Lancet 351 (1998) 467–471.

[10] X. Xu, K. Subbarao, N. Cox, Y. Guo, Genetic characterization of the pathogenic influenza A/Goose/ Guangdong/1/96 (H5N1) virus: similarity of its haemagglutinin gene to those of H5N1 viruses from the 1997 outbreaks in Hong Kong, Virology 261 (1999) 15–19.

[11] N.N. Zhou, K.F. Shortridge, E.J. Claas, S.L. Krauss, R.G. Webster, Rapid evolution of H5N1 influenza viruses in chickens in Hong Kong, J. Virol. 73 (1999) 3366–3374.

International Congress Series 1219 (2001) 195–200

Co-circulation of avian H9N2 and human H3N2 viruses in pigs in southern China

J.S.M. Peiris[a,*], Y. Guan[a], P. Ghose[a], D. Markwell[a], S. Krauss[b], R.G. Webster[b], K.F. Shortridge[a]

[a]*Department of Microbiology, University of Hong Kong, Hong Kong SAR, China*
[b]*Department of Virology and Molecular Biology, St Jude Children's Research Hospital, Memphis, TN, USA*

Abstract

Background: Pigs may be an intermediate host for the adaptation of avian influenza viruses to humans. Avian influenza viruses of multiple lineages, including the precursors of the H5N1 causing the avian flu incident in Hong Kong in 1997 (H5N1/97), are now established in geese and land-based poultry in southern China. It is important to examine whether these avian viruses have undergone inter-species transmission to pigs. *Methods*: Serological and virological surveillance of influenza viruses were carried out in pigs from southern China between 1998 and 2000. Antigenic and molecular characterisation of the virus isolates was done. *Results*: One hundred and ninety influenza A viruses of subtypes H9N2 ($n=4$), H3N2 (A/Sydney/97-like) ($n=13$), H3N2 (A/Victoria/75-like) ($n=15$), and H1N1 (classical swine-like) ($n=158$) were isolated. Seroepidemiology provided independent confirmation of the circulation of each of these viruses. Molecular analysis of all eight gene segments confirmed that the H9N2 viruses belonged to the Duck/HK/Y280/97 lineage. Similarly, the H3N2 Sydney-like viruses were genetically highly homologous to viruses currently circulating in the human population. *Conclusions*: H9N2 subtype viruses co-circulate with contemporary human A/Sydney/97-like viruses and other porcine H1N1 and H3N2 viruses in pigs in southern China, and the potential for the emergence of viruses of pandemic potential needs to be considered. © 2001 Elsevier Science B.V. All rights reserved.

Keywords: Surveillance; Influenza; Pigs

1. Introduction

Southern China is regarded as an epicenter for the emergence of pandemic influenza viruses [1]—the 1957, 1968 and possibly the 1918 pandemics originating in this region [2].

* Corresponding author. Tel.: +852-2855-4888; fax: +852-2855-1241.
E-mail address: malik@hkucc.hku.hk (J.S.M. Peiris).

0531-5131/01/$ – see front matter © 2001 Elsevier Science B.V. All rights reserved.
PII: S 0 5 3 1 - 5 1 3 1 (0 1) 0 0 6 6 7 - 7

It has been proposed that pigs, by being permissive to both avian and human influenza viruses, act as an intermediate host allowing reassortment and adaptation of avian viruses to humans [3]. Over the last three decades, a number of influenza viruses have been isolated from pigs in the south China region. These include classical and avian-like swine H1N1 viruses and H3N2 viruses similar to A/HK/68 and A/Victoria/75, respectively [4–6]. These H3N2 viruses appear to be able to persist in swine for many years with minimal antigenic drift. Some of the early human H3N2 viruses circulating in pigs have undergone reassortment with classical swine H1N1 viruses [7,8] in China, or with avian-like swine H1N1 viruses in Europe [9]. Triple reassortant viruses with gene segments from human, avian and porcine influenza viruses have been reported in the United Kingdom [10], Belgium [11] and the USA [12].

Avian influenza viruses of multiple lineages, including the precursor of the H5N1 virus causing the "bird flu" incident in Hong Kong in 1997 (H5N1/97), are now established in geese and land-based poultry in the southern China region [13,14]. Given the close proximity and interaction between poultry and pigs in this region, it is important to examine whether these avian viruses have undergone inter-species transmission to pigs. It is also important to establish whether there is co-circulation of these avian viruses with current human viruses in the pig population in the south China region.

2. Methods

Sampling of pigs: Tracheal swabs were collected at random from pigs slaughtered at an abattoir in Hong Kong on a monthly basis between March 1998 and June 2000. A total of 4669 tracheal swabs were collected. Serum specimens were also collected during these visits—117 in 1998, 46 in 1999 and 294 in 2000. Approximately 25% of pigs slaughtered in Hong Kong originate from neighbouring Guangdong province, 60% from other Provinces in southern China (predominantly Hunan, Jiangxi, Hubei, and Henan) and the rest are raised in Hong Kong SAR. Those from Mainland China were slaughtered within a day of importation.

Table 1
Antigenic characterization of H9N2 virus isolates in haemagglutination inhibition tests

Virus antigen	Date isolated	HAI tests using ferret antisera[a] to		
		Qu/HK/G1/97	Hk/1073/99	Sw/HK/9/98
Sw/HK/2160/98	Mar-98	<40	<40	80
Sw/HK/9/98	Apr-98	<40	40	640
Sw/HK/10/98	Apr-98	<40	40	320
Sw/HK/3297/99	Oct 99	40	80	320
Qu/HK/G1/97		640	160	<40
Ch/HK/G9/97		<40	<40	640
HK/1073/99[a]		160	640	<40

[a] Reference ferret antisera and HK/1073/99 virus provided by Dr. A. Hay, National Institute for Medical Research, London.

Table 2
Antigenic characterization of representative H3N2 virus isolates in haemagglutination inhibition tests

Virus	Date isolated	HAI tests using ferret antisera[a]						MAb121/1[b]
		A/HK/68	A/PC/73	A/Vic/75	A/Bk/79	A/Ph/82	A/Syd/97	
A/Sw/HK/5190/99	Sep-99	<40	640	1280	<40	160	<40	1600
A/Sw/HK/5200/99	Sep-99	<40	640	2560	<40	80	<40	3200
A/Sw/HK/5212/99	Sep-99	<40	1280	2560	<40	<40	160	800
A/Sw/2422/98	Apr-98	<40	<40	<40	<40	<40	5120	<400
A/Sw/2405/98	Apr-98	<40	<40	<40	<40	<40	2560	<400
A/Sw/2429/98	May-98	<40	<40	<40	<40	<40	5120	<400
A/Hong Kong/68	1968	2560	<40	320	<40	<40	<40	<400
A/Port Chalmers/73	1973	<40	640	640	<40	<40	<40	25,600
A/Victoria/75	1975	<40	<40	2560	<40	<40	<40	12,800
A/Sydney/97	1997	80	<40	40	<40	<40	1280	<400

[a] Reference ferret antisera provided by Dr. N. Cox, Centers for Disease Control, Atlanta.
[b] Monoclonal antibody to A/Port Chalmers/73 provided by Dr. R.G. Webster.

Virus isolation: Tracheal swabs were inoculated into embryonated eggs as described previously [6]. In addition, the swabs were inoculated onto MDCK cell culture tubes in Eagles Minimum Essential Medium without foetal calf serum but containing trypsin (2 μg/ml). Virus isolates were passaged and identified using haemagglutination inhibition (HAI) tests and neuraminidase inhibition (NAI) tests using a panel of reference sera. Re-isolation was attempted from the original swab specimen.

Serology tests: Pig sera were treated with receptor-destroying enzyme and used for haemagglutination inhibition (HAI) tests using turkey erythrocytes. Neutralisation tests were carried out using 100 $TCID_{50}$ of virus on MDCK cells grown in microtitre plates, and cytopathic effect was read under an inverted microscope.

Viral RNA extraction, PCR amplification, nucleotide sequencing and phylogenetic analysis: These were carried out as described previously [14].

3. Results

One hundred and eighty nine influenza A viruses were isolated. Antigenic characterisation of the virus isolates by haemagglutination inhibition (HAI) tests identified H9N2 ($n = 4$), H3N2 (A/Sydney/97-like) ($n = 13$), H3N2 (A/Victoria/75-like) ($n = 15$) and H1N1 (classical swine-like) ($n = 158$) viruses. The antigenic characterisation of representative H9N2 and H3N2 viruses is shown in Tables 1 and 2. These were also used for partial genome sequencing and phylogenetic analysis. All four H9N2 viruses and each of the representative H3N2 and H1N1 viruses used for antigenic analysis and sequencing were re-isolated from the original swab to confirm the validity of the isolates. In addition, serological responses to each of these viruses were demonstrated in porcine sera by HAI tests and neutralisation tests.

a)   b)

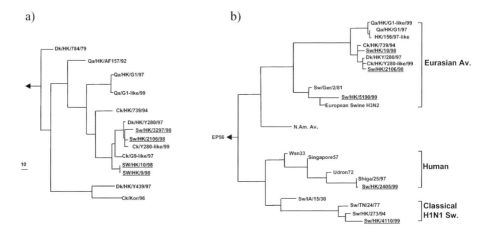

Fig. 1. Cladograms for (a) the HA1 region of H9 from Asia and (b) the M gene of H9, H3 and H1 subtype Eurasian viruses. Nucleotides 88 to 1077 (990 bp) of H9 HA, and 41 to 860 (820 bp) of the M gene of H9, H3 and H1 viruses were used for phylogenetic analysis with PAUP, using the maximum-parsimony algorithm. The HA1 and M phylogenetic trees are rooted to Dk/Alberta/60/76 (H12N5) and Eq/Pra/56/56 (H7N7), respectively.

Phylogenetic analysis of the HA1 gene region (Fig. 1a) of the four porcine H9N2 viruses show that they belong to the Y280/97-lineage. The nucleotide sequence homology of the seven other gene segments (data not shown) confirms that no gene reassortment has taken place.

H3N2 viruses were repeatedly isolated from pigs throughout 1998 and 1999. Most of these were antigenically (Table 1) and genetically (Fig. 1b) similar to A/Sydney/97 that currently circulates in the human population in this region. The other gene segments share close homology with human A/Sydney-like viruses (data not shown). In September 1999, H3N2 viruses antigenically distinct from A/Sydney/97 viruses but more closely related to A/Port Chalmers/73 and A/Victoria/75 were isolated from pigs. Genetic analysis of the M (Fig. 1b) and other genes (data not shown) demonstrates that these viruses belong to the European avian-like swine lineage and were distinct from previous A/Victoria-like viruses isolated in Hong Kong between 1976 and 1982. H1N1 viruses were isolated throughout the study period and were antigenically and genetically classical swine H1N1-like viruses. No viruses similar to the avian-like swine H1N1 or the human-like H1N2 viruses prevalent in Europe were isolated.

4. Discussion

We have found that H9N2 viruses of the Y280/97 lineage, contemporary Sydney-like H3N2 viruses similar to those currently circulating in humans, Port Chalmers-like H3N2 viruses belonging to the European swine lineage and classical swine H1N1 viruses, co-circulate in pigs in southern China. Previous experimental studies had demonstrated that H9 subtype avian viruses (and others) could replicate efficiently in pigs [15].

Current H3N2 viruses circulating in European pigs carry haemagglutinin and neuraminidase antigens derived from human viruses of the 1970s (A/Victoria-like), but have acquired H1N1 internal genes through reassortment with swine H1N1 viruses of the avian lineage [9]. These reassortants are well established in Europe and have rarely been transmitted to humans [16]. Our current data indicate that these viruses may have spread to southern China. Around the time of our isolation of these Port Chalmers-like H3N2 viruses from pigs, a child was diagnosed with a flu-like illness in Hong Kong from whom a similar virus was isolated (Lin, Y.P. and Hay, A., unpublished data).

In contrast, H3N2 viruses isolated from pigs in this region between 1976 and 1982 [4,5] were either nonreassorted early human H3N2 viruses (A/Victoria-like) or reassortants carrying the internal genes of classical swine H1N1 viruses [7,8]. Neither of these viruses was detected in the present study and was not isolated during a similar study carried out between 1993 and 1994 [6]. However, in the latter survey, 2.5% of sera had HAI antibody to A/Victoria/75, suggesting that H3N2 viruses may have circulated at low level through this period.

Although neither H9N2 nor H3N2 Sydney-like viruses were isolated during the first six months of the year 2000, serological evidence suggests that both viruses are still circulating in the pig population. Repeated introductions of avian H9N2 viruses into such an environment offers significant opportunity for the generation of reassortants containing an H9 haemagglutinin and internal genes adapted to replication in human cells. In the context of a human population naïve to the H9 antigen, such a virus would pose a significant pandemic threat.

Acknowledgements

We thank Dr. T. Sit and the Department of Food and Environmental Hygiene, Hong Kong, and Drs. T.M. Ellis and K.C. Dyrting, Department of Agriculture, Fisheries and Conservation, Hong Kong, for facilitating this study. We acknowledge the technical assistance of O.K. Wong, T.Y. Leung, S.K. Ma and C.Y. Cheung. This research was supported by Public Health Research Grant AI95357 from the National Institutes of Allergy and Infectious Diseases and the Wellcome Trust (research grant 057476).

References

[1] K.F. Shortridge, C.H. Stuart-Harris, An influenza epicentre? Lancet ii (1982) 212–213.
[2] K.F. Shortridge, The 1918 "Spanish" flu: pearls from swine? Nature Medicine 5 (1999) 384–385.
[3] C. Scholtissek, H. Burger, O. Kistner, K.F. Shortridge, The nucleoprotein was a possible major factor in determining host specificity of influenza H3N2 viruses, Virology 147 (1985) 287–294.
[4] K.F. Shortridge, R.G. Webster, W.K. Butterfield, C.H. Campbell, Persistence of Hong Kong influenza virus variants in pigs, Science 196 (1976) 1454–1455.
[5] K.F. Shortridge, R.G. Webster, Geographical distribution of swine (swH1N1) and Hong Kong (H3N2) influenza virus variants in pigs in Southeast Asia, Intervirology 11 (1979) 9–15.
[6] Y. Guan, K.F. Shortridge, S. Krauss, P.H. Li, Y. Kawaoka, R.G. Webster, Emergence of avian H1N1 influenza viruses in pigs in China, J. Virol. 70 (1996) 8041–8046.

[7] L.L. Shu, Y.P. Lin, S.M. Wright, K.F. Shortridge, R.G. Webster, Evidence for interspecies transmission and reassortment of influenza A viruses in pigs in Southern China, Virology 202 (1994) 825–833.

[8] K. Nerome, Y. Kanegae, K.F. Shortridge, S. Sugita, M. Ishida, Genetic analysis of procine H3N2 viruses originating in southern China, J. Gen. Virol., (1995) 613–624.

[9] M.R. Castrucci, I. Donatelli, L. Sidoli, G. Barigazzi, Y. Kawaoka, R.G. Webster, Genetic reassortment between avian and human influenza A viruses in Italian pigs, Virology 193 (1993) 503–506.

[10] I.H. Brown, P.A. Harris, J.W. McCauley, D.J. Alexander, Multiple genetic reassortment of avian and human influenza A viruses in European pigs, resulting in the emergence of an H1N2 virus of novel genotype, J. Gen. Virol. 79 (1998) 2947–2955.

[11] K. Van Reeth, I.H. Brown, M. Pensaert, Isolation of H1N2 influenza A viruses from pigs in Belgium, Vet. Rec. 146 (2000) 588–589.

[12] N.N. Zhou, D.A. Senne, J.S. Landgraf, S.L. Swenson, G. Erikson, K. Rossow, L. Liu, K.-J. Yoon, S. Krauss, R.G. Webster, Genetic reassortment of avian, swine and human influenza A viruses in American pigs, J. Virol. 73 (1999) 8851–8856.

[13] Y. Guan, K.F. Shortridge, S. Krauss, R.G. Webster, Molecular characterisation of H9N2 influenza viruses: were they the donors of the "internal" genes of H5N1 viruses in Hong Kong? Proc. Natl. Acad. Sci. U. S. A. 96 (1999) 9363–9367.

[14] Y. Guan, K.F. Shortridge, S. Krauss, P.S. Chin, K.C. Dyrting, T.M. Ellis, R.G. Webster, M. Peiris, H9N2 influenza viruses possessing H5N1-like internal genes continue to circulate in poultry in southeastern China, J. Virol. 14 (2000) 9372–9380.

[15] H. Kida, T. Ito, J. Yasuda, Y. Shimizu, C. Itakura, K.F. Shortridge, Y. Kawaoka, R.G. Webster, J. Gen. Virol. 75 (1994) 2183–2188.

[16] E.C. Claas, Y. Kawaoka, J.C. De Jong, N. Masurel, R.G. Webster, Infection of children with avian–human reassortant influenza viruses from pigs in Europe, Virology 204 (1994) 453–457.

International Congress Series 1219 (2001) 201–211

Influenza surveillance in poultry market and its inter-species transmission in Taiwan

H.-L. Yen[a], M.-C. Cheng[b], J.L. Liu[a], C.-L. Kao[c], S.R. Shih[d],
N.J. Cox[e], R.G. Webster[f], C.-C. King[a,*]

[a]*Institute of Epidemiology, College of Public Health, National Taiwan University (NTU), No. 1,
Jen-Ai Road Section 1, Taipei, Taiwan*
[b]*National Institute for Animal Health, Council of Agriculture, Taipei, Taiwan*
[c]*School of Medical Technology, National Taiwan University, Taipei, Taiwan*
[d]*School of Medical Technology, Chang-Gung University, Taoyuan, Taiwan*
[e]*Influenza Branch, Centers for Disease Control and Prevention, Atlanta, GA, USA*
[f]*St. Jude Children's Research Hospital, Memphis, TN, USA*

Abstract

Background: Since Taiwan has high population density and a similar ecological environment to Mainland China, the epi-center of influenza viruses, it is very important to establish influenza virologic surveillance systems in both animal and human populations. The H5N1 Hong Kong Flu in 1997 and H9N2 in 1999 have showed that avian influenza viruses can cross the receptor of host species boundary and transmit to human. Therefore, the specific aim of this study is to understand the frequency of inter-species transmission in Taiwan. *Methods*: We have established an avian influenza virologic surveillance system in one of the largest live poultry markets in Taipei City from October 1999 to March 2000. Serum samples were collected from 341 blood donors, including veterinarians, poultry farm workers, and market employees. HI and microneutralization were used to detect specific antibody against H6, an endemic virus in chicken farms in southern Taiwan, and antibodies against H3, H4, and H9 viruses. *Results*: Among about 1300 fecal specimens of chickens and ducks collected, we isolated 12 H3 viruses, 14 H4 viruses, and 2 H6 viruses (i.e. 9 serotypes of HA and NA) from ducks. The isolation rates were 0% (0/580) and 7% (28/400) in chickens and ducks, respectively. Phylogenetic analysis of HA from 7 of our 12 H3 isolates showed the highest (93%) homology with A/equine/Jilin/89 (H3N8). Both phylogenetic relationship of HA and NP genes from selected representative strains (7 H3, 7 H4, and 2 H6) found they all fell into Eurasian lineage of avian influenza viruses. Their NP genes were away from the G1 lineage that was found in H5N1 strain isolated in Hong Kong in 1997. In addition, the results of HI and microneutralization tests found that they were all seronegative against two avian influenza virus strains [A/Duck/

---

* Corresponding author. Tel.: +886-2-2341-4347; fax: +886-2-2351-1955.
  E-mail address: a1234567@ccms.ntu.edu.tw (C.-C. King).

Czechoslovakia/56 (H4N6) and A/Shearwater/Australia/1/72 (H6N5)]. *Conclusion*: Continuous efforts by integrating animal, market and human influenza surveillance systems have provided the best early warning signals to detect new influenza virus activities for preventing potential pandemics and providing effective controls. © 2001 Elsevier Science B.V. All rights reserved.

Keywords: Market Surveillance; Influenza; Zoonosis; Taiwan

---

1. Introduction

Avian influenza viruses are considered to be the ancient source of equine, swine, and human influenza viruses' molecular evolution, with aquatic birds as the natural reservoirs of 15 HA and 9 NA serotypes [1]. Although these viruses tend to achieve evolutionary balance and do not lead to disease in their natural reservoirs, they periodically infect domestic poultry. Particularly, H5 and H7 subtypes may result in economic loss [2,3]. On the other hand, interspecies transmission of avian influenza viruses to mammalian animals including horses, pigs, whales, dolphins, and minks occurs less frequently. Pigs with receptors of both avian and humans have been proposed to serve as an intermediate host for reassortant viruses, which could subsequently infect human population and probably cause a pandemic outbreak [4–7]. This concept was challenged in 1997 when avian influenza H5N1 virus was demonstrated to transmit directly from domestic poultry to humans in Hong Kong and resulted in 6 deaths out of 18 confirmed cases, raising the concern that chickens may also be an intermediate host [8–10]. The epidemiologic significance of chickens was further supported in 1999, when avian influenza virus H9N2 serotype caused five human cases in Southern China, and two other cases in Hong Kong [11,12]. In order to prepare for the future pandemic, continuous and collaborative surveillance systems of human, domestic poultry, pigs and wild birds are the most effective prevention strategy.

Extensive studies on animal influenza viruses in domestic poultry in Hong Kong and southern China have been documented by Dr. K.F. Shortridge since the 1970s [13]. Earlier surveillance results found that influenza viruses were predominantly isolated from ducks and less frequently from chickens and other species. However, recent studies have shown a reverse pattern in that influenza virus is endemic in poultry in southern China, especially the H9N2 subtype which predominantly appeared in chickens and quails. Furthermore, genetic analysis of human H5N1 and H9N2 viruses revealed high homology (98%) compared to G1 lineage viruses in their six internal genes [14,15]. These findings indicate that pandemic strains might emerge from reassorted internal genes of those circulating strains, which were derived from avian domestic poultry but could be related to infection and replication in humans.

In Taiwan, domestic poultry influenza surveillance in the past found ducks had higher infection rates than other domestic avian species. Serological surveillance in 1980s showed that the seropositive rates were 3.7% (56/2056) in chickens, 19.8% (845/4274) in ducks, 2.3% (4/177) in turkeys, and 9.1% (1/11) in quails [16]. In addition, the isolation rates of avian influenza viruses among cloacal swabs collected from chickens, ducks, and wild waterfowls in 1986–1988 were 0.53% (7/1322), 0.85% (13/1524), and 1.6% (3/188), respectively, through active virologic surveillance [17]. Moreover, the isolation rate of avian influenza viruses became higher and reached 2.68% among 1420 fecal specimens, trachea and cloacal swabs collected from chicken breeders in middle Taiwan in 1990–1991. However, no active surveillance study has been conducted since 1991. The Hong Kong Flu incident in 1997 accelerated the Council of Agriculture and Poultry Health Centers in Taiwan to initiate an ELISA antibody screening test against nucleoprotein of avian influenza A virus in domestic poultry. However, the avian influenza virologic baseline data were lacking. Therefore, we established a poultry market surveillance system in the largest wholesale market, which sells about 60,000–70,000 chickens and 50,000 ducks per day in Taipei City from October 1999 to March 2000. The specific aims of this study were: (1) to understand current circulating avian influenza viruses in domestic poultry in Taiwan, (2) to investigate the possibility of interspecies transmission of these viruses to Taiwanese population, and (3) to provide more information on the gene pool data base of avian influenza viruses in Asia. Our market influenza active surveillance obtained all 28 avian market virus isolates from ducks that belong to nine serotypes of HA and NA combinations. Phylogenetic relationship of HA and NP genes from selected strains found that they all belong to the Eurasian lineage of avian influenza viruses, and their NP genes were away from the G1 lineage. In addition, further seroepidemiologic investigation among 195 poultry workers and 146 veterinarians distributed all over Taiwan did not find any single seropositive individual against two avian influenza virus strains [A/Duck/Czechoslovakia/56 (H4N6) and A/Shearwater/Australia/1/72 (H6N5)]. Our preliminary virologic surveillance and seroepidemiologic data indicate that the possibility of direct transmission of new avian influenza virus virulent strains to humans in Taiwan during 1999–2000 season was extremely low.

2. Materials and methods

2.1. Poultry market

The wholesale market A located in Taipei city is the main source of chickens and ducks at retail markets in Taipei City and Taipei County. In general, about 60,000–70,000 chickens and 50,000 ducks on average, coming from different counties in Taiwan, were transported to market A every day, except special holidays, according to the Chinese traditional lunar calendar. During the period of sampling, chickens sold in market A involved Simulated Native Chicken, Native Chickens, Silky Chickens, and old layers. The wholesale ducks included Peking Duck, Kaiya Duck and Muscovy Duck. Live chickens are usually sold at different retail markets but all ducks were slaughtered at market A. Those chickens that were not sold on the first arrival day would stay at the market for 2–3 days, while all ducks were slaughtered every day.

2.2. Field specimens

About 100 fresh fecal samples were collected biweekly from cages or trucks that were transported to the poultry market A from October 1999 to March 2000. Every three fecal specimens obtained from the same flock of chickens or ducks were put together into one collection media tube. All of these tubes contained medium 199 (Gibco), 4000 U/ml Penicillin G, 4 mg/ml Streptomycin sulfate, 2000 U/ml Polymyxin B, 500 µg/ml Gentamicin, 500 U/ml Nystatin, 20 µg/ml Ofloxacin HCl, and 200 ug/ml Sulfamethoxazole [obtained from Dr. Robert G. Webster]. In total, about 600 chicken feces and 700 duck fecal specimens were collected. These samples were passaged in allantoic cavity of 10-day-old specific-pathogen-free (SPF) chicken embryonic eggs. Those allantoic fluid samples with a positive result of hemagglutination test were further subtyped by hemagglutination inhibition and neuraminidase inhibition tests with monospecific antisera obtained from Dr. K. Kida and Dr. Robert G. Webster followed standard procedures as described [18].

2.3. RNA extraction and polymerase chain reaction (PCR)

Viral RNA was extracted from allantoic fluid by using RNeasy Mini Kit (Qiagen, Chatsworth, CA). Complement DNA was synthesized with Uni12 and reverse transcriptase (AMV), and cDNA was amplified by PCR using gene specific primers obtained from Dr. Lee, and Xu et al. [19]. PCR products were analyzed by 1% agarose gel electrophoresis and further purified by QIAquick PCR Purification Kit (Qiagen).

2.4. Gene sequencing and phylogenetic analysis

Representative viruses of the same HA subtype and derived from the same geographic location were randomly chosen for further genetic analyses. All the selected strains for HA phylogenetic analysis were also used for obtaining their NP gene sequences. Purified PCR products were sequenced with synthetic oligonucleotides by using Rhodamine Dye-Terminator Cycle Sequencing Kit with AmpliTaq DNA polymerase FS and an ABI model 377 DNA Sequencer (Perkin-Elmer/Applied Biosystems). Sequence data were edited by the computer packages of DNAStar and GeneDoc. The WISCONSIN Sequence Analysis Package, Version 10.0 (GCG) was used for further analyses and comparison. Phylogenetic analysis was performed with Maximum Parsimony method of PAUP (Phylogenetic Analysis Using Parsimony, Version 4.0, Swafford, Illinois Natural History Survey, Champaign, IL, USA).

2.5. Human serum samples

Blood samples and questionnaires were obtained from 195 poultry workers distributed all over Taiwan, including 37 market A workers, 136 and 22 employees from chicken and duck raising farms, respectively, and 146 veterinarians from January 1998 to April 2000. Serum samples were collected after centrifugation of the whole blood at 2000 rpm for 10 min and several aliquots of each sample were stored in $-70\ °C$ refrigerator.

2.6. HI and microneutralization test

Considering the HA subtypes of our market surveillance results and avoiding possible cross reaction of current human NA subtypes (N1 and N2), we chose A/Duck/Czechoslovakia/56 (H4N6) and A/Shearwater/Australia/1/72 (H6N5) viruses to conduct the serology test. HI test was performed as described [18], and microneutralization test was run according to the standard protocols [20]. Briefly, serum samples were incubated at 56 °C for 30 min. Serial dilutions of serum samples were made from 1:10, 1:20, 1:40, to 1:1280 in 96-well tissue culture plates. 100 $TCID_{50}$ virus was added into each well, incubated with the diluted serum samples at 37 °C for 2 h. Then, 1.3×10^5 MDCK cells were added to each well and incubated at 37 °C for 18–22 h. After removing the supernatant and washing each well with 250 µl PBS, the cells were fixed with 80% acetone solution at 4 °C for 10 min, and the plates were air dried at room temperature. ELISA was performed using mouse anti-NP monoclonal antibody (CDC, #VS2208), HRP labeled goat anti-mouse IgG (KPL, cat# 074-1806), and TMB substrate (KPL, cat# 50-76-06) to detect influenza virus nucleoprotein. Optical density (OD) values of each well were read by an ELISA reader with a 450-nm filter. Any well that showed 50% virus reduction was considered as seropositive.

Table 1
List of avian influenza A virus isolates in poultry market in Taipei, Taiwan

Virus isolates	Subtypes	Abbreviation	Source counties	Dates of isolation
A/Duck/Taiwan/7-8/2000	H3N8	dtw7-8	Unknown	13/01/2000
A/Duck/Taiwan/7-17/2000	H3N8	dtw7-17	Unknown	13/01/2000
A/Duck/Taiwan/7-20/2000	H3N8	dtw7-20	Unknown	13/01/2000
A/Duck/Taiwan/7-28/2000	H3N8	dtw7-28	Unknown	13/01/2000
A/Duck/Taiwan/8-4/2000	H3N8	dtw8-4	Ilan	31/01/2000
A/Duck/Taiwan/8-6/2000	H3N8	dtw8-6	Ilan	31/01/2000
A/Duck/Taiwan/8-8/2000	H3N8	dtw8-8	Ilan	31/01/2000
A/Duck/Taiwan/8-12/2000	H3N2	dtw8-12	Unknown	31/01/2000
A/Duck/Taiwan/8-19/2000	H3N1	dtw8-19	Unknown	31/01/2000
A/Duck/Taiwan/8-20/2000	H3N1	dtw8-20	Unknown	31/01/2000
A/Duck/Taiwan/9-3/2000	H4N4	dtw9-3	Yunling	15/02/2000
A/Duck/Taiwan/9-4/2000	H4N4	dtw9-4	Yunling	15/02/2000
A/Duck/Taiwan/9-5/2000	H4N1	dtw9-5	Yunling	15/02/2000
A/Duck/Taiwan/9-6/2000	H4N1	dtw9-6	Yunling	15/02/2000
A/Duck/Taiwan/9-23/2000	H6N1	dtw9-23	Unknown	15/02/2000
A/Duck/Taiwan/10-2/2000	H4N6	dtw10-2	Yunling	06/03/2000
A/Duck/Taiwan/10-3/2000	H4N6	dtw10-3	Yunling	06/03/2000
A/Duck/Taiwan/10-5/2000	H4N6	dtw10-5	Yunling	06/03/2000
A/Duck/Taiwan/10-6/2000	H3N6	dtw10-6	Yunling	06/03/2000
A/Duck/Taiwan/10-8/2000	H3N8	dtw10-8	Yunling	06/03/2000
A/Duck/Taiwan/10-12/2000	H6N1	dtw10-12	Unknown	06/03/2000
A/Duck/Taiwan/10-19/2000	H4N6	dtw10-19	Unknown	06/03/2000
A/Duck/Taiwan/10-21/2000	H4N2	dtw10-22	Changhwa	06/03/2000
A/Duck/Taiwan/10-22/2000	H4N2	dtw10-22	Changhwa	06/03/2000
A/Duck/Taiwan/10-24/2000	H4N2	dtw10-24	Changhwa	06/03/2000
A/Duck/Taiwan/10-25/2000	H4N2	dtw10-25	Changhwa	06/03/2000
A/Duck/Taiwan/10-27/2000	H4N2	dtw10-27	Changhwa	06/03/2000
A/Duck/Taiwan/10-32/2000	H4N2	dtw10-32	Changhwa	06/03/2000

Unknown source counties: feces of market avians were hard to identify due to mixing effect.

3. Results

3.1. Market surveillance

No avian influenza virus was isolated from 600 chicken feces whereas 28 avian influenza viruses were isolated from 700 fecal samples collected through our active market surveillance from October 15, 1999 to March 31, 2000. These 28 isolates were further

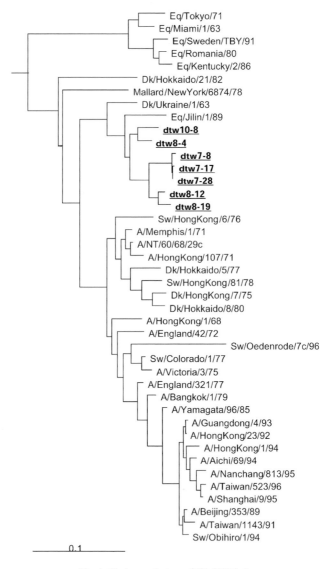

Fig. 1. Phylogenetic tree of H3 (450 bp).

identified as 12 H3 (including 2 of H3N1, 1 of H3N2, 1 of H3N6, 8 of H3N8), 14 H4 (including 2 of H4N1, 6 of H4N6, 2 of H4N4, 4 of H4N6), and 2 H6N1 viruses. The isolation rate were 0% (0/600) in chickens and 4% (25/700) in ducks. Table 1 lists epidemiologic characteristics of all these virus isolates, including dates of isolation, and the source

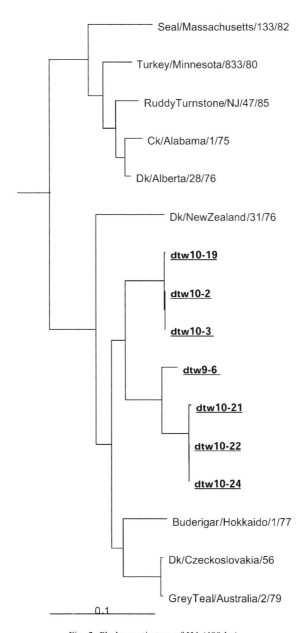

Fig. 2. Phylogenetic tree of H4 (480 bp).

counties of the ducks that carried the viruses. Half (14/28) of our isolates were of H4 serotype, and H3N8 serotype was the most frequent isolate from the market.

3.2. Genetic analysis of HA gene

7 of 12 H3, 7 of 14 H4, and 2 H6 market avian influenza virus isolates were further sequenced. The HA gene sequences of our seven H3 isolates showed homology between 91% and 99%. All of them had the highest homology with A/Equine/Jilin/89 (H3N8). Phylogenetical analysis of H3 found that it involved three subgroups (A, B, C) that were correlated with the dates of isolation (Fig. 1). In particular, group A included two viruses, A/DK/Taiwan/10-8/2000 and A/DK/Taiwan/8-4/2000, that were isolated from different parts of Taiwan at different months. The phylogenetic tree of seven H4 isolates involved

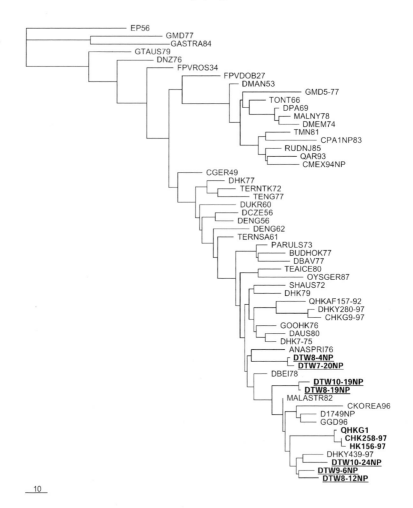

Fig. 3. Phylogenetic tree of NP (586 bp).

three subgroups with homology between 89% and 100% (Fig. 2). Our two additional H6N1 isolates had 90% sequence homology with A/Teal/Hong Kong/W312/97(H6N1), which had seven genes of high homology (97.1–99.8%) with Hong Kong H5N1 virus [21]. Most importantly, none of our 28 isolates had multiple basic amino acids at HA1– HA2 cleavage site, which was found to correlate with virulence of influenza A viruses [22].

3.3. Phylogenetic analysis of NP gene

NP gene sequence data of those seven isolates with the above-mentioned molecular information of HA showed that their homology ranged between 93% and 99%. Phylogenetic analysis of their NP gene involved four subgroups (A, B, C, D) and none of our isolates was in the lineage of G1 group viruses (Fig. 3). Interestingly, A and B groups were located away from C and D groups.

3.4. Serology results

All 195 poultry workers and 146 veterinarians distributed all over Taiwan were seronegative by both HI and microneutralization tests against two avian influenza viruses: A/Duck/Czechoslovakia/56 (H4N6) and A/Shearwater/Australia/1/72 (H6N5).

4. Discussion

This is the first document of active market poultry virologic surveillance system established in Taiwan. Our findings on 9 HA–NA serotypes of 28 duck influenza viruses among 700 fecal specimens, but no isolates obtained from 600 chickens, demonstrated a similar pattern with the surveillance data of Hong Kong and Southern China in 1970s [13]. In addition, further sequence analysis showed that these duck influenza viruses isolated from different counties at different months were located in the same Eurasian lineage, implying that sources of avian influenza viruses in Taiwan should be part of the Eurasian gene pool. In addition, the migrating waterfowl might play an important role in the transmission of these duck influenza viruses. The zero isolation rate among chicken fecal samples derived from different breeding farms located in various counties could again be explained by the following reasons: (1) only healthy chickens were sold in the wholesale market, (2) limitation of the method used in collecting field specimens, and (3) a different domestic poultry raising style in Taiwan from Southern China where an ecological niche of different animals was reported. Considering the endemic status of avian influenza viruses in Southern China and Hong Kong in recent years due to viral adaptation via molecular evolution, it is very important for us to monitor avian influenza viruses in Taiwan continuously by the most efficient prevention strategy using a poultry market surveillance system.

Future efforts on avian influenza virus should improve by: (1) collecting more respiratory swabs through market surveillance, (2) phylogenetic analysis of all eight gene segments especially the internal genes of the our isolates, (3) comparing nucleotide and amino acid sequences with wild bird and domestic avian influenza virus isolates for investigating possible sources and spreading of those market viruses, and (4) conducting serologic tests against the avian viruses recently isolated from Taiwan. A more comprehensive picture of avian influenza viruses through global surveillance network and international collaboration will be very helpful in vaccine development and prevention of future pandemics.

References

[1] R.G. Webster, Influenza: an emerging microbial pathogen, in: R.M. Krause (Ed.), Emerging Infections, Academic Press, New York, 1998, pp. 275–300.

[2] M. Ohuchi, M. Orlich, R. Ohuchi, Mutations at the cleavage site of the hemagglutinin after the pathogenicity of influenza virus A/chick/penn/83 (H5N2), Virology 168 (1989) 274–280.

[3] R.G. Webster, R. Rott, Influenza virus A pathogenicity: the pivotal role of hemagglutinin, Cell 50 (1987) 665–666.

[4] T. Ito, J.N.S.S. Couceiro, S. Kelm, L.G. Baum, S. Krauss, M.R. Castrucci, I. Donatelli, H. Kida, J.C. Paulson, R.G. Webster, Y. Kawaoka, Molecular basis for the generation in pigs of influenza A viruses with pandemic potential, J. Virol. 72 (1998) 7367–7373.

[5] C. Scholtissek, Pigs as "mixing vessels" for the creation of new pandemic influenza A virus, Med. Principles Pract. 2 (1990) 65–71.

[6] M.R. Castrucci, I. Donatelli, L. Sidoli, G. Barigazzi, Y. Kawaoka, R.G. Webster, Genetic reassortment between avian and human influenza A viruses in Italian pigs, Virology 193 (1993) 503–506.

[7] E.C.J. Claas, Y. Kawaoka, J.C. DeJong, N. Masurel, R.G. Webster, Infection of children with avian–human reassortant influenza virus from pigs in Europe, Virology 204 (1994) 453–457.

[8] E.C.J. Claas, A.D.M.E. Osterhaus, R.V. Beek, J.C. Jong, G.F. Rimmelzwaan, D.A. Senne, S. Krauss, K.F. Shortridge, R.G. Webster, Human influenza A H5N1 virus related to a highly pathogenic avian influenza Virus, Lancet 351 (1998) 472–477.

[9] K.F. Shortridge, N.N. Zhou, Y. Guan, P. Gao, T. Ito, Y. Kawaoka, S. Kodihalli, S. Krauss, D. Markwell, K.G. Murti, M. Norwood, D. Senne, L. Sims, A. Takada, R.G. Webster, Characterization of avian H5N1 influenza viruses from poultry in Hong Kong, Virology 252 (1998) 331–342.

[10] K. Subbarao, V. Klimov, J. Katz, H. Regnery, W. Lim, H. Hall, M. Perdue, D. Swayne, C. Bender, J. Huang, M. Hemphill, T. Rowe, M. Shaw, X. Xu, K. Fukuda, N. Cox, Characterization of an avian influenza A (H5N1) virus isolated from a child with a fatal respiratory illness, Science 279 (1998) 393–396.

[11] Y.J. Guo, S. Krauss, D.A. Senne, I.P. Mo, K.S. Lo, X.P. Xiong, M. Norwood, K.F. Shortridge, R.G. Webster, Characterization of the pathogenicity of members of the newly established H9N2 influenza virus lineage in Asia, Virology 267 (2000) 279–288.

[12] M. Peiris, K.Y. Yuen, C.W. Leung, K.H. Chan, P.L.S. Ip, R.W.M. Lai, W.K. Orr, K.F. Shortridge, Human infection with influenza H9N2, Lancet 354 (1999) 916–917.

[13] K.F. Shortridge, Isolation of ortho- and paramyxoviruses from domestic poultry in Hong Kong between November 1977 and October 1978 and comparison with isolations made in the preceding two years, Res. Vet. Sci. 28 (3) (1980) 296–301.

[14] Y. Guan, K.F. Shortridge, S. Krauss, R.G. Webster, Molecular characterization of H9N2 influenza viruses: were they the donors of the "intenal" genes of H5N1 viruses in Hong Kong? Proc. Natl. Acad. Sci. U. S. A. 96 (1999) 9363–9367.

[15] Y.P. Lin, M. Shaw, V. Gregory, K. Cameron, W. Lim, A. Klimov, K. Subbarao, Y. Guan, S. Krauss, K.F. Shortridge, R.G. Webster, N. Cox, A. Hay, Avian-to-human transmission of H9N2 subtype influenza A viruses: relationship between H9N2 and H5N1 human isolates, Proc. Natl. Acad. Sci. U. S. A. 97 (2000) 9654–9658.

[16] C.H. Chan, H.K. Shieh, Y.S. Lu, Y.L. Lee, D.F. Lin, Y.K. Liao, M.C. Cheng, Studies on avain influenza in Taiwan, R.O.C. (I): antibody screening, virus isolation and identification, Taiwan J. Vet. Med. Anim. Husb. 53 (1989) 75–88.

[17] H.K. Shieh, W.J. Huang, J.H. Shien, S.Y. Chiu, L.F. Lee, Y.S. Lu, Studies on avain influenza in Taiwan, R.O.C. (III): isolation, identification, and pathogenicity tests of the virus isolated from breeding chickens, Taiwan J. Vet. Med. Anim. Husb. 59 (1992) 45–55.

[18] A.P. Kendal, M.S. Pereira, J.J. Skehel, Concepts and Procedures for Laboratory-based Influenza Surveillance, Public Health Service, Centers for Disease Control, Atlanta, 1982.

[19] X. Xu, K. Subbarao, N. Cox, Y. Guo, Genetic characterization of the pathogenic influenza a/goose/guangdong/1/96 (H5N1) virus: similarity of its hemagglutinin gene to those of H5N1 viruses from the 1997 outbreaks in Hong Kong, Virology 261 (1999) 15–19.

[20] T. Rowe, R.A. Abernathy, J. Huprimmer, W.W. Thompson, X. Lu, W. Lim, K. Fukuda, N. Cox, J.M. Katz, Detection of antibody to avian influenza A (H5N1) virus in human serum by using a combination of serologic assays, J. Clin. Micobiol. 37 (1999) 937–943.

[21] E. Hoffmann, J. Stech, I. Leneva, S. Krauss, C. Scholtissek, P.S. Chin, M. Peiris, K.F. Shortridge, R.G. Webster, Characterization of the influenza A virus gene pool in avian species in Southern China: was H6N1 a derivative or a precursor of H5N1? J. Virol. 74 (2000) 6309–6315.

[22] J.A. Walker, T. Sakaguchi, Y. Matsuta, T. Yoshida, Y. Kawaoka, Location and character of the cellular enzyme that cleaves the hemagglutinin of a virulent avian influenza virus, Virology 190 (1992) 278–287.

International Congress Series 1219 (2001) 213–223

Analyses of evolutionary and virulence divergency of Hong Kong H5N1 influenza A viruses isolated from humans

Kuniaki Nerome[a,*], Yasuaki Hiromoto[a], Stephen E. Lindstrom[a], Shigeo Sugita[b]

[a]*Laboratory of Respiratory Viruses, Department of Virology I, National Institute of Infectious Diseases, 23-1 Toyama 1-chome, Shinjuku-ku, Tokyo 162-8640, Japan*
[b]*Epizootic Research Station, Equine Research Institute, Japan Racing Association, 1400-4, Shiba, Kokubunji-machi, Shimotuga-gun, Tochigi, Japan*

Abstract

Nucleotide and amino acid sequence homologies of the entire RNA segments of six H5N1 human influenza viruses were divided into two or three variant groups. This result was compatible with that of phylogenetic analysis, which showed that trees of the eight genes were composed of two or three minor branch clusters. The PB2, PA, NP and M proteins of human H5N1 viruses were further characterized by the presence of previously reported amino acid sequences peculiar to those of human strains. The virulence of A/Hong Kong/483/97 (HK483) in mice exhibited a sharp contrast to that of A/Hong Kong/156/97 (HK156). Virulence of the former even remained after constant repeated passage in eggs, while the latter rapidly decreased in virulence for mice after only a few passages in eggs. It became apparent that Madin–Darby canine kidney (MDCK) cell-grown virus (HK156-CK) and its clones derived from mouse brain produced a fatal infection in mice through intranasal (i.n.) or intracerebral (i.c.) routes. Conversely, the pathogenicity shown by the egg-derived parental virus (HK156-E3) and its clones were considerably lower in mice after i.n. or i.c. infection. A series of experimental infections revealed that the marked differences in neurovirulence among viruses could be attributed to whether or not viruses were transmitted from the lung to the brain. In amino acid sequence comparison of the entire proteins, it was suggested that a total of six amino acid differences in the PB1(residues 456 and 712), PA (residue 631), HA (residue 211), NP (residue 127) and NS1 (residue101) proteins related closely to changes in pathogenicity or neurovirulence of the HK156 virus in mice. As a result, it was evident that less pathogenic and neurovirulent strains appeared through adaptation and selection of variants during passage in eggs. © 2001 Elsevier Science B.V. All rights reserved.

Keywords: H5N1 viruses; Evolution; Virulence

---

* Corresponding author.

0531-5131/01/$ – see front matter © 2001 Elsevier Science B.V. All rights reserved.
PII: S 0 5 3 1 - 5 1 3 1 (0 1) 0 0 4 0 2 - 2

1. Introduction

Unlike influenza B virus, influenza A virus has been known to be distributed in many varieties of mammalian and avian species. In particular, this virus is further characterized by the appearance of pandemic strains with a novel hemagglutinin (HA) or neuraminidase (NA) in humans. Three pandemics occurred during the 20th century: Spanish (H1N1) influenza of 1918, Asian (H2N2) influenza of 1957 and the Hong Kong (H3N2) influenza of 1967 [1]. It has been shown that RNA segments of H2N2 and H3N2 pandemic viruses were derived from those of previously circulating human strains and viruses originating in avian species [2,3]. It is of particular interest to know that a large number of H3N2 viruses, which are similar antigenically and genetically to the early and more recent human epidemic H3N2 viruses, have been isolated from pigs in southern China [4]. Subsequent genomic analysis revealed the presence of reassortants between swine H3N2 and H1N1 viruses [4], suggesting an important surveillance site of southern China. In the cause of virological surveillance in the Japanese swine population, we also isolated three authentic antigenic reassortants between human H3N2 and swine H1N1 viruses [5,6].

The first H5N1 virus was isolated from a 3-year-old boy who died of Reye's syndrome on May 21, 1997 in Hong Kong [7]. Subsequently, 17 additional patients were reported to be infected with avian H5N1 virus during November and December 1997 and a total of six deaths were confirmed. [8]. On the basis of nucleotide sequence homology and phylogenetic analysis, it was confirmed that the above human infection was associated with an outbreak of highly pathogenic H5N1 virus infections of chickens [9–12], indicating direct infection of humans by an avian virus. Subsequently, evolutionary analysis revealed that the HA genes of H5N1 viruses isolated from humans and chickens were separated into two groups [10,13]. The remaining internal genes of human H5N1 viruses had not been characterized.

Mouse-adapted human influenza A viruses have been used to study the mechanisms of virulence or neurovirulence since human influenza viruses are generally nonpathogenic in mice without adaptation. It has been reported that virulence in mice is polygenic [14]. Therefore, the fact that HK156 virus exhibited a fatal infection in mice without adaptation [11,15,16] was of great interest. In this study, we describe the evolutionary divergence of Hong Kong H5N1 viruses and the genetic basis in pathogenicity and neurovirulence of these viruses.

2. Methods

2.1. Viruses

The following Hong Kong A H5N1 viruses were grown in Madin–Darby canine kidney (MDCK; M) or fertile 10-day-old hen's eggs (E): A/Hong Kong/481/97 (HK481), A/Hong Kong/482/97 (HK482), A/Hong Kong/483/97 (HK483), A/Hong Kong/485/97 (HK485), A/Hong Kong/486/97 (HK486). The HK156 strain was also used in pathogenicity and neurovirulence studies after passage in MDCK cells or eggs and these parental viruses were also used in the preparation of brain (B)—or egg (L or D)—cloned viruses.

2.2. Nucleotide sequence and phylogenetic analyses

Nucleotide sequences were determined as described previously [17]. The nucleotide sequences used in the phylogenetic analyses are Genebank accession numbers for as follows: AF036363, AF115290, AF084261, AF084262, AF084263, AF115291 AF036359, AF115284, AF084276, AF084277, AF084278, AF115285. All genes examined here were used for construction of phylogenetic trees as described previously [17].

2.3. Animal experiments

Five-week-old specific pathogen-free (SPF) female ddY mice (Japan SLC Shizuoka, Japan) were used in all experimental infections. All technical procedures for experimental infections were described in a previous report [18].

3. Result

3.1. Evolutionary analysis of the PB2, PB1 PA,NP, M and NS genes

As seen in Fig. 1a, the PB2 genes of influenza A viruses have evolved into the major human, swine, equine and avian lineages; the Hong Kong H5N1 PB2 gene apparently belongs to an avian lineage. The PB2 genes of H5N1 viruses, formed a lineage different from other avian viruses. They were characterized by three distinct minor branch clusters, containing HK156 (i: HK482 and HK486), HK483 (ii: HK485 and HK220), and HK481-like strains. Similarly, the PB1 and PB2 genes were also separated into two minor lineages containing HK 156 (i: 482, 486 and 481) and (ii: HK483, HK485 and ckHK220) (data not shown). Also, it was evident that the PA gene of H5N1 viruses, formed two minor clades. For example, HK156, HK481, HK482, HK485 and HK486 were included in the minor lineage i, whereas the remaining two strains (HK483 and ckHK220) were on lineage ii. The NP genes of influenza A virus also form several large branch clusters (Fig. 1b). The NP genes of H5N1 viruses apparently branched off from that of mallard/Astrakhan/2404/82, and were of composed of three minor lineage i (HK156, HK482, and HK486), ii (HK485, ckHK220 and ckHK225) and HK481 strain. The M and NS genes were also divided into two (i and ii) or three (i, ii and HK481) minor lineages, and these results were summarized in Table 1. The gene constellations of H5N1 viruses are presented in Table 1, which indicates that RNA segments of five strains appear to be composed of two minor lineages.

3.2. Amino acid changes in the internal proteins (PB2, PA, NP and M2) of Hong Kong H5N1 viruses in relation to the host range

Specific amino acid changes in the internal (PB2, PA, NP and M2) proteins have been reported to correlate with the host range of influenza virus [19,20]. Quite recently, Zhou et al. [19] have compared the amino acid sequences of Hong Kong H5N1 viruses isolated from chickens with those of other avian and human viruses. In order to examine the amino

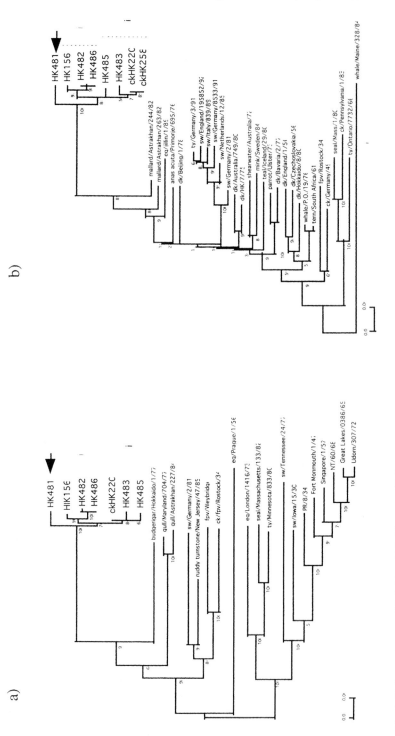

Fig. 1. Phylogenetic trees of PB2 (a) and NP (b) genes of influenza A viruses including those of Hong Kong H5N1 influenza viruses isolated from humans and chickens. Internal branching probabilities were determined by boostrap analysis using 500 replications and are indicated as percentages at each branch point.

Table 1
Genomic constellation and amino acids in the internal genes of Hong Kong H5N1 viruses similar to those of avian or human viruses

Viruses	RNA segments[a]								PB2				Amino acid at position				
	PB2	PB1	PA	HA	NA	NP	M	NS	199	627	661	667	PA	NP	M2		
													409	136	16	28	55
Avian	−[b]	−	−	−	−	−	−	−	A	E	A	V	S	L	E	I	L
Human	−	−	−	−	−	−	−	−	S	K	T[c]	I[d]	N	M	G	V	F
HK156	i	i	i	i	i	i	i	i	S	E	T	I	N	M	G	V	F
HK481	HK481	i	i	i	HK481	i	HK481	A	E	T	I	N	M	G	V	F
HK482	i	i	i	i	i	i	ii	i	S	E	T	I	N	M	G	V	F
HK486	i	i	i	i	i	i	ii	i	S	E	T	I	N	M	G	V	F
HK483	ii	ii	ii	ii	ii	ii	i	ii	A	K	T	I	S	M	G	V	F
HK485	ii	i	ii	ii	ii	ii	i	ii	A	K	T	I	S	M	G	V	F

[a] Symbols i, ii and HK481 indicates evolutionary minor clades represented by HK156-, HK483-, HK481-like viruses.

[b] −, Not examined.

[c] Residue determined in 20 of 22 sequences reported previously.

[d] Residue determined in 21 of 22 sequences reported previously.

acid changes specific for human virus, we also compared amino acid sequences of the PB2, PA, NP and M2 gene products; results are presented in Table 1. Six strains were found to contain three amino acid residues characteristic of the PB2 protein of human viruses at positions 199 (Ser), 661 (Thr) and 667 (Ile). One human specific amino acid was found in the PA protein of four strains at position 409 (Asn), and a further amino acid at position 136 (Met) of the NP protein specific for human virus was observed in all strains. It was of particular interest that the M2 protein of all strains contained human specific amino acid residues at positions 16 (Gly), 28 (Val) and 55 (Phe).

3.3. Attenuation of HK156 virus with passage in egg and tissue tropism between high and less virulent strains

In order to compare the virulence of MDCK- and egg-derived HK156 viruses, five groups of mice were infected through intranasal (i.n.) and intracerebral (i.c.) routes with 2×10^5 plaque-forming unit (PFU) of each virus and monitored for 14 days. MDCK-derived parental virus showed a lethal infection after i.n. or i.c. inoculation on day 8 post-infection (p.i.), killing 100% of mice (data not shown). In contrast, i.n. infection with egg-derived parental virus (HK156-E3) resulted in 60% mortality by day 14 p.i., showing less pathogenicity; and mice infected i.c. with the same virus showed a 100% survival rate even after 13 days p.i., demonstrating disappearance of neurovirulence (data not shown).

To examine the mechanisms of pathogenicity and neurovirulence, two types of variants were prepared in primary chick embryo cells and mouse brains, and they were cloned through plaque purification. Table 2 shows the growth characteristics of the parental and cloned viruses. All viruses prepared in the present study grew well in MDCK cells and eggs based on virus titers, whereas the virulence of egg-derived strains and its clones were

Table 2
Growth comparison and virulence of HK156 and its cloned viruses prepared in the study

Viruses and virulence in mouse	Passage history[a]	MDCK (log 10 PFU/ml)	ELD_{50} (log 10 PFU/ml)	ELD_{50} (PFU/ml)	MLD_{50} (PFU/ml)
High					
HK156-ck	Mx-M2	7.3	7.5	0.6	8.0×10^2
Brain clones					
B-1-1	Mx-Mb1-M4	7.2	7.5	4.0×10^2	3.2
B-1-2	Mx-Mb1-M4	7.7	7.5	4.0×10^4	3.2
B-3-11	Mx-Mb1-M4	7.8	8.0	6.0×10^3	3.2
Low					
HK156-E	Mx-M1-E3	7.3	8.0	0.2	1.3×10^4
Egg clones					
L7-4-1	Mx-M1-E3-C3-E1	7.6	8.2	0.2	$>2.0 \times 10^5$
D5-7-1	Mx-M1-E3-C3-E1	7.8	8.0	0.2	$>2.0 \times 10^5$

[a] Passage history in Hong Kong and our laboratory; Mx, MDCK but unknown history; Mb, mouse brain; C, CE cells; E, Egg. The number following these abbreviation indicates the number of passage. Method for virus cloning is explained in Methods.

considerably higher in eggs than that of MDCK derived virus. For instance, ELD_{50} of brain-derived clones (B1-1-1, B1-1-2 and B3-1-1) were apparently higher (4.0×10^2, 1.0×10^4 and 6.0×10^3) than those of HK156-E3 (0.2) and its cloned viruses (0.2), indicating that virulence of brain-derived clones in eggs was lower than parental HK156-E3 and its cloned viruses.

In contrast, the former brain-derived virus showed MLD_{50} values of 3.2 PFU, 250-fold higher than HK156-CK. It became clear that virulence of parental HK-156-E3 and its cloned viruses in mice were apparently lower than that of HK156-CK and its cloned viruses. These differences in pathogenicity of the above viruses in mice are clearly seen in Table 3. In fact, brain-derived clones appeared to be more pathogenic in mice than other HK156-E3 clones after i.n. or i.c. infection. For example, all mice infected i.n. or i.c. with brain-cloned viruses died on day 7 or day 8 p.i. Parental HK156-E3 and its cloned viruses showed 0% mortality after i.n. infection of mice. Similarly, even after i.c. infection, egg-cloned viruses killed only 20% of mice. The growth of parental and cloned viruses in the lung, brain, liver (data not shown) and kidney (data not shown) of mice was monitored for 6 days p.i. and the results are presented in Table 4. High virus titers were detected on day 2 p.i. in the lung of one mouse infected. i.n. with HK156-CK but not in HK156-E3 virus-infected mice. On day 4 p.i., virus replication was confirmed in the lungs of both groups of mice infected with HK156-CK and HK156-E3 viruses but titers of the latter virus were slightly lower than those of the former. Virus was isolated from the liver and kidney of one mouse on day 4 p.i., but virus could no longer detected at day 6 (data not shown). It was of particular interest that approximately 10^3 PFU/ml were detected in the brains of two mice infected i.n. with MDCK derived parental virus. In contrast, virus could not be detected in the brains of mice infected i.n. with egg-derived parental virus.

Table 3
Comparison of the mortality rate of mouse brain- and chick embryo cell-cloned viruses after I.n. and I.c. infection in mice

Viruses and pathogenicity	Mortality (%) on days p.i.									
	I.n. infection					I.c. infection				
	5	7	9	11	13	5	7	9	11	13
High										
Brain clones										
B1-1-1	40	100	100	100	100	60	80	100	100	100
B1-1-2	20	100	100	100	100	40	100	100	100	100
B3-1-1	0	100	100	100	100	80	100	100	100	100
Low										
CE clones										
L7-4-1	0	0	0	0	0	0	0	20	20	20
D5-7-1	0	0	0	0	0	0	20	20	20	40

Mortality rates of ddY mice infected with each cloned virus were examined using group of mice infected I.n. with 10^5 PFU or I.c. with, 10^4 PFU, respectively.

The brain-cloned viruses (B-1-1, B1-2 and B3-1-1) were further characterized by early replication in the brain when compared with its parental virus (HK156-CK). As these two parental viruses were quite different from each other in the replication in brain, their

Table 4
Comparative growth profiles of HK156 and its cloned viruses in mouse organs after I.n. or I.c. infection[a]

Viruses and virulence in mouse	Virus infectivity (log 10 PFU/ml) on days p.i.								
	I.n. infection						I.c. infection		
	Lung			Brain			Brain		
	2	4	6	2	4	6	2	4	6
High									
HK 156-CK	6.7/8.8	5.8/6.2	4.5/4.9	−/−[b]	−/−	3.3/3.1	nd	4.2/4.3	nd
Clones									
B1-1-1	6.0/6.0	6.3/6.5	nd[c]	−/−	−/−	nd	4.3/4.3	4.7/5.0	nd
B1-1-2	6.9/7.2	6.0/6.8	nd	−/−	1.3/1.7	nd	3.5/4.7	5.2/5.2	nd
B3-1-1	5.9/6.5	6.6/6.8	nd	−/−	1.4/1.6	nd	4.2/4.7	4.9/5.0	nd
Low									
HK 156-E3	−/−	5.3/5.4	3.5/4.0	−/−	−/−	−/−	nd	2.5/2.6	nd
Clones									
L7-4-1	0.7/4.7	5.4/5.4	4.8/5.0	−/−	−/−	−/−	2.7/3.2	3.5/4.5	1.2/2.7
D5-7-1	5.0/5.1	4.4/4.9	4.2/4.3	−/−	−/−	−/−	3.2/3.2	3.5/3.7	−/3.1
Aichi68[d]	nd	nd	nd	nd	nd	nd	nd	−/−	nd

[a] After infection, to determine virus infectivity, two mice were sacrificed on days 2, 4 and 6 p.i. and plaque-titrated in MDCK cells in the presence of trypsin.
[b] −, Virus titer less than 10 PFU/ml.
[c] nd, Not determined.
[d] Aichi68 virus was used a negative control as non-virulent virus.

growth was further compared with i.c. infection in mice. As seen in Table 4, both viruses appeared to replicate in the brains of mice infected i.c. with 10^4 PFU of viruses. The virus titers of HK156-CK virus were higher than those of HK156-E3 virus, indicating marked differences in neurovirulence between parental viruses. Virus was not isolated from mouse brain infected with Aichi68, which was used as a negative control and a non-neurovirulent strain. Thus, virus yield detected in the brains infected i.c. with the above parental viruses was not a reflection of surviving virus inoculate.

3.4. Nucleotide and amino acid sequence comparisons of high pathogenic and low pathogenic strains

To investigate the genetic basis of pathogenicity and neurovirulence, nucleotide sequences of the parental and cloned viruses were determined (Table 5). Interestingly, two distinct nucleotides were determined at positions 464 and 631 of the HA gene and at position 50 of the PB1 gene of HK156-CK, suggesting the existence of two variant populations in the parental virulent strain. These nucleotide changes coded for amino acids Ser and Asn at position 155, and coded for Pro and Thr at position 211 of the HA gene. Ala and an Asp residue were encoded at position 17 of the PB1 protein of the same strain. To confirm these changes, the HA genes of 18 cloned viruses were sequenced. It became clear that 11 clones contained Ser at position 155 of the HA1 domain, whereas the remaining seven possessed Asn.

Table 5
Amino acid changes of HK156 and its cloned viruses in relation to the pathogenicity and neurovirulence

Virus and virulence in mice	Amino acids and (nucleotides) at the following position:										
	HA		NSI	PBI			PA	NP	PB2	NA	
	155 (464)	211 (631)	101 (301)	17 (56)	456 (1366)	712 (2134)	631 (1891)	127 (379)	701 (2101)	54 (161)	83 (248)
High											
HK156-CK	Ser(G)[a] or Asn(A)	Pro(C)[a] or Thr(A)	Asp(G)	Ala(C)[a] or Asp(A)	His(C)	Ser(T)	Gly(G)	Glu(G)	Asn(A)	Asn(A)	Lys(A)
B1-1-1	Ser	*Proc*[b]	*Asp*	Ala	*Tyr*	*Pro*	*Ser*	*Lys*	Asp	Asn	Lys
B1-1-2	Ser	*Pro*	*Asp*	Ala	*Tyr*	*Pro*	*Ser*	*Lys*	Asp	Asn	Lys
B3-1-1	Ser	*Pro*	*Asp*	Ala	*Tyr*	*Pro*	*Ser*	*Lys*	Asp	Asn	Lys
Mouse brain homogenates	Ser	*Pro*	*Asp*	Ala	*Tyr*	*Pro*	*Ser*	*Lys*	Asp	−[c]	−
Low											
HK156-E3	Ser	*Thr*	*Asn*	Ala	His	Ser	Gly	Glu	Asp	Asn	Lys
L7-4-1	Ser	*Thr*	*Asn*	Ala	His	Ser	Gly	Glu	Asp	Ile(G)	Lys
D5-7-1	Ser	*Thr*	*Asn*	Ala	His	Ser	Gly	Glu	Asp	Asn	Arg(G)

[a] Nucleotide mixtures were observed in sequence gel image.
[b] Italic letter indicated specific amino acid changes associated with pathogenecity or neurovirulence.
[c] −, Not sequenced.

The passage of MDCK-derived parental HK156-CK in eggs might lead to the selection of a dominant virus because the egg-derived virus and its clones contained single amino acid residues at positions 155 (Ser) and 211 (Thr) of HA domain as well as at position 17 (Ala) of the PB1 protein. Moreover, two amino acid substitutions were detected in the NS (Asp $\rightarrow^{101}$ Asn) and PB2 (Asn $\rightarrow^{701}$ Asp) proteins.

In order to investigate the amino acid residues in relation to the neurovirulence, we sequenced the entire genome of brain-derived clones as well as infected-brain homogenates, using samples taken at 6 days p.i. This way, it became apparent that replication in the brain led to the selection of Ser at position 155 and Pro at position 211 of the HA protein as well as Ala at position 17 of the PB1 protein. Amino acid substitutions were also detected in the PB1 (His $\rightarrow^{456}$ Tyr and Ser $\rightarrow^{712}$ Pro), PA (Gly $\rightarrow^{631}$ Ser), NP (Glu $\rightarrow^{127}$ Lys) and PB2 (Asn $\rightarrow^{701}$ Asp) proteins of all brain clones and brain homogenates. It was noteworthy that all brain-derived clones appeared to be different from egg-derived clones at the following positions: the HA1 (Pro^{211} vs. Thr), NS (Asp^{101} vs. Asn), PB1(Tyr^{456} vs. His and Pro^{712} vs. Ser), PA(Ser^{631} vs. Gly), and NP (Lys^{127} vs. Glu). Also, all viruses including pathogenic and low pathogenic strains examined here possessed a series of basic amino acids adjacent to the cleavage site of the connecting peptide in the HA molecule, indicating that the above basic amino acids are not determinants of pathogenicity of HK156 virus in mice.

4. Discussion

Influenza A H5N1 viruses isolated from humans in Hong Kong in 1997 are reported to be separated into two serologic groups based on the hemagglutinin-inhibition test [13,15]. In agreement with the above reports, we confirmed the presence of two antigenic groups (data not shown). Through a series of evolutionary analyses, the six internal genes of human Hong Kong H5N1 viruses were found to have diverged generally into two or three distinguishable evolutionary groups, including HK156 (i)-, HK483 (ii)- and HK481-like strains. Indeed, the phylogenetic locations of the PB2, NP and NS genes of HK481 were somewhat divergent from those of the other two groups. In agreement with our analysis of human H5N1 virus, it has been shown that the internal genes of Hong Kong H5N1 viruses isolated from poultry clustered in two minor evolutionary groups. The gene constellations of human H5N1 viruses, which were shown in this study, suggest the frequent occurrence of genetic reassortment among two or three variant groups. Even though it is not clear why avian H5N1virus was able to infect humans in Hong Kong in 1997, one reason may be that human and poultry H5N1 viruses possessed human specific amino acids in the NP, PB2 and M2 proteins [13,15,20].

It has been reported previously that Hong Kong H5N1 viruses were separated into different pathogenic groups, including a less virulent group [15]. In the present study we have shown that differences in pathogenicity may relate to evolutionary divergence and differing gene constellations. In fact, HK483 did not change its pathogenicity even after passage in eggs, whereas virulence HK156 decreased for mice after passage in eggs. Although HK156 strains have been reported to cause lethal infection in mice [11,15,16], we observed that the pathogenicity of this virus was attenuated in mice after few passage in eggs. We also successfully isolated clones with low virulence from the parental egg-derived virus. The growth levels of these viruses in the lung and brain of mice appeared to be lower than those of the parental MDCK-grown virus and its brain clones. Although Lu et al. [16] reported that HK156 virus passaged only in eggs was found to grow in mouse brain and to cause lethal infection in mice even after i.n. infection, in this study, HK156-CK passaged in eggs became less virulent in mice and did not replicate in brain after i.n. infection.

How do differences in pathogenicity in mice relate to changes in the structural proteins of the viruses? Clear amino acid differences in the HA1 domain of the HA, PB1, PA, NP and NS1 proteins were detected between high and low pathogenic, neurovirulent and non-neurovirulent strains. On the basis of amino acids present in HA1 domain (Ser[155] or Asn–Ser, Pro[211] or Thr–Thr) and PB1 (Ala[17] or Asp–Ala) of low pathogenic strains, isolation of these viruses was apparently accompanied by selection from mixed populations in the parental MDCK-grown virus. On the other hand, other mutations in PB1, PA, NP, PB2 and NS1 of pathogenic, neurovirulent and less pathogenic strains may have occurred by adaptation to growth in eggs cells. As a result, one or all mutations at position 211 of the HA1 domain, and/or 101 of the NS protein of HK156 virus correlated with attenuation of this virus in mice. Additionally, amino acid substitutions in the PB1, PA, and NP proteins may be associated with neurovirulence in mice. Even though the Hong Kong outbreak in 1997 has taught us many lessons about surveillance and vaccine strategies, the causative viruses deserve more study from the evolutionary, biological and pathologic points of view.

References

[1] B.R. Murphy, R.G. Webster, Orthomyxoviruses. In: B.N. Fields, D.M. Knipe, P.M. Howley (Eds.), Field Virology, 3rd edn. Lippincott-Raven, Philadelphia, pp. 1397–1445.
[2] Y. Kawaoka, S. Krauss, R.G. Webster, Avian-to-human transmission of the PB1 gene of influenza A virus in the 1957 and 1968 pandemics, J. Virol. 63 (1989) 4603–4608.
[3] C. Scholtissek, W. Rhode, V. Van Hoynigen, R. Rott, On the origin of the human influenza subtypes H2N2 and H3N2, Virology 87 (1978) 13–20.
[4] K. Nerome, Y. Kanegae, K.F. Shortridge, S. Sugita, M. Ishida, Genetic analysis of porcine H3N2 viruses originating in southern China, J. Gen. Virol. 76 (1995) 613–624.
[5] K. Nerome, S. Sakamoto, N. Yano, T. Yamamoto, S. Kobayashi, R.G. Webster, A. Oya, Antigenic character-istics and genome composition of a naturally occurring recombinant influenza viruses isolated from a pig in Japan, J. Gen. Virol. 64 (1983) 2611–2620.
[6] A. Ouchi, K. Nerome, Y. Kanegae, M. Ishida, R. Nerome, K. Hayashi, T. Hashimoto, M. Kazi, Y. Kazi, Y. Inada, Large outbreak of swine influenza in southern Japan caused by reassortant (H1N2) influenza viruses: its epizootic background and characterization of the causative viruses, J. Gen. Virol. 77 (1996) 1751–1759.
[7] J.C. de Jong, E.C. Class, A.D. Osterhaus, R.G. Webster, W.L. Lim, A pandemic warning? Nature 389 (1997) 554.
[8] K.Y. Yuen, P.K. Chan, M. Periris, D.N. Tsang, T.L. Que, K.F. Shortridge, P.T. Cheung, W.K. To, E.T. Ho, R. Sung, A.F. Cheng, Clinical features and viral rapid diagnosis of human diseases associated with avian influenza A H5N1 virus, Lancet 351 (1998) 467–471.
[9] E.C. Class, A.D. Osterhaus, R. van Beek, J.C. de Jong, G.E. Rimmelzwaan, D.A. Senne, S. Lraiss, K.F. Shortridge, R.G. Webster, Human influenza A H5N1 virus related to a highly pathogenic avian influenza virus, Lancet 351 (1998) 472–477.

[10] D.L. Suarez, M.L. Perdue, N. Cox, T. Rowe, C. Bender, J. Huang, D.E. Swayne, Comparison of highly virulent H5N1 influenza A viruses isolated from humans and chickens from Hong Kong, J. Virol. 72 (1998) 6678–6688.

[11] K.F. Shortridge, N.N. Zhou, Y. Guan, P. Gao, T. Ito, Y. Kawaoka, S. Kodihalli, S. Kraus, D. Morkwell, L. Sims, A. Takada, R.G. Webster, Characterization of avian H5N1 influenza viruses from poultry in Hong Kong, Virology 252 (1998) 331–342.

[12] N.N. Zhou, K.F. Shortridge, E.C.J. Class, S.L. Kraus, R.G. Webster, Rapid evolution of H5N1 influenza viruses in chickens in Hong Kong, J. Virol. 73 (1999) 3366–3374.

[13] C. Bender, H. Hall, J. Huang, A. Klimov, N. Cox, A. Hay, V. Gregory, K. Cameron, W. Lim, K. Subarao, Characterization of the surface proteins of influenza A (H5N1) viruses isolated from humans in 1997–1998, Virology 254 (1999) 115–123.

[14] A.C. Ward, Virulence of influenza A virus for mouse lung, Virus Genes 14 (1997) 187–194.

[15] P. Gao, S. Watanabe, T. Ito, H. Goto, K. Wells, M. McGregor, A.J. Cooley, W. Kawaoka, Biological heterogeneity, including systemic replication in mice, of H5N1 influenza A virus isolates from humans in Hong Kong, J. Virol. 73 (1999) 3184–3189.

[16] X. Lu, T.M. Tumpey, T. Morken, J.Rm. Zaki, N.J. Cox, J.M. Katz, A mouse model for the evaluation of pathogenesis and immunity to influenza A (H5N1) viruses isolated from humans, J. Virol. 73 (1999) 5903–5911.

[17] Y. Hiromoto, Y. Yamazaki, T. Fukushima, T. Saito, S.E. Lindstrom, K. Omoe, R. Nerome, W. Lim, S. Sugita, K. Nerome, Evolutionary characterization of the six internal genes of H5N1 human influenza A virus, J. Gen. Virol. 81 (2000) 1293–1303.

[18] Y. Hiromoto, T. Saito, S. Lindstrom, K. Nerome, Characterization of low virulent strains of highly pathogenic A/Hong Kong/156/97 (H5N1) virus in mice after passage in embryonated hen's eggs, Virology 272 (2000) 429–437.

[19] A.J. Buckler-White, B.R. Murphy, Nucleotide sequence analysis of the nucleoprotein gene of an avian and human influenza virus strain identifies two classes of nucleoproteins, Virology 155 (1986) 156–159.

[20] B.R. Murphy, A.J. Buckler-White, W.T. London, M.H. Snyder, Characterization of the M protein and nucleoprotein genes of and avian influenza A virus which are involved in host range restriction in monkeys, Vaccine 7 (1989) 557–561.

International Congress Series 1219 (2001) 225–231

Infection of grey seals and harbour seals with influenza B virus

R.A.M. Fouchier[a,*], T.M. Bestebroer[a], B.E.E. Martina[a,b],
G.F. Rimmelzwaan[a], A.D.M.E. Osterhaus[a,b]

[a]Department of Virology, Erasmus University, PO Box 1738, 3000 DR, Rotterdam, The Netherlands
[b]Seal Rehabilitation and Research Center, Pieterburen, The Netherlands

Abstract

Background: Influenza B virus is exclusively a human pathogen whose origin and possible reservoir in nature are not known. Seals in the wild are known to be susceptible to influenza A as well as other virus infections. *Methods*: PCR-based analyses, virus isolation techniques and serological assays were used for the detection of influenza B virus infection of seals. Sequence analysis and serology were used for virus characterisation. *Results*: An influenza B virus was isolated from a naturally infected harbour seal (*Phoca vitulina*). The infected seal and a second seal, both of which had been admitted to a seal rehabilitation centre in the Netherlands, seroconverted to influenza B virus. Influenza virus B/Seal/Netherlands/1/99 was found to be infectious to seal kidney cells in vitro. Sequence analyses as well as serology indicated that this influenza B virus is closely related to strains that circulated in humans 4 to 5 years earlier. Retrospective analyses of sera collected from 971 seals showed a prevalence of antibodies to influenza B virus in 2% of the animals after 1995, and in none before 1995, suggesting that the virus was introduced in the seal population from a human source around 1995. *Conclusions*: This is the first report on natural influenza B virus infection emerging in a non-human species. The data document that influenza B virus can be maintained in seals. This reservoir, harbouring influenza B viruses that have circulated in the past, may pose a direct threat to humans in the future. © 2001 Elsevier Science B.V. All rights reserved.

Keywords: Animal; Ecology; Reservoir; Epidemiology

* Corresponding author. Tel.: +31-10-4088066; fax: +31-10-4089485.
E-mail address: fouchier@viro.fgg.eur.nl (R.A.M. Fouchier).

1. Introduction

Influenza A viruses have been isolated from many species, and aquatic birds may form the natural reservoir from which pandemics and subsequent epidemics in humans have originated [1]. In contrast, influenza B virus infection is supposed to be restricted to humans. Previous reports on influenza B virus infection of a dog and a pig did not meet the established criteria to prove infection [2,3].

Herpes-, morbili-, calici- and poxviruses have been identified as causes of significant morbidity and mortality among pinniped species [4–9]. In addition, influenza A viruses of avian origin, including four different antigenic subtypes (H3N3, H4N5, H4N6 and H7N7), have caused outbreaks of influenza among seals [10–13].

Seals stranded at the Dutch coast are admitted to the Seal Rehabilitation and Research Center (SRRC) in Pieterburen, the Netherlands for rehabilitation. In the spring of 1999, a number of juvenile harbour seals presented respiratory problems, but were not infected with phocine herpesvirus (PHV) or phocine distemper virus (PDV). We decided to test these seals for influenza virus infection.

2. Materials and methods

All materials and methods have been described elsewhere [14–17].

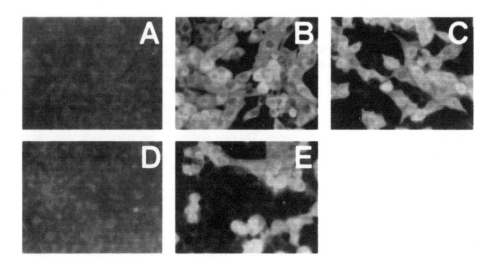

Fig. 1. Replication of influenza virus isolates in seal kidney cells. Seal kidney cells were inoculated with influenza virus B/Seal/Netherlands/1/99 (B), B/Netherlands/429/98 (C), A/Seal/Massachusetts/1/80 (E) or mock-infected (A, D) and stained with anti-influenza B virus (A, B, C) or anti-influenza A virus specific NP antibodies (D, E) 24 h after inoculation. All influenza virus-infected cultures were productively infected, as determined by hemagglutination assays with turkey erythrocytes.

3. Results

3.1. Virus isolation

Upon inoculation of MDCK cells with throat swab samples taken from 12 juvenile harbour seals, cytopathic changes were noted within 3 days of inoculation with one of the samples (seal 99-012). The supernatant of this cell culture agglutinated turkey erythrocytes in a hemagglutination assay. Negative contrast electron microscopic analysis of the hemagglutinin (HA) positive culture supernatant showed the presence of orthomyxovirus-like particles. To our surprise, the presence of influenza B virus was identified by reverse-transcription and polymerase chain reaction (RT-PCR) analysis of RNA isolated from the culture supernatant as well as hemaggultination inhibition assays with influenza B virus-specific ferret sera. This influenza virus, B/Seal/Netherlands/1/99, as well as a human influenza B virus could be readily propagated in primary seal kidney cell cultures (Fig. 1).

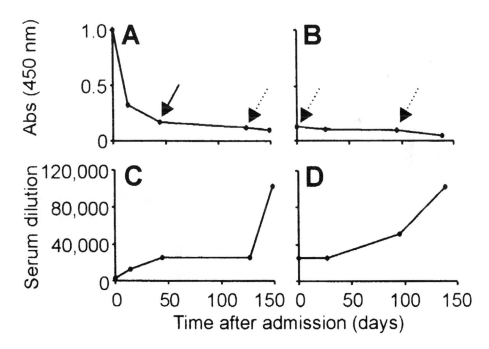

Fig. 2. Antibody response in influenza B virus infected seals. Sera from seals 99-012 (panel A and C) and 99-041 (panel B and D) were tested for the presence of IgM antibodies to NP (panel A and B) and IgG antibodies to HA/NA proteins (panel C and D). Arrows indicate the time-points when virus detection in throat swab samples was attempted, with isolate B/Seal/Netherlands/1/99 represented as a solid arrow and negative results as dotted arrows. Reprinted with permission from Ref. [15], Copyright 2000 American Association for the advancement of Science.

3.2. Serology

To exclude the possibility of sample contamination in our laboratory, serum samples collected from the 8-month-old seal 99-012 taken before and after virus isolation were tested for the presence of hemagglutination inhibiting (HAI) antibodies to B/Seal/Netherlands/1/99. Samples collected 44 days before and at the day of virus isolation were negative (HAI titre <6), whereas the sample collected 83 days after virus isolation showed a HAI titre of 192, confirming that seal 99-012 had been infected with influenza B virus. Sera from seven other juvenile harbour seals, kept in the same basin as seal 99-012, were also tested for the presence of HAI antibodies. The serum of one seal, 99-041, collected 61 days after the day of virus isolation from seal 99-012, showed a HAI titre of 48. All other sera from this and other animals were negative (HAI titre <6). Unfortunately, we were unable to detect influenza B virus by RT-PCR in the throat swabs collected from seal 99-041 at 34 days before and 61 days after virus isolation from seal 99-012.

Quantitative analyses of IgG antibodies to the nucleoprotein (NP) and envelope glycoproteins HA and neuraminidase (HA/NA) of influenza B virus as well as IgM antibodies to NP as an indicator for primary infection were performed by enzyme linked immunosorbent assay (ELISA)(Fig. 2) [17]. In seals 99-012 and 99-041, IgG antibodies to HA/NA and NP were detected, which increased over time and correlated with virus neutralizing and HAI antibodies. Both harbour seals displayed decreasing IgM antibody levels to the NP from the day of admission onward; virus was isolated from the throat swab of seal 99-012 at day 44 after admission. The kinetics of IgM responses generally observed upon primary virus infection in mammals suggest that both seals had been infected days (seal 99-012) or weeks (seal 99-041) before admission.

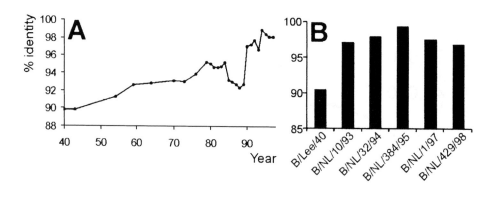

Fig. 3. Comparison of HA of influenza virus B/Seal/Netherlands/1/99 to human influenza B virus. The nucleotide sequences of HA of prototypes of the human influenza B virus epidemics from the past 60 years were compared to the seal influenza B virus, revealing that isolates obtained from humans around 1994 and 1995 displayed the highest resemblance (A). Amino acid homology between influenza virus B/Seal/Netherlands/1/99 and Dutch prototypes of influenza B virus from 1993 to 1998 (B). Sequence data are available from Genbank under accession numbers AF217214-AF217223.

3.3. Sequence analysis

We next amplified the first domain of the hemagglutinin gene (HA1) from B/Seal/ Netherlands/1/99, as well as from the original throat swab by RT-PCR and sequenced the amplified fragments. The sequences from the throat swab and the virus isolate were identical. Comparison of the sequence from B/Seal/Netherlands/1/99 with human influenza B virus sequences revealed that the seal isolate closely resembled B/Harbin/ 7/94-like strains (Fig. 3). In fact, one HA1 sequence in the database (B/Argentina/4105/ 95) proved to be identical to that of B/Seal/Netherlands/1/99. Since this isolate had never been used in our laboratory and no reagents were used which are not fully accounted for in terms of their origin, contamination of our samples by B/Argentina/ 4105/95 is highly unlikely. The high antibody titres to influenza B virus in seal 99-012 support this conclusion. The homology between B/Seal/Netherlands/1/99 and 1995-like strains is surprising as HA from human influenza B undergoes significant antigenic and genetic change over time. This had indeed occurred from 1995 until 1999 in humans. The rapid adaptation of influenza A viruses to their new host, typically observed upon zoonotic transmission, was not obvious from the HA1 sequence of this seal influenza B virus.

A HAI assay was performed with serum from seal 99-012 and B/Seal/Netherlands/1/99 as well as B/Netherlands/384/95 and B/Netherlands/429/98, prototypes of the 1994/1995 and 1998/1999 epidemics. Serum from seal 99-012 consistently showed an approximate twofold better recognition of homologous and 1995 viruses as compared to the 1998 virus in independently repeated HAI assays. Although twofold differences in HAI titres are generally not considered significant, these data do suggest that seal 99-012 was indeed infected with a 1995-like virus.

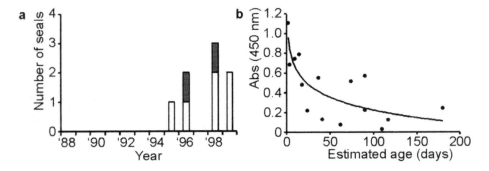

Fig. 4. Frequency of influenza B virus seropositive seals admitted at the SRRC over time and decline of antibody titres in seropositive seals. Serum samples obtained from seals in the past 10 years (580 seals before 1995, 391 seals from 1995 and later) were screened for antibodies against influenza B virus by HAI and confirmed by ELISA with NP and HA/NA proteins (panel a). White bars represent harbour seals; black bars represent grey seals. IgG antibody levels to NP from longitudinal samples obtained from the six seropositive seals admitted to the SRRC from 1995 to 1998 (panel a) were determined by ELISA and plotted against seal age (panel b). Reprinted with permission from Ref. [15], Copyright 2000 American Association for the advancement of Science.

3.4. Epidemiology

As both seals seemed to have been infected in the wild, we tested the hypothesis that a human influenza B virus was introduced in the seal population in 1995, and had circulated since. We screened sera obtained from 580 seals before 1995 and 391 seals during or after 1995 for HAI activity against B/Seal/Netherlands/1/99 and confirmed the findings by ELISA using HA/NA and NP as antigens. For seals stranded in 1995 or later, both the serum sample taken at the moment of admission to the SRRC and the last sample before release in the wild were included, to exclude seroconversion during rehabilitation. None of the seals admitted to the SRRC before 1995 were seropositive, whereas 8 (including 99-012 and 99-041) out of 391 seals admitted from 1995 onward had HAI antibody titres between 24 and 768 ($p < 0.001$) (Fig. 4). The six additional seals were four harbour seal pups and two grey seal (*Halichoerus grypus*) pups. Harbour and grey seals are known to share the same habitat in the Dutch coastal waters. None of these animals had IgM antibodies to NP, and all of them displayed decreasing levels of IgG antibodies to HA/NA and NP (Fig. 4) over time. This decrease correlated with a decrease in virus neutralizing and HAI antibody levels. This is in contrast to seals 99-012 and 99-041, which had decreasing IgM and increasing IgG titres. The estimated half-life of NP-specific antibodies during the first 2 months of life in these six pups of approximately 25 days, is in accordance with the half-life of maternal antibody titres to PDV observed in seal pups, suggesting that the detected antibodies are of maternal origin. On the basis of available seal population data in the Netherlands, it may be estimated that between half and 2% of animals in the wild have experienced influenza B virus infection since 1995.

4. Discussion and conclusions

Our data do not allow conclusions about the pathogenesis of influenza B virus infections in seals. Although the two harbour seals with proven influenza B virus infection displayed respiratory symptoms during their rehabilitation period, this occurred at a time when the admitted juvenile seals suffered from lungworm (*Otostrongylus circumlitus* and *Parafilaroides gymnurus*) infections as well.

The combined serological and virological data obtained from seal 99-012 indicate that influenza B virus shedding in seals was prolonged as compared to shedding in humans and IgG antibody responses to NP and HA/NA were delayed. Possible explanations for this apparent suboptimal immune response upon infection may be associated with xenobiotic-related immunosuppression or the therapeutic use of corticosteroids to combat the lungworm infections. Prolonged virus shedding in addition to the limited spreading of influenza B virus among seals—as shown in the SRRC and indicated by the limited seroprevalence of specific antibodies in the wild—may explain why little or no genetic and antigenic drift of influenza B virus is observed in seals.

Our data not only highlight that influenza B virus infections can emerge in seal populations, but also show that seals may constitute an animal reservoir from which humans may be exposed to influenza B viruses that have circulated in the past.

Acknowledgements

We are grateful to L. van der Kemp, G. de Mutsert, J. Habova and M. van der Bildt for technical assistance, Solvay Pharmaceuticals, Weesp, The Netherlands for providing HA/ NA proteins from B/Harbin/7/94, and the SRRC staff for taking care and sampling of seals. R.F. is a fellow of the Royal Dutch Academy of Arts and Sciences.

References

[1] R.G. Webster, W.J. Bean, O.T. Gorman, T.M. Chambers, Y. Kawaoka, Evolution and ecology of influenza A viruses, Microbiol. Rev. 56 (1) (1992) 152–179.

[2] C.P. Chang, A.E. New, J.F. Taylor, H.S. Chiang, Influenza virus isolations from dogs during a human epidemic in Taiwan, Int. J. Zoonoses 3 (1976) 61–64.

[3] G. Takatsy, J. Romvary, E. Farkas, Susceptibility of the domestic swine to influenza B virus, Acta Microbiol. Acad. Sci. Hung. 14 (3) (1967) 309–315.

[4] C.M. Prato, T.G. Akers, A.W. Smith, Serological evidence of calcivirus transmission between marine and terrestrial mammals, Nature 249 (454) (1974) 255–256.

[5] A.W. Smith, D.E. Skilling, Viruses and virus diseases of marine mammals, J. Am. Vet. Med. Assoc. 175 (9) (1979) 918–920.

[6] A.D. Osterhaus, J. Groen, P. De Vries, F.G. UytdeHaag, B. Klingeborn, R. Zarnke, Canine distemper virus in seals, Nature 335 (6189) (1988) 403–404.

[7] A.D. Osterhaus, H. Yang, H.E. Spijkers, J. Groen, J.S. Teppema, G. van Steenis, The isolation and partial characterization of a highly pathogenic herpesvirus from the harbor seal (*Phoca vitulina*), Arch. Virol. 86 (3–4) (1985) 239–251.

[8] A. Osterhaus, J. Groen, H. Niesters, M. van de Bildt, B. Martina, L. Vedder, J. Vos, H. van Egmond, B. Abou-Sidi, M.E. Barham, Morbillivirus in monk seal mass mortality, Nature 388 (6645) (1997) 838–839.

[9] C.D. Harvell, K. Kim, J.M. Burkholder, R.R. Colwell, P.R. Epstein, D.J. Grimes, E.E. Hofmann, E.K. Lipp, A.D. Osterhaus, R.M. Overstreet, J.W. Porter, G.W. Smith, G.R. Vasta, Emerging marine diseases — climate links and anthropogenic factors, Science 285 (5433) (1999) 1505–1510.

[10] R.G. Webster, V.S. Hinshaw, W.J. Bean, K.L. Van Wyke, J.R. Geraci, D.J. St Aubin, G. Petursson, Characterization of an influenza A virus from seals, Virology 113 (2) (1981) 712–724.

[11] V.S. Hinshaw, W.J. Bean, R.G. Webster, J.E. Rehg, P. Fiorelli, G. Early, J.R. Geraci, D.J. St. Aubin, Are seals frequently infected with avian influenza viruses? J. Virol. 51 (3) (1984) 863–865.

[12] J.R. Geraci, D.J. St. Aubin, I.K. Barker, R.G. Webster, V.S. Hinshaw, W.J. Bean, H.L. Ruhnke, J.H. Prescott, G. Early, A.S. Baker, S. Madoff, R.T. Schooley, Mass mortality of harbor seals: pneumonia associated with influenza A virus, Science 215 (4536) (1982) 1129–1131.

[13] R.J. Callan, G. Early, H. Kida, V.S. Hinshaw, The appearance of H3 influenza viruses in seals, J. Gen. Virol. 76 (1995) 199–203.

[14] R.A. Fouchier, T.M. Bestebroer, S. Herfst, L. van der Kemp, G.F. Rimmelzwaan, A.D. Osterhaus, Detection of influenza A viruses from different species by PCR amplification of conserved sequences in the matrix gene, J. Clin. Microbiol. 38 (2000) 4096–4101.

[15] A.D. Osterhaus, G.F. Rimmelzwaan, B.E.E. Martina, T.M. Bestebroer, R.A. Fouchier, Influenza B virus in seals, Science 288 (5468) (2000) 1051–1053.

[16] G.F. Rimmelzwaan, M. Baars, E.C. Claas, A.D. Osterhaus, Comparison of RNA hybridization, hemagglutination assay, titration of infectious virus and immunofluorescence as methods for monitoring influenza virus replication in vitro, J. Virol. Methods 74 (1) (1998) 57–66.

[17] J.T. Voeten, J. Groen, D. van Alphen, E.C. Claas, R. de Groot, A.D. Osterhaus, G.F. Rimmelzwaan, Use of recombinant nucleoproteins in enzyme-linked immunosorbent assays for detection of virus-specific immunoglobulin A (IgA) and IgG antibodies in influenza virus A- or B-infected patients, J. Clin. Microbiol. 36 (12) (1998) 3527–3531.

International Congress Series 1219 (2001) 233–240

Antigenic and genetic diversity among swine influenza viruses in Europe

S. Marozin[a],*, V. Gregory[a], K. Cameron[a], M. Bennett[a], M. Valette[b], M. Aymard[b], E. Foni[c], G. Barigazzi[c], Y. Lin[a], A. Hay[a]

[a]*National Institute for Medical Research, The Ridgeway, Mill Hill, London NW7 1AA, UK*
[b]*Laboratory of Virology, Université Lyon 1, 8 Avenue Rockefeller, 69373 Lyon Cedex 08, France*
[c]*Istituto Zooprofilattico, Sperimentale della Lombardia e dell'Emilia, Parma, Italy*

Abstract

H3N2 and "avian-like" H1N1 subtypes have circulated in European pigs since the mid- to late 1970s. Following reassortment to acquire six internal genes of the H1N1 viruses in the early 1980s, the H3N2 viruses have evolved to produce antigenically distinguishable variants. Sw/Finistere/127/99, isolated from a pig in January 1999, was shown to be closely related in antigenic and genetic characteristics to contemporary human A/Sydney/5/97-like viruses, and may represent the emergence of another "human-like" virus in European pigs. The H1N1 viruses circulating in pigs in France have evolved gradually over the past 20 years, but are in general closely related to early isolates such as Sw/Finistere/2899/82. An antigenically distinct variant, represented by Sw/Ille et Vilaine/1455/99, represents a significant drift from other recent French H1N1 viruses. Most of the H1N2 reassortant viruses isolated in France and Italy since 1997 were shown to be genetically similar to the H1N2 viruses which have become prevalent in the U.K., but to exhibit significant variation in antigenicity. Genetic reassortment between H1N2 and H1N1 viruses has also contributed to the recent increase in diversity of viruses circulating in pigs in Europe, and emphasizes the potential difficulties in controlling influenza by vaccination. Since most of these swine viruses are resistant to amantadine, they provide an increasing pool of amantadine-resistant M genes for potential incorporation into future human viruses. © 2001 Elsevier Science B.V. All rights reserved.

Keywords: Influenza; European swine; H1N1; H1N2; H3N2; Reassortment

* Corresponding author. Tel.: +44-20-8959-3666x2152; fax: +44-20-8906-4477.
  E-mail address: smarozi@nimr.mrc.ac.uk (S. Marozin).

0531-5131/01/$ – see front matter © 2001 Elsevier Science B.V. All rights reserved.
PII: S0531-5131(01)00390-9

1. Introduction

Similarities in the subtypes of influenza A, H1N1 and H3N2, which circulate in swine and human populations reflect the frequent transmission of viruses between the two species. Classical swine H1N1 viruses and H3N2 viruses similar to contemporary human H3N2 viruses were first isolated from pigs in Europe in the mid-1970s [1,2]. "Avian-like" H1N1 viruses, first isolated from European pigs in 1979 [3] replaced classical H1N1 swine viruses and have since co-circulated with H3N2 viruses. Genetic reassortment between viruses of the two subtypes in 1983–1984 gave rise to H3N2 viruses which contain six internal genes (encoding PB2, PB1, PA, NP, M and NS proteins) corresponding to those of the "avian-like" H1N1 viruses [4]. The subsequent lack of divergence of these genes of the two subtypes indicates frequent exchange of genes between the H1N1 and H3N2 subtypes. Reassortment of the genes encoding the surface antigens to produce H1N2 viruses was observed [5], but these viruses did not become established in Europe. During the 1990s a novel H1N2 subtype emerged in pigs in the U.K, which possessed a haemagglutinin (HA) closely related to the HAs of H1N1 viruses circulating in the human population during the early 1980s [6].

This paper reports the results of studies of viruses recently isolated from pigs in Northern France (Brittany) and Northern Italy and focuses in particular on the characteristics of recent antigenic variants of H1N1 and H1N2 viruses emerging among pigs in continental Europe.

2. Viruses from France and Italy

Of some 111 viruses isolated during 1997 to 2000, 26 were from France, including 2 H3N2, 19 H1N1 and 5 H1N2 viruses, and 85 were from Italy, including 52 H3N2, 29 H1N1 and 4 H1N2 viruses. Whereas H3N2 viruses were prevalent among viruses from Italy, few were obtained from Brittany. Since the initial H1N2 isolate from Brittany in 1997, this "UK-like" subtype appears to be increasing in prevalence.

3. H3N2 viruses

Gradual evolution of the HA gene of H3N2 viruses has resulted in increased genetic heterogeneity with the appearance of antigenic variants, such as those represented by A/swine/Belgium/220/92 and A/swine/Italy/1523/98 (Sw/Italy/1523/98), which are distinguishable in haemagglutination inhibition (HI) tests using post infection ferret antisera. Most recent Italian isolates were antigenically and genetically similar to Sw/Italy/1523/98, although other variants have been identified. The only H3N2 virus from France during 1998 and 1999, A/swine/Finistere/127/99, was similar in its antigenic and genetic (see Fig. 2) characteristics to A/Sydney/5/97-like human viruses. Comparisons of the sequences of the HA and NA components showed that this swine virus was closely related to the contemporary human variant, consistent with the recent introduction of a human virus.

Table 1
Antigenic characterization of swine H1N1 and H1N2 viruses

Haemagglutination inhibition titre[b]

Viruses[a]	Subtype	Rabbit sera		Post-infection ferret sera										
		Sw/Fin 2899/82	A/Brazil 11/78	Sw/Fin 2899/82	Sw/It 15131/98	Sw/IV 1482/99	Sw/CA 1455/99	Sw/It 2064/99	A/Braz 11/78	A/Chile 1/83	A/Taiw 1/86	Sw/Scot /94	Sw/It 1521/98	Sw/CA 604/99
Sw/Fin/2899/82	**H1N1**	**5120**	40	**1280**	160	2560	160	80	<	<	<	<	<	<
Sw/Italy/15131/98	**H1N1**	5120	320	320	**640**	1280	160	320	<	<	<	<	<	<
Sw/CA/1482/99	**H1N1**	5120	160	1280	640	**2560**	320	160	<	<	<	<	<	<
Sw/IV/1455/99	**H1N1**	1280	40	80	40	640	**1280**	40	40	<	<	<	<	<
Sw/Italy/2064/99	**H1N2**	1280	<	160	40	640	40	**1280**	<	<	<	<	<	<
Sw/CA/1488/99	H1N1	1280	40	320	40	640	1280	80	<	<	<	<	<	<
Sw/IV/760/00	H1N1	nd	nd	640	80	nd	1280	80	nd	nd	nd	nd	nd	nd
A/Brazil/11/78	**H1N1**	80	**5120**	<	<	40	80	80	**640**	160	<	160	<	<
A/Chile/1/83	**H1N1**	40	5120	<	<	40	40	40	80	**160**	<	40	<	<
A/Taiwan/1/86	**H1N1**	<	2560	<	<	<	<	<	<	<	**640**	80	<	<
Sw/Scot410440/94	**H1N2**	80	5120	<	<	<	<	<	320	640	80	**2560**	40	80
Sw/Italy/1521/98	**H1N2**	<	5120	<	<	<	<	<	<	<	<	<	**320**	<
Sw/CA/604/99	**H1N2**	80	5120	<	<	<	<	<	160	320	40	320	80	**1280**
Sw/CA/790/97	H1N2	80	5120	<	<	<	<	<	160	160	40	320	80	320
Sw/CA/2433/98	H1N2	160	5120	<	<	<	<	<	160	320	<	320	80	160
Sw/Italy/16541/99	H1N2	40	5120	<	<	<	<	<	40	<	<	<	320	40
Sw/Italy/1081/00	H1N2	<	5120	<	<	<	40	40	<	40	<	40	320	<

[a] Reference viruses are in bold.
[b] Homologous titres in bold; < indicates <40.

4. H1N1 viruses

Although the H1N1 viruses have evolved gradually over the past 20 years, the majority are still closely related in their antigenic characteristics to viruses isolated in the

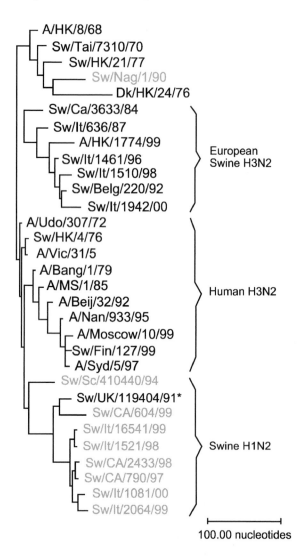

Fig. 1. Phylogenetic relationships between N2 genes of human H3N2 viruses and swine H3N2 and H1N2 viruses. Nucleotides 70 to 1031 of the coding sequences were analysed with PAUP using a maximum parsimony algorithm. The lengths of the horizontal lines are proportional to the number of nucleotide differences (as indicated). Sequences not determined in this study were obtained from GenBank. Abbreviations used include: Beij, Beijing; Belg, Belgium; Bk, Bangkok; CA, Cotes d'Armor; Dk, duck; Fin, Finistere; HK, Hong Kong; It, Italy; Mosc, Moscow; Ms, Mississippi; Nag, Nagasaki; Nc, Nanchang; Sc, Scotland; Sw, swine; Syd, Sydney; Tw, Taiwan; Ud, Uldorn; UK, United Kingdom; Vic, Victoria. H1N2 viruses are in grey.

early 1980s, such as A/swine/Finistere/2899/82 (Sw/Fin/2899/82). A/swine/Ille et Vilaine/ 1455/99 (Sw/IV/1455/99) provided an example of a more clearly distinguishable antigenic variant (Table 1). Two later French isolates A/swine/Cotes d'Armor/1488/99 (Sw/CA/1488/99) and Sw/IV/760/00 were antigenically similar in HI and NI tests to Sw/ IV/1455/99, whereas an Italian variant, Sw/Italy/2064/99, was distinguishable in HI tests (Table 1). Comparisons of the HA gene sequences of these viruses showed that Sw/IV/ 1455/99 and Sw/CA/1488/99 shared 99.5% homology but were distantly related (92% homology) to the majority of other recent French H1N1 swine viruses, represented by, e.g. Sw/CA/1482/99. They were in fact more closely related genetically (94–95% homology) to some of the recent Italian H1N1 isolates and to earlier isolates such as Sw/Germany/8533/91. Sequences of the NA genes of these two variants exhibited a similar divergence from the NA gene sequences of other recent French H1N1 viruses. Although Sw/Italy/2064/99 was antigenically distinguishable in HI tests, its HA gene, which shares only 95% sequence homology, groups phylogenetically with the HA genes of the two French variants. This virus is however of the H1N2 subtype and possesses a NA gene similar to those of several H1N2 viruses recently isolated in France and Italy (Fig. 1).

5. H1N2 viruses

Eight H1N2 viruses isolated in Brittany and Italy were shown to be similar to H1N2 viruses previously isolated in the U.K. HI tests (using rabbit antisera) showed that their HAs were antigenically related to human H1N1 viruses, such as A/Brazil/11/78 (Table 1). The results obtained using post-infection ferret antisera indicated that the French isolates, like A/swine/Scotland/410440/94 (Sw/Sc/410440/94), were more closely related to the early human H1N1 viruses than were the Italian isolates and distinguished the Scottish and French isolates from the three closely related Italian isolates (Table 1). These relationships were to some extent reflected in comparisons of HA sequences. Phylogenetic relationships showed that the HA genes of two of the French and two of the Italian isolates were more closely related (93–97% sequence homology) to the HA gene of Sw/England/690421/95 (H1N2), while the isolate Sw/CA/604/99 was more closely related to Sw/Sc/41440/94. Phylogenetic comparisons of the NA genes (Fig. 1) showed that the N2s of these viruses were closely related to the N2 of the U.K. H3N2 virus Sw/UK/119404/91 (93–95% homology) and distantly related (86–91% homology) to the N2s of swine H3N2 viruses circulating in continental Europe between 1984 and 2000, indicating that, like the HA, the NA of these viruses was derived from the previously identified U.K. H1N2 viruses. Whereas the N2s of most of the French and Italian isolates were closely related to each other and had diverged somewhat from those of U.K. isolates, as for the HA, the N2 of Sw/CA/604/99 was more closely related to the N2s of certain U.K. swine isolates, indicating separate introduction of this, or a related, virus into French pigs.

Comparisons of the sequences of the six internal genes showed that they were closely related to the internal genes of co-circulating H1N1 and H3N2 viruses. Differences in sequence homology between subtypes were comparable to differences between corresponding genes of viruses within the same subtype. This is illustrated in Fig. 2 for the NP

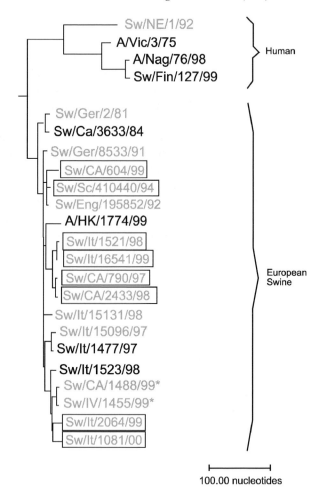

Fig. 2. Phylogenetic relationships between NP genes of human H3N2 viruses and swine H1N1, H1N2 and H3N2 viruses. Nucleotides 442–1422 of the coding sequences were analysed as indicated in Fig. 1. Abbreviations not explained in the legend to Fig. 1 include: Eng, England; Ger, Germany; IV, Ille et Vilaine; Ne, Nebraska. H1N2 viruses are in boxed and H3N2 viruses are in black. The asterisks indicate the antigenically distinguishable H1N1 viruses.

gene where the similarity between the NP genes of Sw/Italy/15096/97 (H1N1) and Sw/Italy/1477/97 (H3N2) contrasts with the differences between each of these genes and another of a virus of the same subtype, Sw/Italy/15131/98 (H1N1) and Sw/Italy/1523/98 (H3N2), respectively. The NP genes of most of the H1N2 viruses, represented by Sw/Italy/1521/98, were similar to each other and distinguishable from the corresponding genes of the two 1999 H1N1 variants, represented by Sw/IV/1455/99. In contrast, as for the HA, NA and other five internal genes, the NP gene of Sw/CA/604/99 was more closely related to the NP gene of Sw/Sc/410440/94.

6. Genetic reassortment

It is apparent that, as for the HA, the NP of Sw/Italy/2064/99 (H1N2) is more closely related to that of the H1N1 virus Sw/IV/1455/99 (Fig. 2); a similar relationship was observed for the PB2, PB1, PA and M genes (Table 2). The NS gene of Sw/Italy/2064/99 was, however, like the N2, more closely related to the NS genes of the other H1N2 viruses (Table 2) indicating that this virus is the product of genetic reassortment between a H1N2 virus and a virus similar to Sw/IV/1455/99. Fig. 2 also indicates that contrary to the other H1N2 viruses, Sw/Italy/1081/00 has an NP gene more closely related to that of Sw/IV/1455/99 than to that of, e.g. Sw/Italy/1521/98. Table 2 indicates the relationships of the various genes of Sw/Italy/1081/00 (H1N2) with the corresponding genes of Sw/Italy/1521/98 (H1N2) and Sw/IV/1455/99 (H1N1). It is apparent that Sw/Italy/1081/00 possesses five genes, PB2, PB1, PA, NP and M, which are more closely related to those of the H1N1 virus than to those of the H1N2 virus (the degree of sequence homology reflects the results of phylogenetic comparisons, not shown) and is the product of genetic reassortment.

7. Amatadine resistance

M gene sequences showed that the M2 proteins of the different subtypes (with the exception of Sw/Fin/127/99), like H1N1 and H3N2 viruses circulating since 1987 [7], possessed asparagine at position 31, indicating resistance to the anti-influenza drugs, amantadine and rimantadine. For several viruses, including Sw/IV/1455/99 and Sw/Italy/1521/98, this was confirmed by drug sensitivity tests.

Table 2
Evidence for genetic reassortment between H1N1 and H1N2 viruses

Gene	Sequence difference (%)[a]			
	Sw/IV/1455/99 (H1N1)		Sw/It/1521/98 (H1N2)	
	Sw/It/2064/99	Sw/It/1081/00	Sw/It/2064/99	Sw/It/1081/00
PB2	**1.2**	**1.4**	3.1	3.5
PB1	**1.5**	**2.1**	4.9	4.5
PA	**2.4**	**2.3**	4.1	3.6
H1	**5.5**	30.8	29.3	**4.3**
NP	**2.3**	**2.5**	5.4	4.9
N2	–	–	**3.7**	**3.2**
M	**2.1**	**2.1**	3.9	3.9
NS	5.7	5.2	**3.2**	**2.4**

[a] Percent difference in sequence between the corresponding genes of reassortant viruses Sw/Italy/2064/99 and Sw/Italy/1081/00 and reference viruses (bold) Sw/IV/1455/99 (H1N1) and Sw/Italy/1521/98 (H1N2). Numbers in bold indicate the closer relationship.

8. Conclusions

The results of these studies (1) showed that the majority of H3N2 and H1N1 influenza A viruses recently circulating in pigs in continental Europe are closely related to previously circulating variants, (2) identified a swine A/Sydney/5/97 (H3N2)-like virus, and (3) revealed the emergence of antigenically distinguishable H1N1 variants and antigenically heterogeneous H1N2 subtype viruses. The genetic similarities and differences between the H1N2 viruses isolated in France and the U.K. indicate that introductions from the U.K. may have occurred on more than one occasion. Two of the H1N2 viruses were shown to be reassortants, apparently deriving genes from H1N2 and H1N1 viruses; Sw/Italy/1081/00 (H1N2) had acquired five internal genes more closely related to the H1N1 viruses, whereas Sw/Italy/2064/99 (H1N2) possessed two genes, NA and NS, of the H1N2 virus. These viruses thus contribute to a significant increase in the diversity of swine influenza viruses in Europe.

References

[1] L. Nardelli, S. Pascucci, G.L. Gualandi, P. Loda, Zentralbl. Veterinaermed., Reihe B 25 (1978) 853–857.
[2] B. Tumova, D. Veznikova, J. Mensik, A. Stumpa, Zentralbl. Veterinaermed., Reihe B 27 (1980) 517–523.
[3] M. Pensaert, K. Ottis, J. Vandeputte, M.M. Kaplan, P.A. Bachmann, Bull. W. H. O. 59 (1981) 75–78.
[4] M.R. Castrucci, I. Donatelli, L. Sidoli, G. Barigazzi, Y. Kawaoka, R.G. Webster, Virology 193 (1993) 503–506.
[5] J.M. Gourreau, C. Kaiser, M. Valette, A.R. Douglas, J. Labie, M. Aymard, Arch. Virol. 135 (1994) 365–382.
[6] I.H. Brown, P.A. Harris, J.W. McCauley, D.J. Alexander, J. Gen. Virol. 79 (1998) 2947–2955.
[7] M. Bennett, S. Grambas, Y. Lin, A. Hay, submitted for publication.

International Congress Series 1219 (2001) 241–249

Evolving H3N2 and emerging H1N2 swine influenza viruses in the United States

Richard J. Webby[a], Sabrina L. Swenson[b], Scott L. Krauss[a],
Sagar M. Goyal[c], Kurt D. Rossow[c], Robert G. Webster[a,d,*]

[a]*Department of Virology and Molecular Biology, St. Jude Children's Research Hospital,
Memphis, TN 38105, USA*
[b]*National Veterinary Services Laboratories, United States Department of Agriculture, Ames, IA 50010, USA*
[c]*Veterinary Diagnostic Medicine, University of Minnesota, St. Paul, MN 55108, USA*
[d]*Department of Pathology, University of Tennessee, Memphis, TN 38105, USA*

Abstract

Background: Reassortant H3N2 influenza viruses have recently become established in swine populations throughout the United States. Viruses of two genotypes (a human and swine virus reassortant and a human, swine, and avian virus reassortant) were isolated from swine during the index disease outbreaks. *Methods*: To identify the genetic composition of the currently circulating viruses, we sequenced the genes of seven isolates from different infected herds. *Results*: Six viruses contained the human/swine/avian gene complex, but the complex was associated with three phylogenetically distinct human H3 haemagglutinins (HA). The remaining virus was an H1N2 reassortant containing seven genes similar to those of swine H3N2 viruses and an HA gene derived from a classical-swine H1N1 virus. The non-HA genes of this H1N2 virus were more similar to those of swine H3N2 viruses than to those of the recently reported H1N2 swine virus from Indiana [J. Clin. Microbiol. 38 (2000) 2453]. This finding suggests that each of the H1N2 viruses were derived through independent reassortment events. *Conclusions*: We conclude that viruses containing the avian-like genes are primarily responsible for the increased prevalence of H3N2 viruses throughout U.S. swine populations. H3N2 viruses have continued to spread and have undergone further reassortment with human and swine viruses resulting in the emergence of viruses with distinct antigenicity and subtype. © 2001 Elsevier Science B.V. All rights reserved.

Keywords: Porcine influenza A virus; Reassortant virus; Antigenic drift

* Corresponding author. Department of Virology and Molecular Biology, St. Jude Children's Research Hospital, 332 N. Lauderdale Street, Memphis, TN 38105-2794, USA. Tel.: +1-901-495-3400; fax: +1-901-523-2622.

E-mail address: robert.webster@stjude.org (R.G. Webster).

1. Introduction

Influenza viruses of the H1N1, H3N2, and more recently H1N2, subtypes circulate widely in pig populations throughout the world. The predominant circulating subtypes differ between geographical regions. The first isolation of influenza in swine was reported in the United States in 1930 [1] and viruses derived from this lineage (classical swine H1N1) have become the cause of endemic disease in this population. Unlike the situation in other parts of the world, where H1N1 and H3N2 subtypes co-circulate, swine influenza in the United States has been predominately confined to H1N1 viruses [2,3].

During a period of 3 months in 1998 influenza-like diseases occurred in four U.S swineherds [4]. The initial outbreak occurred in North Carolina and resulted in severe disease with morbidity approaching 100%. The subsequent outbreaks in Texas, Minnesota, and Iowa were less severe but involved larger numbers of animals. Influenza viruses of the H3N2 subtype were isolated from swine in all four outbreaks. Genetic characterisation of these H3N2 viruses demonstrated the presence of two distinct reassortant genotypes: a double reassortant containing human-like (HA, NA, PB1) and swine-like (PA, PB2, NP, M, NS) genes, and a triple reassortant containing human-like (HA, NA, PB1), swine-like (NP, M, NS), and avian-like (PA, PB2) genes [4]. The double-reassortant virus was isolated from the North Carolina outbreak (Sw/NC/35922/98; Sw/NC/98), whereas the viruses from Texas (Sw/TX/4199-2/98; Sw/TX/98), Minnesota (Sw/MN/90882-2/98; Sw/MN/98), and Iowa (Sw/IA/8548-1/98; Sw/IA/98) belonged to the triple-reassortant genotype. Subsequently, Karasin et al. [5] described a triple-reassortant H3N2 virus isolated from diseased piglets in Nebraska during March 1998. This finding indicates that viruses containing the avian-like gene complement were present and probably spreading throughout the country before the simultaneous disease outbreaks occurred in Texas, Minnesota, and Iowa.

The severity of disease and the spread of H3N2 influenza viruses in swine are issues of concern for the ecologic and epidemiologic factors affecting influenza in the United States. To further address issues concerning the spread and evolution of H3N2 viruses in U.S. swine, we have determined the genetic composition of recently isolated H3N2 viruses and an H1N2 swine reassortant virus.

2. Methods

2.1. Virus strains

All viruses used in this study were obtained from the National Veterinary Services Laboratories (NVSL), Ames, IA, or from the Department of Veterinary Diagnostic Medicine, University of Minnesota, St. Paul, MN. The viruses used were isolated from swine in Oklahoma, Illinois, Colorado, Wisconsin, and North Carolina. When necessary, viruses were grown in the allantoic cavities of 11-day embryonated chicken eggs or in Madin–Darby canine kidney (MDCK) cells before RNA extraction or antigenic analysis.

2.2. Serologic studies

The antigenic similarity among viral isolates was compared in haemagglutination inhibition (HI) assays as previously described [6]. All sera were pretreated with the receptor-destroying enzyme from *Vibrio cholerae* (Denka Seiken, Tokyo) to abolish interference by nonspecific serum inhibitors.

2.3. RNA extraction, RT-PCR, and DNA sequencing

Viral RNA extraction, RT-PCR and DNA sequencing were carried out as described by Zhou et al. [4]. The sequences of oligonucleotide primers and a description of the amplification conditions are available upon request.

2.4. Sequence analysis

DNA sequences were compiled and edited by using the Lasergene sequence analysis software package (DNASTAR, Madison, WI). Multiple sequence alignments were made by using CLUSTAL W [7], and phylogenetic trees were generated by using the neighbor-joining algorithm within the PHYLIP version 3.57C software package [8].

3. Results

3.1. Serologic analysis

We compared the antigenic characteristics of seven swine influenza viruses isolated during 1999 and 2000 to Sw/TX/98 (triple reassortant) and Sw/NC/98 (double reassortant). All viruses, with the exception of A/Swine/Minnesota/40318/00 (Sw/MN/00), were of the H3 subtype although there was considerable heterogeneity among the haemagglutinins (HA) (Table 1).

3.2. 1999 H3N2 swine isolates—characterization of genes encoding internal proteins

To determine whether the increased prevalence of H3N2 swine viruses in the United States is due to the spread of single or multiple lineages of virus we determined the genotypes of the 1999 H3N2 swine viruses. Partial sequencing of the gene segments encoding internal proteins showed that all viruses had nearly identical gene sequences to those of the triple-reassortant viruses Sw/TX/98, Sw/MN/98, and Sw/IA/98 (similarities >98%, data not shown). No additional isolates with the double-reassortant gene complex were found, a finding suggesting that these viruses have not established a stable lineage.

3.3. 1999 H3N2 swine isolates—characterization of genes encoding surface proteins

The immunologic pressure that drives antigenic drift in influenza viruses is considered to be less severe in swine populations than in humans because of the continual availability

Table 1
Antigenic relatedness between swine viruses isolated in 1999 and 2000 and index H3N2 viruses isolated in 1998

Virus	Haemagglutination inhibition assay titres	
	A/Sw/Texas/4199-2/98[a] (triple reassortant H3N2)	A/Sw/N.Carolina/35922/98[a] (double reassortant H3N2)
A/Sw/Texas/4199-2/98	640	<10
A/Sw/N.Carolina/35922/98	20	640
A/Sw/Minnesota/40318/00	<10	<10
A/Sw/Oklahoma/18089/99	80	10
A/Sw/Oklahoma/18717/99	160	10
A/Sw/Wisconsin/14094/99	80	10
A/Sw/N.Carolina/16497/99	640	10
A/Sw/Illinois/ 21587/99	80	10
A/Sw/Colorado/23619/99	40	20

[a] Sera were from experimentally infected pigs.

of naive hosts. However, the results of the HI assay showed that there is significant antigenic variation among the recent H3 swine viruses (Table 1). Consequently, the HA1 region of each isolate was sequenced (Table 2), and this sequence was used in phylogenetic analysis. A phylogenetic tree produced from the predicted amino acid sequences (Fig. 1) shows that three distinct clusters of H3 molecules are associated with viruses of the triple-reassortant genotype. The swine viruses do not form a separate lineage, and the HA genes from each swine cluster are more related to those of human strains than to those of the swine viruses of the other clusters. This finding suggests that the triple-reassortant swine viruses have undergone reassortment with human H3N2 viruses on at least three occasions. Nucleotide identities among the HA genes of the 1999 swine isolates and Sw/TX/98 ranged from 94% (Sw/CO/23619/99) to 99% (Sw/NC/16497/99). The HA gene of Sw/CO/23619/99 shared the highest GenBank similarity to A/

Table 2
Nucleotide sequence homologies of HA and NA genes[a] of recently isolated swine viruses

Virus	Highest nucleotide similarities with sequences in GenBank (percent nucleotide similarity, number of nucleotides compared)	
	HA	NA
A/Sw/Minnesota/40318/00	A/Sw/Indiana/9K035/99 H1N2 (97%, 577)	A/Sw/Texas/4199-2/98 H3N2 (99%, 658)
A/Sw/Oklahoma/18089/99	A/Sw/Texas/4199-2/98 (99%, 987)	A/Sw/Texas/4199-2/98 (99%, 1377)
A/Sw/Oklahoma/18717/99	A/Texas/9/96 H3N2 (99%, 987)	A/Sw/Texas/4199-2/98 (99%, 1377)
A/Sw/Wisconsin/14094/99	A/Texas/9/96 (99%, 987)	A/Sw/Texas/4199-2/98 (99%, 1377)
A/Sw/N.Carolina/16497/99	A/Texas/9/96 (99%, 987)	A/Sw/Texas/4199-2/98 (99%, 1377)
A/Sw/Illinois/ 21587/99	A/Texas/9/96 (99%, 987)	A/Sw/Texas/4199-2/98 (99%, 1377)
A/Sw/Colorado/23619/99	A/Sydney/05/97-like H3N2 (98%, 987)	A/Shiga/25/97 H3N2 (98%, 1377)

[a] All other genes were most similar to those of representatives of the triple reassortant swine virus lineage; the homologies were greater than 98%.

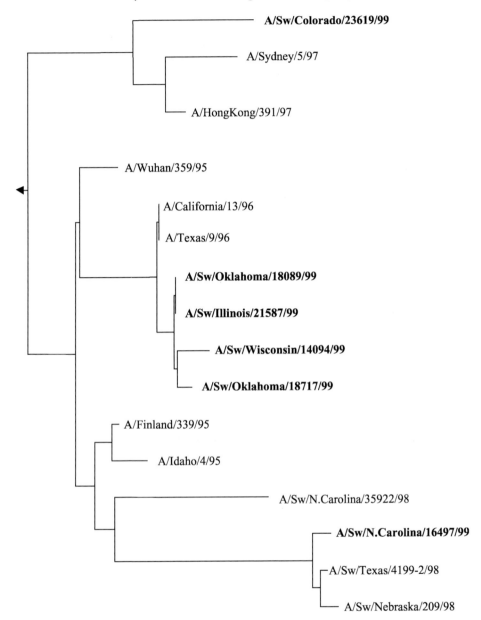

Fig. 1. Distance phylogenetic tree produced from results of our analysis of HA1 amino acid sequences. The tree is rooted to A/Victoria/3/75. Isolates in bold are viruses of the triple-reassortant genotype sequenced in this study. All other virus sequences were obtained from GenBank.

Sydney/5/97-like viruses, with Sw/WI/14094/99, Sw/OK/18089/99, Sw/IL/21587/99, and Sw/OK/18717/99 most similar to those of human viruses circulating in the United States in 1996. The HA1 sequences of the 1996 U.S viruses were more similar to those of A/

Wuhan/359/95-like viruses than to those of A/Sydney/5/97-like. A/Wuhan/359/95-like viruses were the predominant H3N2 virus isolated in the United States before the 1997–1998 influenza season; during that season, the A/Sydney/5/97-like viruses were the influenza virus most commonly isolated from humans [9,10].

The NA genes of the recently isolated swine viruses were also sequenced (Table 2). All viruses were of the N2 subtype. The NA genes were more conserved than the HA genes, although the unavailability of sequence data for recently isolated North American human strains made phylogenetic analysis of the NA genes difficult. Therefore, we were unable to determine whether the reassortment events resulted in the acquisition of human HA genes or of both human HA and NA genes by the swine viruses. The greater similarity of the NA gene of A/Sw/CO/23619/99 to that of a human virus does however suggest that, at least in this virus, both human surface glycoprotein genes were obtained in the reassortment event.

3.4. Identification and characterisation of an H1N2 influenza virus

An additional viral strain was isolated from diseased replacement gilts on a farm in Minnesota. Analysis of convalescent sera showed that approximately 50% of the 220 gilts were infected, with the resulting pneumonia being further complicated by *Pasteurella multocida* and *Streptococcus suis* infections. Retrospective analysis showed that adult sows from the infected herd were seropositive for H1N1 and H3N2 influenza viruses. A strain isolated from this outbreak, Sw/MN/00, was subtyped as H1N2 using haemagglutination and neuraminidase inhibition assays (data not shown). Partial sequencing of two MDCK plaque-purified clones confirmed that the isolate was an H1N2 influenza virus (Table 2). The HA sequences in GenBank that were most similar were the HA gene of A/Swine/Indiana/9K035/99 (Sw/IN/99), which is a recently described H1N2 virus [11], and the HA genes of recently isolated classical swine H1N1 viruses. All remaining gene segments were at least as, or more, similar to those of the triple-reassortant H3N2 swine viruses. The fact that some genes of Sw/MN/00 were more similar to those of the H3N2 swine viruses than to those of Sw/IN/99 suggests that Sw/MN/00 is a novel reassortant virus derived from the reassortment of H1N1 and H3N2 viruses rather than from a clonal isolate of Sw/IN/99.

4. Discussion

The isolation of two distinguishable H3N2 viruses in U.S. swine populations during 1998 represents a significant event in the epidemiology of swine influenza, because the isolation of H3N2 viruses from pigs in North America has been infrequent, unlike the situation in Asia and Europe. Previous serologic studies of U.S. swineherds had identified H3N2 seroprevalence rates of 1.4% in 1976–1977 and of 1.1% in 1988–1989 [2,3]. These rates were significantly lower than the corresponding levels of seroreactivity to H1N1 viruses (average levels of 21% in 1976–1977 and 30% in 1988–1989). In geographical regions where H1N1 and H3N2 viruses have co-circulated reassortant viruses have been identified. These reassortant viruses include H3N2 viruses in Italy, which contain internal protein genes from the avian-like H1N1 swine viruses [12,13], and the emergence of swine–human and swine–human–avian reassortant H1N2 viruses in swine in Japan,

Great Britain, and Europe [14–20]. The H1N2 viruses from Great Britain have become an increasing concern and appear to be replacing both the H1N1 and H3N2 viruses in the British pig population [21]. Recently, an H1N2 virus containing a classical swine-like HA gene and seven gene segments from the triple-reassortant H3N2 viruses was isolated in Indiana [11]. The identification of a second H1N2 virus in Minnesota (Sw/MN/00) raises concerns that H1N2 viruses may also be spreading in U.S. swine. Although the gene composition of both H1N2 viruses was the same, the Sw/MN/00 gene segments, except for the HA gene segment were more similar to those of H3N2 swine viruses than to those of Sw/IN/00. This finding suggests that the two H1N2 viruses arose through independent reassortment events and that they are not clonal isolates of a spreading lineage. It remains to be seen whether these H1N2 viruses will establish stable lineages in U.S. swine and what impact they will have economically.

When human H3N2 viruses have crossed the species barrier and entered the swine population, these viruses have undergone genetic drift and formed phylogenetically distinct swine lineages [22,23]. Because of the continual availability of immunologically naive hosts, this antigenic drift is less marked in viruses circulating in swine than in viruses circulating in human populations. One of the unexpected findings of the current study is the association of the triple-reassortant complex of genes encoding internal proteins with three phylogenetically distinct human HA molecules. The phylogenetic relationships of each of the three swine HA clusters are consistent with the reassortment of swine H3N2 viruses with circulating human viruses rather than with antigenic drift. The HA genes of the viruses responsible for the 1998 swine disease outbreaks were most similar to those of the 1995 human viruses [4]. The 1999 swine isolates can be separated into three groups on the basis of the sequence of their HA genes. The HA gene of A/Sw/NC/16497/99 is similar to that of the initial 1998 swine H3N2 isolates and hence 1995 human strains, the HA genes of a second group are similar to those of U.S. human strains circulating in 1996, and the HA gene of A/Sw/CO/23619/99 is similar to that of A/Sydney/5/97. The similarities of the HAs of the swine viruses to those of human viruses circulating in consecutive years suggest a temporal appearance of the reassortant viruses. The selective pressures that drive the acquisition of different HAs is unknown but it is apparent that only progeny containing the triple-reassortant complex of genes encoding internal proteins emerge from these reassortment events.

Since their emergence during 1998, the triple-reassortant H3N2 influenza viruses have spread throughout the country and have continued to reassort with human and swine viruses. The establishment of the triple-reassortant H3N2 viruses has changed the dynamics of swine influenza in the United States. In addition, the affinity for acquiring different HA genes that has been displayed by this internal gene complex warrants the close surveillance of U.S. swine populations for the emergence of new and potentially pathogenic viral strains.

Acknowledgements

These studies were supported by Public Health Service grants AI29680 and AI95357 and Cancer Center Support (CORE) grant CA-21765 from the National Institutes of Health and by the American Lebanese Syrian Associated Charities (ALSAC).

We thank David Walker and Lijuan Zhang for excellent technical assistance and Julia Cay Jones for editorial assistance.

References

[1] R.E. Shope, Swine Influenza: III. Filtration experiments and aetiology, J. Exp. Med. 54 (1931) 373–385.

[2] T.M. Chambers, V.S. Hinshaw, Y. Kawaoka, B.C. Easterday, R.G. Webster, Influenza viral infection of swine in the United States 1988–1989, Arch. Virol. 116 (1991) 261–265.

[3] V.S. Hinshaw, W.J. Bean Jr., R.G. Webster, B.C. Easterday, The prevalence of influenza viruses in swine and the antigenic and genetic relatedness of influenza viruses from man and swine, Virology 84 (1978) 51–62.

[4] N.N. Zhou, D.A. Senne, J.S. Landgraf, S.L. Swenson, G. Erickson, K. Rossow, L. Liu, K.-J. Yoon, S. Krauss, R.G. Webster, Genetic reassortment of avian, swine, and human influenza A viruses in American pigs, J. Virol. 73 (1999) 8851–8856.

[5] A.I. Karasin, M.M. Schutten, L.A. Cooper, C.B. Smith, K. Subbarao, G.A. Anderson, S. Carman, C.W. Olsen, Genetic characterization of H3N2 influenza viruses isolated from pigs in North America, 1977–1999: evidence for wholly human and reassortant virus genotypes, Virus Res. 68 (2000) 71–85.

[6] D.F. Palmer, M.T. Coleman, W.R. Dowdle, G.C. Schild, Advanced laboratory techniques for influenza diagnosis, Immunol. Ser. (1975) 51–52, U.S. Department of Health, Education, and Welfare.

[7] J.D. Thompson, D.G. Higgins, T.J. Gibson, CLUSTAL W: improving the sensitivity of progressive multiple sequence alignment through sequence weighting, position-specific gap penalties and weight matrix choice, Nucleic Acids Res. 22 (1994) 4673–4680.

[8] PHYLIP (phylogenetic I reference package) version 3.5, Department of Genetics, University of Washington, Seattle, Distributed by the author, 1993.

[9] [No authors listed] Update: influenza activity, United States and worldwide, 1996–97 season, and composition of the 1997–98 influenza vaccine, MMWR Morb. Mortal Wkly. Rep. 1997, 46, 325–330.

[10] [No authors listed] Update: influenza activity, United States and worldwide, 1997–98 season, and composition of the 1998–99 influenza vaccine. MMWR Morb, Mortal Wkly, Rep, 1998, 47, 280–284.

[11] A.I. Karasin, C.W. Olsen, G.A. Anderson, Genetic characterization of an H1N2 influenza virus isolated from a pig in Indiana, J. Clin. Microbiol. 38 (2000) 2453–2456.

[12] L. Campitelli, I. Donatelli, E. Foni, M.R. Castrucci, C. Fabiani, Y. Kawaoka, S. Krauss, R.G. Webster, Continued evolution of H1N1 and H3N2 influenza viruses in pigs in Italy, Virology 232 (1997) 310–318.

[13] M.R. Castrucci, I. Donatelli, L. Sidoli, G. Barigazzi, Y. Kawaoka, R.G. Webster, Genetic reassortment between avian and human influenza A viruses in Italian pigs, Virology 193 (1993) 503–506.

[14] H. Brown, P.A. Harris, J.W. McCauley, D.J. Alexander, Multiple genetic reassortment of avian and human influenza A viruses in European pigs, resulting in the emergence of an H1N2 virus of novel genotype, J. Gen. Virol. 79 (1998) 2947–2955.

[15] J.M. Gourreau, C. Kaiser, M. Valette, A.R. Douglas, J. Labie, M. Aymard, Isolation of two H1N2 influenza viruses from swine in France, Arch. Virol. 135 (1994) 365–382.

[16] T. Ito, Y. Kawaoka, A. Vines, H. Ishikawa, T. Asai, H. Kida, Continued circulation of reassortant H1N2 influenza viruses in pigs in Japan, Arch. Virol. 143 (1998) 1773–1782.

[17] K. Nerome, Y. Yoshioka, S. Sakamoto, H. Yasuhara, A. Oya, Characterization of a 1980-swine recombinant influenza virus possessing H1 hemagglutinin and N2 neuraminidase similar to that of the earliest Hong Kong (H3N2) virus, Arch. Virol. 86 (1985) 197–211.

[18] A. Ouchi, K. Nerome, Y. Kanegae, M. Ishida, R. Nerome, K. Hayashi, T. Hashimoto, M. Kaji, Y. Inaba, Large outbreak of swine influenza in southern Japan caused by reassortant (H1N2) influenza viruses: its epizootic background and characterization of the causative viruses, J. Gen. Virol. 77 (1996) 1751–1759.

[19] T. Sugimura, H. Yonemochi, T. Ogawa, Y. Tanaka, T. Kumagai, Isolation of a recombinant influenza virus (Hsw 1 N2) from swine in Japan, Arch. Virol. 66 (1980) 271–274.

[20] K. Van Reeth, I.H. Brown, M. Pensaert, Isolations of H1N2 influenza A virus from pigs in Belgium, Vet. Rec. 146 (2000) 588–589.

[21] S.H. Done, I.H. Brown, Swine influenza viruses in Europe, in: Proceedings of the Allen D Leman Swine Conference 26, (1999) 263–267, Minneapolis, MN.

[22] J.C. de Jong, A.P. van Nieuwstadt, T.G. Kimman, W.L. Loeffen, T.M. Bestebroer, K. Bijlsma, C. Verweij, A.D. Osterhaus, E.C. Class, Antigenic drift in swine influenza H3 haemagglutinins with implications for vaccination policy, Vaccine 17 (1999) 1321–1328.

[23] K. Nerome, Y. Kanegae, K.F. Shortridge, S. Sugita, M. Ishida, Genetic analysis of porcine H3N2 viruses originating in southern China, J. Gen. Virol. 76 (1995) 613–624.

International Congress Series 1219 (2001) 251–258

Isolation of influenza viruses from wild birds in the Volga River basin and in the North Caspian Region

D.K. Lvov[a,*], S.S. Yamnikova[a], A.S. Gambaryan[b],
I.T. Fedyakina[a], M.N. Matrosovich[b]

[a]*D.I. Ivanovsky Institute of Virology, RAMS, Gamaley Street 16, Moscow, 123098, Russia*
[b]*M.P. Chumakov Institute of Poliomyelitis and Viral Encephalities, RAMS, Moscow, Russia*

Abstract

Background: The North Caspian Region and delta of the Volga River constitute historic flyways and a place of mass congregation of wild birds for most of the year. *Methods*: A total 3513 biological samples from 3229 birds of 37 species were collected, antigenic structure and receptor activity of isolated influenza A viruses were studied. Nucleotide sequences of NS gene PCR fragments were analysed. *Results*: 344 strains of influenza A virus with various combination of hemagglutinin and neuraminidase were isolated: H4N3, H4N6, H5N2, H6N2, H9N2, H13N3, H13N6, H13N8, H14N5, H14N6. The influenza virus A/H13 was isolated annually from the nestlings of *Larus ichthyaetus* and *L. argentatus* species. Isolation of viruses from embryos and young birds suggests the existence of at least two ways of infection: alimentary and transovarial. The studies of the binding of the viruses H13 and H14 with gangliosides GM3, GD1a and 3SPG did not reveal the essential difference from the viruses of H1–H12 subtypes. Among avian HA only HA13 subtype has the substitution at residue 77 DT, A and 228 GS. The substitution 225 GN found in HA14 virus also isolated only in the North of Caspian Sea. Study of NS genes of some isolates revealed significant differences in the structure of genes of influenza viruses isolated at the same time but from various species of birds. *Conclusions*: The ability of the viruses H5, H4, H6, H9 to infect mammals and to provoke epizootics determine the necessity to carry out further monitoring in the Northern Caspian basin and other key points in Northern Eurasia. © 2001 Elsevier Science B.V. All rights reserved.

Keywords: Influenza A subtypes; Hemagglutinin; NS gene

* Corresponding author. Tel.: +7-95-190-2842; fax: +7-95-190-2867.

0531-5131/01/$ – see front matter © 2001 Elsevier Science B.V. All rights reserved.
PII: S0531-5131(01)00378-8

1. Introduction

Emerging and re-emerging infections, which often connect with unpredictable extraordinary epidemic consequences, have great priority on a national and an international level [1–5]. This program stipulates the carrying and monitoring by the studies of: (1) the evolution of the viruses in the process of gene pool changing of the virus populations in nature and among human beings; (2) the geographic, and ecological peculiarities of virus-distribution; (3) the relations between epizootics and epidemics; and (4) tendencies and mechanisms of virus diversity in natural biocenosis and among human beings.

Understanding of such processes with consideration of specific organization of the virus genome and the use of molecular ecology and epidemiology permits the study of movements of the genetic material of a single protected gene pool of the totality of virus populations, particularly influenza A which would be the most dangerous emerging–re-emerging viruses in the future. Such investigations were carried out in Northern Eurasia during a period of more than 20 years in key points of different physico-geographical countries with unique ecosystems [4]. Influenza A viruses of 1–14 types of hemagglutinines and 1–9 types of neuraminidase were isolated from natural biocenoses, including all epidemic viruses. Some of these were dominated and isolated practically every year. Different viruses were dominated at different key points.

2. Materials and methods

The lower part of the Volga basin and North Caspian region is located in one of the four (one of eight in the world) main migratory routes of birds in Eurasia–East European migratory route. Birds nesting on the Eastern Fennoscandia, Northern-Central territories of the Russian Plain, Ural, and part of Western Siberia fly through this key area for over wintering in Africa (93%) and south-western Asia (6.5%). In the period of maximum migration level over 100,000 birds of more than 100 species fly through this region per day. Nesting places of gulls, terns, ducks, herons and other birds, are located in the avan-delta of the Volga and islands of North of the Caspian Sea. Gulls and terns were most often investigated in this region. Cloacal and tracheal swabs from the water birds were collected. The regions of the material's collection are presented in Fig. 1. The isolation of the strains was carried out by inoculation of 9- to 11-day-old chick embryos.

Antigenic structure of isolates was determined by the usage of the set of diagnostic sera to reference-strains of influenza A viruses, H1–H14 and NA1–NA9 according to WHO recommendations [6].

Receptor activity of the strains was studied as described previously [7].

RNA was isolated by the guanidine-sulphocyanide method [8]. To obtain amplification of RDNA fragments the commercial kit of "Promega" Access RT-PCR was used. Various combinations of direct and inverse primers were used to obtain the fragments of different length. The analysis of initial structure was carried out with commercial set "pMol" of the

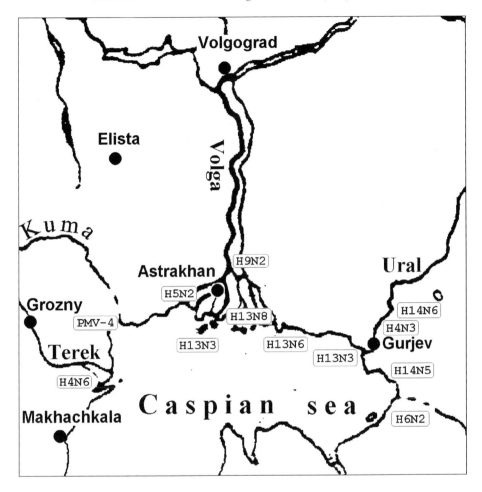

Fig. 1. Places of isolation of influenza viruses in the North of the Caspian basin. Scale 1:8,000,000.

"Promega" firm. The analysis of obtained sequences was carried out by the "Clustalv" method [9].

3. Results and discussion

From 1975 to 1999 in the northern part of the Caspian sea basin, 3513 materials were collected from 3299 birds of 37 species belonging to six families: *Laridae*, *Charadridae*, *Anatidae*, *Ardeidae*, *Phalacrocoracidae*. 344 strains of influenza A virus with various combinations of hemagglutinin and neuraminidase were isolated: H4N3, H4N6, H5N2, H6N2, H9N2, H13N2, H13N3, H13N6, H13N8, H14N5, H14N6 (Table 1). The largest number of strains (190) was isolated from nestling *Larus ichthyaetus*. An isolation of the

Table 1
Isolation of influenza virus A from waterfowl in the Northern Caspian Region and the mouth of the Volga (1979–1999)

Year	Subtype	*Larus ichthyaetus*	*L. argentatus*	*Hydraprogne tcigrava*	Others	Total	Total strains
1979	H13N2	1	4			5	5
1980	H13N6	21	8	3		32	32
1981	H5N2	1		1		2	3
1982	H13N2	6	3	2		11	15
	H14N5			1		1	
	H14N6	1			2	3	
1983	H13N2	18				18	25
	H13N3	1			5	6	
	H13N6	1				1	
1984	H13N6	6	1	3		10	10
1985	H13N3		2			2	17
	H13N6	13	2			15	
1986	H4N3				1	1	10
	H6N2				2	2	
	H9N2			1		1	
	H13N2	3				3	
	H13N3	1	2			3	
1987	H9N2	1				1	3
	H13N2	1	1			2	
1988	H13N6	21				21	21
1989	H13N2	15	4			19	69
	H13N6	41	8	1		50	
1990	H13N6	16	15			31	31
1991	H4N6				1	1	23
	H13N6	21	1			22	
1993	H13N6		4	1		5	5
1998	H13N6		12			12	20
	H13N8		8			8	
Total		190	74	15	9	288	

viruses from embryo *Larus argentatus* presents transovarial transmission of the viruses simultaneously with an alimentary method of infection.

The studies of antigenic structure of influenza viruses A/H13 with polyclonal and monoclonal antibodies showed the variability of the structure of their hemagglutinin. During one period, three to four different variants were isolated, and every year the number of strains rose, and these strains were not identified by antibodies against standard A/gull/Maryland/707/77 (H13N6). Most strains revealed a unilateral relationship. The presence of such antigenic variability was not shown for other avian influenza viruses. Phylogenetic analysis of HA genes of different strains A/H13 is correlated with these data [10].

One of the factors determining a range of the virus hosts is its ability to bind with sialylglycoconjugates arranged on a cellular surface. Most avian viruses had a higher affinity to 3SL than to Neu5Ac. The studies carried out earlier [11] of receptor activity of the largest number of viruses of birds and mammals indicated that avian HA-3-SL complex is stabilized by an energetically favorable interaction of the HA with the lactose moiety of 3-SL. It is significant that this property was absent in human viruses H1 and H3 and slowly manifested in H13 isolates.

Comparison of HA amino acid sequences and modeling of ligand disposition in RBS revealed that amino acid in positions 77, 138, 190, 194, 225, 226 and 228 is very conservative for the avian viruses, unlike the human one, among different HA serotypes. Among avian HA only HA13 subtype has the substitution at residue 77 DT, A and 228 GS. The substitution 225 GN found in HA14 virus is also isolated only in the North of Caspian Sea. A change of 226 QL and 228 GS is a characteristic feature of H2 and H3 human strains, and correlated with the receptor-binding phenotype of these viruses [11]. One of them, 228 GS, is in HA H13. A change of 138, 190, 194, 225 is specific for H1 human viruses.

The studies of the binding of the viruses H13 and H14 with gangliosides GM3, GD1a and 3SPG did not reveal the essential difference from the viruses of H1–H12 subtypes (Fig. 2). Avian strains bound to GM3 and GD1a, exposed on a membrane-like assay surface, suggest that these ganglioside species could serve as receptor for avian viruses in nature.

We compared the abilities of some isolates to bind free Neu5Ac, and gangliosides with the intent of identifying changes in the receptor-binding properties required for a successful interspecies transfer of avian viruses (Table 2).

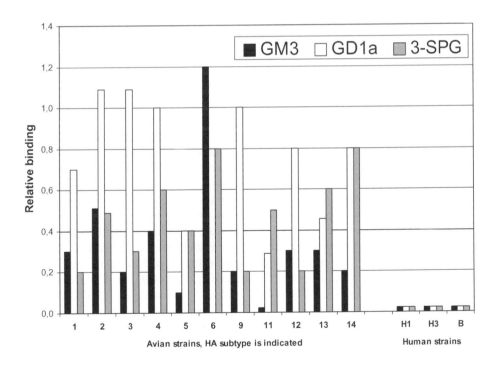

Fig. 2. Binding to gangliosides GM3, GD1a and 3-SPG by avian and human influenza viruses.

Table 2
Binding of influenza viruses to total gangliosides from the bovine brain and alantoic membrane, and K_{aff} to sialyl-3'lactose

No.	Strain	Subtype	Bovine brain	Alantoic membrane	K_{aff} to S-3'-L
Avian strains					
1	A/duck/Ukrain/1/63	H3N8	++	++	0.40
2	A/equine/Maiami/1/63	H3N8	++	++	0.03
3	A/FPV/Rostock/34	H7N1	+	(+)	0.10
4	A/mallard/Primorye/3/82	H9N2	++	++	0.05
5	A/gull/Astrakhan/165/86	H9N2	+	+	0.20
6	A/gull/Maryland/704/77	H13N6	+	+	0.30
7	A/gull/Astrakhan/988/90	H13N6	+	+	0.30
8	A/gull/Astrakhan/227/84	H13N6	(+)	+	0.70
9	A/whale/Main/328/84	H13N9	+	+	0.50
10	A/mallard/Gurjev/244/82	H14N6	++	++	0.05
11	A/mallard/Gurjev/263/82	H14N5	++	++	0.05
12	A/gull/Gurjev/266/82	H14N5	++	++	0.05
13	A/gull/Gurjev/267/82	H14N5	++	+	0.05
Human strains					
14	B/NIB/48/98M	H1N1	–	–	0.20
15	A/NIB/23/89M	H1N1	–	–	1.00
16	A/HIB/44/90M	H3N2	–	–	1.00

The binding with gangliosides isolated from epithelial cells of alantoic membrane of chick embryo was studied. On the alantoic membrane 2–6 sialosides are absent, as a rule, and it can be considered that this preparation is presented only by 2–3 sialosides.

As can be seen in Table 2, human influenza viruses differ from avian strains by their inability to bind the studied gangliosides. Also, the A/H13 viruses normally bind them much weaker than the influenza viruses isolated from ducks.

There is significant data on the studies of structure and functions of HA, NA, NP and polymerase complex. The information on the structure of NS genes is not numerous although it can contribute in the reproductive features of the viruses. The comparison of the structure of gene NS virus A/mallard/Gurjev/244/82 (H14N6) with the structure of the genes H7 viruses revealed maximal homology with the virus A/FPV/Rostok/34. The differences in nucleotide sequence made up 4.3%, in the amino acid sequence − 3%. Minimal relationship was revealed to NS gene A/duck/Alberta/60/76 (H12N5). We studied the structure of partial PCR product from a series of NS genes of isolates (Fig. 3). Genes NS of influenza viruses (H13 and H14) presented one branch of the phylogenetic tree and the second branch was presented with NS genes of H14 and H9, which are sufficiently related to the first group. The position of the virus A/mallard/Gurjev/263/82 (H14N5) isolated from ducks drew our attention. There is a difference in the structure of genes of influenza viruses H14 isolated at the same time and place but from various species of birds. However, only the analysis of the remaining strains will provide the final conclusion. However, it is not excluded that NP and NS genes structure could be a factor which can restrict epidemic potency of probably avian flu viruses.

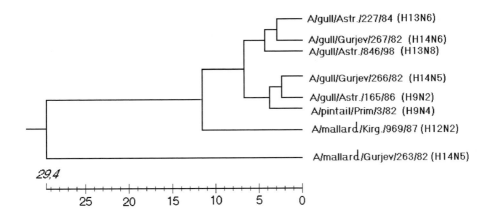

Fig. 3. Phylogenetic tree of NS segments of influenza viruses isolated from gull.

Influenza virus A/H13 has some unique properties: circulating of the virus, mostly among *Laridae* birds, some similarity between RBS with human H3 strains, in contrast to other avian viruses for H13, only one cycle of mutations in PBS position 226 is necessary.

The isolation of influenza viruses H5, H4, H6, H9 should be marked apart [12,13]. The ability of the viruses with this subtype HA to infect mammals and to provoke epizootics determines the necessity to carry out further monitoring in the Northern Caspian basin and at other key points. From this point of view, the data of the isolation of viruses with new 14 subtype hemagglutinin during epizootic promoted by *B. Botulinus C* is crucial [14,15]. More than a million birds have died. The same situation is the appearance of new pathogenic variants and as Kida et al. [15] showed all subtype of influenza viruses should take part in this process.

Acknowledgements

This work was supported by grants from the Russian Foundation of Fundamental Investigation (No. 98-04-48894), the Russian States Scientific and US Civilian Research and Development Foundation (No. RNI-412).

References

[1] J. Lederberg, R.E. Shore, S.C. Oaks, Emerging Infections, National Academic Press, Washington, 1992.
[2] D.K. Lvov, Problem of not registered and not predictable infections, J. Epidemiol. Microbiol. Immunol. 5 (1997) 104–109 (in Russian).
[3] D.K. Lvov, Birds–parasites–viruses: interpopulation interactions, Bull. Scand. Soc. Parasitol. 8 (1998) 29.
[4] D.K. Lvov, The role of emerging and re-emerging infections in extraordinary epidemic situations, Global

D.K. Lvov et al. / International Congress Series 1219 (2001) 251–258

Problems as Source of Extraordinary Situations, Ministry of Extraordinary Situations Russian Federation, Moscow, 1998, pp. 199–207 (in Russian).

[5] S. Morse, Emerging Viruses, Oxford Univ. Press, New York, 1993, pp. 1–317.

[6] W.A. Douwdal, A. Kendal, G.R. Noble, Influenza virus, in: E.N. Lennete, N.J. Schoridt (Eds.), Diagnostic Procedures for Viral, Rickettsial and Chlamydial Infection, American Public Health Association, Washington, 1979, pp. 585–609.

[7] A.S. Gambaryan, M.N. Matrosovich, A solid-phase enzyme-linked assay for influenza virus receptor-binding activity, J. Virol. Methods 39 (1992) 111–123.

[8] P. Chomezynski, N. Sacchi, Single-step method of RNA isolation by acid guanidium thiocyanate-phenol-chloroform extraction, Anal. Biochem. 162 (1987) 156–159.

[9] T.M. Chambers, S.S. Yamnikova, Y. Kawaoka, D.K. Lvov, R.G. Webster, Antigenic and molecular characterization of subtype H13 hemagglutinin of influenza virus, Virology 172 (1989) 180–188.

[10] M.N. Matrosovich, A.S. Gambaryan, S. Teneberg, V.E. Piskarev, S.S. Yamnikova, D.K. Lvov, J.C. Robertson, K.A. Karlsson, Avian influenza A viruses differ from human viruses by recognition of sialyloligosaccarides and gangliosides and by a higher conservation of the HA receptor-binding site, Virology 233 (1997) 224–234.

[11] R.J. Webster, Influenza-lesions from H5N1 in Hong Kong, 11th International Congress of Virology, Sydney, 1999, p. 6.

[12] D.K. Lvov, A.N. Slepushkin, S.S. Yamnikova, E.I. Burtseva, Influenza is still unpredictable infection, Voprosi Virusologii 3 (1998) 141–144 (in Russian).

[13] D.K. Lvov, S.S. Yamnikova, M.N. Matrosovich, R.G. Webster, Persistence of avian virus genes of human and birds' origin in animal population, Option for Control of Influenza III. Cairns, North Queensland, Australia, 1996, p. 198.

[14] Y. Kawaoka, S.S. Yamnikova, T.M. Chambers, D.K. Lvov, R.G. Webster, Molecular characterization of a new hemagglutinin subtype 14 of influenza A virus, Virology 179 (1990) 758–767.

[15] H. Kida, T. Ito, J. Yasuda, C. Itakura, K.F. Shortridge, Y. Kawaoka, R.G. Webster, Potential for transmission of avian influenza viruses to pigs, J. Gen. Virol. 75 (1994) 2183–2188.

International Congress Series 1219 (2001) 259–266

Phylogenetic analysis of the polymerase genes of five equine influenza A(H3N8) viruses isolated in France between 1993 and 1999

J.-C. Manuguerra[a,*], C. Rousseaux[a], S. Zientara[b], C. Sailleau[b], B. Gicquel[b], I. Rijks[a], S. van der Werf[a]

[a]*Unité de Génétique Moléculaire des Virus Respiratoires, URA 1966 CNRS, Institut Pasteur, F-75724 Paris cedex 15, France*
[b]*AFSSAA-Alfort-LCRV, 22 rue Pierre Curie, F-94703 Maisons Alfort, France*

Abstract

The nucleotide sequences of the genes encoding the P proteins (PB2, PB1 and PA) of five A(H3N8) equine influenza viruses isolated in France (one in 1993, one in 1998 and three in 1999) as well as those of the prototype strain A/equine/Miami/63(H3N8) were determined. Phylogenetic analysis was carried out on the deduced amino acid (AA) sequences and their respective evolutionary relationships with AA sequences available in databanks were determined. The phylogenetic trees showed that all equine PB2s, PB1s and PAs were genetically clustered. As shown for human isolates [J. Virol. 72 (1998) 8021], the PA protein had slightly higher variability. However, contrary to human viruses, the number of positions involved in variation was significantly high (35, 30 and 44 for PB2, PB1 and PA, respectively) and our data suggest that some AA changes were not erratic but determine a single evolutionary pathway for each P gene. © 2001 Elsevier Science B.V. All rights reserved.

Keywords: Equine influenza; Polymerase; Phylogeny; H3N8 subtype

* Corresponding author. National Influenza Centre, Institut Pasteur, 25 rue du Docteur Roux, 75724 Paris cedex 15, France. Tel.: +33-1-4061-3354; fax: +33-1-4061-3241.
  E-mail address: jmanugu@pasteur.fr (J.-C. Manuguerra).

1. Introduction

Three kinds of Influenza A viruses (IV) have been isolated from horses: equine-1 in 1956, equine-2 in 1963 and equine-3 in 1989. The equine-1 belongs to the A(H7N7) subtype, whereas the other two belong to the A(H3N8) subtype. Whereas no equine-1 viruses have been isolated since 1980 [1], equine-2 influenza A(H3N8) viruses, which essentially circulate in an enzootic manner, are currently isolated in developed countries such as the USA and those of Western Europe. In France, there has been no real epizootic of equine influenza since 1981 apart from some localised outbreaks. Equine-3 viruses, introduced from the avian reservoir some time around 1989 in Asia, have not been reported in the USA and Europe so far. Equine viruses belong to one of the three established mammalian virus lineages. As the human and swine lineages, the equine lineage shows a progressive accumulation of substitutions in the course of time. However, on the generalised phylogenies of IV genes [2], equine sequences form clusters which are either very much distinct from the sequences of the viruses isolated in all other species or are most closely related to avian virus sequences. For the P genes, these phylogenies are based on a very limited number of sequence data. Concerning equine viruses, the paucity of data was even greater since, at the start of this study, there were only three complete sequences for PB2 (two of equine A(H7N7) and one of equine A(H3N8) viruses), and two complete sequences of PB1 and PA, each corresponding to one of the two equine subtypes A(H3N8) and A(H7N7). The present study had two main objectives. The first one was to detail the relative phylogenetic relationship between the equine IV genes coding for the proteins of the transcriptase/replicase complex (PB2, PB1 and PA) [P genes] and the corresponding genes from viruses isolated in other species. The second objective was to give a basic description of the trends of evolutionary patterns within the equine genes. We therefore sequenced the three P genes of five A(H3N8) equine (Eq) IV isolated in France (one in 1993, one in 1998 and three in 1999) as well as those of the prototype strain A/equine/Miami/63(H3N8) [Mia63]. Phylogenetic analysis was then carried out on the deduced amino acid (AA) sequences of PB2, PB1 and PA and their respective evolutionary relationships with AA sequences available in data-banks were determined.

2. Materials and methods

2.1. Clinical material and virus isolation

Nasal swabs were collected from horses with clinical signs of respiratory disease in 1993, 1998 and 1999, two in the training centre of Boissy-St-Léger (Grosbois) near Paris, one in Normandy (Livarot, France) and one in the French Pyrenees (Miossens, France). Medium was recovered from the swabs and inoculated into two 8-day-old embryonated chicken eggs. The eggs were incubated at 35 °C for 48 h and the allantoic fluids harvested and tested for haemagglutination (HA) activity in microtitre plates as described previously [3]. The five isolates sequenced in this study were named A/

equine/Grosbois/93(H3N8) [GB93], A/equine/Grosbois/98(H3N8) [GB98], A/equine/
Grosbois/1/99(H3N8) [GB99], A/equine/Livarot/36/99 (H3N8) [Liv99], A/equine/Mios-
sens/18/99 (H3N8) [Mio99].

2.2. Viral RNA extraction, RNA purification, reverse transcription and polymerase chain reaction

Total RNA was extracted from allantoic fluid using the RNeasy Mini Kit for total RNA
minipreps (Qiagen), according to the manufacturer's instructions. Reverse transcription
and polymerase chain reaction were carried out as previously described [3].

2.3. Gene sequencing, sequence edition and analysis, phylogenetic analysis

The PCR amplified products were purified with the QIAquick PCR purification kit
according to the manufacturer's instructions (Qiagen). The purified PCR products were
then sequenced as described previously [3]. The nucleotide sequences were assembled
using Complign PPC (U. Priedmuth, H. Horch and V. Schöneberg, 1993–1999), then
edited and translated using the Mac Molly package (version 3.10, Softgene, Germany).
The deduced AA sequences of the whole coding regions of PB2, PB1 and PA were first
aligned using ClustalX (version 1.8). Phylogenetic analyses of the complete protein coding
regions of the three RNA segments were done using the Neighbour Joining (NJ) method of
Saitou and Nei [4] applied to the AA distance matrices. Evolutionary trees for the PB2,
PB1 and PA genes (Fig. 1) were constructed using the Draw NJ option in the ClustalX
package. To evaluate the robustness of the trees, the probabilities of the internal branches
were determined by 1000 bootstrap replications [5]. The trees were drawn using Treeview
(version 1.5.1, Roderic D.M. Page, 1997).

3. Results

3.1. Amino acid differences in the PB2, PB1, and PA proteins of the RNP complex

In this study, we compared the aligned sequences of GB93, GB98, GB99, Liv99,
Mio99, Mia63, which were determined in this work, as well as those of A/equine/London/
1416/73(H7N7) [Lon73], and A/equine/Kentucky/2/86 [Ken86] in the case of PB2 or A/
equine/Tenessee/5/86(H3N8) [Ten86] in the case of PB1 and PA.

Analysis of the PB2 AA sequences of recent equine-2 viruses and of the A(H7N7)
strain (Lon73) available in databanks revealed a significant number of AA changes when
compared with the prototype strain Mia63 (Table 1, panel a). Of the 36 AA positions
involved in variation for the PB2 proteins of viruses from 1963 to 1999, four, at position
461 (V to I), 588 (A to T), 613 (V to A) and 684 (N to A), differed between Mia63 and
all the other viruses. Ten other positions were also different between Mia63 and all the
other strains analysed, but in this case the latter ones were similar, at these positions, to
Prag56. These 10 positions were: 62 (K to R), 65 (G to E), 102 (S to N), 168 (Y to F),
249 (K to E), 298 (R to K), 446 (L to F), 463 (V to I), 507 (H to Q) and 662 (N to T).

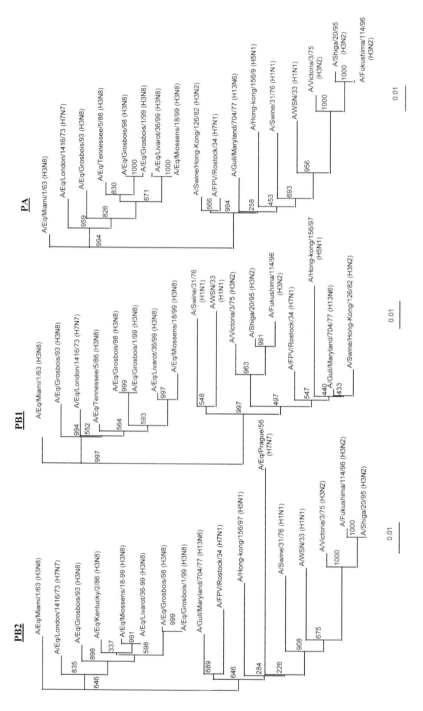

Fig. 1. Phylogenetic trees for the deduced amino acid sequences of the whole coding regions of PB2, PB1 and PA of Mia63, the 1993, 1998 and 1999 French influenza isolates (see text) and of a selection from the databanks of sequences from viruses isolated from humans, swine and various avian species. The trees were constructed using the Neighbour Joining method (see Materials and methods). Mia63 sequences were arbitrarily chosen as the outgroups to root the trees. The bar represents 1% AA substitutions.

Table 1
Number of amino acid (AA) differences within the whole coding regions of PB2, PB1 and PA between the AA sequences of Mia63, the 1993, 1998 and 1999 French influenza isolates and those from the equine strains found in the databanks (see text)

(a) PB2

	Mia63	Lon73	GB93	Ken86	GB98	GB99	Mio99	Liv99
Mia63	0							
Lon73	19	0						
GB93	22	9	0					
Ken86	24	10	6	0				
GB98	27	16	11	7	0			
GB99	27	16	11	7	0	0		
Mio99	25	14	9	6	9	9	0	
Liv99	24	13	8	5	8	8	1	0

(b) PB1

	Lon73	Mia63	Ten86	GB93	GB98	GB99	Mio99	Liv99
Lon73	0							
Mia63	12	0						
Ten86	6	10	0					
GB93	10	13	8	0				
GB98	10	15	7	13	0			
GB99	10	15	7	13	0	0		
Mio99	11	15	7	13	10	10	0	
Liv99	11	15	7	13	10	10	1	0

(c) PA

	Lon73	Mia63	Ten86	GB93	GB98	GB99	Mio99	Liv99
Lon73	0							
Mia63	14	0						
Ten86	18	22	0					
GB93	19	21	14	0				
GB98	20	24	8	17	0			
GB99	21	25	9	18	1	0		
Mio99	20	23	12	21	13	14	0	
Liv99	21	24	13	22	14	15	1	0

The sequences used as reference for comparison in the text are in bold. The A(H7N7) strain appears in italics. The abbreviations are those used in the text.

As compared with Mia63, three AA differences were found in all A(H3N8) PB2s: at position 147 (I to V), 255 (V to I), and 715 (N to K). Two positions (V109I and A717T) distinguished Mia63 from the other viruses with the exceptions of GB98 and GB99 for position 109 and Mio99 and Liv99 for position 717. The PB2 proteins of Ken86, GB98, GB99, Mio99 and Liv99 shared a common substitution at position 590 (G to S). The I67V substitution was specific of the strains isolated in 1998 and 1999. Five positions were specific of GB98 and GB99: T76S, V480I, R555K and I559F. Isolates GB98 and GB99 were similar to Mia63 at position 109 and to Ken86 at position 511 (V to I). Two substitutions were specific of Mio99 and Liv99: 137 (N to S) and 511 (V to M). Mio99 and Liv99 were similar to Lon73 at position 109, and similar to Mia63 at positions 76 and 717. The R368K and R427L changes were specific of GB93. It is noteworthy that GB93 did not show the substitution found in all the viruses isolated since 1986 at position 344 (V to M). The D441G and K443E AA changes were only observed for Lon73. The equine PB2 proteins could thus basically be separated into five groups: (1) Mia63, (2) Lon73, (3) the recent viruses Ken86, GB98 and GB99, (4) Mio99 and Liv99 and (5) GB93.

Analysis of AA sequence changes in the PB1 proteins of recent equine-2 viruses and the prototype strain Mia63 revealed a significant number of AA changes in these proteins as compared with the A(H7N7) strain Lon73, as shown in Table 1, panel b. These changes were often maintained in other strains isolated during subsequent years. Of the 30 AA positions involved in variation between the PB1 proteins from the A(H7N7) strain (Lon73) and the A(H3N8) strains isolated between 1963 and 1999, three distinguished the PB1 proteins of the A(H3N8) equine-2 strains from those of the A(H7N7) strain, at position 94 (S to F), 339 (L to I) and 682 (V to I). The R614E AA change was shared by all equine-2 PB1s except GB98 and GB99 for which the substitution was R614A. The substitution at position 397 (I to V) was shared by all the equine-2 PB1s isolated since 1986 except GB93, similar at this position to Mia63 and Lon73. The substitution at position 198 (K to R) was common to the strains isolated in 1998 and 1999. The GB98 and GB99 sequences were identical and exhibited specific AA changes at four positions: M111I, M179I, K391R and V527I. Mio99 and Liv99 were identical except at positions 749 (T to P for Mio99) and 757 (K to E for Liv99). Four positions showed AA changes found only in this group: V114I, A221T, M317I and E738D. Among the sequences of PB1 analysed in this study, eight positions were characteristic of Mia63 (I61T, M164I, N328H, V451I, T587A, K621Q, A741T and L753F) and six were characteristic of GB93 (I69V, A320T, I325M, R571K, R584Q and K621E).

The PA protein had slightly higher variability, with 44 variable positions observed between isolates. The number of difference in AA sequence between the strains are shown in Table 1, panel c. Five changes were common to all A(H3N8) PAs, at positions 255 (T to A), 277 (Y to H except for Mia63 Y to S), 290 (E to L), 536 (N to K) and 596 (T to I). Four differences with the A(H7N7) strain PA were shared among all A(H3N8) PAs except that of Mia63 at positions: 216 (D to N), 437 (H to Y), 532 (L to F, except for GB93 L to H) and 665 (I to L). Three substitutions were observed in all A(H3N8) PAs except those of Mia63 and GB93 at positions: 231 (A to V), 388 (S to N) and 479 (D to E). Six substitutions were found specifically in the case of Mio99 and Liv99 at positions 62 (I to V), 312 (K to R), 345 (L to I), 354 (I to T), 365 (Q to H) and 450 (V to I). Four positions were specifically observed in the case of GB98 and GB99 at positions 228 (N to S), 355 (P to S), 503 (F to Y) and 535 (H to Y). The substitution R269K was found in the strains isolated in 1998 and 1999. Position 270 carried either the T to M or the T to I substitution. The N321S and V432I substitutions were observed for the A(H3N8) viruses isolated between 1986 and 1999 except Mio99 and Liv99. Thus, the equine PB1 as well as PA proteins could basically be separated into five groups: (1) Mia63, (2) Lon73, (3) the recent viruses Ten86, GB98 and GB99, (4) Mio99 and Liv99 and (5) GB93.

3.2. Evolutionary analyses of the PB2, PB1 and PA proteins

Phylogenetic analyses were carried out on the deduced AA sequences of the P genes from equine viruses and from a selection of Ivs isolated from humans, swine and various avian species (Fig. 1). Results showed that all equine PB2, PB1 and PA were genetically clustered (except for the PB2 from Prag56). In the PB2, PB1 and PA phylogenetic trees, Mia63 sequences were positioned within the equine clusters but always as a separate group, as observed in direct sequence comparison. Mia63 sequences were arbitrarily chosen as the outgroups to root the trees. The horizontal distances between Mia63 sequences and the respective avian clusters indicated that Mia63 PB2, PB1 and PA were more closely related to their avian counterparts. PA has undergone a higher degree of evolution than PB2 and PB1, as observed for human viruses [6]. The construction of the evolutionary trees for the P genes (Fig. 1) revealed a globally similar topology. The P genes of equine viruses were found to evolve generally in a sequential fashion (Fig. 1). However, the PB2, PB1 and PA of one virus, GB93, formed a separate branch on their respective trees and apparently diverged separately. As observed by direct AA sequence comparisons, the P proteins of the 1998 isolate and of the 1999 isolates clustered, further from the root of the tree, into two subgroups, one comprised of GB98 and GB99 and the other one comprised of Mio99 and Liv99.

4. Discussion

Generalised phylogenies published on the basis of data generated about a decade ago, showed that equine P proteins were either the most divergent or the most closely related to avian P proteins [2]. The determination of the phylogeny pathways of the P genes of five IV, isolated between 1993 and 1999, and of the prototype strain Mia63, presented in this study, suggested that the gene segments coding for the P proteins of equine viruses were evolving according to a single evolutionary pathway. The number of variable AA residues within the P proteins of the equine clusters were 35, 30 and 44 for PB2, PB1 and PA, respectively. Within the equine cluster (which represents all equine P genes except for the PB2 from Prag56), all P genes belonged to the same global lineage, including Lon73. This was in accordance with the hypothesis first suggested by Bean [7] of a reassortment between equine-1 and equine-2 viruses between 1964 and 1973 leading to the substitutions of the equine-1 internal genes by equine-2 internal genes. Excluding GB93, globally from 1963 to 1999, the rates of variation per site and per year were 1.82×10^{-3} for PB2, 1.52×10^{-3} for PB1 and 2.36×10^{-3} for PA. Because of the limited data available, it is not yet possible to determine whether the evolution was more rapid until 1986 than in the late 1990s. Contrary to human P genes [6], the AA changes did not appear to be erratic but rather seemed to be cumulative in the course of time. However, two positions in the sequence of PB2 seem to have undergone a subsitution back to the residues observed in Mia63: at position 109 for the GB98 and GB99 group and at position 717 for the Mio99 and Liv99 group. The comparison of the phylogenetic analyses of the HA AA sequences (data not shown) with those of the proteins of the polymerase complex suggested that, for recent equine H3N8 viruses, the evolution of the P proteins were linked to the evolution of the HA1 domain of the HA protein. It is indeed noteworthy that GB98 and GB99 were clustered together and that Mio99 and Liv99 formed another group in all the P proteins phylogenetic trees. Genetic data about the sequence of the HA1 domain of the HA showed that the GB98 and GB99 viruses (Ref. [3] and data not shown) belonged to the recently emerged Eurasian lineage of equine-2 viruses, whereas Mio99 and Liv99 (data not shown) were found within the newly emerged American lineage [8,9].

The data presented in this study confirmed the generalised phylogenies published to date and, with satisfactory bootstrap values, allowed a detailed description of the phylogenetic relationship of the equine P proteins between themselves and with those of viruses isolated from other species. Many more data are needed to go further in the search of the point of entry of P genes of avian origin into horses leading to host specific lineages.

Acknowledgements

The authors wish to thank veterinary surgeons Vincent Ammann, Sébastien Caure, Gérard Tourtoulou, Richard Corde and Fabrice Rossignol for providing the swabs.

References

[1] J. Mumford, J. Wood, WHO/OIE meeting: consultation on newly emerging strains of equine influenza, 18–19 May 1992, Animal Health Trust, Newmarket, Suffolk, UK, Vaccine 11 (11) (1993) 1172–1175.
[2] O.T. Gorman, W.J. Bean, R.G. Webster, Evolutionary processes in influenza viruses: divergence, rapid evolution, and stasis, in: R.W. Compans, M. Cooper, H. Koprowski (Eds.), Genetic Diversity of RNA Viruses, Springer-Verlag, 1992, pp. 75–98 (JHJ Ed. Curr. Top in Microbiol. Immunol., vol. 176).
[3] J.C. Manuguerra, S. Zientara, C. Sailleau, et al., Evidence for evolutionary stasis and genetic drift by genetic analysis of two equine influenza H3 viruses isolated in France, Vet. Microbiol. 74 (1–2) (2000) 59–70.
[4] N. Saitou, M. Nei, The neighbor-joining method: a new method for reconstructing phylogenetic trees, Mol. Biol. Evol. 4 (4) (1987) 406–425.
[5] J. Felsenstein, Confidence limits on phylogenies: an approach using the bootstrap, Evolution 39 (1985) 783–791.
[6] S.E. Lindstrom, Y. Hiromoto, R. Nerome, et al., Phylogenetic analysis of the entire genome of influenza A (H3N2) viruses from Japan: evidence for genetic reassortment of the six internal genes, J. Virol. 72 (10) (1998) 8021–8031.
[7] W.J. Bean, Correlation of influenza A virus nucleoprotein genes with host species, Virology 133 (2) (1984) 438–442.
[8] J.M. Daly, A.C. Lai, M.M. Binns, T.M. Chambers, M. Barrandeguy, J.A. Mumford, Antigenic and genetic evolution of equine H3N8 influenza A viruses, J. Gen. Virol. 77 (1996) 661–671.
[9] S. Lindstrom, A. Endo, R. Pecoraro, S. Sugita, Y. Hiromoto, K. Nerome, Genetic divergency of equine A(H3N8) influenza viruses: cocirculation of earliest and recent strains, in: H. Nakajima, W. Plowright (Eds.), Equine Infectious Diseases VII, Proceedings of the 7th International Conference of Equine Infectious Diseases, vol. 1, R. and W. Publications, Tokyo, 1994, p. 307.

International Congress Series 1219 (2001) 267–273

Molecular methods for diagnosis of influenza

Maria C. Zambon*, Joanna S. Ellis

Enteric, Respiratory and Neurological Virus Laboratory, Central Public Health Laboratory,
Public Health Laboratory Service, 61 Colindale Avenue, Colindale, London NW9 5HT, UK

Abstract

The accurate and reliable diagnosis of transmissible diseases is the first requirement to ensure their control. Several different pathogens can produce respiratory illness with similar clinical symptoms, making an accurate diagnosis of influenza by a physician difficult. The invention and development of polymerase chain reaction (PCR) technology has enabled rapid and sensitive viral diagnostic tests to influence patient treatment. Molecular methods used directly on clinical materials have an important role to play in the diagnosis and surveillance of influenza viruses. © 2001 Elsevier Science B.V. All rights reserved.

Keywords: RT-PCR; Sequence; HMA; Surveillance; Restriction assay

1. Introduction

The application of molecular methodology has had an important impact on the diagnosis and surveillance of influenza viruses. Since influenza viruses continue to circulate and cause significant morbidity and mortality throughout the world, accurate identification and monitoring of circulating strains are essential. The early detection and characterisation of newly emerging variants is one of the aims of the WHO global surveillance network. Both timely and accurate information on the relationship of circulating viruses to current vaccine strains aid optimal vaccine formulation. The sensitivity and specificity of molecular methods such as reverse-transcription polymerase chain reaction (RT-PCR) assays enable the detailed analysis of the molecular epidemiology of circulating strains. While determination of changes in the sequence of the

---

* Corresponding author. Tel.: +44-208-200-4400.
E-mail address: mzambon@phls.nhs.uk (M.C. Zambon).

0531-5131/01/$ – see front matter © 2001 Elsevier Science B.V. All rights reserved.
PII: S0531-5131(01)00338-7

haemagglutinin (HA) gene can give us information on the direction of genetic drift, the effect of specific amino acid changes on antigenicity cannot as yet be predicted. Therefore, virus isolation followed by full characterisation of the antigenic properties of virus isolates still remains the cornerstone of WHO influenza virus surveillance.

2. Application of molecular methods

2.1. Diagnosis

The advent of molecular technology has transformed the diagnosis of a number of diseases, for example HIV and HCV infections [1,2]. This is in contrast to the diagnosis of respiratory infections, where the application of molecular methods to the detection of respiratory pathogens is still in its infancy.

The development of the new neuraminidase inhibitors and the subsequent evaluation of these drugs in clinical trials have provided an excellent source of data on the usefulness of PCR in the diagnosis of influenza infection [3]. In some early phase III trials of zanamivir in Europe and North America, samples were collected from community cases of influenza during periods when influenza virus was circulating from patients who presented within the first or second calendar day of onset of symptoms. Patients were aged between 12 and 81 years (mean 37 years) and had fever together with two symptoms (headache, myalgia, sore throat, cough). The results of the comparison of the percentage of samples positive for influenza A or B virus by virus isolation, serology or PCR show an excellent concordance between PCR and the classical methodology (Fig. 1). Furthermore, there was a significant correlation between the number of tests positive and illness severity. Where all three tests were positive, there was a significant correlation between duration of illness, but not antibiotic use and the risk of complications (data not shown). Although PCR was more sensitive than either culture or paired haemagglutina-

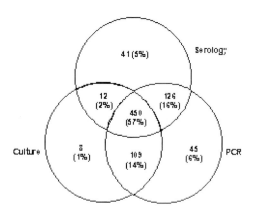

Fig. 1. Concordance of diagnostic test results in 791 patients with positive results from serology, virus culture or PCR.

tion inhibition (HI) serology, PCR positivity alone was not more likely to be associated with severity of illness, development of complications or antibiotic usage. From these analyses, it can be concluded that PCR provides rapid and accurate diagnosis in individual patient diagnosis and is the most sensitive method for detection of cases of influenza in the community.

2.2. Surveillance

The detection and analysis of influenza viruses by molecular methods also have an important role to play in enhancing the surveillance and characterisation of circulating influenza strains. In some national surveillance schemes, the benefit of utilising multiplex RT-PCR has been demonstrated successfully [4]. In Portugal, a comparison of multiplex RT-PCR for the detection of influenza viruses with culture, enzyme immunoassay (EIA) and serology was performed during surveillance over seven influenza seasons from 1992 to 1999 [5]. More samples were found to be positive by RT-PCR than by any of the other methods used. The best correlation was seen between RT-PCR and paired serology, where 43.6% and 38%, respectively, of the total number of individuals sampled were positive for influenza virus, which also reflected the clinical indices of influenza-like illness in the community.

The annual outbreak of influenza activity in Scotland is monitored by a community-based surveillance scheme and from 2000–2001, virological surveillance will be performed by molecular detection alone. This decision was made following the results of a comparison of RT-PCR with culture and serology, which was recently reported [6]. An excellent concordance between diagnosis by RT-PCR and serology was demonstrated, with influenza virus detected in 57% and 61% of samples, respectively. However, whereas, RT-PCR is rapid and can be performed in 36 h, serological methods are usually retrospective. It can be concluded that the use of RT-PCR in surveillance of influenza is more sensitive and rapid than established methods. Molecular methods are able to give a better estimate of the true burden of illness due to influenza in the community. In addition, since multiplex approaches to molecular diagnosis are able to detect more than one respiratory pathogen in a single specimen [7,8], they are more cost-effective than single-target assays.

The exact impact of molecular methodology on surveillance is likely to depend upon the sensitivity of laboratory systems already in place. In both of the above national schemes, culture of influenza viruses was found to be difficult and suboptimal for a number of reasons. Hence, the decision as to whether to use molecular methods, either in addition to or in the place of traditional assays has to be made by each laboratory in each country according to local circumstances.

3. Outbreaks

The investigations of outbreaks of respiratory illness are often hampered by the inability to culture the organism responsible. However, the use of molecular techniques directly on clinical respiratory specimens facilitates the analysis of respiratory outbreaks

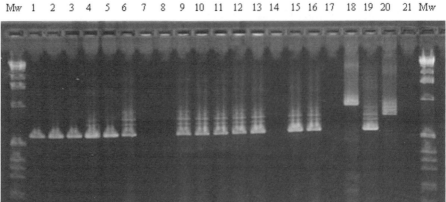

Fig. 2. Comparison of detection of influenza virus by RT-PCR and cell culture in specimens from an outbreak of respiratory illness on a cruise-ship. Lanes 1–7 and 9–16; clinical specimens. Lanes 8, 17, 21; negative controls. Lane 18; A H1N1 positive control. Lane 19; A H3N2 positive control. Lane 20; influenza B positive control. Mw; DNA molecular weight markers.

and can provide rapid identification of an organism and reveal its relationship to currently circulating viruses and vaccine strains. This was demonstrated most recently during the investigation of an outbreak of influenza-like illness on board a cruise-ship in the Mediterranean in 1999 [9]. A total of 55 of 490 crew members and 60 of 590 passengers presented with respiratory tract infection. Of the passengers, two were hospitalised with pneumonia. Respiratory samples were analysed by RT-PCR and culture within 24 h of collection. Of the first 15 throat swabs tested, 13 were positive by RT-PCR for influenza AH3N2 virus (Fig. 2), whereas, virus was isolated by culture from only four of the RT-PCR positive samples. On the basis of these findings, the decision was made to immunise the crew with influenza vaccine. These results highlight the suitability of applying molecular methodology to outbreak situations.

4. Analysis of molecular products

The coupling of amplification by PCR of nucleic acid directly from respiratory samples with typing techniques allows the analysis of circulating lineages of virus genes and enhances rapid tracking of influenza virus evolution. A combination of RT-PCR and enzyme digestion of the PCR product (PCR restriction assay) has been used to differentiate rapidly genetic variants that are antigenically similar [10]. This technique may also differentiate between vaccine strains and currently circulating strains. PCR restriction assays have most recently been used to differentiate the internal genes of human influenza H1N1, H3N2 and H5N1 influenza A viruses [11].

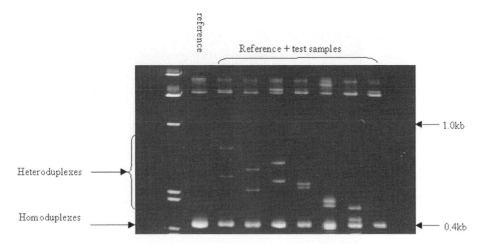

Fig. 3. Characterisation of influenza M gene PCR products by heteroduplex mobility assay (HMA). Lane 1; molecular weight markers, Lane 2; reference PCR amplicon alone (homoduplex), Lanes 3–9; reference PCR amplicon mixed, denatured and annealed with test amplicons of decreasing divergence, which form heteroduplexes of increasing mobility with the reference DNA.

Direct amplification of internal genes from clinical material can also be coupled with heteroduplex mobility assays (HMA) to allow rapid species identification of the origin of influenza viruses, or analysis of variant strains (Fig. 3). Sequence analysis of PCR amplicons is routinely performed in many laboratories, particularly on HA gene products where an association between sequence changes with genetic drift is studied [12,13].

5. Tissue diagnosis

The most important application of RT-PCR and sequencing in tissue analysis to date has been in the genetic analysis of the 1918 pandemic influenza strain in archival material [14]. Influenza RNA fragments were isolated from lung tissue from three victims of the 1918 pandemic and the coding sequences of the genes are being analysed to determine the origin of this virus. Molecular methodology is of particular use in the study of post-mortem specimens (Fig. 4) and may be of extreme value in the diagnosis of influenza in the central nervous system [15,16]. Analysis of other body tissues may help to clarify mechanisms of pathogenesis [17].

6. Approaches

When designing a molecular diagnostic assay, the prospective application of the assay will influence the choice of gene target. For type-specific diagnosis of influenza A, B or C infection, internal genes such as nucleoprotein (NP) and matrix (M) genes

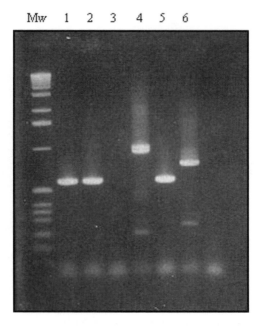

Fig. 4. Detection of influenza AH3N2 by RT-PCR on post-mortem lung tissue samples. Lanes 1 and 2; tissue samples. Lane 3; negative control. Lanes 4–6; influenza A H1N1, A H3N2 and B positive controls, respectively.

are usually chosen, since these are highly conserved within influenza types [18]. If, however, information on the subtype of influenza A is required, then the genes encoding the surface antigens must be targeted. One advantage of assays based on detection of the HA gene is that subsequent sequence information can be determined from the assay products. Multisegment PCR using primers complimentary to the conserved 5′ and 3′ sequences on each gene allows the detection of all segments in a single reaction [19].

7. Predictions for the future

Diagnostic molecular methodology has developed considerably during the past few years. The coupling of automated purification of nucleic acids together with real-time PCR should enable even more rapid identification of viral pathogens such as influenza viruses in clinical material. Quantitative RT-PCR systems are being designed to allow the determination of viral load in infections. Finally, the use of DNA microarrays to identify either multiple gene targets from a single pathogen, or multiple pathogens in a single sample has the capacity to revolutionise influenza diagnosis. Although molecular methods will not replace cell culture for the provision of virus isolates for antigenic characterisation, they will continue to be invaluable in aiding our understanding of the epidemiology of influenza viruses.

Acknowledgements

We would like to acknowledge the excellent work of Carol Sadler and Alex Elliot.

References

[1] K. Christano, A.M. DiBisceglie, J.H. Hoofnagle, S.M. Feinstone, Hepatitis C viral RNA in serum of patients with chronic non-A, non-B hepatitis: detection by the polymerase chain reaction using multiple primer sets, Hepatology 14 (1991) 51–55.

[2] S. Cassol, A. Butcher, S. Kinard, J. Spadoro, N. Lapointe, S. Read, et al., Rapid screening for the early detection of mother-to-child transmission of HIV-1, Journal of Clinical Microbiology 32 (1994) 2641–2645.

[3] M.C. Zambon, J. Hays, A. Webster, R. Newman, Comparison of virus culture, RT-PCR and serology in the diagnosis of influenza, Journal of Antimicrobial Chemotherapy 44 (Supplement A) (1999) 42.

[4] J.S. Ellis, D.M. Fleming, M.C. Zambon, Multiplex reverse transcription-PCR for surveillance of influenza A and B viruses in England and Wales in 1995 and 1996, Journal of Clinical Microbiology 35 (8) (1997) 2076–2082.

[5] H. Rebelo-de-Andrade, M.C. Zambon, Different diagnostic methods for detection of influenza epidemics, Epidemiology and Infection 124 (3) (2000) 515–522.

[6] W.F. Carman, J. Walker, S. McInyyre, A. Noone, P. Christie, J. Millar, et al., Rapid virological surveillance of community influenza infection in general practice, British Medical Journal 321 (2000) 736–737.

[7] J. Stockton, J.S. Ellis, M. Saville, J.P. Clewley, M.C. Zambon, Multiplex PCR for typing and subtyping influenza and respiratory syncytial viruses, Journal of Clinical Microbiology 36 (1998) 2990–2995.

[8] B. Grondahl, W. Puppe, A. Hoppe, I. Kuhne, J.A. Weighl, H.J. Schmitt, Rapid identification of nine microorganisms causing respiratory tract infections by single-tube multiplex reverse transcription-PCR: feasibility study, Journal of Clinical Microbiology 37 (1999) 1–7.

[9] Anonymous. Influenza on a cruise ship in the Mediterranean, Communicable Disease Report 9 (24) (1999) 209, 12.

[10] J.S. Ellis, C.J. Sadler, P. Laidler, H. Rebelo-de-Andrade, M.C. Zambon, Analysis of influenza A H3N2 strains isolated in England during 1995–1996 using polymerase chain reaction restriction, Journal of Medical Virology 51 (1997) 234–241.

[11] L.A. Cooper, K. Subbarao, A simple restriction fragment length polymorphism-based strategy that can distinguish the internal genes of human H1N1, H3N2, and H5N1 influenza A viruses, Journal of Clinical Microbiology 38 (7) (2000) 2579–2583.

[12] N. Cox, C. Bender, Molecular epidemiology of influenza, Seminars in Virology 6 (1995) 359–370.

[13] J.S. Ellis, P. Chakraverty, J.P. Clewley, Genetic and antigenic variation in the haemagglutinin of recently circulating influenza A (H3N2) viruses in the United Kingdom, Archives of Virology 140 (1995) 1889–1904.

[14] J.K. Taubenberger, A.H. Reid, A.E. Krafft, K.E. Bijwaard, T.G. Fanning, Initial genetic characterisation of the 1918 "Spanish" influenza virus, Science 275 (5307) (1997) 1793–1796.

[15] S. Fujimoto, M. Kobayashi, O. Uemura, M. Iwasa, T. Ando, T. Katoh, et al., PCR on cerebrospinal fluid to show influenza-associated acute encephalopathy or encephalitis, The Lancet 352 (1998) 873–875.

[16] J.A. McCullers, S. Facchini, P.J. Chesney, R.G. Webster, Influenza B virus encephalitis, Clinical Infectious Diseases 28 (4) (1999) 898–900.

[17] H. Xu, O. Yasui, H. Tsuruoka, K. Kuroda, K. Hayashi, A. Yamada, et al., Isolation of type B influenza virus from the blood of children, Clinical Infectious Diseases 27 (1998) 654–655.

[18] E.J.C. Claas, M.J.W. Sprenger, G.E.M. Kleter, R. van Beek, W.G.V. Quint, N. Masurel, Type-specific identification of influenza viruses A, B and C by the polymerase chain reaction, Journal of Virological Methods 39 (1992) 1–13.

[19] D.E. Wentworth, M. McGregor, M.D. Macklin, V. Neumann, V.S. Hinshaw, Transmission of swine influenza virus to humans after exposure to experimentally infected pigs, Journal of Infectious Diseases 175 (1997) 7–15.

International Congress Series 1219 (2001) 275–282

PCR-based influenza A virus surveillance in European birds

Ron A.M. Fouchier[a,*], Björn Olsen[b], Theo M. Bestebroer[a],
Sander Herfst[a], Liane van der Kemp[a], Guus F. Rimmelzwaan[a],
Albert D.M.E. Osterhaus[a]

[a]*National Influenza Center, Department of Virology, Erasmus University, P.O. Box 1738,
3000 DR, Rotterdam, The Netherlands*
[b]*Kalmar County Hospital, Kalmar, Sweden*

Abstract

Background: The recently raised awareness of the threat of a new influenza pandemic has stimulated the interest in detection of influenza A viruses in animal secretions. Virus isolation alone is unsatisfactory for this purpose because of the inherent limited sensitivity and the lack of host cells that are universally permissive to all influenza A viruses. Previously described PCR methods are more sensitive, but are targeted predominantly at virus strains currently circulating in humans, since the primer sets display considerable numbers of mismatches to animal influenza A viruses. *Methods*: Classical virus isolation approaches were compared with an RT-PCR based screening approach for the detection of influenza A virus in cloacal swabs and droppings collected from wild birds. *Results*: A new set of primers, based on highly conserved regions in the matrix gene, was designed for single tube reverse transcription PCR for the detection of influenza A viruses from multiple species. This PCR proved to be fully reactive with a panel of genetically diverse virus isolates obtained from birds, humans, pigs, horses and seals and including all known subtypes of influenza A virus. It was not reactive with other RNA viruses tested. *Conclusions*: Comparative tests using fecal and cloacal swab samples from birds confirmed that the new PCR is faster and up to 100-fold more sensitive than classical virus isolation procedures. PCR-based pre-testing of specimens enables high throughput screening for influenza A virus in wild animals. © 2001 Elsevier Science B.V. All rights reserved.

Keywords: Animal; Ecology; Reservoir; Epidemiology

---

* Corresponding author. Tel.: +31-10-4088066; fax: +31-10-4089485.
E-mail address: fouchier@viro.fgg.eur.nl (R.A.M. Fouchier).

1. Introduction

Migratory birds and waterfowl are thought to serve as the reservoir for influenza A viruses in nature [1]. To date, influenza A viruses representing 15 hemagglutinin (HA) and 9 neuraminidase (NA) subtypes have been detected in wild birds and poultry throughout the world [1,2].

Although the routine diagnostic procedures for influenza A virus described to date, including in vitro virus isolation, immunofluorescence (IF) and PCR-based assays, are powerful tools for the detection of human influenza A viruses, they may be less effective for detection of influenza viruses of avian and porcine origin. The phenotypic and genetic heterogeneity of the latter viruses may result in false negative diagnosis of influenza A virus infection using in vitro cell culture or previously described primer sets for PCR analysis.

The aim of this study was to set up a rapid and sensitive PCR method for screening specimens for the presence of phenotypically and genotypically diverse influenza A viruses. To this end, we have designed a primer-set for PCR-based detection of influenza A viruses that was validated with a panel of influenza A virus strains representing all known HA and NA subtypes obtained from a variety of host species and from different geographical locations. The efficacy of this PCR-based screening of samples from avian origin was compared with classical isolation of influenza A virus in embryonated chicken eggs. We conclude that this PCR, based on the detection of gene segment 7 of influenza A virus, is fast, sensitive and specific and suitable for all genetic variants of influenza A virus known to date.

2. Materials and methods

2.1. Design of oligonucleotides

PCR primers were designed on the basis of sequence information obtained from the Influenza Sequence Database at Los Alamos National Laboratories, Los Alamos NM (http://www.flu.lanl.gov) as described elsewhere [3].

2.2. Specimens

Cloacal swabs or fresh droppings were collected from wild birds in the Netherlands and Sweden in 1998 and 1999. Cotton swabs were used for sampling and subsequently stored in transport media [4]. Samples were stored at 4 °C for a few days, at − 20 °C for less than a week, or at − 70 °C for extended periods of time. Transport media consisted of Hanks balanced salt solution supplemented with 10% glycerol, 200 U/ml penicillin, 200 μg/ml streptomycin, 100 U/ml polymyxin B sulphate, 250 μg/ml gentamicin and 50 U/ml nystatin (all from ICN, Zoetermeer, The Netherlands).

2.3. RNA isolation

RNA was isolated using a high pure RNA isolation kit (Roche Molecular Biochemicals) according to the instructions from the manufacturer, with minor modifications.

0.2 ml sample was homogenized by vortexing and subsequently lysed with 0.4 ml lysis/binding buffer to which poly-A (Roche Molecular Biochemicals) was added as a carrier to 1 μg/ml. After binding to the column, Dnase I digestion and washing, the RNA was eluted in 50 μl nuclease-free double-distilled water.

2.4. PCR

Samples were amplified in a one-step RT-PCR in 25 μl final volume, containing 50 mM Tris–HCl pH 8.5, 50 mM NaCl, 7 mM MgCl$_2$, 2 mM DTT, 1 mM each dNTP, 0.4 μM each oligonucleotide, 2.5 U recombinant RNAsin, 10 U AMV reverse transcriptase, 2.5 U Ampli-Taq DNA polymerase (all enzymes from Promega Benelux, Leiden, The Netherlands) and 5 μl RNA. Thermo-cycling was performed in an MJ PTC-200 apparatus using the following cycling conditions: 30 min at 42 °C, 4 min at 95 °C once and 1 min at 95 °C, 1 min at 45 °C, 3 min at 72 °C repeated 40 times. Reactions were analyzed by agarose gel electrophoresis and ethidium–bromide staining, Southern blot hybridization or dot–blot hybridization.

2.5. Hybridization

Blots were prehybridized for 5 min at 55 °C in 2 × SSPE (0.3 M NaCl, 20 mM NaH$_2$PO$_4$, 2 mM EDTA, pH 7.4) and 0.1% SDS, after which biotinylated oligonucleotide probe Bio-M93C was added to 2 pmol/ml and hybridization was continued for 45 min at 55 °C. Blots were washed twice for 10 min at 55 °C with hybridization buffer, transferred to 2 × SSPE with 0.5% SDS after which streptavidin–peroxidase (Roche Molecular Biochemicals) was added to 0.125 U/ml and incubated for 45 min at 42 °C. Blots were washed 10 min at 42 °C in 2 × SSPE, 0.5% SDS, 10 min at 42 °C in 2 × SSPE, 0.1% SDS and 10 min at room temperature in 2 × SSPE, after which the samples were visualized using ECL detection reagents and exposure to hyperfilm (Amersham Pharmacia Biotech Benelux, Roosendaal, The Netherlands) for 5–60 s.

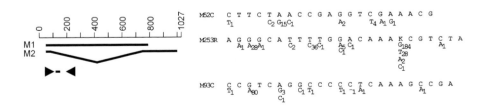

Fig. 1. Position of the M gene primer set, and conservation of the oligonucleotides. (A) Primers M52C (▶) and M253R (◀) amplify a 244-nucleotide fragment of the M1 protein of influenza A virus that is detected using biotinylated oligonucleotide M93C (—). (B) The variation in influenza A virus sequences was compared to each of the oligonucleotides and is displayed below its sequence, where numbers in subscript refer to the number of strains in the database in which the mutation is found. For M52C, M253R and M93C, 175, 215 and 189 influenza A virus sequences, respectively, were available for analysis.

2.6. Virus isolation and propagation

Influenza A viruses used for validation studies have been described earlier and were kindly provided by Dr. R.G. Webster [2,5]. All of these viruses had been isolated and propagated in the allantoic cavities of 11-day-old embryonated chicken eggs [6]. HA titers in virus stocks were determined with turkey erythrocytes using standard procedures [7]. Virus isolates were characterized by hemagglutination inhibition assays with subtype-specific hyper-immune rabbit antisera raised against HA/NA preparations of a panel of virus isolates including all HA and NA subtypes.

3. Results

3.1. Design of oligonucleotides for PCR detection of influenza A viruses

We have designed a new set of three oligonucleotides for the detection of influenza A virus (Fig. 1). The oligonucleotide sequences are based on highly conserved sequences in the matrix (M) gene of influenza A virus. These oligonucleotides display very little variability compared to the influenza A virus M sequences found in nature, and therefore may be more suitable for the detection of influenza A virus as compared to previously described sets of primers.

3.2. Sensitivity and specificity of influenza A virus PCR

RNA was isolated from virus stocks of a panel of influenza A viruses, which was used for amplification by PCR with primer-set M52C–M253R (Fig. 2). For each of the virus strains tested, a band of 244 bp was amplified, which was easily visualized on a 1% agarose gel stained with ethidium–bromide. Hybridization of dot–blots with the internal biotinylated oligonucleotide probe M93C also resulted in clear signals for each of the influenza A virus strains tested.

Using titrated stocks of influenza A viruses, we found that PCR-based detection was up to 100-fold more sensitive as compared to virus isolation in cell culture and embryonated

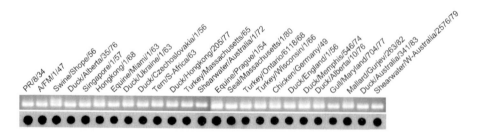

Fig. 2. PCR analysis of a panel of influenza A virus isolates, originating from different hosts and geographical locations. RNA was isolated from influenza A viruses grown in embryonated chicken eggs, followed by PCR analysis and agarose gel electrophoresis (top panel) or dot–blot analysis (bottom panel).

chicken eggs [3]. Moreover, PCR and dot–blot analysis using RNA from a panel of RNA viruses revealed that the procedure is specific for influenza A virus; no hybridization signals were observed with any of the other 11 RNA viruses tested [3].

3.3. Detection of influenza A virus in bird samples

We next tested the suitability of the PCR for avian influenza A virus screening of cloacal swabs and droppings from ducks, geese and other wild birds collected in the Netherlands and Sweden. The screening procedure is outlined in Fig. 3. Because PCR screening appeared to be up to 100-fold more sensitive than virus isolation, and to reduce cost and workload, the number of RNA isolations and PCR analyses were reduced by making pools of five samples each (40 μl per sample). Between each five pooled samples, a negative control consisting of transport media was inserted to check for contamination during processing of the samples.

From 235 pools of samples representing 1175 individual specimens, 19 revealed the presence of influenza A virus upon RNA isolation, PCR and hybridization (a typical result is shown in Fig. 4). RNA was then isolated from each of the individual samples present in these 19 pools, revealing that each pool contained a single positive bird sample except for one pool, which contained two positive samples.

Each of the 20 positive individual samples were used to inoculate two to four embryonated chicken eggs, from which the allantoic fluids were collected, pooled and inoculated a second time in duplicate in embryonated chicken eggs (blind passage). From 15 out of 20 PCR-positive samples we were able to isolate influenza A virus in eggs. From the other five samples, which appeared to contain less virus as judged by the intensity of signals on dot–blots, no influenza A virus could be isolated even upon blind passage in embryonated chicken eggs.

To test the possibility that the PCR analysis would give false negative results as compared to virus isolation in eggs, 243 individual PCR-negative cloacal swabs and dropping samples were inoculated in two to four embryonated chicken eggs each, followed by a blind passage of the pooled allantoic fluids in duplicate. We were unable to isolate influenza A virus from these PCR-negative samples, indicating that no false negative results were obtained by PCR analysis. Inoculation of tertiary monkey kidney

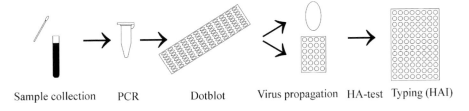

Sample collection   PCR   Dotblot   Virus propagation HA-test Typing (HAI)

Fig. 3. Screening procedure for detection of influenza A virus in avian specimens. Cloaca swabs or fresh dropping samples are collected in the field and stored in transport media at − 70°C. Upon RNA isolation, RT-PCR and dot–blot hybridization, samples are selected for virus isolation in embryonated chicken eggs or cell cultures. The subtype of the virus isolates is subsequently determined using HAI assays.

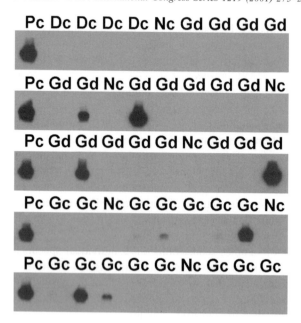

Fig. 4. PCR-based detection of influenza A virus in a representative set of avian cloacal swabs and droppings. RNA was isolated from 0.2 ml of 38 pooled samples, each consisting of five individual bird samples, and used for PCR and Southern blot analysis. Pc: positive control; Nc: negative control; Dc: duck cloacal swabs: Gd: goose droppings; Gc: goose cloacal swabs.

cells and MDCK cell cultures with 212 random PCR-negative individual bird samples also did not reveal additional influenza A virus-positive samples. In fact, these cell lines were found to be less susceptible to avian influenza A virus as compared to embryonated chicken eggs.

4. Discussion and conclusions

PCR-based methods for virus detection have been described for many clinically relevant viruses. The sensitivity and specificity of PCR-based methods are most critically determined by the choice of primer sequences. Primer-sets described earlier for PCR-based detection of influenza A virus may be appropriate for the detection of virus strains currently circulating in humans, but display considerable numbers of mismatches when compared with animal influenza A viruses [3,8–10]. Primers M52C and M253R and probe M93C span conserved sequences in gene segment 7 of influenza A virus and have no homology to nucleotide sequences from other species available from GenBank. Our experimental data confirmed that PCR amplification and dot blot analyses with this set of primers does not pick up cross-reacting host-derived sequences or other RNA viruses and is suitable for detection of a wide variety of influenza A virus strains. The limited variability in influenza A virus sequences spanning the primer sequences is mostly confined to the 5′ ends of the oligonucleotides and therefore unlikely to obscure PCR amplification. Indeed, we successfully amplified the genome of virus isolates with mismatches in these primer sequences that were included in the viruses shown in Fig. 2.

Based on titration experiments as well as on analyses of avian specimens, we conclude that the PCR-based method is more sensitive (up to 100-fold) than virus isolation in eggs or mammalian cell cultures. This is not surprising in view of the sensitivity of PCR-based assays in general, and the low ratio of infectious units to physical particles for RNA viruses such as influenza A virus.

Using the PCR-based method, we have detected many influenza A viruses in bird samples that could not be isolated in mammalian cell cultures and some that could not be isolated in embryonated chicken eggs. Presumably, this failure was due to a combination of low virus titers in the original specimens and limited susceptibility of target cells to certain influenza A virus strains.

Taken together, our data indicate that the newly designed PCR offers a more sensitive and faster tool for the diagnosis of human influenza A virus infection than virus isolation. Because of the better matching primers, it can be expected that for the detection of animal influenza A viruses this PCR is also more suitable than previous PCR protocols [8–10].

Acknowledgements

The authors wish to thank John de Boer, Hans Zantinge, Dick Jonkers, and their colleagues for collection of bird samples, and Rob Webster for providing influenza A virus isolates. R.F. is a fellow of the Royal Dutch Academy of Arts and Sciences. This work was made possible in part through a grant from the Dutch Ministry of Agriculture and from the Foundation for Respiratory Virus Infections (SRVI).

References

[1] R.G. Webster, W.J. Bean, O.T. Gorman, T.M. Chambers, Y. Kawaoka, Evolution and ecology of influenza A viruses, Microbiol Rev 56 (1) (1992) 152–179.

[2] C. Rohm, N. Zhou, J. Suss, J. Mackenzie, R.G. Webster, Characterization of a novel influenza hemagglutinin, H15: criteria for determination of influenza A subtypes, Virology 217 (2) (1996) 508–516.

[3] R.A.M. Fouchier, T.M. Bestebroer, S. Herfst, L. van der Kemp, G.F. Rimmelzwaan, A.D. Osterhaus, Detection of influenza A viruses from different species by PCR amplification of conserved sequences in the matrix gene, J Clin Microbiol 38 (2000) 4096–4101.

[4] G.B. Sharp, Y. Kawaoka, S.M. Wright, B. Turner, V. Hinshaw, R.G. Webster, Wild ducks are the reservoir for only a limited number of influenza A subtypes, Epidemiol Infect 110 (1) (1993) 161–176.

[5] M. Matrosovich, N. Zhou, Y. Kawaoka, R.G. Webster, The surface glycoproteins of H5 influenza viruses isolated from humans, chickens, and wild aquatic birds have distinguishable properties, J Virol 73 (2) (1999) 1146–1155.

[6] V.S. Hinshaw, R.G. Webster, B. Turner, Novel influenza A viruses isolated from Canadian feral ducks: including strains antigenically related to swine influenza (Hsw1N1) viruses, J Gen Virol 41 (1) (1978) 115–127.

[7] G.F. Rimmelzwaan, M. Baars, E.C. Claas, A.D. Osterhaus, Comparison of RNA hybridization, hemagglutination assay, titration of infectious virus and immunofluorescence as methods for monitoring influenza virus replication in vitro, J Virol Methods 74 (1) (1998) 57–66.

[8] R.L. Atmar, B.D. Baxter, E.A. Dominguez, L.H. Taber, Comparison of reverse transcription-PCR with tissue culture and other rapid diagnostic assays for detection of type A influenza virus, J. Clin. Microbiol. 34 (10) (1996) 2604–2606.

[9] T. Cherian, L. Bobo, M.C. Steinhoff, R.A. Karron, R.H. Yolken, Use of PCR-enzyme immunoassay for identification of influenza A virus matrix RNA in clinical samples negative for cultivable virus, J. Clin. Microbiol. 32 (3) (1994) 623–628.

[10] E.C. Claas, M.J. Sprenger, G.E. Kleter, R. van Beek, W.G. Quint, N. Masurel, Type-specific identification of influenza viruses A, B and C by the polymerase chain reaction, J Virol Methods 39 (1–2) (1992) 1–13.

International Congress Series 1219 (2001) 283–289

Antibodies from lymphocytes used as diagnostic markers: a novel approach

Lars R. Haaheim[a,b,*], Margrethe W. Ibsen[a], Monica Skogstrand[b,c], Rebecca J. Cox[c]

[a]*Department of Microbiology and Immunology, University of Bergen, Bergen, Norway*
[b]*PlasmAcute AS, Bergen, Norway*
[c]*Department of Molecular Biology, University of Bergen, Bergen, Norway*

Abstract

Background: Serodiagnosis frequently depends on comparing acute and convalescent serum samples. We present a simple and novel general approach using antibodies from disrupted purified peripheral blood lymphocytes to obtain a more precise picture of the acute antibody production. *Methods*: A case of natural infection is presented, as well as data from clinical influenza vaccine trials. Influenza antibodies from disrupted lymphocytes were tested by enzyme-linked immunoassay (ELISA) and compared with serum ELISA and HI antibodies. *Results*: Trace amounts of contaminating plasma antibodies in the cellular pellet did not interfere with the test. Vaccine trials showed that serum ELISA antibodies were usually detected prior to vaccination, rising gradually to elevated and sustained levels during the next 2 weeks. In contrast, only negligible quantities of lymphocyte antibodies were detected pre-vaccination, rising to peak levels at days 7–12, and subsequently declining to background levels. Lymphocyte antibodies appeared earlier than HI antibodies. *Conclusions*: As lymphocyte antibodies will be detected at an earlier stage than serum antibodies, the seronegative time-window will be reduced. Using cells from capillary blood taken from finger tip, ear lobe or heel, our method could also facilitate detailed kinetic studies (e.g. clinical vaccine trials), and be useful for analysing perinatal infections, avoiding the interference of passively transferred maternal antibodies. © 2001 Elsevier Science B.V. All rights reserved.

Keywords: Antibodies; Lymphocytes; Diagnostics; Acute; Kinetics; ELISA

---

* Corresponding author. Department of Microbiology and Immunology, Bergen High Technology Centre, University of Bergen, POB 7800, N-5020 Bergen, Norway. Tel.: +47-5558-4505; fax: +47-5558-4512.
E-mail address: lars.haaheim@gades.uib.no (L.R. Haaheim).

0531-5131/01/$ – see front matter © 2001 Elsevier Science B.V. All rights reserved.
PII: S 0 5 3 1 - 5 1 3 1 (0 1) 0 0 3 3 9 - 9

1. Introduction

Nucleic acid amplification tests have brought a new dimension into diagnostics. Still, there are many instances where material from the offending microbe cannot be obtained or the infectious agent may only be transiently available. Therefore, both in the short- and long-term future, antibody-based diagnostic procedures will continue to play an important role.

Following the introduction of solid-phase enzyme-linked immunoassay (ELISA) three decades ago [1], antibody assays have been brought to a high level of sophistication and automation. The need to reduce the "silent window" between exposure and seroconversion has become urgent, both for general diagnostic routines and to ensure the safety of blood products. The enzyme-linked immunospot assay (ELISPOT), developed two decades ago, is an advanced and labour-intensive research procedure used for enumerating antibody-secreting cells (ASC) spontaneously producing antibodies against the test antigen in question [2]. This method has been successfully used to observe the detailed and real-time kinetic profile of antibody development following infection or vaccination, without the interference of pre-existing serum antibodies, and avoiding the time-lag between antibody synthesis and the ensuing detection in serum.

A simple and novel procedure is presented for measuring the acute antibody production, using lymphocytes obtained from microvolumes of peripheral blood, combining the advantages of the ELISA and ELISPOT techniques.

2. Materials and methods

2.1. Case LOH

Male, 25 years, gave a heparinised blood sample on day 9 after his first day of influenza-like illness. A mixed epidemic of influenza A and B had been recorded in the local community. Lymphocytes were separated by Lymphoprep (Nycomed Pharma, Oslo) according to the manufacturer's instructions. Disruption of lymphocytes was done using standard lysis buffer with protease inhibitors.

2.2. Influenza vaccine trial A

Nine healthy subjects (six females aged 24–27 years, mean 26.2, and three males aged 24–31 years, mean 28.3) were given licensed inactivated influenza vaccine (Vaxigrip; Mérieux Sérum and Vaccines) containing 15 µg HA of each of the strains A/Sydney/5/97(H3N2)-like virus, A/Beijing/262/95(H1N1)-like virus, and B/Beijing/184/93-like virus. Heparinised blood samples were taken at intervals as indicated. Lymphocytes were isolated as described under case LOH, whereas lymphocytes were disrupted by two cycles of freezing–thawing.

2.3. Influenza vaccine trial B

This trial is described previously in this volume [3]. The lymphocytes were separated from plasma antibodies through a simple three-cycle washing procedure by centrifugation, resulting in a purified blood cell pellet that was subsequently disrupted as described under case LOH above.

2.4. Serological tests

ELISA procedures, using purified surface antigens kindly provided by Solvay Pharmaceuticals, Holland, and HI tests were done essentially as described earlier [4]. All ELISA testing of disrupted lymphocyte antibodies used lysates from 300-μl blood.

2.5. Storage of blood

Male subject (EJAa, 20 years) was given inactivated licensed influenza vaccine (as for trial B). Heparinised blood samples were taken at days 0 and 9 post-vaccination. Parallel blood samples were processed either immediately or after storage at 4 °C for 4 days, followed by 4 h at room temperature. Subsequent analyses were as described under trial B.

3. Results

3.1. Case LOH: natural infection

Table 1 shows that plasma IgG contamination of the purified cell pellet was negligible and that the proportion of serum IgG antibodies to the surface antigens from the prevalent A and B strains was 4.8% and 3.0%, respectively. Using this single blood sample, it was not possible to identify which of the two influenza virus types, A or B, was responsible for the current infection. However, the IgG antibodies released from purified lymphocytes provided a conclusive picture. More than 15% of the total IgG antibody population was against influenza A, whereas less than 1% was against influenza B, strongly suggesting that the offending influenza virus was of type A.

3.2. Influenza vaccine trial A

Of the nine vaccinated subjects, four did not elicit HI antibodies ≥ 40 at day 7, whereas significant quantities of H3N2 IgG antibodies from the lymphocytes were detected for all subjects, ranging from 55 to 713 ng/ml. Fig. 1a shows the results for four representative subjects.

3.3. Influenza vaccine trial B

Generally, for all subjects, significant levels of serum ELISA antibodies were detected on day 0, showing varying degree of rising antibody levels during the following 15 days. In contrast, antibodies from disrupted lymphocytes were absent or at very low levels at day 0, rising more sharply and peaking at day 12, showing a falling trend at day 15. HI antibody titres to the vaccine strains were generally absent at day 0. Most subjects

Table 1

Relationship between IgG antibodies in serum and from disrupted lymphocytes post-infection measured by ELISA

Specificity	Number of lymphocytes (10^3) in 100-µl well	IgG detected in well (ng)	Serum IgG contamination of cells (ng)	Net IgG from lymphocytes in well (ng)	Net IgG from each lymphocyte (10^{-5} ng)
Influenza A	50	1.06	2.5×10^{-3}	1.06	2.12
	200	10.72	10.0×10^{-3}	10.71	5.35
Influenza B	200	0.38	nd[a]	0.38	0.19
	800	1.29	nd[a]	1.29	0.16
IgG general	50	13.29	8×10^{-2}	13.21	26.42
	200	44.60	32×10^{-2}	44.28	22.14

	Serum[b]	IgG (µg/ml)	%	Each lymphocyte average (10^{-5} ng)	%
	Influenza A	112	4.8	3.74	15.4
	Influenza B	70	3.0	0.18	0.7
	IgG general	2365	100.0	24.28	100.0

[a] Not detectable.
[b] Plasma 1:2.

elicited protective HI titres (≥ 40) at day 7 or 12 post-vaccination, depending on the virus strain used.

Data from subject #16 is presented in Fig. 1b, showing a varied pattern of antibody kinetics, depending on the vaccine strain used.

3.3.1. H3N2 virus

The levels of serum ELISA antibodies were present at day 0 and only slowly rose to slightly higher levels for the subsequent samples. The initial HI titre of ≤ 20 reached the protective titre of 40 on day 12. In contrast, antibodies from disrupted lymphocytes showed a significant rise on day 5, and falling on day 12.

3.3.2. H1N1 virus

Serum ELISA antibodies were evident on day 0, reaching high levels on day 7. Serum HI antibodies reached protective levels on day 7, whereas lymphocyte antibodies were clearly evident at day 5, peaking at day 12.

Fig. 1. Antibodies in serum and from disrupted lymphocytes measured at intervals post-vaccination. (a) Vaccine trial A. Subjects 6, 7, 4, and 8. Blood samples from days 0, 7 and 13 post-vaccination were analysed for lymphocyte IgG antibodies (nanograms) against A/Sydney/5/97(H3N2). (b) Vaccine trial B. Subject #16. Serum ELISA antibodies (top panel) and serum HI and antibodies from disrupted lymphocytes (lower panel) tested at days 0, 5, 7, 9, 12 and 15 post-vaccination against the three strains A/Sydney/5/97(H3N2), A/Beijing/262/95(H1N1) and B/Yamanashi/166/98. ELISA antibody response is recorded as optical density at 492 nm.

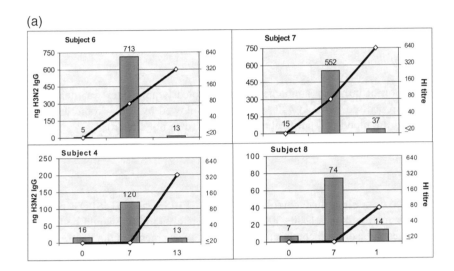

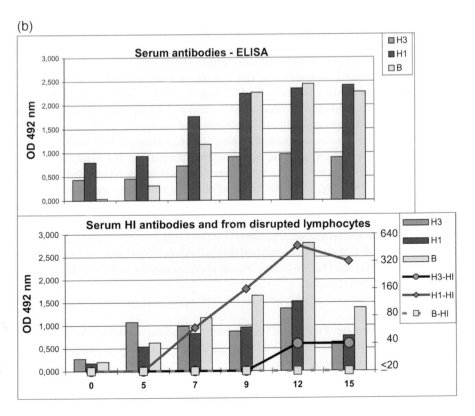

3.3.3. B virus

No serum ELISA antibodies were detected at day 0, and significant levels were reached on day 7. No HI antibodies against influenza B were detected throughout the observation period. Again, antibodies from disrupted lymphocytes were evident on day 5, peaking at very high levels on day 12.

3.4. Storage of blood

The detection of influenza antibodies from disrupted lymphocytes was unaffected by storing the unprocessed blood at 4 °C for 4 days, followed by 4 h at room temperature, before starting the blood cell purification procedure (data not shown).

4. Discussion

Our method is a simplified combination of the ELISA and ELISPOT procedures, requiring only microvolumes (100–300 μl) of peripheral blood that could be taken from the finger tip, ear lobe or heel, combining the quantitative elements of the ELISA technique and the real-time features of the ELISPOT procedure. The precise kinetic profile for antibody development varied slightly between the two clinical trials. This may partly be due to the fact that in trial A, the actual nanogram quantities of influenza antibodies were calculated, whereas for trial B, antibody activity was presented as crude ELISA read-outs (optical density). The two trials were also performed in different winter seasons, implying use of different vaccine batches and a different priming history for the vaccines.

Initially, we used live lymphocytes in cell culture medium in antigen-coated ELISA wells, subsequently incubating the cells for 1–3 h at 37 °C to allow the lymphocytes to synthesise the acute antibodies to be measured by standard ELISA methods. Based on the current knowledge on immunoglobulins synthesis and secretion by B lymphocytes, requiring intracellular processing and assembly of immunoglobulin chains [5], we unexpectedly found that disrupting the lymphocytes and placing the lysate in ELISA wells generated enough functional IgG antibodies that specifically recognised the solid-phase target antigen. Presently, we do not know whether the antibodies we measure by this approach are released in a completely or sufficiently processed form from the cytoplasmic B-cell membrane, or whether functional but not fully processed immunoglobulin chains are released from intracellular compartments.

A useful practical feature of our method is that whole blood can be stored under refrigeration for several days before processing, or alternatively, the cellular pellet or lysate can be kept frozen until required.

Using our method several advantages can be envisaged:

- Measure the precise kinetics of the immune response enabling the distinction between "old" serum antibodies and those generated by B-cells as a consequence of the ongoing immune stimulation.
- Monitor the effect of therapeutic intervention, taking advantage of the fall in numbers of antibody-secreting cells when the offending agent is being cleared [6,7].

- Enable clinical vaccine trials with daily blood samples.
- Conveniently measure perinatal infections without the interference of passively acquired maternal antibodies.
- Reduce the "window-period" between time of infection and seroconversion.

Acknowledgements

This work was supported in part by a start-up industrial grant from the Research Council of Norway (#120572/213).

References

[1] D.M. Kemeny, S. Chantler, An introduction to ELISA, in: D.M. Kemeny, S.J. Challacombe (Eds.), ELISA and Other Solid Phase Immunoasays, Wiley, Chichester, 1988, pp. 1–30.

[2] C. Czerkinsky, L.-Å. Nilsson, A. Tarkowski, W.J. Koopman, J. Mestecky, Ö. Ouchterlony, The solid phase enzyme-linked immunospot assay (ELISPOT) for enumerating antibody-secreting cells: methodology and applications, in: D.M. Kemeny, S.J. Challacombe (Eds.), ELISA and Other Solid Phase Immunoasays, Wiley, Chichester, 1988, pp. 217–239.

[3] R.J. Cox, E. Mykkeltvedt, H. Sjursen, L.R. Haaheim, The effect of Relenza treatment on the early immune response induced after influenza vaccination, This volume.

[4] K.A. Brokstad, R.J. Cox, J. Olofsson, R. Jonsson, L.R. Haaheim, Parenteral influenza vaccination induces a rapid systemic and mucosal immune response, J. Infect. Dis. 171 (1995) 198–203.

[5] F. Melchers, Biosynthesis, transport and secretion of immunoglobulin in plasma cells, Histochem. J. 3 (1971) 389–397.

[6] L. Morris, J.M. Binley, B.A. Clas, S. Bonhoeffer, T.P. Astill, R. Kost, A. Hurley, Y. Cao, M. Markowitz, D.D. Ho, J.P. Moore, HIV-1 antigen-specific and -nonspecific B cell responses are sensitive to combination antiretroviral therapy, J. Exp. Med. 188 (2) (1998) 233–245.

[7] I.L. Tabidze, F.K. Lee, P. Tambe, E. Rocha, S.A. Larsen, B.J. Stoll, M.E. St. Louis, A.J. Nahmias, Enzyme-linked immunospot assay for the diagnosis of active *Treponema pallidum* infection during the various stages of syphilis, Sex. Transm. Dis. 26 (8) (1999) 426–430.

Insight into host defence mechanisms

International Congress Series 1219 (2001) 293–300

Memory and recall CD8$^+$ T cell responses to the influenza A viruses

Peter C. Doherty[a,*], Janice M. Riberdy[a], Jan P. Christensen[b]

[a]*Department of Immunology, St. Jude Children's Research Hospital, 332 North Lauderdale, Memphis, TN 38104, USA*
[b]*Institute of Medical Microbiology and Immunology, The Panum Institute, 3c Blegdamsvej, DK-2200 Copenhagen N, Denmark*

Abstract

The recent development of tetrameric complexes of MHC class I glycoprotein + peptide (tetramers) enables, for the first time, accurate quantitation of CD8$^+$ T cell responses. The characteristics of the cellular immune response following primary, secondary or even tertiary challenge with serologically distinct influenza A viruses can now be understood much more clearly. The prevalence of H-2D^b-restricted CD8$^+$ memory T cells specific for the immunodominant NP$_{366-374}$ peptide that stains with the D^{b}NP$_{366}$ tetramer increases from undetectable levels in naïve mice, to frequencies of 0.2–0.5% (of the CD8$^+$ set) following i.p. exposure to an H1N1 virus. This is boosted to >10% when these H1N1-immune mice are exposed intranasally to an H3N2 virus. Further respiratory challenge of these H1N1- or H3N2 → H1N1-primed mice with a virulent H7N7 virus shows very clearly that the rate of virus clearance is a direct function of the size of the available CD8$^+$ memory T cell pool. However, though established CD8$^+$ T cell memory always provides a measure of protection against the development of clinical disease, replicative infection is still established in the face of massive numbers of virus-specific CD8$^+$ memory T cells. The implications of these findings for immunization against both influenza and other viruses are discussed. © 2001 Elsevier Science B.V. All rights reserved.

Keywords: Protection; Vaccines; Epitopes; Tetramers

1. Historical background

The recognition [1] that virus-specific CD8$^+$ T cells are specific both for some component(s) of an infecting virus and for self class I MHC glycoproteins (MHC

---

* Corresponding author.

restriction) broke open the analysis of cell-mediated immunity (CMI). Prior to that, we knew [2,3] that the specific T cell response was central to virus clearance (ectromelia) and immunopathology (lymphocytic choriomeningitis virus, LCMV), but had not realized that the specificity profiles of T cells and B cells were radically different. Following the initial finding with LCMV [4,5], analysis with the spectrum of MHC class I recombinant and mutant mice that had been developed by transplant immunologists allowed the rapid genetic mapping of MHC restriction. The effect was remarkably precise, with T cell recognition being totally disrupted by a single-point mutation in the particular MHC class I gene [6]. The next big question was obviously the nature of the viral component that was being seen in association with the MHC class I glycoprotein. Several groups seized on the obvious possibilities that the great variety of antigenically "drifted" and recombinant influenza A viruses seemed to offer for dissecting this key question of viral specificity. The results were surprising [7–9], and even disturbing for those who had been involved in the long term in influenza research.

The discovery that the CD8$^+$ T cell response is highly cross-reactive for serologically different influenza A viruses was greeted initially with considerable scepticism. Why, if this were the case, would prior infection with an H1N1 virus not protect against subsequent challenge with an H3N2 virus? Still, the basic observation proved to be correct, leading first to the finding that most influenza-specific CD8$^+$ T cells are specific for components derived from the relatively conserved internal proteins [10,11], then to the demonstration by Townsend et al. [12] that CD8$^+$ T cells recognize peptides that associate with MHC class I glycoproteins in the endoplasmic reticulum. Dissection of CD8$^+$ T cell specificity profiles for the influenza A viruses, thus, led directly to the identification of the cytoplasmic processing pathway, and to the initiation of a new area of research in basic and applied immunology.

Even so, the various experiments that have analyzed the protective effect of this cross-reactive, influenza-specific CD8$^+$ T cell response have generally been rather disappointing [13–17]. At best, there has been a shortening of 1–2 days in the duration of the infectious process in the lungs of mice with established CD8$^+$ T cell memory. This could, as suggested by an early study by McMichael et al. [18], lead to a less severe disease process in humans, but may still allow the development of a substantial episode of clinical influenza.

2. Measuring virus-specific CD8$^+$ T cell responses

The dissection of virus-specific CMI has been revolutionized by the development of tetrameric complexes of MHC class I glycoprotein + peptide (tetramers) for the direct staining of virus-specific CD8$^+$ T cells [19]. This approach allows accurate quantitation of primary, memory and recall CD8$^+$ T cell responses [20]. Prior to that, the effector phase of acute CD8$^+$ T CMI was analyzed by the convenient, but minimally quantitative, cytotoxic T lymphocyte (CTL) ^{51}Cr release assay. The best measurement that we had of immune memory was the cumbersome and tedious limiting dilution analysis (LDA), which required 6 days of in vitro microculture followed by assay for CTL activity [21].

We knew from these approaches that influenza-specific CTL effectors are found at greatest potency in the site of virus-induced pathology in the lung [22]. Long-term LDA studies established that CD8$^+$ T cell memory following both myxovirus and para-myxovirus infection lasts for the life of a laboratory mouse and is, subsequent to the virus replication phase, antigen-independent. Also, the phenotype of CD8$^+$ T cell memory was determined by flow cytometric sorting and subsequent LDA [21]. The memory populations were found to be CD44^{hi}CD62L^{lo} soon after the initial encounter with antigen, with at least some cells reverting to a CD44^{hi}CD62L^{hi} phenotype at later stages. The idea that the size of the memory T cell pool was determined by the magnitude of the antigen-driven clonal burst was also developed from LDA experiments [23].

These observations and interpretations are currently being refined by studies with the tetramers [24,25]. The difference is that the magnitude of the response measured by tetramer (Tet) staining is generally in the region of 10-fold greater than that detected by LDA [26]. Part of the reason for this discrepancy is that the CTL precursors (CTLp) need to go through 10–15 cycles of division before the microclones can be detected by cytotoxicity [27], while the tetramers stain every CD8$^+$ T cell that binds the complex of MHCI+peptide. We know that the great majority, if not all, of the CD8$^+$ Tet$^+$ lymphocytes can be induced to synthesize γ-interferon (IFN-γ) when stimulated for 5 h with the cognate peptide in the presence of Brefeldin A (which inhibits protein secretion), but are otherwise unclear about the extent of functional diversity [24,26] within this population. Even so, the ability to measure CD8$^+$ T cell responses by accurate quantitation of lymphocytes taken directly from the in vivo situation has greatly enhanced our understanding of the nature of CMI.

3. Characteristics of primary, secondary and tertiary influenza-specific CD8$^+$ T cell responses

3.1. Primary response

Influenza-specific CD8$^+$ T cells specific for the immunodominant nucleoprotein (NP$_{366-374}$) peptide presented by H-2D^b cannot be detected in immunologically competent C57BL/6J (B6, H-2^b) naïve mice, and are first found in numbers sufficient to be measured by staining with the D^{b}NP$_{366}$ tetramer at about 6–7 days after primary intranasal (i.n.) challenge with a high dose of the A/HK × 31 (H3N2) influenza virus [24]. The counts for CD8$^+$D^{b}NP$_{366}$$^+$ T cells reach levels of about 2–3% of the CD8$^+$ set in the regional mediastinal lymph nodes (MLN) and the spleen, and are then maintained at about 0.3–0.5% into long-term memory. The latter values are at the limit of detection by flow cytometry. Accurate measurement of lower CD8$^+$ T cell frequencies requires the use of an IFN-γ ELISA spot (ELISPOT) assay, subsequent to in vitro restimulation of diluted lymphocyte populations [28]. The ELISPOT approach is currently the best available technique for measuring virus-specific CD4$^+$ T cell responses [29,30].

The surprising finding for the primary influenza-specific CD8$^+$ T cell response was that the D^{b}NP$_{366}$$^+$ set eventually constitutes approximately 15% of the CD8$^+$ population that can be recovered by bronchoalveolar lavage (BAL) of the infected lung [24]. More recently, the discovery of a prominent new epitope [31] derived from one of the polymerases (D^bPA_{224}) means that, together with the minor responses to peptides from the influenza NS2 and M proteins, >30% of the CD8$^+$ T cells in the BAL of mice with influenza pneumonia could be shown to be specific for the inducing virus. This value has risen to >40% with the finding of a further epitope (G. Belz and P.C. Doherty, manuscript in preparation) from one of the other polymerases (PB1).

The earlier perception (derived from LDA experiments) that the majority of the CD8$^+$ T cells in any virus-induced inflammatory exudate are passively recruited "bystanders" is clearly incorrect, though it is the case that memory T cells of unrelated specificity do localize to such sites of pathology [25,32]. The divergence between the LDA and tetramer results presumably reflects that most of the highly activated CTL in the lungs of mice with influenza pneumonia are driven to apoptosis in the LDA microcultures and, thus, fail to give clones that can be detected 6 days later in the cytotoxicity assay. We had suspected that this was the case, but had totally underestimated the magnitude of the effect.

3.2. Secondary response

Mice that are primed by intraperitoneal (i.p.) inoculation with the A/PR8/34 (PR8) H1N1 influenza virus develop a massive secondary response following i.n. challenge with the H3N2 HK × 31 virus [24,25]. This was very apparent following immunization 7 months previously, representing about 25% of the normal life span of a laboratory mouse. There can, thus, be no doubt that influenza-specific CD8$^+$ T cell memory is long-lived in the absence of continued exposure to the cognate peptide. The prevalence of D^bNP_{366}-specific T cells in the spleen increases from <0.5% in "resting" memory to 15–25% at the height of the recall response. These very high numbers decline progressively, but are still elevated above the levels found following primary exposure at 100 days after secondary challenge. Evidence of clonal expansion is also found for the $D^bPA_{224}^+$ population, but at a much lower level than that recognized for the immunodominant $D^bNP_{336}^+$ set [31]. This difference in the magnitude of the recall response is intriguing, as these two epitopes are equally prominent in the primary response and the numbers of memory T cells in the H1N1-immune mice looked to be approximately equivalent for D^bNP_{366} and D^bPA_{224} prior to infection with the H3N2 virus.

The CD8$^+$ component of the inflammatory exudate recovered by BAL of the infected lung is also dominated by D^bNP_{366}-specific T cells, with frequencies reaching >70% at this site. Despite this massive recall response, however, enhanced numbers of virus-specific CD8$^+$ T cells are not detected in the respiratory tract for 4–5 days and virus clearance is only enhanced by 2–3 days [24,25]. Even so, shortening the duration of the active disease process to this extent would still be expected to diminish the severity of lung pathology. The prior exposure of humans to serologically different influenza A viruses is, thus, likely to provide some degree of protection against the development of lethal pneumonia.

The reason that secondarily stimulated T cells take so long to appear in significant numbers at the site of virus-induced pathology in the lung seems to be that the lymphocytes must again, as following primary exposure, be stimulated in organized lymphoid tissue [24]. The process of clonal expansion, followed by migration from the lymph nodes and spleen (via the blood) to the lung, takes time. The problem is not, therefore, with the inducability of the individual CD8$^+$ memory T cells, which make significant amounts of IFN-γ following in vitro stimulation with the cognate peptide, but with the physiology of the immune response.

3.3. Tertiary response

The next question was whether challenging mice that had D^{b}NP$_{366}$$^+$ memory T cells at levels in excess of 10% (the situation following the H3N2 → H1N1 secondary response, see above) would develop a more limited infectious process following infection with a third, serologically distinct influenza A virus [33]. These experiments were done with an extremely virulent, mouse-adapted A/Equine/london/72 virus. This H7N7 virus causes both lethal pneumonia and dissemination to the central nervous system (CNS) following low-dose i.n. infection of naïve, adult B6 mice [34].

As with the secondary H3N2 → H1N1 challenge, mice that had been primed i.p. with the H1N1 virus were protected against lethal H7N7-induced influenza pneumonia, though there was still a protracted virus growth phase in the lung. The H7N7 virus also became established in the respiratory tract (to an extent equivalent to that following primary infection), and spread to the CNS, in mice that had been given the H1N1 virus i.p, challenged i.n. with the H3N2 virus, then rested for at least a month prior to the tertiary H7N7 exposure. However, the duration of the virus growth phase was dramatically shortened following this tertiary challenge.

4. Discussion

The presence of large numbers of virus-specific CD8$^+$ memory T cells provides substantial protection against lethal challenge with an extremely virulent H7N7 influenza A virus. However, the infectious process still becomes established in the lung, though the virus growth phase is dramatically shortened. Comparable experiments with a murine gammaherpesvirus (γHV) gave similar results [35]. High level CD8$^+$ T cell memory substantially abrogated the lytic phase in the respiratory tract, the site of virus challenge. However, the γHV still became established as a latent infection of B cells and macrophages and, within several weeks, the magnitudes of these persistently infected populations were essentially equivalent in previously unprimed and immune individuals. The results [35] from both the influenza and the γHV model, thus, raise real questions about the ultimate efficacy of vaccination protocols that aim to exploit CD8$^+$ T cell memory as the sole protective mechanism against, for example, infection with the human immunodeficiency viruses.

Even so, if achieving a measure of protection against clinical disease is the aim (rather than sterilizing immunity), enhancing the numbers of cross-reactive, influenza-specific CD8$^+$ memory T cells can clearly be of benefit. This suggests that we should be thinking more in terms of using live, attenuated influenza vaccines. One concern with live vaccines is that cross-reactive antibodies may rapidly neutralize the virus and diminish the effectiveness of the priming regime. However, limited virus replication was still found to occur following low-dose challenge of H3N2-immune mice with a virulent H3N8 avian virus [29]. This much-diminished infectious process also boosted virus-specific CD8$^+$ T cell numbers.

The case for using DNA vaccines [36], or recombinant viruses expressing a spectrum of influenza peptides recognized in the context of the major HLA class I MHC glycoproteins [37], would also seem to be reasonable. This could provide some degree of protection in the face of a massive pandemic caused by a novel influenza strain that had recently emerged from a domestic animal reservoir. Should we be thinking in terms of having such vaccine preparations in reserve for emergency use?

Acknowledgements

These experiments were supported by NIH grants CA21765, AI29759 and AI38359, and by the American Syrian Lebanese Associated Charities (ALSAC). We thank Kristin Branum for technical assistance, and Vicki Henderson for help with the manuscript. J.P.C. was the recipient of a fellowship from the Alfred Benzon Foundation, Denmark.

References

[1] P.C. Doherty, R.M. Zinkernagel, A biological role for the major histocompatibility antigens, Lancet 1 (1975) 1406–1409.

[2] R.V. Blanden, T cell response to viral and bacterial infection, Transplant. Rev. 19 (1974) 56–88.

[3] P.C. Doherty, R.M. Zinkernagel, T-cell-mediated immunopathology in viral infections, Transplant. Rev. 19 (1974) 89–120.

[4] R.M. Zinkernagel, P.C. Doherty, Immunological surveillance against altered self components by sensitised T lymphocytes in lymphocytic choriomeningitis, Nature 251 (1974) 547–548.

[5] R.M. Zinkernagel, P.C. Doherty, Restriction of in vitro T cell-mediated cytotoxicity in lymphocytic chorio-meningitis within a syngeneic or semiallogeneic system, Nature 248 (1974) 701–702.

[6] R.M. Zinkernagel, P.C. Doherty, MHC-restricted cytotoxic T cells: studies on the biological role of poly-morphic major transplantation antigens determining T-cell restriction-specificity, function, and responsive-ness, Adv. Immunol. 27 (1979) 51–177.

[7] R.B. Effros, P.C. Doherty, W. Gerhard, J. Bennink, Generation of both cross-reactive and virus-specific T-cell populations after immunization with serologically distinct influenza A viruses, J. Exp. Med. 145 (1977) 557–568.

[8] H.J. Zweerink, S.A. Courtneidge, J.J. Skehel, M.J. Crumpton, B.A. Askonas, Cytotoxic T cells kill influenza virus infected cells but do not distinguish between serologically distinct type A viruses, Nature 267 (1977) 354–356.

[9] T.J. Braciale, Immunologic recognition of influenza virus-infected cells, I. Generation of a virus-strain specific and a cross-reactive subpopulation of cytotoxic T cells in the response to type A influenza viruses of different subtypes, Cell Immunol. 33 (1977) 423–436.

[10] J.R. Bennink, J.W. Yewdell, G.L. Smith, B. Moss, Anti-influenza virus cytotoxic T lymphocytes recognize the three viral polymerases and a nonstructural protein: responsiveness to individual viral antigens is major histocompatibility complex controlled, J. Virol. 61 (1987) 1098–1102.

[11] J.W. Yewdell, J.R. Bennink, G.L. Smith, B. Moss, Influenza A virus nucleoprotein is a major target antigen for cross-reactive anti-influenza A virus cytotoxic T lymphocytes, Proc. Natl. Acad. Sci. U. S. A. 82 (1985) 1785–1789.

[12] A.R. Townsend, J. Rothbard, F.M. Gotch, G. Bahadur, D. Wraith, A.J. McMichael, The epitopes of influenza nucleoprotein recognized by cytotoxic T lymphocytes can be defined with short synthetic peptides, Cell 44 (1986) 959–968.

[13] M.E. Andrew, B.E. Coupar, G.L. Ada, D.B. Boyle, Cell-mediated immune responses to influenza virus antigens expressed by vaccinia virus recombinants, Microb. Pathog. 1 (1986) 443–452.

[14] M.E. Andrew, B.E. Coupar, D.B. Boyle, G.L. Ada, The roles of influenza virus haemagglutinin and nucleoprotein in protection: analysis using vaccinia virus recombinants, Scand. J. Immunol. 25 (1987) 21–28.

[15] P.C. Doherty, W. Allan, D.B. Boyle, B.E. Coupar, M.E. Andrew, Recombinant vaccinia viruses and the development of immunization strategies using influenza virus, J. Infect. Dis. 159 (1989) 1119–1122.

[16] S.L. Epstein, C.Y. Lo, J.A. Misplon, C.M. Lawson, B.A. Hendrickson, E.E. Max, K. Subbarao, Mechanisms of heterosubtypic immunity to lethal influenza A virus infection in fully immunocompetent, T cell-depleted, β_2-microglobulin-deficient, and J chain-deficient mice, J. Immunol. 158 (1997) 1222–1230.

[17] C.M. Lawson, J.R. Bennink, N.P. Restifo, J.W. Yewdell, B.R. Murphy, Primary pulmonary cytotoxic T lymphocytes induced by immunization with a vaccinia virus recombinant expressing influenza A virus nucleoprotein peptide do not protect mice against challenge, J. Virol. 68 (1994) 3505–3511.

[18] A.J. McMichael, F.M. Gotch, D.W. Dongworth, A. Clark, C.W. Potter, Declining T-cell immunity to influenza, 1977–82, Lancet 2 (1983) 762–764.

[19] J.D. Altman, P.A.H. Moss, P.J.R. Goulder, D.H. Barouch, M.G. McHeyzer-Williams, J.I. Bell, A.J. McMichael, M.M. Davis, Phenotypic analysis of antigen-specific T lymphocytes, Science 274 (1996) 94–96.

[20] P.C. Doherty, The numbers game for virus-specific CD8$^+$ T cells, Science 280 (1998) 227.

[21] P.C. Doherty, D.J. Topham, R.A. Tripp, Establishment and persistence of virus-specific CD4$^+$ and CD8$^+$ T cell memory, Immunol. Rev. 150 (1996) 23–44.

[22] P.C. Doherty, W. Allan, M. Eichelberger, S.R. Carding, Roles of alpha beta and gamma delta T cell subsets in viral immunity, Annu. Rev. Immunol. 10 (1992) 123–151.

[23] S. Hou, L. Hyland, K.W. Ryan, A. Portner, P.C. Doherty, Virus-specific CD8$^+$ T-cell memory determined by clonal burst size, Nature 369 (1994) 652–654.

[24] K.J. Flynn, G.T. Belz, J.D. Altman, R. Ahmed, D.L. Woodland, P.C. Doherty, Virus-specific CD8$^+$ T cells in primary and secondary influenza pneumonia, Immunity 8 (1998) 683–691.

[25] K.J. Flynn, J.M. Riberdy, J.P. Christensen, J.D. Altman, P.C. Doherty, In vivo proliferation of naive and memory influenza-specific CD8$^+$ T cells, Proc. Natl. Acad. Sci. U. S. A. 96 (1999) 8597–8602.

[26] K. Murali-Krishna, J.D. Altman, M. Suresh, D. Sourdive, A.J. Zajac, JjD. Miller, J. Slansky, R. Ahmed, Counting antigen-specific CD8 T cells: a reevaluation of bystander activation during viral infection, Immunity 8 (1998) 177–187.

[27] A.J. McMichael, C.A. O'Callaghan, A new look at T cells, J. Exp. Med. 187 (1998) 1367–1371.

[28] E.A. Butz, M.J. Bevan, Massive expansion of antigen-specific CD8$^+$ T cells during an acute virus infection, Immunity 8 (1998) 167–175.

[29] J.M. Riberdy, K.J. Flynn, J. Stech, R.G. Webster, J.D. Altman, P.C. Doherty, Protection against a lethal avian influenza A virus in a mammalian system, J. Virol. 73 (1999) 1453–1459.

[30] J.P. Christensen, P.C. Doherty, Quantitative analysis of the acute and long-term CD4$^+$ T-cell response to a persistent gammaherpesvirus, J. Virol. 73 (1999) 4279–4283.

[31] G.T. Belz, W. Xie, J.D. Altman, P.C. Doherty, A previously unrecognized H-2D(b)-restricted peptide prominent in the primary influenza A virus-specific CD8$^+$ T-cell response is much less apparent following secondary challenge, J. Virol. 74 (2000) 3486–3493.

[32] P.G. Stevenson, G.T. Belz, J.D. Altman, P.C. Doherty, Virus-specific CD8(+) T cell numbers are maintained during gamma-herpesvirus reactivation in CD4-deficient mice, Proc. Natl. Acad. Sci. U. S. A. 95 (1998) 15565–15570.

[33] J.M. Riberdy, J.P. Christensen, K. Branum, P.C. Doherty, Diminished primary and secondary influenza-specific CD8$^+$ T cell responses in CD4-depleted Ig$^{-/-}$ Mice, J. Virol. 74 (2000) 9762–9765.

[34] Y. Kawaoka, Equine H7N7 influenza A viruses are highly pathogenic in mice without adaptation: potential use as an animal model, J. Virol. 65 (1991) 3891–3894.

[35] P.G. Stevenson, G.T. Belz, M.R. Castrucci, J.D. Altman, P.C. Doherty, A gamma-herpesvirus sneaks

through a CD8[+] T cell response primed to a lytic-phase epitope, Proc. Natl. Acad. Sci. U. S. A. 96 (1999) 9281–9286.

[36] Y. Chen, R.G. Webster, D.L. Woodland, Induction of CD8[+] T cell responses to dominant and subdominant epitopes and protective immunity to Sendai virus infection by DNA vaccination, J. Immunol. 160 (1998) 2425–2432.

[37] S.A. Thomson, S.L. Elliott, M.A. Sherritt, K.W. Sproat, B.E.H. Coupar, A.A. Scalzo, C.A. Forbes, A.M. Ladhams, X.Y. Mo, R.A. Tripp, P.C. Doherty, D.J. Moss, A. Suhrbier, Recombinant polyepitope vaccines for the delivery of multiple CD8 cytotoxic T cell epitopes, J. Immunol. 157 (1996) 822–826.

International Congress Series 1219 (2001) 301–309

Shaping the T cell response to influenza virus

Anne Kelso*, Barbara J. Johnson

The Cooperative Research Centre for Vaccine Technology and the Queensland Institute of Medical Research, Post Office Royal Brisbane Hospital, Brisbane, Queensland 4029, Australia

Abstract

Primary T cell responses to viral and other infections are guided by factors acting at each stage of the host response, during the initial inflammatory reaction to infection, during T cell priming in the regional lymph nodes (LN), and after recruitment of activated T cells to the site of infection. The factors that shape the functional phenotype of activated T cells in vivo include the strength and character of signals delivered by antigen-presenting cells and other cells in the lymph nodes that in turn reflect the nature of the pathogen and the tissue from which they have migrated. It has not been clear, however, whether effector T cells are programmed entirely in the lymph nodes or whether they could differentiate further following recruitment to the effector site. When mice were infected with influenza virus, marked differences were observed in levels and types of cytokine expression by T cells from the mediastinal lymph nodes and lung, and cytolytic T lymphocytes (CTL) were only detected in the lung. PCR-based single-cell assays for perforin and granzyme B expression suggested that some CTL completed their differentiation in the lymph nodes and that their selective detection was mainly due to higher effector cell numbers in the infected lung. Some activated CD8$^+$ T cells in the lung could nevertheless undergo further differentiation to express an altered cytokine profile, indicating that the T cell response can also be shaped after recruitment to the effector site. © 2001 Elsevier Science B.V. All rights reserved.

Keywords: Cytokines; CTL; Perforin; Granzyme B

1. Introduction

Rapid progress is being made in understanding how the innate and adaptive immune responses interact to protect the host against infection by viruses and other pathogens.

---

* Corresponding author. Tel.: +61-7-3362-0382; fax: +61-7-3362-0105.
E-mail address: anneK@qimr.edu.au (A. Kelso).

0531-5131/01/$ – see front matter © 2001 Elsevier Science B.V. All rights reserved.
PII: S0531-5131(01)00342-9

Properties of pathogens or vaccines designed to mimic them play a critical role in shaping the differentiation of T lymphocytes into cells with appropriate effector functions for host protection. Here, we discuss the early events that lead to the development of effector T cells following immune stimulation in vivo and summarize our recent studies on this process in a murine model of influenza virus infection.

2. Host barriers to infection

Pathogens and other immunogens, such as vaccines, must breach a series of barriers to enter host tissues (Fig. 1). The first are physical barriers: the epithelial cells of the skin and mucosal surfaces, and host products such as mucous, that form the boundary between the host and the outside world. The breaching of these barriers usually causes tissue damage and inflammation and this, along with subsequent inflammation triggered by infection or other properties of the immunogen, activates the innate immune response. This early antigen-nonspecific response is mediated by macrophages, neutrophils and other leukocytes, which infiltrate the injured tissue, responding to and releasing cytokines, chemokines, reactive oxygen species and other products that may destroy or inhibit spread of the foreign agent. Pre-existing antibodies or infiltrating T cells with cross-reactivity against antigens of the immunogen may also contribute to this early protective response.

When the innate response fails to eliminate the immunogen, host protection depends on the additional barrier of the adaptive immune response mediated by antigen-specific T and B cells activated over the first week or two after infection or immunization. This primary response declines when the infection is resolved, ideally leaving a pool of memory T and B cells, which can be rapidly re-activated on subsequent challenge.

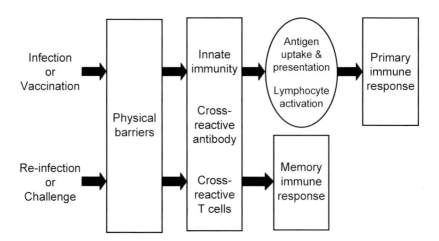

Fig. 1. Host barriers to infection. The figure shows the major mechanisms that successively protect the host from infection or re-infection.

3. The primary T cell response

Efficacy of the adaptive immune response to pathogens depends on two crucial events. The first is the activation and expansion of lymphocytes able to recognize antigens of the infectious agent. The second is activation of an appropriate class of response: namely, synthesis of immunoglobulin isotypes that contribute to pathogen destruction, for example through binding to Fc receptors on inflammatory cells; synthesis of cytokines by T cells and other cells that stimulate isotype switching in B cells and activate relevant effector functions in lymphocytes and inflammatory cells; and, where required, activation of cytolytic T lymphocytes (CTL) that limit pathogen replication by killing infected host cells.

Both these events are initiated at the site of infection or vaccine delivery (Fig. 2). The early inflammatory response to infection or vaccination activates local dendritic cells (DC), specialized antigen-capturing cells that form a network throughout most tissues [1]. This initial activation triggers DC to take up extracellular material by macropinocytosis, phagocytosis and receptor-mediated endocytosis, then migrate via the lymphatics to the regional lymph nodes (LN). They concomitantly switch from a state of high antigen uptake, high turnover of class II major histocompatibility complex (MHC) molecules and low expression of costimulatory molecules, to a state of low antigen uptake, stable peptide/MHC display and high costimulator expression. Naive T cells of all antigen specificities trafficking through the LN from the blood have the opportunity to "scan" the surface of these DC. If they recognize class I or II MHC/peptide complexes on the DC surface via

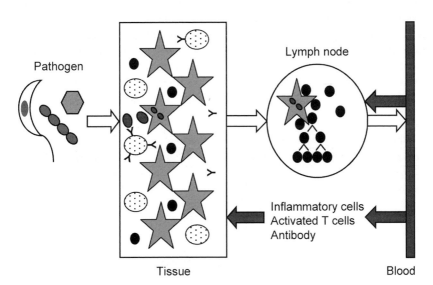

Fig. 2. The primary immune response to infection. Infection causes uptake of pathogens and other material by DC (represented by stars) which are activated to migrate to the draining LN. Here, DC present peptide/MHC complexes to naive T cells, stimulating their activation and clonal expansion. Tissue damage at the site of infection causes an influx of inflammatory cells from the blood, followed later by activated T cells, which have left the LN and returned to the blood, and by specific antibody.

their antigen receptors and receive costimulatory signals, their primary activation and clonal expansion is initiated.

At some point during their differentiation, these newly activated T cells leave the LN and rejoin the circulating lymphocyte pool in the blood, from which they traffic freely throughout the tissues. When they encounter the relevant peptide/MHC complexes on cells in the tissues, they are triggered to secrete cytokines and/or lyse antigen-presenting cells. Since these effector functions largely depend on antigen recognition but do not require costimulation, T cell effector activity is generally greater at the site of infection or vaccination than in the priming LN and, whereas DC regulate the early stages of specific T cell priming and proliferation, effector functions can be triggered by any type of antigen-presenting cell.

The class of the T cell response is also shaped during T cell activation in the LN, at least in part by DC as the cellular messengers of events at the site of antigen deposition. Most attention has been paid to the development of polarized type 1 and type 2 cytokine responses. Type 1 cytokines (IFN-γ, IL-2 and TNF-β) are often associated with viral immunity and type 2 cytokines (IL-4, IL-5, IL-6 and IL-10) with responses to helminths and allergens [2]. Although some primary responses are strongly polarized to type 1 or type 2 cytokine synthesis, many responses (and indeed many individual T cells in these responses) display mixed cytokine profiles [3,4]. These profiles may also differ between different tissue sites (see below).

Naive T cells display marked plasticity, having the potential to give rise to effector cells that secrete type 1 and/or type 2 cytokines [5,6] depending on various factors and signals they receive during activation (Table 1). Host genotype is a significant factor and many polymorphisms and mutations (for example, in cytokine and cytokine receptor genes) can modulate the tendency to type 1 or type 2 polarization of an immune response. Against this genetic background, properties of the immunogen and the tissue site are the key determinants of immune response class. Many microbial and viral structures act as adjuvants in stimulating antigen-nonspecific inflammatory responses that lead to type 1

Table 1
Factors and signals that promote polarization of cytokine responses

Factor or signal	Type 1 responses	Type 2 responses
Genetic background	various	various
Properties of immunogen	LPS, lipopeptides	cholera toxin
	CpG in bacterial DNA	alum-precipitated protein
	double-stranded RNA	
Cytokines	IL-12	IL-4
	IFN-α (human)	IL-10
	IFN-γ	IL-1
	IL-18	
Cells	dendritic cells (DC1) (IL-12)	dendritic cells (DC2) (?)
	macrophages (IL-12)	mast cells (IL-4)
	NK cells (IFN-γ)	NKT cells (IL-4)
	type 1 T cells (IFN-γ)	type 2 T cells (IL-4)
Antigen and costimuli	dose/density	dose/density
Death molecules	?	Fas ligand

polarization: bacterial lipoproteins and lipopolysaccharides which interact with members of the Toll-like receptor family on DC, macrophages and other cells [7], nonmethylated CpG-containing motifs in bacterial DNA [8] and double-stranded viral DNA [9] are important examples. Less is known about the properties of helminths and allergens that lead to type 2 polarization.

Cytokines themselves are the best-understood regulators of polarization [10]. While no single cytokine is absolutely required, IL-12 strongly promotes type 1 T cell differentiation and IL-4 is a key inducer of type 2 differentiation in most circumstances, in both cases by direct action on the T cell. IL-10, on the other hand, promotes type 2 differentiation indirectly by inhibiting IL-12 production by antigen-presenting cells. Some of the effects of microbial structures are mediated by induction of synthesis of IL-12 and other proinflammatory cytokines. Similarly, some effects of antigen-presenting cells and other cells present during T cell differentiation can be attributed to their secretion of regulatory cytokines. DC are obvious candidates to guide the early polarization of T cell cytokine profiles and indeed several recent studies have suggested that distinct DC subsets drive type 1 and type 2 differentiation [11,12], although the underlying molecular mechanisms have not yet been defined.

There is evidence in several systems that various determinants of signal strength, such as antigen dose, peptide/MHC density, peptide/MHC-T cell receptor affinity and the type of costimulatory molecule (e.g., CD80 versus CD86), influence cytokine polarization [13,14]. The mechanisms are likely to be diverse, sometimes due to effects on antigen-presenting cells and sometimes on T cells themselves. One possible mechanism is by regulation of T cell division number. The finding that IFN-γ tends to be produced after fewer cell divisions than IL-4 when CD4$^+$ T cells are first activated [15] may explain why high signal strength or persistent stimulation increases the likelihood of type 2 polarization in some situations. The cell density of an activated T cell population can also influence the dominance of type 1 or type 2 polarized effector cells because of the relative resistance of type 2-polarized CD4$^+$ cells to fratricidal killing by Fas–Fas ligand interaction [16].

The T cell must therefore integrate multiple signals that regulate its initial activation, the probability of de novo expression of IFN-γ, IL-4 and/or other cytokine genes, cell division number, and survival or death. Although this complex process is initiated in the regional LN when T cells are first activated by antigen-presenting DC, it is not known whether it is completed at this site or can continue after recruitment to the site of infection where most T cell effector activity is manifested. The following sections summarize work from the authors' laboratory that addresses this question in a murine model of influenza virus infection.

4. Development of effector T cells in the response to influenza virus infection

We have characterized the phenotypes and functions of the CD4$^+$ and CD8$^+$ T cell populations isolated from key tissues following intranasal infection of BALB/c mice with the H3N1 Mem71 reassortant virus: the mediastinal LN (MLN) that drain the respiratory tract, the lung parenchyma and, in some experiments, the bronchoalveolar lavage fluid (BAL). The restriction of viral replication to the epithelial cells of the lung makes this a useful model in which to distinguish the T cell priming site (MLN) from the effector site (lung parenchyma and BAL).

Table 2 summarizes some differences between T cell populations freshly isolated by fluorescence-activated cell sorting from MLN, lung parenchyma and BAL at the peak of the cellular response in the lung 1 week after infection [17–19]. Whereas CD4:CD8 ratio, proliferative responsiveness to polyclonal stimuli and the capacity to provide help to B cells in vitro were highest in MLN, virus-specific CTL activity and expression of several cytokines (assessed by reverse-transcription PCR) were markedly higher per T cell in the lung parenchyma and BAL. The CD4$^+$ and CD8$^+$ populations in MLN displayed a more mixed type 1/type 2 cytokine profile than in the lung where IFN-γ was expressed at very high levels by both populations and IL-4 expression was only occasionally detected, despite the presence of measurable IL-5 mRNA.

The striking difference between CTL activity in MLN and lung raised the question whether this was due to a difference in their quantity or their quality: were effector CTL numbers simply too low to detect in the LN by conventional ^{51}Cr-release assay without in vitro restimulation, or did they leave the MLN before completing their differentiation? Cell purification experiments showed that CD8$^+$ cells of activated phenotype were responsible for the measurable lytic activity of lung parenchymal cells for syngeneic target cells infected with Mem71 virus or loaded with the major nucleoprotein epitope NP$_{147-155}$ (Johnson and Kelso, unpublished observations). Cells of this phenotype were four- to fivefold more frequent among lung than MLN CD8$^+$ cells, suggesting that quantitative differences in the number of activated CD8$^+$ cells accounted for much of the difference in lytic activity between the two tissues.

Because of the insensitivity of the ^{51}Cr-release assay, we developed PCR assays for the mRNAs encoding the two crucial mediators of CTL function, the pore-forming protein perforin and the serine protease, granzyme B (Johnson, Costelloe, Fitzpatrick and Kelso, unpublished observations). Previous work in this laboratory showed that PCR was sufficiently sensitive to detect cytokine mRNAs at high frequency in single activated T cells [4,20]. This proved also to be true for perforin and granzyme B, which were expressed at significant frequencies by CD8$^+$ cells of activated phenotype both from lung parenchyma and MLN. Although some differences were noted in the frequencies of

Table 2
Functional differences between T cells from different regions of the respiratory tract during influenza virus infection

Function	Mediastinal lymph nodes	Lung parenchyma	Bronchoalveolar lavage fluid
CD4:CD8 ratio	2	1	0.5
Proliferation	+++	++	++
B cell help	+++	+	not tested
Activated T cells	+	++	+++
Effector CTL	−	++	++
Cytokine	+	++	++
IFN-γ	+	+++	+++
IL-4	+	+/−	−
IL-10	+	++	+

expression between these two cell sources, the data suggested that qualitative differences were minor compared with differences in effector cell number between MLN and lung.

Collectively, the data suggest that at least some CD8$^+$ T cells complete their differentiation into effector CTL during priming in the regional LN but are difficult to detect by ^{51}Cr-release assay because of their low numbers. Although their phenotype and perforin/granzyme expression frequencies are comparable in the lung parenchyma, their abundance in the lung allows their detection by conventional assays without restimulation and expansion in vitro.

5. Reshaping of the effector T cell response

While these data and the earlier cytokine analyses indicate that effector cell differentiation can be completed in the MLN, it was not known whether further differentiation could occur after migration to the infected lung. To address this question, we used paired daughter analysis to assess the flexibility of individual activated CD8$^+$ cells isolated from the lungs of virus-infected mice to alter their cytokine profile in response to a new signal [21].

Initial work established that CD8$^+$ T cells from the infected lung were type 1-polarized with high IFN-γ and negligible IL-4 expression. Most of this cytokine synthesis was due to cells in the CD44^{high} CD11a^{high} fraction (abbreviated as influenza lung^{high}), whereas cells of the opposite phenotype (influenza lung^{low}) were depleted in effector activity [19]. Paired daughter analysis was undertaken with these two populations and control CD44^{low} CD11a^{low} CD8$^+$ cells from LN of uninfected BALB/c mice (normal LN^{low}). Individual cells from each population were cultured under conditions of polyclonal stimulation that support the activation and proliferation of most naive CD8$^+$ cells [6] with some modification to maximize cloning frequencies from the two lung-derived populations. Cloning efficiencies of influenza lung^{high} cells were nevertheless only $\sim 25\%$, compared with $\sim 75\%$ and $\sim 80\%$ for influenza lung^{low} and normal LN^{low} cells, respectively, suggesting that effector cell differentiation was associated with significant loss of proliferative potential.

When the cultured single cells had divided once or twice, individual daughter or granddaughter cells were transferred by micromanipulation into new cultures with or without IL-4 as an inducer of type 2 cytokine expression. The resultant subclones were analysed by RT-PCR for expression of IFN-γ and IL-4. Most subclones generated from cells of all three starting populations expressed IFN-γ mRNA, regardless of their exposure to IL-4. As expected, few subclones grown in the absence of IL-4 expressed IL-4 mRNA. However, significant differences in IL-4 expression were noted between the three groups of subclones grown with IL-4. These frequencies followed the hierarchy: normal LN^{low} > influenza lung^{low} > influenza lung^{high}. Among those cells which cloned and could therefore be analysed by this approach, the calculated average frequencies of "flexible" (IL-4-responsive) cells were 51% for normal LN^{low}, 25% for influenza lung^{low} and 17% for influenza lung^{high} cells [21].

We conclude that the flexibility of CD8$^+$ cells to express new cytokines in response to IL-4 declines as the cells differentiate into effector cells, consistent with the conclusions of bulk culture studies of CD4$^+$ T cells [22,23]. Nevertheless, a significant proportion of highly activated cells in the type 1-polarized effector CD8$^+$ fraction in the infected lung retains both proliferative potential and the capacity to switch on the expression of a type 2 cytokine gene. This indicates that the functional programming of effector T cells is not completed in the priming LN. Instead, some cells can undergo further differentiation after recruitment to an effector site in response to signals in their new environment.

Acknowledgements

The financial support of the Cooperative Research Centre for Vaccine Technology, the Queensland Institute of Medical Research Trust and the National Health and Medical Research Council is gratefully acknowledged.

References

[1] J. Banchereau, R.M. Steinman, Dendritic cells and the control of immunity, Nature 392 (1998) 245–252.

[2] A.K. Abbas, K.M. Murphy, A. Sher, Functional diversity of helper T lymphocytes, Nature 383 (1996) 787–793.

[3] A. Kelso, Th1 and Th2 subsets: paradigms lost?, Immunol. Today 16 (1995) 374–379.

[4] A. Kelso, P. Groves, L. Ramm, A.G. Doyle, Single-cell analysis by RT-PCR reveals differential expression of multiple type 1 and 2 cytokine genes among cells within polarized CD4$^+$ T cell populations, Int. Immunol. 11 (1999) 617–621.

[5] S. Sad, T.R. Mosmann, Single IL-2-secreting precursor CD4 T cell can develop into either Th1 or Th2 cytokine secretion phenotype, J. Immunol. 153 (1994) 3514–3522.

[6] A. Kelso, P. Groves, A single peripheral CD8$^+$ T cell can give rise to progeny expressing type 1 and/or type 2 cytokine genes and can retain its multipotentiality through many cell divisions, Proc. Natl. Acad. Sci. U. S. A. 94 (1997) 8070–8075.

[7] A. Aderem, R.J. Ulevitch, Toll-like receptors in the induction of the innate immune response, Nature 406 (2000) 782–787.

[8] K.J. Stacey, D.P. Sester, M.J. Sweet, D.A. Hume, Macrophage activation by immunostimulatory DNA, Curr. Top. Microbiol. Immunol. 247 (2000) 41–58.

[9] M. Cella, M. Salio, Y. Sakakibara, H. Langen, I. Julkunen, A. Lanzavecchia, Maturation, activation, and protection of dendritic cells induced by double-stranded RNA, J. Exp. Med. 189 (1999) 821–829.

[10] A. O'Garra, Cytokines induce the development of functionally heterogeneous T helper cell subsets, Immunity 8 (1998) 275–283.

[11] M.-C. Rissoan, V. Soumelis, N. Kadowaki, G. Grouard, F. Briere, R. de Waal Malefyt, Y.-J. Liu, Reciprocal control of T helper cell and dendritic cell differentiation, Science 283 (1999) 1183–1186.

[12] B. Pulendran, J.L. Smith, G. Caspary, K. Brasel, D. Pettit, E. Maraskovsky, C.R. Maliszewski, Distinct dendritic cell subsets differentially regulate the class of immune response in vivo, Proc. Natl. Acad. Sci. U. S. A. 96 (1999) 1036–1041.

[13] S.L. Constant, K. Bottomly, Induction of Th1 and Th2 CD4$^+$ T cell responses: the alternative approaches, Annu. Rev. Immunol. 15 (1997) 297–322.

[14] V.K. Kuchroo, M.P. Das, J.A. Brown, A.M. Ranger, S.S. Zamvil, R.A. Sobel, H.L. Weiner, N. Nabavi, L.H. Glimcher, B7-1 and B7-2 costimulatory molecules activate differentially the Th1/Th2 developmental pathways: application to autoimmune disease therapy, Cell 80 (1995) 707–718.

[15] A.V. Gett, P.D. Hodgkin, Cell division regulates the T cell cytokine repertoire, revealing a mechanism underlying immune class regulation, Proc. Natl. Acad. Sci. U. S. A. 95 (1998) 9488–9493.

[16] F. Ramsdell, M.S. Seaman, R.E. Miller, K.S. Picha, M.K. Kennedy, D.H. Lynch, Differential ability of Th1

and Th2 cells to express Fas ligand and to undergo activation-induced cell death, Int. Immunol. 6 (1994) 1545–1553.

[17] N. Baumgarth, L. Brown, D. Jackson, A. Kelso, Novel features of the respiratory tract T-cell response to influenza virus infection: lung T cells increase expression of gamma interferon mRNA in vivo and maintain high levels of mRNA expression for interleukin-5 (IL-5) and IL-10, J. Virol. 68 (1994) 7575–7581.

[18] N. Baumgarth, A. Kelso, Functionally distinct T cells in three compartments of the respiratory tract after influenza virus infection, Eur. J. Immunol. 26 (1996) 2189–2197.

[19] N. Baumgarth, M. Egerton, A. Kelso, Activated T cells from draining lymph nodes and an effector site differ in their responses to TCR stimulation, J. Immunol. 159 (1997) 1182–1191.

[20] A.B. Troutt, A. Kelso, Enumeration of lymphokine mRNA-containing cells in vivo in a murine graft-versus-host reaction using the PCR, Proc. Natl. Acad. Sci. U. S. A. 89 (1992) 5276–5280.

[21] A.G. Doyle, K. Buttigieg, P. Groves, B.J. Johnson, A. Kelso, The activated type 1-polarized CD8 [+] T cell population isolated from an effector site contains cells with flexible cytokine profiles, J. Exp. Med. 190 (1999) 1081–1091.

[22] E. Murphy, K. Shibuya, N. Hosken, P. Openshaw, V. Maino, K. Davis, K. Murphy, A. O'Garra, Reversibility of T helper 1 and 2 populations is lost after long-term stimulation, J. Exp. Med. 183 (1996) 901–913.

[23] M. Assenmacher, M. Lohning, A. Scheffold, A. Richter, S. Miltenyi, J. Schmitz, A. Radbruch, Commitment of individual Th1-like lymphocytes to expression of IFN-γ versus IL-4 and IL-10: selective induction of IL-10 by sequential stimulation of naive Th cells with IL-12 and IL-4, J. Immunol. 161 (1998) 2825–2832.

International Congress Series 1219 (2001) 311–318

Roles of CD4⁺ T and B cells in influenza virus infection

Walter Gerhard*, Krystyna Mozdzanowska

Immunology Program, The Wistar Institute, 3601 Spruce Street, Philadelphia, PA 19114-4268, USA

Abstract

Studies in mice have shown that influenza virus infection induces vigorous CD4⁺ T (Th) and B cell responses which are quite effective in controlling the infection in the absence of a concomitant CD8⁺ T (Tc) cell response. The Th-dependent (TD) antibody (Ab) response appears to play an important role in the control of the infection in this situation, but Th and B cells also contribute significantly to anti-viral defense by mechanisms that are independent of each other. The role of the TD Ab response was investigated by systemic treatment of infected severe combined immunodeficiency (SCID) mice with monoclonal Abs (MAbs). In vivo, Abs may control the infection by suppressing the release of progeny virus from infected host cells (yield reduction [YR]) and/or by preventing released progeny virus from infecting new host cells (virus neutralization [VN]). MAbs to NA and M2, which exhibited only YR, suppressed virus growth in the lung but failed to resolve the infection. They appeared to operate primarily by directing innate defenses against infected host cells. By contrast, HA-specific MAbs, which displayed both YR and VN, were capable of clearing the infection, indicating that VN is essential for Ab-mediated recovery. YR and VN appeared to act additively in these MAbs. Some HA-specific MAbs that lacked measurable VN in vitro appeared to require the presence of innate defense mechanisms for VN in vivo. © 2001 Elsevier Science B.V. All rights reserved.

Keywords: Innate defense; Antibody; Neutralization; Yield reduction

1. Introduction

Studies have shown that influenza virus infection can be controlled quite effectively in mice that lack either Tc or Th cells but not both of these T cell subsets. Control and

* Corresponding author. Tel.: +1-215-898-3840; fax: +1-215-898-3868.
E-mail address: gerhard@mail.wistar.upenn.edu (W. Gerhard).

0531-5131/01/$ – see front matter © 2001 Elsevier Science B.V. All rights reserved.
PII: S 0 5 3 1 - 5 1 3 1 (0 1) 0 0 6 4 4 - 6

Table 1
Roles of Th and B cells in the control and resolution of PR8 virus infection in mice that lack Tc cells

Host defense				Activities	Contribution to control (evidence)	Resolution of infection
Innate	Tc	Th	B			
+	−	−	−	Innate (IFNα/β, MΦ, collectins, etc.)	Yes (decreased resistance of mice with defects in innate immunity)	No
+	−	+	−	Cytokines → highly activated innate defense, cytotoxicity (cl II-restricted)	Yes (enhanced therapeutic activity of passive Ab in presence of Th)	No, often increased pathology
+	−	−	+	TI Ab (natural and virus-induced)	Yes (improved resistance of mice with Tc and B cells)	No
+	−	+	+	All of the above plus TD Ab	Yes	Yes
+	−	−	−	Passive Ab	Yes, depending on Ab specificity and isotype	Yes, depending on Ab

resolution of the infection in the absence of either Tc or Th appear to be based largely on distinct mechanisms. In the case of Th cell-deficient mice, activated virus-specific Tc cells control the infection mainly through perforin/granzyme and Fas ligand (FasL)/Fas-mediated killing of infected host cells upon cognate interaction [1]. In the following, evidence regarding the efficacy of Th and B cells in controlling the infection in the absence of Tc cells is discussed. The focus is on experimental findings obtained in the mouse and addressing mainly the question how Th and B cells control and resolve a primary infection of the lower respiratory tract (RT) that has been initiated with a small dose (~50 MID$_{50}$, 50% mouse infectious dose) of the relatively pathogenic virus strain A/PR/8/34(H1N1) (PR8). The three principle types of activities that will be discussed are Th cell-mediated, B cell-mediated and collaborative Th−B cell activities (Table 1).

1.1. Protective activities of Th cells

Infection with PR8 results in a rapid and massive increase in the cellularity of the mediastinal lymph nodes (MedLN), which drain the lower RT, and in the lung parenchyma. For instance, the cell number in MedLNs increased from $\sim 0.5 \times 10^6$ to $\sim 10^7$ within 3−4 days of infection and peaked at $15-20 \times 10^6$ by 6−7 days. The cellularity of the lung (viz. number of lymphoid cells released from total lung by digestion with collagenase) increased from $\sim 25 \times 10^6$ before infection to $\sim 7 \times 10^6$/lung around days 10−11. At the peak of the response, CD4$^+$ cells made up approximately 1/3 of the cells in MedLN and 1/4 of the cells in the lung. Functionally, the Th cells appear mainly to be of type 1, secreting IFN-γ, TNF-α, etc. The specificity of the response has not been studied in much detail but appears to be directed to many different viral protein determinants [2]. Based on limiting dilution analyses [3] and by analogy to the Tc response, it is likely that a substantial faction of the Th response is virus-specific. The Th cell response may conceivably contribute to the control of the infection, e.g., by activation of innate defenses (inflammatory cell response, enhancement of cellular antiviral state) and by killing infected host cells through FasL/Fas- and/or TNF-mediated pathways.

Analysis of the course of infection in mice that lacked both Tc and B cells, and thus depended entirely on Th cells and innate defense to control the infection, revealed a rather surprising ineffectiveness of Th cells in dealing with the infection [4], even if the virus was of low pathogenicity [5,6]. In fact, the Th cell response tended to enhance morbidity and shorten mean survival time [7]. However, while Th cell-mediated activities were ineffective on their own in controlling the infection, they were often found to be highly beneficial in the context of other cells or products of the adaptive immune system, like Tc and B cells or passive Ab. For instance, the therapeutic activity of passive Ab was found to be higher in mice that made an endogenous Th cell response than in mice that did not (our unpublished observation). This may be due to increased inflammation-related transudation of passive Ab into the lumen of the RT and/or a general enhancement of Ab-mediated therapeutic activity inasmuch as it operated by directing innate defense mechanisms against infected host cells (see below). Thus, on their own, Th cells are poorly effective in controlling the infection; they appear to operate primarily by enhancing other anti-viral effector mechanisms of the adaptive immune system.

1.2. Th cell-independent (TI) protective activities of B cells

As found with other polyvalent bacterial and viral particles [8], i.v. or i.p. injection of influenza virus into mice lacking T cells induced TI Ab of IgM isotype (our unpublished observation). By contrast and analogous to the low TI response seen after subcutaneous injection of antigen [8], RT infection induced only a minimal TI response, at least when assessed by Ab titer in serum, and most important, in the present context, many studies have shown that this TI Ab response is not effective enough to control and resolve the infection on its own [9]. Nevertheless, the finding that B cells greatly improved the control of the infection in mice that contained Tc but lacked Th cells [10] showed that B cells could make a significant TI contribution to virus control. It is presently not known what type of TI B cell activities is involved. Treatment of infected B and Th cell-deficient mice with normal serum Ig (to provide natural Ab) and virus-specific Ab of IgM isotype (to mimic the virus-induced TI Ab response) did not measurably improve recovery from infection [10]. This finding argued against TI and natural virus-specific Ab of IgM isotype as having a major protective role but needs to be confirmed, e.g., by testing BCR-transgenic B cells, which cannot produce virus-specific Ab, for protective activity in Tc containing mice. Baumgarth et al. [11] recently showed that IgM increased resistance to infection. However, in this case, the protective effect of IgM may have been due to subsequent enhancement of the antiviral IgG response [11]. An alternative explanation for the protective TI B cell activity in Th-deficient mice would be a role of B cells in the induction or recruitment of the virus-specific Tc response. However, we found no evidence for such an activity, and this possibility would also run against findings made in other experimental systems showing that B cells tend to suppress rather than enhance Tc responses.

1.3. A major histocompatibility complex (MHC) class-II restricted Th–B cell interaction is required for control and resolution of the infection

As shown in Table 1, mice that possess both Th and B cells and thus can make a TD Ab response are quite effective in controlling the infection, in contrast to mice containing only Th or B cells. While this observation is consistent with the idea that the TD Ab response plays an important role, it does not prove it because the alternative explanation, i.e., that the combined action of independent Th and B cell-mediated activities is sufficient for controlling the infection, is not excluded. To differentiate between these possibilities, the course of the PR8 infection was studied in B cell-deficient Tc-depleted (μMT[-CD8]) mice of C57BL/6 background, which had been injected i.v. 1 day prior to infection with 15–20 million splenic B cells from naive C57BL/6-IA($-/-$) mice, that fail to express MHC class II protein, or from BALB/c mice, that express MHC class II of allogeneic haplotype. Since the TD Ab response is dependent on the cognate interaction between virus-specific Th and B cell, which is mediated by the TCR of the Th cell recognizing syngeneic MHC class II–peptide complex on the B cell, these mice cannot produce a TD Ab response but generate the independent Th and B cell-mediated activities. As positive controls, μMT($-$CD8) mice of C57BL/6 background were reconstituted with B cells from normal C57BL/6 mice. These experiments showed that the mice containing Th and class II ($-/-$) or allogeneic B cells failed to control the infection while all mice in the control group readily resolved it (our unpublished observations). Thus, a cognate Th–B cell interaction is necessary for controlling the infection and the combined effects of independent Th and B cell-mediated activities are insufficient. The relevant activity resulting from the cognate Th–B cell interaction is presumably the TD Ab response, but other activities like improved cytokine/chemokine secretion are not formally excluded.

1.4. The therapeutic activity of passive Abs in PR8 virus-infected SCID mice

Ab-mediated anti-viral activities were investigated by passive transfer of Abs into SCID mice several hours or days after they had been infected with PR8. SCID mice, which lack both T and B cells, were used to avoid contributions by the adaptive immune response to the course of the infection. The status of the infection was usually assessed by determination of the virus titer in trachea and/or lung 1–3 weeks after infection. It is important to note also that the infection was initiated with a small dose of virus, typically in the range of 20–50 MID_{50}, from which immunologically intact mice recovered without mortality but not SCID mice, which usually died in the second to third week of infection. The initial infection typically involved the lower RT (trachea, bronchial tree) and only rarely the upper RT (nasal epithelium). Accordingly, these experiments addressed only the therapeutic activity of passive Ab in the lower RT. Evidence from various experimental systems indicates that systemically administered passive Ab is therapeutically less effective in the upper RT [12].

To avoid outgrowth of viral escape mutants in Ab-treated mice, initial studies [13] used a pool of HA-specific MAbs directed to distinct HA sites for treatment. These studies showed that PR8-infected SCID mice could readily be cured of the infection by i.p. treatment with 170–280 μg of the MAb pool and that Ab treatment with 280 μg was fully effective even when administered 7 days after infection, when the pulmonary virus load is massive. Interestingly, the Ab dose required for resolution of infection was not much different if Ab was administered 1 (175 μg cured 100% of mice) or 7 days (280 μg cured 100% of mice) after initiation of infection. Although the virus load was much greater on day 7 than on day 1, this is probably compensated by increased inflammation-induced transudation of serum Ab into RT secretion at day 7 compared to day 1. Subsequent experiments used individual purified HA-specific MAbs that were administered 6–24 h after infection to minimize outgrowth of viral escape mutants. These studies showed that the infection could be resolved in 50% of the SCID mice by treatment with 40 μg of an HA-specific Ab (resulting in an Ab concentration in serum of ~ 15 μg/ml after 1 day of equilibration) [14]. This Ab was directed to the HA site Sb/B (H1[15]/H3 [16,17] designations, respectively), displayed high VN activity in vitro and was of IgG2a isotype. Other MAbs of similar specificity and VN activity but of IgG3, IgG1 and IgG2b isotype were used in the form of ascites fluid. They were also effective in clearing the infection but their therapeutic efficacy was not determined. MAbs of IgM and IgA isotype failed to cure the infection, even when administered repetitively at high dose [13]. The reason for the low therapeutic activity of IgA and IgM isotypes is still incompletely understood. Treatment with NA- and M2-specific MAbs, both of IgG2a isotype, reduced the lung virus titer but failed to clear the infection, and NP- and M1-specific were without therapeutic effect [18].

In immunologically intact mice, therapeutically effective serum Ab titers were generated by the active Ab response in the second to third week of infection, when virus had already been cleared, but were larger than those seen around days 7–10, when the infection was actually being cleared [13]. However, this does not exclude an important role of Ab in virus clearance in immunocompetent mice. First, the above comparison could not take into account the possible contribution by Ab secreted by B cells located in the lamina propria of the airways; such locally secreted Ab would be expected to contribute more effectively to the Ab concentration in RT secretion than serum Ab. Second, as mentioned above, the concomitant Th response in immunocompetent mice would be expected to enhance the therapeutic activity of Ab. Thus, the data are consistent with the conclusion that the TD Ab response is the activity responsible for resolution of the infection in the absence of Tc.

1.5. How do Abs operate in vivo?

There are two distinct stages in virus replication at which Abs may act. First, by reacting with intact infectious virus, they may reduce the virions ability to spread the infection. The various mechanisms operating at this stage are collectively referred to as virus neutralization (VN). Second, by reacting with live infected host cells prior to completion of virus release, they may reduce the total yield of progeny virus through various mechanisms which are collectively referred to in the following as YR. As the ectodomains of HA, NA, and M2 are the viral target structures for both types of activities, the same Abs can potentially operate at both stages. We have determined these activities in vitro and in vivo for several Abs that differed in specificity but shared the same heavy chain isotype, IgG2a. VN in vitro was expressed as Ab concentration at which 50% of MDCK micro-cultures were protected from infection by ~ 100 TCID$_{50}$ of PR8 virus. VN in vivo was expressed as the total Ab dose or the resulting serum concentration which protected 50% of mice against challenge with a similar dose of virus as used in vitro. As prophylaxis typically required less passive Ab than therapy, it is clear that Ab operated in prophylaxis by preventing the initial virus inoculum from initiating an infection rather than by resolving an infection after it had been initiated. YR activity in vitro and in vivo could only be assessed with Abs that lacked VN activity. In vitro, YR activity was determined by measuring virus yield in MDCK cultures that were incubated in the presence of non-neutralizing concentrations of Ab. YR in vivo was similarly assessed by the determination of the virus titer in the lung of mice that had been treated with subneutralizing Ab doses. Some findings from these studies are summarized below.

(1) The VN activity of HA-specific Abs varied greatly, apparently depending largely on their fine specificity. Sa,Sb/B-specific Abs showed generally very high VN activity (1 unit activity at ~ 0.001 μg/ml) and Cb/E-specific Abs low activity (~ 1 μg/ml). NA- and M2-specific Abs exhibited no VN activity at 10 μg/ml.

(2) VN activity in vivo could hardly be predicted from the Abs VN activity in vitro. For instance, while a HA(Sa,Sb/B)-specific Ab exhibited VN activity at the concentration of $1-2$ μg/ml serum (i.e., ~ 1000-fold larger than concentration required in vitro), two HA(Cb/E)-specific Abs exhibited VN activity at $10-20$ μg/ml (~ 10-fold larger than effective concentration in vitro). Because these Abs were of the same isotype (IgG2a) and presumably transudated at the same rate from serum into RT secretion, the findings indicated that factors in vivo either inhibited VN of the HA(Sa,Sb/B)-specific Ab or enhanced VN of HA(Cb/E)-specific Abs. The latter is supported by preliminary studies showing that heat-sensitive serum components enhanced the HI activity of HA(Cb/E)-specific Abs on average by 20-fold, but had no significant effect on HA(Sa,Sb/B)-specific Abs. The enhancement was consistently seen with IgG2a, sporadically with IgG3 and never with IgG1. NA- and M2-specific Abs exhibited no VN activity at the highest concentration tested (~ 80 μg/ml serum), indicating that mere binding of IgG2a Ab to virus at the density provided by the NA- and M2-specific Abs was not sufficient for VN. Although only one NA- and one M2-specific Ab were tested, the lack of VN activity of Abs specific for these proteins is consistent with studies showing that NA- [19] and M2-specific [20,21] immunity is "infection-permissive."

(3) As reported by Zebedee and Lamb [22], the M2-specific Ab failed to exhibit YR activity in vitro against PR8 virus-infected cells at 20 μg/ml, in spite of its strong reaction with M2 expressed on the plasma membrane of live infected cells. Yet, the same Ab was capable of suppressing virus titers in the lung by 100–1000-fold at a serum concentration of 10–40 μg/ml [18]. Since this Ab exhibited no VN activity at this concentration, it follows that the suppression in pulmonary virus titer resulted from Ab-mediated YR activity in vivo. Furthermore, because reaction of this Ab with infected cells in vitro did not result in detectable YR, it appears that the M2-specific Ab operated in vivo by directing innate defense activities, such as complement, FcγRI-, FcγRIII-, CRI- and CRII-expressing cells, against the infected host cells. The additional finding that anti-M2 Ab of IgG2a isotype was therapeutically more effective than the anti-M2 Ab of IgG1 isotype, both Abs having the same V regions, is consistent with the above proposition since these

innate defense activities are known to have isotypic preferences [23–25]. The VN-negative NA-specific Ab suppressed virus titer in the lung at a serum concentration of 20–80 μg/ml. Although this Ab exhibited YR activity in vitro, it required a high Ab concentration (20 μg/ml) and solely delayed virus release by 1–2 days but did not suppress it permanently, as seen in vivo. Therefore, the NA-specific Ab-mediated YR activity in vivo was probably also due to targeting innate defense activities against infected host cells, and thus, killing them prior to the release of the entire load of progeny virus.

(4) The ability of HA-specific Abs to resolve the infection if given therapeutically correlated with the Ab's VN activity in vivo [14], and Abs that lacked measurable VN activity failed to resolve the infection [18]. Thus, VN activity appears to be required for clearance of the PR8 virus infection and YR activity alone is not powerful enough to achieve it.

2. Concluding remarks

Current evidence indicates that the TD anti-viral Ab response makes an important contribution to the control and resolution of influenza virus infection not only in the absence of Tc, as discussed here, but also in their presence. The latter is most clearly shown by the significant decrease in the resistance to infection of mice that lack B cells [12,26]. The TD Ab response is equally, if not more important, in the immune host. Unlike memory Tc cells, which persist as resting cells that need to be reactivated by infection before they generate effector cells with therapeutic activity, B cell memory persists not only at the level of resting memory B cells but also at the level of Ab secreting cells which can maintain a level of circulating Ab. The limitation of Ab-mediated protection is obviously the propensity of the influenza virus to mutate the target structures recognized by protective HA- and NA-specific Abs. An important exception to this may be the highly conserved ectodomain of M2 which has recently been used to induce heterosubtypic protection in mice [20,21]. The data presented here suggest that in addition to its specificity, the Abs' heavy chain isotype and perhaps also their avidity may be of importance for their protective activity.

Acknowledgements

The work described here was supported by Grant AI-13989 from NIAID.

References

[1] D.J. Topham, R.A. Tripp, P.C. Doherty, CD8[+] T cells clear influenza virus by perforin or fas-dependent processes, J. Immunol. 159 (1997) 5197–5200.

[2] A.J. Caton, W. Gerhard, The diversity of the CD4[+] T cell response in influenza, Sem. Immunol. 4 (1992) 85–90.

[3] D.J. Topham, R.A. Tripp, A.M. Hamilton-Easton, S.R. Sarawar, P.C. Doherty, Quantitative analysis of the influenza virus-specific CD4[+] T cell memory in the absence of B cells and Ig., J. Immunol. 157 (1996) 2947–2952.

[4] K. Mozdzanowska, M. Furchner, K. Maiese, W. Gerhard, CD4$^+$ T cells are ineffective in clearing a pulmonary infection with influenza type A virus in the absence of B cells, Virology 239 (1997) 217–225.

[5] D.J. Topham, P.C. Doherty, Clearance of an influenza A virus by CD4$^+$ T cells is inefficient in the absence of B cells, J. Virol. 72 (1998) 882–885.

[6] S.L. Epstein, C.-Y. Lo, J.A. Misplon, J.R. Bennink, Mechanisms of protective immunity in mice without antibodies, J. Immunol. 160 (1998) 322–327.

[7] K.N. Leung, G.L. Ada, Different functions of subsets of effector T cells in murine influenza virus infection, Cell. Immunol. 67 (1982) 312–324.

[8] A.F. Ochsenbein, D.D. Pinschewer, B. Odermatt, A. Ciurea, H. Hengartner, R.M. Zinkernagel, Correlation of T cell independence of antibody responses with antigen dose reaching secondary lymphoid organs: implications for splenectomized patients and vaccine design, J. Immunol. 164 (2000) 6296–6302.

[9] P.A. Scherle, G. Palladino, W. Gerhard, Mice can recover from pulmonary influenza virus infection in the absence of class I-restricted cytotoxic T cells, J. Immunol. 148 (1992) 212–217.

[10] K. Mozdzanowska, K. Maiese, W. Gerhard, Th cell-deficient mice control influenza virus infection more effectively than Th- and B cell-deficient mice: evidence for a Th-independent contribution by B cells to virus clearance, J. Immunol. 164 (2000) 2635–2643.

[11] N. Baumgarth, O.C. Herman, G.C. Jager, L.E. Brown, L.A. Herzenberg, J. Chen, B-1 and B-2 cell-derived immunoglobulin M antibodies are nonredundant components of the protective response to influenza virus infection, J. Exp. Med. 192 (2000) 271–280.

[12] W. Gerhard, K. Mozdzanowska, M. Furchner, G. Washko, K. Maiese, Role of the B-cell response in recovery of mice from primary influenza virus infection, Immunol. Rev. 159 (1997) 95–103.

[13] G. Palladino, K. Mozdzanowska, G. Washko, W. Gerhard, Virus-neutralizing antibodies of immunoglobulin G (IgG) but not of IgM or IgA isotypes can cure influenza virus pneumonia in SCID mice, J. Virol. 69 (1995) 2075–2081.

[14] K. Mozdzanowska, M. Furchner, G. Washko, J. Mozdzanowski, W. Gerhard, A pulmonary influenza virus infection in SCID mice can be cured by treatment with hemagglutinin-specific antibodies that display very low virus-neutralizing activity in vitro, J. Virol. 71 (1997) 4347–4355.

[15] A.J. Caton, G.G. Brownlee, J.W. Yewdell, W. Gerhard, The antigenic structure of the influenza virus A/PR/ 8/34 hemagglutinin (H1 subtype), Cell 31 (1982) 417–427.

[16] D.C. Wiley, J.J. Skehel, The structure and function of the hemagglutinin membrane glycoprotein of influenza virus, Annu. Rev. Biochem. 56 (1987) 366–394.

[17] I.A. Wilson, N.J. Cox, Structural basis of immune recognition of influenza virus hemagglutinin, Annu. Rev. Immunol. (1990) 8737–8771.

[18] K. Mozdzanowska, K. Maiese, M. Furchner, W. Gerhard, Treatment of influenza virus-infected SCID mice with nonneutralizing antibodies specific for the transmembrane proteins matrix 2 and neuraminidase reduces the pulmonary virus titer but fails to clear the infection, Virology 254 (1999) 138–146.

[19] B.E. Johansson, D.J. Bucher, E.D. Kilbourne, Purified influenza virus hemagglutinin and neuraminidase are equivalent in stimulation of antibody response by induce contrasting types of immunity to infection, J. Virol. 63 (1989) 1239–1246.

[20] A.M. Frace, A.I. Klimov, T. Rowe, R.A. Black, J.M. Katz, Modified M2 proteins produce heterotypic immunity against influenza A virus, Vaccine 17 (1999) 2237–2244.

[21] S. Neirynck, T. Deroo, X. Saelens, P. Vanlandschoot, W. Min Jou, W. Fiers, A universal influenza A vaccine based on the extracellular domain of the M2 protein, Nat. Med. 5 (1999) 1119–1157.

[22] S.L. Zebedee, R.A. Lamb, Influenza A virus M2 protein: monoclonal antibody restriction of virus growth and detection of M2 in virions, J. Virol. 62 (1988) 2762–2772.

[23] M.S. Neuberger, K. Rajewsky, Activation of mouse complement by monoclonal mouse antibodies, Eur. J. Immunol. 11 (1981) 1012–1016.

[24] J.V. Ravetch, J.P. Kinet, Fc receptors, Annu. Rev. Immunol. 9 (1991) 457–492.

[25] M.D. Hulett, P.M. Hogarth, Molecular basis of Fc receptor function, Adv. Immunol. 57 (1994) 1–96.

[26] M.B. Graham, T.J. Braciale, Resistance to and recovery from lethal influenza virus infection in B lymphocyte-deficient mice, J. Exp. Med. 186 (1997) 2063–2068.

International Congress Series 1219 (2001) 319–326

H2M- and MHC class II recycling-independent loading of a hemagglutinin-derived epitope

D. Rajagopal, M. Tewari, N. Yeh, L.C. Eisenlohr*

Thomas Jefferson University, Philadelphia, PA, USA

Abstract

Background: Helper T Cells are stimulated by antigenic peptides (epitopes) displayed at the cell surface by major histocompatibility complex (MHC) class II molecules. Thus far, two pathways for peptide loading have been defined. The first requires the participation of a chaperonin-like protein, H2M but not the ability of class II molecules to traffic from the cell surface to early endosomes. The second is the reverse in not requiring H2M expression but requiring class II internalization. The studies described here were undertaken to test the hypothesis that loading of an epitope, termed S3, within the A/PR/8/34 influenza (PR8) hemagglutinin (HA) molecule is via this second pathway, as we previously determined its presentation to be H2M-independent. *Methods*: Genes encoding the α and β 1 chains of the murine I-E^d class II molecule were truncated to remove putative internalization motifs in the cytosolic tails. Loss of internalization was confirmed by confocal immunofluorescence microscopy. COS cells were transiently transfected with wild-type or truncated genes and tested for the ability to present the S3 epitope to an S3-specific T cell hybridoma that expresses β-galactosidase upon activation. *Results*: Removal of the recycling motif had no discernable impact upon the presentation of S3. *Conclusions*: Results suggest the existence of a third route of class II-restricted antigen processing, one that requires neither H2M expression nor class II recycling. Future experiments are aimed at further defining this pathway. © 2001 Elsevier Science B.V. All rights reserved.

Keywords: Antigen presentation; Antigen processing; MHC class II

* Corresponding author. Department of Microbiology and Immunology, Jefferson Medical College, BLSB Room 726, 233 South 10th Street, Philadelphia, PA, 19107, USA. Tel.: +1-215-503-4540; fax: +1-215-923-4153.
E-mail address: L_Eisenlohr@lac.jci.tju.edu (L.C. Eisenlohr).

1. Introduction

CD4$^+$ T cells respond to antigen in the form of short peptides (epitopes) bound to MHC class II molecules. It appears that the majority of epitopes load onto class II molecules situated in a late endocytic compartment having been guided to that location by invariant chain (Ii), a polypeptide that nascent class II molecules associate with. Within the late endocytic compartment invariant chain is digested by proteases, sparing only a short peptide (termed CLIP) that resides in the antigen-binding groove. Ingested antigens are also digested and the resulting fragments replace CLIP, a step that is mediated in many cases by a late endosome-resident heterodimer termed H2M. Recently, evidence has accumulated for the existence of a second loading pathway that appears to take place in the early endosome. In this case, H2M function is not necessary and the pool of class II molecules used for loading is delivered from the plasma membrane. The internalization step is mediated by a dileucine sequence situated in the cytosolic tail of the β chain though some influence of the α chain has been suspected.

We have focused for several years upon the presentation of two HA-derived epitopes, S1 (residues 109–119) and S3 (residues 302–313). Though restricted to the same class II molecule, I-E^d, these epitopes display strikingly different presentation phenotypes, including: (1) their expression kinetics at the cell surface, (2) the effect that acidification has on epitope accessibility, and (3) the extent to which expression of endogenous HA increases epitope availability. We suspect that these differences are due not to the primary sequence of the epitopes but rather their relative locations within HA. S3 resides in the "stalk" region of HA, which unfolds in response to acidification while S1 resides in the globular domain, a region that does not undergo radical change upon acidification. Recently, we utilized monoclonal antibodies specific for S1 and S3 and confocal immunofluorescence microscopy to show that S3 becomes available for antibody (and presumably class II) binding in an early endosome, soon after internalization of influenza virions, a step that coincides with the acid-induced conformational change. In contrast, S1 is not revealed until much later after uptake in a late endosomal compartment. Furthermore, as might be predicted, we demonstrated that presentation of S1 depends upon expression of H2M while presentation of S3 does not. Based upon these findings, we expected to confirm that S3 presentation depends upon recycling of class II molecules. Interestingly, our results contradict this prediction.

2. Materials and methods

2.1. Chemicals/antigens/viruses

All chemicals were obtained from Sigma (St. Louis, MO, USA) unless noted. PR8 stocks were generated and titered by hemagglutination assay as previously described. For all assays, 5×10^6 cells were pulsed for 1 h with 2000 hemagglutinating units (HAU) of live or UV-inactivated PR8, diluted with balanced saline solution $+0.1\%$ bovine serum albumin in a volume of 250 μl.

2.2. Genes and constructs

The class II α and β genes were the generous gift of Dr. Jim Miller, (University of Chicago, Chicago, IL, USA) and were cloned into pBlueScript (SK+). Truncations were made via PCR-based site-directed mutagenesis. For both chains, truncation was achieved by utilizing downstream primers that eliminated the final 12 codons of each gene. The PCR products were then cloned into the eukaryotic expression vector, pRC-CMV.

2.3. Cell lines

The COS7 cell line used for transfection was the kind gift from Dr. Bice Perussia (Thomas Jefferson University, Philadelphia, PA, USA). The BWZ.36 used as fusion partner for generation of the lacZ based T cell hybrids was kindly provided by Dr. Nilabh Shastri (University of California, Berkeley, CA, USA). S1- and S3-specific T hybridomas that express β-galactosidase upon activation were generated by fusion of peptide-specific CD4+ cytotoxic T cell clones with the fusion partner BWZ.36. Clones were screened for specific recognition by coincubation with I-E^d-expressing A20 B lymphoma cells infected with either PR8 or B/Lee (whose HA contains neither S1 nor S3). β-galactosidase production by individual cells was monitored using X-gal as the chromogenic substrate.

2.4. Transfections

Transient transfection of COS cells was performed with DEAE–dextran solution. Prior to transfection, 6×10^6 cells were washed well in serum-free medium and incubated with a transfection mix containing 80–120 μg of maxi-prep plasmid for each transfection, 1.4 mg/ml DEAE–dextran (mol. wt. 500 K), 10 mM HEPES, pH 7.4, 0.1 μM chloroquine for 4 h at 37 °C following which the cells were subjected to a 10% DMSO shock for 2 min. The cells were incubated in complete medium (RPMI supplemented with 10% FCS, 0.05 mM 2-mercaptoethanol, and 0.01 mg/ml gentamycin) for 96 h. Cells were then harvested by trypsinization and the efficiency of transfection was assessed by flow cytometry and/or immunostaining using the I-E^d-specific monoclonal antibody, 14.4.4 S.

2.5. Assessment of class II recycling

Transfected cells were labeled with purified, I-E^d-specific monoclonal, 14.4.4 S, for 1 h on ice. Cells were then washed thrice with ice-cold PBS containing 0.2% BSA and subsequently incubated with fluorescein labeled anti-mouse IgG, for 1 h on ice. The cells were washed thrice with ice-cold PBS and incubated in internalization buffer (RPMI containing 5 mM HEPES, pH 7.4) and either fixed with 2% paraformaldehyde immediately or allowed to incubate at 37 °C for various intervals of time prior to fixation. The cells were then washed and mounted on coverslips using anti-fade mounting medium (Molecular Probes, Eugene, Oregon, USA), after permeabilization using 0.1% Triton X-100 in PBS for 2 min at room temperature. All images were viewed at the Kimmel Cancer Center confocal facility.

2.6. Presentation assays

Transfected COS cells, used as APC in presentation assays, were infected with live PR8 or pulsed with UV-inactivated PR8 as described earlier. APC were plated at twofold dilutions starting from 5×10^4 cells/well. S1- and S3-specific T hybrids were incubated overnight with APC. The extent of activation was determined using the fluorescent substrate, methyl-umbelliferyl-β-D galactoside (MUG) as has been described elsewhere.

3. Results

3.1. Phenotypes of recycling versus nonrecycling class II in transfected COS cells

We utilized PCR-directed mutagensis to remove the 12 amino acids at the N-termini of both the α and β genes as described in Section 2. These manipulations eliminated the 12 carboxy-terminal amino acids from the cytosolic domains of each chain, including the dileucine motif within the tail of the β chain. To test the effect of these manipulations, COS cells were cotransfected with eukaryotic expression vectors containing the four possible combinations of wild type and mutant class II α and β genes. After 96 h, the cells were harvested and cooled to 0 °C by incubation on ice, a measure that prevents internalization of cell surface proteins. Surface class II molecules were then labeled by coincubation of the cells with an I-E^d-specific monoclonal antibody followed by FITC-labeled rabbit anti-mouse Ig. Cells were fixed immediately or shifted to 37 °C for 1 h before fixation and analysis by confocal immunofluorescence microscopy. Fig. 1A shows the result when the two wild-type genes were employed. As expected, nearly the entire FITC label has been internalized. In contrast, cotransfection with the truncated versions of the α and β genes lead to staining that remained almost entirely at the cell surface (panel D). Interestingly, the transfectants bearing one of the truncations showed drastically reduced recycling rates (panels B and C), however, the presence of wild-type α chain did permit internalization to a marginal extent (Fig. 1B), in conformity to the earlier described reports. We refer here and below to the product of a wild-type gene as recycling (RC) and the product of a truncated gene as nonrecycling (NRC).

3.2. Generation and titration of lacZ-transduced S1- and S3-specific T hybridomas

Shastri et al. have developed a scheme for generating T cell hybridomas that produce β-galactosidase upon antigen-specific activation, allowing for a very convenient and sensitive readout of antigen presentation. Following the protocol established by this group, we generated S1- and S3-specific hybridomas using as fusion partners S1- and S3-specific T cell clones that have been previously described. For each epitope, several rounds of limiting dilution subcloning were required to obtain stable hybridomas. Fig. 2A shows the response of these two hybridomas to different concentrations of synthetic peptide. The assay shows that they are specific for peptide and, importantly, that they respond to different doses of peptide in a graded manner. Panel B further emphasizes the ability of the hybrids (in this case the S1-specific hybrid) to respond to graded doses of peptide. In this

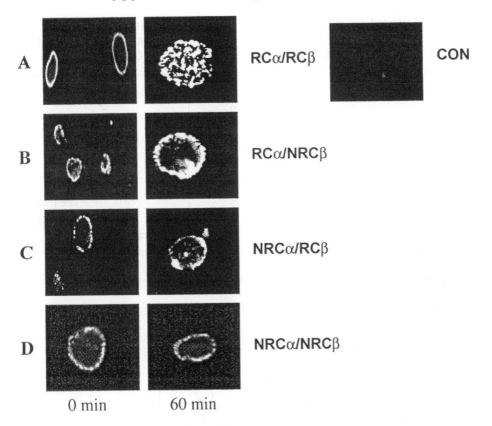

Fig. 1. Recycling phenotypes of class II in COS cells transiently transfected with intact and/or truncated class II α and β chains in various combinations. COS cells were cotransfected with combinations of (A) wild type (WT) α and β, (B) WT α and truncated β, (C) truncated α and WT β or (D) both truncated α and β constructs, as described in Section 2. The transfectants were harvested after 96 h, chilled on ice and surface-labeled with I-E^d-specific monoclonal antibody, 14.4.4 S. Cells were washed with ice-cold PBS and incubated for an additional hour with rabbit anti-mouse IgG–FITC conjugate. After washing, cells were either fixed immediately for the zero time point or shifted to 37 °C for 1 h prior to fixation. The recycling phenotype was assessed by confocal immunomicroscopy. Control refers to cells mock transfected with plasmid vector alone.

case, A20 B cell lymphoma cells were pulsed with different concentrations of the S1 peptide and then diluted in wells prior to addition of the S1-specific T hybridoma. The "two-dimensional" dose titration that we observed further strengthens the conclusion that the hybridomas are capable of reporting small differences in the level of peptide presentation. As will be seen, this becomes critical in evaluating the results shown in the final figure.

3.3. Presentation of S1 versus S3 occurs equally efficiently on RC or NRC class II

To assess the role of recycling class II in the presentation of S1/S3, COS cells were transfected with either RC or NRC α and β chains (as in Fig. 1A,D), pulsed with UV-

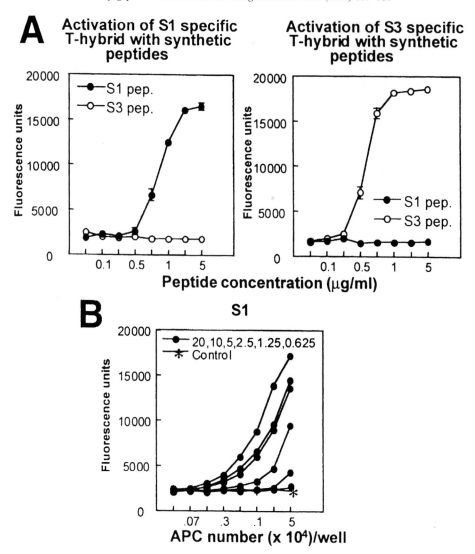

Fig. 2. Titration of S1- and S3-specific T cell hybridomas. (A) A20 cells (5×10^4/well) were pulsed with the indicated concentrations of S1/S3 peptide for 1 h at 37 °C. Peptide-pulsed cells were overlaid with S1- or S3-specific T cell hybrids and incubated overnight. Extent of activation was determined using the MUG assay and represented as arbitrary fluorescence units. (B) A20 cells were pulsed with indicated concentrations (µg/ml) of S1 peptide, plated as twofold dilutions starting from 5×10^4 cells/well, and incubated overnight with S1-specific T hybrids. Extent of activation was determined using the MUG assay. Control indicates cells pulsed with medium alone.

inactivated PR8 and then tested for the ability to present the S1 and S3 epitopes to the β-galactosidase-producing T hybridomas. As anticipated, presentation of S1 (Fig. 3A) is independent of the recycling ability of class II. The epitope is presented equally well by

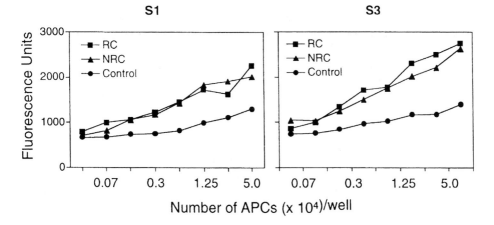

Fig. 3. Presentation assay for S1 and S3. COS cells cotransfected transiently with RC, or NRC combinations of α and β chains were used as antigen presenting cells for presentation assays. Cells were pulsed with UV-inactivated PR8 (as described in Section 2), and indicated twofold dilutions of these APC were overlaid with S1- (A) or S3- (B) specific T cell hybrids and incubated overnight. T cell activation was measured by MUG assay and data represented as arbitrary fluorescence units. Cells transfected with plasmid vector alone were used as control.

either form of class II. Unexpectedly, a similar presentation pattern was observed when S3 presentation was monitored (Fig. 3B), a finding that was consistent in several independent experiments. Thus, S3 appears to be an epitope whose presentation is independent of both H2M function and class II recycling.

4. Discussion

Indeed, different antigens even regions within the same antigen vary in their suscept-ibility to degradation. Thus, various epitopes are first available for class II binding within different endocytic compartments. Our published experiments described above show this to be true for S1 and S3. A reasonable explanation for class II internalization is that it allows for the acquisition of epitopes that, like S3, are revealed in an early endocytic compartment and might be largely degraded prior to reaching a compartment where loading of nascent class II molecules with epitopes like S1, can occur. This mechanism would serve to broaden the spectrum of determinants that could trigger an immune response. However, although presentation of S3 is not dependent upon expression of DM, whose presence appears to be critical for peptide exchange in the more acidic environment of the late endosome, neither does its presentation appear to be dependent upon class II internalization. The data suggest that, at least in the cell type tested, nascent class II molecules are able to reach the early endosome where they can acquire peptide in a DM-independent fashion. To our knowledge, our data are the first to support the existence of such a pathway.

Several aspects of this proposed model should be discussed. First, COS cells have a fairly rapid rate of membrane trafficking and, as a result, nascent class II molecules may gain compartments, such as early endosomes, that are not accessible in other cell types. We are in the process of testing additional cell types to determine if this suspicion is correct. We note, however, that the immature dendritic cell, a cell type highly relevant to class II-restricted responses, also has a very dynamic plasma membrane and may therefore permit such class II trafficking. Overexpression of class II, as may have been achieved using the CMV-based vectors, might also expand the intracellular distribution of class II. A second issue is how Ii might be efficiently removed from class II in an early endosome where proteolytic activity is relatively low. We have not evaluated our COS cells for expression of functional Ii but note that expression of Ii, via cotransfection with an appropriate vector, had no impact upon the RC versus NRC results shown in Fig. 3 (unpublished observations). Perhaps nascent class II molecules travel first to a late endosome where most Ii is removed before traveling to the early endosome where exchange of S3 for CLIP might be possible. Alternatively, the cathepsins required for removal of Ii have been detected in the early endosomes of some cell types, suggesting the possibility that all the steps required for peptide loading could occur in early endosomes, at least in some cases. Again, future experiments will be required to determine the finer, but critical details of the proposed pathway. Third, it is possible that H2M dependence/independence differs when COS cells are employed instead of the B cell lymphoma that we have used in the past to address this issue. This could be due, again, to differences in membrane dynamics. However, if there is any variability in DM dependence/independence, it seems likely given the various points that have been discussed, that presentation of S1 might be H2M-independent in some cell types, while presentation of S3, the focus of the work, is uniformly H2M-independent. Finally, we have made attempts to characterize in other ways the compartment in which S3 loads. Recently, a novel recycling compartment, distinct from the standard transferrin receptor-positive recycling compartment, has been described. This compartment contains the ADP-ribosylation factor, ARF6 and expression of dominant-negative ARF-6 mutants prevents membrane flow between the compartment and the plasma membrane. We have tested the effect that these ARF-6 mutants have upon presentation of the S3 epitope but have observed no impact. Thus, we continue to gain important information about the presentation of these two epitopes, similar in some ways yet dissimilar in many others, but many key aspects remain to be elucidated.

Acknowledgements

This work was funded by a grant from the National Institute of Health (AI36331). We thank the Kimmel Cancer Institutes Nucleic Acid Facility for the synthesis of oligonucleotides and sequencing and the Confocal Microscopy Facility for the help in generating the images shown. We thank Sinnathamby Gomathinayagam for the critical reading of this manuscript.

International Congress Series 1219 (2001) 327–332

Susceptibility and immunity to influenza A strains in Ig−/−mice

Kimberly A. Benton*, Julia A. Misplon, Chia-Yun Lo, Suzanne L. Epstein

Laboratory of Immunology and Developmental Biology, Division of Cellular and Gene Therapies, Center for Biologics Evaluation and Research, Food and Drug Administration, Bethesda, MD, USA

Abstract

Background: Broad cross-protection to influenza strains of different subtypes, termed heterosubtypic immunity, can be observed in animal models and is the goal of new approaches to human vaccines. Knockout mouse models, such as doubly inactivated (DI) mice lacking B cells and Ig, can be used to focus on the role of T cells in heterosubtypic immunity. We previously demonstrated that DI mice immunized with influenza B/Ann Arbor were protected from homologous challenge. We wished to identify influenza A strains that could be used in DI mice to examine the contributions of T-cell subsets to heterosubtypic immunity. *Methods*: DI mice were infected intranasally (i.n.) under anesthesia with influenza strains at varying doses. Mice were monitored for mortality, and lung titers were assessed for non-lethal strains. *Results*: Commonly used mouse-tropic influenza A strains were lethal to DI mice, even at low doses. Several other isolates were found to replicate to high titers in the lungs for several days until being cleared to undetectable levels. *Conclusion*: Non-lethal strains that replicate in the lungs can be used to study heterosubtypic protection in DI mice measured as reduction in lung virus titers. Published by Elsevier Science B.V.

Keywords: Viral immunity; In vivo animal models; T lymphocytes

1. Introduction

Infection with a strain of one influenza A subtype can elicit protection against strains of other subtypes, which is called heterosubtypic immunity. Although numerous studies have examined the roles of T cells [1] and cross-reactive antibodies [2,3], many questions

---

* Corresponding author. FDA/CBER, 1401 Rockville Pike, HFM 521, Rockville, MD 20852, USA. Tel.: +1-301-827-0461; fax: +1-301-827-0449.

E-mail address: bentonk@cber.fda.gov (K.A. Benton).

0531-5131/01/$ – see front matter. Published by Elsevier Science B.V.
PII: S0531-5131(01)00343-0

remain about the basis of heterosubtypic immunity. The use of animal models, such as mice with defined immunodeficiencies, can help to clarify the contributions of different immune mechanisms. Our laboratory and others have used Ig $-/-$ mice to examine the role of T cells in protection against secondary infections with the same strain or strains of the same subtype, in the absence of pre-existing Abs. In DI mice, we observed that both CD4+ and CD8+ T cells were required for protection against homologous secondary infection with influenza B/Ann Arbor [4]. Others have demonstrated a greater role of CD8 + T cells in protection against primary or homologous secondary infection with influenza A strains [5–7].

Studies with Ig $-/-$ mice have been complicated by the lethality of most mouse-tropic influenza A strains to these mice. We present here the identification of influenza A isolates that are non-lethal but replicate to high titers in the lungs, and thus, can be used in our studies of heterosubtypic immunity in DI mice.

2. Materials and methods

Materials and methods have been previously described [4]. Influenza virus strains used are listed in Table 1. The mouse strain used in these studies, DI (doubly inactivated, $\Delta J_H/\Delta J_H$, $\Delta C_\kappa/C_\kappa$) that lacks mature B cells and Ig was obtained from Dr. Aya Jakobovits under a Materials Transfer Agreement. Immunization and challenge was performed with live influenza virus in a volume of 50 μl of PBS, administered intranasally (i.n.) under light anesthesia with methoxyflurane, which permits infection of the full respiratory tract. Intraperitoneal (i.p.) immunization was performed by injection of live virus in volume of 0.2 ml PBS. Influenza virus was quantitated by titration on Madin–Darby canine kidney

Table 1
Characteristics of influenza A strains tested in DI mice

Strain	Subtype	Lethal (dose tested)[a]	Replicates in the lungs	Enhanced clearance of lung virus after homologous challenge
A/Puerto Rico/8/34	H1N1	Yes (25 TCID$_{50}$)	N.T.[b]	No
A/Philippines/2/82/X-79	H3N2	Yes (25 TCID$_{50}$)	N.T.	No
A/Japan/305/57	H2N2	No (10^5 TCID$_{50}$)	No	N.T.
A/Japan/305/57 mouse-passed[c]	H2N2	Yes (10^2 TCID$_{50}$)	N.T.	N.T.
A/Udorn/307/72	H3N2	No (10^5 TCID$_{50}$)	Yes	Yes
A/Udorn/307/72 mouse-passed[c]	H3N2	Yes (10^2 TCID$_{50}$)	N.T.	N.T.
A/AA/Marton/43	H1N1	No (10^5 TCID$_{50}$)	No	No[d]
A/Texas/36/91	H1N1	No (5×10^2 TCID$_{50}$)	Yes	Yes
A/Taiwan/1/86	H1N1	No (10^4 TCID$_{50}$)	Yes	Yes
A/Johannesburg/82/96	H1N1	No (10^2 TCID$_{50}$)	Yes	Yes
A/Kawasaki/6/86	H1N1	No (10^2 TCID$_{50}$)	No	N.T.

[a] Indicated doses are minimum tested for lethal strains or maximum tested for non-lethal strains.
[b] N.T., not tested.
[c] Mouse-passed 10 times.
[d] Challenged with homosubtypic virus A/PR/8 at a dose of 25 TCID$_{50}$.

cells (MDCK) using cytopathic effect as the indicator of presence of virus, and titer was expressed as the tissue culture 50% infectious dose per milliliter ($TCID_{50}$/ml).

3. Results

DI mice express no Ig due to the disruption of the heavy and light chain loci, in contrast to μMT mice that have been reported to produce low levels of Ig [6]. In order to find virus combinations for heterosubtypic immunization and challenge, we studied influenza A strains in DI mice. The results are summarized in Table 1.

We initially studied A/Puerto Rico/8/34 (A/PR/8) and A/Philippines/2/82/X-79 (A/Phil), strains that we routinely use in immunocompetent mice. A/Phil is a reassortant virus with the HA and NA genes of A/Philippines/2/82 origin. The stock of A/Phil used has been mouse-adapted [8]. Intranasal infection with A/PR/8 was 100% lethal even at doses

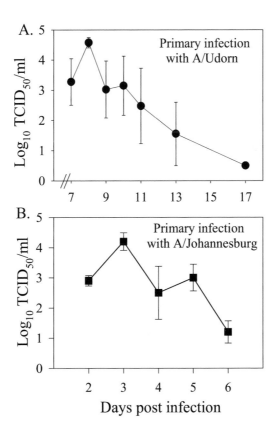

Fig. 1. Kinetics of virus clearance during primary infection of DI mice with A/Udorn or A/Johannesburg. The mean virus titers (log_{10} $TCID_{50}$/ml) ± standard error are shown for lung homogenates from DI mice infected with 10^4 $TCID_{50}$ A/Udorn (A) or 10^6 $TCID_{50}$ A/Johannesburg (B). All groups contained four mice, except for the A/Udorn infection group at day 17 that contained three mice. The limit of detection was 0.5 $TCID_{50}$/ml.

of 25 $TCID_{50}$, and A/Phil was 50% lethal at 25 $TCID_{50}$. The few survivors of infection with these low doses of A/PR/8 were challenged with 10^4 $TCID_{50}$ A/Phil, but no protection was observed. We also performed i.p. immunization with live virus to avoid infecting the respiratory tract yet achieve systemic priming. Intraperitoneal immunization with 10^4 $TCID_{50}$ A/PR/8 or A/Phil was not lethal but did not protect against homologous i.n. challenge.

Several other influenza isolates were tested by i.n. administration. A/Japan, A/Udorn, A/AA/Marton, A/Johannesburg, A/Texas, A/Taiwan, and A/Kawasaki were all non-lethal at the doses indicated in Table 1. We then tested whether i.n. immunization with these non-lethal strains could protect against lethal challenge with mouse-adapted challenge viruses. Mice immunized with non-lethal A/Japan and challenged with mouse-adapted (lethal) A/Japan were not protected; mortality was greater than 50% even at doses as low as 10^2 $TCID_{50}$. The same was true for non-lethal A/Udorn priming followed by mouse-adapted A/Udorn challenge.

Reduction in lung titers is an indicator of immune control of influenza virus replication. The strains identified as non-lethal were assessed for their ability to replicate in the lungs after i.n. infection. A/Udorn, A/Texas, A/Taiwan, and A/Johannesburg were observed to replicate in the lungs. In order to determine the best time point(s) post-infection to assess immunologically specific reduction in lung virus titers, we assessed the kinetics of replication and clearance of two selected viruses, A/Udorn and A/Johannes-burg, in naive DI mice. As shown in Fig. 1A, A/Udorn was cleared slowly, being found at titers of 10^3 $TCID_{50}$/ml or greater for up to 10 days post challenge. A/Johannesburg was cleared more rapidly, with levels of nearly 10^3 $TCID_{50}$/ml for 5 days (Fig. 1B). A/Udorn and A/Johannesburg were selected for studies of heterosubtypic immunity in DI mice (Benton et al., submitted for publication).

4. Discussion

A robust immune response to influenza infection involves multiple effector mechanisms, many of which likely contribute to the response to a subsequent heterosubtypic infection. Knockout mouse models with defined immunodeficiencies can be used to study the roles of specific effector mechanisms, which may aid in the development and evaluation of new vaccines.

DI mice lacking all Ig and B cells provide one such model. We found that most influenza strains were highly lethal in DI mice, so much so that we were unable to identify strains for use in studies of protection against mortality. However, we were successful in identifying several influenza A strains that persist and replicate in the lungs and can be used to measure immune clearance of lung virus.

The susceptibility of DI mice to influenza A strains is similar to that observed in μMT mice [5,7,9,10] and $J_HD -/-$ mice [11]. In addition to the absence of Ig, other potential factors in the vulnerability of Ig $-/-$ mice include T-cell defects resulting indirectly from the disruption of the Ig loci, or a function of B cells other than Ig production. Although one study reported suboptimal T-cell function in μMT mice [12], multiple studies have shown that Ig $-/-$ mice have relatively normal total T-cell numbers and T-cell function

[4,5,10,13,14]. Functions of B cells other than Ig production have been demonstrated to contribute to recovery from influenza infection by an undefined mechanism [10]. Thus, functions of B cells, both Ig production and other functions, are possible factors in the increased susceptibility of Ig $-/-$ mice to influenza A.

The DI mouse model can be used to study the roles of T cells acting alone, in the absence of contributions of B cells. The results presented here identify influenza A strains of different subtypes for use in such studies of heterosubtypic immunity.

Acknowledgements

We thank Anthony Ferrine and other staff in the CBER animal facility for expert animal care, and Drs. Zhiping Ye and Carolyn Wilson for critical review of the manuscript. This project was supported in part by a grant from the National Vaccine Program Office to S.L.E. K.A.B. was supported by an appointment to the Research Participation Program at the CBER administered by the Oak Ridge Institute for Science and Education.

References

[1] S. Liang, K. Mozdzanowska, G. Palladino, W. Gerhard, Heterosubtypic immunity to influenza type A virus in mice: effector mechanisms and their longevity, J. Immunol. 152 (1994) 1653–1661.

[2] I.N. Mbawuike, H.R. Six, T.R. Cate, R.B. Couch, Vaccination with inactivated influenza A virus during pregnancy protects neonatal mice against lethal challenge by influenza A viruses representing three subtypes, J. Virol. 64 (1990) 1370–1374.

[3] S. Neirynck, T. Deroo, X. Saelens, P. Vanlandschoot, W.M. Jou, W. Fiers, A universal influenza A vaccine based on the extracellular domain of the M2 protein, Nat. Med. 5 (1999) 1157–1163.

[4] S.L. Epstein, C.-Y. Lo, J.A. Misplon, J.R. Bennink, Mechanism of protective immunity against influenza virus infection in mice without antibodies, J. Immunol. 160 (1998) 322–327.

[5] M.B. Graham, T.J. Braciale, Resistance to and recovery from lethal influenza virus infection in B lymphocyte-deficient mice, J. Exp. Med. 186 (1997) 2063–2068.

[6] K. Mozdzanowska, M. Furchner, K. Maiese, W. Gerhard, CD4+ T cells are ineffective in clearing a pulmonary infection with influenza type A virus in the absence of B cells, Virology 239 (1997) 217–225.

[7] D.J. Topham, P.C. Doherty, Clearance of an influenza A virus by CD4+ T cells is inefficient in the absence of B cells, J. Virol. 72 (1998) 882–885.

[8] K.-S. Chen, G.V. Quinnan Jr., Induction, persistence and strain specificity of haemagglutinin-specific secretory antibodies in lungs of mice after intragastric administration of inactivated influenza virus vaccines, J. Gen. Virol. 69 (1988) 2779–2784.

[9] J.M. Riberdy, K.J. Flynn, J. Stech, R.G. Webster, J.D. Altman, P.C. Doherty, Protection against a lethal avian influenza A virus in a mammalian system, J. Virol. 73 (1999) 1453–1459.

[10] K. Mozdzanowska, K. Maiese, W. Gerhard, Th cell-deficient mice control influenza virus infection more effectively than Th-and B cell-deficient mice: evidence for a Th-independent contribution by B Cells to Virus Clearance, J. Immunol. 164 (2000) 2635–2643.

[11] A. Bot, A. Reichlin, H. Isobe, S. Bot, J. Schulman, W.M. Yokoyama, C.A. Bona, Cellular mechanisms involved in protection and recovery from influenza virus infection in immunodeficient mice, J. Virol. 70 (1996) 5668–5672.

[12] D. Homann, A. Tishon, D.P. Berger, W.O. Weigle, M.G. von Herrath, M.B.A. Oldstone, Evidence for an underlying CD4 helper and CD8 T-cell defect in B-cell-deficient mice: failure to clear persistent virus infection after adoptive immunotherapy with virus-specific memory cells from μMT/μMT mice, J. Virol. 72 (1998) 9208–9216.

[13] M.M. Epstein, F. DiRosa, D. Jankovic, A. Sher, P. Matzinger, Successful T cell priming in B cell-deficient mice, J. Exp. Med. 182 (1995) 915–922.

[14] D.J. Topham, R.A. Tripp, A.M. Hamilton-Easton, S.R. Sarawar, P.C. Doherty, Quantitative analysis of the influenza virus-specific CD4+ T cell memory in the absence of B cells and Ig, J. Immunol. 157 (1996) 2947–2952.

International Congress Series 1219 (2001) 333–340

Mechanism of heterosubtypic immunity to influenza A virus infection

Huan H. Nguyen*, Frederik W. van Ginkel, Huong L. Vu,
Jerry R. McGhee, Jiri Mestecky

*Department of Microbiology and the Immunobiology Vaccine Center, University of Alabama,
Birmingham, AL 35294-2170, USA*

Abstract

Heterosubtypic immunity (HSI) is defined as protective cross-reactive immune responses to lethal infection with influenza A virus of a different serotype than the virus initially encountered, and is thought to be mediated by serotype cross-reactive cytotoxic T lymphocytes (CTL). These CTL recognize conserved epitopes of internal proteins, such as nucleoprotein (NP) or matrix (M) protein shared by influenza A virus subtypes. Despite extensive studies, the precise effector mechanism for HSI remains elusive. For example, our recent studies and those of others reported HSI in T cell-depleted, β_2-microglobulin-deficient, and CD8 cell-deficient mice. The role for humoral immune responses in HSI is also unclear. Passive transfer of heterosubtypic immune serum did not provide protection against lethal heterosubtypic challenge, while B cell-deficient mice failed to develop HSI. Our recent findings and those of others now allow us to suggest a two-tiered HSI. Early after heterosubtypic challenge, a number of factors including subtype-specific CTL as well as antibody (Ab) responses and other as yet not well characterized host factors are able to minimize temporarily the virus spread, but are unable to clear the infection. In the later phase, the development of virus-neutralizing (VN) antibodies is important for virus clearance resulting in complete host recovery. © 2001 Elsevier Science B.V. All rights reserved.

Keywords: Influenza virus; Heterosubtypic immunity; Knockout mice

1. Introduction

Influenza type A is an acute respiratory disease that causes epidemics affecting between 20 and 40 million people per year and is responsible for about 20,000 infection-related

---

* Corresponding author. Tel.: +1-205-934-1737; fax: +1-205-934-3894.
E-mail address: nghuan@uab.edu (H.H. Nguyen).

0531-5131/01/$ – see front matter © 2001 Elsevier Science B.V. All rights reserved.
PII: S 0 5 3 1 - 5 1 3 1 (0 1) 0 0 3 4 4 - 2

deaths in the U.S. [1]. While influenza vaccines are available, the disease is still largely uncontrolled due to the virus's ability to mutate. For example, inactivated vaccines were effective against homologous challenge, but usually failed to develop immunity against virus undergoing heterologous drift. On the other hand, natural infections usually afford complete protection against homologous virus as well as strong immunity against infection with virus of a different subtype [2]. This cross-protection between different subtypes of influenza A virus is mediated by heterosubtypic immunity (HSI) in the absence of pre-existing virus-specific antibodies (Abs) that recognize the outer membrane proteins [3]. For years, HSI was thought to be mediated by subtype cross-reactive cytotoxic T lymphocytes (CTL) [4–7]. However, recent studies indicate that the role for CTL in HSI is ambiguous. Here we report new evidence for a role of subtype-specific CTL and humoral immune responses in HSI and suggest a two-tiered HSI.

2. Subtype-specific CD8$^+$ CTL in HSI

The role of CD8$^+$ CTL in HSI was suggested by the observations that passive transfer of large numbers of in vitro-cloned T cells possessing subtype-specific cytotoxic activity to influenza virus-infected mice can reduce pulmonary virus titers, promote their recovery, and provide protection under certain circumstances [8–13]. We have reported recently that subtype-specific CTL responses induced in mediastinal lymph nodes (MLN), a mucosa-associated lymphoid tissue (MALT), are associated with host recovery after lethal infection with heterosubtypic influenza A virus [14]. In contrast, immunization with recombinant vaccinia virus expressing a NP epitope recognized by CD8$^+$ T cells readily induced primary pulmonary NP-specific CD8$^+$ CTL. However, no protection by these T cells was observed after challenge with virus, as determined by virus titers, clearance kinetics, or survival [15]. Furthermore, in vivo depletion of CD8$^+$ T cells by monoclonal Abs led to partial, but not complete reduction of HSI [16] and HSI was also observed in β_2-microglobulin-deficient [17–19], T cell-depleted [19] mice. Using mice with a targeted disruption in the α chain of the CD8 molecule (CD8$^+$ T cell-deficient) we have demonstrated that cross-reactive CD8$^+$ CTL are not required for HSI, since CD8$^+$ T

Table 1
Induction of HSI in naive mice by passive transfer

Transfer of	HSI	Note
Cloned subtype-specific CTL	Yes	Requires enormous number of in vitro-cloned virus specific CD8$^+$ CTL
Lymphocytes isolated from mucosa-associated lymphoid tissue (MALT) of heterosubtypically immune mice	No	No dose effect
Lymphocytes isolated from systemic lymphoid tissue (spleen) of heterosubtypically immune mice	No	No dose effect
Serum of heterosubtypically immune mice	No	No dose effect

Table 2
Induction of HSI in transgenic mice

Mice	CD8$^+$ CTL	Antibodies	Th1/Th2	HSI
WT	+	+	> *	+
CD4$^{-/-}$	+	−	NA	−
CD8$^{-/-}$	−	+	< **	+
β2-microglobulin$^{-/-}$	−	+	<	+
μ$^{-/-}$	+	−	>	−
γ$^{-/-}$	+	+	<	+

NA: Not applicable.
 * Switched to Th1-type cytokines.
 ** Switched to Th2-type cytokines.

cell-deficient mice developed full immunity to heterosubtypic challenge. In contrast, B cell-deficient mice failed to develop protective HSI to lethal influenza A virus challenge, although they developed significant cross-reactive CTL responses [20]. Thus, the role for CD8$^+$ CTL as an effector mechanism for HSI remains controversial (Tables 1 and 2). It is noteworthy that adoptive transfer usually requires enormous numbers (e.g., 10^7 cells per mouse) of in vitro-cloned virus-specific CD8$^+$ CTL to achieve protection against heterosubtypic challenge, raising questions of effectiveness of virus-specific CD8$^+$ CTL responses for heterosubtypic protection.

3. Humoral immune responses

Early studies have shown that HSI occurs in the absence of virus-specific Abs that recognize predominantly the outer membrane proteins [3]. Adoptive transfer of a large amount of heterosubtypically immune serum that contains a high titer of subtype-specific Ab failed to protect naive recipients against subsequent challenge with heterosubtypic virus [19]. However, other studies suggest that HSI is mediated, in part, by cross-reactive Abs [21]. For example, Abs specific for viral internal proteins expressed on the surface of infected cells reduced production of progeny virus and inhibited the spread of primary infection in SCID mice [22]. We have used mice with a targeted disruption in the immunoglobulin μ heavy chain (B cell-deficient) and we have demonstrated that these mice failed to develop protective HSI to lethal influenza A virus challenge [20]. Although a lack of B cells reduces immunity against primary infection with influenza virus [23–26], we have observed that B cell-deficient mice survived the primary infection with the same dose that is used for induction of HSI in immunocompetent mice. Furthermore, the primary infection evoked vigorous heterosubtypic CTL responses in B cell-deficient, as well as in immunocompetent mice. However, the latter, but not B cell-deficient developed complete HSI. Thus, our study demonstrates that while CD8$^+$ CTL are less efficient in HSI B cells appeared to be important for complete HSI [20] (Tables 1 and 2).

In addition to the absence of HSI in B cell-deficient mice, severely impaired HSI, along with a lack of specific Abs, were observed in CD4$^+$ T cell-deficient mice [20]. As reported earlier, CD4$^+$ T cells alone were unable to clear virus and promote recovery from primary infection [27,28] but they were important for provision of help for B cells and Ab responses by secretion of cytokines (for review see Ref. [29]). Lack of specific Abs is most likely responsible for impaired HSI in CD4$^+$ T cell-deficient mice [20]. Cytokine analysis revealed that Th1- and Th2-type cytokine secretion in the lungs was not significantly altered in either B cell- or CD8$^+$ T cell-deficient mice [20]. Furthermore, we observed earlier that IFN-γ, which is thought to be a first line of host defense in the control of viral infection, is not necessary for heterosubtypic immunity and either Th1- or Th2-biased responses could provide heterosubtypic protection [30] (Table 2).

4. Two-tiered HSI

In addition to these studies of the mechanisms of HSI, we have observed recently that passive transfer of T cells, B cells or unseparated mononuclear cells isolated from MALT or systemic lymphoid organs, such as spleen of HSI mice, did not provide protection against heterosubtypic challenge (our unpublished observations). This indicates that memory heterosubtypically immune cells (B and T cells) may function as secondary effector cells. The primary pre-exposed antigen presenting cells (APC), such as dendritic cells (DC) [31] or other undefined regulatory cells may play an important role in the initiation of memory adaptive immune responses mediated by B and T cells. It is possible that pre-exposed APC may produce undefined antiviral factor(s) that result directly in low

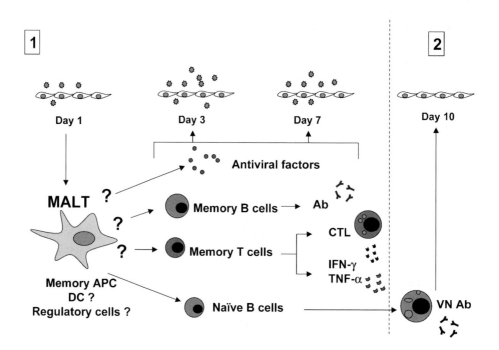

Fig. 1. A model for two-tiered HSI.

virus titer during the first phase of HSI (Fig. 1). It is noteworthy that pre-exposed DC localized in MALT may be critical for HSI, since the immune responses observed in systemic lymphoid organs may not reflect the events occurring at the site of infection, i.e., the mucosal surface [14]. The same observation is true for influenza virus as for other pathogens that initiate infection at the mucosal surface of the respiratory tract.

Thus, our findings and those of others now allow us to suggest a two-tiered HSI. Early after heterosubtypic challenge, APC such as pre-exposed DC or other regulatory cells in MALT recognize subtype-specific viral internal proteins expressed on the surface of infected cells. Upon activation, the Hg pre-exposed APC are able to produce specific cytokines for memory B and T cell activation and undefined soluble antiviral cytokine(s). The complex of factors that include subtype-specific CD8$^+$ CTL as well as non-neutralizing Ab responses and soluble antiviral cytokine(s) is able to minimize temporarily virus spread and replication, but does not clear the virus. During a second later phase, induction of virus-neutralizing (VN) Ab is required for virus clearance resulting in complete host recovery (Fig. 1).

Indeed, the two-tiered HSI explains why heterosubtypically immune mice, but not naive mice, survived a subsequent lethal challenge with a heterologous virus strain. After challenge of naive mice, primary antigen-specific CTL appear on day 3 and reach their maximal number on day 6 [32] (for review see Ref. [33]). At this time point, a lethal dose usually resulted in death of infected mice, i.e., before VN Abs are produced to clear the virus [34] (Fig. 2). After heterosubtypic challenge of immune mice, memory subtype-specific CTL differentiate into activated CTL effectors as early as 2 days after challenge [14] (possibly with help provided by pre-exposed DC). In addition to pre-existing subtype-specific Abs [14,19] differentiation of memory B cells to plasma cells subsequently increase the level of subtype-specific Abs upon challenge with heterosubtypic but not homotypic virus. Thus, subtype-specific CTL as well as Ab responses and soluble antiviral

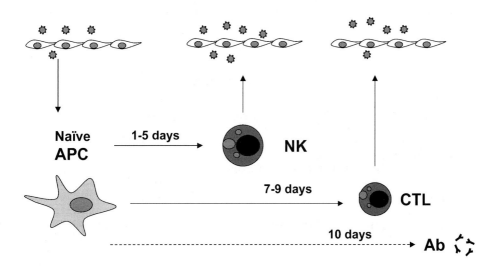

Fig. 2. Primary immune responses of naive mice to virus challenge.

factors released by pre-exposed DC suppress virus spread (but do not clear the virus) and keep the virus titer at a level similar to that observed during a primary infection with a sublethal dose. As a result, mice with HSI survive the first 7 days after the lethal challenge with heterologous virus and are comparable with naive mice receiving a sublethal dose. VN Ab responses are induced within next 7 days [34] and are responsible for complete host recovery from heterosubtypic challenge. This may explain why heterosubtypically immune mice exhibit only modest reductions in lung virus titer at day 5 after the challenge, but a significant increase in host survival [19].

In conclusion, our observations and those of others led us to postulate two-tiered HSI that provides new insight into the effector mechanisms responsible for immunity. The effectiveness of either Ab- or CTL-mediated immune responses, and possibly other additional host factors involved in the early phase of HSI, remains to be determined, and studies along these lines are underway.

Acknowledgements

This work was supported in part by US PHS grants AI 28147, AI 43197, AI 18958, P30DK54781, T32 AI 07150 and T32 HL 07553, and contracts AI 65298 and AI 65299.

References

[1] L. Simonson, L.B. Schonberger, D.F. Stroup, N.H. Arden, N.J. Cox, The impact of influenza on mortality in the USA, in: L.E. Brown, A.W. Hampson, R.G. Webster (Eds.), Options for the Control of Influenza III, Elsevier, Amsterdam, 1996, pp. 26–33.

[2] R.G. Webster, B.A. Askonas, Cross-protection and cross-reactive cytotoxic T cells induced by influenza virus vaccines in mice, Eur. J. Immunol. 10 (1980) 396–401.

[3] J.L. Schulman, E.D. Kilbourne, Induction of partial specific heterotypic immunity in mice by a single infection with influenza virus, J. Bacteriol. 89 (1965) 170–174.

[4] P.M. Taylor, J. Davey, K. Howland, J.B. Rothbard, B.A. Askonas, Class I MHC molecules rather than other mouse genes dictate influenza epitope recognition by cytotoxic T cells, Immunogenetics 26 (1987) 267–272.

[5] A.R.M. Townsend, A.J. McMichael, N.P. Carter, J.A. Huddleston, G.G. Brownlee, Cytotoxic T cell recognition of the influenza nucleoprotein and hemagglutinin expressed in transfected mouse L cells, Cell 9 (1984) 13–25.

[6] D.C. Wraith, A.E. Vessey, B.A. Askonas, Purified influenza virus nucleoprotein protects mice from lethal infection, J. Gen. Virol. 68 (1987) 433–440.

[7] J.W. Yewdell, J.R. Bennink, G.L. Smith, B. Moss, Influenza virus nucleoprotein is a major target antigen for cross-reactive anti-influenza A virus cytotoxic T lymphocytes, Proc. Natl. Acad. Sci. U. S. A. 82 (1985) 1785–1789.

[8] T.M. Fu, L. Guan, A. Friedman, T.L. Schofield, J.B. Ulmer, M.A. Liu, J.J. Donnelly, Dose dependence of CTL precursor frequency induced by a DNA vaccine and correlation with protective immunity against influenza virus challenge, J. Immunol. 162 (1999) 4163–4170.

[9] Y.L. Lin, B.A. Askonas, Biological properties of an influenza A virus-specific killer T cell clone. Inhibition of virus replication in vivo and induction of delayed-type hypersensitivity reactions, J. Exp. Med. 154 (1981) 225–234.

[10] A.E. Lukacher, V.L. Braciale, T.J. Braciale, In vivo effector function of influenza virus-specific cytotoxic T lymphocyte clones is highly specific, J. Exp. Med. 160 (1984) 814–826.

[11] P.M. Taylor, B.A. Askonas, Influenza nucleoprotein-specific cytotoxic T-cell clones are protective in vivo, Immunology 58 (1986) 417–420.

[12] M.A. Wells, S. Daniel, J.Y. Djeu, S.C. Kiley, F.A. Ennis, Recovery from a viral respiratory tract infection: IV. Specificity of protection by cytotoxic T lymphocytes, J. Immunol. 130 (1983) 2908–2914.

[13] K.L. Yap, G.L. Ada, I.F. McKenzie, Transfer of specific cytotoxic T lymphocytes protects mice inoculated with influenza virus, Nature 273 (1978) 238–239.

[14] H.H. Nguyen, Z. Moldoveanu, M.J. Novak, F.W. van Ginkel, E. Ban, H. Kiyono, J.R. McGhee, J. Mestecky, Heterosubtypic immunity to lethal influenza A virus infection is associated with virus-specific CD8(+) cytotoxic T lymphocyte responses induced in mucosa-associated tissues, Virology 254 (1999) 50–60.

[15] C.M. Lawson, J.R. Bennink, N.P. Restifo, J.W. Yewdell, B.R. Murphy, Primary pulmonary cytotoxic T lymphocytes induced by immunization with a vaccinia virus recombinant expressing influenza A virus nucleoprotein peptide do not protect mice against challenge, J. Virol. 68 (1994) 3505–3511.

[16] S. Liang, K. Mozdzanowska, G. Palladino, W. Gerhard, Heterosubtypic immunity to influenza type A virus in mice. Effector mechanisms and their longevity, J. Immunol. 152 (1994) 1653–1661.

[17] B.S. Bender, W.E. Bell, S. Taylor, P.A. Small Jr, Class I major histocompatibility complex-restricted cytotoxic T lymphocytes are not necessary for heterotypic immunity to influenza, J. Infect. Dis. 170 (1994) 1195–1200.

[18] M. Eichelberger, W. Allan, M. Zijlstra, R. Jaenisch, P.C. Doherty, Clearance of influenza virus respiratory infection in mice lacking class I major histocompatibility complex-restricted CD8+ T cells, J. Exp. Med. 174 (1991) 875–880.

[19] S.L. Epstein, C.Y. Lo, J.A. Misplon, C.M. Lawson, B.A. Hendrickson, E.E. Max, K. Subbarao, Mechanisms of heterosubtypic immunity to lethal influenza A virus infection in fully immunocompetent, T cell-depleted, beta 2-microglobulin-deficient, and J chain-deficient mice, J. Immunol. 158 (1997) 1222–1230.

[20] H.H. Nguyen, F.W. van Ginkel, H.L. Vu, J.R. McGhee, J. Mestecky, Heterosubtypic immunity to Influenza A virus infection requires B cells, but not CD8+ cytotoxic T lymphocytes (CTL), J. Infect. Dis. 183 (2001) 368–376.

[21] W. Gerhard, K. Mozdzanowska, M. Furchner, The nature of heterosubtypic immunity, in: L.E. Brown, A.W. Hampson, R.G. Webster (Eds.), Options or the Control of Influenza III, Elsevier, Amsterdam, 1996, pp. 235–243.

[22] K. Mozdzanowska, K. Maiese, M. Furchner, W. Gerhard, Treatment of influenza virus-infected SCID mice with nonneutralizing antibodies specific for the transmembrane proteins matrix 2 and neuraminidase reduces the pulmonary virus titer but fails to clear the infection, Virology 254 (1999) 138–146.

[23] S.L. Epstein, C.Y. Lo, J.A. Misplon, J.R. Bennink, Mechanism of protective immunity against influenza virus infection in mice without antibodies, J. Immunol. 160 (1998) 322–327.

[24] M.B. Graham, T.J. Braciale, Influenza virus clearance in B lymphocyte deficient mice, in: L.E. Brown, A.W. Hampson, R.G. Webster (Eds.), Options for the Control of Influenza III, Elsevier, Amsterdam, 1996, pp. 166–169.

[25] M.B. Graham, T.J. Braciale, Resistance to and recovery from lethal influenza virus infection in B lymphocyte-deficient mice, J. Exp. Med. 186 (1997) 2063–2068.

[26] K. Mozdzanowska, M. Furchner, G. Washko, J. Mozdzanowski, W. Gerhard, A pulmonary influenza virus infection in SCID mice can be cured by treatment with hemagglutinin-specific antibodies that display very low virus-neutralizing activity in vitro, J. Virol. 71 (1997) 4347–4355.

[27] K. Mozdzanowska, M. Furchner, K. Maiese, W. Gerhard, CD4+ T cells are ineffective in clearing a pulmonary infection with influenza type A virus in the absence of B cells, Virology 239 (1997) 217–225.

[28] D.J. Topham, P.C. Doherty, Clearance of an influenza A virus by CD4+ T cells is inefficient in the absence of B cells, J. Virol. 72 (1998) 882–885.

[29] P.C. Doherty, D.J. Topham, R.A. Tripp, R.D. Cardin, J.W. Brooks, P.G. Stevenson, Effector CD4+ and CD8+ T-cell mechanisms in the control of respiratory virus infections, Immunol. Rev. 159 (1997) 105–117.

[30] H.H. Nguyen, F.W. van Ginkel, H.L. Vu, M.J. Novak, J.R. McGhee, J. Mestecky, IFN-gamma is not required for mucosal cytotoxic T lymphocyte responses or heterosubtypic immunity (HSI) to influenza A virus infection, J. Virol. 74 (2000) 5495–5501.

[31] D. Qin, J. Wu, K.A. Vora, J.V. Ravetch, A.K. Szakal, T. Manser, J.G. Tew, Fc gamma receptor IIB on follicular dendritic cells regulates the B cell recall response, J. Immunol. 164 (2000) 6268–6275.

[32] K.L. Yap, G.L. Ada, Cytotoxic T cells in the lungs of mice infected with influenza A virus, Scand. J. Immunol. 7 (1978) 73–80.

[33] P.C. Doherty, W. Allan, M. Eichelberger, S.R. Carding, Roles of $\alpha\beta$ and $\gamma\delta$ T cell subsets in viral immunity, Annu. Rev. Immunol. 10 (1992) 123–1151.

[34] R.A. Yetter, S. Lehrer, R. Ramphal, P.A.J. Small, Outcome of influenza infection: effect of site of initial infection and heterotypic immunity, Infect. Immun. 29 (1980) 654–662.

International Congress Series 1219 (2001) 341–345

Lack of cross-protection between European H1N1 and H1N2 swine influenza viruses

Kristien Van Reeth*, Sophie De Clercq, Maurice Pensaert

Laboratory of Virology, Faculty of Veterinary Medicine, Ghent University, Salisburylaan 133, 9820 Merelbeke, Belgium

Abstract

Background: Swine influenza viruses (SIVs) of H1N2 subtype have recently become established in several European countries, and they cocirculate with H1N1 and H3N2 viruses. The H1N2 virus haemagglutinin (HA) appears to be of human origin and fails to cross-react with avian-like H1N1 SIVs in vitro. This study examines whether in vivo cross-protection occurs between H1N1 and H1N2 viruses isolated in Belgium. *Methods*: Influenza virus-seronegative pigs were inoculated first with Sw/Gent/7625/99 (H1N2) or Sw/Belgium/1/98 (H1N1), or left uninoculated. Four weeks later, all pigs were challenged with the H1N2 virus. We examined H1N2 antibody titres prior to challenge, and clinical signs and virus replication after challenge. *Results*: H1N2 antibodies were found exclusively in the pigs previously infected with H1N2, and these were protected against disease and infection. Fever and respiratory signs typical of H1N2 infection developed in the challenge control pigs and the H1N1-immune pigs. In both groups, all pigs had H1N2 virus in the lungs at 24 h and in nasal swabs during the first week after challenge. In H1N1-immune pigs, however, the mean virus titre in the lungs was 1.9 $\log_{10}$ EID_{50}/g lower than in the challenge controls. Similarly, the total amount of virus excreted was significantly reduced and virus excretion was on the average 1.4 days shorter. *Conclusions*: Pigs immune after H1N1 subtype infection are not protected against H1N2 infection and disease. This is in agreement with the antigenic difference in the HAs of these viruses. Our data, however, suggest partial heterosubtypic immunity between H1N1 and H1N2, which may be mediated by the cytotoxic T lymphocyte response. © 2001 Elsevier Science B.V. All rights reserved.

Keywords: Swine influenza; Virus subtypes; Cross-immunity; Pigs; Virus replication; Disease

1. Introduction

A novel influenza A virus subtype, H1N2, has been associated with swine influenza outbreaks in Great Britain since 1994 [1]. This virus is probably a double genetic

---

* Corresponding author. Tel.: +32-9-264-73-66; fax: +32-9-264-74-95.
E-mail address: kristien.vanreeth@rug.ac.be (K. Van Reeth).

reassortant, with the haemagglutinin (HA) gene of human H1N1 viruses from the early 1980s, the neuraminidase (NA) gene of 'human-like' swine H3N2 viruses and the internal protein genes of 'avian-like' swine H1N1 viruses [2]. Starting in 1998, similar H1N2 viruses have been diagnosed in Italy, France and Belgium, and they may already be widespread in other European countries [3,4]. Swine H1N2 viruses in Europe coexist with avian-like H1N1 and human-like H3N2 viruses and, importantly, there is growing evidence that all three subtypes are pathogenic [1,3,5]. There is no cross-protection between H1N1 and H3N2 and these subtypes can sequentially hit a swine herd. It is less clear, however, whether cross-protection exists between H1N1 and H1N2. These viruses are of the same HA subtype, but they show little, if any, cross-reaction in haemagglutination-inhibition (HI) tests. Still, the in vivo immune response to influenza infection is complex and the true impact of antigenic variation has to be addressed by in vivo challenge studies. Here, we have studied clinical and virological protection against Sw/Gent/7625/99 (H1N2) challenge in pigs immune against a prototype avian-like H1N1 influenza virus.

2. Materials and methods

Nineteen conventional pigs were used. At the age of 15 weeks, six pigs (H1N2–H1N2 group) were inoculated intranasally with 7.0 $\log_{10}$ EID_{50} of the Sw/Gent/7625/99 (H1N2) virus, seven pigs (H1N1–H1N2 group) were inoculated similarly with the Sw/Belgium/1/98 (H1N1) virus, and six pigs (H1N2 challenge controls) were left uninoculated. Four weeks later, all pigs were challenged intranasally (7.0 $\log_{10}$ EID_{50}) and intratracheally (7.5 $\log_{10}$ EID_{50}) with the Sw/Gent/7625/99 (H1N2) isolate. All pigs were monitored for HI antibody titres to H1N1 and H1N2 subtypes before challenge, and for body temperatures and respiratory signs at 24 h post challenge (h PC). Three pigs from each group were euthanized 24 h PC for virus titration of lung tissue homogenates. In the remaining three (H1N2 challenge controls and H1N2–H1N2 group) or four (H1N1–H1N2 group) pigs, nasal swabs were collected daily between 0 and 7 days (d) PC and used in virus titrations.

HI tests were performed with 0.5% chicken erythrocytes according to standard procedures. Due to the different pretreatments of sera in H1N1 and H1N2 (treatment with a receptor destroying enzyme) serology, starting dilutions were 1:4 and 1:20, respectively. Virus titrations were performed by inoculation in the allantoic cavity of 10-day-old embryonated hens' eggs.

3. Results

3.1. Serology at challenge

Pigs were negative for antibodies against Sw/Belgium/1/98 (H1N1) and Sw/Gent/7625/99 (H1N2) at the start of the experiment. At the time of the H1N2 challenge, the control group was still negative and the H1N2–H1N2 (anti-H1N2 titres 80–320) and H1N1–

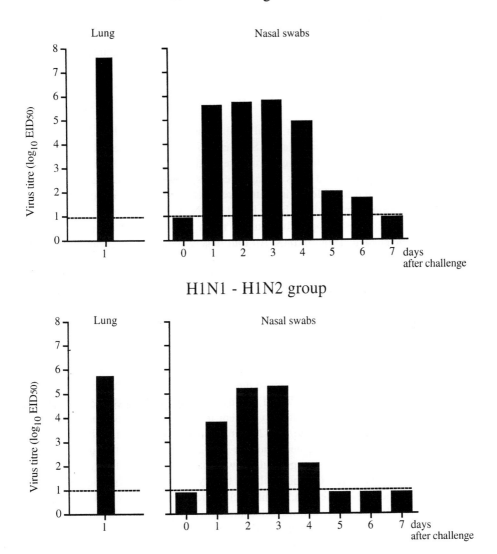

Fig. 1. H1N2 influenza virus titres in lungs and nasal swabs of challenge control pigs and pigs immune against H1N1. Virus was undetectable in the homologous challenge group (not shown). Data represent means of at least three pigs. Virus titres are expressed per g lung tissue and per 100 mg nasal secrete. Detection limits were $10^{1.1}$ EID_{50}/g lung tissue and $10^{0.9}$ EID_{50}/100 mg nasal secrete.

H1N2 groups (anti-H1N1 titres 16–128) only had antibodies against the strain with which they had been inoculated 4 weeks earlier.

3.2. Clinical protection

Twenty-four hours after the H1N2 challenge, fever (body temperature * (40°C) and laboured abdominal breathing were recorded in three and four of the six challenge control pigs, respectively. In contrast, all six pigs of the H1N2–H1N2 group showed evidence of clinical protection. Morbidity rates and disease severities in the H1N1–H1N2 group were similar to those in the challenge controls, with prominent fever and breathing difficulties in six and five of the seven pigs, respectively.

3.3. Virological protection

Virus isolated from lung tissue or nasal swabs was identified as H1N2 influenza by using monospecific swine serum against Sw/Gent/7625/99. The three H1N2 challenge control pigs sacrificed 24 h PC had high virus titres in their lungs (mean 7.6 $\log_{10}$ EID$_{50}$/g) (Fig. 1). All three pigs excreted virus during five consecutive days PC, and 1/3 pigs was still virus-positive at 6 d PC. Mean virus titres were between 4.9 and 5.8 $\log_{10}$ EID$_{50}$/100 mg nasal secrete from 1 until 4 d PC. In the H1N1–H1N2 group, the lungs of all three pigs euthanized 24 h PC were virus-positive, but the mean virus titre (5.7 $\log_{10}$ EID$_{50}$/g) was lower than in the challenge control pigs. All four pigs excreted virus 1, 2 and 3 d PC, but only 3/4 and 1/4 pigs were virus-positive at 4 and 5 d PC, respectively. Mean virus titres in nasal secretions were comparable to those in the challenge controls at 2 and 3 d PC (5.2–5.3 $\log_{10}$ EID$_{50}$/100 mg), but lower thereafter.

4. Discussion

This study demonstrates that pigs immune after infection with an avian-like H1N1 influenza virus still excrete large amounts of the H1N2 virus upon challenge. What's more, H1N1 immune pigs were not protected against H1N2-induced disease. Neutralizing antibodies against the HA are essential to prevent influenza virus infection. The lack of cross-protection between H1N1 and H1N2, therefore, is in agreement with the antigenic difference in their HAs. On the other hand, the H1N2 virus titres in the lungs and nasal swabs of H1N1-immune pigs were generally lower than in H1N2 challenge controls, and virus excretion was shortened. One possibility is that cytotoxic T lymphocytes, which have been primed by the H1N1 infection, facilitate clearance of H1N2-infected cells from the respiratory tract. Interestingly, cell-mediated immunity is primarily directed against the more conserved internal viral proteins and frequently cross-reactive between different subtypes [6].

It remains to be seen whether a previous H3N2 infection can influence the replication of H1N2. The NA antigen is closely related in H1N2 and H3N2 [2] and, though less important than the HA in immunity, anti-neuraminidase antibodies may affect the spread of virus. Overall, however, our data further support the notion that pigs may experience infection and, theoretically, disease with three different influenza viruses throughout their lifetime. The emergence of a third virus subtype in the European swine population has implications for diagnosis and vaccination.

Acknowledgements

This work was supported by the Belgian Ministry of Agriculture and the Fund for Scientific Research (FWO)-Flanders (postdoctoral fellowship K. Van Reeth). The authors thank Lieve Sys and Fernand De Backer for excellent technical assistance.

References

[1] I.H. Brown, P. Chakraverty, P.A. Harris, D.J. Alexander, Disease outbreaks in pigs in Great Britain due to an influenza A virus of H1N2 subtype, Vet. Rec. 136 (1995) 328–329.

[2] I.H. Brown, P.A. Harris, J.W. McCauley, D.J. Alexander, Multiple genetic reassortment of avian and human influenza A viruses in European pigs, resulting in the emergence of an H1N2 virus of nove genotype, J. Gen. Virol. 79 (1998) 2947–2955.

[3] M. Ferrari, A. Scalvini, E. Foni, A. Corradi, R. DiLecce, S. Gozio, E. Bignotti, G. Marruchella, Experimental infection of pigs with a H1N2 influenza virus isolated from a swine herd in Italy, Proceedings of the 4th Congress of the European Society for Veterinary Virology, August, Brescia, Italy, 2000, pp. 311–312.

[4] K. VanReeth, I.H. Brown, M. Pensaert, Isolations of H1N2 influenza A virus from pigs in Belgium, Vet. Rec. 146 (2000) 588–589.

[5] K. Van Reeth, G. Labarque, M. Pensaert, Pathogenicity of an H1N2 swine influenza virus isolated in Belgium, Proceedings of the 4th Congress of the European Society for Veterinary Virology, August, Brescia, Italy, 2000, pp. 313–314.

[6] J.L. Schulman, E.D. Kilbourne, Induction of partial specific heterotypic immunity in mice by a single infection with influenza A virus, J. Bacteriol. 85 (1965) 170–174.

International Congress Series 1219 (2001) 347–351

Analysis of influenza specific CTL responses in children using fibroblasts as stimulator and target cells

Peter F. Wright[a,*], Huan H. Nguyen[b], Mine R. Ikizler[a],
Jay A. Werkhaven[c], Sandra M. Yoder[a], Hiroshi Kiyono[b]

[a]*Division of Pediatric Infectious Diseases, Departments of Pediatrics and Microbiology and Immunology,
Respiratory Pathogens Research Unit, Vanderbilt University School of Medicine, Nashville, TN, USA*
[b]*Department of Microbiology, University of Alabama, Birmingham, AL, USA*
[c]*Department of Otolaryngology, Vanderbilt University, Nashville, TN, USA*

Abstract

Determination of cytotoxic T lymphocyte (CTL) responses in humans by traditional assays have been restricted by the volumes of blood needed and the nature of the target cells used for the assays. A number of technological advances have recently been described which improve quantitation and sensitivity of the assays. We are developing the concept of using fibroblasts as permissive targets for respiratory viruses in CTL assays. *Methods*: Fibroblasts can be grown from dispersed nasal epithelium obtained from adenoids. These cells infected with influenza are used as a stimulator layer for lymphocytes. They also can form the target for CTLs in a chromium release assay. *Results*: Comparison showed fibroblasts to be comparable to influenza infected lymphocytes as stimulators and to EBV transformed lymphocytes as targets. Cells from 25 adenoids have been explored in the fibroblast CTL system with about half of the cryoperserved peripheral blood lymphocytes showing CTL activity and mucosally associated CTLs being found in one patient. *Conclusions*: Exploration of new CTL targets that may be adapted not only to chromium release assays but to newer CTL assays offers the promise of developing a practical way of defining the CTL response in young children to natural infection and to varying immunization strategies. This may allow us to put in perspective CTLs as a correlate of immunity to influenza in humans. © 2001 Elsevier Science B.V. All rights reserved.

Keywords: CTL response; Children; Influenza A virus

* Corresponding author. Tel.: +1-615-322-2250; fax: +1-615-343-9723.
E-mail address: peter.wright@mcmail.vanderbilt.edu (P.F. Wright).

0531-5131/01/$ – see front matter © 2001 Elsevier Science B.V. All rights reserved.
PII: S 0 5 3 1 - 5 1 3 1 (0 1) 0 0 6 6 3 - X

1. Introduction

The cytotoxic T lymphocyte (CTL) response has a well-characterized role in protection against heterologous influenza challenge and in recovery from primary influenza infection in the murine model [1]. In humans, particularly in children, a CTL response has been harder to measure and interpret [2,3]. Also in question in man is the role of mucosal CTLs in the respiratory tract, although again studies in the murine model suggest their importance [4]. To determine the most effective strategy for stimulation of antigen specific CTL responses to influenza A, a traditional CTL assay using EBV transformed lymphocytes was compared with the use of autologous fibroblasts as stimulators and targets. The fibroblasts were derived from respiratory tract tissue and hence got closer to what is the physiologic CTL target, the respiratory epithelial cell, which is the sole target for influenza replication. One of the authors has previously shown that influenza CTLS will recognize antigen presented on infected murine epithelial cell line [5]. In the present study, we have shown that fibroblasts offer significant advantages in decreasing the volume of blood needed for the assay and in lowering background chromium release. Using fibroblasts and mucosal associated lymphocytes obtained from children at the time of adenoidectomy, CTLs could be demonstrated from about 50% of cryopreserved peripheral blood mononuclear cells from young children and were present, though less frequently, in adenoidal lymphocytes.

2. Methods

With approval of the Vanderbilt Institutional Review Board, adenoidal tissue and 5 cm^3 of heparinized peripheral blood (PBMC) were obtained at the time of previously scheduled adenoidectomy for established medical indications in 25 children. Fibroblasts were prepared from dispersed epithelial tissue, grown to confluency and subsequently passaged in MEM with 10% fetal bovine serum. Lymphocytes were cryopreserved after separation on a Ficoll–Hypaque gradient. Stimulation using fibroblasts was carried at in 24-well plates with fibroblasts infected with A/Udorn (H3N2) or A/PR8 (HINI). After initiation of infection the cells were irradiated and PBMC or adenoidal lymphocytes were added at a ratio of 20:1 for secondary stimulation. IL-2 was added on day 3 and the total stimulation interval was 6 days, after which the cells were washed and tested in a ^{51}Cr release assay as previously described [5]. In brief, fibroblasts were seeded in a 96-well plate and infected with influenza A/Udorn or A/PR8. The cells were labeled with chromium overnight and the stimulated lymphocytes added as effector cells in effector to target, E/T, ratios anging from 20:1 to 5:1 for 4 h after which specific ^{51}Cr release was calculated and compared to maximum release using Triton X-100. This assay format was compared to that using Epstein–Barr virus, EBV, transformed lymphocytes as targets.

3. Results

It was initially shown that the fibroblasts of respiratory origin had extensive and uniform expression of influenza proteins although infectious virus was not released and

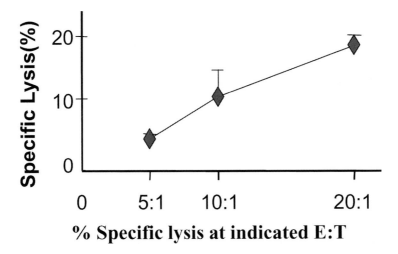

% Specific lysis at indicated E:T

Fig. 1. Reproducibility of the CTL assay based on fibroblasts as stimulators and targets from a single adult's PBMC. The mean values are shown with the standard deviation of four to six determinations.

cytopathic effect was minimal. The assay using fibroblasts and stimulators and targets was highly reproducible with adult peripheral blood lymphocytes (Fig. 1). The use of fibroblasts was compared with infected PBMC from the same individual as stimulators and with autologous EBV-transformed B cells as target cells. The irradiated fibroblasts were as effective as autologous lymphocytes in stimulating a secondary CTL response. The fibroblasts were also as sensitive as EBV transformed lymphocytes as targets and had a lower nonspecific release of chromium.

The assay was then undertaken with 25 consecutive attempts at deriving fibroblasts and systemic and mucosal lymphocytes from children undergoing adenoidectomy. The children averaged 4 years of age and all but one had experienced infection with one or more influenza A strains based on HAI antibody. The success in obtaining fibroblasts and viable lymphocytes from adenoids and from the small available volume, 5 ml or less, of peripheral blood is shown in Table 1. Adequate viability of lymphocytes from adenoids depended on their prompt separation from the tissue after surgery, a factor in the lower success initially with this tissue.

Table 1
Success in establishing influenza specific CTL assays in children

	PBMC	Adenoids
Total number of subjects	25	25
Number of successfully studied	17	12
Non-viable fibroblasts	5	5
Low lymphocyte viability[a]	–	6
Other technical problems	3	2

[a] Initial problems with viability until adenoid lymphocytes promptly separated and frozen.

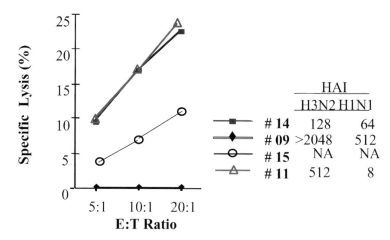

Fig. 2. Cytotoxicity of PBMC from four children using fibroblasts as stimulators and targets. The serum HAI titers are indicated where available.

Fig. 2 demonstrates the dose response by E/T ratio in three children with CTLs and the negative response seen in one child who had serologic evidence of past influenza. Overall CTLs with a specific immune release of > 10% were seen in PBMC from 8/17 children successfully tested but in only 1/12 adenoidal lymphocytes. In this individual, there was a very clear response with a SIR of 32% with an E/T ratio of 20:1. In three instances there were positive CTLs in the peripheral blood and not in the adenoidal lymphocytes in seropositive children. The seronegative child had neither systemic nor local CTL responses.

4. Discussion

The detection of influenza specific CTLs in children has been difficult for technical reasons and thus it has been impossible to put into perspective their role in protection from influenza or in resolution of infection. The heterologous immunity so well defined in the murine model has thus remained a supposition in man. Indeed, the virologic and immunologic response to a live, attenuated influenza vaccine was almost indistinguishable between naïve children and those with prior heterologous infection [6]. As different vaccine approaches to the prevention of influenza are developed, e.g. live, attenuated intranasal vaccine, a comparison of the complexity of the humoral, cell-mediated and mucosal immune response at the local and systemic level is needed to derive correlates of immunity.

The current report defines a secondary CTL response in the PBMCs of young children (average age 4 years) at intervals that are indeterminately removed from their naturally acquired influenza. A response in adenoidal lymphocytes appears to be seen less frequently but was detectable in a single individual of 12 tested. CD8-T lymphocytes are seen in the intraepithelial and subepithelial layers of adenoids but constitute only about 6% of the mucosal cells in the adenoid [7].

There are steps in validation of the assay that remain to be undertaken including demonstrating that the response is uniquely CD-8 mediated, influenza A restricted, and HLA restricted. Ultimately newer CTL techniques such as intracellular cytokines, interferon gamma Elispots and tetramer technology with mapping of peptide epitopes might be undertaken using this system. Meanwhile, fibroblasts have been shown to offer significant advantages over autologous lymphocytes as stimulators and EBV transformed lymphocytes as targets in a CTL assay adaptable to use in children.

Future directions of our research will be towards the detection of specific CTL immune responses in adenoid lymphocytes and PBMC in children intentionally immunized with live, attenuated influenza vaccine prior to adenoidectomy and to compare the PBMC CTL response in seronegative children receiving inactivated parenteral or live intranasal influenza vaccine.

Acknowledgements

The support for the Respiratory Pathogens Research Unit by NIAID contract NO1-AI-65298 is gratefully acknowledged.

References

[1] P.C. Doherty, D.J. Topham, R.A. Tripp, R.D. Cardin, J.W. Brooks, P.G. Stevenson, Effector CD4+ and CD8+ T-cell mechanisms in the control of respiratory virus infections, Immunol. Rev. 159 (1997) 105–117.

[2] A.J. McMichael, F.M. Gotch, Recognition of influenza A virus by human cytotoxic T lymphocytes, Adv. Exp. Med. Biol. 257 (1989) 109–114.

[3] I.N. Mbawuike, P.A. Piedra, T.R. Cate, R.B. Couch, Cytotoxic T lymphocyte responses of infants after natural infection or immunization with live cold-recombinant or inactivated influenza A vaccine, J. Med. Virol. 50 (1996) 105–111.

[4] H.N. Nguyen, Z. Moldoveanu, M.J. Nokav, F.W. van Ginkel, E. Ban, H. Kiyono, J.R. McGhee, J. Mestecky, Heterosubtypic immunity to lethal influenza A virus infection is associated with virus-specific cytotoxic T lymphocyte reponses induced in mucosa-associated tissues, Virology 254 (1999) 50–60.

[5] H.N. Nguyen, P.N. Boyaka, Z. Moldoveanu, M.J. Novak, H. Kiyono, J.R. McGhee, J. Mestecky, Influenza virus-infected epithelial cells present viral antigens to antigen-specific CD8+ cytotoxic T lymphocytes, J. Virol. 72 (1998) 4534–4536.

[6] P.F. Wright, P.R. Johnson, D.T. Karzon, Clinical experience with live, attenuated vaccines in children. Options of the control of Influenza, in: A.P. Kendal, P.A. Patriarca (Eds.), UCLA Symposia on Molecular and Cellular Biology 36 (1986) 243–253.

[7] P.N. Boyaka, P.F. Wright, M. Marinaro, H. Kiyono, J.E. Johnson, R. Gonzales, M.R. Ikizler, J.A. Werkhaven, R.J. Jackson, K. Fujihashi, S. Di Fabio, H.F. Staats, J.R. McGhee, Human nasoparygeal-associated lymphoreticular tissues: functional analysis of subepithelial and intraepithelial B and T cells from adenoids and tonsils, Am. J. Pathol. (In press).

International Congress Series 1219 (2001) 353–359

The basal level of influenza specific antibody-secreting cells in healthy subjects

Karl Albert Brokstad[a,*], Rebecca Jane Cox[b],
Jens-Christian Eriksson[c], Jan Olofsson[c], Roland Jonsson[a],
Åke Davidsson[a,c,d]

[a]*Broegelmann Research Laboratory, University of Bergen, Armauer Hansen Bldg., N-5021 Bergen, Norway*
[b]*Department of Molecular Biology, University of Bergen, Bergen, Norway*
[c]*Department of Otolaryngology/Head and Neck Surgery, Haukeland University Hospital, Bergen, Norway*
[d]*Department of Otolaryngology, Örebro Medical Centre Hospital, Örebro, Sweden*

Abstract

Background: In the absence of true efficacy markers, the serum haemagglutination inhibition titre has been correlated with protection against influenza infection. Serum antibody does not, however, play a direct role in protection against infection. Two important factors that may be involved in protection against influenza infection are the number of influenza specific activated B-cells and the specificity of the secreted antibodies in the epithelial mucosa of the respiratory tract. *Methods*: Nineteen patients scheduled for tonsillectomy were enrolled in this study. Tonsils, blood, saliva and a biopsy from the inferior turbinate in the nasal cavity were collected from the patients. None of the patients had been infected or vaccinated with influenza in the previous year. ELISPOT and ELISA assays were used to examine the basal level of antibody-secreting cell (ASC) levels and antibodies in the collected samples, respectively. *Results*: We found low numbers of influenza specific ASC in the blood and tonsils, but there were much higher numbers of specific ASC in the nasal tissue despite no recent influenza exposure or vaccination. *Conclusion*: We found antibody-secreting B-cells in the nasal mucosa tissue, which probably results in secretion of specific antibody at the mucosal surfaces and protection from influenza infection. © 2001 Elsevier Science B.V. All rights reserved.

Keywords: Basal level; ASC; Protection

---

[*] Corresponding author. Tel.: +47-55-97-46-22; fax: +47-55-97-58-17.
E-mail address: karl.brokstad@gades.uib.no (K.A. Brokstad).

0531-5131/01/$ – see front matter © 2001 Elsevier Science B.V. All rights reserved.
PII: S0531-5131(01)00346-6

1. Introduction

The majority of human pathogens initiate infection via the mucosal surfaces. Mucosal immunity of the upper respiratory tract confers the first line of defence against a number of pathogens of both viral and bacterial origin. Concurrently, this local immune system is also central in development of allergic reactions, tolerance and in some instances, autoimmune disease. The quantity of foreign antigens and micro-organisms passing through the mouth and upper respiratory tract every day is enormous and has to be dealt with by an effective natural and acquired immune system. The tonsils and nasal associated lymphoid tissue (NALT) play an important role in trapping foreign antigens, neutralising them and inducing local immune reactions. After immune stimulation, a high number of immune-competent cells leave the lymph nodes and home to the mucosal surfaces in the upper respiratory tract to fight invading pathogens.

Influenza is a major respiratory pathogen causing high morbidity in the general population and high mortality in high-risk groups. Despite the fact that most pathogens enter the body via the mucosal route, the majority of vaccines are administered parenterally. Mucosal immunity mediated by secretory IgA (SIgA) and or systemic IgG is associated with protection from influenza. We have previously used parenterally administered influenza vaccine as a model to investigate the systemic and local immune responses induced after influenza vaccination in healthy human volunteers [1–5]. The local immune response was examined in tonsils and oral fluid by vaccinating subjects at various time intervals prior to tonsillectomy. We have shown a rapid homing of influenza specific B-cells to the tonsils after influenza vaccination [2]. We found that parenteral influenza vaccination induced a significant IgA response in peripheral blood, which correlated with the appearance of IgA producing B-cells in the tonsils and SIgA in the oral fluid of adults.

The aim of this study was to examine the basal level of influenza specific ASC in blood (circulation, periphery), in tonsils (local lymphoid organ) and in nasal tissue (local mucosa).

2. Material and methods

2.1. Patients and samples

Nineteen patients (9 males and 10 females, mean age 28 years) scheduled for tonsillectomy at the Department of Otolaryngology at Haukeland University Hospital, Bergen were enrolled in this study. All patients fulfilled the medical criteria for tonsillectomy, but were otherwise healthy with no acute bacterial infection of the tonsils, no history of allergy and no known influenza infection in the previous year. Tonsils, a biopsy sample from the mid-portion of the caudal medial part of the inferior turbinate, peripheral blood and oral fluid (Orasure, Epitope, Beaverton, USA) were collected. This study was approved by the Regional Ethical Committee.

2.2. Influenza virus antigens

Purified surface glycoproteins were from the following viruses; A/New Caledonia/20/99 (H1N1); A/Panama/2007/99 (H3N2) and B/Yamanashi/166/98 were used as antigens in the ELISA and ELISPOT. These purified HA antigens were a generous gift from Medeva Pharma (Surrey, UK). Viruses (A/Beijing/262/95 (H1N1); A/Sydney/5/97 (H3N2) and B/Yamanashi/166/98) were propagated in embryonated hen eggs and used in the haemagglutination inhibition test (HI).

2.3. Immunological tests

Lymphocytes were isolated from the blood, tonsils and nasal tissue using Lymphoprep (Nycomed Pharma, Oslo, Norway) and were analysed by the ELISPOT method [2]. Antibodies in the oral fluid and serum were quantified by ELISA [2]. All capture and detector antibodies were purchased from Sigma (St. Louis, MO, USA). In addition, the level of serum antibody to the test viruses was analysed by the HI test [1].

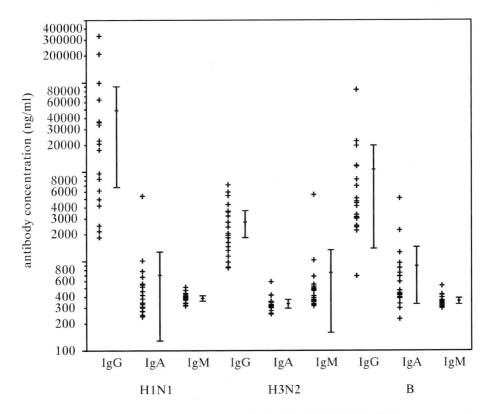

Fig. 1. The influenza specific serum antibody concentrations in 19 healthy individuals. The data are presented as the individual serum antibody concentrations (ng/ml) of the three major subtypes of immunoglobulin to the current influenza viruses. The bars represent the mean and standard deviation, and n is the number of subjects.

3. Results

The 19 subjects had not had an episode of tonsilitis for at least 3 months prior to operation, had no history of allergy and had not experienced influenza infection during the previous year. Blood samples from the subjects were analysed for immunoglobulin levels and allergy at the routine laboratory at the hospital and the tests confirmed the healthy status of the volunteers (data not shown).

3.1. Serum antibody levels

All subjects had haemagglutination inhibition test (HI) titers below the level of detection (<10) to the H1N1 and B viruses (data not shown). A serum titer equal or above 40 HI units has been correlated with protection against influenza infection. Nine subjects had detectable HI titers (>10) to the H3N2 virus, but only two of these subjects had protective levels. These results indicate that the subjects had not recently been infected with influenza, which otherwise may have had an adverse effect on the study.

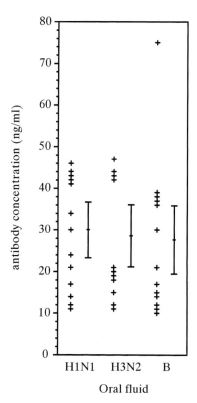

Fig. 2. The influenza specific antibody concentrations in the oral fluid of 19 healthy individuals. The data are presented as the individual antibody concentrations (ng/ml) in the oral fluid to the current influenza viruses. The bars represent the mean and standard deviation.

The serum antibody levels assayed by the ELISA method (Fig. 1) shows the presence of the three main immunoglobulin (Ig) subtypes (IgG, IgA and IgM) to the influenza surface glycoproteins in all subjects. The mean IgG titers varies between 2800 ng/ml to the H3N2 virus and 49,000 ng/ml to the H1N1 virus. The mean titers for IgA and IgM varies between 340 and 890 ng/ml. The overall serum response is lowest to the H3N2 virus. An explanation for this might be that the H3N2 virus has undergone more extensive drift than the other viruses. These serum antibodies are comparable with the pre-vaccination levels reported in our previous work [2], except for the IgG response to the H1N1 virus, which is higher, due to a high base level in a few subjects.

3.2. Oral fluid antibody levels

Due to the limitation of available oral fluid, the samples were only tested for total Ig levels, although we know from previous work that it mainly contains the IgA subclass,

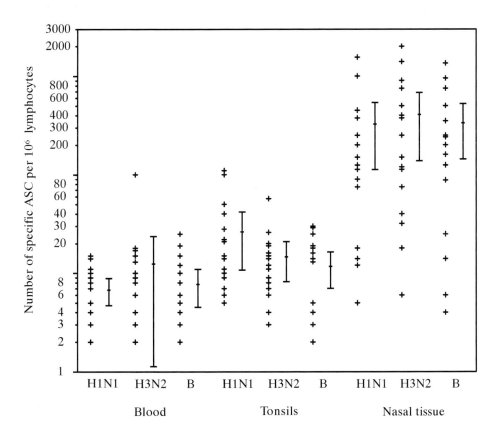

Fig. 3. The basal level of influenza specific ASC in 18 healthy individuals. The graph shows the individual number of specific ASC per 10^6 lymphocytes for the blood, tonsils and nasal tissue to the current influenza viruses. The bars represent the mean and standard deviation.

specifically IgA1 [3]. We found a low but detectable basal level of anti-influenza antibodies in the oral fluid (Fig. 2). The level of influenza specific antibodies in oral fluid varies between 10 and 47 ng/ml, with one exception of 75 ng/ml, with an average of 28–30 ng/ml against the three vaccine strains. These results are also comparable with previously reported pre-vaccination levels [2,3]. Even if the antibody levels in oral fluid are considerable lower than in serum, we have to consider that the serum levels represent an accumulated production over several days, while oral fluid level represent the production for only a very short time period.

3.3. Influenza specific antibody-secreting cells (ASC)

Fig. 3 shows the level of influenza specific ASC in blood (circulation), tonsils (lymphoid organ) and nasal tissue (mucosa) against the influenza strains. We tested only for total Ig due to limited sample material. The level of influenza specific ASC in blood and tonsils are low and similar to what we have reported previously [2]. The detected number of influenza specific ASC in blood and tonsils varied from 2 to 110 per million lymphocytes, with an average of 7–12 in blood, and slightly higher with an average of 12–26 cells in the tonsils. The number of influenza specific ASC in the nasal tissue are from 10 to 100 times higher than in blood or tonsils, with an average between 327 and 410 cells per million lymphocytes. If the number of influenza specific ASC in the nasal tissue are related to the total area of mucosa surface in the upper respiratory tract, this may represent an incredible army of anti-influenza B-cells.

4. Discussion

With the lack of proper markers, the serum haemagglutination inhibition titre has been correlated with protection against influenza infection. Serum antibodies do not play a direct role in protection against influenza infection on upper respiratory tract infection. What are the factors which result in susceptibility or protection from influenza infection? Two important factors which may be involved in protection against influenza infection are the number of influenza specific activated B-cells and the specificity (affinity/avidity) of the secreted antibodies in the epithelial mucosa of the respiratory tract.

In previous vaccination studies, we have observed a low but detectable level of influenza specific B-cells and immunoglobulins prior to vaccination in blood and tonsils [2]. The methodological difficulties involved in assessing the immune response in the upper airway mucosa have resulted in a paucity of data on the local antibody secreting cell response to influenza virus infection or vaccination.

In this study, we have detected a considerable level of activated influenza specific B-cells in the nasal mucosal tissue in a period of low influenza activity. These high levels, which are 10–100 times higher than in blood and tonsils, are probably more or less constant throughout the whole year and not dependent on influenza stimulation. The constant production of secretory antibodies probably has an important role in protecting an individual from influenza infection. The level of antibodies in oral fluid are apparently low, but the accumulated production of secreted anti-influenza antibodies represent an impressive protection mechanism against infection.

We hypothesise that not only is the match (affinity/avidity) between the produced antibodies virus important for influenza protection, but also the overall basal level of activated influenza specific B-cells in the mucosa of the upper respiratory tract and the level of secreted influenza specific SIgA. These levels may drop gradually after several years without a proper local stimulation (infection) and make the subject more vulnerable to influenza infection.

Acknowledgements

We would like to thank Lars R. Haaheim for valuable discussion, Turid Tynning and Hilde Garverg for technical assistance, and the Norwegian Research Council for financial support. Special thanks go to Medeva Pharma for providing the purified influenza virus antigens.

References

[1] R.J. Cox, K.A. Brokstad, M.A. Zuckerman, J.M. Wood, L.R. Haaheim, J.S. Oxford, An early humoral immune response in peripheral blood following parenteral inactivated influenza vaccination, Vaccine 12 (11) (1994) 993–999.
[2] K.A. Brokstad, R.J. Cox, J. Olofsson, R. Jonsson, L.R. Haaheim, Parenteral influenza vaccination induces a rapid systemic and local immune response, J. Infect. Dis. 171 (1) (1995) 198–203.
[3] K.A. Brokstad, R.J. Cox, J.S. Oxford, L.R. Haaheim, IgA, IgA subclasses and secretory component levels in oral fluid collected from subjects after parenteral influenza vaccination, J. Infect. Dis. 171 (4) (1995) 1072–1074.
[4] K.A. Brokstad, R.J. Cox, D. Major, J.M. Wood, L.R. Haaheim, Cross-reaction but no avidity change of the serum antibody response after influenza vaccination, Vaccine 13 (16) (1995) 1522–1528.
[5] A.S. El-Madhun, R.J. Cox, A. Søreide, J. Olofsson, L.R. Haaheim, Systemic and mucosal immune responses in young children and adults after parenteral influenza vaccination, J. Infect. Dis. 178 (1998) 933–938.

Insights into the structure and replication of the virus

International Congress Series 1219 (2001) 363–367

Changes in the HA and NA genes prior to the emergence of HPAI H7N1 avian influenza viruses in Italy

J. Banks[a,*], E.M. Speidel[a], I. Capua[b], A. Fioretti[c], A. Piccirillo[a,c], E.H. Moore[a], L. Plowright[a], D.J. Alexander[a]

[a]VLA-Weybridge Addlestone, Surrey, KT15 3NB, UK
[b]IZS, Padua, Italy
[c]Universita di Napoli, Italy

Abstract

Background: Outbreaks of avian influenza due to an H7N1 virus of low pathogenicity (LP) occurred in domestic poultry in Northern Italy from May 1999 until December 1999 when a highly pathogenic avian influenza (HPAI) virus emerged. *Methods*: Nucleotide sequences for HA1 and the stalk region of the NA gene were determined for viruses from the outbreak. *Results*: The HPAI viruses have an unusual HA cleavage site motif, PEIPKGSRVRRGLF. Phylogenetic analysis showed that the HPAI viruses arose from LP viruses and that they are most closely related to a wild bird isolate. Additional glycosylation sites (GSs) were seen at position 149 of the HA for two separate lineages, 123 for all HPAI and some LP viruses. Other viruses had no additional GSs. All viruses from the outbreak have a 22 amino acid deletion in the NA stalk that is not present in the N1 genes of the wild bird viruses examined. *Conclusion*: The Italian HPAI viruses arose from LP strains, and additional glycosylation at the globular head of HA1, together with a deletion in the NA stalk, may be an adaptation of H7 viruses to a new host species, i.e. domestic poultry. Crown Copyright © 2001 Published by Elsevier Science B.V. All rights reserved.

Keywords: Poultry; Glycosylation; Host specificity

1. Introduction

In March 1999, an H7N1 virus of LP for chickens was isolated from turkeys in the northern region of Italy [1]. Following this initial isolation, 199 outbreaks were

---

* Corresponding author. Tel.: +44-1932-357-307; fax: +44-1932-357-239.
E-mail address: jbanks.cvl.wood@gtnet.gov.uk (J. Banks).

reported and in December 1999, a HPAI H7N1 virus was isolated. Between December 1999 and April 2000, a total of 413 HPAI outbreaks occurred in poultry in Italy. In the present study, we have analysed the molecular changes occurring in the HA1 and the NA of H7N1 AI viruses isolated prior to and during this major outbreak of HPAI in poultry.

2. Materials and methods

The complete coding sequences for the HA1 of 56 H7N1 subtype influenza viruses isolated from poultry during AI outbreaks in Italy between March 1999 and February 2000 were determined. Partial sequences on the NA gene were determined for eight Italian isolates and four other viruses held in the repository at VLA-Weybridge. Additional published HA and NA sequences were obtained from Genbank. Phylogenetic analysis was performed for the first 1000 nucleotides of the HA1 coding region [2] and is presented as an unrooted maximum likelihood phylogram, where the horizontal branch lengths are proportional to the nucleotide differences between the sequences (Fig. 1).

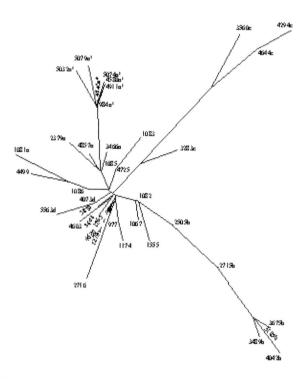

Fig. 1. Maximum likelihood phylogenetic tree for 1000 nucleotides of the HA1 of the 1999/2000 Italian H7N1 influenza viruses. Key; (a) = viruses with glycosylation site 123, (b) and (c) = viruses with glycosylation site 149, (d) = viruses with PEVPK cleavage site motif, (*) = HPAI.

3. Results

The deduced amino acid cleavage site motif obtained for the 1999 Italian LP viruses was PEIPKGRGLF, two viruses had the unusual motif PEVPKGRGLF. All the HPAI isolates had an insertion of four amino acids (underlined), giving the motif PEIPKGSRVRRGLF.

Phylogenetic analysis revealed three lineages that appear to be emerging from a common pool of viruses possibly originating from a single introduction to poultry from the wild bird reservoir. The distinguishing feature for viruses in all three lineages is the acquisition of an additional GSs at the globular head of the HA1. Viruses marked with letter 'a' in Fig. 1 all share a GSs at position 123 (H7 numbering). At the 'root' of this lineage, the viruses are LP, by the end of the lineage all the viruses are HPAI. Viruses in the other two lineages, although divergent, share the acquisition of a GS at position 149 (viruses marked 'b' and 'c' in Fig. 1), none are HPAI. Clustered around the divergence point for the lineages are viruses without additional GSs, again none are HPAI. They do, however, have a range of nucleotide or amino acid changes consistent with a pattern of non-cumulative change.

Nucleotide sequences for the region spanning the NA protein stalk were obtained for Italian viruses selected to represent viruses without additional GSs in the HA1 (the earliest isolate), viruses with GS 149, and viruses with GS 123 of both low and high pathogenicity. All eight Italian viruses shared an identical 22 amino acid deletion in the NA stalk, corresponding to amino acids 54–75, as compared with the six viruses with full-length stalks (A/fairy-bluebird/Singapore/F92/94, A/teal/Taiwan/WB2-32-2TPFE2/98, A/conure/England/766/94, A/parrot/Northern Ireland/VF-73-67/73A/waterfowl/Hong Kong/306/97, A/goose/Guangdong/1/96). Other viruses with NA stalk deletions were nine viruses from the H5N1 HPAI outbreak in Hong Kong in 1997, including the Human virus A/Hong Kong/156/97, the HPAI viruses A/ty/Eng/50-92/91 (H5N1), and A/FPV/Rostock/34 (H7N1) and the LP virus A/chicken/Taiwan/7-5/99 (H6N1), missing 19, 23, 22, and 12 amino acids, respectively.

4. Discussion

Phylogenetic analysis has shown the Italian 1999/2000 H7N1 viruses to be most closely related to a wild bird isolate A/teal/Taiwan/WB2-32-2TPFE2/98 within a group of Eurasian and South African viruses isolated since 1994 [3]. Most of the Italian outbreaks occurred in the regions of Veneto and Lombardia where 65% of Italy's intensively reared poultry population is concentrated. This area in northern Italy is on a main migratory flyway for waterfowl and these birds are probably the source for the initial introduction of LP virus to poultry.

All the 1999/2000 Italian H7N1 influenza viruses have the three GSs conserved among H7 viruses at amino acid positions 12, 28 and 231 (H7 numbering). Some have an additional GS at either amino acid position 123 or 149, both these sites lie close to the receptor binding site (RBS) in the globular head of the HA and can affect the affinity of the RBS for its cellular receptor [4]. In the phylogenetic analysis (Fig. 1), viruses without additional GSs are concentrated around the divergence point of the three main lineages. This is consistent with a pattern of non-cumulative mutations soon after the initial virus introduction into poultry, followed by divergence into lineages when the mutations become fixed [5]. Viruses with a GS at position 149 account for two branches. Acquisition of this mutation could have occurred independently or at an early stage followed by divergence. The evidence supports the former because the 'roots' and early isolates of both phylogenetic branches do not share the 149 GS. A third branch shows the progression of mutations from low to high pathogenicity with this change preceded by the acquisition of a GS at position 123. This evidence suggests that there is a selective pressure in the poultry host for acquisition of GS in the proximity of the RBS, and that these mutations occur relatively readily. Changes in glycosylation at the sites adjacent to the RBS have been reported to be an important determinant for cell tropism and host range [4,6,7].

A 22 amino acid deletion was present in the NA stalk of all eight Italian viruses examined, regardless of the pathogenicity or the GS status of the HA. This deletion results in the removal of three potential GSs from the NA. The effect this may have upon NA function is not clear, but viruses with different stalk lengths have been shown to have different growth characteristics in different host cells [6,7]. All the viruses with NA stalk deletions had a domestic poultry origin, while those with full-length stalks were isolated from wild or captive cage birds. The origin of the latter is not always known, however, most had been wild or had been in contact with wild birds. It is likely that a deletion in the NA stalk followed by the acquisition of additional glycosylation at the RBS of the HA, in the Italian viruses, is an adaptation to a new host, i.e. domestic poultry. Whether these changes also influenced the subsequent change to HPAI in the Italian viruses is unknown. The HPAI virus A/goose/Guangdong/1/96 has a long NA stalk with a 123 HA phenotype, and the H6N1 virus A/chicken/Taiwan/7-5/99 has a NA deletion suggesting that these events are probably unrelated. However, although not a prerequisite, there does seem to be a trend for viruses with the GS 123 phenotype to become HPAI.

5. Conclusion

The Italian HPAI viruses arose from non-pathogenic strains, and additional GSs at the globular head of HA1 together with a deletion in the NA stalk may be an adaptation of H7 viruses to a new host species, i.e. domestic poultry.

Acknowledgements

This work was funded by the Ministry of Agriculture Fisheries and Food UK.

References

[1] I. Capua, S. Marangon, The avian influenza epidemic in Italy, 1999–2000: a review, Avian Pathol. 29 (2000) 289–294.
[2] J. Felsenstein, Evolutionary trees from DNA sequences: a maximum likelihood approach, J. Mol. Evol. 17 (1981) 368–378.
[3] J. Banks, E.C. Speidel, J.W. McCauley, D.J. Alexander, Phylogenetic analysis of H7 haemagglutinin subtype influenza A viruses, Arch. Virol. 145 (2000) 1047–1058.

[4] M. Ohuchi, R. Ohuchi, A. Feldmann, H.D. Klenk, Regulation of receptor binding affinity of influenza virus hemagglutinin by its carbohydrate moiety, J. Virol. 71 (1997) 8377–8384.

[5] W.M. Fitch, R.M. Bush, C.A. Bender, N.J. Cox, Long term trends in the evolution of H(3) HA1 human influenza type A, Proc. Natl. Acad. Sci. U. S. A. 94 (1997) 7712–7718.

[6] J.M. Katz, M. Wang, R.G. Webster, Direct sequencing of the HA gene of influenza (H3N2) virus in original clinical samples reveals sequence identity with mammalian cell grown virus, J. Virol. 64 (1990) 1808–1811.

[7] M. Matrosovich, N. Zhou, Y. Kawaoka, R. Webster, The surface glycoproteins of H5 influenza viruses isolated from humans, chickens, and wild aquatic birds have distinguishable properties, J. Virol. 73 (1999) 1146–1155.

International Congress Series 1219 (2001) 369–374

Hemagglutinin residues of recent human A(H3N2) viruses that affect agglutination of chicken erythrocytes

Rita Medeiros, Nicolas Escriou, Nadia Naffakh, Jean-Claude Manuguerra, S. van der Werf*

Unité de Génétique Moléculaire des Virus Respiratoires, URA 1966 CNRS, Institut Pasteur 25, rue du Dr Roux, 75724 Paris Cedex 15, France

Abstract

Background: The hemagglutination remains crucial in diagnosis of influenza virus and for the antigenic characterization of the hemagglutinin (HA) and neuraminidase. However, the human influenza viruses A(H3N2) isolated recently appear to have lost the ability to agglutinate chicken erythrocytes (ER) (RBC). The molecular determinants of this phenomenon are not known. *Methods*: Two viruses isolated in Paris were studied, since their ability to agglutinate chicken RBC was observed after serial passages either in Madin Darby canine kidney (MDCK) cells or embryonated hen's eggs. Sequencing analyses and hemadsorption assays were performed to demonstrate the role of amino acid substitutions in the HA gene. *Results*: Sequencing of the HA gene revealed the presence of either the Leu194Ile or the Val226Ile mutation following the phenotypic change. Hemadsorption assays performed following transfection of COS-1 cells, with plasmids expressing wild-type or mutated HA molecules, showed that the Leu194Ile and Val226Ile mutations were responsible for the ability of the HA to bind chicken RBCs. *Conclusion*: These findings suggest that a valine at position 226 in the HA molecule, found in recent clinical isolates of human A(H3N2) viruses, could be responsible for their inability to agglutinate chicken erythrocytes. © 2001 Elsevier Science B.V. All rights reserved.

Keywords: Influenza; Hemadsorption; Receptor; Sialic acid

---

* Corresponding author. Tel.: +33-1-45-68-87-25; fax: +33-1-40-61-32-41.
E-mail address: svdwerf@pasteur.fr (S. van der Werf).

0531-5131/01/$ – see front matter © 2001 Elsevier Science B.V. All rights reserved.
PII: S 0 5 3 1 - 5 1 3 1 (0 1) 0 0 6 5 0 - 1

1. Introduction

The ability of human influenza viruses to agglutinate the erythrocytes (ER) of different animal species has been studied since its recognition in 1941 [1]. Since then, chicken, human, turkey or guinea-pig erythrocytes have commonly been used in hemagglutination assays for detection of influenza viruses and antigenic characterization of the hemagglutinin (HA) and neuraminidase glycoproteins. However, recent clinical isolates of human A(H1N1) and A(H3N2) influenza viruses appear to have lost the ability to agglutinate chicken erythrocytes. For the A(H1N1) viruses, it has been noted that changes in the presumed receptor-binding pocket are responsible for the loss of ability of recent isolates to agglutinate chicken erythrocytes [2]. Changes in the receptor-binding residues in recent influenza A(H3N2) viruses have also been noted, although the correlation between amino acid changes and binding specificity has not yet been identified [3]. On the other hand, it has been reported that agglutination properties of influenza virus isolates can be altered upon passage in embryonated chicken eggs or in MDCK cells [4,5].

Ito et al. [6] have shown that the ability of influenza viruses to agglutinate erythrocytes from different animal species correlates with their receptor specificity. Indeed, the distribution of specific sialic acids differs among animal species. For example, erythrocytes from horse and cow display mainly the sialic acid-$\alpha2,3$-galactose (SA$\alpha2,3$Gal). In contrast, those from chicken and human display both SA$\alpha2,6$Gal and SA$\alpha2,3$Gal. There are no data available about guinea-pig erythrocytes.

In this report, we present evidence that two amino acid changes in the hemagglutinin molecule are responsible for the inability of recent human A(H3N2) viruses to agglutinate chicken erythrocytes.

2. Material and methods

2.1. Viruses and cells

Human influenza A(H3N2) viruses A/Paris/906/97 and A/Paris/908/97 used in this study were isolated in Madin Darby canine kidney (MDCK) cells directly from clinical specimens and passaged 14 times in these cells or twice in embryonated eggs. The collected infectious allantoic and culture fluids were stored at $-80\ °C$. The viruses were antigenically and genetically related to the A/Nanchang/933/95 H3N2 reference strain, like all the influenza A viruses which circulated in France during the 1996/1997 season. COS-1 cells were cultured in Dulbecco's modified Eagle Medium (DMEM, Gibco) supplemented with 5% fetal calf serum. The MDCK cells were cultivated in Eagle's minimal essential medium (MEM) containing 5% FCS.

2.2. Hemagglutination test

The hemagglutination test was performed at room temperature with a 0.5% suspension in PBS of guinea-pig, chicken, human, horse or sheep erythrocytes.

2.3. Cloning of the HA genes

Viral RNA was extracted from allantoic fluids or cell culture supernatants using the guanidium extraction method. Full-length cDNAs of the H3 gene segments were amplified by PCR with oligonucleotides 5'-AAGCAGGGGATAATTCTATTAACC-3' and 5'-AGAAACAAGGGTGTTTTTAATTACT-3' and the AmpliTaq enzyme (Perkin Elmer). The PCR products were purified with the QIAquick PCR Purification Kit (Qiagen), and sequenced using H3-specific primers and an automated sequencer (ABI Prism 377, Perkin Elmer). In addition, the PCR products were cloned between the *Mlu*I and *Sal*I restriction enzyme sites of the pCI expression vector downstream of the CMV immediate–early enhancer/promoter (Promega).

2.4. Hemadsorption assay on HA expressing cells

The procedures for the hemadsorption assay have been described previously [2,7]. Briefly, COS-1 cells (60% confluency) were transfected with 2 μg of purified plasmid DNA using the Fugene reagent (Roche) and incubated for 15 min at room temperature, and for 40 h at 37 °C. After removal of the medium, cells were washed twice with PBS, treated with *Vibrio cholerae* sialidase (5.5 mU/ml, Roche) for 1 h at 37 °C, washed twice again with PBS and incubated for 1 h at 4 °C with chilled 1% erythrocyte suspension (chicken or guinea-pig, Charles River) in PBS. The cells were washed five times with PBS and rinsed with methanol. After being air dried, the cells were stained with a 1:20 dilution of Giemsa solution (Reactifs RAL).

Table 1
Hemagglutination of erythrocytes from different animal species and amino acid changes in the HA upon passage of recent A(H3N2) isolates in eggs or MDCK cells

Viruses	Passage number in:		Hemagglutination with erythrocytes from:[a]					Change in HA aa[b]	
			Guinea-pig	Human	Chicken	Sheep	Horse	194	226
906/97	MDCK	C1	256	256	<2	<2	<2	Leu	Val
		C14	128	64	<2	<2	<2	Leu	Val
	Eggs	C1E1[c]	256	2048	512	<2	<2	*Ile*	Val
		C1E2	256	1024	256	32	<2	*Ile*	Val
908/97	MDCK	C1	128	128	<2	<2	<2	Leu	Val
		C5	128	128	4	NT	NT	Leu	Val[d]
		C7	64	128	32	NT	NT	Leu	Val[e]
		C8	64	128	32	NT	NT	Leu	*Ile*
		C10	128	64	16	<2	<2	Leu	*Ile*
		C14	64	64	16	NT	NT	Leu	*Ile*
	Eggs	C1E1	16	32	<2	NT	NT	NT	NT
		C1E2	128	128	128	NT	NT	Leu	*Ile*

[a] Titers are expressed as the reciprocal of the highest virus dilution producing hemagglutination.
[b] Amino acid.
[c] C*x*E*y*, where *x* refers to the number of passages in MDCK cells, and *y* to the number of passages in eggs.
[d] Ile in 3.5% of individual cDNA clones.
[e] Ile in 33.5% of individual cDNA clones.

3. Results

As the first part of this study, we investigated how the adaptation to growth in MDCK cells or in embryonated chicken eggs of two human influenza viruses, isolated in Paris during the 1996/1997 season, altered their binding to chicken erythrocyte receptors. These viruses were not capable to agglutinate chicken erythrocytes after isolation in MDCK cells. However, this property was restored upon five passages in MDCK cells (for A/Paris/ 908/97), or after one passage in eggs (for A/Paris/906/97) (Table 1). Comparison of the nucleotide sequences of the HA, NA and M gene segments allowed us to identify mutations that were likely to be correlated with the observed phenotype in the HA gene segment at residues 226 (Val → Ile) or 194 (Leu → Ile) localized within the receptor binding site. Thus, the L194I change could be related to the ability of A/Paris/906/97 to agglutinate chicken erythrocytes after one passage in eggs. For A/Paris/908/97, the V226I change was detected upon eight passages in MDCK cells or two passages in eggs (Table 1), whereas the change of phenotype was already detected after five passages in MDCK cells. Indeed, molecular cloning and sequence analysis of individual clone revealed the presence of the V226I substitution for a small proportion of the viral population (Table 1).

To confirm that these mutations were indeed responsible for the observed phenotype, we cloned the HA gene of the two A(H3N2) viruses from primary isolates as well as after a number of passages in MDCK cells or in eggs that conferred the ability to the virus to agglutinate chicken erythrocytes. The HA sequences, cloned in plasmid pCI, were

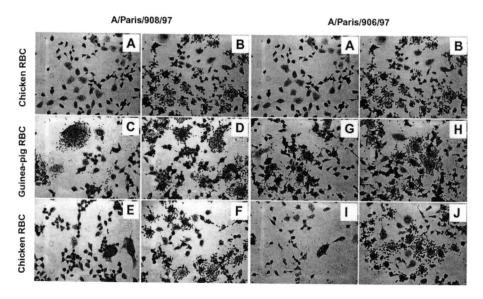

Fig. 1. Effect of mutations at positions 194 or 226 on the hemadsorption activity of the HA from A/Paris/906/97 and A/Paris/908/97. COS-1 cells were transfected with pCI (A) or with pCI–HA plasmids that expressed the HA from viruses A/Nanchang/933/95 (B); A/Paris/908/97 after 1 (C, E) or 10 passages (D, F) in MDCK cells; A/ Paris/906/97 after one passage in MDCK cells (G, I) or an additional passage in eggs (H, J). The hemadsorption assay was performed as described in Material and methods using chicken or guinea-pig erythrocytes as indicated.

expressed to high levels at the surface of transiently tranfected COS-1 cells, as determined by FACSCAN analysis (data not shown). Using an hemadsorption assay, we demonstrated that the V226I and L194I changes were indeed correlated with the ability to agglutinate chicken erythrocytes and did not alter the capacity to agglutinate guinea-pig erythrocytes (Fig. 1). Moreover, this result confirmed that the observed phenotype could be attributed to the sole characteristics of the HA.

Its has been shown previously [7,8] that residues at positions 226 and 228 are involved in the ability of the HA to interact with α2,3Gal or α2,6Gal-linked sialic acids, depending on the nature of the linkage of the sialic acid with the underlying β-galactose harbored by the sialoconjugates present at the surface of erythrocytes. However, the nature of the SA linkage at the surface of erythrocytes did not seem to be involved in the phenotype analyzed here, as suggested by FACSCAN analysis using linkage-specific lectins (data not shown). The results of this assay showed that the relative amounts of SAα2,3Gal and SAα2,6Gal linkages were similar for chicken, human and guinea-pig erythrocytes. Unlike previously reported for human and chicken erythrocytes [6], although SAα2,6Gal seemed to be present in reduced amount on chicken erythrocytes as compared to human or guinea-pig erythrocytes. In contrast, sheep erythrocytes, which were not agglutinated by the viruses, displayed only SAα2,3Gal. These observations suggested that the phenotypic changes observed here were not strictly correlated with receptor specificity.

4. Conclusions

A V226I or L194I change in the HA was sufficient to confer the ability to the glycoprotein to bind chicken erythrocytes. These observations suggested that a valine at position 226 in the HA molecule, found in recent clinical isolates of human A(H3N2) viruses, could be responsible for loss of the ability to agglutinate chicken erythrocytes, and that a change at residue 194 (Leu $\rightarrow$ Ile) after passage in eggs could restore this ability.

The phenotypic change was not correlated with receptor specificity but could however reflect differences in affinity for α2,6Gal-linked sialic acid.

Acknowledgements

This study was supported in part by the Ministère de l'Education Nationale, de la Recherche et de la Technologie (EA 302) and by grants for R.M. from CAPES, Brasilia-Brazil.

References

[1] G.K. Hirst, Agglutination of red cells by allantoic fluid of chick embryos infected with influenza virus, Science 94 (1941) 22–23.

[2] T. Morishita, et al., Studies on the molecular basis for loss of the ability of recent influenza A (H1N1) virus strains to agglutinate chicken erythrocytes, J. Gen. Virol. 77 (Pt. 10) (1996) 2499–2506.

[3] S. Lindstrom, et al., Evolutionary characterization of recent human H3N2 influenza A isolates from Japan and China: novel changes in the receptor binding domain, Arch. Virol. 141 (7) (1996) 1349–1355.

[4] A. Azzi, et al., The haemagglutinins of influenza A (H1N1) viruses in the 'O' or 'D' phases exhibit biological and antigenic differences, Epidemiol. Infect. 111 (1) (1993) 135–142.

[5] F.M. Burnet, D.R. Bull, Changes in influenza virus associated with adaptation to passage in chick embryo, Aust. J. Exp. Biol. Med. Sci. 21 (1941) 55–69.

[6] T. Ito, et al., Receptor specificity of influenza A viruses correlates with the agglutination of erythrocytes from different animal species, Virology 227 (2) (1997) 493–499.

[7] A. Vines, et al., The role of influenza A virus hemagglutinin residues 226 and 228 in receptor specificity and host range restriction, J. Virol. 72 (9) (1998) 7626–7631.

[8] R.J. Connor, et al., Receptor specificity in human, avian, and equine H2 and H3 influenza virus isolates, Virology 205 (1) (1994) 17–23.

International Congress Series 1219 (2001) 375–382

N-glycans attached to hemagglutinin in the head region and the stem domain control growth of influenza viruses by different mechanisms

R. Wagner[a],*, D. Heuer[a], T. Wolff[b], H.-D. Klenk[a]

[a]*Institute of Virology, Philipps-Universität Marburg, Postfach 2360, 35011 Marburg, Germany*
[b]*Robert-Koch-Institute, Berlin, Germany*

Abstract

Background: The hemagglutinin (HA) of fowl plague virus A/FPV/Ro/34 (H7N1) contains seven *N*-glycans, two of which are flanking the receptor binding site and three being located in the stem domain. In the present study, we have elucidated the functional role of these five glycans in the course of virus replication in different hosts. *Methods*: Using a RNA polymerase I-based reverse genetics system, we generated recombinant viruses in which the HA mutants were stably incorporated in the background of the influenza reassortants WSN-HK and HK-WSN. *Results*: Growth of viruses lacking the glycans from the HA head region was impaired in MDCK cells as well as in embryonated chicken eggs. This restriction was due to limited release of progeny viruses from host cells as a result of the enhanced receptor affinity of the mutated HA. Accordingly, the high activity N2-subtype neuraminidase (NA) was able to partly overcome this effect, while the low activity N1-subtype NA was not. Thus, HA and NA activities need to be highly balanced to promote influenza viruses growth. When glycans were eliminated from the HA stem, the resulting viruses showed temperature sensitive growth in cell culture and in chicken eggs. The degree of growth restriction was dependent on the position from which the glycan had been removed. The viruses had a decreased pH stability, indicating that the stem glycans might maintain the HA in a fusion competent conformation. Viruses lacking the stem glycan from Asn 28 could not be rescued, indicating that this glycan is essential for the formation of replication competent viruses. *Conclusions*: Our results demonstrate that *N*-glycans linked to distinct HA domains regulate influenza virus growth at different stages of the replication cycle. Moreover, the deletion of glycan attachment sites from HA represents a powerful experimental strategy for the generation of attenuated influenza viruses. © 2001 Elsevier Science B.V. All rights reserved.

Keywords: Receptor binding; Virus release; Metastabile conformation; Fusion activity

---

* Corresponding author. Tel.: +49-6421-2865146; fax: +49-6421-2868962.
E-mail address: wagnerr@mailer.uni-marburg.de (R. Wagner).

0531-5131/01/$ – see front matter © 2001 Elsevier Science B.V. All rights reserved.
PII: S 0 5 3 1 - 5 1 3 1 (0 1) 0 0 3 4 7 - 8

1. Introduction

Influenza A and B viruses contain two spike glycoproteins, the hemagglutinin (HA) and the neuraminidase (NA). Both glycoproteins fulfill distinct functions during the viral replicative cycle (for a review, see Ref. [1]). Influenza virus infection is initiated by binding of HA to sialic acid containing receptors on the surface of target cells. Following internalization of bound viruses by endocytosis HA induces fusion of the viral envelope with the endosomal membrane. This fusion reaction is an absolute requirement for the delivery of viral nucleocapsids into the cytoplasm, thus triggering the generation of progeny viruses. In the late stage of infection, NA acts as receptor-destroying enzyme catalyzing the removal of sialic acids from viral and cellular components to promote the release of progeny viruses from host cells and to prevent virion aggregation [2].

HA is the prototype of a class I transmembrane glycoprotein and is embedded in the viral membrane as a homotrimer [3]. It consists of a globular head region connected to a fibrous stalk domain. Both regions carry N-linked oligosaccharide side chains, with those attached to the head of the molecule showing considerable variation in number and structure among different influenza A viruses [4]. The HA of fowl plague virus (FPV) carries two N-glycans at the tip of the molecule in close proximity of the receptor binding site [5]. Previously, we were able to demonstrate that these tip glycans regulate receptor affinity of HA expressed from a SV40 vector [6]. A balance of receptor-binding (HA) and receptor-destroying (NA) activity seems to be crucial for a productive influenza virus infection. This notion was promoted by the observation that in natural or laboratory derived influenza viruses, some combinations of HA and NA occurred quite frequently, while others were never detected [7]. However, direct experimental proof for this concept of matching HA and NA activities is still lacking.

N-glycans linked to the HA stem are extremely conserved [8]. Glycosylation sites at Asn 12 and Asn 28 (H7 numbering) are present in all HA sequences and the site at Asn 478 appears in most strains analyzed to date. The high conservation of these three sites suggested that the respective N-glycans may serve an important structural or functional role. Correspondingly, loss of all three glycans from FPV–HA was found to cause temperature sensitivity and a complete transport block at the nonpermissive temperature [9]. Further analysis of HA mutants lacking individual glycans from the stem region revealed that these glycans contribute to the maintenance of the metastabile form of HA required for fusion activity [10]. Despite their ubiquitous presence, no data are yet available addressing the function of these HA stem glycans during the process of a viral infection.

Here, we report on the generation of recombinant influenza viruses stably expressing HA mutants lacking individual N-glycans either from the tip or the stem of the molecule. By this approach, we were able to precisely attribute specific functions to individual HA-glycans. Evidence is presented that N-glycans can be regarded as potent regulators of influenza virus replication in different host systems. Furthermore, we show that N-glycans attached to either the tip or the stem of the HA molecule exert their function by different mechanisms.

2. Results

2.1. Generation of recombinant viruses

To investigate effects of oligosaccharides on the growth of intact influenza viruses, glycan attachment sites at Asn 123 and 149 (for head glycans) and at Asn 12, Asn 28, and Asn 478 (for stem glycans) (see Fig. 1) were abolished from the HA sequence by site directed mutagenesis. Resulting HA cDNAs were inserted in a plasmid vector between RNA Polymerase I promoter and hepatitis delta virus ribozyme sequences. When transfected in CV1 cells, RNA polymerase I-based transcription produces a virus-like HA RNA gene that is amplified by proteins of the influenza virus polymerase complex translated from expression plasmids, which had been cotransfected along with the *Pol*I vector [11].

To obtain recombinant viruses, CV1 cells were then infected with helper viruses. Two influenza virus reassortants were chosen for that purpose. The HK-WSN (H3N1) reassortant contains all WSN genes except for the H3-subtype HA from Hong Kong strain and the WSN-HK (H1N2) reassortant contains all WSN genes except for the N2-subtype NA from Hong Kong virus. When using the HK-WSN reassortant as helper, selection for recombinant viruses was achieved by applying a neutralizing H3-HA-specific antiserum which blocks growth of helper viruses, while leaving the recombinant FPV–HA-carrying viruses unaffected. To select for recombinant viruses produced with the WSN-HK helper strain, CV1 cell supernatants were passaged on MDBK cells in the absence of trypsin. Since FPV–HA is activated by the cellular protease furin [12] only, recombinant virus is propagated under these conditions, whereas helper virus growth is inhibited. By this approach, we generated two series of recombinant viruses expressing the

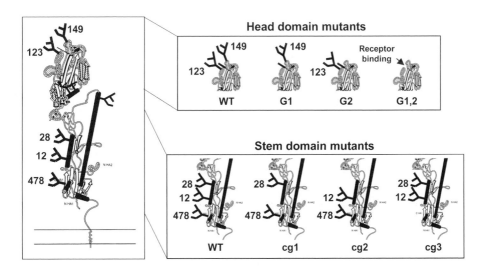

Fig. 1. Schematic representation of the FPV-HA molecule with special emphasis on *N*-glycans decorating the head region and the stem domain. Phenotypes of HA glycosylation mutants generated in this study are illustrated.

head glycosylation mutants of FPV–HA. Both series carried FPV–HA in the WSN background and only differed by containing either N1- or N2-subtype NA. HA mutants lacking the stem glycans were introduced only in the background of the WSN-HK helper virus. Interestingly, it was not possible to rescue recombinant viruses expressing the cg2 mutant HA, where the glycan attachment site at Asn 28 had been deleted. This strongly suggests that this glycan is indispensable for the generation of replication competent influenza viruses.

The recombinant identity of all rescued viruses was confirmed by RT-PCR analysis of viral RNA (data not shown) and by SDS-PAGE examination of the HA protein profile (Fig. 2; data are shown for head glycosylation mutants with N2-NA only). HA1 subunits from G1 and G2 mutant viruses showed a reduced molecular mass compared to wild-type HA1. An even larger reduction was observed with the G1,2 recombinant. PNGase F treatment confirmed that these differences resulted from loss of oligosaccharides.

2.2. Replication of viruses lacking N-glycans from the HA head domain

MDCK cells were infected with recombinant viruses and cultivated at 33 and 37 °C, respectively. Three days post-infection virus titers in cell supernatants were determined by plaque assay. Within the N2-NA series, wild-type and G1 viruses grew nearly equally well (Table 1). Growth of the G2 and G1,2 mutants was weakly reduced. However, with viruses of the N1-NA group, the loss of oligosaccharides from the HA tip had marked effects on virus growth, depending on the number and position of deleted glycans. Titers obtained with G2 mutants were reduced about 20-fold compared to those reached by wild-type viruses. With a more than 100-fold reduction in titer, the G1,2 virus exhibited an attenuated phenotype in MDCK cells. Virus titers obtained in the allantoic fluid of embryonated chicken eggs 3 days after infection with N2-NA-carrying mutant viruses

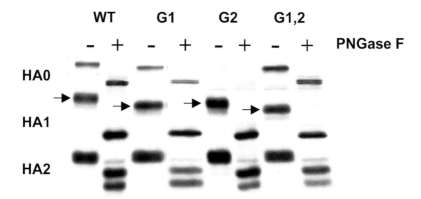

Fig. 2. Analysis of the glycosylation pattern of radiolabeled FPV-HA immunoprecipitated from recombinant viruses. One-half of the material was treated with PNGase F (+), while the other half remained untreated (−). The protein profile was analyzed by SDS-PAGE and visualized by fluorography. Arrows point to HA1 bands displaying a reduced molecular mass compared to wild-type (WT) HA.

Table 1
Growth of recombinant viruses lacking either the head or stem glycans in MDCK cells and allantoic fluids of embryonated chicken eggs at 33 and 37 °C

Virus	Growth in MDCK cells (33 °C/37 °C)	Growth in embryonated chicken eggs (33 °C/37 °C)
Head domain mutants		
WT/N1	$1.5 \times 10^9/1.4 \times 10^9$	$1.8 \times 10^9/1.2 \times 10^9$
G1/N1	$1.2 \times 10^9/1.2 \times 10^9$	$1.2 \times 10^5/8.5 \times 10^4$
G2/N1	$6.5 \times 10^7/8.1 \times 10^7$	$2.4 \times 10^5/6.2 \times 10^4$
G1,2/N1	$3.6 \times 10^6/4.0 \times 10^6$	$2.0 \times 10^4/2.0 \times 10^4$
WT/N2	$1.7 \times 10^9/1.2 \times 10^9$	$1.2 \times 10^9/8.5 \times 10^8$
G1/N2	$1.5 \times 10^9/1.0 \times 10^9$	$5.8 \times 10^8/1.5 \times 10^8$
G2/N2	$5.1 \times 10^8/6.0 \times 10^8$	$3.4 \times 10^8/9.6 \times 10^7$
G1,2/N2	$7.4 \times 10^7/8.5 \times 10^7$	$4.2 \times 10^8/1.1 \times 10^8$
Stem domain mutants		
cg1/N2	3.5×10^6/no growth	1.8×10^4/no growth
cg3/N2	$1.0 \times 10^9/7.5 \times 10^8$	$3.5 \times 10^8/6.9 \times 10^6$

Titers were determined by plaque assay and are given as PFU/ml.

revealed no evidence for a significant influence of glycans on virus yield in this host system. Yet, the situation was remarkably different in the case of eggs infected with viruses of the N1-NA series. Here, the loss of any of the two glycans seriously interfered with virus replication. These results show that *N*-glycans at the HA tip promote influenza replication growth in cell culture and embryonated chicken eggs to a different extent. Moreover, from these results, it is obvious that NA also has a crucial impact on virus growth. This is evident from the finding that N2-NA, but not N1-NA, was capable of abrogating the downregulating effects of missing *N*-glycans. We have shown previously that enzymatic activity of Hong Kong virus NA (N2 subtype) is about sixfold higher than that of WSN virus NA (N1 subtype) [13]. In view of this, it appeared that the restrictions caused by the loss of glycans from the tip are due to an incomplete release of progeny viruses from host cells. This concept is strengthened by our previous finding that *N*-glycans at the HA tip reduce receptor binding activity [6]. Incomplete release of progeny viruses from infected cells might be overcome by treatment with *Vibrio cholerae* NA (VCNA). Therefore, infected MDCK cells were treated with VCNA prior to virus harvest to elute viruses from the cell surface. Virus titers were then determined by plaque assay. Compared to release in the presence of VCNA, untreated G2 and G1,2 viruses of the N1-NA group were released to only 20% and 5%, respectively (Fig. 3). Within the N2-NA group, only the elution of the G1,2 viruses was impeded.

2.3. Replication of viruses lacking N-glycans from the HA stem domain

As above, growth of these viruses was monitored in MDCK cell culture and embryonated chicken eggs. Titers obtained in MDCK cells with cg3 mutant viruses (lacking the *N*-glycan at Asn 478) were quite similar to those of wild-type viruses (Table 1). In chicken

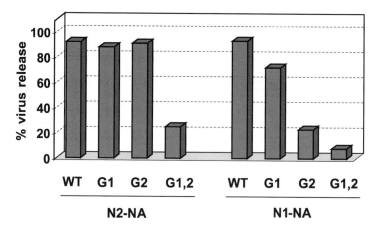

Fig. 3. Release of recombinant viruses from MDCK cells. Cells were infected at an MOI of 5 and incubated at 37 °C overnight. One hour before virus harvest, VCNA was added to the culture medium of one-half of the samples. Titers of progeny viruses released into the medium were determined by plaque assay. Levels of virus release in the absence of VCNA are presented as a percentage of the virus titers released after VCNA treatment.

eggs, we observed a weak temperature sensitivity of cg3 viruses in that growth at 37 °C was decreased about 100-fold when compared to that at 33 °C. However, loss of the N-glycan from Asn 12 (in cg1 viruses) had striking effects on virus replication in MDCK cells and chicken eggs. In both systems growth of these viruses was totally blocked at 37 °C. At 33 °C, virus yield from chicken eggs was strongly reduced, while yields from MDCK cells were only slightly affected.

Thus, loss of the N-glycan at Asn 12 caused a pronounced temperature sensitivity of the respective virus mutants. We then tested the pH-stability of the cg mutant viruses by preincubation with buffers of different pH ranging from 5.0 to 6.0. Remaining infectivity was subsequently determined by plaque assay (data not shown). Tested viruses showed distinct differences in their response to acid preincubation. Inactivation of wild-type viruses was observed only at pH values lower than 5.5, whereas cg mutant viruses displayed a higher pH lability with inactivation starting already at pH 5,6. This effect was very distinct with cg1 viruses and less pronounced with cg3 viruses.

3. Discussion

FPV–HA contains seven N-linked oligosaccharide side chains [5]. When HA was expressed using a simian virus 40 vector, it was found that the two glycans flanking the receptor binding site [6] and the three confined to the stem region [10] rule functional properties of HA. It was now of interest to examine the role of these glycans for influenza virus replication. To this end. we applied a recently described reversed genetics system [13] to stably incorporate mutants lacking either the glycans from the head or the stem of HA in recombinant influenza viruses.

We found that loss of *N*-glycans from the HA tip interfered with virus replication both in MDCK cells and embryonated chicken eggs. This effect could be attributed to a restricted release of progeny viruses from host cells caused by the enhanced receptor affinity of the mutant HA. It was interesting to see that the high activity N2-subtype NA, but not the low-activity N1-subtype NA, was able to partly overcome this restriction. Taken together, our data clearly point out that for the establishment of a productive infection influenza viruses are strictly dependent on a balanced action of HA and NA. The need for such a match of HA and NA activities had so far only been deduced from studies analyzing natural virus isolates or laboratory-generated reassortants [4,14,15]. Hence, we present here the first concise study of the functional interrelationship of distinct HA and NA species and provide experimental evidence for the strict requirement of a fine tuning of HA receptor binding and NA receptor-destroying activity in order to allow efficient influenza virus propagation.

The data obtained from replication studies with stem glycosylation mutants were even more striking. While growth of cg3 mutant viruses (lacking the glycan at Asn 478) were only marginally affected, that of cg1 viruses (lacking the glycan at Asn 12) was totally blocked at 37 °C and considerably reduced at 33 °C. These findings impressively illustrated the pivotal role of the *N*-glycan at Asn 12 for FPV replication and at the same time raised the interesting question at which stage of the replicative cycle this glycan exerts its crucial function. Previously, we showed that stem glycans do not contribute to receptor binding activity of HA, but maintain the metastabile conformation required for fusion activity [10]. Accordingly, it seemed unlikely that growth restriction of stem mutant viruses originated from a mechanism similar to that outlined for viruses lacking the head glycans. Rather, in intact viruses, these glycans also preserve the fusion competent conformation of HA. This concept was confirmed when we found that loss of stem glycans significantly lowered the pH stability of the respective viruses, most probably as a result of premature acid induced denaturation of HA. Therefore, stem glycans can be considered effective stabilizers of the metastabile HA conformation with the glycan at Asn 12 being dominant and that at Asn 478 being less important.

In summary, our results demonstrate that *N*-glycans of FPV–HA efficiently regulate virus replication in cell culture and chicken eggs. The extent of growth restrictions conferred by eliminating individual *N*-glycans may vary among different host systems. Furthermore, our data reveal that glycans attached to the head domain and the stem region of HA exert their important functions during the viral replication cycle by totally different mechanisms. Accordingly, *N*-glycans can be regarded as very powerful and versatile regulators of the function of viral proteins.

Acknowledgements

We are grateful to Peter Palese and Adolfo Garcia-Sastre for kindly providing the anti-H3-HA serum, the reassortant helper viruses, and the *Pol*I-*Sap*I vector.This work was supported by grants from the Deutsche Forschungsgemeinschaft (SFB 286) and from the Fonds der Chemischen Industrie. T. W. was a recipient of a fellowship of the Deutsches Krebsforschungszentrum (Infektionsforschung, AIDS-Stipendienprogramm).

References

[1] R.A. Lamb, R.M. Krug, Orthomyxoviruses: the viruses and their replication, in: B.N. Fields, P.M. Howley (Eds.), Virology, Lippincott-Raven, Philadelphia, 1996, pp. 1353–1395.

[2] P. Colman, Structure and function of the neuraminidase, in: K.G. Nicholson, R.G. Webster, A.J. Hay (Eds.), Textbook of Influenza, Blackwell, London, 1998, pp. 65–73.

[3] D.C. Wiley, J.J. Skehel, The structure and function of the hemagglutinin membrane glycoprotein of influenza viruses, Annu. Rev. Biochem. 56 (1987) 365–394.

[4] M. Mastrosovich, N. Zhou, Y. Kawaoka, R. Webster, The surface glycoproteins of H5 influenza viruses isolated from humans, chickens, and wild aquatic birds have distinguishable properties, J. Virol. 73 (1999) 1146–1155.

[5] W. Keil, R. Geyer, J. Dabrowski, U. Dabrowski, H. Niemann, S. Stirm, H.D. Klenk, Carbohydrates of influenza virus: structural elucidation of the individual glycans of the FPV hemagglutinin by two-dimensional ^{1}H n.m.r. and methylation analysis, EMBO J. 4 (1985) 2711–2720.

[6] M. Ohuchi, R. Ohuchi, A. Feldmann, H.D. Klenk, Regulation of receptor binding affinity of influenza virus hemagglutinin by its carbohydrate moiety, J. Virol. 71 (1997) 8377–8384.

[7] E.D. Kilbourne, Influenza, Plenum, New York, 1987.

[8] E. Nobusawa, T. Aoyama, H. Kato, Y. Suzuki, Y. Tateno, K. Nakajima, Comparison of complete amino acid sequences and receptor-binding properties among 13 serotypes of hemagglutinins of influenza A viruses, Virology 182 (1991) 475–485.

[9] P.C. Roberts, W. Garten, H.D. Klenk, Role of conserved glycosylation sites in the maturation and transport of influenza A virus hemagglutinin, J. Virol. 67 (1993) 3048–3060.

[10] R. Ohuchi, M. Ohuchi, W. Garten, H.D. Klenk, Oligosaccharides in the stem region maintain the influenza virus hemagglutinin in the metastabile form required for fusion activity, J. Virol. 71 (1997) 3719–3725.

[11] S. Pleschka, R. Jaskunas, O.G. Engelhardt, T. Zürcher, P. Palese, A. Garcia-Sastre, A plasmid-based reverse genetics system for influenza A virus, J. Virol. 70 (1996) 4188–4192.

[12] A. Stieneke-Gröber, M. Vey, H. Angliker, E. Shaw, G. Thomas, C. Roberts, H.D. Klenk, W. Garten, Influenza virus hemagglutinin with multibasic cleavage site is activated by furin, a subtilisin-like endoprotease, EMBO J. 11 (1992) 2407–2414.

[13] R. Wagner, T. Wolff, A. Herwig, S. Pleschka, H.D. Klenk, Interdependence of hemagglutinin glycosylation and neuraminidase as regulators of influenza virus growth: a study by reverse genetics, J. Virol. 74 (2000) 6316–6323.

[14] L.J. Mitnaul, M.N. Matrosovich, M.R. Castrucci, A.B. Tuzikov, N.V. Bovin, D. Kobasa, Y. Kawaoka, Balanced hemagglutinin and neuraminidase activities are critical for efficient replication of influenza A virus, J. Virol. 74 (2000) 6015–6020.

[15] N.V. Kaverin, A.S. Gambaryan, N.V. Bovin, I.A. Rudneva, A.A. Shilov, O.M. Khodova, N.L. Varich, B.V. Sinitsin, N.V. Makarova, E.A. Kropotkina, Postreassortment changes in influenza A virus hemagglutinin restoring HA-NA functional match, Virology 244 (1998) 315–321.

International Congress Series 1219 (2001) 383–387

Multiple lineages co-circulation and genetic reassortment of the neuraminidase and hemagglutinin genes within influenza viruses of the same type/subtype

X. Xu*, J. Shaw, C.B. Smith, N.J. Cox, A.I. Klimov

*Influenza Branch, G-16, Centers for Disease Control and Prevention,
1600 Clifton Road, NE, Atlanta, GA 30333, USA*

Abstract

Background: Analysis of the hemagglutinin (HA) and neuraminidase (NA) genes of influenza A and B viruses revealed worldwide circulation of multiple genetic lineages within the same type/subtype. Genetic reassortment between distinct genetic lineages was examined in this study. *Methods*: Nucleotide sequencing, polymerase chain reaction (PCR) and restriction fragment length polymorphism (RFLP) were used. Phylogenetic studies were used to analyze sequence data. *Results*: Influenza A (H3N2). The NA genes of H3N2 viruses were found to have evolved as three distinct lineages represented by A/Sydney/5/97, A/Panama/2007/99, and A/Moscow/10/99, respectively. Similar genetic groups were also found among the HA genes of these viruses. PCR/RFLP data of strains isolated between June 1999 and June 2000 showed that 122 of 141 viruses examined (87%) had their NA genes closely related to that of A/Moscow/10/99 virus; 14 of 141 viruses (10%) had A/Panama/2007/99-like NA genes, and only 5 strains (3%) had A/Sydney/5/97-like NA genes. Viruses bearing A/Panama/2007/99-like HA, and either A/Moscow/10/99-like, or A/Sydney/5/97-like NA were detected, indicating that genetic reassortments of the NA genes among different lineages of H3N2 viruses had occurred. Influenza A (H1N1). Analyses showed that the NA and HA genes of the current strains each evolved as two genetically distinct lineages, represented by A/Bayern/7/95 and A/Beijing/262/95, respectively. The NA genes of the majority of circulating H1N1 viruses were closely related to that of the current vaccine strain A/New Caledonia/20/99 virus (A/Beijing/262/95 lineage). Influenza B. The NA genes of influenza B viruses, similar to their HA genes, were found to have diverged into two genetically and antigenically distinguishable lineages represented by B/Yamagata/16/88 (recently B/Yamanashi/166/98) and B/Victoria/2/87 (recently by B/Shandong/7/97) strains. Reassortants bearing the B/Yamagata-like HA and B/Victoria-like NA were isolated from

---

* Corresponding author. Tel.: +1-404-639-2747; fax: +1-404-639-2334.
  E-mail address: xxu@cdc.gov (X. Xu).

several countries. *Conclusion*: Monitoring both HA and NA genes/antigens is important for appropriate vaccine strain selection. © 2001 Elsevier Science B.V. All rights reserved.

Keywords: Neuraminidase; Hemagglutinin; Reassortment

1. Introduction

Influenza viruses are enveloped and have two surface glycoproteins, hemagglutinin (HA) and neuraminidase (NA). The HA performs two crucial roles, receptor binding and membrane fusion, during the early stages of virus replication [1]. NA functions primarily in the final stage of virus replication [2]. NA prevents formation of virus aggregates and releases newly assembled virus particles from the cell surface by removing sialic acid from the virus envelope proteins [2]. Antibodies to HA neutralize the infectivity of influenza virus [3], while antibodies to NA may modify the disease and play a role in the epidemiology of influenza [4]. In this study, NA and HA genes of recent influenza A (H3N2), (H1N1) and influenza B epidemic strains were analyzed to determine the evolutionary patterns of influenza viruses and to assist in vaccine strain selection.

2. Material and methods

Viruses. Influenza viruses examined were propagated in embryonated eggs or MDCK cells. *PCR, RFLP and nucleotide sequencing.* Viral RNAs were amplified by PCR and sequenced as described previously [5]. Phylogenetic studies were performed to analyze viral sequences [5].

PCR-amplified N2 NAs were digested by restriction enzymes *Aci*I and *Hga*I. Restriction digestion patterns were examined by electrophoresis [6].

3. Results

3.1. Influenza A (H3N2)

Antigenic variants of influenza A (H3N2) virus, represented by A/Sydney/5/97, emerged in 1997 and caused significant influenza activity in many countries. Viruses antigenically similar to or slightly drifted from A/Sydney/5/97 continued to circulate

Fig. 1. Evolutionary trees of influenza viruses: (A) HA1 domains of HA genes of (H3N2) viruses; (B) neuraminidase genes of (H3N2) viruses; (C) HA1 domains of HA genes of influenza B viruses; (D) neuraminidase genes of influenza B viruses. The sequence data were analyzed using version 8.0 of the sequence analysis software package of the University of Wisconsin Genetics Computer Group. Version 3.5 of PHYLIP with the neighbor-joining program was used to estimate phylogenies from nucleotide sequences. Vaccine strains are underlined.

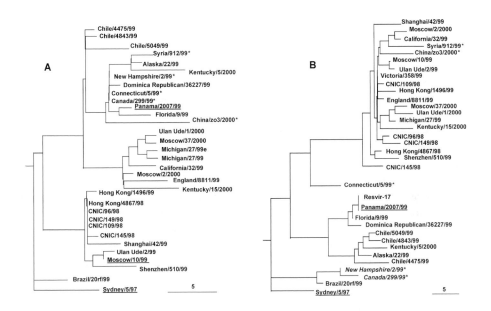

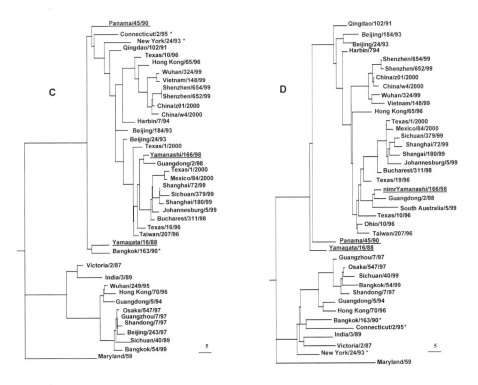

worldwide. NA genes of 32 strains of H3N2 viruses isolated between 1997 and 2000 were sequenced. Phylogenetic analysis showed that the NA genes of these viruses have evolved as three distinct lineages, represented by A/Sydney/5/97, A/Panama/2007/99 and A/Moscow/10/99, respectively (Fig 1B). Similar genetic groups were found in the HA genes, except that viruses with HAs that are genetically closely related to that of A/California/32/99 viruses formed a separate group (Fig. 1A). Four strains labeled with a " * " had HA genes located on the same branch as that of A/Panama/2007/99 (Fig. 1A), but had NA genes located either on the same branch as that of A/Moscow/10/99, or as that of A/Sydney/5/97 (Fig. 1B). The HA gene of A/Connecticut /5/99 was located on the same branch as A/Panama/2007/99 virus (Fig. 1A); its NA gene, however, was located between the NAs of the A/Moscow/10/99-like viruses and A/Panama/2007/99-like viruses (Fig. 1A and B). This finding indicates that genetic reassortments of the NA genes among different lineages of H3N2 viruses have occurred. Data obtained from the PCR/RFLP analysis reveals that the NA genes of 122 out of 141 (87%) viruses examined belong to the A/Moscow/10/99-like genetic lineage; 14 (10%) strains belong to the A/Panama/2007/99-like genetic lineage, and only 5 strains (3%) belong to the A/Sydney/5/97-like lineage (data not shown). By comparing NA and HA data, we found that a total of 16 strains have an A/Panama/2007/99-like HA and an A/Moscow/10/99-like NA; one strain has an A/Panama/2007/99-like HA and an A/Sydney/7/97-like NA, and one strain has an A/Moscow/10/99-like HA but an A/Panama/10/99-like NA (data not shown).

3.2. Influenza A (H1N1)

H1N1 viruses diverged into two antigenically and genetically distinct lineages in 1995. One lineage was represented by A/Bayern/7/95 virus, an antigenic variant of A/Taiwan/1/86, while another lineage was represented by A/Beijing/262/95 virus, which had an amino acid deletion in the HA gene at residue 134. The nucleotide sequences of the NA genes were obtained for 33 strains of H1N1 viruses. A phylogenetic study reveals that the NA genes of the A/Beijing/262/95-like viruses were located on a separate branch of the evolutionary tree from that of A/Bayern/7/95-like viruses (data not shown). The NA genes of the majority of circulating H1N1 viruses were closely related to that of the current vaccine strain A/New Caledonia/20/99 virus.

3.3. Influenza B

Between 1986 and 1987, two lineages of antigenically and genetically distinguishable influenza B viruses were isolated, which were represented by B/Yamagata/16/88 and B/Victoria/2/87 [7]. These two lineages of influenza B viruses have co-circulated in humans since that time. From the middle of the 1990s, B/Victoria/2/87 or B/Shandong/7/97-like (a recent B/Victoria/2/87-like representative strain) viruses were isolated only from Asia. NA sequences of 39 influenza B viruses isolated between 1986 and 2000 were obtained. Phylogenetic analysis revealed that NA genes of influenza B viruses, like their HA genes, have evolved as two distinct lineages (Fig. 1C and D). Three strains labeled with a " * " (B/Bangkok/163/90, B/Connecticut/2/95 and B/New York 24/93) had HA genes located on the same branch as that of the B/ Yamagata/16/88 (Fig. 1C), but their NA genes were located on the same branch as that of the B/Victoria/2/87 (Fig. 1D). Our findings provided further evidence that genetic reassortment of the NA genes between the two lineages of influenza B viruses has occurred [8]. The NA genes of the majority of influenza B viruses circulating recently were closely related to that of the vaccine strain B/Yamanashi/166/98, a variant from the B/Yamagata/16/88 lineage.

4. Discussion

In the current study, we used PCR/RFLP, sequence, and phylogenetic analyses to examine the evolution of the NA genes of influenza A (H3N2), (H1N1), and influenza B epidemic strains. Data obtained from this study showed that the co-circulation of multiple lineages and genetic reassortment of NA genes has occurred in both influenza A and B viruses. Genetic reassortants were isolated from different countries. Our results demonstrated that molecular analysis of influenza virus genes is useful for studying virus evolution and emphasized the need to sequence both the HA and NA genes of field strains to achieve as close a match as possible for both surface antigens between vaccine and circulating strains.

References

[1] R. Lamb, Genes and proteins of influenza viruses, in: R. Krug, H. Fraenkel-Conrat, R. Wagner (Eds.), The Influenza Viruses, Plenum, New York, 1989, pp. 1–88.
[2] G. Air, W. Laver, The neuraminidase of influenza virus, Proteins: Struct., Funct., Genet. 6 (1989) 341–356.
[3] R. Couch, J. Kasel, Immunity to influenza in man, Annu. Rev. Microbiol. 37 (1983) 529–549.
[4] J. Schulman, in: E. Kilbourne (Ed.), The Influenza Viruses and Influenza, Academic Press, New York, 1975, pp. 373–393.
[5] X. Xu, N.J. Cox, C. Bender, H. Regnery, M.W. Shaw, in: Genetic variation in neuraminidase genes of influenza A (H3N2) viruses, Virology 224 (1996) 175–183.
[6] A.I. Klimov, N.J. Cox, PCR restriction analysis of genome composition and stability of cold-adapted re-assortant live influenza vaccine, J. Virol. Methods 52 (1995) 41–49.
[7] P.A. Rota, T.R. Wallis, M.W. Harmon, J.S. Rota, A.P. Kendal, K. Nerome, Cocirculation of two distinct evolutionary lineages of influenza type B viruses since 1983, Virology 175 (1990) 59–68.
[8] J.A. McCullers, G.C. Wang, S. He, R.G. Webster, Reassortment and insertion-deletion are strategies for the evolution of influenza B viruses in nature, J. Virol. 73 (1999) 7343–7348.

International Congress Series 1219 (2001) 389–396

Structure–function relationship of the M_2 ion channel of influenza A virus

Jorgen A. Mould[a], Kevin Shuck[b], Jason E. Drury[a],
Stephan M. Frings[c], U. Benjamin Kaupp[c], Andrew Pekosz[b],
Robert A. Lamb[b,d], Lawrence H. Pinto[a,*]

[a]*Department of Neurobiology and Physiology, Hogan Hall, 2153 North Campus Drive, Northwestern University, Evanston, IL 60208-3500, USA*
[b]*Department of Biochemistry, Molecular Biology and Cell Biology, Northwestern University, Evanston, IL 60208-3500, USA*
[c]*Institut Für Biologische Informationsverarbeitung, Forschungszentrum, 52425 Jülich, Germany*
[d]*Howard Hughes Medical Institute, Northwestern University, Evanston, IL 60208-3500, USA*

Abstract

The use of oligomers comprised of amantadine-sensitive and -resistant forms demonstrated that the active oligomeric state of the channel is a tetramer. Cysteine scanning mutagenesis followed by evaluation of the ability of sulfhydryl-specific reagents to inhibit the channel demonstrated that each monomer is a coiled coil and that the pore-lining residues are Val-27, Ala-30, Gly-34, His-37 and Trp-41. Under oxidizing conditions, mutant proteins containing cysteine at or close to these residues form dimers, but do so less readily at low pH for residues near #41, supporting the notion that a pH-induced conformational change occurs in this region of the protein. A functional change in state was detected by comparing the efflux of H^+ from acid-loaded cells expressing M_2 protein with those treated with the protonophore FCCP: the efflux was high for FCCP-treated cells, but not M_2-expressing cells when pH_{out} was elevated. The current of the wild-type protein is carried by H^+ and is increased by low pH_{out}, but replacement of the His-37 results in pH-independent currents of other ions as well, suggesting that the selectivity and activation of the channel might result from the action of His-37. The C-terminus is needed for sustained function of the channel, as truncation mutants are abnormal and that they pass H^+ for only a short time. © 2001 Elsevier Science B.V. All rights reserved.

Keywords: Amantadine; Ion channels

---

* Corresponding author. Tel.: +1-847-491-7915; fax: +1-847-491-5211.
E-mail address: larry-pinto@northwestern.edu (L.H. Pinto).

0531-5131/01/$ – see front matter © 2001 Elsevier Science B.V. All rights reserved.
PII: S 0 5 3 1 - 5 1 3 1 (0 1) 0 0 6 4 1 - 0

1. Introduction

The M_2 protein of influenza A virus is thought to function as an ion channel that permits protons to enter virus particles during virion uncoating in endosomes. In addition, in influenza virus-infected cells, the M_2 protein causes the equilibration of pH between the acidic lumen of the trans-Golgi network and the cytoplasm (reviewed in Refs. [1,2]). The activity of the M_2 ion channel is inhibited by the antiviral drug amantadine [3–5]. The mature M_2 protein consists of a 23-residue N-terminal extracellular domain, a single internal hydrophobic domain of 19 residues which acts as a transmembrane domain and forms the pore of the channel, and a 54-residue cytoplasmic tail [6].

Despite the small size of the active M_2 oligomer, several lines of evidence indicate that ion channel activity is intrinsic to the M_2 protein. First, ion channel activity has been observed in three different expression systems, Xenopus oocytes [3,7,8], mammalian cells [5,9] and yeast [10]. Second, M_2 channel activity has also been recorded in artificial lipid bilayers from a reconstituted peptide corresponding to the transmembrane domain of the M_2 protein [11] and from purified M_2 protein [12]. Thus, due to its structural simplicity, the M_2 ion channel is a potentially useful model for the study of ion channels in general.

2. Active oligomeric state and pore-lining residues

2.1. Active oligomeric state

Chemical cross-linking studies showed the M_2 protein exists minimally as a homotetramer [13–15]. Statistical analysis of the ion channel activity of mixed oligomers also indicated that a homotetramer is the minimal active oligomeric form of the protein [16].

2.2. Identification of pore-lining residues

To determine which residues line the aqueous pore of the M_2 ion channel, a set of mutants was generated in which each residue of the M_2 TM domain (residues 25–44) was substituted for cysteine [17]. The accessibility of the cysteine residues to aqueous sulfhydryl-specific reagents applied both extracellularly and intracellularly was tested [18]. Oocytes were injected with mRNA for a given M_2 mutant, and membrane currents were recorded after the pH of the bath medium was lowered from pH 7.5–6.2 to activate the M_2 ion channel. A sulfhydryl-specific reagent was then added to the bath and its effect on current was recorded. After the membrane current reached a new steady-state amplitude, the reagent was washed out. Finally, amantadine (100 μM) was added to determine M_2-specific currents. As a control, the currents were recorded from an M_2 ion channel that did not contain a cysteine residue. The effect of extracellular MTSEA application on mutant channels with cysteines substituted at every position in the putative transmembrane domain was tested. The conductances of only two mutants, M_2-A30C and M_2-G34C, decreased ($34 \pm 3\%$, $n = 7$ and $20 \pm 3\%$, $n = 7$, respectively; $p < 0.05$, according to one-way ANOVA using the Student–Newman–Keuls test). The currents of the M_2-G34C ion channel were also inhibited by the sulfhydryl-specific reagents MTSET (2 mM) and NEM (1 mM), although the inhibition observed was less ($14 \pm 5\%$, $n = 3$ and $7 \pm 2\%$, $n = 5$, respectively). No other mutant ion channels were inhibited in this way, although two could not be tested (M_2-L26C and M_2-H37C) because they had very low currents, even when measured at very low pH. These results are consistent with Ala-30 and Gly-34 lining the channel pore. In order to determine the accessibility to intracellular sulfhydryl-specific reagent, oocytes expressing 10 individual M_2 mutant proteins (M_2-G34C to M_2-W41C) were injected with a concentrated MTSET solution (40 mM, yielding a final cytoplasmic concentration of approximately 2 mM), and the effects on currents were measured. Only the currents of oocytes expressing the M_2-W41C mutant decreased, although again, we were not able to test His-37 because of its low activity when substituted with cysteine. Injection with water had no effect on the observed currents, indicating that the decreased current observed with the M_2-W41C mutant was a specific effect of the reagent and was not due to the diminution of the leakage current, increase of oocyte volume, or other non-specific mechanical effects. Importantly, M_2-G34C was not affected by internal MTSEA, in contrast to the results obtained when the reagent was applied extracellularly. These results are consistent with Trp-41 lining the channel pore, and the data for M_2-G34C indicate that the reagent is not able to permeate through to the outer membrane region of the pore.

The possibility that His-37 is a pore-lining residue was tested by measuring membrane currents of oocytes expressing the M_2 protein in a bathing solution containing various transition metals [19]. Membrane currents were strongly and reversibly inhibited by Cu^{2+} involving a fast-binding peripheral site with low specificity for divalent metal ions, as well as a high-affinity site ($K_{diss} = \sim 3$ μM) that lies deep within the pore and shows rather slow-binding kinetics ($k_{on} = 20 \pm 5$ M^{-1} s^{-1}). The pH-dependence of the interaction with the high-affinity Cu^{2+}-binding site parallels the pH dependence of inhibition by amantadine, which has previously been ascribed to the protonation of His-37. The voltage-dependence of the inhibition at the high-affinity site indicates that the binding site lies within the transmembrane region of the pore. Further, the inhibition by Cu^{2+} could be prevented by prior application of the reversible blocker of M_2 channel activity, BL-1743, providing further support for the location of the site within the pore region of the M_2 protein. Finally, substitutions of His-37 by alanine or glycine eliminated the high-affinity site, and resulted in membrane currents that were only partially inhibited at millimolar concentrations of Cu^{2+}. These results are consistent with the interpretation that His-37 lines the channel pore.

3. Functional studies

3.1. Mechanism for proton conduction

We have confirmed the high proton selectivity of the channel ($1.5 - 2.0 \times 10^6$) in both oocytes and mammalian cells that occur under naturally occurring conditions by using four methods: (1) comparison of V_{rev} with proton equilibrium potential; (2) measurement of pH_{in} and V_{rev} while Na_{out}^+ was replaced; (3) measurements with limiting external buffer concentration to limit proton currents specifically; and (4) comparison of measurements of

M_2-expressing cells with cells exposed to a protonophore [20]. However, the M_2 ion channel is also capable of conducting ammonium and hydroxylamine ions when these ions are present in the bathing solution [8,20]. M_2 ion channel activity is increased when the pH of the extracellular domain is lowered [3,5,21]. This increase in activity occurs within the range of pH values expected for titration of histidine [22]. The only amino acid in the transmembrane domain of the M_2 protein with a titratable group in this pH range is His-37, and when His-37 is replaced by Ala, Gly or Glu, the proton selectivity of the channel is greatly reduced, and the channel is conductive over a wider range of pH [3,5]. It has been proposed that His-37 forms a selectivity filter for protons [17]. Two possible mechanisms could account for the high proton selectivity of the M_2 ion channel. First, it is possible that certain residues of the pore form a narrow selectivity filter through which only hydronium ions can pass. Second, a residue in the pore region might form part of a conducting pathway, perhaps a proton wire [23], by providing a site highly favorable for interactions with protons. We distinguished between these possibilities by replacing the water solvent with D_2O. To test the possibility that protons interact directly with the M_2 ion channel protein when traversing its pore region, we took advantage of some differences in the physical properties of H_2 and D_2. First, D_2O is 1.25 times more viscous than H_2O. If protons pass through the M_2 channel as hydronium ions, then only a modest decrease in current on changing from H_2O to D_2O solvent would be expected according to the ratio of their viscosities. On the other hand, if protons traverse the M_2 channel via a proton wire, involving the exchange of protons between H_2O molecules occupying the channel pore, or if protons interact directly with the channel, then a larger conductance decrease upon changing from H_2O to D_2O should occur since there exists a large difference in both the mobility and the zero point energies of protons and deuterons, respectively [23,24]. To test between these possibilities, we compared the conductance and reversal voltage of M_2-expressing oocytes bathed in water and D_2O solvents. The water permeability of the oocyte membrane is very high, and it has been demonstrated [23] that the external solvent will determine the internal solvent of the cell in these experiments. An alteration of the internal solvent would be expected to modify the internal hydrogen ion concentration of the cell since the dissociation constant for many buffers is lower for protons than for deuterons. Thus, simply changing the external solvent from H_2O to D_2O at constant pL_{out} (pH_{out} or pD_{out}) would be expected to increase the pL_{in} of the ooplasm. We compared the conductance of M_2-expressing oocytes at three or more values of pL_{out} in the same oocyte between $pL_{out} = 5.0$ and $pL_{out} = 7.5$. For every value of pL_{out} tested, the current–voltage relationship of the amantadine-sensitive current had the same overall shape in both solvents, with a higher slope conductance for more negative membrane voltages. Also, for every value of pL_{out} tested, the relationship shifted to more positive voltages and its slope decreased (by 50–60%) when D_2O was substituted for H_2O. This comparison of the conductance measured in water and D_2O suggests that hydrogen ions do not pass through the channel in the form of hydronium ions. If this were the case, only a modest decrease in conductance would be expected due the greater viscosity of D_2O, about 20%. Instead, we found that the slope conductance, measured over a range of ~ 1.5 pH units, decreased by 40–50%. The greater decrease in conductance could be explained by either deuterons having a greater affinity than protons for a titratable group lining the M_2 channel pore [24], or by the large difference in the mobilities of protons in H_2O and deuterons in D_2O [23].

Several lines of evidence indicate that one of the ionizable groups of the channel that binds the conducting protons lies within the electric field of the membrane. First, the slope conductance of the current–voltage relationship increases for negative voltages. The voltage-dependence that we measured is similar to that found previously in MEL cells [5]. Secondly, site-directed mutagenesis experiments have shown that residue His-37 is essential for the activation of the current of the M_2 channel by low pH [22]. The experiments described above have shown that the channel can be inhibited with Cu^{2+} and that the high-affinity site for inhibition results from coordination of Cu^{2+} with residue His-37 [19]. This inhibition is strongly voltage-dependent, indicating that residue His-37 lies within the electric field of the membrane. It thus seems likely that residue His-37 binds protons as they traverse the pore of the channel [17].

3.2. Evidence for a conformational change in the M_2 ion channel protein under conditions experienced during the viral life cycle

High ion selectivity and activation are the two hallmarks of ion channel proteins. The process of activation is accompanied by structural changes that have been observed by the movement of charged elements of several ion channels as they open (activate) and close (deactivate) when an activating stimulus is presented [25–27]. The suggestion that the M_2 ion channel undergoes activation has been obtained by examination of the current–voltage relationship of the channel under conditions where the pH of the medium in the ectodomain is lower than that of the cytoplasmic domain [3–5]. If the channel did not undergo activation, the slope of this relationship would be significantly greater for the current passing from the region of high $[H^+]$ to low $[H^+]$ than for current passing from the opposite direction, i.e., greater for inward than for outward current. However, the slope of the relationship is found to be nearly equal under these conditions, a finding that could be explained by the occurrence of a conformational change that increases the permeability for protons in both directions (activation). This conclusion has been supported by several models of the channel obtained by molecular dynamic simulation [28,29]. Although the H^+ current of the M_2 ion channel protein in both the inward and outward directions is increased by elevated $[H^+]$ in the extracellular medium, this increased current might also be due to an increased abundance of the conducting species, in addition to the activation of the channel at low pH. One way to distinguish pH-dependent changes in the activity from the effects of increased abundance of H^+ at low pH is to compare the efflux of H^+ from acidified cells that express the M_2 protein to the efflux from acidified cells treated with the electrogenic protonophore FCCP, which is not believed to undergo a conformational change similar to that of ion channel proteins undergoing activation. Cell acidification can be achieved by lowering the pH of the medium bathing M_2-expressing or FCCP-treated cells. If the M_2 ion channel is indeed activated by low pH_{out} and conversely deactivated by neutral or alkaline pH_{out}, then the efflux of H^+ should be greater for FCCP-treated cells than for M_2-expressing cells upon return to a bathing solution of neutral or alkaline pH [20]. The inward current of FCCP-treated cells normally appeared within 1 min of exposing cells to FCCP, a delay that was probably due to the time required for incorporation of FCCP into the oocyte plasma membrane. The pH_{in} of oocytes treated with FCCP did not begin to decrease until about 100 s after the increase of inward current.

One important difference was noted between the behavior of oocytes expressing the M_2 protein and those into which FCCP had been incorporated. When the pH of the bathing solution of FCCP-treated oocytes was returned to pH 8.5 following oocyte acidification, a large, transient outward current appeared. This was in contrast with the measurements of M_2-expressing oocytes for which no outward current flowed upon return to bathing medium of pH 8.5 after prolonged bathing in low pH medium. The incorporation of FCCP into the plasma membrane appeared to be reversible, as re-exposure of oocytes to a medium of pH 5.8 following washout of FCCP in the medium of pH 8.5 failed to produce an inward current. These results support the conclusion that the M_2 ion channel is activated by low pH of the extracellular domain of the protein.

4. Conclusions

Our model for the function of the M_2 ion channel is that its aqueous pore is lined by residues Val-27, Ala-30, Gly-34, His-37 and Trp-41. Upon lowering the pH of the medium bathing the extracellular domain, a conformational change occurs in the protein that promotes the ready access of H_3O^+ to an imidazole nitrogen atom of His-37. The imidazole moieties are normally facing the lumen of the channel and obstruct the flow of ions other than the proton, thus, explaining the high proton selectivity of the channel. Because the channel is activated by lowered pH of the extracellular domain, the efflux of protons is not favored when the pH of the cytoplasmic domain is low but the pH of the extracellular domain is high. We expect that structural studies with solid state NMR [30–32] and site-directed spin labeling [33] will provide direct evidence of the structure of the pore-lining domain, and that unnatural amino acid mutagenesis [34,35] will provide further insight into the mechanism for proton transport by the transmembrane His residue. It is very likely that the inhibitory action of the antiviral drug amantadine requires the interaction of the imidazole nitrogen atoms with the amine nitrogen of amantadine. A better understanding of this interaction may allow the design of more useful and effective inhibitors of the channel.

References

[1] A.J. Hay, The action of adamantanamines against influenza A viruses: inhibition of the M_2 ion channel protein, Sem. Virol. 3 (1992) 21–30.
[2] R.A. Lamb, L.J. Holsinger, L.H. Pinto, The influenza A virus M_2 ion channel protein and its role in the influenza virus life cycle, in: E. Wimmer (Ed.), Receptor-Mediated Virus Entry into Cells, Cold Spring Harbor Press, Cold Spring Harbor, NY, 1994, pp. 303–321.
[3] L.H. Pinto, L.J. Holsinger, R.A. Lamb, Influenza virus M_2 protein has ion channel activity, Cell 69 (3) (1992) 517–528.
[4] C. Wang, K. Takeuchi, L.H. Pinto, R.A. Lamb, The ion channel activity of the influenza A virus M_2 protein: characterization of the amantadine block, J. Virol. 67 (9) (1993) 5585–5594.
[5] I.V. Chizhmakov, F.M. Geraghty, D.C. Ogden, A. Hayhurst, M. Antoniou, A.J. Hay, Selective proton permeability and pH regulation of the influenza virus M_2 channel expressed in mouse erythroleukemia cells, J. Physiol. 494 (1996) 329–336.
[6] R.A. Lamb, S.L. Zebedee, C.D. Richardson, Influenza virus M_2 protein is an integral membrane protein expressed on the infected cell surface, Cell 40 (1985) 627–633.

[7] L.J. Holsinger, D. Nichani, L.H. Pinto, R.A. Lamb, Influenza A virus M_2 ion channel protein: a structure–function analysis, J. Virol. 68 (3) (1994) 1551–1563.

[8] K. Shimbo, D.L. Brassard, R.A. Lamb, L.H. Pinto, Ion selectivity and activation of the M_2 ion channel of influenza virus, Biophys. J. 70 (1996) 1336–1346.

[9] C. Wang, R.A. Lamb, L.H. Pinto, Direct measurement of the influenza A virus M_2 protein ion channel in mammalian cells, Virology 205 (1994) 133–140.

[10] S. Kurtz, G. Luo, K.M. Hahnenberger, C. Brooks, O. Gecha, K. Ingalls, et al., Growth impairment resulting from expression of influenza virus M_2 protein in *Saccharomyces cerevisiae*: identification of a novel inhibitor of influenza virus, Antimicrob. Agents Chemother. 39 (1995) 2204–2209.

[11] K.C. Duff, R.H. Ashley, The transmembrane domain of influenza A M_2 protein forms amantadine-sensitive proton channels in planar lipid bilayers, Virology 190 (1992) 485–489.

[12] M.T. Tosteson, L.H. Pinto, L.J. Holsinger, R.A. Lamb, Reconstitution of the influenza virus M_2 ion channel in lipid bilayers, J. Membr. Biol. 142 (1) (1994) 117–126.

[13] L.J. Holsinger, R.A. Lamb, Influenza virus M_2 integral membrane protein is a homotetramer stabilized by formation of disulfide bonds, Virology 183 (1) (1991) 32–43.

[14] P.P. Panayotov, R.W. Schlesinger, Oligomeric organization and strain-specific proteolytic modification of the virion M_2 protein of influenza A H1N1 viruses, Virology 186 (1992) 352–355.

[15] R.J. Sugrue, A.J. Hay, Structural characteristics of the M_2 protein of influenza A viruses: evidence that it forms a tetrameric channel, Virology 180 (2) (1991) 617–624.

[16] T. Sakaguchi, Q. Tu, L.H. Pinto, R.A. Lamb, The active oligomeric state of the minimalistic influenza virus M_2 ion channel is a tetramer, Proc. Natl. Acad. Sci. U. S. A. 94 (1997) 5000–5005.

[17] L.H. Pinto, G.R. Dieckmann, C.S. Gandhi, M.A. Shaughnessy, C.G. Papworth, J. Braman, et al., A functionally defined model for the M_2 proton channel of influenza A virus suggests a mechanism for its ion selectivity, Proc. Natl. Acad. Sci. U. S. A. 94 (1997) 11301–11306.

[18] K. Shuck, R.A. Lamb, L.H. Pinto, Analysis of the pore structure of the influenza A virus M(2) ion channel by the substituted cysteine accessibility method [in process citation], J. Virol. 74 (17) (2000) 7755–7761.

[19] C.S. Gandhi, K. Shuck, J.D. Lear, G.R. Dieckmann, W.F. DeGrado, R.A. Lamb, et al., Cu(II) inhibition of the proton translocation machinery of the influenza A virus M_2 protein, J. Biol. Chem. 274 (9) (1999) 5474–5482.

[20] J.A. Mould, J.E. Drury, S.M. Frings, U.B. Kaupp, A. Pekosz, R.A. Lamb, et al., Permeation and activation of the M_2 ion channel of influenza A virus, J. Biol. Chem 37 (2000) 31038–31050.

[21] Q. Tu, L.H. Pinto, G. Luo, M.A. Shaughnessy, D. Mullaney, S. Kurtz, et al., Characterization of inhibition of M_2 ion channel activity by BL-1743, an inhibitor of influenza A virus, J. Virol. 70 (1996) 4246–4252.

[22] C. Wang, R.A. Lamb, L.H. Pinto, Activation of the M_2 ion channel of influenza virus: a role for the transmembrane domain histidine residue, Biophys. J. 69 (1995) 1363–1371.

[23] T.E. DeCoursey, V.V. Cherny, Deuterium isotope effects on permeation and gating of proton channels in rat alveolar epithelium, J. Gen. Physiol. 109 (4) (1997) 415–434.

[24] A. Fersht, Enzyme Structure and Mechanism, Freeman, New York, 1985.

[25] C.M. Armstrong, F. Bezanilla, Charge movement associated with the opening and closing of the activation gates of the Na channels, J. Gen. Physiol. 63 (5) (1974) 533–552.

[26] A. Cha, G.E. Snyder, P.R. Selvin, F. Bezanilla, Atomic scale movement of the voltage-sensing region in a potassium channel measured via spectroscopy, Nature 402 (6763) (1999) 809–813.

[27] K.S. Glauner, L.M. Mannuzzu, C.S. Gandhi, E.Y. Isacoff, Spectroscopic mapping of voltage sensor movement in the Shaker potassium channel, Nature 402 (6763) (1999) 813–817.

[28] K.J. Schweighofer, A. Pohorille, Computer simulation of ion channel gating: the M(2) channel of influenza A virus in a lipid bilayer, Biophys. J. 78 (1) (2000) 150–163.

[29] Q. Zhong, D.M. Newns, P. Pattnaik, J.D. Lear, M.L. Klein, Two possible conducting states of the influenza A virus M_2 ion channel, FEBS Lett. 473 (2) (2000) 195–198.

[30] F.A. Kovacs, J.K. Denny, Z. Song, J.R. Quine, T.A. Cross, Helix tilt of the M_2 transmembrane peptide from influenza A virus: an intrinsic property, J. Mol. Biol. 295 (1) (2000) 117–125.

[31] Z. Song, F.A. Kovacs, J. Wang, J.K. Denny, S.C. Shekar, J.R. Quine, et al., Transmembrane domain of M_2 protein from influenza A virus studied by solid-state (15)N polarization inversion spin exchange at magic angle NMR [in process citation], Biophys. J. 79 (2) (2000) 767–775.

[32] F.A. Kovacs, T.A. Cross, Transmembrane four-helix bundle of influenza A M_2 protein channel: structural implications from helix tilt and orientation, Biophys. J. 73 (5) (1997) 2511–2517.

[33] R. Mollaaghababa, H.J. Steinhoff, W.L. Hubbell, H.G. Khorana, Time-resolved site-directed spin-labeling studies of bacteriorhodopsin: loop-specific conformational changes in M, Biochemistry 39 (5) (2000) 1120–1127.

[34] P.M. England, Y. Zhang, D.A. Dougherty, H.A. Lester, Backbone mutations in transmembrane domains of a ligand-gated ion channel: implications for the mechanism of gating, Cell 96 (1) (1999) 89–98.

[35] M.W. Nowak, J.P. Gallivan, S.K. Silverman, C.G. Labarca, D.A. Dougherty, H.A. Lester, In vivo incorporation of unnatural amino acids into ion channels in *Xenopus* oocyte expression system, Methods Enzymol. 293 (1998) 504–529.

International Congress Series 1219 (2001) 397–404

Role of influenza virus M1 protein in the viral budding process

Rob Ruigrok*, Florence Baudin, Isabelle Petit, Winfried Weissenhorn

EMBL Grenoble Outstation, BP 181, 38042 Grenoble cedex 9, France

---

Abstract

The initial step in the influenza virus budding process involves most likely the organisation of the glycoproteins in semi-crystalline membrane structures called "rafts". M1 protein then binds to the lipids and the cytoplasmic tails in these rafts (work by Kai Simons, Bob Lamb and Debi Nayak). In a next step, ribonucleoproteins (RNPs) bind to this initial scaffold. Here, we will discuss biochemical and structural data on M1 protein and its interactions with synthetic liposomes and viral RNPs. In solution, intact M1 is a monomeric, elongated protein. A recent neutral pH crystal structure of the N-terminal domain confirms the monomeric nature of M1 in solution. M1 seems to interact with negatively charged membranes though its N-terminal domain. This interaction has an important electrostatic component. The C-terminal domain binds to the RNPs in vitro. In relation to our work on the Ebola virus VP40 matrix protein, we suggest that there might be two conformations of M1 in the infected cell: one that is soluble and has a low affinity for membranes and RNP and one that polymerises easily and that has a high affinity for membranes and RNPs. © 2001 Elsevier Science B.V. All rights reserved.

Keywords: M1 protein; Budding; Membrane binding; RNP binding; M1 polymerisation

---

1. Introduction

Influenza virus particles have a genetic and a transport component. The genetic component consists of the segmented RNA genome complexed with the viral nucleoprotein and the RNA-dependent RNA polymerase, forming 8 ribonucleoprotein (RNP) particles. These RNPs are autonomous biological machines active in transcription and replication. The transport component consists of the lipid membrane and its embedded

---

* Corresponding author. EMBL Grenoble Outstation, 6 rue Jules Horowitz, 38000 Grenoble, France. Tel.: +33-4-76-20-72-73; fax: +33-4-76-20-71-99.

E-mail address: ruigrok@embl-grenoble.fr (R. Ruigrok).

0531-5131/01/$ – see front matter © 2001 Elsevier Science B.V. All rights reserved.
PII: S0531-5131(01)00637-9

glycoprotein spikes, haemagglutinin and neuraminidase, instrumental for virus entry and for release of newly formed virus from the infected cell. Embedded in the lipid membrane is a further transport component, the M2 protein, that forms an ion channel needed for acidification of the virus interior during the cell entry process [1,2]. The M1 protein forms the bridge between these transport and genetic components. The protein is situated beneath the viral membrane [3–6] and makes contact with this membrane, with the cytoplasmic tails of the glycoproteins and with the RNPs.

M1 can either be seen in end-on view or in side view in electron microscopy images when the virus is negatively stained and the stain has penetrated the viral membrane. In end-on view, M1 appears as small dots that form lines, which associate in a two-dimensional array without apparent symmetry (Fig. 1A). The dots in the lines are about 4-nm apart and the lines themselves are also about 4-nm apart [7]. In the side view M1 is

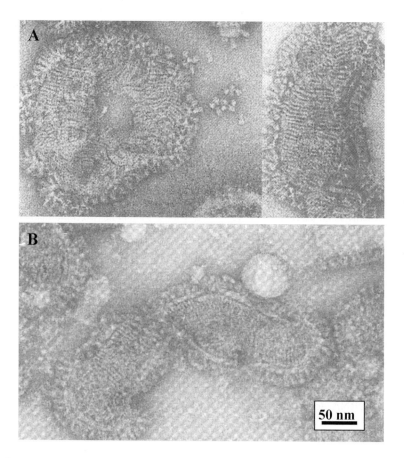

Fig. 1. Electron micrographs of influenza virus negatively stained with 1% sodium silicotungstate. The stain has penetrated the virus particles and outlines the M1 layer underneath the lipid membrane. The particles in A show M1 mainly in end-on views and the particle in B shows M1 in side views lying against the inside of the viral membrane as a thin, light rod. The bar in B represents 50 nm.

seen as a thin rod, 6-nm long, that touches the viral membrane with one of its ends (Fig. 1B). In these side views, M1 seems to make contact with the membrane but does not seem to enter it to any significant extent [8].

Fig. 2 shows the primary sequence of influenza A virus M1 protein with some of its functional domains. The protein can bind zinc through the 148-CCHH-162 sequence [9,10]. A small fraction of M1 in the virus indeed contains zinc but up to now, the

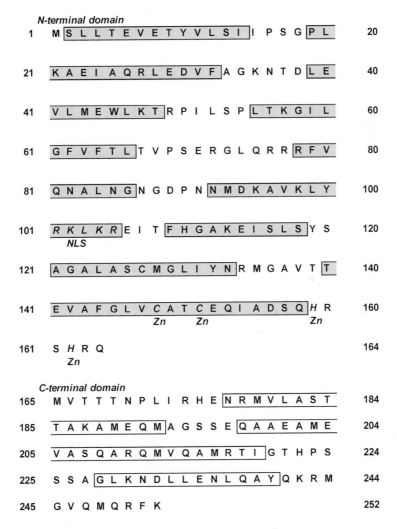

Fig. 2. Sequence of influenza virus A/PR/8/34 M1 protein. The sequence is divided into two parts, the N-terminal domain from amino acid residue 1–164 and the C-terminal domain from residue 165–252. The grey boxed bars in the N-terminal part represent the *known* α-helices observed in the crystal structure and the open boxes in the C-terminal part represent *predicted* α-helices. Two functional sequences in the N-terminal domain are in italics and noted below the sequence; the nuclear localisation sequence (*NLS*) and the zinc binding sequence (*HHCC* indicated by *Zn*).

significance of this activity, conserved between A and B viruses, is not known. The protein also has a nuclear localisation signal, the 101-RKLKR-105 sequence [11]. This sequence is also responsible for the in vitro binding activity of M1 to naked RNA [12,13]. Again, the significance of the binding activity of M1 to naked RNA is not known. In the virus, virtually all of the viral RNA is bound to the nucleoprotein that covers the sugar–phosphate backbone of the RNA and has a 10-fold higher affinity for naked RNA than the M1 protein [13,14]. For this reason, it is unlikely that the binding of M1 to the viral RNA is important for the budding process. It is possible that binding to viral or cellular RNA is necessary when M1 is localised in the nucleus. Fig. 2 shows another important feature of the M1 protein that is observed when the protein is either isolated from virus or from a recombinant source: in solution, the protein is cleaved between glutamine 164 and methionine 165. The nature of the protease responsible for this cleavage is unknown and the specificity of glutamine–methionine is only known for certain plant virus proteases. This cleavage occurred during the incubation process for crystallisation of virus-isolated M1 protein and as a result of this, only the N-terminal part of the protein was found in the crystals [15,16]. We have independently observed the same phenomenon in crystallising recombinant protein and in many of the biochemical and physical measurements and experiments described below. This cleavage suggests that the M1 protein in solution consists of two domains connected by a protease accessible linker.

2. Shape of M1 in crystal and in solution

The N-terminal domain of M1 was first crystallised at pH 4 [15,16]. This domain is highly structured with two bundles of four α-helices that pack together with a hydrophobic interface (see schematic representation in Fig. 3). In the low-pH crystal, two monomers of M1 are packed as a dimer and it was suggested that M1 was dimeric in solution based on the abnormal behaviour of the protein on gel exclusion columns. However, when we crystallised the N-terminal fragment at neutral pH, the molecule in the crystal was a monomer and the crystal packing suggested that the protein was monomeric when it crystallised (Arzt et al., submitted for publication). Otherwise, the structures of M1 at low-pH and at neutral pH are identical. A particular feature that we further observed is that one side of M1 is strongly positively charged and one side is negatively charged. The molecules in the crystal pack with their positive side onto the negative side of their neighbour. The solubility of isolated, intact M1 is strongly dependent on the salt concentration and on the pH, which may be related to these surface charges.

We then decided to study the shape and oligomeric structure of intact M1 protein and its N-terminal domain in solution, by using a variety of biophysical techniques. In gel exclusion chromatography, intact M1 (28 kDa) behaved as a protein with an apparent molecular weight of 38 kDa. The N-terminal fragment (18 kDa) ran indeed as a protein of 18 kDa but the C-terminal domain (10 plus 2 kDa His-tag) eluted as a protein with a molecular weight of 20 kDa. Thus, in our hands, the intact M1 protein seems to be an elongated monomeric protein. The elongated shape may be caused by the addition of an elongated C-terminal domain to a spherical N-terminal domain. We also employed small angle neutron scattering (SANS) that gives information on the shape as well as on the

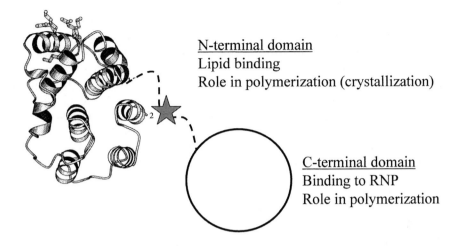

N-terminal domain
Lipid binding
Role in polymerization (crystallization)

C-terminal domain
Binding to RNP
Role in polymerization

Fig. 3. Schematic representation of the structure and function of M1 protein. The structure of the N-terminal domain is shown with the NLS pointing out of the α-helix at the top. The last ordered residue in the crystal structure is Q-158 with the C-terminal six amino acids not visible because of disorder in the crystal. The N-terminal domain is connected in a flexible manner to the C-terminal domain whose structure is not known, although circular dichroism measurements have indicated that this domain contains 40% α-helix. The functions are written next to the domains. The five-pointed star indicates the naturally occurring cleavage site at 164Q–165M.

molecular weight of the particular species in solution. This technique also clearly indicated that both at pH 4 and 7, the N-terminal domain has the same monomeric structure in solution as in the crystal. In addition, we again found that the intact M1 protein is an elongated monomer in solution (Arzt et al., submitted for publication). We obtained similar results for M1 protein isolated from virus as for recombinant M1. Finally, there does not seem be any obvious symmetry in the M1 layer underneath the viral membrane (Fig. 1). This is also an indication that the M1 protein participates in budding as a monomer.

From the SANS data, we were able to estimate the length of M1 in solution to be 8 nm, slightly longer than the 6 nm observed on the electron micrographs of M1 inside virus. However, it is possible that the relative orientation of the N- and C-terminal domains of M1 inside virus is different from that of M1 in solution.

3. Activities of M1: lipid and RNP binding and M1–M1 polymerisation

A number of interactions of M1 with other viral components need to take place during the formation of a virus particle. Some of these interactions could be tested in vitro.

The first activity that was tested was the interaction of M1 with lipid membranes. For 20 years, it had been assumed that M1 was an integral membrane protein [17,18] and that interaction of M1 with the membrane took place through hydrophobic stretches of amino acids. However, in the crystal structure of the N-terminal domain, these stretches of hydrophobic amino acids were found to be present in the hydrophobic core of the protein [15]. Kretzschmar et al. [19] found that M1 mutant proteins that lacked these hydrophobic sequences still interacted with membranes. Hydrophobic photolabelling of intact virus particles showed labelling of the transmembrane region of HA2 but no clear labelling of M1, suggesting that M1 is not inserted into the membrane to any significant extent. Then, we tested the interaction of M1 protein with liposomes in vitro. We found that M1 binds to negatively charged but not to neutrally charged liposomes and that this binding could be inhibited by high salt and high pH [8]. However, after the initial binding of M1 to the negatively charged liposomes, the interaction had become less sensitive to salt. This lipid binding behaviour is very similar to that of the vesicular stomatitis virus M protein [20]. We then tested the intact M1 protein and its N- and C-terminal domains separately for liposome binding and found that both intact M1 and the N-terminal domain bound to lipid but not the C-terminal part (Baudin et al., submitted for publication).

The second activity we tested was RNP binding, again for intact M1 as well as its two subdomains, in a cosedimentation assay of RNP plus added protein. Both intact M1 and its C-terminal domain bound to RNPs but not the N-terminal domain (Baudin t al., submitted for publication; see also Ref. [21]). However, for in vitro transcription inhibition, only the intact M1 protein was active.

The third activity is the M1–M1 polymerisation activity needed for building the M1 network underneath the viral membrane. One of the clear observations we made is that both the isolated intact M1 protein and its C-terminal domain were very difficult to concentrate. When the concentration was higher than 2–3 mg/ml, the protein aggregated/ polymerised. We also observed phenomena of seeded polymerisation of oversaturated protein solutions, as if the protein wants to polymerise, which is what it is designed to do during virus formation. In contrast, under the right salt conditions, the N-terminal domain could easily be concentrated to the high concentrations needed for crystallisation. Under the right conditions, large crystals grew within 10 min. Therefore, we would like to suggest that both the N-terminal and C-terminal domains of M1 are involved in the polymerisation process.

4. Model for M1 shape and activities; role in budding process

Fig. 3 shows a model for M1 protein in solution with the attributed activities for the N- and C-terminal domains. The star indicates the site at which proteolytic digestion occurs. This model depicts the M1 protein after isolation from virus and also as it is isolated in recombinant form. The protein has two domains connected by a flexible linker. It is probable that the relative orientation of the two domains in solution is different from that when M1 is assembled inside the virus particle. The N-terminal domain binds to negatively charged liposomes and the C-terminal domain binds to RNP. This would define the orientation of the M1 rods inside the virus particle; the thin end that touches the membrane is probably the N-terminal part of M1.

It is interesting to compare the shape and activities of influenza virus M1 protein with those of the matrix protein of Ebola virus. Although the structures of the two proteins are totally different [15,22], the roles that the two proteins have to play during the budding process may be similar. The intact Ebola virus VP40 matrix protein is a soluble and monomeric protein [22]. However, when the protein is destabilised with urea or when the protein is placed in the presence of negatively charged liposomes, it self-associates into hexameric complexes and at the same time, it acquires affinity for negatively charged membranes. These hexameric molecules clearly have two domains that seem to be flexibly linked (Scianimanico et al., submitted for publication). When the C-terminal part of VP40 is removed from the intact protein, the N-terminal part also forms hexameric rings that can no longer associate with membranes [23]. These rings, however, do not have the second, flexibly linked domain. So it seems that for Ebola virus VP40, the protein is first produced in monomeric, soluble form, but the protein can undergo a conformational change upon which two domains are separated. The N-terminal domain of the Ebola VP40 is needed for oligomerization and probably also nucleocapsid binding and the C-terminal domain is needed for membrane association.

Based on the presented data on M1 and Ebola VP40, we suggest that influenza virus M1 is synthesised as a soluble protein that might undergo a conformational change at the site for virus budding, exposing the interfaces for M1–M1 polymerisation, M1–lipid binding and M1–RNP binding. Although there is as yet no proof for such a soluble, inactive conformation, coexpressed M1 and nucleoprotein do not form hetero-oligomers in BHK-21 cells [24]. Further, for a number of negative strand RNA viruses, it has been described that the matrix protein has two different conformations [25–27]. For influenza virus matrix protein, the zinc binding sequence is right in the middle between the N- and C-terminal domains. The presence of zinc would certainly have an effect on the conformation of the 6 C-terminal residues of the N-terminal domain that are invisible in the crystal structure and would probably also have an effect on the orientation of the two domains with respect to each other.

References

[1] R.A. Lamb, R.M. Krug, Orthomyxoviridae: the viruses and their replication, in: B.N. Fields, D.M. Knipe, P.M. Howley, et al. (Eds.), Fields Virology, 3rd edn., Lippincot-Raven Publishers, Philadelphia, 1996.

[2] R.W.H. Ruigrok, Structure of influenza A, B, and C viruses, in: K.G. Nicholson, R.G. Webster, A.J. Hay (Eds.), Textbook of Influenza, Blackwell, Oxford, 1998, pp. 29–42.

[3] M.V. Nermut, Further investigation on the fine structure of influenza virus, J. Gen. Virol. 17 (1972) 317–331.

[4] J.S. Oxford, D.J. Hockley, Orthomyxoviridae, in: M.V. Nermut, A.C. Steven (Eds.), Animal Virus Structure, Elsevier, Amsterdam, 1987, pp. 213–232.

[5] I.T. Schulze, The structure of influenza virus: II. A model based on the morphology and composition of subviral particles, Virology 47 (1972) 181–196.

[6] N.G. Wrigley, Electron microscopy of influenza virus, Br. Med. Bull. 35 (1979) 35–38.

[7] R.W.H. Ruigrok, L.J. Calder, S.A. Wharton, Electron microscopy of the influenza virus submembranal structure, Virology 173 (1989) 311–316.

[8] R.W.H. Ruigrok, A. Barge, P. Durrer, J. Brunner, K. Ma, G.R. Whittaker, Membrane interaction of influenza virus M1 protein, Virology 267 (2000) 289–298.

[9] L. Wakefield, G.G. Brownlee, RNA-binding properties of influenza A virus matrix protein M1, Nucleic Acids Res. 17 (1989) 8569–8580.

[10] C. Elster, E. Forest, F. Baudin, K. Larsen, S. Cusack, R.W.H. Ruigrok, A small percentage of influenza virus M1 protein contains zinc but zinc does not influence in vitro M1–RNA interaction, J. Gen. Virol. 75 (1994) 37–42.

[11] Z. Ye, D. Robinson, R.R. Wagner, Nucleus-targeting domain of the matrix protein (M1) of influenza virus, J. Virol. 69 (1995) 1964–1970.

[12] K. Watanabe, H. Handa, K. Mizumoto, K. Nagata, Mechanism for inhibition of influenza virus RNA polymerase activity by matrix protein, J. Virol. 70 (1996) 241–247.

[13] C. Elster, K. Larsen, J. Gagnon, R.W.H. Ruigrok, F. Baudin, Influenza virus M1 protein binds to RNA through its nuclear localisation signal, J. Gen. Virol. 78 (1997) 1589–1596.

[14] F. Baudin, C. Bach, S. Cusack, R.W.H. Ruigrok, Structure of influenza virus RNP: I. Influenza virus nucleoprotein melts secondary structure in panhandle RNA and exposes the bases to the solvent, EMBO J. 13 (1994) 3158–3165.

[15] B. Sha, M. Luo, Structure of a bifunctional membrane-RNA binding protein, influenza virus matrix protein M1, Nat. Struct. Biol. 4 (1997) 239–244.

[16] B. Sha, M. Luo, Crystallization and preliminary X-ray crystallographic studies of type A influenza virus matrix protein M1, Acta Crystallogr., Sect. D. 53 (1997) 458–460.

[17] D.J. Bucher, I.G. Kharitonenkov, J.A. Zakomirdin, V.B. Grigoriev, S.M. Klimenko, J.F. Davis, Incorporation of influenza virus M-protein into liposomes, J. Virol. 36 (1980) 586–590.

[18] A. Gregoriades, B. Frangione, Insertion of influenza M protein into the viral lipid bilayer and localization of site of insertion, J. Virol. 40 (1981) 323–328.

[19] E. Kretzschmar, M. Bui, J.K. Rose, Membrane association of influenza virus matrix protein does not require specific hydrophobic domains or the viral glycoproteins, Virology 220 (1996) 37–45.

[20] J.J. Zakowski, W.A. Petri Jr., R.R. Wagner, Role of matrix protein in assembling the membrane of vesicular stomatitis virus: reconstitution of matrix protein with negatively charged phospholipid vesicles, Biochemistry 20 (1981) 3902–3907.

[21] Z. Ye, T. Liu, D.P. Offringa, J. McInnis, R.A. Levandowski, Association of influenza virus matrix protein with ribonucleoproteins, J. Virol. 73 (1999) 7467–7473.

[22] A. Dessen, V. Volchkov, O. Dolnik, H.D. Klenk, W. Weissenhorn, Crystal structure of the matrix protein VP40 from Ebola virus, EMBO J. 15 (19) (2000) 4228–4236.

[23] R.W.H. Ruigrok, G. Schoehn, A. Dessen, E. Forest, V. Volchkov, O. Dolnik, H.-D. Klenk, W. Weissenhorn, Structural characterization and membrane binding properties of the matrix protein VP40 of Ebola virus, J. Mol. Biol. 300 (2000) 103–112.

[24] H. Zhao, M. Ekström, H. Garoff, The M1 and NP proteins of influenza A virus form homo- but not heterooligomeric complexes when co-expressed in BHK-21 cells, J. Gen. Virol. 79 (1998) 2335–2446.

[25] Y. Gaudin, C. Tuffereau, A. Benmansour, A. Flamand, Fatty acylation of rabies virus proteins, Virology 184 (1991) 441–444.

[26] A. Hirano, A.H. Wang, A.F. Gombart, T.C. Wong, The matrix proteins of neurovirulent subacute sclerosing panencephalitis virus and its acute measles virus progenitor are functionally different, Proc. Natl. Acad. Sci. U. S. A. 89 (1992) 8745–8749.

[27] M. De Melo, G. Mottet, C. Orvell, L. Roux, Sendai virus M protein is found in two distinct isoforms defined by monoclonal antibodies, Virus Res. 24 (1992) 47–64.

International Congress Series 1219 (2001) 405–410

The crystal structure of the influenza matrix protein M1 at neutral pH: M1-M1 protein interfaces can rotate in the oligomeric structures of M1

Audray Harris, Farhad Forouhar, Shihong Qiu, Bingdong Sha[1], Ming Luo*

Department of Microbiology and Center for Biophysical Sciences and Engineering, University of Alabama at Birmingham, Birmingham, AL 35294, USA

Abstract

Matrix protein (M1) of influenza virus is a bifunctional protein that mediates the encapsidation of RNA-nucleoprotein cores into the membrane envelope. Therefore, M1 must bind to both membrane and RNA simultaneously. The matrix protein, M1, of influenza virus strain A/PR/8/34 has been purified from virions and crystallized. The crystals consist of a stable fragment (18 kd) of the M1 protein. X-ray diffraction studies indicated that the crystals have a space group of P3121, with a=68.74 Å, c=136.57 Å. Vm calculations showed that there are two monomers in asymmetric unit. The success in crystallization will lead to the solution of the three-dimensional structure of the M1 protein. The X-ray crystal structure of a type A influenza virus M1 at pH 4.0 has been determined at 2.08-Å resolution. It consists of a stable N-terminal fragment from amino acid residue 2–158 in a dimeric form. A highly positively charged region on the dimmer surface is suitably positioned to bind RNA while the hydrophobic surface opposite the RNA binding region may be involved in interactions with membrane. The membrane-binding surface might have specific binding sites for accommodation of charged groups, hydrophobic parts or interactions with the envelope proteins. The structure of M1 was also determined at neutral pH. This structure showed conformational changes and a different mode of association compared to the pH 4.0 structure. Another protein (NS2) that may be associated with the M1 protein during assembly has been shown to be involved in nuclear export. Examination of its structure indicates that this protein has a flexible conformation. © 2001 Elsevier Science B.V. All rights reserved.

Keywords: Matrix protein; Influenza virus; RNA

---

* Corresponding author. Tel.: +1-205-934-4259; fax: +1-205-975-9578.
E-mail address: ming@cmc.uab.edu (M. Luo).
[1] Current address: Department of Cell Biology, University of Alabama at Birmingham, Birmingham, AL 35294, USA.

0531-5131/01/$ – see front matter © 2001 Elsevier Science B.V. All rights reserved.
PII: S 0 5 3 1 - 5 1 3 1 (0 1) 0 0 3 4 9 - 1

The assembly of influenza virus (IV) takes place at the plasma membrane where the ribonucleoprotein–RNA complex (RNP) is associated with the membrane and the envelope proteins, hemagglutinin and neuraminidase. In order to package the RNP and the polymerase into the infectious virions, a membrane associating matrix protein (M1) is required to target the RNP to the plasma membrane. Some other viral proteins may also be involved, such as the NS2 protein of IV which has been proposed to be the nuclear export protein [1], M1 is a phosphorylated 252 amino acid protein encoded by segment 7, which also encodes M2, a transmembrane proton channel. In the virion, M1 is tightly associated with RNP cores while interacting with the membrane envelope and the cytoplasmic tails of the spike glycoprotein [2]. Cleavage by formic acid produced two polypeptides, an N-terminal fragment (9 kd, residues 1–89), and a C-terminal fragment (15 kd, residues 90–252) [3]. The 9 kd fragment is readily bound to DPPC (dipalisitoylphosphatidylcholine) vesicles, equivalent to that of intact M1, while the C-terminal fragment does not show significant binding to lipids. This demonstrates that the N-terminal one third of M1 is the major domain responsible for M1 interaction with lipid bilayers. On the other hand, the C-terminal two thirds of M1 has a strong ability to inhibit the in vitro transcription of the RNPs. The 15 kd fragment of formic acid digestion can inhibit the transcription of RNP cores by ~70%, and the inhibition can be reversed by prebinding monoclonal antibody (289/6) to the 15 kd fragment [4]. An Arg–Lys rich region (residues 95–105 CKAV-KLYRKLKR) was also suggested to form charge interactions with the phosphate backbone in RNP [5], M1 also plays a role in nucleus transport of RNP [6]. By electron microscopy, Helenius et al. [6] demonstrated that after penetration, M1 was dissociated from RNP upon acidification of the endosome. This dissociation is inhibited by amantadine, the drug which blocks the function of the M2 proton channel [7]. RNP depleted M1 is actively transported through the nuclear pores to the nucleus where transcription/replication takes place. The released M1 passively diffuses into the nucleus at a lower efficiency. In later stages of virus infection, a large number of RNP particles are assembled in the nucleus. However, these RNP particles are confined to the nucleus if M1 is absent in the nucleus. Upon entering the nucleus, M1 promotes the transport of RNPs to the cytosol.

The crystal structure of this stable M1 fragment (which corresponds to amino acid 2–158 of the 252 amino acids in the intact M1) consists of nine α helices (H1–H9), eight loop regions (L1–L8) and no beta strands (Fig. 1). H1, H2, H3 and H4 form the first domain (N(-terminal) domain, amino acids 2–67) and H6, H7, H8 and H9 form the second domain (M(iddle) domain, amino acids 91–158). The missing amino acids 159–252 should form at least another domain (C-terminal domain). The first two domains are linked by a coil which contains a short helix H5. A half turn left-handed helix was found between H5 and H6. H1, H2, H3 and H4 form a so called "up and down" anti-parallel helix bundle, while anti-parallel H6, H7, H8 and H9 are crossed at H7. The linker, H5, connects the two domains via H4 and H6 which are parallel to each ether. A search for structurally homologous proteins in the Protein Data Bank by DALI 2.0 did not reveal any protein with a fold similar to M1 [8]. M1 forms a dimer in the asymmetric unit of the pH 4.0 crystal with an interface between the two monomers of 1620 $\overset{\circ}{A}{}^{2}$. The dimerization is maintained by the hydrophobic interactions between two antiparallel H6 helices from monomer A (residues A90 Pro, A93 Met and A97 Val) and B (residues B90 Pro, B93 Met

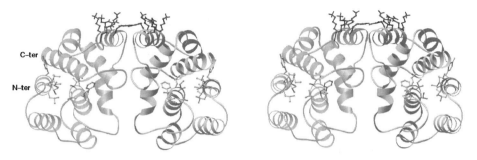

Fig. 1. The ribbon drawings of a stereo view of the M1 dimer in the pH 4.0 crystal asymmetric unit. The blue colored residues are those of the positively charged amino acids exposed at the boundary of the dimer. The green colored residues are those in the hydrophobic core of the M1 monomer.

and B97 Val), and a hydrogen bond network involving L4, H5, L5 from monomer A and L4, H5, L8 from monomer B, as well as bound water molecules. Ten positively charged groups within the RNA binding region reported by previous studies (A95 Lys, A98 Lys, A101 Arg, A102 Lys, A105 Arg in monomer A and their counterparts in monomer B) are exposed on a platform surface formed by helices H6 and H7. This sequence also corresponds to the nuclear targeting signal. The geometry of the N-terminal domain and the M-domain is consistent with that the N-terminal domain facing the membrane and the M-domain (perhaps also the C-terminal domain) facing the RNP.

The M1 protein was recently crystallized at pH7.0 and its crystal structure showed a different dimer arrangement, which is more consistent with the polymerization of the M1 protein under the membrane and/or on the RNP [9]. Further refinement and analysis is required to derive information with regard to the association of M1 in the influenza virus virion.

Another important protein associated with the assembly of the RNP is NS2. NS2 binds to the RNP only when M1 is associated with RNP [26,27]. Therefore, both proteins are essential for transport of the RNP to the assembly site at the plasma membrane. In an in vivo model system, it was shown that vRNP export was sufficiently induced by expression of recombinant M1 [28]. However, NS2 expression was required if efficient production of infectious virus-like particles was to be maintained [29]. We were able to establish a protocol to produce a large amount of purified NS2 from *Escherichia coli* expression (> 14 mg/l culture). The isolated protein appeared as one band of ca. 11 kDa on reducing SDS-PAGE similar to that previously found in cells infected with influenza virus. The N-terminal 5 amino acids were determined to be MDPNT by N-terminus sequencing, identifying the expressed protein as NS2. The ability of recombinant NS2 to bind matrix protein M1 was confirmed by a far Western blot assay. Characterization of the recombinant NS2 was carried out by several methods, including ANS binding, protease digestion, near UV CD spectrum, and thermal denaturation. The results indicated that NS2 is a two-domain protein with a very flexible conformation. Not only the linker of the two domains is flexible, but also the two domains themselves are not very stable (data not shown).

Based on the structural knowledge and literature results, we have proposed a model for the role of M1 in influenza virus assembly/disassembly (Fig. 2). When the virion enters the

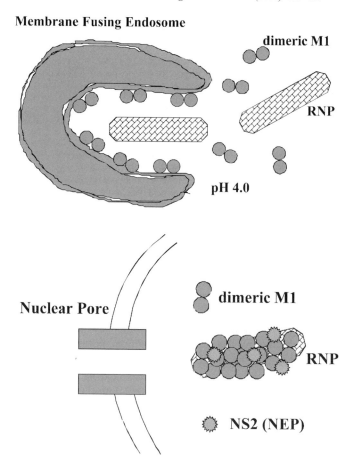

Fig. 2. The model of the role of M1 in the assembly/disassembly of influenza virus. (A) The disassociation of M1 from the RNP by acidification during fusion in the endosome. (B) Assembly of an export competent M1–RNP–NS2 complex in the nucleus.

infected cell, the interior of the virion in the endosome will be acidified, which will dissociate M1 from the RNP [Zhirnov, 1992 #32][Sha, 1997 #73]. After the viral membrane is fused with the cellular membrane, the RNP will be released to the cytosol without any M1 attached. Thus, the nuclear targeting signal will be unveiled, which directs the RNP to the nucleus. During the phase of assembly, M1 targets itself into the nucleus with its own nuclear targeting signal. Upon entering the nucleus, M1 switches the RNP–polymerase complex from transcription to replication, and becomes associated with the RNP. The M1-RNP is readied to bind NS2, which chaperones the export of the M1–RNP complex through the nuclear pore. The newly formed M1–RNP–NS2 can target to the plasma membrane to interact with the cytoplasmic tails of hemagglutinin and neuraminidase. A complete virion could be produced through budding. M1 plays a critical role directing the movement of the RNP in and out of the nucleus.

Matrix protein is universally present in all negative stranded RNA viruses, even in retroviruses [Lenard, 1996 #44]. In addition to similar functions between the matrix protein from negative stranded RNA viruses and retroviruses, there seem to be many structural similarities between the two families of proteins. However, we find that the N-terminal domain of M1 could be superimposed very well with that of MA from human immunodeficiency virus while the M-domain could be superimposed with CA, the capsid protein (Fig. 3) [Harris, 1999 #76]. The structural similarity between the HIV matrix and capsid proteins and influenza virus M1 protein may indicate remnants of a common ancestry. As the structure of more matrix or capsid proteins from enveloped retro and negative stranded viruses become available, more similarities may be identified to support this notion. The recent observation of structural similarities in the gp41 glycoprotein of HIV and the hemagglutinin of influenza virus provides an additional indication that retrovirus may have a common evolutionary origin with influenza virus. The 18 kd M1

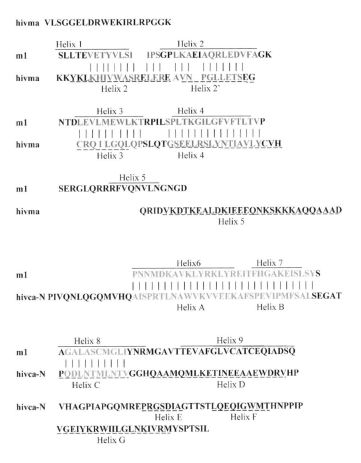

Fig. 3. The amino acid sequence alignment between M1 of influenza virus MA (A) and CA (B) of human immunodeficiency virus. The secondary structural elements are labeled under or above each sequence.

protein can be viewed as a fusion of a membrane binding N domain and a RNA binding M domain with similar folds and functions corresponding to the matrix protein and the capsid protein of HIV, respectively. This is particularly interesting since the HIV matrix and capsid proteins are initially joined in the GAG protein. Comparisons of the electrostatics of the M1 and the capsid dimers imply that the HIV capsid may have a different mode of binding the RNA/nucleocapsid complex, even though the electrostatic interaction may still play a minor role. Based on these results, we may suggest that similar folds could be present in the functionally similar matrix and capsid proteins of other enveloped retro or negative strand RNA viruses.

References

[1] R.E. O'Neill, J. Talon, P. Palese, The influenza virus NEP (NS2 protein) mediates the nuclear export of viral ribonucleoproteins, EMBO J. 17 (1998) 288–296.

[2] A. Gregoriades, Interaction of influenza M protein with viral lipid and phosphatidylcholine vesicles, J. Virol. 36 (1980) 470–479.

[3] Z. Ye, et al., Functional and antigenic domains of the matrix (M1) protein of influenza A virus, J. Virol. 61 (1987) 239–246.

[4] Z. Ye, N.W. Baylor, R.R. Wagner, Transcription–inhibition and RNA-binding domains of influenza A virus matrix protein mapped with anti-idiotypic antibodies and synthetic peptides, J. Virol. 63 (1989) 3586–3594.

[5] G. Winter, S. Fields, Cloning of influenza cDNA in M13: the sequence of the RNA segment encoding the A/PR/8/34 matrix protein, Nucleic Acids Res. 8 (1980) 1965–1974.

[6] K. Martin, A. Helenius, Transport of incoming influenza virus nucleocapsids into the nucleus, J. Virol. 65 (1991) 232–244.

[7] L.H. Pinto, R.A. Lamb, Understanding the mechanism of action of the anti-influenza virus drug amantadine, Trends Microbiol. 3 (1995) 271.

[8] L. Holm, C. Sander, Searching protein structure databases has come of age, Proteins 19 (1995) 165–173.

[9] R.W.H. Ruigrok, et al., Membrane interaction of influenza virus M1 protein, Virology 267 (2000) 289–298.

International Congress Series 1219 (2001) 411–419

The influenza B virus BM2 protein may be involved in the ribonucleoprotein complexes through the binding with membrane protein M1

Takato Odagiri[a,b,*], Hiroaki Kariwa[c], Yoshiro Ohara[a]

[a]*Department of Microbiology, Kanazawa Medical University, Uchinada, Ishikawa 920-0293, Japan*
[b]*Department of Virology 1, National Institute of Infectious Diseases, Tokyo 162-8640, Japan*
[c]*Department of Environmental Veterinary Sciences, Graduate School of Veterinary Medicine, Hokkaido University, Sapporo 060-0818, Japan*

Abstract

Background: The influenza B virus genome RNA segment 7 encodes M1 and BM2 proteins. We have shown previously that in virus-infected MDCK cells, the BM2 is synthesized as a cytoplasmic product, and thereafter, transported from the outside of the nuclear membrane to the virion budding site on the plasma membrane, resulting in the incorporation into virion. *Methods*: The interactions of virus proteins were analyzed by immunoprecipitation, mammalian two-hybrid system and indirect immunofluorescence. *Results*: By two-hybrid analysis, the BM2 was shown to interact with the M1 and the nuclear export protein NS2, but not with NP. Fractionation of viral ribonucleoprotein (vRNP) complexes extracted from the cytoplasm of infected cells indicated that the BM2 was detected in the vRNP complexes containing M1, but not in the M1-free vRNP complexes. Moreover, the localization of BM2 in the cytoplasm was highly correlated with that of vRNP complexes in the late phase of infection. *Conclusion*: The BM2 protein might be involved in vRNP complexes through binding with M1 protein, which is a component of vRNP complex. © 2001 Elsevier Science B.V. All rights reserved.

Keywords: BM2 protein; Two-hybrid assay; vRNP complexes; Influenza B virus

* Corresponding author. Department of Virology 1, National Institute of Infectious Diseases, Tokyo 162-8640, Japan. Tel.: +81-3-5285-1111; fax: +81-3-5285-1155.
  E-mail address: todagiri@nih.go.jp (T. Odagiri).

0531-5131/01/$ – see front matter © 2001 Elsevier Science B.V. All rights reserved.
PII: S0531-5131(01)00638-0

1. Introduction

Influenza A and B viruses contain eight RNA segments of negative-polarity. These viruses are similar to each other structurally and biochemically in their life cycles. However, the coding strategy and features of the proteins encoded by RNA segments 6 and 7 of these viruses are quite different. The RNA segment 6 of influenza A virus encodes only neuraminidase (NA), whereas the segment of influenza B virus encodes NA and a virion-associated integral membrane protein NB with an ion channel activity [1] using a bicistronic mRNA containing overlapping open reading frames (ORFs) [2,3].

The RNA segment 7 of influenza A virus encodes the membrane protein M1, which is translated from a collinear mRNA [4], and the ion channel glycoprotein M2 [5,6], which is translated from a spliced mRNA [7]. On the other hand, the RNA segment 7 of influenza B virus encodes the M1 with 248 amino acids and the BM2 with 109 amino acids in the +0 ORF and in the +2 ORF, respectively, of a bicistronic mRNA [4]. The BM2 is synthesized from the overlapping translational stop–start codons, TAATG, at nucleotides 769–773 [8]. We have recently showed that the BM2 is a phosphoprotein synthesized in the late phase of infection, and that it is detected in the cytoplasm throughout the infection cycle [9]. Moreover, we demonstrated that the BM2 protein is incorporated into virions [9].

In the present study, we aimed to clarify the features and the functions of the BM2 protein in infected cells. Our data suggested that the BM2 was involved in vRNP complexes through the binding with M1 protein, and that the interaction may occur at the periphery of the nuclear membrane immediately after the nuclear export of vRNP complexes.

2. Materials and methods

2.1. Cells and viruses

MDCK cells were cultured in Eagle's minimal essential medium supplemented with 10% fetal calf serum (FCS). Influenza virus B/Yamagata/1/73 was propagated in MDCK cells in Opti-MEM I (Gibco) containing 4 μg/ml N-acetyl trypsin.

2.2. Virus protein–protein interaction

Virus protein(s), which interacted with BM2 protein, was identified by mammalian two-hybrid system using the pBIND and the pACT vectors containing the ORFs of BM2, M1, NP and NS2, and pG5luc reporter vector containing firefly and *Renilla* luciferase genes (Promega). These vectors were transfected into COS-1 cells with LipofectAmine Plus reagent (Gibco) and the luciferase activity in the cell lysates was measured at 48-h post-transfection (p.t.) by using a luminometer.

2.3. Isolation of vRNP complexes from infected cells

vRNP complexes, synthesized in infected cells, were purified by the methods described previously [10] with modifications. To isolate pure vRNP core complex without other viral proteins associated with the complexes, the RNP pellet was purified by centrifugation at 35,000 rpm for 24 h in an SW50.1 rotor through two consecutive CsCl–glycerol gradients. To isolate vRNP complexes associated with M1 and probably NS2 proteins, the RNP pellet was centrifuged at 45,000 rpm for 4 h in an SW50.1 rotor on a glycerol gradient with four steps of 33% glycerol, 40% glycerol, 50% glycerol and 70% glycerol containing 50 mM Tris–HCl pH 7.8 and 150 mM NaCl. The gradient was fractionated and each fraction was examined by SDS-PAGE followed by Western blotting using anti-B/ Yamagata and anti-BM2#3 antibodies as described previously [9].

2.4. Indirect immunofluorescence

MDCK cells on glass coverslips were infected with B/Yamagata virus or transfected with the expression vectors, pCAGGS/B-NP and pCAGGS/BM2 [9], and the virus proteins were detected by indirect immunofluorescence as described previously [9]. The fluorescence signals were detected by confocal microscopy.

3. Results

3.1. Detection of BM2 protein in vRNP complexes

We previously observed that in noninfectious virus produced by COS-1 cells, the BM2 protein and vRNP, which contains polymerase, NP and vRNA segments, were not efficiently packaged into the virion, although all vRNAs and virus proteins including those components were synthesized in infected cells (unpublished data). The finding led us to speculate that the BM2 protein might be involved in the vRNP complexes. To examine this, [^{35}S]methionine/cysteine labeled MDCK cells infected with virus were immunopre-

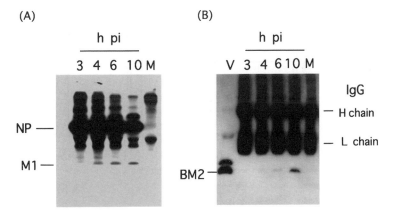

Fig. 1. Immunoprecipitation of virus-infected cells labeled with [^{35}S] methionine/cystein at various times p.i. with anti-NP antibody (A). The precipitates were then subjected to Western blotting using anti-BM2 antibody for detection of BM2 protein (B). Lanes M and V indicate mock-infected cells and whole virion, respectively.

cipitated with anti-NP antibody at various times post-infection (p.i.) (Fig. 1A). The major immunoprecipitate was NP, but a small amount of M1 coprecipitated with NP in the late phase of infection. A part of M1 protein is known to form a complex with vRNP by binding to vRNA [11,12]. Therefore, the immunoprecipitates obtained late in infection were thought to be the mixture of NP and vRNP complexes. Since the BM2 protein is not detected by a metabolic labeling of infected cells [9], the immunoprecipitates were then subjected to Western blotting using anti-BM2 antibody (Fig. 1B). A small amount of BM2 protein coprecipitated with the precipitates containing M1 protein, implying that the BM2 protein was also involved in vRNP complex.

3.2. Virus protein–protein interaction

Computer analysis using the program of Motif Libraries in the GenomeNet (ICR, Kyoto University) indicated that the BM2 protein did not contain an RNA binding motif. This finding suggested that the BM2 protein should bind to a certain protein(s) of vRNP complexes, i.e. NP, M1 and NS2, rather than vRNA segments. To identify the virus protein which is associated with BM2 protein, an analysis of protein–protein interactions was carried out by using the mammalian two-hybrid system with a reporter vector containing dual luciferase genes as described in Materials and methods. Prior to the two-hybrid analysis, the expression level of the inserted gene in each vector was ascertained by Western blotting using virus protein specific antisera and an anti-Gal4DNA-BD monoclonal antibody (Clontech).

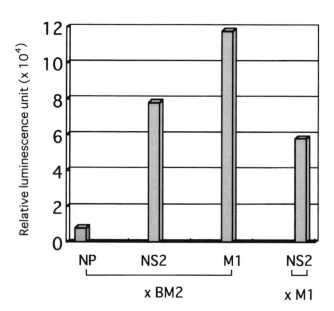

Fig. 2. Identification of virus protein which interacts with BM2 protein. Interaction between the BM2 protein and the virus protein present in vRNP complex, i.e. NP, M1 or NS2, was examined by mammalian two-hybrid system. The extent of the interaction against the BM2 protein is shown as luminescence unit. Similarly, the interaction between M1 and NS2 proteins was also examined as a positive control.

Fig. 2 shows the luciferase activity, which indicates the magnitude of interaction between proteins. In the combination of BM2 and M1 proteins, a very high level of luciferase activity was obtained. Similarly, the high activity was also obtained in the combination of BM2 and NS2 proteins, although it was approximately 70% of the activity induced by the former combination. In contrast, in the combination of BM2 and NP, the activity remained at a background level. Consequently, the BM2 protein was shown to interact with M1 and NS2 proteins, but not with NP. In influenza A virus the NS2 is known to bind to the M1 protein [13]. To ensure that our two-hybrid system represented the innate virus protein–protein interaction in infected cells, we also examined the interaction between M1 and NS2 proteins of influenza B virus as a positive control. As shown in Fig. 2, their interaction was confirmed, although the extent was much weaker than the interactions of BM2–M1 and BM2–NS2.

3.3. Fractionation of vRNP complexes extracted from the cytoplasm of infected cells

On the basis of the above findings, it was speculated that the BM2 protein was involved in vRNP complexes by binding to M1 and/or NS2 proteins. To demonstrate this, the vRNP complexes were purified from the cytoplasm of infected MDCK cells by two different fractionation methods as described in Materials and methods. We first separated the vRNP complexes by centrifugation through two consecutive CsCl–glycerol step gradients and

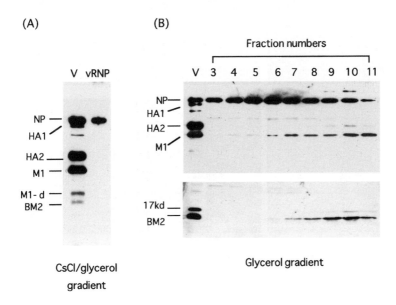

Fig. 3. Fractionation of vRNP complexes by two consecutive CsCl–glycerol gradient centrifugations (A) and by a glycerol step gradient centrifugation (B). (A) The highly purified NP enriched fraction was analyzed by Western blotting with a mixture of anti-B/Yamagata and anti-BM2 antibodies. Lane V indicates whole virion as a marker. (B) The vRNP complexes were fractionated from the top (small number on the lane) to the bottom (large number on the lane). Virus proteins present in fractions 3 to 11 were analyzed by Western blotting using anti-B/Yamagata (upper panel) and anti-BM2 (lower panel) antibodies.

isolated the NP enriched fractions. By Western blot analysis with a mixture of anti-B/ Yamagata antibody, which was raised against the whole virion, and anti-BM2 antibody, the vRNPs were shown to be free of M1 and BM2 proteins (Fig. 3A). This indicates that the segregation of M1 protein from the vRNP complexes resulted in the loss of BM2 protein. The second fractionation of vRNP complexes was carried out by centrifugation through a glycerol step gradient for isolation of vRNP complexes containing M1 protein. Fig. 3B shows virus proteins in each fraction collected from the top to the bottom of the gradient. The top five fractions contained the vRNPs without M1 protein (lanes 3 to 5) and the middle to bottom fractions contained the vRNPs with M1 protein (lanes 6 to 11). As expected, these lower fractions also contained the BM2 protein and the peak of the content was found in the M1 enriched fraction 10. The results together with those of two-hybrid

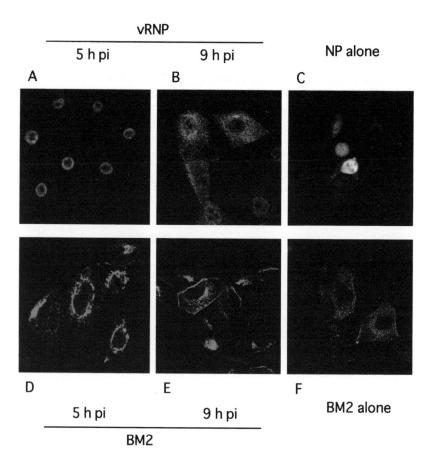

Fig. 4. Localization of vRNP, NP and BM2 proteins in MDCK cells infected with virus and transfected with plasmid vector. The localization of vRNP (panels A and B) and BM2 protein (panels D and E) at 5 and 9 h p.i. was analyzed by indirect immunofluorescence with anti-NP and anti-BM2 antibodies, respectively, as a first antibody. The localization of NP and BM2, which were solely expressed by pCAGGS/B-NP and pCAGGS/BM2, respectively, was detected 30 h post transfection (panels C and F).

assay indicated that the BM2 protein was included in vRNP complexes through the binding with M1 protein.

3.4. Localization of vRNP complex and BM2 protein in MDCK cells

We previously showed that the BM2 protein was found at the periphery of the nuclear membrane immediately after the synthesis, and thereafter, moved to the plasma membrane [9]. These observations were also confirmed in the present immunofluorescence study (Fig. 4, panels D and E). We next examined whether the localization of vRNP complexes correlated with that of BM2 protein. The vRNP complexes were detected 5 and 9 h p.i. by anti-NP antibody. At 5 h p.i., the vRNP complexes were detected exclusively in the nucleus, whereas at 9 h p.i., they were found in the entire region of the cytoplasm and partly along the plasma membrane (Fig. 4, panels A and B). To ensure that these signals represented the vRNP complexes, but not free molecules of NP, the NP was solely expressed by transfection of the pCAGGS/B-NP vector, which contained the NP-ORF of B/Yamagata virus, and was examined in the same manner. The free NP was detected only in the nucleus even when the expression level reached maximum (Fig. 4, panel C). This was consistent with the recent report that the nuclear export of NP was caused by the interaction with M1 protein [14]. Therefore, the signals shown in Fig. 4B represented the vRNP complexes. From these results, it was clearly indicated that the localization of vRNP and BM2 protein was correlated well at the late phase of infection, but not at the early phase of infection. It is noteworthy that the BM2 protein expressed solely by the pCAGGS/BM2 expression vector [9] was detected in the cytoplasm (Fig. 4, panel F), suggesting that the BM2 protein itself was capable of moving to the cytoplasm.

4. Discussion

In the present study, we showed that the BM2 protein interacts with M1 and NS2 proteins and that the BM2 protein might be involved in the vRNP complexes through binding to the encapsidated M1 and/or NS2 proteins. The newly synthesized vRNP of influenza A virus has been known to form complexes in the nucleus by association with M1 through the two putative RNA binding sites [15,16] and with NS2 protein [13]. In the case of influenza B virus, on the other hand, the vRNP complexes were further associated with BM2 protein. However, it is not likely that this association is direct binding with the genome RNA and the NP molecules. This is based on the data that the BM2 protein did not possess RNA binding motifs and that by two-hybrid assay, the BM2 protein did not interact with NP (Fig. 2). However, the immunoprecipitation and the fractionation of vRNP complexes suggested that the BM2 protein associated with the complex (Figs. 1 and 3). Moreover, the BM2 protein was shown to interact with M1 and NS2 proteins by two-hybrid analysis (Fig. 2). Since the M1 and NS2 proteins are involved in vRNP to form the complexes [12,13], our data suggest that the BM2 protein was involved in the vRNP complexes through binding with the M1 and/or NS2 protein. In fact, the BM2 protein was detected in the vRNP complexes containing M1 protein, but not in the M1 free-vRNP complexes (Fig. 3). The consistent results have also been obtained from fractionation of the detergent-disrupted virion; the BM2 protein was detected in the fractions containing M1 protein, but not in the fractions containing NP and polymerase proteins [9]. A similar association has been found with NS2 protein, which binds to M1 protein [13].

The question arises whether BM2 protein associates with unencapsidated M1 proteins present in the cytosol. The M1 protein is the most abundant product synthesized in virus-infected cells and underlays the plasma membrane to form the virus envelope. In addition, M1 binds to vRNP to form the complex. In contrast, BM2 protein is synthesized as a minor component [9], and the molar ratio of BM2 to M1 synthesized in infected cells was greatly different. Furthermore, when the M1 protein in virions was immunoprecipitated with anti-M1 antibody under conditions where vRNP did not coprecipitate with M1, only a trace amount of BM2 protein coprecipitated with M1 protein [9]. This amount was less than 3.1% of the amount of BM2 in the intact virion. It is likely, therefore, that most M1 protein free from vRNP was not associated with BM2 protein.

The complex formation among vRNP, M1 and NS2 molecules is known to be required for the nuclear export of the vRNP molecules [17,18]. The interaction between the vRNP complexes and the BM2 protein, however, might not be involved in the step of nuclear export of vRNP. The BM2 protein did not enter the nucleus during the infection cycle (Fig. 4). This is consistent with the prediction that the BM2 protein does not have a nuclear localization signal [9]. Furthermore, the localization of vRNP and BM2 protein was completely different in the early phase of infection and their correlation was found after the nuclear export of vRNP complexes (Fig. 4). Since the BM2 protein accumulated along the nuclear membrane immediately after synthesis (Fig. 4D), the association of these components should occur at the periphery of the nuclear membrane. Although no counterpart of BM2 protein has been found in influenza A virus, the vRNP complexes are normally transported to the virion budding site on the plasma membrane. However, it is possible to speculate that a certain virus protein(s) possesses a similar function to the BM2 protein of influenza B virus. Further analysis of the function of BM2 is required to address the question.

Acknowledgements

We thank M. Arai for excellent technical assistance. This work was supported in part by grants-in-aid for Scientific Research from the Ministry of Science, Education and Culture; a grant from the Ministry of Public Welfare; and a grant for Collaborative Research from Kanazawa Medical University (C99-2).

References

[1] N.A. Sunstrom, L.S. Premkumar, A. Premukumar, G. Ewart, G.B. Cox, P.W. Gage, Ion channels formed by NB: an influenza B virus protein, J. Membr. Biol. 150 (1996) 127–132.

[2] T. Betakova, M.V. Nermut, A.J. Hay, The NB protein is an integral component of the membrane of influenza B virus, J. Gen. Virol. 77 (1996) 2689–2694.

[3] M.A. Williams, R.A. Lamb, Effect of mutations and deletions in a bicistronic mRNA on the synthesis of influenza B virus NB and NA glycoproteins, J. Virol. 63 (1989) 28–35.

[4] R.A. Lamb, Genes and proteins of the influenza viruses, in: R.M. Krug (Ed.), The Influenza Viruses, Plenum, New York, 1989, pp. 1–87.

[5] K.C. Duff, R.H. Ashley, The transmembrane domain of influenza A M2 protein forms amantadine-sensitive proton channels in planar lipid bilayers, Virology 190 (1992) 485–489.

[6] M.S. Sansom, I.D. Kerr, Influenza virus M2 protein: a molecular modelling study of the ion channel, Protein Eng. 1 (1993) 65–74.

[7] R.A. Lamb, P.W. Choppin, Identification of a second protein (M2) encoded by RNA segment 7 of influenza virus, Virology 112 (1981) 729–737.

[8] C.M. Horvath, M.A. Williams, R.A. Lamb, Eukaryotic coupled translation of tandem cistrons: identification of the influenza B virus BM2 polypeptide, EMBO J. 9 (1990) 2639–2647.

[9] T. Odagiri, J. Hong, Y. Ohara, The BM2 protein of influenza B virus is synthesized in the late phase of infection and incorporated into virions as a subviral component, J. Gen. Virol. 80 (1999) 2573–2581.

[10] J. Martin, C. Albo, J. Ortin, J.A. Melero, A. Portela, In vitro reconstitution of active influenza virus ribonucleoprotein complexes using viral proteins purified from infected cells, J. Gen. Virol. 73 (1992) 1855–1859.

[11] C. Eister, K. Larsen, J. Gagnon, R.W. Ruigrok, F. Baudin, Influenza virus M1 protein binds to RNA through its nuclear localization signal, J. Gen. Virol. 78 (1997) 1589–1596.

[12] Z. Ye, T. Liu, D.P. Offrenga, J. McInnis, R.A. Levandowski, Association of influenza virus matrix protein with ribonucleoproteins, J. Virol. 73 (1999) 7467–7473.

[13] J. Yasuda, S. Nakada, A. Kato, T. Toyoda, A. Ishihama, Molecular assembly of influenza virus: association of the NS2 protein with virion matrix, Virology 196 (1993) 249–255.

[14] M. Bui, E.G. Wills, A. Helenius, G.R. Whittaker, Role of the influenza virus M1 protein in nuclear export of viral ribonucleoproteins, J. Virol. 74 (2000) 1781–1786.

[15] E.H. Nasser, A.K. Judd, A. Sanchez, D. Anastasiou, D.J. Bucher, Antiviral activity of influenza virus M1 zinc finger peptides, J. Virol. 70 (1996) 8639–8644.

[16] L. Wakefield, G.G. Brownlee, RNA-binding properties of influenza A virus matrix protein M1, Nucleic Acids Res. 17 (1989) 8569–8580.

[17] K. Martin, A. Helenius, Nuclear transport of influenza virus ribonucleoproteins: the viral matrix protein (M1) promotes export and inhibits import, Cell 67 (1991) 117–130.

[18] R.E. O'Neill, J. Talon, P. Palese, The influenza virus NEP (NS2 protein) mediates the nuclear export of viral ribonucleoproteins, EMBO J. 17 (1998) 288–296.

International Congress Series 1219 (2001) 421–426

Identification of the functional domains of the matrix protein of influenza A/WSN/33 virus

Zhiping Ye*, Teresa Liu, Xiaoyuan Huang, Daniel P. Offringa, Jonathan McInnis, Roland A. Levandowski

Laboratory of Pediatric and Respiratory Viral Diseases, Division of Viral Products, Office of Vaccines Research and Review, Center for Biologics and Evaluation and Research, Food and Drug Administration, Bethesda, MD, USA

Abstract

Background: The matrix protein (M1) of influenza virus plays a central role in viral replication and has been ascribed a variety of functions including association with viral RNA and ribonucleoprotein (RNP). It is essential to understand the binding mechanism by identification of the functional domains of M1. *Methods*: The RNA and RNP-binding domains of M1 protein were identified by introducing amino-acid substitutions and deletions. The RNA–protein interaction was investigated by measuring the binding of radiolabeled RNA to immobilized M1 protein. Reconstitution of M1 with RNP was studied by incubation of radiolabeled M1 with purified RNP. *Results*: We characterized RNA-binding domains of M1 protein by mutating M1, and show that M1 binds to RNA through two independent domains, a zinc-finger motif and a series of basic amino acids (RKLKR). One of the RNA-binding domains consisting of a series of basic amino acids is also involved in RNP binding. An independent domain located in the N-terminal 76 amino acids of M1 also participates in RNP-binding activity. *Conclusions*: The data suggest that M1 interacts with both the RNA and protein components of RNP in assembly/disassembly of influenza A viruses. © 2001 Elsevier Science B.V. All rights reserved.

Keywords: M1 protein; RNP binding; RNA binding

* Corresponding author. Room 2B17, Building 29A, 8800 Rockville Pike, Bethesda, MD 20982, USA. Tel.: +1-301-435-5197; fax: +1-301-402-5128.
  E-mail address: yez@cber.fda.gov (Z. Ye).

0531-5131/01/$ – see front matter © 2001 Elsevier Science B.V. All rights reserved.
PII: S 0 5 3 1 - 5 1 3 1 (0 1) 0 0 3 5 0 - 8

1. Introduction

The M1 of influenza A virus is a major structural protein located between the RNP complex and the inner surface of the lipid envelope in the intact virion [1,5,8]. The interaction of M1 and RNP is required for transport of M1/RNP complexes from the nucleus into the cytoplasm [6]. Two domains in M1 have been shown to affect the disposition of RNA. One domain residing in a palindromic stretch of basic amino acids (101–RKLKR–105) has been shown to bind viral RNA [4,10,11], fulfilling a prediction based on X-ray crystallographic data [9], and to serve also as a nuclear translocation signal for M1 [11,13]. The other RNA-binding domain containing a zinc-finger motif (148C–C–H–H162) has been shown to associate with zinc molecules [3] and to inhibit viral replication [7], but its role in binding RNA is less certain. In this report, we describe binding of radiolabeled RNA to immobilized M1 protein and the association of purified RNPs with ^{35}S-labeled M1 translated from cDNAs coding for either M1 or for substitution and deletion mutants of M1. The effects of reconstituting these M1 and mutant M1s with RNP under conditions of altered pH, ionic strength, and added detergent were used to further define the interacting domains of M1 and to explore mechanisms of the M1–RNP interaction.

2. Materials and methods

2.1. Virus and DNA constructs

Influenza virus A/WSN/33 (WSN) was propagated in the allantoic cavities of 9-day-old embryonic eggs and was concentrated and purified by banding in 15% to 60% sucrose gradient [12].

Plasmids to express the mutant M1 genes with deletions or substitutions were constructed from a wild-type WSN M1 (wt M1) gene recombinant vaccinia vector pTFM21 [3] as described previously [2,11]. pTFM21 [3] was employed to create substitution mutations of WSN M1 corresponding to the RNA-binding amino acids 101–RKLKR–105 and the zinc finger motif (amino acids 148–162). The substitution of 101–RKLKR–105 by 101–SNLNS–105 (designated M101–SNLNS–105) was constructed by PCR. The zinc finger motif (148C–151C–159H–162H) in amino acids 148–162 was altered to S–C–H–H in PCR reaction using the primer 456-5'GGC CTG GTA TCC GCA ACCT3'-474 and a primer corresponding to the vector sequence. Deletion mutants of the M1 gene were constructed using restriction enzyme digestion and PCR. All of the altered M1 cDNA sequences were confirmed by DNA sequence analysis.

2.2. Protein–RNA interaction assay

The interaction of M1 with RNA was analyzed as described previously [11] with minor modifications. Viral RNA (vRNA) was labeled by growing influenza virus in cell cultures containing ^{32}P orthophosphate (15 µCi/ml, radioactivity concentration 8 mCi/ml, Amersham), and was purified from virus by phenol extraction. The M1s used for RNA-binding assays were derived by expression in a coupled transcription–translation system (Promega) from the specific plasmids described above.

2.3. In vitro reconstitution of M1 protein with RNPs

The analysis of association of M1 and RNP was carried out as follows: 50 μg purified RNP [9] was incubated with labeled M1 (10,000 cpm). The negative control containing the same activity of ^{35}S methionine (10,000 cpm) was derived from the translation product of the same plasmid without M gene insertion. A 20 μl aliquot of the RNP-^{35}S-labeled M1 suspension was centrifuged through a 150 μl cushion of 20% sucrose at 10,000 rpm for 15 min in a 0.5 ml of Eppendorf tube, and the resulting pellet was collected. The amount of ^{35}S-labeled M1 associated with RNP was determined by autoradiographic densitometry of proteins separated by SDS-PAGE. The percentage of M1 bound to RNP was calculated from more than three individual experiments by comparing to the total input ^{35}S-labeled M1.

3. Results and discussion

3.1. A basic amino-acid domain (101–RKLKR–105) and the zinc-finger motif of M1 participate in RNA-binding activity

Table 1 includes the RNA-binding activities of M1 (M1–252) and mutant M1 proteins determined by measuring the binding of ^{32}P-labeled RNA (extracted from A/WSN/33 virions) to wt M1 immobilized on nitrocellulose membrane. Deletion of the C-terminal 52 amino acids (M1–200) had little effect on the RNA-binding capacity of the protein (about an 8% reduction in RNA binding compared to M1). Altering the zinc finger motif (MC148S) resulted in moderate reduction of RNA binding (31%). Substitution of amino acids RKLKR (M101–SNLNS–105) reduced binding activity by 44% compared to the M1. Deletions of amino acids (Mdel111–202, M1–112, or M135–240) that eliminated one of the two RNA-binding domains decreased RNA-binding activity by 50–58%. However, the M1 expressed from Mdel77–202 missing both the RNA-binding domains bound RNA only weakly if at all (>90% reduction in RNA binding). These results indicate that in vitro translated M1s retained RNA-binding capacity provided by both of the RNA-binding domains, and the two RNA-binding domains of M1 bind independently to RNA.

3.2. An RNA-binding domain located in the middle region of the M1 amino-acid sequence had RNP-binding activity

Further studies were conducted to determine the association of M1 with RNP (Table 1). Reconstitution of M1 and mutant M1s with this RNP was carried out at pH 7.0 and 0.15 M NaCl. The association of M1 with RNP was about 88% of total input M1 translated from the wt M1. Similarly, 71–86% of each of the mutant M1s (M1–200,

Table 1
Functional domains of M1 of influenza A/WSN/33 virus

Protein or peptide[a]	RNA-binding domain		N-terminal hydrophobic domain	RNA-binding activity[b]	RNP binding[c]		
	RKLKR[d]	Zinc-finger[e]			NaCl 0.15 M[f]	Rnase[g]	1% Triton[h]
M1–252	+	+	+	100	88 (100)	41 (47)	85 (97)
M1–200	+	+	+	92	86 (98)	50 (57)	ND[i]
MC148S	+	−	+	69	85 (97)	46 (52)	80 (91)
Mdel111–202	+	−	+	50	71 (81)	50 (57)	90 (102)
M1–112	+	−	+	42	80 (91)	40 (46)	85 (97)
M101– SNLNS– 105	−	+	+	56	50 (57)	36 (41)	20 (23)
M135–240	−	+	−	44	11 (13)	6 (7)	ND
Mdel77–202	−	−	+	<10	42 (48)	43 (49)	15 (17)

  [a] Amino acid sequences from M1 and mutant M1s.
  [b] The percentage of RNA bound to M1 calculated by comparison to the total input ^{32}P-RNA.
  [c] The number was quantified by comparison to the percentage of RNP association of M1.
  [d] A basic amino acid sequence between 101 and 105 of M1.
  [e] A zinc-finger motif within amino acids148C–C–H–H162 of M1.
  [f] The percentage of RNP association quantified by comparison to the total input ^{35}S-M1 proteins at pH 7.0 and 0.15 M of NaCl.
  [g] The RNP was pretreated with 3μg/ml of ribonuclease A (RNase) for 30 min at 37 °C before association assay. The percentage of RNP association quantified by comparison to the total input ^{35}S-M1 proteins.
  [h] The association was performed in presence of 1% Triton. The percentage of RNP association quantified by comparison to the total input ^{35}S-M1 proteins.
  [i] ND, Not determined.

MC148S, Mdel111–202, and M1–112), containing both RKLKR and N-terminal 76 amino acids, was associated with RNP. However, the RNP-binding activity of M1 with substitution in the RNA-binding domain (M101–SNLNS–105) was reduced to 50%. RNP-binding activity of M1 missing both RNA-binding domains (Mdel77–240) was 42%. However, M135–240, which contains the zinc finger motif but is missing the N-terminal portion of M1 including the basic amino-acid site (101–RKLKR–105), had only 11% of RNP-binding activity. These results indicate that of the two RNA-binding domains of M1, only the basic amino-acid domain (101–RKLKR–105) is involved in RNP-binding activity. The zinc-finger participates in RNA binding, but is not involved in RNP association.

Reconstitution of M1 and mutant M1s with this RNP was also characterized by increasing the salt concentration and lowering pH. Increasing the salt concentration from 0.15 to 0.30 M reduced approximately half of the association of M1 (M1–252) and mutant M1s (MC148S, M1–200, Mdel111–202 and M1–112)(data not shown). Under the same conditions, the RNP-binding activity of M101–SNLNS–105 was reduced by 20%. Further increase in salt concentration to 0.60 M NaCl had proportionally little additional effect on the RNP binding (17% at 0.60 M NaCl). Reconstitution at pH 5.0 essentially abolished M1/RNP association in vitro for all mutant M1s including M1. These experiments also showed that in vitro translated M1 binds to RNP efficiently at pH 7.4, but is inhibited at lower pH.

3.3. The RNP-binding activity of M1 partially due to interaction with RNA molecules of RNP complex

In order to further understand the role of RNA binding in the M1/RNP association, M1-depleted RNPs of A/WSN/33 virus were enzymatically treated with ribonuclease A to digest unprotected RNA. To assay association, ^{35}S-labeled M1 and mutant M1s were reconstituted with RNPs that had been preincubated with ribonuclease A. The results of reconstitution of M1 protein (M1–252) and substitution mutants (M101–SNLNS–105, and MC148S) with ribonuclease A-treated RNP are shown in Table 1. When RNP was treated with ribonuclease A, binding of M1 was only 47% relative to RNP not treated with ribonuclease. M1s with substitution in the RNA-binding domain (M101–SNLNS–105) or in the zinc finger motif (MC148S) did not further reduce RNP-binding activity compared to M1 (41% and 52%), nor did deletion of the C-terminal 52 amino acids, 46%, (M1–200). M1s with deletion of the C-terminal 140 amino acids (M1–112) or amino acids 77 to 202 (Mdel77–202) also exhibited 46% and 49% association. RNP treated with high concentrations of ribonuclease A (30 µg/ml) showed approximately 20% binding in all cases. However, the deletion mutant containing amino acids 135 to 240 (M135–240) exhibited only background RNP binding at all ribonuclease A concentrations. These results suggest that the RNP-binding activity of M1 is partially due to the interaction of the basic amino-acid domain of M1 with RNA molecules of RNP complex.

3.4. The M1 may bind to RNP via a hydrophobic domain

Although the association of M1 with RNPs was reduced by the addition of salt or pretreatment of RNP with ribonuclease A, deletion or substitution in the RNA-binding domain did not completely abolish RNP-binding activity. However, removal of the N-terminal amino acids including the RNA-binding domain resulted in the complete elimination of RNP binding (M135–240). All of the M1 mutants retaining the N-terminal 76 amino acids exhibited RNP-binding capacity even when RNA-binding site were deleted.

In order to explore the RNP-binding properties of the N-terminal 76 amino acids, M1 and mutant M1s were reconstituted with RNP in buffer containing 1% Triton X-100 in 0.05 M NaCl. As shown in Table 1, addition of Triton X-100 to the reconstitution mixture did not affect association of M1 to RNP (approximately 97% (M1–252)). Substitution in the zinc finger motif (MC148S) did not further reduce the association of M1 with RNP (same as that from the wt M1, approximately a 9% reduction comparing binding with and without Triton X-100). Other deletions affecting the zinc finger motif (Mdel111–202 or M1–112) did not alter M1–RNP association (102% and 97%). However, substitution in the RNA-binding domain (M101–SNLNS–105) resulted in a 77% reduction of M1/RNP association in the presence of Triton X-100. The deletion of both RNA-binding domains (Mdel77–202) resulted in a similar 83% reduction of RNP association. These data suggest that a detergent-labile element located in the N-terminal 76 amino acids of M1 is involved in RNP binding and that it is independent of RNA-binding domains.

The data suggest that M1 interacts with both the RNA and protein components of RNP in assembly/disassembly of influenza viruses.

References

[1] H. Allen, J. McCauley, M. Waterfield, M.J. Gething, Influenza virus RNA segment 7 has the coding for two polypeptides, Virology 107 (1980) 548–551.

[2] N.W. Balyor, Y. Li, Z. Ye, R.R. Wagner, Transient expression and sequence of the matrix (M1) gene of WSN influenza virus in a vaccinia vector, Virology 163 (1988) 618–621.

[3] C. Elster, E. Fourest, F. Baudin, K. Larsen, S. Cusack, R.W. Ruigrok, A small percentage of influenza virus M1 protein contains zinc but zinc does not influence in vitro M1–RNA interaction, J. Gen. Virol. 75 (1994) 37–42.

[4] C. Elster, K. Larsen, J. Gagnon, R.W.H. Ruigrok, F. Baudim, Influenza virus M1 protein binds to RNA through its nuclear localization signal, J. Gen. Virol. 78 (1997) 1589–1596.

[5] R.A. Lamb, P.W. Choppin, The structure and replication of influenza virus, Annu. Rev. Biochem. 52 (1983) 467–506.

[6] K. Martin, A. Helenius, Nuclear transport of influenza virus ribonucleoproteins: the viral matrix protein (M1) promotes export and inhibits import, Cell 67 (1991) 117–130.

[7] E.H. Nasser, A.K. Judd, A. Sanchez, D. Anastasiou, D.J. Bucher, Antiviral activity of influenza virus M1 zinc finger peptides, J. Virol. 70 (1996) 8639–8644.

[8] I.T. Schulze, The structure of influenza virus: II. A model based on the morphology and composition of subviral particles, Virology 47 (1972) 181–196.

[9] B. Sha, M. Luo, Structure of a bifunctional membrane-RNA binding protein, influenza virus matrix protein M1, Nat. Struct. Biol. 4 (1997) 239–244.

[10] L. Wakefield, G.G. Brownlee, RNA binding properties of influenza virus matrix protein M1, Nucleic Acids Res. 17 (1989) 8569–8580.

[11] Z. Ye, N.W. Baylor, R.R. Wagner, Transcription-inhibition and RNA-binding domains of influenza virus matrix protein mapped with anti-idiotype antibodies and synthetic peptides, J. Virol. 63 (1989) 3586–3594.

[12] Z. Ye, R. Pal, J.W. Fox, R.R. Wagner, Functional and antigenic domains of the matrix (M1) protein of influenza virus, J. Virol. 61 (1987) 239–246.

[13] Z. Ye, D. Robinson, R.R. Wagner, Nucleus-targeting domain of the matrix protein (M1) of influenza virus, J. Virol. 69 (1995) 1964–1970.

International Congress Series 1219 (2001) 427–434

Transcription of influenza A virus genes

Ervin Fodor, Leo L.M. Poon[1], Andrea Mikulasova[2],
Louise J. Mingay, George G. Brownlee[*]

Sir William Dunn School of Pathology, University of Oxford, South Park Road, Oxford, OX1 3RE, UK

Abstract

Background: Polyadenylation of eukaryotic mRNAs occurs by cleavage of the pre-mRNA downstream of a conserved AAUAAA hexamer, followed by polyadenylation of the upstream cleavage product by a poly(A) polymerase in a template-independent manner. By contrast, polyadenylation of influenza virus mRNA molecules is performed by the viral RNA polymerase by reiterative copying of a U_{5-7} sequence near the $5'$ end of the vRNA template. *Methods*: We used both in vitro and in vivo transcription assays to demonstrate that replacement of the viral U_6 poly(A) site with a A_6 sequence in vRNA results in transcription products with poly(U) tails. A recombinant influenza A/WSN/33 virus has been generated, by using a helper virus-dependent rescue method, in which the U_6 poly(A) site of the neuraminidase (NA) gene has been modified so that the virus expressed a poly(U)-tailed NA mRNA. The growth properties of the virus were characterised in cell culture and in an animal model. A plasmid-based transcription/replication assay was used to study whether influenza RNA polymerase transcripts are substrates for cleavage and polyadenylation by the eukaryotic $3'$ end processing machinery. *Results and Conclusions*: Our studies show, firstly, that the U_{5-7} sequence near the $5'$ end of vRNA acts directly as a template for poly(A) addition. Secondly, we show that a recombinant virus expressing a poly(U)-tailed mRNA for the NA gene is attenuated in cell culture and in mice, suggesting a novel strategy for designing live attenuated influenza virus vaccines. Thirdly, we show that a poly(U)-tailed NA influenza RNA polymerase transcripts containing a eukaryotic poly(A) site, could be processed by the cellular polyadenylation machinery even although such molecules are not synthesized by the host RNA polymerase II. © 2001 Elsevier Science B.V. All rights reserved.

Keywords: Polyadenylation; Poly(U)-tail; 3′ End processing; Attenuated virus; Vaccine

[*] Corresponding author. Tel.: +44-1865-275559; fax: +44-1865-275556.
E-mail address: George.Brownlee@path.ox.ac.uk (G.G. Brownlee).
[1] Present address: Department of Microbiology, The University of Hong Kong, Queen Mary Hospital, Hong Kong SAR, China.
[2] Present address: Mount Sinai School of Medicine, 1 Gustave L Levy Place, Box 1124, New York, NY 10029, USA.

0531-5131/01/$ – see front matter © 2001 Elsevier Science B.V. All rights reserved.
PII: S0531-5131(01)00645-8

1. Introduction

The synthesis of eukaryotic messenger RNAs is performed by RNA polymerase II (pol II). The maturation of eukaryotic mRNAs is a complex, multi-step process, which involves capping, splicing, and polyadenylation of pre-mRNAs [1,6,17]. Polyadenylation occurs by endonucleolytic cleavage of the pre-mRNA at 10–30 nucleotides downstream of a conserved AAUAAA sequence [16], followed by the addition of a poly(A) tail to the upstream cleavage product. According to the current model, polyadenylation is coupled to cellular RNA pol II transcription; thus, only RNAs synthesised by pol II are believed to be efficiently polyadenylated [2,9].

Influenza virus mRNAs, synthesised by the viral RNA-dependent RNA polymerase, are also polyadenylated at their 3′ end [7], but the mechanism of influenza mRNA polyadenylation differs from the mechanism which is used to polyadenylate eukaryotic mRNAs. The poly(A) tail of influenza mRNAs is synthesised by reiterative copying of a

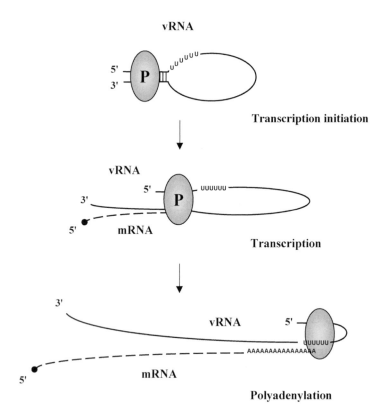

Fig. 1. Proposed mechanism for polyadenylation of influenza virus mRNA molecules [3,19]. Transcription is initiated by RNA polymerase bound to both the 5′ and 3′ ends of the vRNA template. Throughout transcription, the polymerase remains attached to the 5′ end of the template. As a result, the polymerase is unable to transcribe the site to which it is bound. Instead, polyadenylation of mRNA occurs by reiterative copying of the U_6 sequence [12].

5–7 nt long U sequence about 16 nt from the 5′ end of the viral RNA (vRNA) template [12,13,18]. Polyadenylation is performed by a *cis*-acting polymerase, which is bound to the 5′ end of the vRNA template [3,11,14,15,19] (Fig. 1). If the polymerase remains bound to the 5′ end of the vRNA template during transcription, when it reaches the U sequence near the 5′ end, the polymerase pauses, because of steric hindrance, and adds a poly(A) tail by a slippage mechanism.

In this article, we review recent evidence from our laboratory that the U sequence near the 5′ end of the vRNA template acts directly as a template for poly(A) addition [12,13]. In addition, we show that a recombinant influenza virus synthesising a poly(U)-tailed "mRNA" is attenuated in an animal model, suggesting a new strategy for generating live attenuated influenza virus vaccines. Finally, we use a influenza-like mRNA to address the question whether RNAs synthesised by the influenza RNA polymerase could undergo cleavage and polyadenylation by the cellular 3′ end processing machinery.

2. Results and discussion

2.1. The U sequence near the 5′ end of the vRNA acts directly as a template for poly(A) addition

Although the reiterative copying model has been widely accepted as a plausible model for the polyadenylation of influenza virus mRNA as well as mRNAs synthesised by other negative-strand RNA viruses [18], there was no direct experimental evidence to show definitively that the U sequence is the template for poly(A) synthesis. In particular, a model in which the U sequence participates indirectly in polyadenylation, in a way analogous to the conserved AAUAAA hexamer in the case of eukaryotic RNAs, has not been excluded. In theory, the U sequence could act as a pause signal for the polymerase, allowing the influenza RNA polymerase to become a template-independent poly(A) polymerase.

The first direct evidence that the U sequence is a template for poly(A) addition came from in vitro transcription studies with model influenza-like vRNAs [12]. Mutating the U_6 sequence of a 49 nt long vRNA-like template into a A_6 sequence resulted in the synthesis of transcription products with poly(U) tails. In addition, these in vitro findings were validated in vivo by using a plasmid-based CAT-reporter assay [10] for influenza transcription and replication. A vRNA-like CAT gene containing a A_6 sequence instead of the U_6 poly(A) site was transcribed by a recombinant influenza RNA polymerase into "mRNA" with poly(U) tail at its 3′ end [12]. About $3 \pm 1.5\%$ CAT-activity was observed in cells synthesising poly(U)-tailed CAT mRNA compared to cells producing wild-type poly(A)-tailed CAT mRNA, suggesting that the poly(U)-tailed mRNA could be translated, although at low efficiency [13].

2.2. Poly(U)-tailed "mRNA" synthesised by a recombinant influenza virus is defective in nuclear export

We extended the above studies by constructing a recombinant influenza A/WSN/33 virus containing a neuraminidase (NA) vRNA which has its U_6 poly(A)-site mutated into a

A_6 sequence [13]. Instead of synthesising poly(A)-tailed NA mRNA, this engineered virus (the A_6 mutant virus) produced poly(U)-tailed NA mRNA, providing further evidence that the U sequence in the vRNA acts simply as a template for poly(A) addition. Analysis of NA-specific vRNA, complementary RNA (cRNA), and mRNA levels in cells infected with the A_6 mutant virus showed that the synthesis of both NA vRNA and mRNA was reduced about twofold, while NA cRNA levels were not significantly affected. On the other hand, the A_6 mutant virus synthesised significantly reduced amounts of neuraminidase (8% compared to the wild-type virus) and consequently, was attenuated in cell culture. It showed about one log reduction of maximum plaque titre compared to that of the wild-type virus, both on MDBK and MDCK cells.

Although the A_6 mutant virus synthesised about twofold less NA mRNA than the wild-type virus, the dramatic reduction in NA synthesis (more than tenfold) was primarily due to the retention of poly(U)-tailed NA mRNA in the cell nucleus [13]. Poly(U)-tailed NA mRNA was predominantly detected in the nuclei of infected cells, while control polyadenylated NA mRNA was transported to the cytoplasm, suggesting that the poly(U)-tailed mRNA is defective in nuclear export. Our findings are in agreement with the idea that the poly(A) tail is required for nuclear export.

2.3. The A_6 mutant virus is attenuated in mice

Due to the retention of poly(U)-tailed NA mRNA in the nucleus of infected cells, the A_6 mutant virus produced reduced amounts of NA and showed an attenuated phenotype in cell culture [13]. This suggested that manipulating the U_6 poly(A) site might represent a novel strategy which could be considered for generating live attenuated influenza virus

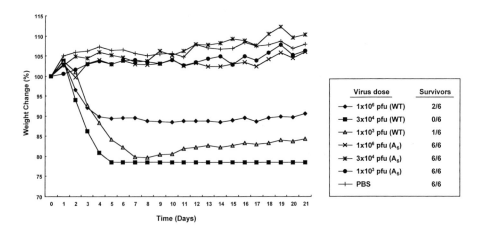

Fig. 2. Pathogenicity of the A_6 mutant virus in mice. Groups of six mice were infected i.n. with three different doses (1×10^6, 3×10^4, or 1×10^3 pfu) of wild-type influenza A/WSN/33 virus or with A_6 mutant virus. A control group of six mice was inoculated with PBS. Following infection, animals were weighed daily and body weights were compared to those on the day of infection. The average body weight percentages of surviving animals per group are represented. Numbers of survivors per group are indicated in the panel next to the graphics.

vaccines. To test this possibility further, we tested the pathogenicity and immunogenicity of the A_6 mutant virus in mice.

Groups of six BALB/c mice were infected intranasally (i.n.) with 1×10^6, 3×10^4, or 1×10^3 plaque forming units (pfu) of the A_6 mutant or A/WSN/33 wild-type virus. The seventh group (non-infected control) received i.n. inoculation of phosphate-buffered saline (PBS). Mice were observed for clinical symptoms and body weight changes were monitored daily. Any mice showing advanced symptoms, of pneumonia or any mice losing 20% or more of their body weight were euthanized following Home Office regulations. All mice in the three groups infected with the wild-type virus exhibited signs of illness and lost weight (Fig. 2). Fifteen of the 18 mice in these three groups were euthanized by day 7 post-infection. On the other hand, mice in all three groups infected with the A_6 mutant virus gained weight. Signs of illness were only observed in the group infected with the highest dose (1×10^6 pfu) of A_6, but all mice recovered and survived. The non-infected group (PBS control) also gained weight and survived.

These results demonstrate that the A_6 mutant virus is attenuated in mice. Infection with wild-type A/WSN/33 caused definitive signs of illness, weight loss, and death, while infection with the A/WSN/33 A_6 mutant caused mild illness only at the 1×10^6 pfu dose.

2.4. The A_6 mutant virus confers protection against a lethal challenge with wild-type influenza virus

On day 21 post-infection, mice infected with the A_6 mutant virus and the non-infected control group were challenged with more than 1000 LD_{50} of the wild-type A/WSN/33 virus (Fig. 3). Although mice in all three groups immunised with the A_6 mutant virus developed signs of illness and initially lost weight, by day 14 after the challenge, the groups immunised with 1×10^6 or 3×10^4 pfu of A_6 mutant gained back more than all their lost weight and the group immunised with 1×10^3 pfu of A_6 mutant gained back nearly all of their lost weight. Only one mouse died in the group immunised with the lowest dose of A_6 mutant. In contrast, mice in the control group (PBS) lost more weight and only two mice survived.

These results show that mice immunised with the A_6 mutant virus were protected against a lethal dose of wild-type A/WSN/33 virus corresponding to more than 1000 LD_{50}. A dose–response was observed in weight loss when comparing groups receiving different doses of A_6 mutant indicating that higher titres of mutant virus prior to wild-type infection are more effective at preventing illness. We conclude that the A_6 mutant virus exhibits signs of being an effective vaccine in reducing the intensity of infection with the wild-type A/WSN/33 virus. Further experimentation with other viral strains, in different animal models and ultimately in humans will be required to assess the potential of poly(A) site mutants as live attenuated influenza virus vaccines.

2.5. Poly(U)-tailed mRNA synthesised by the influenza RNA polymerase is a substrate for cleavage and polyadenylation by the cellular 3' end processing machinery

In order to determine whether synthesis by the cellular RNA polymerase II (pol II) is an absolute requirement for 3' end processing of RNA transcripts in vivo, we used the

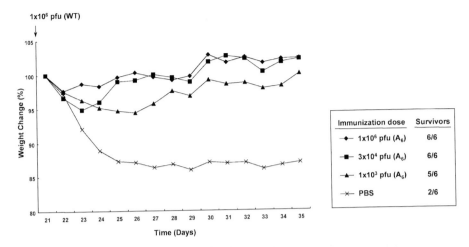

Fig. 3. Immunisation of mice with A_6 mutant virus confers protection against a lethal challenge with wild-type influenza A/WSN/33 virus. Three groups of six mice were immunised i.n. with A_6 mutant virus, using the doses indicated in the panel next to the graphics. As a negative control, one group of six mice was immunised with PBS. Twenty-one days post-immunisation, animals were challenged by i.n. infection with 1×10^6 pfu of wild-type influenza A/WSN/33 virus. Following challenge, animals were weighed daily and their body weights were compared to those on the day of challenge. The average body weight percentages of surviving animals per group are represented. Numbers of survivors per group are indicated in the panel next to the graphics.

poly(U)-tailed influenza RNA polymerase transcript as a model RNA to test whether it could undergo cleavage and polyadenylation by the cellular $3'$ end processing machinery [5]. Here, we briefly review this recent work.

We generated a modified version of the NA vRNA containing a A_6 sequence instead of its U_6 poly(A) site by inserting a negative-sense eukaryotic poly(A) site (SPA) (modified from Levitt et al. [8]) next to the A_6 sequence (Fig. 4). This mutant vRNA was transcribed by RNA polymerase I (pol I) from pPOLI-NA-SPA, a plasmid containing a pol I promoter and a ribozyme sequence as described [4,10]. The vRNA could be transcribed by a recombinant influenza RNA polymerase into a poly(U)-tailed SPA-containing NA mRNA in vivo. We asked the question whether the poly(U)-tailed influenza transcripts were $3'$ end processed. By RT-PCR, sequencing, and S1 nuclease mapping of NA-specific RNA transcripts from transfected cells, we found that the SPA-containing poly(U)-tailed influenza NA mRNA molecules were cleaved and polyadenylated at the cellular poly(A) site. The synthesis of polyadenylated NA-specific RNA transcripts was dependent on the presence of a recombinant influenza RNA polymerase and nucleoprotein (NP) in the cells. In addition, it was also dependent on the presence of the conserved hexamer AAUAAA in the poly(U)-tailed NA mRNA transcript, confirming that polyadenylation occurred through the cellular polyadenylation machinery.

According to the current model, $3'$ end processing of cellular pre-mRNAs is coupled to cellular RNA polymerase II transcription; thus, only RNA products synthesised by pol II are believed to be efficiently polyadenylated. Our results show that the cellular polyadenylation machinery is nevertheless able to recognise and process RNA transcripts,

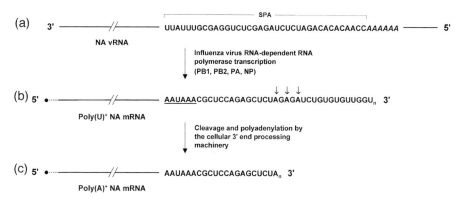

Fig. 4. Schematic representation of NA vRNA, containing a negative-sense eukaryotic poly(A) site (SPA) and a A_6 sequence, and RNA transcripts derived from it. The NA vRNA (a) transcribed by pol I from pPOLI-NA-SPA (not shown) is transcribed into poly(U)-tailed mRNA (b) by a recombinant influenza RNA polymerase in the presence of the nucleoprotein, derived from pcDNA-PB1, pcDNA-PB2, pcDNA-PA, and pcDNA-NP protein expression plasmids. The sequence of the SPA (modified from Levitt et al. [8]) is shown. The conserved hexamer of the SPA is underlined. The A_6 sequence replacing the viral U_6 poly(A) site is shown in italics. Potential cleavage sites in the SPA are indicated by arrows. Only the poly(A)$^+$ NA mRNA (c) cleaved at position 14 downstream of the AAUAAA hexamer is shown.

which are not synthesised by pol II. This indicates that synthesis by pol II is not an absolute requirement for efficient 3′ end processing. In addition, our results suggest that influenza transcription might be intimately coupled to pol II transcription.

Acknowledgements

We thank Retroscreen Virology for performing and ISIS Innovation for sponsoring some of the experiments. This work was supported by the MRC (programme grant G9523972 to G.G.B.), the FEMS (fellowship to A.M.), and the Croucher Foundation (L.L.M.P.).

References

[1] S.M. Barabino, W. Keller, Last but not least: regulated poly(A) tail formation, Cell 99 (1999) 9–11.
[2] D. Bentley, Coupling RNA polymerase II transcription with pre-mRNA processing, Curr. Opin. Cell Biol. 11 (1999) 347–351.
[3] E. Fodor, D.C. Pritlove, G.G. Brownlee, The influenza virus panhandle is involved in the initiation of transcription, J. Virol. 68 (1994) 4092–4096.
[4] E. Fodor, L. Devenish, O.G. Engelhardt, P. Palese, G.G. Brownlee, A. García-Sastre, Rescue of influenza A virus from recombinant DNA, J. Virol. 73 (1999) 9679–9682.
[5] E. Fodor, A. Mikulasova, J.L. Mingay, L.L.M. Poon, G.G. Brownlee, Messenger RNAs that are not synthesised by RNA polymerase II can be 3′ end cleaved and polyadenylated, EMBO Reports 1 (2000) 513–518.
[6] Y. Hirose, J.L. Manley, RNA polymerase II and the integration of nuclear events, Genes Dev. 14 (2000) 1415–1429.

[7] R.M. Krug, F.V. Alonso-Caplen, I. Julkunen, M.G. Katz, Expression and replication of the influenza virus genome, in: R.M. Krug (Ed.), The Influenza Viruses, Plenum, New York, 1989, pp. 89–152.

[8] N. Levitt, D. Briggs, A. Gil, N.J. Proudfoot, Definition of an efficient synthetic poly(A) site, Genes Dev. 3 (1989) 1019–1025.

[9] L. Minvielle-Sebastia, W. Keller, mRNA polyadenylation and its coupling to other RNA processing reactions and to transcription, Curr. Opin. Cell Biol. 11 (1999) 352–357.

[10] S. Pleschka, S.R. Jaskunas, O.G. Engelhardt, T. Zürcher, P. Palese, A. García-Sastre, A plasmid-based reverse genetics system for influenza A virus, J. Virol. 70 (1996) 4188–4192.

[11] L.L.M. Poon, D.C. Pritlove, J. Sharps, G.G. Brownlee, The RNA polymerase of influenza virus, bound to the 5′ end of virion RNA, acts in cis to polyadenylate mRNA, J. Virol. 72 (1998) 8214–8219.

[12] L.L.M. Poon, D.C. Pritlove, E. Fodor, G.G. Brownlee, Direct evidence that the poly(A) tail of infuenza A virus mRNA is synthesized by reiterative copying of a U track in the virion RNA template, J. Virol. 73 (1999) 3473–3476.

[13] L.L.M. Poon, E. Fodor, G.G. Brownlee, Polyuridylated mRNA synthesized by a recombinant influenza virus is defective in nuclear export, J. Virol. 74 (2000) 418–427.

[14] D.C. Pritlove, L.L.M. Poon, E. Fodor, J. Sharps, G.G. Brownlee, Polyadenylation of influenza virus mRNA transcribed in vitro from model virion RNA templates: requirement for 5′ conserved sequences, J. Virol. 72 (1998) 1280–1286.

[15] D.C. Pritlove, L.L.M. Poon, L.J. Devenish, M.B. Leahy, G.G. Brownlee, A hairpin loop at the 5′ end of influenza A virus virion RNA is required for synthesis of poly(A)$^+$ mRNA in vitro, J. Virol. 73 (1999) 2109–2114.

[16] N.J. Proudfoot, G.G. Brownlee, 3′ Non-coding region sequences in eukaryotic messenger RNA, Nature 263 (1976) 211–214.

[17] N.J. Proudfoot, Connecting transcription to messenger RNA processing, Trends Biochem. Sci. 25 (2000) 290–293.

[18] J.S. Robertson, M. Schubert, R.A. Lazzarini, Polyadenylation sites for influenza mRNA, J. Virol. 38 (1981) 157–163.

[19] L.S. Tiley, M. Hagen, J.T. Matthews, M. Krystal, Sequence-specific binding of the influenza virus RNA polymerase to sequences located at the 5′ ends of the viral RNAs, J. Virol. 68 (1994) 5108–5116.

International Congress Series 1219 (2001) 435–450

Influenza virus RNA encapsidation: discrimination for vRNA versus cRNA molecules

Svetlin Tchatalbachev, Gerd Hobom*, Ramon Flick[1]

Institut für Mikrobiologie und Molekularbiologie der Justus Liebig Universität Giessen, Frankfurter Str. 107, D-35392 Giessen, Germany

Abstract

The packaging signal of influenza viral RNA is shown to reside within the 5′ bulged promoter structure, caused by the central unpaired residue A10 in its 5′ branch. Upon insertion of two uridine residues in the 3′ branch opposite A10, the minus-strand vRNA promoter is converted into a 3′ bulged structure, while the plus-strand cRNA promoter adopts the 5′ bulged conformation. The cRNA is packaged exclusively in the progeny virions of this promoter variant. Upon insertion of a single uridine nucleotide opposite A10, the two de-bulged structures of the vRNA and cRNA promoters are rendered identical, and both vRNA and cRNA molecules are packaged indiscriminately, in a 1:1 ratio. We propose that interaction of viral polymerase with the two differently bulged vRNA and cRNA promoter structures results in either of two conformations of the protein, which in turn are recognized in a two-step procedure by matrix protein M1. While both, viral nucleoprotein particles (vRNPs) and cRNPs, are exported from the nucleus in association with M1, attachment to only the 5′ bulged vRNPs is maintained during encapsidation at the plasma membrane. © 2001 Elsevier Science B.V. All rights reserved.

Keywords: Packaging signal; Bulged promoter structure; Corkscrew conformation; M1–RNA polymerase interaction; RNA polymerase I

1. Introduction

Incorporation of viral RNAs into progeny virions must rely on specific structural feature(s) in that RNA, but at the same time remain independent of most of their nucleotide sequence. Recognition of the packaging signal, during morphogenesis of enveloped

---

* Corresponding author. Fax: +49-641-99-41209.
E-mail address: gerd.hobom@mikro.bio.uni-giessen.de (G. Hobom).
[1] Current address: Ludwig Institute for Cancer Research, Nobelsväg 3, S-17177 Stockholm, Sweden.

viruses, is also a central element in the merger of two separately synthesized constituents, the viral glycoproteins and the viral RNP complexes at the appropriate cellular membrane, plasma membrane or other site. Packaging signals have been identified so far only for retroviruses [27,10] and for hepatitis B viruses [23], and are not known for nucleoprotein-covered minus strand RNA viruses including influenza virus.

The genome of influenza virus consists of eight single-stranded RNA molecules, which in association with the viral polymerase complex and a large number of nucleoprotein subunits, together constitute the viral nucleoprotein particles (vRNPs). During assembly of the progeny virions at the plasma membrane [17], RNP molecules containing negative-stranded viral RNAs are incorporated exclusively, while all other RNA species present in the infected cell are selected against, including complementary plus-strand viral RNAs, which constitute the cRNP particles.

In the assembly process, a vRNP core complex becomes enveloped by the cellular plasma membrane, which contains the separately synthesized viral spike glycoproteins hemagglutinin (HA), neuraminidase (NA), and M2. Each of these proteins interacts with the viral matrix protein M1, which densely lines the inside of the plasma membrane [11,13]. While M1–vRNA sequence recognition had been proposed earlier as the vRNP recognition step in budding [28], this has been ruled out because of its 10-fold lower RNA binding affinity as compared to NP, through partial structural resolution of M1, and through determination of its basic peptide sequence, a possible core element in membrane attachment [25,26]. Protein–vRNA recognition are unlikely at this stage also because of the sequence heterogeneity and variability among the vRNA molecules over most of their lengths in different viral isolates, and a tight coverage by viral RNA polymerase at their constant 5' and 3' termini, which are physically brought together in that protein-binding reaction [2,5,6,9,14].

Instead, protein–protein interactions in encapsidation are likely to be conformation-dependent, since both vRNPs and cRNPs constitute the same viral proteins in equal arrangements. While M1–NP interactions have frequently been proposed in this regard, no such interaction could be detected in vivo in a model experiment between M1 and NP (associated with cellular RNAs) [33]. This leaves M1–polymerase interactions as the remaining candidate, since the difference to be recognized by M1 in discriminating between the vRNP and cRNP conformation has to result from subtle differences in interaction of viral polymerase with the 5' and 3' ends of vRNAs versus the 5' and 3' ends of cRNAs. M1–RNP interactions have been described before with regard to M1-mediated nuclear export of viral RNPs [3,15], but without differentiation between M1–NP and M1–polymerase interactions.

The 5' and 3' terminal sequences of influenza vRNAs as well as cRNAs show a section of complete complementarity (in vRNA for positions 11–16 from the 5' end versus from the 3' end) embedded in a region of partial complementary sequence, which is also largely conserved over the first 13 or 12 residues among all eight viral RNA segments. These terminal 16 and 15 nucleotides constitute the functional promoter structure both for the vRNA and cRNA molecules, and the adapted conformation in its binding interaction with viral polymerase has been described as the "corkscrew" structure [4,5]. RNA polymerase I-mediated synthesis of viral RNAs in vivo [21] has made it possible to perform detailed viral mutagenesis studies within the promoter structure. Among the promoter variants created in this way, several constructs such as the original pHL1104 [20] have been converted into complete complementarity between the 5' and 3' branches within the promoter region, with the single exception of a remaining extra, unpaired adenosine nucleotide in 5' position 10 of the vRNA promoter, and correspondingly, the uridine residue in 3' position $\overline{10}$ of the cRNA promoter. All of these constructs remain active or become enhanced in transcription and replication as well as packaging.

In this report, we show that it is the specific conformation of the viral polymerase, conferred through interaction with an overall "bulged" vRNA promoter structure that is recognized by M1 during viral morphogenesis at the plasma membrane. This process results in exclusion of the otherwise identical cRNA molecules.

2. Materials and methods

2.1. Plasmid constructions

Plasmids constructed for in vivo expression of influenza virus vRNA molecules by RNA polymerase I had inserted either the murine or the human rDNA core promoter region (-251 to -1 or -411 to -1), along with the terminator sequence from murine rDNA [21]. Between these two elements, influenza cDNA constructs were exactly incorporated in antisense orientation, with the reporter gene chloramphenicol acetyltransferase (CAT) substituting for the influenza gene coding sequence. In a single case, pHL2971, CAT was inserted in sense orientation, while the flanking influenza non-coding regions containing the promoter and packaging signals remained, i.e. in antisense orientation.

All of the plasmid constructs carried three point mutations in the 3' viral promoter sequence (3'-G $\overline{3}$ A, U $\overline{5}$ C, C $\overline{8}$ U : 3'-UC*A*UC*U*U*U*GUCCCCAU), as originally introduced into plasmid pHL1104 or pHL2024 [5,20], but in addition carried other insertions or deletions as well as substitutions elsewhere in the promoter region, see Fig. 1. Constructs controlled by the murine RNA polymerase I promoter were inserted into plasmid vector pHL1261 [4], while the human RNA polymerase I promoter constructs were made using cloning vector pHH21 [8]. Upon restriction by enzyme *Bsm*BI, these vector plasmids will incorporate in an oriented way PCR fragments that are restricted by *Bsa*I and extend across the entire CAT gene; the promoter sequence mutants designed for each construct were carried in the flanking PCR primers. All plasmid constructs were verified either by sequencing across the mutated flanking regions or by sequencing across the entire CAT insert.

2.2. Cells and viruses

Influenza A/FPV/Bratislava (H7/N7) virus was grown in Madin–Darby canine kidney (MDCK) cells. B82 mouse fibroblast cells [16] and human 293T cells were used for DNA transfection and consecutive superinfection with FPV helper virus, for constructs containing the murine or human RNA polymerase I promoter, respectively. The resulting recombinant influenza viruses were propagated in MDCK cells. All cell lines were grown

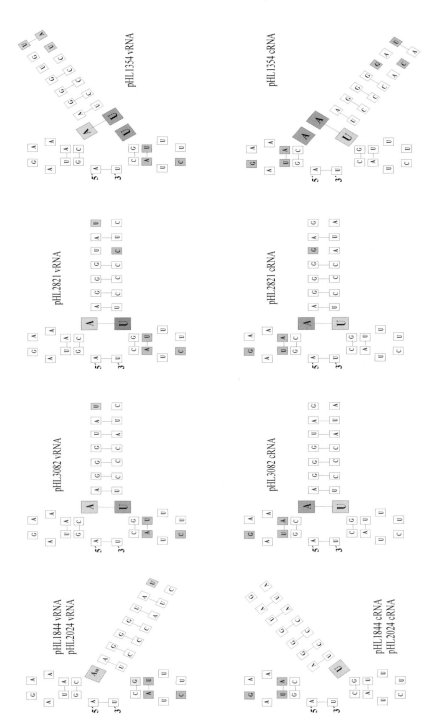

in Dulbecco's modified Eagle's Medium (DMEM; GIBCO/BRL), supplemented with 10% fetal calf serum and antibiotics.

2.3. DNA transfection and influenza virus infection

For DNA transfection, we used $\sim 3.6 \times 10^6$ subconfluent B82 or 293T cells. Briefly: 3 μg of plasmid DNA in 186 μl serum-free DMEM was gently mixed with 6 μl Lipofectamine and 8 μl of Lipofectamine Plus (GIBCO/BRL) and incubated for 30 min at room temperature. In the meantime, cells were washed with serum-free medium, and the transfection mix diluted to 3 ml with medium was carefully dispensed over the cells. After 6 h of incubation, the medium was changed to DMEM containing 10% FCS and further incubated for 15 h. The transfected cells were washed very carefully with PBS+ (2.5 mM $MgCl_2$; 3.4 mM$CaCl_2$ added) and superinfected with FPV helper virus at an m.o.i. of two to three in 1 ml of PBS+. After 1 h, the cells were washed and finally resupplied with DMEM containing 10% FCS for another 8 h of incubation. A complete replication cycle of the virus takes place in this period.

2.4. Serial passage of virus containing supernatants

After 8 h of viral propagation, the supernatant containing the progeny virus was collected, and after a brief centrifugation step (10 000 rpm, 5 min) for cell debris removal, it was used for passaging the recombinant virus mixture onto confluent MDCK cells as described previously [5].

2.5. CAT assay

Cell extracts of 110 μl were prepared as described by Gorman et al. [7]. In an initial series, 50 μl of each cell lysate, and depending on the data obtained, serially diluted amounts of the various cell lysates (always including material from one or more reference reactions) were mixed with 10 μl of 4 mM acetyl-CoA and 8 μl of fluorescent-labeled chloramphenicol (borondippyrromethane difluoride fluorophore: BODIPY CAM substrate, FLASH CAT kit, Stratagene). Samples were incubated at 37 °C for 3 h. For extracting the reaction products, 0.5 ml of ethyl acetate was added, and after a centrifugation step for 3 min at 13 000 rpm, the upper phase containing the acetylated products was transferred into new Eppendorf tubes and vacuum dried.

The resulting pellet was resuspended in 20 μl ethylacetate, and the reaction products were separated by thin layer chromatography (TLC plates 20/20 cm, Silica gel 60) using a

---

Fig. 1. Enzyme-adapted vRNA and cRNA promoter structures of reference constructs pHL1844 and pHL2024, of two variants constructed by insertion of a single extra U (dark gray) residue in the 3′ branch of the promoter sequence opposite standard residue A10 (light gray) in the 5′ branch, inserted into the promoter sequence of segment 5 (pHL3082) or segment 4 (pHL2821), and of variant pHL1354 carrying two inserted U residues in that position. All promoter sequences differ from wild type by three nucleotide substitutions (light gray) in the vRNA 3′ branch: 3′-G $\bar{3}$ A, U $\bar{5}$ C, C $\bar{8}$ U, and correspondingly, in the cRNA 5′ branch. pHL2971 is identical in its promoter structure with pHL1844 or pHL2024.

solvent mixture (mobile phase) of chloroform and methanol (87:13). Finally, the reaction products were visualized by UV illumination, documented by photography and evaluated using the WinCam system (Cybertech, Berlin). Ratios of activity have been calculated relative to reference constructs: pHL2024 and pHL1844, in the murine (B82) or human (293T) series, respectively, based on three independent sets of serial dilutions of cell lysates down to 30–50% of product formation each.

2.6. Virus purification and concentration by hemeadsorption

Virus particles were isolated from infected tissue culture supernatants obtained from the first or second passage on MDCK cells. After 10-h post-infection, the culture medium from infected plates was collected on ice, and cell debris was removed at 5000 rpm for 5 min. Freshly prepared chicken red blood cells in a 50% suspension in PBS+ were added to a final concentration of 2%. After 60 min of adsorption at 0 °C on a rocking platform at 200 rpm, the red blood cells were washed twice with ice-cold PBS. Virus was eluted in 0.1 vol of PBS for 60 min at 37 °C by gentle shaking. Finally, the red blood cells were removed by low speed centrifugation.

2.7. RNA isolation and RT-PCR analysis

RNA from infected cells was isolated using the RNeasy Mini kit (QIAGEN) procedure according to the manufacturer's protocol. Isolation of RNA from purified virions employed the QIAamp Viral RNA kit (QIAGEN) using 560 µl of concentrated virus suspension. Reverse transcription was performed with MMLV reverse transcriptase (Stratagene) as follows: 0.5 or 1 µg of cytoplasmic or viral RNA was mixed with 2 µl of 10 × RT-Buffer (500 mM Tris–HCl, pH: 8.3; 750 mM KCl; 100 mM DTT; 30 mM MgCl$_2$; Stratagene), 50 units of reverse transcriptase, 1 µl RNasin (Promega), 500 µM of dNTPs and 100 pmol of the first strand primer to a final volume of 20 µl; the reaction mix was incubated at 42 °C for 1 h. Primers SN-I (5′-AATCACTGGATATACCACCGTTGA-TAT ATC-3′) or SN-V (5′-TCAGTCAGTTGCTCAATGTACCTATAACC-3′) were used for reverse transcription of vRNA containing the antisense strand of CAT, and primer SN-II (5′-CCTGCCACTCATCGCAGTACTGTTGTAATTC-3′) for annealing to the sense strand of CAT containing cRNA molecules. PCR reactions were done consecutively using the SN-I/SN-II or SN-V/SN-II primer pairs in a GeneAmp 2400 PCR system (Perkin-Elmer) in the following programmed cycle: 1 × 94 °C: 1.5 min; 30 × 94 °C: 15 s/57.5 °C: 45 s/72 °C: 50 s; 1 × 72 °C: 5 min. Recombinant *Taq* DNA polymerase, (GIBCO/BRL) was used for carrying out the polymerase chain reaction: 5 µl of the reverse transcription reaction volume was mixed with 0.2 µl of *Taq* DNA polymerase, 5 µl of 10 × PCR-buffer (200 mM Tris-HCl, pH: 8.4; 500 mM KCl), followed by addition of 50 pmol each of the two primers, 200 µM of dNTPs, 1.5 mM MgCl$_2$ in a final volume of 50 µl. PCR products were then separated on 2% agarose gels (Agarose NEEO, Carl Roth) and visualized by ethidium bromide staining. Semi-quantitative RT-PCR for determination of CAT RNA relative to HA viral RNA sequences in the recombinant virus/helper virus mixture following the same overall procedure required a primer ratio of 100:10 for the CAT-specific primers such as SN-V and SN-II relative to the hemagglutinin-specific primers:

H7-HA-III (5′-ATGAACACTCAAATCCTGG TTTTCGC-3′) and H7-HA-IV (5′-GCA-TAGAATGAAGACCCTGATCTTC-3′).

2.8. RNA isolation from separated nuclear and cytoplasmic fractions

A modified, gentle procedure including cell lysis with digitonin (Sigma) was performed for a separate isolation of nuclear and cytoplasmic RNAs [1]. MDCK cells, grown to 100% confluence on 6-cm tissue culture dishes for 36 h in order to prevent further cell divisions, were infected with virus containing supernatant from the second passage as described above. After 5 h of incubation, the cells were washed twice with PBS, collected using a rubber policeman in 500 μl PBS in Eppendorf tubes, and briefly sedimented at 2000 rpm for 2 min. The supernatant was removed and cells were gently resuspended in 200 μl lysis medium (MDEM, containing 10% FCS; 50 μg/ml digitonin; Sigma). After incubation for another 15 min at 37 °C, the lysate was centrifuged at 3000 rpm for 2 min. The upper phase represents the cytoplasmic fraction, while the pellet containing the nuclei and some cell debris is called here the nuclear fraction. The pellet as well as the supernatant was used for RNA isolation according to the RNeasy Mini Kit instructions (QIAGEN).

2.9. RT-PCR analysis of viral CAT and cellular p53 RNAs

For detecting the presence of pHL1844 and pHL2971 RNAs in the nuclear and cytoplasmic fractions, RT reactions were done with primer 1844-5′ (5′ CAAGGG-TATTTTTC TTTACCTAG-3′). This primer constitutes nucleotides 9 to 31 from the 5′ terminus of pHL1844 vRNA and consequently anneals to the 3′ terminus of the cRNA, while it does not bind tightly to the 3′ end of the corresponding mRNAs. Reverse transcription reactions were run separately for nuclear and cytoplasmic fractions, and consecutive PCRs were done together with primers SN-V for pHL1844 or SN-II for pHL2971, respectively. Due to the different lengths of the flanking regions the expected PCR products for pHL2971 and pHL1844 have a size of 736 and 808 bp, respectively.

Similarly, pHL1354 vRNA was identified using primer 1354-3′N(5′-AGGGGATAATT CTATTAATCATGG-3′) for reverse transcription, and added primer SNII for PCR amplification resulting in a product with the size of 668 bp.

Parallel reactions, directed at the flanking regions to the left and right of intron 7 of the p53 tumor suppressor hnRNA [12], were performed in order to verify the purity of the isolated nuclear and cytoplasmic fractions. While the nucleus should contain both unspliced and spliced mRNA molecules, only the completely spliced mRNAs are expected to have passed the nuclear pores and present the cytoplasm. Reverse transcription reactions were run separately for nuclear and cytoplasmic fractions using primers p53-I (5′-AAGTACC TGGACGACAGAAACAC-3′) and p53-II (5′-GGTGGCTCAGGA-CAAGGCTCC-3′) flanking intron 7 of the p53 tumor suppressor gene at positions 620 and 909, respectively, which were employed for reverse transcription as an internal control. For nuclear fractions, two RT-PCR products 551 and 289 bp in length were expected, corresponding to the spliced mRNA and unspliced hnRNA of p53, respectively. In a pure cytoplasmic fraction, RT-PCR should result in the shorter cDNA fragments only, as produced by the spliced p53 mRNA species.

3. Results

3.1. Template recognition by viral polymerase relies on 16 and $\bar{1}\bar{5}$ terminal nucleotides, in an enzyme-adapted conformation

For the in vivo analysis of influenza vRNA variants carrying substitutions, insertions or deletions within their terminal 5′ and 3′ sequences RNA polymerase I transcription were employed, which gives rise to the respective RNA molecules after DNA transfection of the corresponding plasmid constructs. Murine or human rDNA core promoter segments together with a murine rDNA terminator signal precisely fused onto influenza cDNA templates served to determine the exact influenza 5′ and 3′ vRNA ends [21,35]. A reporter gene read-out for the promoter variant was constructed by exchanging the influenza gene reading frame for the chloramphenicol acetyltransferase (CAT) gene coding sequence, again in antisense orientation. The influenza vRNA non-coding regions as present in these RNA polymerase I transcription products were derived either from segment 4 (HA) or from segment 5 (NP). All constructs carried three substitutions in the 3′ branches of their promoter structures [20], which also were introduced into both reference plasmids pHL2024 and pHL1844: 3′-G $\bar{3}$ A, U $\bar{5}$ C, and C $\bar{8}$ U. Further individual rearrangements are also shown in Fig. 1. Sequence variation provided increased transcription and replication activity upon superinfection by FPV helper virus, making any selection for recombinant viruses unnecessary. It also removed heterogeneities existing in the wild-type sequence between the vRNA and cRNA promoter structures.

Two structural differences between vRNA and cRNA molecules remain within the 5′ and 3′ terminal sequences of 22 and 15 nucleotides, respectively, that constitute the minimum requirement for viral propagation. One of them is the vRNA promoter-adjacent U_{5-6} element (U17–U22) that is known to be responsible for viral mRNA polyadenylation [24]; in cRNA molecules that 5′ oligo U element is converted into a 3′ oligo A element (A$\bar{1}\bar{7}$–A$\bar{2}\bar{2}$). The second element of divergence, and the only one remaining in the promoter itself, is an unpaired, extra nucleotide A10 in the 5′ vRNA sequence, in cRNA converted into 3′ unpaired U$\bar{1}\bar{0}$.

Either element of divergence or both, together, may be involved in the vRNP versus cRNP discrimination step(s) during RNP encapsidation. No influence upon encapsidation or progeny maturation in general has been observed by the three substitutions introduced into the two reference promoter-up variants and into all other constructs used in this study (see below), or indeed by any other substitution in the proximal or distal element of the influenza promoter structure, provided the promoter variant stays functional.

Since the unpaired 5′ residue A10 in the vRNA promoter structure or the corresponding 3′ nucleotide U$\bar{1}\bar{0}$ in the cRNA promoter structure are located between two rigid, double-stranded elements in the enzyme-adapted "corkscrew" conformation (see Fig. 1), they may either be freely exposed or buried because of stacking interactions and cause a bulged overall structure. According to the first model, an exposed A10 (and U$\bar{1}\bar{0}$) residue might be expected to be recognized specifically by viral polymerase as a major element of discrimination against other RNA molecules in the cell. That prediction was analyzed in constructing a series of single nucleotide substitution variants regarding 5′ position 10, see

Fig. 2. Since variant A10G left CAT, expression rates unaffected and variant A10C and A10U only caused moderate reductions in activity and no defect in packaging efficiency, we conclude that an unpaired residue A10 cannot be recognized directly and specifically by viral polymerase, but appears to exert structural influence, only indirectly, i.e. according to the second model. A buried position of A10 is supported also through results obtained for variants carrying an inserted uridine nucleotide in the 3′ branch opposite A10 (or G10), i.e. potentially involving A10 in basepairing, which were still recognized by polymerase and active in transcription, replication and packaging, even if at somewhat lower levels (see below).

Since the constellation of two neighboring 5′ adenosine residues, A10 and A11, opposite a single 3′ uridine residue, U$\overline{10}$ left some doubt, whether U$\overline{10}$ in its basepair formation would interact with A11 or possibly instead with A10, the same series of substitution variants has also been constructed for A11, but here all single substitution variants lost activity (see Fig. 2). Complementary double exchange in A11/U$\overline{10}$ regained activity, thereby, proving an A11–U$\overline{10}$ basepairing interaction (not shown). Therefore, it is the unpaired vRNA residue A10 (and similarly the unpaired cRNA residue U$\overline{10}$), which caused a bulged overall structure and served as a characteristic element for promoter recognition by viral polymerase.

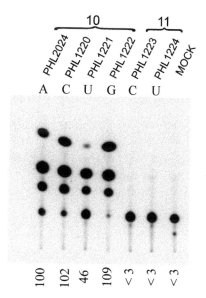

Fig. 2. Promoter and packaging activity of A10 and A11 substitution derivatives. CAT activity measurements for 50 µl of cell lysates obtained at 8-h post-infection from MDCK cells of the first viral passage. Cells were infected with supernatant containing recombinant progeny viruses derived from plasmid DNA transfected and FPV superinfected B82 cells. CAT activities have been calculated relative to the results obtained for diluted samples of reference construct pHL2024.

3.2. Encapsidation of RNA molecules carrying nucleotide insertions opposite unpaired residue A10

To investigate the recognition requirement during virion assembly for a polymerase binding structure carrying an A10 vRNA bulge, we constructed several variants carrying an inserted uridine residue in the 3′ promoter branch opposite residue A10 in the 5′ branch, i.e. inserted in-between G9̄ and U1̄0̄ of the 3′ branch, see Fig. 1. CAT assays following DNA transfection and FPV super infection of pHL3082 and pHL2821 in 293T cells showed reduced activity of these de-bulged promoter constructs (Fig. 3). The same result has been repeated in viral transfer of pHL3082 and pHL2821 recombinants, and also, in using related constructs carrying a de-bulged promoter structure due to insertion of a single U residue, plus additional variations in the adjacent non-coding regions (data not shown).

In a further step, not one, but two uridine residues were inserted into the 3′ branch opposite 5′ residue A10. Consequently, the resulting vRNA and cRNA molecules are expected to have their structural shapes exchanged, i.e. in pHL1354, it is the sense strand which carries an extra nucleotide in the 5′ branch, while it is the antisense strand of pHL1354 that is characterized by an extra nucleotide in the 3′ branch (Fig. 1). In spite of the severe structural deformation, pHL1354 was active after DNA transfection as well as in viral passage, a step requiring recognition in the encapsidation process (Fig. 3). Another variant, pHL1246, proved to be inactive in both regards due to insertion of an extra A

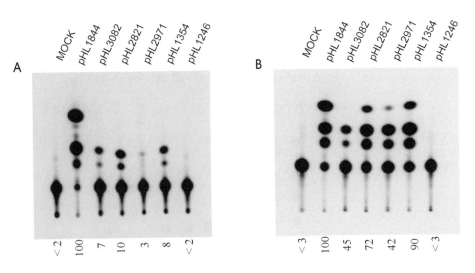

Fig. 3. Promoter and packaging activity of nucleotide insertion variants. (A) CAT activity measurements of 50-μl cell lysates obtained from plasmid DNA transfected and FPV helper virus infected cells at 8-h post-infection of 293T cells (pHL1844–pHL2971) or B82 cells (pHL1354 and pHL1246). CAT activities have been calculated relative to diluted samples of human rDNA promoter reference construct pHL1844, or to murine rDNA promoter reference construct pHL2024 (not shown). (B) CAT activity measurements of 50-μl cell lysates obtained from MDCK cells at 8-h post-infection with recombinant virus containing supernatants from reactions shown in (A) at an m.o.i. of two to four. CAT activities have been calculated relative to diluted samples of reference construct pHL1844.

residue next to A10 in the 5' branch, which is expected to create a 5' double-sized bulge (structure not shown).

3.3. vRNP/cRNP discrimination during encapsidation

The polarity of the CAT-RNA molecules packaged into progeny virions was analyzed by RT-PCR reactions. For this purpose, the virus-containing supernatants obtained from MDCK cells infected in a first step of viral passage, i.e. containing second step viral progeny were purified by hemadsorption. RNAs obtained from these viruses were employed for reverse transcription with oligonucleotide primers binding either to the CAT-containing vRNA or to the CAT-containing cRNA, followed in each case by a PCR reaction together with the other primer, yielding CAT-cDNAs of 573 bp. The results confirm an exclusive incorporation of the vRNA minus strand for recombinant viruses obtained from basic promoter variants such as pHL1844. The same is true for construct pHL2971, which contains an inverted CAT reading frame in sense orientation while the flanking regions are maintained in their vRNA orientation, confirming that the packaging signal is located in the external sequences.

Only the cRNA of PHL1354, which carries an inverted bulge in its promoter sequence, is found incorporated in the virions. In contrast, both species of RNA molecules are found encapsidated (for the constructs which have the bulged promoter conformation eliminated through insertion of a single uridine residue) (Fig. 4A). This result is in agreement with identical structures over the terminal $16 + \bar{1}\bar{6}$ nucleotides for both the vRNA and cRNA molecules. The results of double RT-PCR experiments, using the concomitant HA vRNA template amplification as an internal reference, confirmed an approximate 1:1 ratio for packaging of pHL3082 and pHL2821 vRNAs or cRNAs (Fig. 4B). It has been measured to be 1:0.89 for pHL2821 and 1.2:1 for pHL3082, in relation to a standardized HA cDNA fragment yield after a limited number of amplification cycles. However, the level of incorporation of both recombinant CAT segments together was estimated to be in the range of 1:20 relative to the helper virus HA vRNA segment for these two constructs, attributable to their irregular promoter structure. The results obtained for pHL1354 also excluded the promoter-adjacent U_5 element to be (part of) the vRNA packaging signal, since it is the A_5-containing cRNA that becomes packaged in this case. That result has further been confirmed independently, since U5 deletion and substitution (A_5 instead of U_5) variants of an otherwise standard 5' bulged vRNA promoter were packaged in the regular asymmetric way (not shown). All PCR fragments were identified by restriction cleavage.

3.4. Localization of the M1–vRNP recognition reaction in the cell

The influenza matrix protein M1 is known to be translated late in the infection cycle. While association of the majority of M1 with the plasma membrane appears to be an intrinsic property of this protein [32], a fraction of it is found in the nucleus of the infected cells, in association with viral RNPs [3,15]. This divergent behaviour of M1 has been related to (fractional) modification by phosphorylation, since hyperphosphorylation observed for a variant of M1 caused its retention in the nucleus [30].

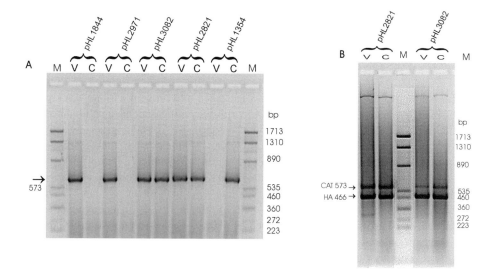

Fig. 4. RT-PCR analyses for viral strand polarity in virions isolated from second viral passage. (A) Progeny viruses isolated from supernatants of infected MDCK cells by hemadsorption were used for two reverse transcription reactions each, specific for CAT containing vRNA (v) and CAT containing cRNA (c), respectively, followed by PCR amplification. The expected size of the CAT-PCR fragments is marked at the left margin, while the fragment sizes of the marker lanes (M) are indicated at the right margin. (B) Semiquantitative assay for the packaging ratios between vRNAs and cRNAs in pHL2821 and pHL3082 virions, relative to internal standard segment 4 (HA) vRNA. Reverse transcription reactions were done simultaneously for pHL2821 or pHL3082 vRNA and for the internal reference vRNA of segment 4 (HA), and for pHL2821 or pHL3082 cRNA and again for viral segment 4 vRNA at primer ratios 10:1, followed by 25 cycles of PCR amplification.

Interaction of M1 with RNP in the nucleus is believed to facilitate nuclear export of M1–RNP complexes [19]. Only vRNP complexes, and cRNA complexes with M1, become a constituent of virus particles; the step responsible for discriminating between the two is unresolved. Discrimination during initial interaction of M1 with the RNPs in the nucleus or during nuclear export would exclude the cRNPs from export into the cytoplasm, and so we analyzed the cytoplasmic fraction of cells infected with recombinant influenza viruses for the presence or absence of cRNA molecules. In cells infected with pHL1354 recombinant influenza virus, vRNP complexes must be selected against a nuclear discrimination step. Infected cells were fractionated at 5-h post-infection using a gentle lysis procedure with digitonin [1]. In order to characterize the nuclear versus cytoplasmic fractions a control RT-PCR was run employing p53 mRNA/hnRNA, or more specifically its intron 7 region, by using an antisense primer to the right of the intron boundary for reverse transcription, and a sense primer to the left of intron 7 for consecutive PCR amplification. The resulting cDNA bands of 289 bp representing the spliced p53 mRNA, and 551 bp indicating unspliced p53 hnRNA (see Fig. 5) allowed us to characterize the nuclear and cytoplasmic fractions; both were analyzed by DNA sequencing for their identity.

Reverse transcription of influenza pHL1844 and pHL2971 cRNAs was initiated with a primer complementary to cRNA nucleotides $\bar{9}$ to $\bar{3}\bar{1}$, i.e. extending across the viral poly-

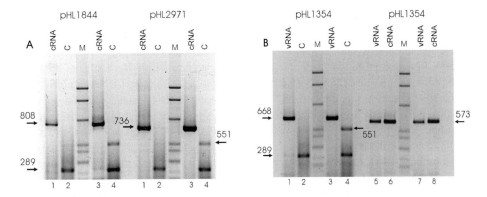

Fig. 5. RT-PCR analysis for the presence of vRNA and cRNA in the cytoplasm of infected cells, at 5-h post-infection. Reverse transcription for CAT specific vRNAs and cRNAs followed by PCR amplification was done similar to Fig. 3. As a control (lanes C), presence of spliced and unspliced p53 mRNA/hnRNA was amplified across intron 7 by RT-PCR. (A) Cytoplasmic (1, 2) and nuclear (3, 4) fractions of MDCK cells infected by pHL1844 or pHL2971 recombinant viruses; analysis for the presence of non-packaged cRNA molecules. (B) Cytoplasmic (1, 2, 5, 6) and nuclear (3, 4, 7, 8) fractions of MDCK cells infected by pHL1354 recombinant viruses; lanes 5, 6, 7, 8: analyses for packaged and non-packaged cRNA and vRNA molecules in the cytoplasm via RT-PCR with CAT internal primers.

adenylation signal. Their specificity for cRNA and also viral mRNA was confirmed in its inability to yield RT-PCR products with vRNA from virions or from mRNA fractions isolated from infected cells via oligo-dT adsorption, while in both cases control reactions with the appropriate primers yielded the expected products. In addition, the primer used for pHL1354 vRNA RT-PCR analysis, complementary to vRNA positions $\overline{12}-\overline{35}$, was unable to give rise to RT-PCR products with the mRNA template. Consecutive PCR amplification was done using a CAT internal oligonucleotide of the respective polarity; the resulting cDNA fragments were confirmed for their identity by restriction enzyme cleavage.

The data obtained for all recombinant influenza viruses analyzed in this way, see Fig. 4, quite clearly demonstrate the presence of both, vRNPs and cRNPs in both the nuclear and cytoplasmic fractions, irrespective of encapsidation of only one of these species. This is also true for double insertion mutant pHL1354 with its observed encapsidation of only the cRNPs. In this case, the observed presence of vRNA (CAT-antisense sequences) in the cytoplasm could not be attributed to irregular antisense mRNA transcription, since oligo-dT primed reverse transcription did not yield any product in consecutive PCR amplification, together with the same CAT-specific primer as used in vRNA specific amplification.

4. Discussion

As a consequence of the experimental results obtained, we conclude that the packaging signal of influenza vRNA is not a separate entity as demonstrated for other structural elements in this category [10,27], but instead constitutes part of the vRNA promoter structure. While viral RNA polymerase is recognizing and binding to both, the 5′ A10 bulged vRNA promoter structure and the 3′ U$\overline{10}$ bulged cRNA promoter structure, either interaction will exert a different conformational stress upon that protein, presumably diverting the conformation across the entire molecule including its surface domains. This is expected to change the potential for specific interaction of viral polymerase with other proteins. Since no more than a double nucleotide insertion within the center of the rather small promoter structure (16 plus 15 terminal nucleotides within the vRNA or cRNA) will reverse the packaging specificity from vRNP packaging to cRNP packaging, it must be the 280-kDa polymerase itself, which recognizes the promoter structure and its sequence variations. Viral polymerase, and in particular the PB1 subunit are known to interact with both branches of the promoter structure and to undergo allosteric conformational changes upon binding [6,14]. Only polymerase in its binding to the structurally adapted pair of terminal sequences could detect the conversion of a 5′ bulged to a 3′ bulged vRNA, and a 3′ bulged to a 5′ bulged cRNA; recognition by any of the NP subunits appears to be extremely unlikely.

In addition to the 5′ bulged and 3′ bulged promoter structures, viral polymerase is also able to recognize the de-bulged structure resulting from insertion of a single uridine residue opposite A10, even if at lower affinity. In this case, it is possible that interaction with viral polymerase will squeeze out that inserted 3′ extra nucleotide, and in this way create a conformationally 5′ bulged structure inspite of the uridine insertion. At least, it has been shown that recognition of a de-bulged promoter is restricted to constructs carrying an inserted U residue opposite A10, while those carrying an inserted C nucleotide opposite a (substituted) G10 residue are inactive, i.e. to resist that proposed conformational adaptation. This is opposed to the result obtained with the G10 substitution variant itself, which is shown to have full-level activity [5].

The obvious candidate for specifically interacting with viral RNA polymerase in its vRNP conformation, and discriminating against viral polymerase in its cRNP conformation during encapsidation is the viral matrix protein M1. Late in the replication cycle, M1 associates tightly with influenza RNPs in the nucleus, and facilitates nuclear export of M1-bound RNPs, possibly with assistance of viral NS2 [3,22], but its binding to polymerase or NP has not been differentially analyzed so far. Based on our data, which indicate M1 recognition of RNP-bound viral polymerase instead of RNP-bound NP, we propose that nuclear M1 interacts with viral polymerase in its promoter-bound state and interferes with initiation of further rounds of transcription or replication. It is known that M1 inhibits the various polymerase activities in vivo, and blocks the corresponding initiation steps [29]; inhibition of transcription in vitro also has been described [31]. M1-recognition of polymerase in the resting state, i.e. bound to the vRNA or cRNA promoter structure in its adapted "corkscrew" conformation, followed by nuclear export of M1-associated, arrested RNPs is in agreement with the time course of M1 synthesis late in the infection cycle, and avoids export of replication intermediates into the cytoplasm and consequent encapsidation.

As M1–vRNPs as well as M1–cRNPs are exported from the nucleus, but only M1–vRNPs are incorporated into the virion (in the wild-type case), we are proposing a second step of M1–RNP recognition which ought to take place at the plasma membrane. Discrimination of M1–vRNPs versus M1–cRNPs, i.e. an increased binding affinity of M1 to vRNPs and/or a decreased binding affinity to cRNPs, is likely to require another conformational change in M1. This change may occur through additional interactions of

M1 with other partners present in plasma membrane. Likely candidates are either an interaction of the RNP-bound M1 subunit with the negatively charged phospholipid membrane itself [25], or interactions of M1 with the cytoplasmic tails of the glycoproteins HA and NA [18,34] as well as M2. Such interactions are known to bring about conformational changes in M1 during budding, while their absence causes aberrant influenza particle shapes [11].

Acknowledgements

We thank U. Ruppert and S. Heck for their expert technical assistance, Dr. A. Vlachou for the helpful advise regarding the digitonin lysis procedure, and Prof. R. Rott for the critical comments. This work was supported by the Deutsche Forschungsgemeinschaft through SFB 535. This work was done in partial fulfillment of the requirements for the PhD degree of S.T., University of Giessen.

References

[1] S.A. Adam, R. Stern-Marr, L. Gerace, Nuclear protein import in permeabilized mammalian cells requires soluble cytoplasmic factors, J. Cell Biol. 111 (1990) 807–816.

[2] F. Baudin, C. Bach, S. Causack, R.W.H. Ruigrok, Structure of influenza RNP: I. Influenza virus nucleoprotein melts secondary structure in panhandle RNA and exposes the bases to the solvent, EMBO J. 13 (1994) 3158–3165.

[3] M. Bui, E.G. Wills, A. Helenius, G.R. Whittaker, Role of the influenza virus M1 protein in nuclear export of viral ribonucleoproteins, J. Virol. 74 (2000) 1781–1786.

[4] R. Flick, G. Hobom, Interaction of Influenza virus polymerase with viral RNA in the "corkscrew" conformation, J. Gen. Virol. 80 (1999) 2565–2572.

[5] R. Flick, G. Neumann, E. Hoffmann, E. Neumeier, G. Hobom, Promoter elements in the influenza vRNA terminal structure, RNA 21 (1996) 1046–1057.

[6] S. Gonzalez, J. Ortin, Distinct regions of influenza virus PB1 polymerase subunit recognize vRNA and cRNA templates, EMBO J. 18 (1999) 3767–3775.

[7] M. Gorman, L. Moffat, B. Howard, Recombinant genomes which express chloramphenicol acetyltransferase in mammalian cells, Mol. Cell. Biol. 2 (1982) 1044–1057.

[8] E. Hoffmann, PhD thesis, Justus Liebig University, Giessen, Germany, 1997.

[9] M. Hsu, J.D. Parvin, S. Gupta, M. Krystal, P. Palese, Genomic RNAs of influenza viruses are held in circular conformation in virions and in infected cells by a terminal panhandle, Proc. Natl. Acad. Sci. U. S. A. 84 (1987) 8140–8144.

[10] J.A. Ippolito, T.A. Steitz, The structure of the HIV-1 RRE high affinity rev binding site at 1.6 A resolution, J. Mol. Biol. 295 (2000) 711–717.

[11] H. Jin, J.P. Leser, J. Zhang, R.A. Lamb, Influenza virus hemagglutinin and neuraminidase cytoplasmic tails control particle shape, EMBO J. 16 (1997) 1236–1247.

[12] A.S. Johnson, C.G. Couto, C.M. Weghorst, Mutant of the p53 tumor suppressor gene in spontaneously occurring osteosarcomas of the dog, Carcinogenesis 19 (1998) 213–217.

[13] R.A. Lamb, R.M. Krug, Orthomyxoviridae: the viruses and their replication, in: B.N. Fields, D.M. Knipe, P.M. Howley (Eds.), Virology, 3rd edn., Raven Press, New York, 1996, pp. 1353–1394.

[14] M. Li, B.C. Ramirez, R.M. Krug, RNA-dependent activation of primer RNA production by influenza virus polymerase: different regions of the same protein subunit constitute the two required RNA binding sites, EMBO J. 17 (1998) 5844–5852.

[15] K. Martin, A. Helenius, Nuclear transport of influenza virus ribonucleoproteins: the viral matrix protein (M1) promotes export and inhibits import, Cell 67 (1991) 117–130.

[16] J.K. McDougall, T.H. Masse, D.A. Galloway, Location and cloning of the herpes virus type 2 thymidine kinase gene, J. Virol. 33 (1980) 1221–1224.

[17] H. Meier-Ewert, R.W. Compans, Time course of synthesis and assembly of influenza virus proteins, J. Virol. 186 (1974) 1083–1091.

[18] L.J. Mitnaul, M.R. Castrucci, K.G. Murti, Y. Kawaoka, The cytoplasmic tail of influenza A virus neuraminidase (NA) affects NA incorporation into virions, virion morphology, and virulence in mice but is not essential for virus replication, J. Virol. 70 (1996) 873–879.

[19] K.G. Murti, P.S. Brown, W.J. Bean Jr., R.G. Webster, Composition of the helical internal components of influenza virus as revealed by immunogold labeling/electron microscopy, Virology 186 (1992) 294–299.

[20] G. Neumann, G. Hobom, Mutational analysis of influenza virus promoter elements in vivo, J. Gen. Virol. 76 (1995) 1709–1717.

[21] G. Neumann, A. Zobel, G. Hobom, RNA polymerase I mediated expression of influenza viral RNA molecules, Virology 202 (1994) 477–479.

[22] R.E. O'Neill, J. Talon, P. Palese, The influenza virus NEP (NS2 protein) mediates the nuclear export of viral ribonucleoproteins, EMBO J. 17 (1998) 288–296.

[23] J.R. Pollack, D. Ganem, An RNA stem-loop structure directs hepatitis B virus genomic RNA encapsidation, J. Virol. 67 (1993) 3245–3263.

[24] L.L. Poon, D.C. Pritlove, E. Fodor, G.G. Brownlee, Direct evidence that the poly(A) tail of influenza A virus mRNA is synthesized by reiterative copying of a U track in the virion RNA template, J. Virol. 73 (1999) 3473–3476.

[25] R.W.H. Ruigrok, A. Barge, P. Durrer, J. Brunner, K. Ma, G.R. Whittaker, Membrane interaction of influenza virus M1 protein, Virology 267 (2000) 289–298.

[26] B. Sha, M. Luo, Structure of a bifunctional membrane-binding protein, influenza virus matrix protein M1, Nat. Struct. Biol. 4 (1997) 239–244.

[27] L.S. Tiley, M.H. Malim, H.K. Tewary, P.G. Stockley, B.R. Cullen, Identification of a high-affinity RNA binding site for the human immunodeficiency virus type 1 Rev protein, Proc. Natl. Acad. Sci. U. S. A. 89 (1992) 758–762.

[28] L. Wakefield, G.G. Brownlee, RNA-binding properties of influenza A virus matrix protein M1, Nucleic Acids Res. 17 (1989) 8569–8580.

[29] K. Watanabe, H. Hanada, K. Mizumoto, K. Nagata, Mechanism for inhibition of influenza virus RNA polymerase activity by matrix protein, J. Virol. 70 (1996) 241–247.

[30] G. Whittaker, I. Kemler, A. Helenius, Hyperphosphorylation of mutant influenza virus matrix protein, M1, causes its retention in the nucleus, J. Virol. 69 (1995) 439–445.

[31] Z. Ye, R. Pal, J.W. Fox, R.R. Wagner, Functional and antigenic domains of the matrix (M) protein of influenza A virus, J. Virol. 61 (1987) 239–246.

[32] J. Zhang, R.A. Lamb, Characterization of the membrane association of the influenza virus matrix protein in living cells, Virology 225 (1996) 255–266.

[33] H. Zhao, M. Ecström, H. Garoff, The M1 and NP proteins of influenza A virus form homo- but not heterooligomeric complexes when coexpressed in BHK-21 cells, J. Gen. Virol. 79 (1998) 2435–2446.

[34] Y. Zhou, M. König, G. Hobom, E. Neumeier, Membrane-anchored incorporation of a foreign protein in recombinant influenza virions, Virology 246 (1998) 83–94.

[35] A. Zobel, G. Neumann, G. Hobom, RNA polymerase I catalyzed transcription of inserted viral cDNA, Nucleic Acids Res. 21 (1993) 3607–3614.

International Congress Series 1219 (2001) 451–456

Structure of the RNA inside influenza virus RNPs

Florence Baudin, Isabelle Petit, Rob W.H. Ruigrok*

EMBL Grenoble Outstation, c/o ILL, BP181, 38042 Grenoble Cedex 9, France

Abstract

Influenza virus nucleoprotein binds to the phosphate sugar backbone of the viral RNA and exposes the nucleotide bases to the solvent. In viral RNP, all nucleotide bases are exposed apart from those at the conserved 3′ and 5′ ends of the vRNA whose Watson–Crick (W–C) positions are protected against modification by chemical reagents. However, when the polymerase is removed from the RNP, the bases and the polymerase in the conserved ends become available for chemical attack. So the presence of the polymerase is correlated with protection of the vRNA ends, either by direct contact between the nucleotide bases and the polymerase or by inducing base pairing between the ends. We also present our latest results on the footprint of the polymerase on the vRNA ends in the intact RNPs, in particular the protection of the N7 positions of the guanine and adenine residues in this region. Our results on the structure of the ends of the RNA and the footprint of the polymerase on these ends are compared with other models from the literature. © 2001 Elsevier Science B.V. All rights reserved.

Keywords: Influenza virus; Transcription; Replication; RNA structure; Polymerase footprint; Panhandle

1. Introduction

Influenza virus RNPs are RNA–protein complexes intricately designed for transcription and replication. Here, we will describe the molecular contacts between the RNA nucleotide bases and the protein components. Our experiments used RNPs in intact virus particles, isolated RNPs, isolated RNPs that had the polymerase complex removed by deoxycholate treatment and reconstituted RNA–nucleoprotein (NP–RNA) complexes. The methods for producing these components and the techniques that were used for these experiments have been described in Baudin et al. [1] and Klumpp et al.

---

* Corresponding author. Delivery address: EMBL Grenoble Outstation, 6 rue Jules Horowitz, 38000 Grenoble, France. Tel.: +33-4-76-20-72-73; fax: +33-4-76-20-71-99.
  E-mail address: ruigrok@embl-grenoble.fr (R.W.H. Ruigrok).

[2]. In short, the various substrates (virus, RNP±pol, reconstituted NP–RNA) were incubated with small chemical probes that bind to specific atomic sites on the nucleotide bases. If these sites are involved in base pairing with another nucleotide, the chemical modification cannot take place. These particular sites involve the Watson–Crick (W–C) positions such as N1 of adenine, N3 of cytidine, N1 and N2 of guanine and N3 of uridine. However, non-reactivity of these sites does not necessarily mean that they are involved in base pairing. It is also possible that a protein is bound to this site since a hydrogen bond between a nucleotide base and an amino acid would also prevent modification. After the probing experiment, the viral RNA is deproteinated and the modified positions are revealed by using a reverse transcription (RT) reaction with a primer 3′ to the site under study. At modified W–C positions, the RT will stop leading to a band on a sequencing gel. When in parallel a similar RT reaction is done on non-modified RNA, the stops on the modified RNA that are not found in the control RNA indicate that this particular site has been modified and that the specific W–C position was neither base paired nor hydrogen bonded to a protein. We have used this method to probe the reactivities of the W–C positions of the nucleotide bases at the conserved 3′ and 5′ ends of the viral RNA. By choosing a specific sequence for the RT primer, one can look at any single viral RNA in the mixture of all eight. This method allows easy evaluation of nucleotide residues near the 5′ end of the viral RNA but information on the 3′ end can only be obtained by direct methods [1].

We have also probed the N7 positions on A and G. These positions are often found to be involved in hydrogen bonding to proteins specifically bound to RNA. In particular, we looked at these positions to determine the foot print of the polymerase on the RNA inside intact RNPs. Modified residues cannot be detected directly by the reverse transcription method described above. The modified RNA has first to undergo another chemical treatment in order to cut in the RNA chain and then a similar reverse transcription reaction can be performed [1].

2. Chemical modification of the nucleotide bases at the conserved 3′ and 5′ ends of intact RNP and RNP without polymerase

The 3′ and 5′ terminal sequences of all eight viral RNA segments are conserved and partially complementary. It has been proposed that these sequences form a double stranded structure in the viral RNP [3]. This panhandle structure has been proposed to be important for viral transcription initiation and termination and for polyadenylation [4–9]. First, we produced a small, virus-like RNA molecule of 81 nucleotides long and containing the conserved 3′ and 5′ RNA ends and we determined the secondary structure of this molecule in solution [1]. We found that the 3′ and 5′ ends of the RNA were base paired, i.e. except for two bulges at A4 (nucleotide 4 from the 5′ end) and A10 all W–C positions were non-reactive to the probing chemicals (see Fig. 1a). A similar experiment was also performed on naked viral RNA segment 8 but here the ends were not base paired (not shown), probably because the ends are further apart in the sequence. Then we added purified NP, which complexed with the naked model RNA. Using a chemical probe that specifically modifies the phosphates, we could determine that the protein binds to the

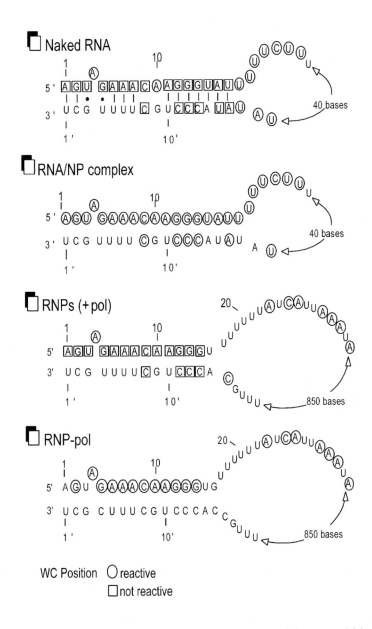

Fig. 1. Schematic representation of the reactivities of the nucleotide bases at their Watson–Crick positions on: Naked 81 nt model RNA (top); the same model RNA complexed with nucleoprotein (second from top); intact RNPs (second from bottom) and RNPs without their polymerase complex (bottom). The squares indicate absence of reactivity and the circles indicate that the bases are reactive. Note that in the figure of the naked RNA (top), the vertical lines and the dots indicate base pairing. These lines and dots are not shown in the RNP + pol figure since in that case we do not know whether absence of reactivity is due to base pairing or to direct interaction of the W–C positions with the polymerase.

sugar-phosphor backbone of the RNA [1]. However, the major effect of the binding of NP to the panhandle sequence was that all base pairing was disrupted and all W−C positions were free for chemical attack (Fig. 1b): The binding of NP to RNA destroys secondary RNA structures and exposes the nucleotide bases to the solvent [1].

We then looked at the solvent accessibility of the nucleotide bases inside viral RNPs, RNA segment 8. All experiments on intact RNPs were paralleled with experiments using intact virus since the chemical probes could penetrate the viral membrane [2]. The results on the intact RNPs are shown in Fig. 1c that shows that the ends are not solvent accessible, either through base pairing or through interaction with the polymerase complex. However, when the polymerase was removed, the bases were available for chemical attack and, thus, were not base paired [2] (Fig. 1d). This result was confirmed by electron microscopy experiments that showed supercoiled circular structures for intact RNPs but linear structures for polymerase-free RNPs [2]. This means that in the viral RNP the ends of the RNA are not base paired when the polymerase is not present, just like the reconstituted synthetic NP-RNA complexes in Fig. 1b.

3. Footprint of polymerase on 5′ conserved end

The footprint of the polymerase on the RNA inside RNP was determined on the N7A and N7G positions of the nucleotide bases as described above. By choosing specific primer sequences for the RT reaction, we were able to test this footprint on the 5′ ends of all RNA segments. Fig. 2a shows that the footprint extends to G13 for segment 8 RNA inside RNP. However, in segments where residue 14 is not a G but an A or otherwise, G13 is not protected by the polymerase. This means that the binding of the polymerase to the RNA is modulated by the non-conserved sequences. This surprising result was confirmed by another finding that specific RNP segments lost their polymerase complex more easily upon purification than others, leading to relatively high reactivities for the W−C positions in the RNPs that were not treated with deoxycholate (not shown). It would appear that there exists a variation in the stability of binding of the polymerase to the 3′ and 5′ ends of the different RNA segments. RNPs containing segment 8 RNA were among the most stable RNPs. Using the RT technique, we found protection of the N7 positions on G5, A8, A10, A11, and G13. These protections were removed when the polymerase was removed by deoxycholate treatment. Using a direct approach, we found that G9′ at the 3′ end was not protected. We could not obtain information on the only other G residue at the 3′ end.

In Fig. 2, our data are compared with models derived by other groups [6,10,11]. These models show the proposed secondary structure of the panhandle plus the binding site for the polymerase complex by gray dots. Note that in Fig. 2a, we do not imply that our data suggests a panhandle structure. The non-reactivity of the bases could be due either to a double stranded RNA structure, to direct binding of the 5′ and 3′ end bases to the polymerase or to non-accessibility of the probe due to the presence of the proteins (charge or hydrophobic effects). However, for those 3′ residues that are not reactive at their W−C positions, a conformational change of the polymerase would be needed for transcription to proceed, allowing base pairing with the incoming nucleotide. Our data correspond best

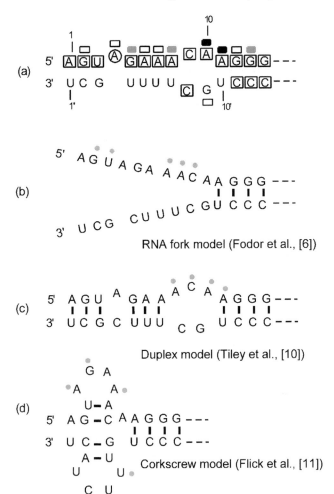

Fig. 2. Summary of the chemical probing experiments on intact segment 8 RNPs on the Watson–Crick positions (same symbols as in Fig. 1) and of the N7 probing experiments (top). The rectangles above the 5′ nucleotides and below the 3′ nucleotides indicate their N7 reactivity. Open rectangles indicate that the N7 position is not protected (so no interaction with the polymerase), black rectangles indicate positions that are fully protected in the presence of the polymerase and reactive in its absence, gray rectangles indicate residues that are only slightly reactive in the presence of the polymerase but much more reactive in its absence. The lower three panels represent results published in the literature with base pairing indicated by vertical lines and positions of interaction with the polymerase by gray dots.

with those of the Krystal group [10,12] and also with the results of Li et al. [13] but perhaps this is correlated to the fact that these groups and we have used (bio)chemical approaches. The models by Fodor et al. [6] and Flick et al. [11] were not determined directly by biochemical methods but more indirectly from functional analysis of the activity of mutant sequences.

References

[1] F. Baudin, C. Bach, S. Cusack, R.W.H. Ruigrok, Structure of influenza virus RNP. I. Influenza virus nucleoprotein melts secondary structure in panhandle RNA and exposes the bases to the solvent, EMBO J. 13 (1994) 3158–3165.

[2] K. Klumpp, R.W.H. Ruigrok, F. Baudin, Roles of the influenza virus polymerase and nucleoprotein in forming a functional RNP structure, EMBO J. 16 (1997) 1248–1257.

[3] M.T. Hsu, J.D. Parvin, S. Gupta, M. Krystal, P. Palese, Genomic RNAs of influenza viruses are held in a circular conformation in virions and in infected cells by a terminal panhandle, Proc. Natl. Acad. Sci. U. S. A. 84 (1987) 8140–8144.

[4] C. Cianci, L. Tiley, M. Krystal, Differential activation of the influenza virus polymerase via template RNA binding, J. Virol. 69 (1995) 3995–3999.

[5] E. Fodor, D.C. Pritlove, G.G. Brownlee, The influenza virus panhandle is involved in the initiation of transcription, J. Virol. 68 (1994) 4092–4096.

[6] E. Fodor, D.C. Pritlove, G.G. Brownlee, Characterization of the RNA-fork model of virion RNA in the initiation of transcription in influenza A virus, J. Virol. 69 (1995) 4012–4019.

[7] E. Fodor, P. Palese, G.G. Brownlee, E. García-Sastre, Attenuation of influenza A virus mRNA levels by promoter mutations, J. Virol. 72 (1998) 6283–6290.

[8] G.X. Luo, W. Luytjes, M. Enami, P. Palese, The polyadenylation signal of influenza virus RNA involves a stretch of uridines followed by the RNA duplex of the panhandle structure, J. Virol. 65 (1991) 1867–2861.

[9] X. Li, P. Palese, Characterization of the polyadenylation signal of influenza virus RNA, J. Virol. 68 (1994) 1245–1249.

[10] L.S. Tiley, M. Hagen, J.T. Matthews, M. Krystal, Sequence-specific binding of the influenza virus RNA polymerase to sequences located at the 5′ ends of the viral RNAs, J. Virol. 68 (1994) 5108–5116.

[11] R. Flick, G. Neumann, E. Hoffmann, E. Neumeier, G. Hobom, Promotor elements in the influenza vRNA terminal structure, RNA 2 (1996) 1046–1057.

[12] M. Hagen, T.D. Chung, J.A. Butcher, M. Krystal, Recombinant influenza virus polymerase: requirement of both 5′ and 3′ viral ends for endonuclease activity, J. Virol. 68 (1994) 1509–1515.

[13] M.L. Li, B.C. Ramirez, R.M. Krug, RNA-dependent activation of primer RNA production by influenza virus polymerase: different regions of the same protein subunit constitute the two required RNA-binding sites, EMBO J. 17 (1998) 5844–5852.

International Congress Series 1219 (2001) 457–462

Type specificity of the viral RNA extremities of the human influenza A and C viruses

Bernadette Crescenzo-Chaigne, Sylvie van der Werf*

Unité de Génétique Moléculaire des Virus Respiratoires, URA 1966 CNRS, Institut Pasteur, 25, rue du Dr Roux, F-75724 Paris Cedex 15, France

Abstract

Background: Previously, we showed that a type C RNA template is transcribed and replicated with equal efficiency by types A and C proteins, whereas a type A RNA template is less efficiently transcribed and replicated by type C than A proteins. This may be related to type-specific recognition of the transcription/replication signals at the extremity of the viral RNA. *Methods*: By making use of an expression system that allows transcription and replication of a reporter RNA template bearing type A or C extremities, the effect of mutations introduced alone or in combination at the 3′ or 5′ end of the type A or C templates were studied in the presence of type A or C polymerase complex. *Results*: The nature of the nucleotides at position 5 and to a lesser extent 6′ was found to contribute to type specificity. Moreover, we showed the importance of base pairs 3′:8′ as well as 2:9 and 3:8 for RNA recognition by the type C proteins. *Conclusions*: The nature of the nucleotides as well as the stability of the hairpin structure at the 5′ end thus appeared as important determinants of type specificity. Also, sequence requirements seemed more stringent for recognition by the type C than type A polymerase complex. © 2001 Elsevier Science B.V. All rights reserved.

Keywords: Polymerase complex; Transcription; Replication; Promoter

1. Introduction

The precise structure of the promoter that serves for the initiation of transcription and replication of the viral RNA segments has been the subject of numerous studies mainly for influenza virus type A. Based on in vitro studies of RNA transcription and on in vivo studies of transcription and replication of model RNA templates, site-directed mutagenesis studies established that the promoter is made of two distinct elements: (i) a distal base-paired element that involves interactions of residues 10–15 of the 3′ end with residues

---

* Corresponding author. Tel.: +33-1-45-68-87-25; fax: +33-1-40-61-32-41.
E-mail address: svdwerf@pasteur.fr (S. van der Werf).

0531-5131/01/$ – see front matter © 2001 Elsevier Science B.V. All rights reserved.
PII: S 0 5 3 1 - 5 1 3 1 (0 1) 0 0 3 5 2 - 1

$11'–16'$ of the $5'$ end of the vRNA; (ii) a proximal element that consists of the extreme terminal sequences of the vRNA which can be folded into two hairpin loops according to the so-called "corkscrew" model [1]. The $5'$ hairpin loop is required for mRNA but not for cRNA synthesis [2], whereas, the $3'$ hairpin loop is not necessary for mRNA synthesis but seems to be required at some stage of RNA replication [1–3].

Having shown that the influenza A and C RNA templates were transcribed and replicated with the same efficiency by the influenza A polymerase complex, but that the type A RNA template was amplified by the influenza C polymerase with a dramatically reduced efficiency [4], we analyzed the nucleotides involved in the type-specific interaction of the types A and C polymerase with the viral promoter, by making use of the genetic system initially described by Pleschka et al. [5] for the reconstitution of functional RNPs.

2. Material and methods

2.1. Plasmids for the expression of wild-type and mutated types A and C model RNA templates

The pA/PRCAT and pC/PRCAT plasmids [4], which direct the expression of model reporter RNA templates derived from the NS segments of A/WSN/33 and C/JHB/66 viruses, were used as the basis for the introduction of mutations within the extremities of the model RNA templates. Mutations were generated by PCR amplification of the CAT gene and NS noncoding sequences in the presence of primers harboring appropriate nucleotide substitutions.

2.2. Transfections and CAT assays

As described previously [4], subconfluent monolayers of COS-1 cells were transfected using the Fugene-6-mediated method with a mixture of plasmids pHMG-PB1, -PB2, -PA/P3 and -NP (1, 1, 1, and 4 µg) derived from the A/Puerto Rico/8/34 or C/Johannesburg/1/66 viruses, together with 1 µg of pPRCAT plasmid harboring wild-type or mutated type A or C extremities. The efficiency of transcription/replication of the reconstituted RNPs was evaluated 48 h after transfection by measuring the levels of CAT in cell extracts.

3. Results

3.1. Effect of mutations at positions 5 and/or 6' of the type A or C model RNA templates

Nucleotides 5 and $6'$ at the $3'$ and $5'$ ends, respectively (the prime notation is used for $5'$ end nucleotides), are among the four positions that differ between types A and C within the proximal promoter element. According to the hairpin loop model of the vRNA [1,2] nucleotides, 5 and $6'$ are not base-paired and thus, are likely to be accessible for interactions with the polymerase complex. As shown in Table 1, for the type A RNA template harboring mutations at position 5 and/or 6′, the levels of CAT were found to be reduced with the type A polymerase. However, in the presence of the type C polymerase, the introduction of either mutation resulted in a four- to five-fold increase of the CAT levels with respect to the type A wild-type RNA template. When both mutations were present, the level of CAT reached a level that corresponds to about half the activity obtained for the type C wild-type RNA template with the type C polymerase. In the case of the type C RNA templates mutated at position 5 and/or 6′, similar or slightly higher levels of CAT activity were obtained with the type C polymerase, whereas with the type A polymerase, introduction of the mutation at position 5 resulted in a significant increase of

Table 1

Effect of mutations within the conserved extremities of types A and C model RNA templates on transcription/replication by the type A or C polymerase complexes

nt position	Type A model RNA		Polymerase complex		Type C model RNA		Polymerase complex	
		5 6′	A	C		5 6′	C	A
5 6′ mutants	A wt	U A	100 (4347)[a]	100 (208)[a]	C wt	C U	100 (2192)[a]	100 (1168)[a]
		C A	59	564		U U	115	182
		U U	73	435		C A	97	92
		C U	52	739		U A	85	164
	C wt	C U	54	1862	A wt	U A	4	168
nt position		3′–8′	A	C		3′–8′	C	A
3′:8′ mutants	A wt	U–A	100 (3450)[a]	100 (182)[a]	C wt	C–G	100 (3353)[a]	100 (1288)[a]
		C A	<	5		C A	<	<
		U:G	22	12		U:G	<	8
		C–G	70	924		G–C	82	73
		G–C	69	368		U–A	64	143
	C wt	C–G	78	2000	A wt	U–A	4	183
nt position		3–8	A	C		3–8	C	A
3:8 mutants	A wt	G–C	100 (2536)[a]	100 (50)[a]	C wt	G–C	100 (3829)[a]	100 (1797)[a]
		A C	<	<		A C	<	16
		G:U	<	<		G:U	<	1
		A–U	48	5		A–U	5	50
		C–G	17	<		C–G	34	49
nt position		2–9	A	C		2–9	C	A
2:9 mutants	A wt	C–G	100 (2536)[a]	100 (50)[a]	C wt	C–G	100 (3829)[a]	100 (1797)[a]
		U:G	<	<		U:G	3	5
		C A	<	<		C A	7	3
		U–A	17	<		U–A	2	18
		G–C	5	<		G–C	3	24

[a] CAT levels were expressed as percentage values of those measured with the indicated wild-type model RNAs. Numbers in parentheses represent CAT values expressed in nanograms per milliliter.

the level of CAT activity that reached a level comparable to that achieved with the cognate type A wild-type RNA template (Table 1).

3.2. Effect of mutations of base pair 3′:8′ at the 5′ end of the type A or C model RNA templates

In order to determine to what extent the hairpin loop structure at the 5′ end is implicated in type-specific interactions with the polymerase complex, and since nucleotides at positions 3′ and 8′ are different in the types A and C RNA templates, mutations were introduced at these positions and their effect on transcription and replication of the RNA templates were studied (Table 1). Disruption of the 3′:8′ base pair drastically reduced or completely abolished transcription and replication of the RNA. When a non-canonical $U_{3'}$:$G_{8'}$ base pair was created, the level of CAT activity remained very low or undetectable in the case of the type C RNA, whereas a low albeit significant level of CAT activity was observed with both types A and C polymerase complexes, in the case of the type A RNA. In contrast, when alternative 3′:8′ base pair sequences were restored, in the presence of the homotypic polymerase, CAT levels reached 70–80% of that obtained with the homotypic wild-type template. In addition, in the presence of the heterotypic polymerase, the levels of CAT increased significantly, reaching a level of 20–80% of that achieved with the homotypic wild-type template. Thus, as reported for type A vRNA [2,3], base pairing between the nucleotides at positions 3′ and 8′ was found to be required for efficient transcription and replication of type A or C vRNA by both types A and C polymerase complexes. Whereas the nature of the 3′:8′ base pair at the 5′ end had only a marginal effect on the efficiency with which the type A vRNA was transcribed and replicated by the type A polymerase, a type A like $U_{3'}$:$A_{8'}$ base pair was preferred over $G_{3'}$:$C_{8'}$ or $C_{3'}$:$G_{8'}$ base pairs for efficient transcription and replication of the type C RNA template by the type A polymerase. In addition, a marked preference for a type C like $C_{3'}$:$G_{8'}$ base pair was revealed for the transcription and replication of the type C or A model RNAs by the type C polymerase complex.

3.3. Effect of mutations of base pairs 2:9 and 3:8 at the 3′ end of the type A or C model RNA templates

In order to determine whether a hairpin loop structure at the 3′ end of the vRNA was required at some stage of the replication process of type C RNA as shown for type A [1–3], mutations were introduced to probe the 2:9 and 3:8 base pairs at the 3′ end of type A or C model RNA and their effect on transcription and replication was analyzed (Table 1). Disruption of the 3:8 or 2:9 base pairs in both the types A and C RNAs drastically reduced or completely abolished transcription and replication by either type of polymerase complexes. When alternative base pair sequences were restored, significant levels of transcription/replication of both types A and C RNAs were observed in most instances with the type A polymerase. In contrast, in the case of the type C polymerase, none of the substitutions of the 2:9 base pair were tolerated, and for the 3:8 base pair, only the G:C → C:G substitution within the type C but not the type A RNA template resulted in a significant level of transcription/replication.

4. Discussion

Site-directed mutagenesis of the influenza A promoter has shown that residues 5 and 6′ can be substituted without significantly affecting transcription and replication of the vRNA [1,6–8]. Indeed, as shown here, substitution of residues 5 and/or 6′ within the vRNA promoter did not significantly affect the efficiency of transcription and replication of either type A or C RNA by the homotypic polymerase complex. However, when type A- or C-like nucleotides were introduced at these positions within the type C or A promoter, respectively, this resulted in a substantial increase of the efficiency of transcription and replication of RNA by the heterotypic polymerase. Thus, overall, our observations suggest that both for influenza A and C, nucleotide 5 contributes to specific recognition of the promoter by the polymerase complex, and furthermore, that nucleotide 6′ may also participate to some extent in efficient recognition of the promoter in the case of the type C polymerase.

Analysis of the 3′:8′ base pair of the 5′ hairpin loop structure allowed us to show that, as previously demonstrated for type A [1,3], a hairpin loop structure at the 5′ end of the vRNA is required for efficient recognition of the viral promoter in the case of influenza C virus. However, in contrast to the type A polymerase, for which a weakly interacting base pair was preferred both in the context of the type A or C promoter, a strongly interacting base pair, with additional preference for C:G over G:C at positions 3′:8′ seemed to be required both in the context of the type A or C vRNA for optimal transcription and replication by the type C polymerase.

A similar hairpin loop structure at the 3′ end of the vRNA and/or at the 5′ end of the cRNA was found to be required at some stage of replication of the type C RNA as suggested for type A [3]. Overall, more stringent sequence requirements at the 5′ end and even more so at the 3′ end within the proximal promoter element seemed to prevail for the type C as compared to the type A polymerase, which may account for the fact that the type C promoter could be used quite efficiently by the type A polymerase, but not reciprocally [4].

Acknowledgements

The authors are very grateful to J. Pavlovic for providing the A/pHMG-PB1, -PB2, -PA and -NP recombinant plasmids. We thank Nicolas Escriou and Nadia Naffakh for helpful discussions. This work was supported in part by the Ministère de l'Education Nationale, de la Recherche et de la Technologie (EA 302).

References

[1] R. Flick, et al., Promoter elements in the influenza vRNA terminal structure, RNA 2 (10) (1996) 1046–1057.
[2] D.C. Pritlove, et al., A hairpin loop at the 5′ end of influenza A virus virion RNA is required for synthesis of poly(A)+ mRNA in vitro, Journal of Virology 73 (3) (1999) 2109–2114.
[3] R. Flick, G. Hobom, Interaction of influenza virus polymerase with viral RNA in the 'corkscrew' conformation, Journal of General Virology 80 (1999) 2565–2572 (Pt. 10).
[4] B. Crescenzo-Chaigne, N. Naffakh, S. van der Werf, Comparative analysis of the ability of the polymerase

complexes of influenza viruses type A, B and C to assemble into functional RNPs that allow expression and replication of heterotypic model RNA templates in vivo, Virology 265 (2) (1999) 342–353.

[5] S. Pleschka, et al., A plasmid-based reverse genetics system for influenza A virus, Journal of Virology 70 (6) (1996) 4188–4192.

[6] E. Fodor, D.C. Pritlove, G.G. Brownlee, The influenza virus panhandle is involved in the initiation of transcription, Journal of Virology 68 (6) (1994) 4092–4096.

[7] L.L. Poon, et al., The RNA polymerase of influenza virus, bound to the 5′ end of virion RNA, acts in cis to polyadenylate mRNA, Journal of Virology 72 (10) (1998) 8214–8219.

[8] N. Kimura, et al., An in vivo study of the replication origin in the influenza virus complementary RNA, Journal of Biochemistry 113 (1) (1993) 88–92.

International Congress Series 1219 (2001) 463–469

Fine mapping of the subunit binding sites of influenza virus RNA polymerase

Yasushi Ohtsu[a], Yoshikazu Honda[b], Tetsuya Toyoda[a],*

[a]*Department of Virology, Kurume University School of Medicine, 67 Asahimachi, Kurume,*
Fukuoka 830-0011, Japan
[b]*International Livestock Research Institute, Nairobi, Kenya*

Abstract

Background: Influenza virus RNA polymerase consists of three subunits, PB1, PB2 and PA, and catalyzes both transcription and replication of the RNA genome. PB1 is a catalytic subunit of RNA polymerization and a core of subunit assembly. Previously, we mapped the PB1–PB2 binding sites (1–259 of PB2 and 501–757 of PB1), and the PB1–PA binding sites (1–140 of PB1 and 201–716 of PA). In order to determine the fine map of the subunit binding sites, we continued the same line of experiments. *Methods*: Serial deletion mutants of each subunit were expressed with N-terminal HA-tag, and co-immunoprecipitated with the non-tagged wild-type subunits by anti-HA or subunit-specific antibodies. *Results*: PB1N599 and PB1C10 were co-immunoprecipitated with PB2wt, but PB1N625 and PB1N700 were weakly co-immunoprecipitated with PB2wt. PB1C25 or PB1C40 were not co-immunoprecipitated with PB2wt. PB2N50 and PB2N75 were co-immunoprecipitated with PB1wt. However, PB2N104 or PB2N150 were not co-immunoprecipitated with PB1wt. PB1C535 and PB1C617 were co-immunoprecipitated with PAwt, but PB1N25 was not. PAN300, PAN400, PAN500 and PA501–692 were co-immunoprecipitated with PB1wt, but PAC49 was not. *Conclusions*: PB1–PB2 binding sites are mapped in PB1(600–747) and PB2(76–104), and PB1–PA binding sites are in PB1(1–25) and PA(668–692). © 2001 Elsevier Science B.V. All rights reserved.

Keywords: Immunoprecipitation; HA-tag; Anti-HA; T7 RNA polymerase

* Corresponding author. Tel.: +81-942-31-7549; fax: +81-942-32-0903.
E-mail address: ttoyoda@supernig.nig.ac.jp (T. Toyoda).

0531-5131/01/$ – see front matter © 2001 Elsevier Science B.V. All rights reserved.
PII: S 0 5 3 1 - 5 1 3 1 (0 1) 0 0 3 9 5 - 8

1. Introduction

Influenza virus RNA polymerase catalyzes both transcription and replication of the RNA genome [1–5]. The viral RNA polymerase also catalyzes polyadenylation at the 3^e termini of mRNA [6], and performs template-dependent capped RNA cleavage [7,8] and apparent proofreading of nascent RNA chains [9].

The RNA polymerase purified from influenza virus consists of one part each of the three subunits, PB1, PB2 and PA [10]. In vitro reconstitution studies of enzymatically active RNA polymerase using individual P proteins purified either from baculovirus infected cells [11], *Pichia pastoris* cells [12] or by SDS-polyacrylamide gel electrophoresis of virions [13] confirmed the subunit structure.

Recently, we and other groups mapped the subunit binding sites of the influenza virus RNA polymerase, which demonstrated that PB1 is the core subunit of polymerase assembly [14–18]. However, the results are somehow contradictory to each other and the subunit binding sites remain still ambiguous. For detailed analysis of the biding sites, we continued the same co-immunoprecipitation experiments of the subunits in various combinations.

2. Materials and methods

2.1. Cell culture

RK-13 cells and COS-7 cells were maintained in Dulbecco's modified minimal essential medium (DMEM; Liftech) containing 5% fetal bovine serum (FBS; JRC Scientific).

2.2. Construction of T7pro/HA-tagged polymerase mutants

A nested set of cDNA for PB1, PB2 and PA mutants was constructed by PCR amplification using pAPR206 (EMBL, GenBank, DDBJ Accession no. J02151), pAPR102 (J02152) and pAPR303 (J02153) as templates (Fig. 1) [19]. The resulting N-terminal HA-tagged mutants of each subunit were constructed. They were cloned into BlueScript II KS (+) (Stratagene) or pSP72 (Promega) under the control of T7 promoter. For construction of non-tagged wild-type subunits, the PCR fragments were cloned into BlueScript II SK (+).

Fig. 1. Construction scheme and the binding activity of deletion mutants of the influenza virus RNA polymerase subunits. Maps of the deletion mutants of PB1 and PB2 (A), and PB1 and PA (B), and the results of co-immunoprecipitation experiments are indicated on the right. Numbers on the bars indicate the position of the first and the last amino acid. Only the fragments which were co-immunoprecipitated by both antibodies were indicated as " + + ", and those were not co-immunoprecipitated by either antibodies were indicated as " − ". " + " indicated weak interaction of the subunits.

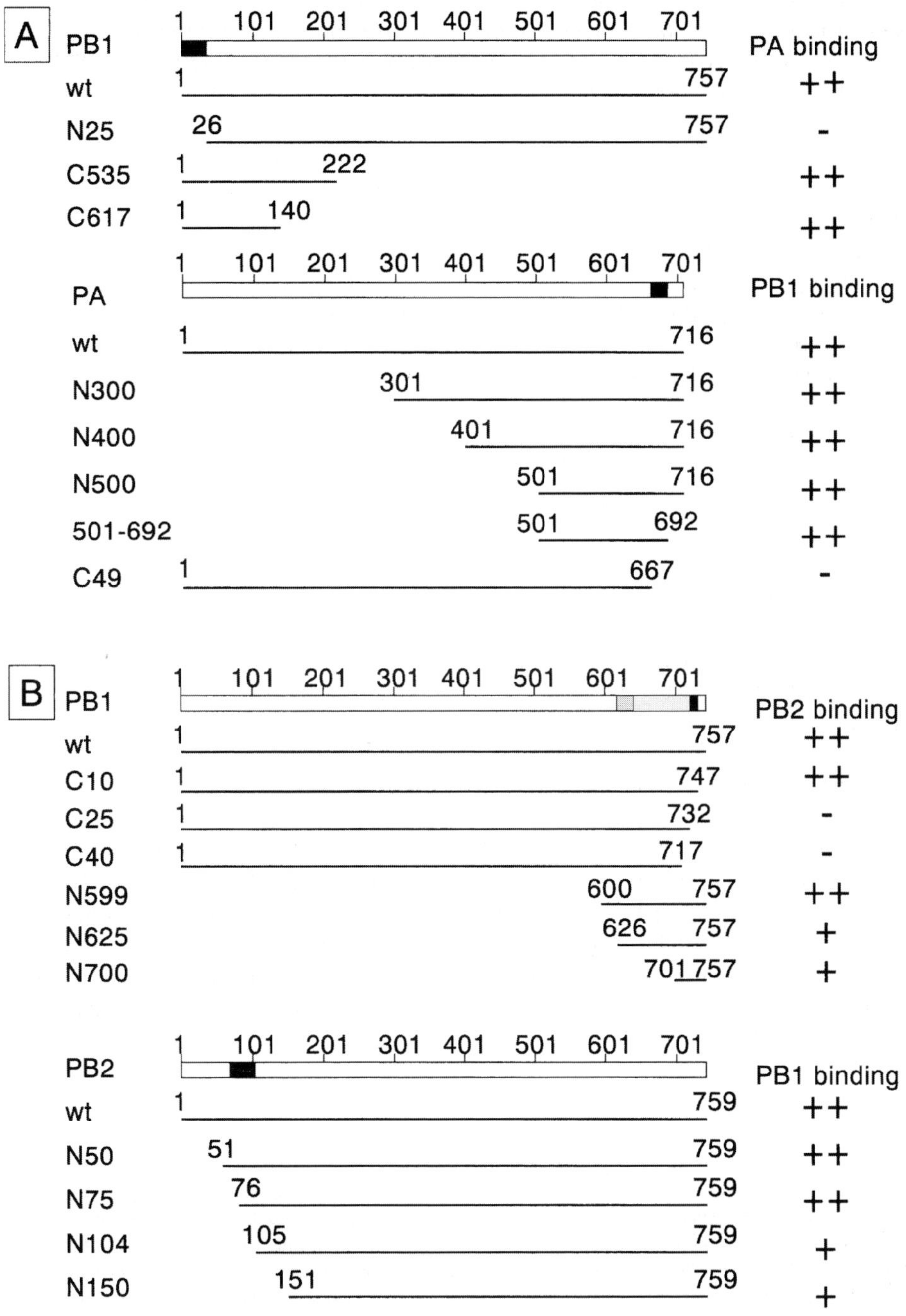
A
PB1
1 101 201 301 401 501 601 701
PA binding
wt 1 757 ++
N25 26 757 -
C535 1 222 ++
C617 1 140 ++
PA
1 101 201 301 401 501 601 701
PB1 binding
wt 1 716 ++
N300 301 716 ++
N400 401 716 ++
N500 501 716 ++
501-692 501 692 ++
C49 1 667 -
B
PB1
1 101 201 301 401 501 601 701
PB2 binding
wt 1 757 ++
C10 1 747 ++
C25 1 732 -
C40 1 717 -
N599 600 757 ++
N625 626 757 +
N700 701 757 +
PB2
1 101 201 301 401 501 601 701
PB1 binding
wt 1 759 ++
N50 51 759 ++
N75 76 759 ++
N104 105 759 +
N150 151 759 +

2.3. Recombinant vaccinia virus expressing the bacteriophage T7 RNA polymerase

Recombinant vaccinia virus, rVVT7, expressing bacteriophage T7 RNA polymerase was generated using pHA vector, which contained the vaccinia virus HA gene and modified 7.5-kDa promoter [20] and T7 RNA polymerase gene (M38308) from pAR1173 [21]. rVVT7 was obtained by homologous recombination from vaccinia virus, Lister 16m0 strain [22].

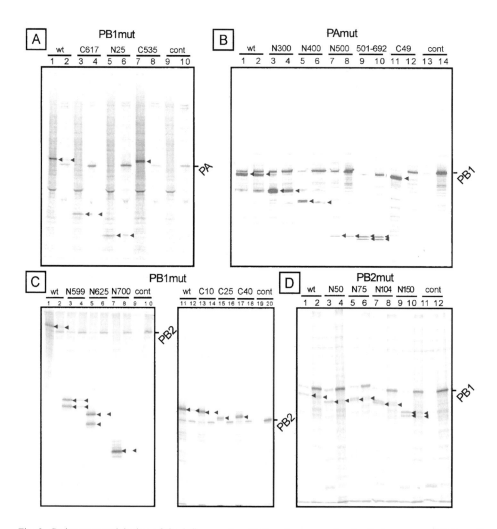

Fig. 2. Co-immunoprecipitation of the influenza virus RNA polymerase subunits. Co-immunoprecipitation of PB1 deletion mutants and PAwt (A), PA deletion mutants and PB1wt (B), PB1 deletion mutants and PB2wt (C), and PB2 deletion mutants and PB1wt (D) are shown. Expressed subunits were co-immunoprecipitated with anti-HA (odd lanes) and subunit-specific antibodies (even lanes). The positions of the intact (non-tagged) wild-type subunits were indicated on the right and those of deletion mutants were indicated by arrowheads.

2.4. Co-transfection and co-immunoprecipitation

COS-7 cells were first infected with vvT7 (m.o.i = 2) for 1 h. The cells were incubated for 4 h in Opti-MEM I containing 2% Lipofectin (Lifetech Orientals), combinations of the P protein expression plasmids and 40 µg/ml of cytosine-1-β-D(+)-arabinofuranoside (Ara-C, Wako). After transfection, the cells were incubated overnight in DMEM containing 5% FBS and 40 µg/ml Ara-C. The cells were pulse-labeled with 1 µCi/ml of [^{35}S]methionine and [^{35}S]cystin (Amersham) for 4 h in methionine-free MEM containing 40 µg/ml Ara-C. The pulse-labeled cells were processed for co-immunoprecipitation with anti-HA or anti-subunit specific antibodies as previously mentioned [17].

3. Results

3.1. PB1–PA binding sites

PB1C535 and PB1C617 were co-immunoprecipitated with PAwt, but PB1N25 and PAwt were not co-immunoprecipitated (Fig. 2A,B). PAN300, PAN400, PAN500 and PA501-692 were co-immunoprecipitated with PB1wt, but PAC49 was not co-immunoprecipitated with PB1wt.

3.2. PB1–PB2 binding sites

PB1N599 and PB2wt were co-immunoprecipitated (Fig. 2C,D). However, the PB2 bands co-immunoprecipitated with PB1N625 and PB1N700 were weak. The signals of PB1N625 and PB1N700 co-immunoprecipitated with PB2 were also weak. PB1C10 and PB2wt were co-immunoprecipitated, but PB1C25 or PB1C40 were not co-immunoprecipitated with PB2wt. Then, the PB1 binding site on PB2 N-terminal 1–259 was determined. PB2N50 and PB2N75 were co-immunoprecipitated with PB1wt, but PB2N104 or PB2N150 were not co-immunoprecipitated with PB1wt.

4. Discussion

In the subunit binding sites determined by four groups, only the fact that PB1 binds with PB2 and PA is consistent [14–18].

From the co-immunoprecipitation experiment using the N-terminal deletion mutants of PB2 and PB1wt, the binding domain was mapped in 76–104 amino acids of PB2 (Fig. 2D). However, internal deletion mutant PB2del76–104 bound with PB1 (data not shown), indicating that the N-terminal region of PB2 also contributed to the binding or the conformation of the N-terminal structure of PB2, which affected the structure of the subunit.

PB1N599 and PB1C10 bound with PB2, but PB1N625 and PB1N700 weakly bound. PB1C25 did not bind with PB2 (Fig. 2C). These results indicated that critical region of PB2 binding was localized on 600–747 amino acids of PB1 and 732–747 of PB1. Amino

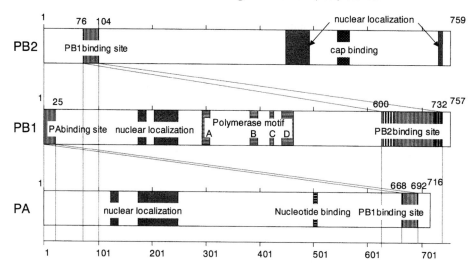

Fig. 3. Fine mapping of the subunit binding sites of influenza virus RNA polymerase.

acids 626–747 of PB1 could weakly bind with PB2, while amino acids 600–625 bound strongly.

From the co-immunoprecipitation experiment (Fig. 2A), we concluded that the PB1 binding region of PA mapped in the C-terminal 49 amino acids (668–692). When the N-terminal 25 amino acids were deleted from PB1, PB1 did not bind with PA (Fig. 2B). However, we failed to identify the responsible amino acid(s) for binding in this region (data not shown).

The subunit binding sites of influenza virus RNA polymerase were mapped in Fig. 3. The subunit binding sites were mapped in independent regions of the other functional domains of each subunit. PB1 and PB2 bound using relatively wide region(s) and PB1 and PA bound to each other alone a 25-amino acid length. This may be the reason why the PB1–PB2 binary complex was tightly formed in a short period (less than 10 m), but the recruitment of PA into the PB1–PB2 complex took more than 3 h when the three subunits were expressed and pulse-labeled in transfected cells [17].

Acknowledgements

The authors are grateful to Dr. H. Shida and Dr. Studier for pHA and pAR1173, respectively. This work was supported partly by a grant-in aid from the Naito Foundation, the Ishibashi Foundation, the Fukuoka Cancer Society and Yakult Honsha Co. Ltd.

References

[1] A. Honda, A. Ishihama, The molecular anatomy of influenza virus RNA polymerase, Biol. Chem. 378 (1997) 483–488.

[2] A. Ishihama, A multi-functional enzyme with RNA polymerase and RNase activities: molecular anatomy of influenza virus RNA polymerase, Biochimie 78 (1997) 1097–1102.

[3] A. Ishihama, K. Nagata, Viral RNA polymerases, CRC Crit. Rev. Biochem. 23 (1988) 27–76.

[4] R.M. Krug, F.V. Alonso-Caplen, I. Julkunen, M.G. Katze, Expression and replication of the influenza virus genome, in: RM. Krug (Ed.), The Influenza Viruses, Plenum, New York, NY, 1989, pp. 89–152.

[5] T. Toyoda, Y. Ohtsu, K. Hara, K. Masunaga, N. Hamada, M. Koga, K. Kashiwagi, J. Iwahashi, Molecular dissection of influenza virus RNA polymerase, Rec. Res. Dev. Virol. 1 (1999) 839–847.

[6] D.C. Pritlove, L.L. Poon, E. Fodor, J. Shares, G.G. Brownlee, Poladenylation of influenza virus m RNA transcribed in vitro from model virion RNA templates: requirement for 5′ conserved sequences, J. Virol. 72 (1998) 1280–1286.

[7] K. Kawakami, K. Mizumoto, A. Ishihama, RNA polymerase of influenza virus, IV. Catalytic properties of the capped RNA endonuclease associated with the RNA polymerase, Nucleic Acids Res. 11 (1983) 3637–3649.

[8] S.J. Plotch, M. Bouloy, I. Ulmanen, R.M. Krug, Initiation of influenza viral RNA transcription by capped RNA primers: a unique cap (m⁷GpppXm)-dependent virion endonuclease generates 5′ terminal RNA fragment that prime transcription, Cell 23 (1981) 847–858.

[9] A. Ishihama, K. Mizumoto, K. Kawakami, A. Kato, A. Honda, Proofreading function associated with the RNA-dependent RNA polymerase from influenza virus, J. Biol. Chem. 261 (1986) 10417–10421.

[10] A. Honda, J. Mukaigawa, A. Yokoiyama, A. Kato, S. Ueda, K. Nagata, M. Krystal, D.P. Nayak, A. Ishihama, Purification and molecular structure of RNA polymerase from influenza virus A/PR8, J. Biochem. 107 (1990) 624–628.

[11] M. Kobayashi, K. Tuchiya, K. Nagata, A. Ishihama, Reconstitution of influenza virus RNA polymerase from three subunits expressed using recombinant baculovirus system, Virus Res. 22 (1992) 235–245.

[12] J.-H. Hwang, K. Yamada, A. Honda, K. Nakade, A. Ishihama, Expression of functional influenza virus RNA polymerase in the methylotropic yeast *Pichia pastoris*, J. Virol. 74 (2000) 4074–4084.

[13] B. Szewczyk, W.G. Laver, D.F. Summers, Purification, thioredoxin renaturation and reconstituted activity of the three subunits of the influenza A virus RNA polymerase, Proc. Natl. Acad. Sci. U. S. A. 85 (1988) 7907–7911.

[14] S.K. Biswas, D.P. Nayak, Influenza virus polymerase basic protein 1 interacts with influenza virus polymerase basic protein at multiple sites, J. Virol. 70 (1996) 6716–6722.

[15] S. González, T. Zürcher, J. Ortín, Identification of two separate domains in the influenza virus PB1 protein involved in the interaction with the PB2 and PA subunits: a model for the viral RNA polymerase structure, Nucleic Acids Res. 24 (1996) 4456–4463.

[16] D. Pérez, R.O. Donis, A 48-amino-acid region of influenza A virus PB1 protein is sufficient for complex formation with PA, J. Virol. 69 (1995) 6932–6939.

[17] T. Toyoda, D.M. Adyshev, M. Kobayashi, A. Iwata, A. Ishihama, Molecular assembly of the influenza virus RNA polymerase: determination of the subunit–subunit contact sites, J. Gen. Virol. 77 (1996) 2149–2157.

[18] T. Zürcher, S. de la Luna, J.J. Sanz-Ezquerro, A. Nieto, J. Ortín, Mutational analysis of the influenza virus A/Victoria/3/75 PA protein L studies of interaction with PB1 protein and identification of a dominant negative mutant, J. Gen. Virol. 77 (1996) 1745–1749.

[19] J.F. Young, U. Desselberger, U. Graves, P. Palese, A. Shatzman, M. Rosenburg, Cloning and expression of influenza virus genes, in: W.G. Laver (Ed.), The Origin of Pandemic Influenza Viruses, Elsevier, New York, NY, 1983, pp. 129–138.

[20] H. Shida, T. Tochikura, T. Sato, T. Konno, K. Hirayoshi, Y. Ito, M. Hatanaka, Y. Hinuma, M. Sugimoto, F. Takahashi-Nishimaki, T. Maruyama, K. Miki, K. Suzuki, M. Morita, H. Sashiyama, N. Yoshimura, M. Hayami, Effect of the recombinant vaccinia viruses that express HTLV-I envelop gene on HTLV-I infection, EMBO J. 6 (1987) 3379–3384.

[21] J.J. Dunn, B. Krippl, K.E. Bernstein, H. Westphal, F.W. Studier, Targeting bacteriophage T7 RNA polymerase to the mammalian cell nucleus, Gene 68 (1988) 259–266.

[22] H. Shida, Y. Hinuma, M. Hatanaka, M. Morita, M. Kidokoro, K. Suzuki, T. Maruyama, F. Takahashi-Nishimaki, M. Sugimoto, R. Kitamura, Effects and virulences of recombinant vaccinia viruses derived from attenuated strains that express the human T-cell leukemia virus type I envelope gene, J. Virol. 62 (1988) 4474–4480.

International Congress Series 1219 (2001) 471–477

Cold-sensitivity of polymerase complexes from human or avian influenza A viruses

Pascale Massin, Nadia Naffakh, Sylvie van der Werf*

Unité de Génétique Moléculaire des Virus Respiratoires, URA 1966 CNRS, Institut Pasteur, 25 rue du Dr Roux, 75724 Paris Cedex 15, France

Abstract

Background: Human influenza A viruses replicate in the upper respiratory tract at about 33 °C, whereas avian viruses replicate in the intestinal tract at a temperature close to 410 °C. *Methods*: The influence of low temperature on virus growth and RNA replication of avian and human viruses was analyzed in MDCK cells. The influence of temperature on the functional efficiency of homo- or heterospecific polymerase complexes derived from human or avian viruses, was examined by making use of a genetic system for the in vivo reconstitution of functional ribonucleoproteins. *Results*: Virus growth, RNA replication kinetics as well as the functional efficiency of the polymerase complex were found to be impaired at 33 °C as compared to 37 °C in the case of the avian A/FPV/Rostock/34 or A/Mallard/NY/6750/78 viruses, whereas they were comparable in the case of the human A/Puerto Rico/8/34 virus. The polymerase complex from the human virus A/Hong Kong/156/97 of avian origin exhibited an intermediate cold-sensitivity. The cold-sensitivity of the complexes of avian origin was determined mostly by residue 627 of PB2. *Conclusions*: Our results suggest that a reduced ability of the polymerase complex of avian viruses to ensure replication of the viral genome at 33 °C could contribute to their inability to grow efficiently in humans. © 2001 Elsevier Science B.V. All rights reserved.

Keywords: Transcription/replication; Host-specificity; PB2 protein

---

* Corresponding author. Tel.: +33-1-45-68-87-25; fax: +33-1-40-61-32-41.
E-mail address: svdwerf@pasteur.fr (S. van der Werf).

0531-5131/01/$ – see front matter © 2001 Elsevier Science B.V. All rights reserved.
PII: S 0 5 3 1 - 5 1 3 1 (0 1) 0 0 3 9 9 - 5

1. Introduction

Human influenza viruses do not spread in birds and avian influenza viruses generally do not replicate efficiently nor cause disease in humans [1]. This may, at least in part, be related to the fact that the temperature at the site of infection of human or avian viruses differs. In humans, influenza viruses initiate replication in the upper respiratory tract at a temperature around 33 °C and induce an acute respiratory illness; whereas in aquatic birds, influenza viruses primarily infect the intestinal tract at a temperature close to 41 °C and give no clinical symptoms. Adaptation of an avian virus to the human host may occur either through genetic reassortment, as has been the case in 1957 and 1968 [2], or following direct transmission, as recently documented in Hong Kong, where human cases of influenza, due to avian A(H5N1) or A(H9N2) viruses were identified in 1997 and in 1999, respectively [3–5]. The molecular bases for the host-specificity of human or avian influenza A viruses are not fully understood. The HA and NA are considered as possible determinants of host-restriction because of different receptor specificities between avian and human viruses [6–11]. In addition, genetic studies have indicated that gene segments encoding internal proteins, and especially the PB2 segment, were determinant for host-range [12–16]. Noteworthy, the A(H5N1) and A(H9N2) viruses isolated from humans were found to share internal genes that are highly related genetically [17].

In the present study, we addressed the question of whether natural temperature-dependence of influenza A viruses could contribute to their host-specificity by comparing the abilities of human and avian influenza A viruses to replicate at the temperature of the upper respiratory tract (33 °C).

2. Materials and methods

2.1. Virus multiplication and plaque assays

The avian viruses A/Mallard/NY/6750/78 (MAL) and A/FPV/Rostock/34 (FPV), the human viruses A/Puerto-Rico/8/34 (PR8) and A/Paris/908/97 (P908), were grown at 35 °C, either in 11-day-old embryonated chicken eggs (for MAL, FPV, PR8) or on Madin-Darby canine kidney (MDCK) cells (for P908). For plaque assays, MDCK cells were infected with 0.4 ml of serial dilutions of the virus stocks. After adsorption for 1 h at 33 °C, cells were incubated at 33 or 37 °C for 72 h (for MAL and P908 viruses) or 96 h (for PR8 and FPV viruses) and stained with crystal violet.

2.2. Transfections and CAT assays

As described previously [16], subconfluent monolayers of COS-1 cells were transfected using the Fugene-6-mediated method with a mixture of plasmids pHMG-PB1, -PB2, -PA and -NP (1, 1, 1, and 2 µg) derived from the PR8, MAL, FPV or HK strains, together with plasmid pPolI-CAT-RT (1 µg). Cells were incubated for 48 h at 37 or 33 °C. The efficiency of transcription/replication of the reconstituted RNPs was then evaluated by measuring the

levels of CAT in cell extracts using the CAT ELISA Kit (Roche), which allowed detection
of 0.05 ng/ml CAT.

3. Results

3.1. Temperature dependence of multiplication of avian and human influenza viruses

When virus multiplication of avian and human influenza viruses was analyzed by plaque
assays on MDCK cells, virus titers were found to be slightly reduced at 33 °C as compared
to 37 °C in the case of the avian FPV or MAL viruses, but not in the case of the human PR8
or P908 viruses. However, the plaque size appeared to be strongly reduced at 33 °C as
compared to 37 °C in the case of avian viruses, and only slightly in the case of human PR8
or P908 viruses (Fig. 1). Analysis of the kinetics of RNA synthesis in MDCK cells
indicated that the kinetics of replication of the NP-RNA segment of the human virus PR8 at
37 or 33 °C were identical. In contrast, replication of the MAL or FPV virus appeared
delayed at 33 °C and the overall levels of NP-RNA synthesized in the infected cells at 33 °C
represented less than 50% of those produced at 37 °C (data not shown).

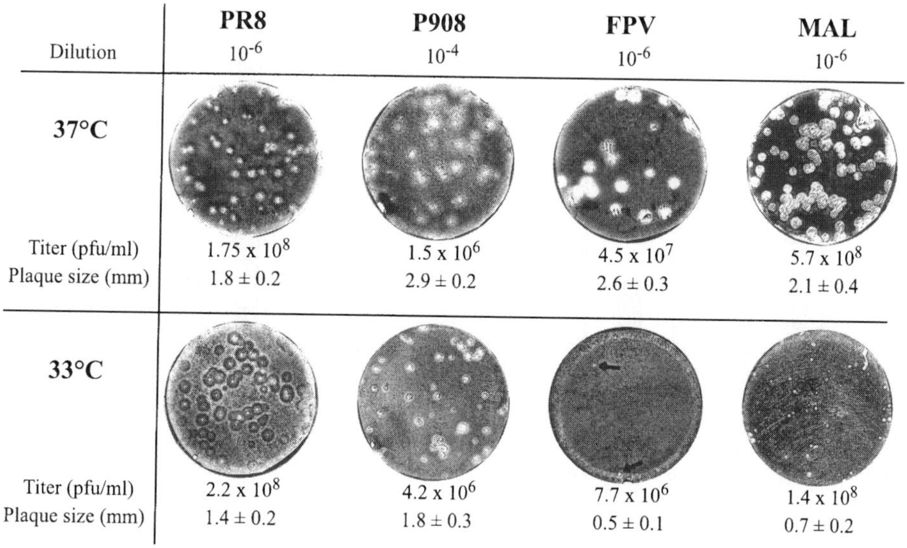

Dilution	**PR8** 10^{-6}	**P908** 10^{-4}	**FPV** 10^{-6}	**MAL** 10^{-6}
37°C				
Titer (pfu/ml)	1.75×10^8	1.5×10^6	4.5×10^7	5.7×10^8
Plaque size (mm)	1.8 ± 0.2	2.9 ± 0.2	2.6 ± 0.3	2.1 ± 0.4
33°C				
Titer (pfu/ml)	2.2×10^8	4.2×10^6	7.7×10^6	1.4×10^8
Plaque size (mm)	1.4 ± 0.2	1.8 ± 0.3	0.5 ± 0.1	0.7 ± 0.2

Fig. 1. Plaque assays on human and avian influenza viruses at 37 °C and 33 °C. MDCK cells were infected in
duplicate with various dilutions of human A/Puerto-Rico/8/34 (PR8) or A/Paris/908/97 (P908), or avian A/FPV/
Rostock/34 (FPV) or A/Mallard/NY/6750/78 (MAL) influenza viruses. For each virus, MDCK cells infected with
the same dilution at either 37 °C or 33 °C are shown. Titers were determined from dilutions that gave a minimum
of 10 plaques. The mean plaque diameters were determined by the measurement of a minimum of 16 plaques. The
results of one representative experiment out of two are shown.

3.2. Temperature-dependence of the polymerase complex of avian and human influenza viruses

In order to determine whether the lower efficiency of viral multiplication observed at 33 °C for MAL and FPV viruses was linked to a defect in the polymerase complex, we made use of a plasmid-based genetic system as initially described by Pleschka et al. [18] that allows the in vivo reconstitution of functional ribonucleoproteins derived from human or avian influenza viruses [16]. The efficiency of transcription/replication of the recon- stituted RNPs was then evaluated by measuring the levels of CAT in cell extracts (see Materials and methods). The efficiency of transcription/replication of the reconstituted RNPs was found to be comparable at 33 °C and 37 °C in cells expressing the PB1, PB2, PA and NP proteins derived from the human PR8 strain, but was significantly reduced at 33 °C as compared to 37 °C in cells expressing the FPV-derived proteins (Fig. 2). An even more drastic reduction was observed in the case of the MAL-derived proteins (data not shown). This indicated that the polymerase complex ensured transcription/replication of the viral- like reporter RNA with similar efficiencies at both temperatures in the case of the human PR8 virus, but much less efficiently at 33 °C in the case of avian viruses. Interestingly, in

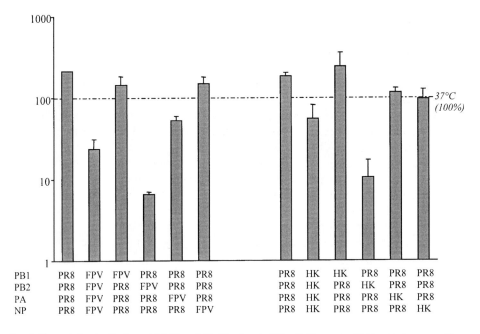

Fig. 2. Transcription/replication at 37 °C and 33 °C of a viral-like CAT reporter RNA with homospecific or heterospecific polymerase complexes. COS-1 cells were co-transfected in duplicate with pPolI-CAT-RT and four plasmids expressing the PB1, PB2, PA and NP proteins derived either from the PR8, FPV, or HK viruses. Cell extracts were prepared and tested for CAT expression following 48 h of incubation at 37 °C or 33 °C. For a given combination of PB1, PB2, PA and NP, the CAT levels measured at 33 °C were compared to the CAT levels measured at 37°C (100%, dashed line). The results are expressed as percentage values, and as the average ± SD of two independent experiments.

the case of the HK-derived polymerase complex, the level of transcription/replication of the viral-like reporter RNA at 33 °C relative to 37 °C was found to be intermediate as compared to the PR8 and FPV-derived polymerase complexes (Fig. 2).

3.3. The cold-sensitivity of the polymerase complex of avian viruses is mainly determined by PB2 residue 627

To determine whether cold-sensitivity could be attributed to one or another of the proteins of the polymerase complex, each of the PB1, PB2, PA or NP proteins derived from FPV was tested in combination with the three other proteins derived from PR8, at 37 °C and 33 °C. In cells expressing the FPV-PB2 or FPV-PA protein in association with PR8 proteins, the CAT levels measured at 33 °C represented about 6% and 60% of those measured at 37 °C, whereas they were slightly higher at 33 °C when the FPV-PB1 or FPV-NP proteins were expressed in association with PR8 proteins (Fig. 2). When each of the P or NP proteins from the HK virus was tested in combination with the PR8-derived proteins, a significant reduction of the CAT levels measured at 33 °C as compared to 37 °C was only observed in cells expressing the HK-PB2 in association with PR8 proteins (Fig. 2). These observations suggested that the proteins responsible for the cold-sensitivity of the transcription/replication complexes derived from viruses of avian origin were mainly PB2, and to a lesser extent PA in the case of FPV.

Residue 627 of PB2 (Glu in PB2 proteins of avian origin, Lys in PB2 proteins of human origin) had previously been identified as an important determinant of the species-specificity of influenza viruses [15,16]. We therefore made use of plasmids encoding mutant FPV- or MAL-PB2 proteins with a Lys instead of a Glu at position 627 (E627K-PB2 proteins) to determine whether or not residue 627 of PB2 was also involved in cold-sensitivity of the polymerase complex. Using western-blot analysis we first established that the steady-state levels of expression of wild-type or mutant PB2 proteins of human or avian origin were similar at 33 °C and 37 °C (data not shown). When functional RNPs were reconstituted in cells expressing the FPV or MAL polymerase complexes including an E627K-PB2 protein, the CAT levels measured at 33 °C represented about 67% and 38% of those measured at 37 °C. In contrast, in cells expressing the FPV- or MAL complexes including a wild-type PB2 protein, the CAT levels measured at 33 °C represented only 16% and 3% of those measured at 37 °C. This identified residue 627 of PB2 as a major determinant with respect to cold-sensitivity of the transcription/replication activity of the polymerase complex.

4. Discussion

Here, we showed that restriction of the multiplication of avian influenza viruses at 33 °C as compared to 37 °C could be related to impaired transcription/replication of the viral RNA. Furthermore, the cold-sensitivity of the avian derived polymerase complex could be attributed mainly to PB2 and to a lesser extent to PA. Remarkably, residue 627 of PB2 (a Lys in all human-derived proteins, and a Glu in all avian-derived proteins), found here to be determinant for natural cold-sensitivity of avian influenza A viruses, has already been identified as a major determinant of the ability of influenza A viruses to replicate in mammalian (MDCK) cells [15], and of the activity of the polymerase complexes reconstituted into mammalian (COS-1) cells [16]. One hypothesis could be that the determination of host-range and cold-sensitivity both rely on the same molecular interactions between PB2 and cellular proteins. In mammalian cells, these interactions would be strong at 37 °C as well as at 33 °C when PB2 is derived from a human virus, while they would be weaker (at 37 °C and even more so at 33 °C) when PB2 is derived from an avian virus. Interestingly, the polymerase complex derived from the human A/Hong Kong/156/97 strain of avian origin exhibited intermediate cold-sensitivity as compared to the human (PR8)- and avian (FPV or MAL)-derived complexes. The cold-sensitivity of the HK-derived polymerase complex was found to be determined by PB2, which harbors a Glu at position 627 as for all avian viruses, but not by PA. This suggested that determinants that contribute to the cold-sensitivity of the avian-derived polymerase complexes are lacking in the case of the HK-derived PA, or alternatively that mutations specific of the HK-PA abolish its cold-sensitivity. These determinants remain to be identified.

On the whole, our results suggest that a reduced ability of the polymerase complex of avian viruses to ensure replication of the viral genome at 33 °C could contribute to their inability to grow efficiently in humans.

Acknowledgements

The authors are very grateful to J. Pavlovic (Institut für Medizinische Virologie, Zurich, Switzerland) for providing the expression plasmids for PR8 proteins, to P. Palese for providing plasmid pPolI-CAT-RT (Mount Sinaï Medical Center, New York, USA), and to J. Ortin (Universidad Autonoma de Madrid, Spain) for providing a polyclonal serum specific for PB2 protein. The technical assistance of Ida Rijks, Claudine Rousseaux and Maryse Tardy-Panit for the production of influenza viruses is gratefully acknowledged.

This work was supported in part by the Ministère de l'Education Nationale, de la Recherche et de la Technologie (EA 302).

References

[1] A.S. Beare, R.G. Webster, Replication of avian influenza viruses in humans, Arch. Virol. 119 (1–2) (1991) 37–42.
[2] C. Scholtissek, et al., On the origin of the human influenza subtype H2N2 and H3N2, Virology 87 (1978) 13–20.
[3] E.C. Claas, et al., Human influenza A H5N1 virus related to a highly pathogenic avian influenza virus, Lancet 351 (9101) (1998) 472–477 [see comments] [published erratum appears in Lancet 351 (9111) (Apr 25 1998) 1292].
[4] K. Subbarao, et al., Characterization of an avian influenza A (H5N1) virus isolated from a child with a fatal respiratory illness, Science 279 (5349) (1998) 393–396 [see comments].
[5] M. Peiris, et al., Human infection with influenza H9N2, Lancet 354 (1999) 916–917.
[6] G.N. Rogers, J.C. Paulson, Receptor determinants of human and animal influenza virus isolates: differences in receptor specificity of the H3 hemagglutinin based on species of origin, Virology 127 (2) (1983) 361–373.

[7] G.N. Rogers, B.L. D'Souza, Receptor binding properties of human and animal H1 influenza virus isolates, Virology 173 (1989) 317–322.

[8] R.J. Connor, et al., Receptor specificity in human, avian, and equine h2 and h3 influenza virus isolates, Virology 205 (1) (1994) 17–23.

[9] A. Vines, et al., The role of influenza A virus hemagglutinin residues 226 and 228 in receptor specificity and host-range restriction, J. Virol. 72 (9) (1998) 7626–7631.

[10] D. Kobasa, et al., Amino acid residues contributing to the substrate specificity of the influenza A virus neuraminidase, J. Virol. 73 (1999) 6743–6751.

[11] T. Ito, et al., Recognition of *N*-glycolylneuraminic acid linked to galactose by the α2,3 linkage is associated with intestinal replication of influenza A virus in ducks, J. Virol. 74 (2000) 9300–9305.

[12] S.F. Tian, et al., Nucleoprotein and membrane protein genes are associated with restriction of replication of influenza A/Mallard/NY/78 virus and its reassortants in squirrel monkey respiratory tract, J. Virol. 53 (3) (1985) 771–775.

[13] M.L. Clements, et al., Evaluation of avian-human reassortant influenza A/Washington/897/80 x A/Pintail/119/79 virus in monkeys and adult volunteers, J. Clin. Microbiol. 24 (1) (1986) 47–51.

[14] M.H. Snyder, et al., The avian influenza virus nucleoprotein gene and a specific constellation of avian and human virus polymerase genes each specify attenuation of avian–human influenza A/Pintail/79 reassortant viruses for monkeys, J. Virol. 61 (9) (1987) 2857–2863.

[15] E.K. Subbarao, W. London, B.R. Murphy, A single amino acid in the PB2 gene of influenza A virus is a determinant of host range, J. Virol. 67 (4) (1993) 1761–1764.

[16] N. Naffakh, et al., Genetic analysis of the compatibility between polymerase proteins from human and avian strains of influenza A viruses, J. Gen. Virol. 81 (2000) 1283–1291.

[17] Y.P. Lin, et al., Avian-to-human transmission of H9N2 subtype influenza A viruses : Relationship between H9N2 and H5N1 human isolates, Proc. Natl. Acad. Sci. U. S. A. 97 (2000) 9654–9658.

[18] S. Pleschka, et al., A plasmid-based reverse genetics system for influenza A virus, J. Virol. 70 (6) (1996) 4188–4192.

International Congress Series 1219 (2001) 479–485

Protease activity of influenza virus RNA polymerase PA subunit

Koyu Hara[a,1], Mayumi Shiota[b,1], Hiroshi Kido[b],
Yasushi Ohtsu[a], Tetsuya Toyoda[a,*]

[a]Department of Virology, Kurume University School of Medicine, 67 Asahimachi, Kurume,
Fukuoka 830-0011, Japan
[b]Division of Enzyme Chemistry, Institute for Enzyme Research, University of Tokushima,
Tokushima 770-8503, Japan

Abstract

Influenza virus RNA polymerase is a multifunctional enzyme that catalyzes both transcription and replication of the RNA genome. The function of the influenza virus RNA polymerase PA subunit in viral replication is poorly understood although the enzyme is known to be required for cRNA → vRNA synthesis. Protease related activity of PA has been discussed ever since protease-inducing activity was demonstrated in transfection experiments. PA protein was highly purified from baculovirus-infected insect cells and a novel chymotrypsin-type serine protease activity with serine624 as an active site was identified in the protein. These results constitute the first demonstration of protease activity in RNA polymerase complexes. © 2001 Elsevier Science B.V. All rights reserved.

Keywords: Serine protease; Influenza virus; PA; Chymotrypsin

1. Introduction

Influenza A virus encodes its own RNA-dependent RNA polymerase consisting of three subunits, PB1, PB2, and PA. All three subunits are required for transcription and replication of the viral RNA genome [1,2]. The PB1 subunit is a core of polymerase assembly and involved in RNA polymerization. The PB2 subunit endonucleolytically cleaves the cap structure of host cell mRNA for utilization as primers for synthesis of the viral mRNA. The PA subunit is implicated in replication of the viral RNA genome and suggested to be

---

* Corresponding author. Tel.: +81-942-31-7549; fax: +81-942-32-0903.
E-mail address: ttoyoda@supernig.nig.ac.jp (T. Toyoda).
[1] These authors equally contributed.

essential for the cRNA-dependent vRNA synthesis. Protease activity related with PA was first identified in an experiment in which the N-terminal one-third of PA induced degradation of coexpressed proteins [3,4]. However, no direct evidence was provided regarding the protease activity of PA and it still remains unknown whether the PA protein has intrinsic protease activity. In this report, we describe the identification and characterization of a unique chymotrypsin-type serine protease activity in highly purified PA in vitro and determined its active site serine residue.

2. Materials and methods

2.1. Purification of PA and its mutants

Native PA (PA-WT) and its mutants (PA-S616T, PA-S624T, PA-S616/624T, PA-ΔC99), derived from influenza virus A/PR8/34 (H1N1), were expressed using a baculovirus expression vector system (Phermingen). The cytoplasmic extracts from *Spodoptera frugiperda* (Sf21) cells infected with recombinant baculoviruses were loaded onto a phosphocellulose column and the passed through fractions were loaded on a Mono Q column (Pharmacia Biotech). The column was eluted with a linear gradient (0.05–0.5 M) of NaCl in 20 mM Tris/HCl, pH 7.6, 0.2 mM EDTA, 1 mM DTT and 10% glycerol. They were further fractionated on a HiLoad 16/60 Superdex 200 pg column (Pharmacia Biotech) in 20 mM Tris/HCl, pH 7.6, 200 mM NaCl, 0.2 mM EDTA, 5% glycerol, 1 mM DTT. The fractions containing PA were dialyzed against BC100 (20 mM Tris/HCl, pH 7.9, 100 mM NaCl, 0.2 mM EDTA, 20% glycerol, and 1 mM DTT). After dialysis, PA was re-chromatographed and concentrated on a Mono Q column and stored at − 80 °C until used. As a control, cytoplasmic extracts of mock infected Sf21 cells were fractionated exactly as outlined above.

2.2. Protease assay

Protease activity of PA was analyzed with a fluorescence spectrophotometer (Hitachi Model 650-10 MS) by measuring the amount of 7-amino-4-methylcoumarin released upon hydrolysis of various MCA peptides as described previously [5]. Five synthetic substrates, Suc-LLVY-MCA, Suc-AAPF-MCA, Boc-FSR-MCA, Boc-GRR-MCA and Boc-VLK-MCA, were used in this study. The reaction was initiated by adding the indicated amount of PA or its mutants to 0.1 mM substrate in the standard protease buffer (50 mM Hepes/NaOH, pH 8.0, 10 mM $CaCl_2$, 1 mM DTT). One unit of protease activity was defined as the amount degrading 1 μmol substrate/min.

3. Results

3.1. Purification of PA and its mutant proteins

For a detailed analysis of the protease activity of PA, we purified 1 mg of PA protein from a 2-l culture of Sf21 cells infected with baculovirus carrying PA cDNA.

This sample revealed a single protein band with a molecular mass of 82.4 kDa on SDS-PAGE, which was consistent with that of PA in virions. The PA protein exhibited over 95% purity (Fig. 1C, PA-WT). Immunoblot analysis using polyclonal antibodies against PA confirmed that the 82.4-kDa protein specifically reacted with the antibodies. The mutant proteins of PA were purified using the same procedure.

3.2. Characterization of PA protease

In order to investigate the protease activity of PA, the amidolytic activity of purified PA was first measured using five synthetic substrates Suc-LLVY-MCA, Suc-AAPF-MCA,

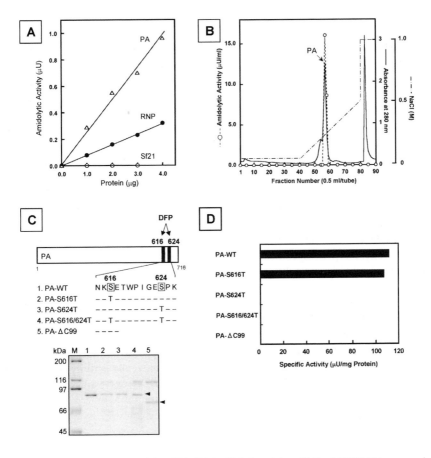

Fig. 1. Characterization of protease activity of PA. (A) Amidolytic activity with Suc-LLVY-MCA measured using the indicated amount of purified PA (open triangle), RNP (closed circle) and uninfected Sf21 cells (open circle). (B) The elution profile of MonoQ column chromatography at the final purification step of PA and amidolytic activity with Suc-LLVY-MCA of each fraction (open circle). Amidolytic activity was measured using aliquots (100 μl each) of the indicated fractions. (C) SDS-PAGE of the purified wild type and mutant PA proteins. The positions of PA proteins are indicated by arrowheads. (D) Amidolytic activity of the wild type and mutant PA proteins with Suc-LLVY-MCA.

Boc-FSR-MCA, Boc-GRR-MCA and Boc-VLK-MCA. PA showed an amidolytic activity against a certain substrate used and the activity was co-eluted with PA at the final purification step (Fig. 1A and B). Of the substrates used, PA preferentially cleaved only Suc-LLVY-MCA but did not cleave Suc-AAPF-MCA, both of which are good substrates for α-chymotrypsin. PA could not cleave any other substrates for trypsin-like protease, such as Boc-FSR-MCA, Boc-GRR-MCA and Boc-VLK-MCA. These results indicated that PA had unique chymotrypsin-like properties with a limited substrate specificity. The specific activities of the purified PA were in the range of 0.1–0.4 mU/mg protein (Fig. 1D, PA-WT), indicating that the turnover number of this enzyme was about 1/700–1/175 of that of α-chymotrypsin from bovine pancreas. This amidolytic activity was also observed in the fraction of ribonucleoprotein complex purified from virions, which contains PB1, PB2, PA and NP, but not in the equivalent fractions of uninfected cells (Fig. 1A). The optimal pH for the activity was found to be 8.0, which was consistent with that of ordinary chymotrypsin-type serine proteases. The amidolytic activity was enhanced by 10 mM Ca^{2+} (280%). It was, however, not affected by heavy metal ions, such as Zn^{2+} and Mg^{2+}, and slightly inhibited by Cu^{2+} (85%). Moreover, PA could digest not only peptides but also large protein, [^{14}C]casein (data not shown). The amount of digested products increased with the amount of added PA in a dose-dependent manner. Essentially, the same results were observed when RNP was used instead of purified PA (data not shown).

3.3. Determination of an active site serine residue in the PA protease

Since the catalytic properties of PA suggest that it was a chymotrypsin-like serine protease, we further examined whether PA was labeled with [^{3}H] diisopropylfluorophosphate (DFP), which specifically binds the active serine residue irreversibly and inhibits the catalytic activity. [^{3}H]DFP specifically cross-linked with not only purified PA but also the peptides corresponding to PA/PB2 in RNP from purified virions (data not shown). The positions of Ser cross-linked with [^{3}H]DFP in PA amino acid sequence were found to be both 616 and 624. In order to determine which serine residue was the active site of PA, we created four mutants of PA and purified these proteins. S616, S624, and both serines were substituted by Thr (PA-S616T, PA-S624T, PA-S616/624T, respectively). The C-terminal 99 amino acids were deleted (PA-ΔC99) (Fig. 1C). The specific amidolytic activity of PA-S616T was retained and identical to that of PA-WT, whereas the activity was completely lost in PA-S624T, PA-S616/624T and PA-ΔC99 (Fig 1D). These results demonstrate that the protease active site of PA is S624.

4. Discussion

Influenza virus RNA polymerase PA subunit has been implicated in viral RNA genome replication by analysis of temperature-sensitive (ts) mutations in the PA gene [6–10], and by expression experiments although no direct evidence of the activity has been obtained [11,12]. In the present study, we detected a unique chymotrypsin-like serine protease activity from purified PA and confirmed that its active site is S624. No specific motif(s) around S624 distinct from the highly conserved active site sequence, GDSGGP, was observed in the ordinary serine proteases. This might be one reason for the low turnover number of PA protease. Although we found Suc-LLVY-MCA to be a substrate of PA protease, the natural substrate may have a sequence different from LLVY.

What is the PA protease activity for? Recently, some factors in proteasome were found also in transcription and DNA repair apparatus in yeast [13,14]. SUG1 is an ATPase of proteasome, and binds to TATA-binding protein (TBP) to form a complex with TFIIH [15–17]. Yeast Rad23, which promotes the assembly of various repair factors and interacts with TFIIH and Rad14, carries ubiquitin-like domains and interacts with proteasome [18–22]. A putative ATPase, SUG1, is both a transcriptional mediator, a DNA helicase and a 26S proteasome in yeast and it is hypothesized that proteasomal ATPases are involved in transcriptional regulation in addition to proteolysis [23–25]. These factors may contribute to recycling of the repair and transcription complexes.

Influenza virus PA is the first case in which protease activity has been demonstrated in a subunit of the RNA polymerase complex. We propose a new function for PA. RNA polymerase complex was extracted from influenza A virus infected cells with high salt buffer [26]. RNA polymerase may be released from the nuclear skeletal fraction with high salt extraction. We speculate that the PA protease works to release the newly assembled RNP complex from the nuclear skeletal fraction into the cytosol. Influenza A virus M1 protein is required for transporting newly assembled RNP from nuclei to the cytosol fraction [27]. M1 bound with RNA and inhibited transcription [28]. M1 also bound to trypsin and chymotrypsin, and inhibited their activity [29], indicating M1 may interact with PA like RNA. In RNP with M1, PA protease may be inactivated.

Elucidation of the tertiary structure of PA and target proteins of PA protease in infected cells will further the development of inhibitors for PA protease as new anti-influenza drugs.

Acknowledgements

We thank Mr. Imamura for his excellent technical assistance. This work was supported by Grants-in-Aid (10670291, 11770163) from the Japan Society for the Promotion of Science.

References

[1] R.A. Lamb, Genes and proteins of the influenza viruses, in: R.M. Krug (Ed.), The Influenza Viruses, Plenum, New York, 1989, pp. 1–87.

[2] T. Toyoda, Y. Ohtsu, K. Hara, K. Masunaga, N. Hamada, M. Koga, K. Kashiwagi, J. Iwahashi, Molecular dissection of influenza virus RNA polymerase, Rec. Res. Dev. Virol. 1 (1999) 839–847.

[3] J.J. Sanz-Ezquerro, S. De La Luna, J. Ortín, A. Nieto, Individual expression of influenza virus PA protein induces degradation of coexpressed proteins, J. Virol. 69 (1995) 2420–2426.

[4] J.J. Sanz-Ezquerro, T. Zürcher, S. De La Luna, J. Ortín, A. Nieto, The amino-terminal one-third of the influenza virus PA protein is responsible for the induction of proteolysis, J. Virol. 70 (1996) 1905–1911.

[5] H. Kido, Y. Yokogoshi, K. Sakai, M. Tashiro, Y. Kishino, A. Fukutomi, N. Katunuma, Isolation and characterization of a novel trypsin-like protease found in rat bronchiolar epithelial Clara cells. A possible activator of the viral fusion glycoprotein, J. Biol. Chem. 267 (1992) 13573–13579.

[6] R.M. Krug, M. Ueda, P. Palese, Temperature-sensitive mutants of influenza WSN virus defective in virus-specific RNA synthesis, J. Virol. 16 (1975) 790–796.

[7] C. Scholtissek, A.L. Bowles, Isolation and characterization of temperature-sensitive mutants of fowl plague virus, Virology 67 (1975) 576–587.

[8] C. Scholtissek, E. Harms, W. Rhode, M. Orlich, R. Root, Correlation between RNA fragments of fowl plague virus and their corresponding gene functions, Virology 74 (1976) 322–344.

[9] B.W.J. Mahy, T. Barrett, S.T. Nichol, C.R. Penn, A.J. Wolstenholme, Analysis of the functions of influenza virus genome RNA segments by use of temperature-sensitive mutants of fowl plaque virus, in: D.H.L. Bishop, R.W. Compans (Eds.), The Replication of Negative Stranded Viruses, Elsevier/North Holland, New York, 1981, pp. 379–387.

[10] S.L. Mowshowitz, RNA synthesis of temperature-sensitive mutants of WSN influenza virus, in: D.H.L. Bishop, R.W. Compans (Eds.), The Replication of Negative Stranded Viruses, Elsevier/North Holland, New York, 1981, pp. 317–323.

[11] M. Kobayashi, T. Toyoda, A. Ishihama, Influenza virus PB1 protein is the minimal and essential subunit of RNA polymerase, Arch. Virol. 141 (1996) 525–539.

[12] Y. Nakagawa, K. Oda, S. Nakada, The PB1 subunit alone can catalyze cRNA synthesis, and the PA subunit in addition to the PB1 subunit is required for viral RNA synthesis in replication of the influenza virus genome, J. Virol. 70 (1996) 6390–6394.

[13] D.M. Rubin, O. Coux, I. Wefes, C. Hengartner, R.A. Young, A.L. Goldberg, D. Finley, Identification of the gal4 suppressor Sug1 as a subunit of the yeast 26S proteasome, Nature 379 (1996) 655–657.

[14] Y. Makino, T. Yoshida, S. Yogosawa, K. Tanaka, M. Muramatsu, T.A. Tamura, Multiple mammalian proteasomal ATPases, but not proteasome itself, are associated with TATA-binding protein and a novel transcriptional activator, TIP120, Genes Cells 4 (1999) 529–539.

[15] J.C. Swaffield, K. Melcher, S.A. Johnston, A highly conserved ATPase protein as a mediator between acidic activation domains and the TATA-binding protein, Nature 374 (1995) 88–91.

[16] E. vom Baur, C. Zechel, D. Heery, M.J. Heine, J.M. Garnier, V. Vivat, B. Le Douarin, H. Gronemeyer, P. Chambon, R. Losson, Differential ligand-dependent interactions between the AF-2 activating domain of nuclear receptors and the putative transcriptional intermediary factors mSUG1 and TIF1, EMBO J. 15 (1996) 110–124.

[17] G. Weeda, M. Rossignol, R.A. Fraser, G.S. Winkler, W. Vermeulen, L.J. van't Veer, L. Ma, J.H. Hoeijmakers, J.M. Egly, The XPB subunit of repair/transcription factor TFIIH directly interacts with SUG1, a subunit of the 26S proteasome and putative transcription factor, Nucleic Acids Res. 25 (1997) 2274–2283.

[18] S.M. Guzder, V. Bailly, P. Sung, L. Prakash, S. Prakash, Yeast DNA repair protein RAD23 promotes complex formation between transcription factor TFIIH and DNA damag recognition factor RAD14, J. Biol. Chem. 170 (1995) 8385–8388.

[19] S.N. Guzder, Y. Habraken, P. Sung, L. Prakash, S. Prakash, Reconstitution of yeast nucleotide excision repair with purified Rad proteins, replication protein A, and transcription factor TFIIH, J. Biol. Chem. 270 (1995) 12973–12976.

[20] D. Mu, D.S. Hsu, A. Sancar, Reaction mechanism of human DNA repair excision nuclease, J. Biol. Chem. 271 (1996) 8285–8294.

[21] J.T. Reardon, T. Mu, A. Sancar, Overproduction, purification and characterization of the XPC subunit of the human DNA repair excision nuclease, J. Biol. Chem. 271 (1996) 19451–19456.

[22] K. Sugasawa, C. Masutani, A. Uchida, T. Maekawa, P.J. van der Spek, D. Bootsma, J.H. Hoeijmakers, F. Hanaoka, Related Articles HHR23B, a human Rad23 homolog, stimulates XPC protein in nucleotide excision repair in vitro, Mol. Cell Biol. 16 (1996) 4852–4861.

[23] R.A. Fraser, M. Rossignol, D.J. Heard, J.M. Egly, P. Chambon, SUG1, a putative transcriptional mediator and subunit of the PA700 proteasome regulatory complex, is a DNA helicase, J. Biol. Chem. 272 (1997) 7122–7126.

[24] Y.J. Kim, S. Bjorklund, Y. Li, M.H. Sayre, R.D. Kornberg, A multiprotein mediator of transcriptional activation and its interaction with the C-terminal repeat domain of RNA polymerase II, Cell 77 (1994) 599–608.

[25] Y. Makino, T. Yoshida, S. Yogosawa, K. Tanaka, M. Muramatsu, T.A. Tamura, Multiple mammalian proteasomal ATPases, but not proteasome itself, are associated with TATA-binding protein and a novel transcriptional activator, TIP120, Genes Cells 4 (1999) 529–539.

[26] T. Toyoda, M. Kobayashi, A. Ishihama, Replication in vitro of the influenza virus genome: selective dissociation of RNA replicase from virus-infected cell ribonucleoprotein complexes, Arch. Virol. 136 (1994) 269–286.

[27] K. Martin, A. Helenius, Nuclear transport of influenza virus ribonucleoproteins: the viral matrix protein (M1) promotes export and inhibits import, Cell 67 (1991) 117–130.

[28] K. Watanabe, H. Handa, K. Mizumoto, K. Nagata, Mechanism for Inhibition of influenza virus RNA polymerase activity by matrix protein, J. Virol. 70 (1996) 241–247.

[29] O.P. Zhirnov, A.L. Ksenofontov, H.D. Klenk, The matrix protein M1 of influenza A virus has a protease inhibitor domain, Abstract for XI the International Congress of Virology (Sydney) (1999) p. 25.

International Congress Series 1219 (2001) 487–502

Evaluation of influenza A virus receptors

Stephen J. Stray, Gillian M. Air*,1

*Department of Biochemistry and Molecular Biology and Oklahoma Center for Medical Glycobiology,
University of Oklahoma Health Sciences Center, PO Box 26901, Oklahoma City, OK 73190, USA*

Abstract

Sialic acid has long been considered the sole cellular receptor for influenza viruses, but it has been demonstrated that influenza can infect cells independently of surface sialic acid [Glycobiology 10 (2000) 649]. Here, we evaluate possible alternative influenza virus receptors, and find evidence for specific virus-binding-proteins in vitro and mediation of entry by carbohydrates containing terminal α-N-acetylgalactosamine. Characterization of such receptors may lead to identification of alternative targets for the design of anti-influenza drugs. © 2001 Elsevier Science B.V. All rights reserved.

Keywords: Influenza A virus receptor; Sialic acid; Terminal α–N-acetylgalactosamine

1. Introduction

The binding of influenza virus to a molecule, which is also a substrate for a viral enzymatic activity, was one of the earliest receptor–ligand relationships identified in biology [1,2]. The substrate for both of these activities was later determined to be sialic acid [3,4]. Many studies have concentrated on the role of sialic acid in virus binding, and these have demonstrated that certain virus strains prefer some forms of sialic acid over others [5–7]. The vast majority of studies into the binding of influenza virus have been performed using either red blood cells, which are not permissive for virus entry, or purified components in vitro. We have recently examined virus entry into a permissive cell line,

*   Corresponding author. Tel.: +1-405-271-2227x1250; fax: +1-405-271-3205.
    E-mail address: gillian-air@ouhsc.edu (G.M. Air).
1   Present address: Department of Molecular Immunogenetics, Oklahoma Medical Research Foundation, 825 NE 13th Street, Oklahoma City, OK 73104, USA.

MDCK, and found that influenza viruses can infect sialidase-treated cells, in which there is no detectable surface sialic acid [8,9].

On the basis of these data, we have proposed that sialic acid acts in viral infection either to recruit virus particles to the cell surface, where they are then able to interact with a rarer entry determinant, akin to Burnet's "browsing" model [10], or that separate sialic acid-mediated and sialic acid-independent pathways of virus uptake exist. Both models require the existence of receptors in addition to sialic acid. Here, we assess the potential of carbohydrates and proteins to mediate viral uptake, and find evidence that both classes of molecules may be involved. We have determined that MDCK cell membrane fractions contain proteins which are bound by influenza hemagglutinin (HA) in vitro, and that molecules containing terminal α-linked N-acetylgalactosamine (α-GalNAc) may mediate virus uptake in vivo.

2. Materials and methods

2.1. Viruses and antisera

Viruses were grown in MDCK cells (ATCC) as previously described [8]. Virus strains were reassortants A/NWS/33$_{HA}$-Tokyo/67$_{NA}$ (H1N2, designated NWS-Tok), A/NWS/33$_{HA}$-tern/Australia/G70c/75$_{NA}$ (NWS-G70c, H1N9), and A/NWS/33$_{HA}$-G70cΔ_{NA}MviA (NWS-Mvi, H1N9$^-$) [8]. NWS-G70c and NWS-Tokyo have been extensively passaged in eggs, but also grow well in MDCK cells without adaptation. Antisera used were rabbit anti-A/PR/8/34 HA and anti-NWS HA (H1, kind gifts from Prof. W.G. Laver, Australian National University, Canberra, Australia), rabbit anti-A/Mem-Bel (H3N1, kind gift from Dr. R.G. Webster, St. Jude's Hospital, Memphis, TN), and goat anti-B/HK (HG) (R.G. Webster). Monoclonal antibody BMA-FOG, specific for the Forssman glycolipid, was obtained from Accurate Chemical, Westbury, NY.

2.2. Preparation of cellular membrane fractions

MDCK cells were harvested by scraping cells from tissue culture dishes (approximately 10^8 cells) and washed with PBS. Cell pellets were frozen at -80 °C prior to further processing. Upon thawing, cells were resuspended in one volume (400–600 μl) ice-cold hypotonic relaxation buffer (100 mM KCl, 3 mM NaCl, 3.5 mM MgCl$_2$, 10 mM PIPES pH 7.3) [11] and incubated on ice for 40 min before Dounce homogenization on ice (at least 40 strokes). The suspended cell lysate (approximately 1.0 ml) was then loaded onto a cushion of 40% sucrose in relaxation buffer (1.0 ml) and centrifuged at 45,000 rpm (Beckman TLS 55 rotor) for 35 min. After centrifugation, the lysate partitioned into a clear upper layer (soluble proteins), a pearlescent band below the top of the sucrose cushion (membrane fragments), and a pellet (undisrupted cells and insoluble debris). The "membrane" band was harvested using a needle and syringe. The protein concentrations of the membrane fractions were in the range of 1.5–3.0 mg/ml. Where indicated, the MDCK membrane preparation was treated with TPCK-treated trypsin in the presence of Triton X-100 (1%) at 37 °C overnight prior to separation by SDS-PAGE and transfer to nitrocellulose.

2.3. Preparation of virus rosettes

To achieve high protein concentration, we prepared viral glycoprotein rosettes from egg-grown virus. Gradient-purified egg-grown virus (200 μl in CaMg saline) was treated with 10 mM NaIO$_4$ (on ice, 20 min) to eliminate binding by cell lectins to egg-specific surface oligosaccharides on the virus in the overlay assay. Periodate treatment was stopped by addition of glycerol (15 mM), and aldehyde functional groups generated by periodate treatment were quenched by the addition of ethanolamine (10 mM). Low molecular weight material (products of periodate oxidation) were removed from the virus by gel filtration over a 2 ml column of Sephadex G25 resin (Sigma) in CaMg saline. Eluate was collected in 0.1 ml fractions and HA-positive fractions were pooled. Virus was disrupted by the addition of *n*-octyl-β-D-glucoside to a final concentration of 2%, which was sufficient to turn the milky virus preparation clear. This material was dialyzed against CaMg saline overnight (at least 200 volumes) to remove detergent, so that the viral glycoproteins aggregate via their hydrophobic transmembrane domain [12]. Precipitated material present after dialysis (viral M protein and RNP complexes) were removed by centrifugation (14,000 rpm, Eppendorf microfuge). Protein concentrations in the final "rosette" fractions ranged from 1.5 to 3.0 mg/ml. The use of HA rosettes was considered preferable in attempting to release HA trimers from virus by protease cleavage [13] because NWS HA is readily degraded by protease digestion, and the presence of multiple HA trimers in the rosettes allows multivalent binding [14].

2.4. Virus overlay

The membrane fraction from MDCK cells (15–50 μg) was separated by polyacrylamide gel electrophoresis in the presence of sodium dodecyl sulfate (SDS-PAGE) and proteins electrophoretically transferred to nitrocellulose membranes. Non-specific binding was blocked by 2% non-fat dry milk powder in CaMg saline, and membranes were then incubated with virus rosettes diluted 1:100 in blocking buffer for 1–2 h at room temperature. After washing with CaMg saline (for least 5 × 5 min), the membranes were incubated with anti-hemagglutinin polyclonal antiserum diluted 1:1000 in blocking buffer, washed, then incubated with anti-rabbit or anti-goat secondary antibody conjugated to horseradish peroxidase, diluted 1:4000 in blocking buffer (at least 30 min). After further washing in CaMg saline, blots were developed with Sigma Fast DAB.

2.5. Use of lectins to inhibit virus infection

Lectins used were agglutinins from *Wisteria floribunda* (WFA), *Helix pomatia* (HPA), *Bandeiraea simplicifolia* (BSA-I-B4), *Lotus tetragonolobus* (*purpureus*) (TPA), all from Sigma, and *Maackia amurensis* (MAL), and *Sambucus nigra* (SNA), from Vector Laboratories. Each was maintained as 10 mg/ml stock solution. Lectins were preincubated with cells in CaMg PBS, approximately at 37 °C for 30 min prior to infection, then removed by washing with CaMg PBS where described, after which virus infection was carried out as usual. Where indicated, virus stocks were pretreated by the addition of lectin (2–10 μg) to 50 μl (16 HAU) virus stock. Of this treated virus mixture, 1 μl (1.6 HAU) was used for infection, allowing the lectin to be diluted to below the level seen to affect virus entry when preincubated with cells. HA titers of the virus after lectin treatment were not determined as some of the lectins used also agglutinate human red blood cells. Infected cells were harvested at 6 h post-infection (p.i.) and RNA quantitated by ribonuclease protection.

2.6. Ribonuclease protection assay (RPA)

MDCK cells (1.5 cm well, approximately 2.5×10^5 cells) were infected with 0.6–1.6 HAU virus (two to five particles per cell, 1 HAU is approximately 10^6 particles [9]). Stocks used were from MDCK cells and grew to 320 HAU/ml (10^8 TCIU/ml). RNA was assayed by ribonuclease protection [15] at 7 h p.i. Total RNA was harvested in 50 µl harvest/hybridization buffer (0.5 M NaCl, 50 mM PIPES pH 6.4, 1.25 mM EDTA in formamide), to which a probe (approximately 5×10^5 cpm) was added directly prior to overnight hybridization at 50 °C. Probe (negative sense) was transcribed from NWS HA cDNA (nt 1517–1746, cloned into pBluescript (Stratagene)) using T7 polymerase (Promega). Ribonuclease T1 digestion was performed by diluting the hybridized RNA in 250 µl RNase T1 digestion buffer (10 mM Tris pH 7.5, 5 mM EDTA, 200 mM sodium acetate pH 7.5, RNase T1 [Life Technologies] 250–750 U) and allowed to digest for approximately 30 min. After hybridization and RNase T1 digestion, products were treated with SDS and proteinase K to remove RNase, then ethanol precipitated and separated by gel electrophoresis (6% polyacrylamide, 0.5 × TBE, 42% urea). Hybridization with RNAs from the infected cell is expected to protect fragments of 215 (mRNA) and 230 nt (cRNA, the positive strand replication intermediate) from RNase cleavage. Product size was initially verified by comparison to denatured, end-labeled DNA fragments of φX174

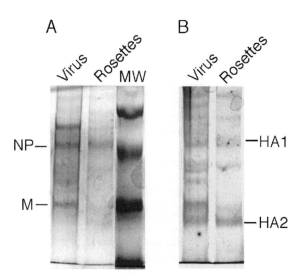

Fig. 1. SDS polyacrylamide gel electrophoresis of the "HA rosettes" preparation. (A). Coomassie blue-stained gel of intact virus, the rosettes, and MW markers. (B) Silver stained gel of the virus and rosettes.

derived by HaeIII endonuclease digestion. Quantitation was performed using Molecular Dynamics PhosphorImager SI.

3. Results

3.1. Virus binds to proteins in MDCK cell membrane extracts in vitro

An overlay assay, in which immobilized membrane proteins from MDCK cells were probed with virus "HA rosettes," was used to identify potential virus receptors. SDS-PAGE analysis revealed that HA (HA1 + HA2) was the major protein constituent of the "rosette" preparation (Fig. 1). Blocking conditions were found to be critical. For nitrocellulose membranes, 2% non-fat dry milk powder in CaMg saline was sufficient to reduce background binding to an acceptable level while allowing detection of virus-specific bands. Typical overlay blots are shown in Fig. 2. Binding of HA rosettes to an 85-kDa protein, designated p85, was consistently observed in overlays with NWS (H1) HA. This protein was not bound by influenza B or A/Mem/31/98 (H3) rosettes. Other proteins at approximately 30 and 39 kDa were variably bound by H1, H3, and influenza B HA rosettes; these are presumably the sialylated proteins previously observed [16,17]. The p85 binding to NWS (H1) rosettes was detected both in low passage (freshly revived) and higher passage MDCK cells.

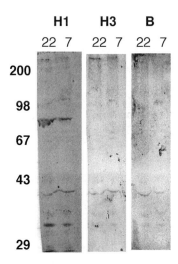

Fig. 2. Virus overlay of blotted MDCK cell proteins. The rosettes were from NWS-G70c (lane H1). The lane designated "H3" was probed with rosettes from A/Memphis/31/98 (H3N2), but was detected with polyclonal antibody against A/Memphis/1/71, which binds only weakly to the 1998 HA. Thus, the negative result may be due to poor reagent. Lane "B" shows binding by B/HK/8/73 (B) HA rosettes detected by a goat anti-B/HK/73 antiserum. Partially purified membranes of MDCK cells at either passage 22 or passage 7 from revival were compared.

To determine whether viral binding is to protein alone, carbohydrate, some other form of protein modification, or a recognition complex combining multiple elements, we examined the ability of the virus to bind to tryptic digestion products of the MDCK cell membrane fractions (Fig. 3A). There was no binding after trypsin digestion confirming that p85 is indeed a protein. Low molecular weight product bands did not bind virus, although it is not known how efficiently the very small peptides were transferred to the membrane. Thus, we found no evidence that specific N- or O-linked carbohydrates or linear polypeptide determinants were the virus targets under these binding conditions. Prominent Coomassie Blue-positive bands appear at 45 and 60 kDa upon trypsin digestion. These may be the digestion products of mucins, which tend to be protease-resistant due to the presence of multiple O-linked carbohydrate side chains, which are usually highly sialylated. Indeed, a polypeptide of approximately 45 kDa in the trypsin-digested membrane fraction bound virus weakly in the overlay assay. Considering the diversity of proteins on cell surfaces that contain sialic acid [18,19], we conclude that the specific binding we see involves proteins. This was confirmed since sialidase treatment of the membrane preparations before gel electrophoresis did not shift the mobility of p85, and virus still bound (Fig. 3B).

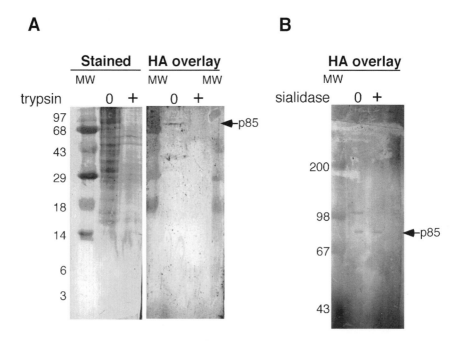

Fig. 3. Effect of in vitro trypsin or sialidase digestion on purified membrane proteins and virus binding. (A) Partially purified MDCK membrane fractions were either mock-treated (0) or digested with trypsin (+) overnight. Digests were separated by electrophoresis (15% polyacrylamide gel) and transferred to membranes. Lanes were run in duplicate, allowing membrane to be cut into sections which were either stained with Coomassie brilliant blue (stained) or subjected to virus overlay with NWS hemagglutinin rosettes (H1). (B) Virus overlay assay of membrane fractions that were mock-treated (0) or treated with Mvi sialidase (+), then blotted from an 8% polyacrylamide SDS gel.

3.2. Carbohydrates as influenza virus receptors

To assess the role of carbohydrate in influenza virus uptake, we tested the ability of various lectins (carbohydrate-binding proteins) to block virus infection. The properties of agglutinins used are listed in Table 1. Additionally, we examined the effect of treatment with monoclonal antibody BMA-FOG, specific for the Forssman glycolipid (GalNAcα-1,3-GalNAcβ-1,3-Galα-1,4-Galβ-1,4Glcβ-1,1′-ceramide), which we had identified in the glycolipids of MDCK cells by thin-layer chromatography. The results are shown in Fig. 4. Of the sialic acid-binding lectins, MAL was strongly inhibitory while treatment with SNA had no effect on NWS-G70c and little effect on NWS-Tokyo virus infection, suggesting that the α2,3-linked sialic acid is more important than the α2,6. The early H1 HAs recognize both types of sialic acid linkage [20]. We previously showed that treatment of red cells with sialidase from *Salmonella typhimurium* (which hydrolyzes α2,3-linked sialic acid 200-fold faster than the α2,6 linkage) abolishes agglutination by NWS-Tokyo but not by NWS-G70c [21,22]. These data emphasize our previous conclusions that binding of virus to red cells is not the same as the binding of virus to permissive cells that leads to productive infection [9]. No inhibition was seen upon treatment with BSA-I-B4 or TPA (data not shown), eliminating α-Gal and fucose as receptors. HPA was a potent inhibitor of virus entry (Fig. 4), whereas WFA had little effect on virus uptake, implicating αGalNac as a receptor determinant. However, there was little if any inhibition by monoclonal antibody specific for the Forssman antigen (FOG). Thus, we conclude that αGalNAc, as found in O-linked glycans on proteins, is important in virus infection.

Table 1
Properties of lectins used in this study

Lectin	Source	Target	Ka (M^{-1})	Comments	Reference
BSA-I-B4	*B. simplicifolia*	αGal > βGal > αGalNAc	2.06×10^4 1.87×10^3 1.26×10^2	Ka given is for methylglycoside	[66]
WFA	*W. floribunda*	βGalNAc > αGalNAc	3.4×10^6	Ka for binding to sheep red blood cells; β1,4-GalNAc preferred to β1,3-GalNAc or α-GalNAc	[67]
HPA	*H. pomatia*	α-GalNAc	8.4×10^7	Ka for binding to sheep red blood cells	[67]
TPA	*L. tetragonolobus purpurea*	α-L-fucose		Binding inhibited by sialic acid	[68]
MAL I	*M. amurensis*	Neu5Ac α3Galβ4-GlcNAc	10^6	Ka for oligosaccharide. MAL shows > 40-fold preference for α2,3-linked Neu5Ac	[69,70]
SNA	*S. nigra*	Neu5Ac α6-Gal or GalNAc	10^5	Ka for 6′sialyllactose; α2,3-linked Neu5Ac binds 20–150 more weakly	[70,71]

Note: The binding of lectins to oligosaccharides has been measured to be 36- to 3000-fold stronger than to monosaccharides (hapten sugars) [72].

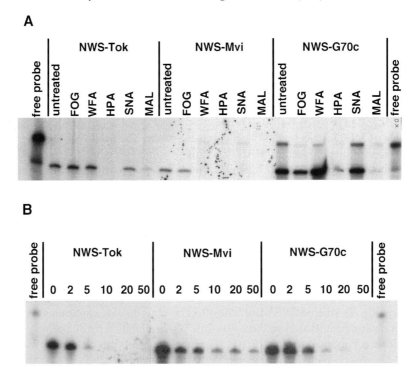

Fig. 4. Effect of lectin treatment on virus infection. (A) Cells were preincubated with anti-Forssman glycolipid monoclonal antibody (FOG), or agglutinins of *W. floribunda* (WFA), *H. pomatia* (HPA), *S. nigra*, (SNA), or *M. amurensis* (MAL); 10 μg of antibody or agglutinin were used per well (approximately 2.5×10^5 cells). After incubation with lectin for 30 min at 37 °C, cells were infected with 1.6 HAU of NWS-Tok, NWS-Mvi, or NWS-G70c virus. Infections were allowed to proceed for 6 h, when cells were disrupted and HA mRNA quantitated by ribonuclease protection (RPA). See Table 1 for lectin specificities. Note that free probe markers represent 500-fold less labeled probe than was present in RPA hybridizations and is used solely to indicate size of input probe. (B) MDCK cells were incubated with increasing doses of *H. pomatia* lectin (HPA) at 37 °C for 30 min. Doses (μg) are indicated above lanes. Cells were washed to remove unbound lectin, then infected with 1.6 HAU of the indicated virus. Cells were harvested at 7 h post-infection and the amount of HA mRNA present was determined by ribonuclease protection.

3.3. Carbohydrate on both virus and cell may be involved in virus entry

To test whether the lectins are blocking infection by binding to the virus or to the cell surface, we preincubated either cells or virus preparations with HPA, FOG, or a preparation of glycopeptides derived from MDCK cells. Unbound lectin was washed from cells prior to infection. Virus–lectin mixes were diluted 1:50 prior to infection to a level of lectin we determined had no effect on virus uptake (Fig. 5).

Pretreatment of either cells or virus with HPA reduced infectivity. The results are dose-dependent and highly reproducible. Treatment of virus with HPA prior to infection may cause agglutination of the viral particles by the lectin, which would reduce infectivity. At the moment, we cannot distinguish between this and the possibility that the carbohydrate incorporated into the viral membrane may be bound by cell surface carbohydrate receptors

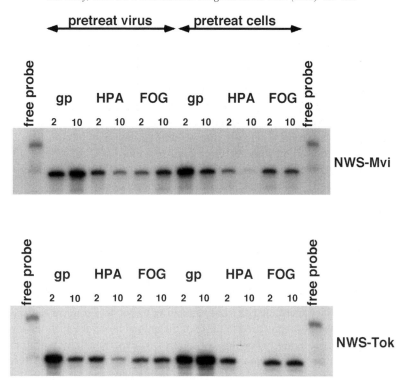

Fig. 5. Carbohydrates of either virus particle or target cell may be involved in virus entry. Cells or virus were pre-treated with 2 or 10 μg lectin as described in the text, then the infection carried out with unbound lectin either washed away (cells) or diluted to a level that is non-inhibitory (virus). The "untreated" lanes are shown in Fig. 4B.

(lectins) of which the natural function may be in cell adhesion. Addition of HPA to the growth medium during virus adsorption and growth inhibited both NWS-Tok and NWS-Mvi infection of MDCK cells. These data strongly suggest that oligosaccharides, particularly those containing terminal α-linked GalNAc, act as cellular receptors for influenza A viruses.

4. Discussion

4.1. Cellular receptors for viruses

A molecule must satisfy several criteria to be considered as a credible virus receptor: it must bind some part of the surface of the virus particle and such a binding event must lead eventually to virus entry into the cell; and the removal or sequestration of the candidate molecule must have a deleterious effect upon virus infection. Ideally, cell lines lacking the candidate receptor due either to lack of expression or chemical or enzymatic removal should not be infectable by virus, and antibodies recognizing the receptor or soluble forms of the same molecule should be able to compete for virus binding to the cell. Several virus receptors, such as those for some retroviruses, are very restricted in distribution and presumably play important roles in tissue tropism. Others are molecules such as heparan sulfate, widely distributed throughout different tissues and organisms. It is now understood that some viruses require sequential interactions with different molecules for entry. For example, HIV initially binds the lymphocyte surface marker CD4 [23,24], but requires subsequent interactions with lineage-specific chemokine receptors to mediate virus entry [25–29]. Adenoviruses 2 and 5 initially interact with an immunoglobulin family protein designated CAR, also used by some Coxsackie virus strains [30], but require subsequent interaction with RGD-binding integrins for internalization [31,32], while others such as herpesviruses apparently use multiple determinants independently [33–36].

4.2. Receptors for influenza viruses

To date, studies to identify receptors for influenza virus have concentrated on molecules containing sialic acids. It has been clearly demonstrated for influenza A that some virus strains have the capability to discriminate between sialic acids in different linkages. Over time, the usage of a particular linkage by variants of the same subtype may drift from that originally seen [37,38], interpreted as viral adaptation to better recognize the sialic acids available in the human host compared to those of the animal hosts in which the viruses are thought to originate. However, when this was addressed experimentally with transfectant viruses, the specificity of NA drove the adaptation of HA specificity [39]. HA recognition of sialic acid may simply serve to recruit viruses to the cell surface indiscriminately in order to facilitate interaction with a specific molecule required to mediate entry [9,10]. Other viruses binding sialic acids have been shown to discriminate between receptor and "pseudoreceptor" sialic acids [40], with important consequences for virulence in tissue culture systems and tissue tropism in animal hosts. As sialic acid is a ubiquitous modification of both glycoproteins and glycolipids, it is likely that some sialylated molecules will have long residence times on the cell surface, while others may be internalized rapidly. Indeed, the half-life of sialic acid on the cell surface is greater than 8 h for some cell lines [41], suggesting that sialic acids would be poor targets to mediate rapid internalization. Since the 1940s [42–47], work to define influenza virus receptors has concentrated on virus binding without attempts to address virus uptake, much less productive entry events leading to initiation of infection.

4.3. Receptors for hemagglutination and infection are different

As early as 1947, it was noted that at least some virus strains showed discrepancies between their binding to red blood cells and infectivity in chick embryo and mouse lung: for example, hemagglutination by B/Lee/40 was completely abrogated by treatment of red cells with a variety of viral and bacterial sialidases [2,48]. However, treatment of mouse lungs or chick allantoic cavities with sialidase failed to completely protect against B/Lee/40 or some influenza A virus strains [42–44]. More recently, we have demonstrated that at least some virus strains grow to high titers in tissue culture in the presence of excess sialidase, although hemagglutination is abolished [21], and viruses can efficiently initiate infection in desialylated cells, although the yield of virus from multicycle growth may be low [9]. Thus, the receptors for influenza-mediated agglutination of red blood cells and those for infection of tissue culture cells or animal tissues must be distinct.

When reassortant viruses having mismatched specificities of HA (α2,6) and NA (α2,3) were passaged in ovo, variant viruses were selected with reduced HA affinity, thus compensating for the residual sialic acid that aggregated virions [39]. Similar results are seen when mutant viruses are selected in the presence of NA inhibitors. Some viruses selected for growth in the presence of NA inhibitors have lower affinity for red blood cell receptors [49,50]. A mutant virus generated by reverse genetic means (H3 Y98F) has no measurable hemagglutinating ability, but is infectious in tissue culture [51]. Thus, tight binding to sialic acids is not required (and is possibly deleterious) for infection, and indeed, there are no electrostatic interactions between HA-binding site residues and the C1 carboxylate [52], and some influenza viruses require NA activity to mediate infection [53]. This is a requirement of Burnet's "browsing" model for virus entry [10], in which virus particles are recruited to the cell surface by low affinity interactions, allowing the particle to roll across the cell surface in search of a suitable partner to mediate high affinity binding and thence uptake. HA selectivity in influenza A and B viruses seems to be driven by the ability of the NA of the virus to cleave the prevalent sialic acid, rather than directing the virus to specific cell types [54] or surface molecules to mediate entry [55] as is seen for influenza C.

TLC overlay assays showed binding of human influenza viruses to a series of gangliosides having terminal sialyllactosamine residues, with some difference between viruses in preference for 3' and 6' sialyllactosamine [6]. Similar methodology showed that virus can bind sulfatide, a non-sialylated glycolipid which is acidic by virtue of sulfate groups on the terminal galactose residue [56]. Sulfatide inhibits viral infection, but the mechanism has not been further investigated, so it is unknown whether this glycolipid binds to the same site as sialic acid, to a separate site on HA, or binds and inhibits by other means.

4.4. The need to understand influenza binding and entry

Although influenza is one of the best-studied of all viral diseases, it has also proven to be one of the most refractory of common, readily transmissible viruses to prevention and therapy. Amantadine is useful in preventing infection by influenza A viruses, but resistant viruses emerge readily [57,58]. Inhibitors of NA enzyme activity became commercially available in the United States in 1999, but these drugs act only at the end of the virus life-cycle to reduce the efficiency of virus propagation and mutations have been observed in vitro [59,60]. Even when NA inhibitors can still block NA activity, viable viruses arise in vitro with altered receptor affinity or specificity to circumvent the requirement for active NA.

4.5. Identification of potential alternative receptors

Identification of virus-binding proteins or lipids from membranes of permissive cell lines will lead to a better understanding of how influenza infection is established in target cells. If a true high affinity receptor for influenza virus can be found, or routes for influenza virus entry independent of sialic acids can be identified, understanding how these are utilized by the virus may aid in the design of the next generation of anti-influenza therapeutics.

4.5.1. Influenza-binding proteins

We have used virus overlay blots to detect H1 influenza-binding molecules found in MDCK cell membrane preparations. A similar approach was previously used to identify annexin V as a receptor for several influenza virus strains including fowl plague virus (FPV) [16,17]. We found that when BSA or polyvinylpyrrolidone were used as blocking reagents, many proteins, including several proteins in the 33–36 kDa range expected for the known MDCK annexins [61,62], bound primary or secondary antibody, even in the absence of virus. Only when dry milk (2%) was used did we observe convincing virus-specific binding. Since the bovine milk proteins contained sialic acid (we measured approximately 2.5 nmol/mg, or 0.1% by weight), our binding assay probably biases detection in favor of proteins which interact with influenza virus by means other than low-affinity interactions with sialic acid. Our overlay system consistently identified a protein of approximately 85 kDa in molecular weight as a ligand for H1 HA. Work to identify this protein is ongoing.

4.5.2. Oligosaccharides as alternative virus receptors

Our data suggest that oligosaccharides, particularly those containing terminal α-linked GalNAc, may act both as cell surface receptors for the virus and as potential ligands on the virus for cell surface lectins. Crystallographic evidence exists of a secondary binding site on the surface of H3 HA, which is apparently capable of binding oligosaccharides without requiring direct interaction with sialic acid, in addition to the more conserved site at the tip of the molecule that binds sialic acid [63]. This secondary binding site is not well-conserved at the level of protein sequence and has not been further characterized. The involvement of cell surface oligosaccharide-binding proteins has already been demonstrated to be important in the uptake of virus by macrophages, where the mannose receptor, a type C lectin, mediates uptake of virus apparently by binding mannose-containing oligosaccharide linked to the HA and NA glycoproteins of the virus [64]. Similar binding by soluble lectins (collectins) such as mouse lung surfactant protein-D and mouse serum mannose-binding lectin has been observed [65]. Binding of virus by soluble lectins and lectin-mediated internalization of virus by macrophages is thought to represent innate immunity to the virus, but similar molecules may function in productive virus infection of permissive cells. Virus binding and inhibition of virus infection by sulfatide, a sulfated glycolipid, have been previously observed [56], but our data open the possibility that the use of carbohydrates other than sialic acid may be widespread.

Our data suggest that in addition to sialic acid, other receptors exist to which influenza viruses may bind and which may be involved in mediating virus uptake into the cell. We have demonstrated specific binding to an immobilized, apparently non-sialylated protein molecule in vitro, and that HPA, a lectin recognizing terminal α-linked N-acetylgalactos-amine (GalNAc), interferes with virus infection in a dose-dependent manner. A deeper understanding of the interactions between influenza virus and host cells may lead to the identification of further potential targets for prophylactic or therapeutic drugs for this, one of the most common and historically most deadly of the world's diseases.

Acknowledgements

This work was supported by NIH Grant AI18203 (to GMA) and a studentship from the OUHSC Department of Biochemistry and Molecular Biology (SJS). We thank Dr. Lalitha Venkatramani for characterizing the rosettes, and Dr. Richard Cummings, OUHSC Biochemistry and Molecular Biology, for many helpful discussions.

References

[1] G.K. Hirst, The agglutination of red cells by allantoic fluid of chick embryos infected with influenza virus, Science 94 (1941) 22–23.

[2] F.M. Burnet, J.F. McCrea, J.D. Stone, Modification of human red cells by virus action: I. The receptor gradient for virus action in human red cells, Br. J. Exp. Pathol. 27 (1946) 228–236.

[3] A. Gottschalk, Carbohydrate residue of a urine mucoprotein inhibiting influenza virus haemagglutination, Nature 170 (1952) 662–663.

[4] A. Gottschalk, The specific enzyme of influenza virus and *Vibrio cholerae*, Biochim. Biophys. Acta 23 (1957) 645–646.

[5] G.N. Rogers, J.C. Paulson, R.S. Daniels, J.J. Skehel, I.A. Wilson, D.C. Wiley, Single amino acid substitutions in influenza haemagglutinin change receptor binding specificity, Nature 304 (1983) 76–78.

[6] Y. Suzuki, T. Nakao, T. Ito, et al., Structural determination of gangliosides that bind to influenza A, B, and C viruses by an improved binding assay: strain-specific receptor epitopes in sialo-sugar chains, Virology 189 (1) (1992) 121–131.

[7] M.N. Matrosovich, A.S. Gambaryan, S. Teneberg, et al., Avian influenza A viruses differ from human viruses by recognition of sialyloligosaccharides and gangliosides and by a higher conservation of the HA receptor-binding site, Virology 233 (1997) 224–234.

[8] C. Liu, G.M. Air, Selection and characterization of a neuraminidase-minus mutant of influenza virus and its rescue by cloned neuraminidase genes, Virology 194 (1993) 403–407.

[9] S.J. Stray, R.D. Cummings, G.M. Air, Influenza virus infection of desialylated cells, Glycobiology 10 (2000) 649–658.

[10] F. Burnet, Principles of Animal Virology, Academic Press, New York, 1955.

[11] K.L. Moore, N.L. Stults, S. Diaz, et al., Identification of a specific glycoprotein ligand for P-selectin (CD62) on myeloid cells, J. Cell Biol. 118 (1992) 445–456.

[12] N.G. Wrigley, W.G. Laver, J.C. Downie, Binding of antibodies to isolated hemagglutinin and neuraminidase molecules of influenza virus observed in the electron microscope, J. Mol. Biol. 109 (1977) 405–421.

[13] I.A. Wilson, J.J. Skehel, D.C. Wiley, Structure of the hemagglutinin membrane glycoprotein of influenza virus at 3Å resolution, Nature 289 (1981) 366–373.

[14] D.K. Takemoto, J.J. Skehel, D.C. Wiley, A surface plasmon resonance assay for the binding of influenza virus hemagglutinin to its sialic acid receptor, Virology 217 (1996) 452–458.

[15] K. Zinn, D. DiMaio, T. Maniatis, Identification of two distinct regulatory regions adjacent to the human β-interferon gene, Cell 34 (1983) 865–879.

[16] M. Otto, A. Günther, H. Fan, O. Rick, R.T.C. Huang, Identification of annexin 33 kDa in cultured cells as a binding protein of influenza viruses, FEBS Lett. 356 (1994) 125–129.

[17] R.T.C. Huang, B. Lichtenberg, O. Rick, Involvement of annexin V in the entry of influenza viruses and role of phospholipids in infection, FEBS Lett. 392 (1996) 59–62.

[18] P. Stanley, T. Sudo, J.P. Carver, Differential involvement of cell surface sialic acid in wheat germ agglutinin

binding to parental and wheat germ agglutinin-resistant Chinese hamster ovary cells, J. Cell Biol. 85 (1980) 60–69.

[19] C.G. Gahmberg, M. Tolvanen, Nonmetabolic radiolabeling and tagging of glycoconjugates, Methods Enzymol. 230 (1994) 23–44.

[20] G.N. Rogers, B.L. D'Souza, Receptor binding properties of human and animal H1 influenza virus isolates, Virology 173 (1989) 317–322.

[21] P. Yang, A. Bansal, C. Liu, G.M. Air, Hemagglutinin specificity and neuraminidase coding capacity of neuraminidase-deficient influenza viruses, Virology 229 (1997) 155–165.

[22] G.M. Air, W.G. Laver, Red cells bound to influenza virus N9 neuraminidase are not released by the N9 neuraminidase activity, Virology 211 (1995) 278–284.

[23] A.G. Dalgleish, P.C.L. Beverly, P.R. Clapham, P.H. Crawford, M.F. Greaves, R.A. Weiss, The CD4 (T4) antigen is an essential component of the receptor for the AIDS retrovirus, Nature 312 (1984) 763–767.

[24] D. Klatzmann, E. Champagne, S. Chamaret, et al., T-lymphocyte T4 molecule behaves as the receptor for human retrovirus LAV, Nature 312 (1984) 767–768.

[25] Y. Feng, C.C. Broder, P.E. Kennedy, E.A. Berger, HIV-1 entry cofactor: functional cDNA cloning of a seven-transmembrane G protein-coupled receptor, Science 272 (1996) 872–876.

[26] H. Deng, R. Liu, W. Ellmeier, et al., Identification of a major co-receptor for primary isolates of HIV-1, Nature 381 (1996) 661–666.

[27] T. Dragic, V. Litwin, G.P. Allaway, et al., HIV-1 entry into CD4+ cells is mediated by the chemokine receptor CC-CKR-5, Nature 381 (1996) 667–673.

[28] G. Alkhatib, C. Combadiere, C.C. Broder, et al., CC CKR5: A RANTES, MIP-1α, MIP-1β receptor as a fusion cofactor for macrophage-tropic HIV-1, Science 272 (1996) 1955–1958.

[29] H. Choe, M. Farzan, Y. Sun, et al., The β-chemokine receptors CCR3 and CCR5 facilitate infection by primary HIV-1 isolates, Cell 85 (1996) 1135–1148.

[30] J.M. Bergelson, J.A. Cunningham, G. Droguett, et al., Isolation of a common receptor for Coxsackie B viruses and adenoviruses 2 and 5, Science 275 (1997) 1320–1323.

[31] T.J. Wickham, P. Mathias, D.A. Cheresh, G.R. Nemerow, Integrins $\alpha_v\beta_3$ and $\alpha_v\beta_5$ promote adenovirus internalization but not virus attachment, Cell 73 (1993) 309–319.

[32] C.Y. Chiu, P. Mathias, G.R. Nemerow, P.L. Stewart, Structure of adenovirus complexed with its internalization receptor, $\alpha_v\beta_5$ integrin, J. Virol. 73 (1999) 6759–6768.

[33] D. WuDunn, P.G. Spear, Initial interaction of herpes simplex virus with cells is binding to heparan sulfate, J. Virol. 63 (1) (1989) 52–58.

[34] M. Shieh, D. WuDunn, R. Montgomery, J. Esko, P. Spear, Cell surface receptors for herpes simplex virus are heparan sulfate proteoglycans, J. Cell Biol. 116 (5) (1992) 1273–1281.

[35] R. Montgomery, M. Warner, B. Lum, P. Spear, Herpes simplex virus-1 entry into cells mediated by a novel member of the TNF/NGF receptor family, Cell 87 (1996) 427–436.

[36] R. Geraghty, C. Krummenacher, G. Cohen, R. Eisenberg, P. Spear, Entry of alphaherpesviruses mediated by poliovirus receptor-related protein 1 and poliovirus receptor, Science 280 (1998) 1618–1620.

[37] G.N. Rogers, J.C. Paulson, Receptor determinants of human and animal influenza virus isolates: differences in the receptor specificity of the H3 hemagglutinin based on species of origin, Virology 127 (1983) 361–373.

[38] L.G. Baum, J.C. Paulson, The N2 neuraminidase of human influenza virus has acquired a substrate specificity complementary to the hemagglutinin receptor specificity, Virology 180 (1991) 10–15.

[39] N.V. Kaverin, A.S. Gambaryan, N.V. Bovin, et al., Postreassortment changes in influenza A virus hemagglutinin restoring functional HA–NA match, Virology 244 (1998) 315–321.

[40] P.H. Bauer, C. Cui, T. Stehle, S.C. Harrison, J.A. DeCaprio, T.L. Benjamin, Discrimination between sialic acid-containing receptors and pseudoreceptors regulates polyomavirus spread in the mouse, J. Virol. 73 (1999) 5826–5832.

[41] J.S. Reichner, S.W. Whitehart, G.W. Hart, Intracellular trafficking of cell surface sialoglycoconjugates, J. Biol. Chem. 263 (1988) 16316–16326.

[42] J.D. Stone, Enzymic modification of the reaction between influenza virus and susceptible tissue cells, Nature 159 (1947) 781.

[43] J.D. Stone, Prevention of virus infection with enzyme of V. cholerae: I. Studies with viruses of mumps–influenza group in chick embryos, Aust. J. Exp. Biol. 26 (1948) 53–64.

[44] J.D. Stone, Prevention of virus infection with enzyme of *V. cholerae*: II. Studies with influenza virus in mice, Aust. J. Exp. Biol. 26 (1948) 287–297.

[45] S. Fazekas de St. Groth, Destruction of influenza virus receptors in mouse lung by an enzyme from *V. cholerae*, Aust. J. Exp. Biol. 26 (1948) 29–36.

[46] S. Fazekas de St. Groth, Regeneration of virus receptors in mouse lungs after artificial destruction, Aust. J. Exp. Biol. 26 (1948) 271–285.

[47] S. Fazekas de St. Groth, Viropexis, the mechanism of influenza virus infection, Nature 162 (1948) 294–295.

[48] F.M. Burnet, W.I.B. Beveridge, J. McEwin, W.C. Boake, Studies on the Hirst haemagglutination reaction with influenza and Newcastle disease viruses, Aust. J. Exp. Biol. 23 (1945) 177–182.

[49] S. Bantia, A.A. Ghate, S.L. Ananth, S. Babu, G.M. Air, G.M. Walsh, Generation and characterization of a mutant of influenza A virus selected with the neuraminidase inhibitor BCX-140, Antimicrob. Agents Chemother. 42 (1998) 801–807.

[50] J.L. McKimm-Breschkin, T.J. Blick, A. Sahasrabudhe, et al., Generation and characterization of variants of NWS/G70c influenza virus after in vitro passage in 4-amino-Neu5Ac2en and 4-guanidino-Neu5Ac2en, Antimicrob. Agents Chemother. 40 (1996) 40–46.

[51] J. Martín, S.A. Wharton, Y.P. Lin, et al., Studies of the binding properties of influenza hemagglutinin receptor site mutants, Virology 241 (1998) 101–111.

[52] N.K. Sauter, J.E. Hanson, G.D. Glick, et al., Binding of influenza virus hemagglutinin to analogs of its cell-surface receptor, sialic acid: analysis by proton nuclear magnetic resonance spectroscopy and X-ray crystallography, Biochemistry 31 (40) (1992) 9609–9621.

[53] M. Ohuchi, A. Feldmann, R. Ohuchi, H.-D. Klenk, Neuraminidase is essential for fowl plague virus hemagglutinin to show hemagglutinating activity, Virology 212 (1995) 77–83.

[54] A. Klein, M. Krishna, N.M. Varki, A. Varki, 9-*O*-acetylated sialic acids have widespread but selective expression: analysis using a dual function probe derived from influenza C hemagglutinin-esterase, Proc. Natl. Acad. Sci. U. S. A. 91 (1994) 7782–7786.

[55] G. Zimmer, H.-D. Klenk, G. Herrler, Identification of a 40-kDa cell surface sialoglycoprotein with the characteristics of a major influenza C virus receptor in a Madin Darby canine kidney cell line, J. Biol. Chem. 270 (1995) 17815–17822.

[56] T. Suzuki, A. Sometani, G. Horiike, et al., Sulphatide binds to human and animal influenza A viruses, and inhibits the viral infection, Biochem. J. 318 (1996) 389–393.

[57] J.R. La Montagne, G.J. Galasso, Report of a workshop on clinical studies of the efficacy of amantadine and rimantadine against influenza virus, J. Infect. Dis. 138 (1978) 928–931.

[58] T. Bektimimov, R.J. Douglas, R. Dolin, G. Galasso, V. Krylov, J. Oxford, Current status of amantadine and rimantadine as anti-influenza A agents: memorandum from a WHO meeting, Bull. W. H. O. 63 (1985) 51–56.

[59] T.J. Blick, T. Tiong, A. Sahasrabudhe, et al., Generation and characterization of an influenza virus neuraminidase mutant with decreased sensitivity to the neuraminidase-specific inhibitor 4-Guanidino-Neu5Ac2en, Virology 214 (1995) 475–484.

[60] K.A. Staschke, J.M. Colacino, A.J. Baxter, et al., Molecular basis for the resistance of influenza viruses to 4-guanidino-Neu5Ac2en, Virology 214 (2) (1995) 642–646.

[61] K. Fiedler, F. Lafont, R.G. Parton, K. Simons, Annexin XIIIb: a novel epithelial specific annexin is implicated in vesicular traffic to the apical plasma membrane, J. Cell Biol. 128 (1995) 1043–1053.

[62] T. Harder, V. Gerke, The annexin II2p11(2) complex is the major protein component of the triton X-100-insoluble low-density fraction prepared from MDCK cells in the presence of Ca^{2+}, Biochim. Biophys. Acta 1223 (1994) 375–382.

[63] N.K. Sauter, G.D. Glick, R.L. Crowther, et al., Crystallographic detection of a second ligand binding site in influenza virus hemagglutinin, Proc. Natl. Acad. Sci. U. S. A. 89 (1) (1992) 324–328.

[64] P.C. Reading, J.L. Miller, E.M. Anders, Involvement of the mannose receptor in infection of macrophages by influenza virus, J. Virol. 74 (2000) 5190–5197.

[65] P.C. Reading, L.S. Morey, E.C. Crouch, E.M. Anders, Collectin-mediated antiviral host defense of the lung: evidence from influenza virus infection of mice, J. Virol. 71 (1997) 8204–8212.

[66] I. Goldstein, D. Blake, S. Ebisu, T. Williams, M. La, Carbohydrate binding studies on the *Bandeiraea simplicifolia* I isolectins, J. Biol. Chem. 256 (1981) 3890–3893.

[67] B. Torres, D. McCrumb, D. Smith, Reactivity of lectins from *Helix pomatia*, *Wisteria floribunda*, and

S.J. Stray, G.M. Air / International Congress Series 1219 (2001) 487–502

Dolichos biflorus with glycolipids containing *N*-acetylgalactosamine, Arch. Biochem. Biophys. 262 (1988) 1–11.

[68] R.D. Cummings, Use of lectins in analysis of glycoconjugates, Methods Enzymol. 230 (1994) 66–85.

[69] W.-C. Wang, R.D. Cummings, The immobilized leukoagglutinin from the seeds of *Maackia amurensis* binds with high affinity to complex-type Asn-linked oligosaccharides containing terminal sialic acid linked a-2,3 to penultimate galactose residues, J. Biol. Chem. 263 (1988) 4576–4585.

[70] S.R. Haseley, P. Talaga, J.P. Kamerling, J.F.G. Vliegenthart, Characterization of the carbohydrate binding specificity and kinetic parameters of lectins by using surface plasmon resonance, Anal. Biochem. 274 (1999) 203–210.

[71] N. Shibuya, I. Goldstein, W. Broekaert, M. Nsimba-Lubaki, B. Peeters, W. Peumans, The elderberry (*Sambuccus nigra* L.) bark lectin recognizes the Neu5Ac Gal/GalNAc sequence, J. Biol. Chem. 262 (1987) 1596–1601.

[72] H. Lis, N. Sharon, Lectins as molecules and as tools, Annu. Rev. Biochem. 55 (1986) 35–67.

International Congress Series 1219 (2001) 503–512

Interaction of the influenza virus nucleoprotein with F-actin

Paul Digard*, Debra Elton, Martha Simpson-Holley, Elizabeth Medcalf

Division of Virology, Department of Pathology, University of Cambridge, Tennis Court Road, Cambridge CB2 1QP, UK

Abstract

Introduction: The influenza virus genome is transcribed in the nucleus of infected cells but assembled into progeny virions in the cytoplasm. This is reflected in the cellular distribution of the virus nucleoprotein (NP), a protein which encapsidates genomic RNA to form ribonucleoprotein (RNP) structures: at the early stage post-infection, NP is found in the nucleus, but later it is found predominantly in the cytoplasm. The purpose of this study was to examine the possibility that cytoplasmic NP interacts with actin microfilaments. *Methods*: Bacterially expressed NP was tested for the ability to interact with filamentous (F)-actin in a variety of in vitro assays, and the localisation of actin and exogenously expressed NP in mammalian cells was examined microscopically. *Results*: Purified NP bound actin filaments in vitro and showed partial colocalisation with β-actin in vivo. Electron microscopy showed that NP induced bundling of actin fibres in vitro. In confirmation of this, NP caused a dramatic increase in the low-shear viscosity and light-scattering properties of F-actin suspensions. *Conclusions*: NP binds F-actin in vitro and can alter the mechanical properties of actin filaments. This raises the possibility that influenza virus may use the host-cell cytoskeleton during virus replication. © 2001 Elsevier Science B.V. All rights reserved.

Keywords: Microfilaments; Ribonucleoprotein; Bundling

1. Introduction

The influenza A virus genome consists of eight segments of negative sense single-stranded RNA (vRNA), which are transcribed in infected cells to yield two types of positive

---

* Corresponding author. Tel.: +44-1223-336918; fax: +44-1223-336926.
E-mail address: pd1@mole.bio.cam.ac.uk (P. Digard).

0531-5131/01/$ – see front matter © 2001 Elsevier Science B.V. All rights reserved.
PII: S0531-5131(01)00628-8

sense transcripts: capped and polyadenylated mRNAs, and exact complements (cRNA) which serve as replicative intermediate RNAs for the production of further vRNAs [1]. Four viral proteins are necessary and sufficient to carry out this process [2]: the three subunits of an RNA-dependent RNA polymerase, (PB1, PB2 and PA) and a 55-kDa single strand RNA-binding nucleoprotein (NP). Indeed, the v- and cRNA segments are always associated with these polypeptides to form ribonucleoprotein (RNP) structures [1].

Unusually for an RNA virus, influenza transcription occurs in the nuclei of infected cells [3]. Thus, on initiation of infection, incoming RNPs enter the nucleus, and during infection, newly synthesised RNP proteins also undergo nuclear import. However, progeny virions are assembled in the cytoplasm at the apical plasma membrane and at later times, this is reflected in the cytoplasmic accumulation of NP, generally assumed to be in the form of RNPs [1]. This changing pattern of RNP localisation necessitates regulatory mechanisms and evidence points to the involvement of at least three viral polypeptides; the virion matrix (M1) protein, the minor virion component NS2 and NP itself. M1 is capable of binding to membranes, RNA, NS2 and RNPs, and in the virion is thought to act as the link between the lipid envelope and the packaged RNPs [4]. Moreover, M1 partially localises to the nucleus, where it promotes the export of RNPs [5,6]. NS2, which binds to RNPs via the M1 protein [7], possesses a nuclear export signal, and it has been proposed that NS2 is the viral factor directly responsible for the export of RNPs from the nucleus [8]. In addition, NP possesses the ability to locate to both cytoplasm and nucleus and in the absence of other viral proteins, it shuttles between the two compartments [6], suggesting that it interacts with the cellular nuclear export apparatus in the absence of M1 and NS2. Indeed, we have recently found evidence that NP interacts with the cellular CRM1-mediated nuclear export pathway and that this pathway is important for RNP export during virus infection [9]. However, the question remains: which mechanisms prevent the nuclear re-import of exported RNPs? One well documented method of modulating nuclear import is through interactions with cytoplasmic anchoring proteins [10], and recent work involving cell fractionation and fluorescent staining experiments has suggested that cytoplasmic NP is associated with the cytoskeleton [11,12]. The purpose of the experiments described here was to examine the possibility that NP might directly interact with the actin cytoskeleton.

2. Materials and methods

2.1. Plasmids and protein expression

A plasmid containing the native A/PR/8/34 NP gene under the control of a bacteriophage T7 RNA polymerase promoter (pKT5) has previously been described [13]. A plasmid containing the NP gene fused to *Escherichia coli* maltose-binding protein (pMAL–NP) has also been reported [14]. Maltose-binding protein (MBP) or MBP fused to NP (MBP–NP) were purified from extracts of *E. coli* cultures containing plasmids pMAL-c2 (New England Biolabs) or pMAL–NP by affinity chromatography on amylose resin columns (New England Biolabs) as previously described [14]. The maltose-binding protein (MBP) moiety of MBP–NP was removed by the addition of 2 mM CaCl$_2$ and 0.5% (w/w) of factor Xa protease (New England Biolabs) in an overnight incubation at 14 °C. NP was then purified by ion-exchange chromatography on a MonoQ column (Pharmacia) or a heparin III agarose column (Affinity Chromatography, Isle of Man). Samples were clarified by centrifugation at 390,000 × g$_{av}$ for 15 min before use. For in vitro RNA binding assays, a 178-nucleotide synthetic RNA target was generated by in vitro transcription of plasmid pKT8-Δ 3'5' as previously described [14].

2.2. Actin-binding assays

Purified rabbit muscle actin [14] was polymerised in 100 mM NaCl, 10 mM Tris–Cl pH 8.0, 1 mM MgCl$_2$, 0.1 mM ATP, 0.2 mM EGTA, 1 mM sodium azide (F-buffer). Sedimentation assays contained 3 μM actin in 50 mM NaCl, 10 mM Hepes pH 7.6, 1 mM MgCl$_2$, 10% glycerol, 0.1 mM EDTA, 0.1 mM ATP in a final volume of 100 μl. After mixing, the samples were centrifuged at 200,000 × g$_{av}$ for 20 min at 20 °C before separation into pellet and supernatant fractions. Equivalent amounts of each fraction were analysed by SDS-PAGE and stained with Coomassie brilliant blue dye. For electron microscopy, actin (1 μM) and MBP or MBP–NP were mixed in F-buffer and left on ice for 20 min. Drops (30 μl) were applied to carbon-coated grids for 1 min, rinsed with five drops of F-buffer and five drops of 1% uranyl acetate before blotting dry and viewing in a Philips 208S electron microscope at 20K or 30K × magnification. Light scattering experiments were performed in an LS50B spectrophotometer (Perkin Elmer) using excitation and emission wavelengths of 520 nm (2.5-nm slit widths), with 4 μM actin either in the form of F-actin (in F-buffer), or starting as G-actin (in 5 mM Tris–Cl pH 8.0, 0.1 mM ATP, 0.2 mM CaCl$_2$ [G buffer]) with polymerisation induced by the addition of 100 mM NaCl, 1 mM MgCl$_2$, 1 mM ATP. Reactions were performed at 20 °C. For low-shear viscosity assays, 5 μM G-actin was induced to polymerise in capillary tubes by the addition of 100 mM NaCl, 1 mM MgCl$_2$, 1 mM ATP in the presence and absence of varying molar ratios of NP polypeptides. After overnight incubation at 4 °C, the speed at which a small steel ball fell through the solution was measured [15].

2.3. Transfection of tissue culture cells and indirect immunofluorescence

HeLa cells were infected with a recombinant vaccinia virus encoding T7 RNA polymerase (VTF7; Ref. [16]) at a multiplicity of infection of 5 for 2 h at 37 °C. The cells were washed three times with serum-free medium before transfection with plasmid DNA encoding NP using a cationic liposome mixture (Lipofectin; Gibco), as previously described [14]. After 4-h incubation at 37 °C, the cells were washed with PBS containing 1% newborn calf serum, fixed in PBS containing 4% formaldehyde, and stained for NP using anti-RNP serum as previously described [14] or for β-actin using monoclonal antibody AC-74 (Sigma). Fluorescence was viewed and images captured on an MRC 1024 confocal microscope. Control experiments, where cells were stained with individual fluorescent reagents (as well as untransfected cells), confirmed that the labelling was channel-specific (data not shown).

3. Results

3.1. Binding of NP to F-actin

We tested whether purified NP bound filamentous (F)-actin in vitro using a cosedimentation assay, where F-actin is readily separated from monomeric protein by centrifugation. As shown in Fig. 1a, most of the actin sedimented after centrifugation (lane 2), and only the expected critical monomer concentration of actin (0.1–0.2 μM) remained in the supernatant (lane 1). The bacterially expressed NP purified as a major band of the expected electrophoretic mobility and three shorter NP polypeptides that presumably resulted from proteolytic cleavage of the authentic molecule (lane 5). In the absence of actin, only trace amounts of NP sedimented (lanes 5 and 6). However, when NP was sedimented after mixing with F-actin, the greater proportion of the NP now partitioned into the pellet fraction (lanes 3 and 4), demonstrating its association with actin filaments. Furthermore, NP fused to MBP or to glutathione-*S*-transferase (GST) also cosedimented with actin filaments, while MBP and GST alone did not [14]. The binding of NP to actin filaments was also visualised directly by electron microscopy. Actin filaments incubated with two molar equivalents of MBP formed an essentially random distribution of fibres (Fig. 1b). However, the addition of a similar ratio of MBP–NP to actin induced massive bundling of the filaments (Fig. 1c). Thus, we conclude that NP binds F-actin in vitro.

Previous work has shown that a proportion of NP in influenza virus infected cells colocalises with peripheral F-actin [11,12]. We therefore tested whether similar colocalisation of NP and actin could be observed in the absence of other influenza virus polypeptides. HeLa cells were infected with vaccinia virus vTF7-3 expressing T7 RNA polymerase [16], transfected with plasmid pKT5 containing the NP gene under the control of a T7 RNA polymerase promoter, and 4 h later, examined for NP and β-actin distribution by indirect immunofluorescence. A relatively high dose of PKT5 was transfected ($\sim$0.3

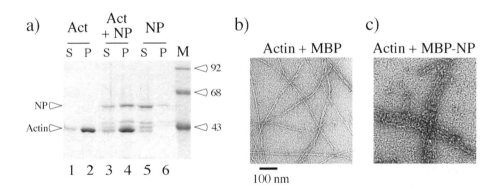

Fig. 1. F-actin-binding activity of NP. (a) Cosedimentation of NP and actin. NP (1.5 μM), actin (Act; 3 μM) and an NP–actin mixture as labelled were centrifuged and separated into supernatant (S) and pellet (P) fractions before analysis by SDS-PAGE and staining with Coomassie brilliant blue. Arrows indicate the named polypeptides and molecular mass markers (M; kDa) are shown on the right. (b, c) Electron microscopy of actin filaments mixed with three-fold molar excesses of MBP (b) and MBP–NP (c). Scale bar: 100 nm.

μg4 × 10^4 cells) to bias NP towards cytoplasmic accumulation [14]. As expected, β-actin was largely peripheral and concentrated in areas of membrane ruffling (Fig. 2b, arrows). NP was diffusely distributed throughout the cytoplasm but also showed areas of concentration at the periphery of the cell in membrane ruffles, which in many cases colocalised with β-actin (Fig. 2a, arrows). In addition, colocalisation of transfected NP was also observed with actin stress fibres [14]. This is consistent with the ability of NP to bind F-actin in vivo as well as in vitro.

Electron microscopic examination of NP–actin complexes suggested that NP is an actin-bundling polypeptide (Fig. 1c). To examine this further, we followed the physical size of actin fibres in solution by light scattering. The ability of F-actin to scatter light is dependent on filament length and is further enhanced by filament bundling [15]. In the absence of actin, 0.5 μM MBP–NP showed a low level ($\sim$100 U) of light scattering that was relatively consistent over 20 min (Fig. 3; NP). A similarly stable signal of around 170 U was obtained from a 4 μM suspension of F-actin that had previously been allowed to polymerise to equilibrium (data not shown, but see G → F trace in Fig. 3). However, when 0.5 μm MBP–NP was added to this F-actin suspension, a very rapid increase in light scattering to around 500 U was observed (Fig. 3; F + NP), suggesting bundling of the actin filaments. Similar results were obtained when G-actin was allowed to polymerise into F-actin in the presence of NP. In the absence of NP, a 4-μM solution of G-actin showed low-level light scattering that after the addition of salt, ATP and MgCl$_2$ to induce polymerisation, increased over time with the characteristic sigmoidal curve (Fig. 3; G → F), indicative of the lag phase imposed by the initially rate-limiting step of the formation of nucleation centres [15]. However, when G-actin was allowed to polymerise in the presence of 0.5 μM MBP–NP, no lag phase was evident and the steady-state scattering intensity reached after 20 min was much higher (Fig. 3; G → F + NP). This indicates that NP causes the polymerisation of longer and/or bundled actin filaments.

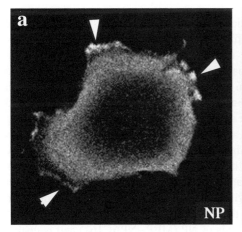
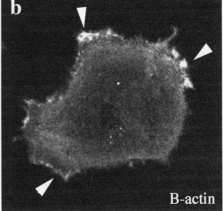

Fig. 2. Colocalisation of NP and β-actin. HeLa cells were transfected with 0.3 μg of pKT5 and analysed 4 h later by confocal microscopy after fixation and indirect immunofluorescent staining for (a) NP and (b) β-actin.

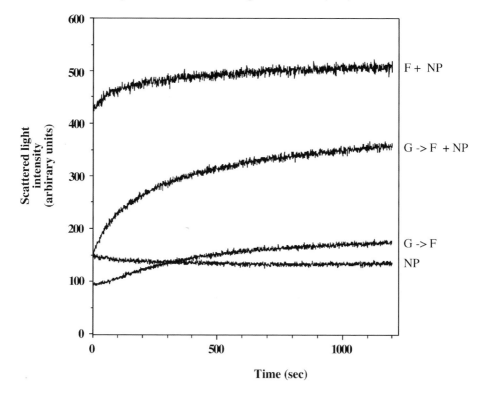

Fig. 3. Light scattering analysis of actin and NP. The scattering intensity at 520 nm of solutions of MBP–NP and actin (4 μM) in the indicated mixtures was followed over 1200 s. In certain cases, actin was added as F-actin (F), in others, as G-actin (G) and induced to polymerise by the addition of NaCl, ATP and MgCl$_2$ to the buffer.

The finding that NP induced the formation of actin bundles suggested that it might change the mechanical properties of microfilaments. To test this hypothesis, we investigated the effects of NP addition on the apparent viscosity of actin filaments. The viscosity of an F-actin solution is proportional to the length and number of filaments and these properties can be altered by the addition of actin-binding proteins [15]. The approach used was to allow the polymerisation of G-actin in capillary tubes in the presence and absence of MBP–NP and then measure the apparent viscosity of the solution by falling ball viscometry [15]. In the absence of NP, relatively low viscosity solutions of F-actin were formed, as assessed by the speed at which a ball bearing fell through the capillary (Fig. 4a). However, the apparent viscosity of the solutions increased as increasing amounts of MBP–NP were included in the polymerisation reactions. Low molar ratios of NP–actin (<0.4:1) caused only modest increases in viscosity, but higher ratios caused a dramatic increase (Fig. 4a). As a control, we tested the effects of adding a truncated version of MBP–NP which lacks the C-terminal two-thirds of NP (MBP–NPΔC161) and is unable to bind actin (data not shown). No significant increase (or decrease) in apparent viscosity of the actin solution was seen, even with equimolar ratios of this mutant NP polypeptide

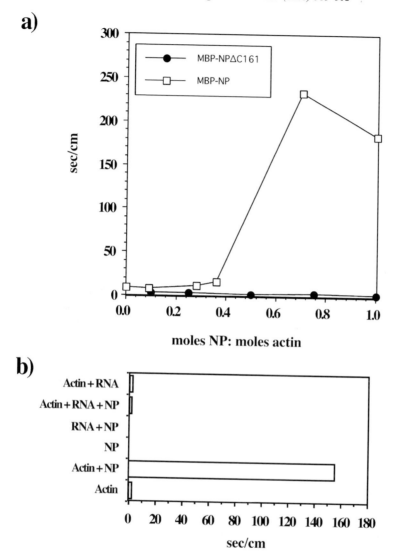

Fig. 4. Low-shear viscosity analysis of actin and NP. (a) Titration of WT MBP–NP and MBP–NPΔC161. Solutions (5 μM) of G-actin were allowed to polymerise overnight at 4 °C in the presence of increasing amounts of MBP–NP polypeptides before analysis by falling-ball viscometry. (b) The indicated mixes of actin (5 μM), MBP–NP (3.5 μM) and a 178-nucleotide transcript (0.4 μM) were analysed as above.

(Fig. 4a). Thus, NP can alter the mechanical properties of an actin gel, again consistent with its ability to bundle actin fibres.

Much of the NP in infected cells exists in the form of a complex with viral RNA. Previously, we have shown that the RNA- and actin-binding activities of NP are separate and that ternary complexes of NP, RNA and actin can form [14]. We therefore tested whether NP–RNA complexes also increased the viscosity of F-actin solutions. Polymerisation reactions were set up containing various combinations of actin, MBP–NP and a 178-nucleotide RNA transcript corresponding to influenza virus segment 8 with the coding sequences deleted. Solutions of NP or NP and RNA had no measurable apparent viscosity in the absence of actin (Fig. 4b). Actin alone showed relatively low viscosity and this was not altered by the addition of RNA (Fig. 4b). As before, a mixture of NP and actin showed a dramatic increase in apparent viscosity, but this was abolished by the further addition of RNA (Fig. 4b). This suggests that NP–RNA complexes interact with F-actin in a different manner to free NP.

4. Discussion

Two recent studies suggested that influenza virus NP interacts with microfilaments of the host cell cytoskeleton late in virus infection [11,12]. Both reports found that NP partitioned into cytoskeleton-containing pools during biochemical fractionation of infected cells, that NP colocalised with microfilaments, especially at the cell periphery and that disruption of microfilaments with cytochalasins altered the distribution of NP. Here, we confirm and extend these observations by showing that NP binds directly to F-actin in vitro and is capable of inducing filament bundling (Figs. 1, 3 and 4). We also provide evidence that NP associates with actin filaments in vivo in the absence of other influenza proteins (Fig. 2). Furthermore, in an extension of the study reported here, we have shown that complexes containing F-actin, NP and RNA could be formed and have identified point mutations in NP, which specifically weaken the NP–actin interaction [14].

The question therefore arises as to what role(s) the NP–actin interaction might play in the virus lifecycle. The finding that NP induces actin bundling in vitro (Figs. 1, 3 and 4) raises the possibility that the virus might specifically modify the actin cytoskeleton during infection. However, influenza virus infection does not cause major alterations in the microfilament network until very late in infection when the cells begin to apoptose (data not shown). More subtle modifications have not yet been ruled out, and this is a worthwhile area for further experimentation. We note though, that most of the NP in infected cells is thought to be bound to RNA [1] and that NP did not cause the dramatic changes in actin viscosity when in the presence of RNA (Fig. 4).

From analogy with the ways other viral and intracellular pathogens subvert the actin cytoskeleton [17] roles in intracellular trafficking of viral components, viral transcription and assembly and release of virions are possible. The hypothesis that influenza uses microfilaments for the purpose of directing the intracellular localisation of RNPs is perhaps supported by the behaviour of NP mutants with weakened affinity for actin: we have shown that in the absence of other influenza virus polypeptides, these mutant NP molecules displayed an increased propensity to accumulate in the nucleus. This suggested the possibility that actin-binding might serve to retain RNPs in the cytoplasm [14]. The RNP particles of some paramyxoviruses are associated with the actin cytoskeleton, and in the case of human parainfluenza virus type 3, actin stimulates virus transcription [18]. However, the ability of NP mutants to support transcription and replication of a model influenza virus segment did not correlate with their affinity for F-actin [14], arguing against actin playing a significant role in influenza virus transcription. The question of whether actin plays a role during influenza virus budding is an interesting one. Although disruption of microfilaments with cytochalasins does not inhibit the assembly and release of spherical influenza virions, an intact actin cytoskeleton is necessary for the formation of filamentous virus particles [19]. Recent work from our laboratory suggests that actin microfilaments are involved in maintaining the correct organisation of the plasma membrane lipid rafts that the virus is thought to bud from (unpublished experiments). However, it remains to be determined whether microfilaments play other roles during the assembly of filamentous particles.

The ultimate determination of the role(s) of the actin cytoskeleton in influenza virus infection requires further experimentation. An interesting avenue will be to try and create mutant viruses containing NP mutants deficient for actin-binding, using the recently described systems for influenza virus reverse genetics [20,21].

Acknowledgements

We are grateful to Drs. B. Pope and A. Weeds for the gift of actin and their expertise. This work was supported by grants from the Royal Society, Wellcome Trust (nos. 048911 and 059151) and Medical Research Council (no. G9901213) to PD. PD is a Royal Society University Research fellow.

References

[1] R.A. Lamb, R.M. Krug, Orthomyxoviridae: the viruses and their replication, in: B.N. Fields, D.M. Knipe, P.M. Howley (Eds.), Fields Virology, Lippincott-Raven, Philadelphia, 1996, pp. 1353–1396.

[2] T.-S. Huang, P. Palese, M. Krystal, Determination of influenza virus proteins required for genome replication, J. Virol. 64 (1990) 5669–5673.

[3] C. Herz, E. Stavnezer, R.M. Krug, Influenza virus, an RNA virus, synthesizes its messenger RNA in the nucleus of infected cells, Cell 26 (1981) 391–400.

[4] G. Whittaker, M. Bui, A. Helenius, The role of M1 in nuclear import and export in influenza virus infection, Trends Cell Biol. 6 (1996) 67–71.

[5] K. Martin, A. Helenius, Nuclear transport of influenza virus ribonucleoproteins: the viral matrix protein (M1) promotes export and inhibits import, Cell 67 (1991) 117–130.

[6] G. Whittaker, M. Bui, A. Helenius, Nuclear trafficking of influenza virus ribonucleoproteins in heterokaryons, J. Virol. 70 (1996) 2743–2756.

[7] J. Yasuda, S. Nakada, A. Kato, T. Toyoda, A. Ishihama, Molecular assembly of influenza virus: association of the NS2 protein with virion matrix, Virology 196 (1993) 249–255.

[8] R.E. O'Neill, J. Talon, P. Palese, The influenza virus NEP (NS2 protein) mediates the nuclear export of viral ribonucleoproteins, EMBO J. 17 (1998) 288–296.

[9] D. Elton, M. Simpson-Holley, K. Archer, L. Medcalf, R. Hallam, J. McCauley, P. Digard, Interaction of the influenza virus nucleoprotein with the cellular CRM1-mediated nuclear export pathway. J. Virol. 75 (2001) 408–419.

[10] E.A. Nigg, Nucleocytoplasmic transport: signals, mechanisms and regulation, Nature 386 (1997) 779–787.

[11] R.T. Avalos, Z. Yu, D.P. Nayak, Association of influenza virus NP and M1 proteins with cellular cytoskeletal elements in influenza virus infected cells, J. Virol. 71 (1997) 2947–2958.

[12] M. Husain, C.M. Gupta, Interactions of viral matrix protein and nucleoprotein with the host cell cytoskeletal actin in influenza viral infection, Curr. Sci. 73 (1997) 40–47.

[13] V. Blok, C. Cianci, K.W. Tibbles, S.C. Inglis, M. Krystal, P. Digard, Inhibition of the influenza virus RNA-dependent RNA polymerase by antisera directed against the carboxy-terminal region of the PB2 subunit, J. Gen. Virol. 77 (1996) 1025–1033.

[14] P. Digard, D. Elton, K. Bishop, E. Medcalf, A. Weeds, B. Pope, Modulation of nuclear localization of the influenza virus nucleoprotein through interaction with actin filaments, J. Virol. 73 (1999) 2222–2231.

[15] J.A. Cooper, Actin filament assembly and organization in vitro, in: K.L. Carraway, C.A.C. Carraway (Eds.), The Cytoskeleton: A Practical Approach, IRL Press, Oxford, 1992, pp. 47–71.

[16] T.R. Fuerst, P.L. Earl, B. Moss, Use of a hybrid vaccinia virus-T7 RNA polymerase system for expression of target genes, Mol. Cell Biol. 7 (1987) 2538–2544.

[17] S. Cudmore, I. Reckman, M. Way, Viral manipulations of the actin cytoskeleton, Trends Biochem. Sci. 5 (1997) 142–148.

[18] B.P. De, A. Lesoon, A.K. Banerjee, Human parainfluenza virus type 3 transcription in vitro: role of cellular actin in mRNA synthesis, J. Virol. 65 (1991) 3268–3275.

[19] P.C. Roberts, W.R. Compans, Host cell dependence of viral morphology, Proc. Natl. Acad. Sci. U. S. A. 95 (1998) 5746–5751.

[20] G. Neumann, T. Watanabe, H. Ito, H. Watanabe, S. Goto, P. Gao, M. Hughes, D.R. Perez, R. Donis, E. Hoffmann, G. Hobom, Y. Kawaoka, Generation of influenza A viruses entirely from cloned cDNAs, Proc. Natl. Acad. Sci. U. S. A. 96 (1999) 9345–9350.

[21] E. Fodor, L. Devenish, O.G. Engelhardt, P. Palese, G.G. Brownlee, A. García-Sastre, Rescue of influenza A virus from recombinant DNA, J. Virol. 73 (1999) 9679–9682.

International Congress Series 1219 (2001) 513–520

Virus versus host: modulation of the host α/β interferon pathways by the influenza A virus NS1 protein

Mirella Salvatore, Adolfo García-Sastre*

Department of Microbiology, Mount Sinai School of Medicine, Box 1124, One Gustave Levy Place, New York, NY 10029, USA

Abstract

α/β Interferons (IFN) represent one of the first host responses against viral infection. IFN activates a signaling cascade involving multiple genes and pathways leading to the stop of viral replication. However, many viruses have developed mechanisms to overcome this first line of the host defense. We studied the IFN antagonist properties of the NS1 protein of influenza A virus. The NS1 protein is a dsRNA binding protein. Since dsRNAs produced during viral infection are potent activators of the IFN cascade, sequestering of dsRNA by the NS1 protein might prevent the IFN response during influenza virus infection. To test in vivo the anti-IFN activity of NS1, we investigated the biological properties of a recombinant influenza virus lacking the NS1 gene (delNS1). delNS1 virus replication is highly compromised in IFN competent hosts. However, this mutant virus replicates efficiently in IFN deficient hosts. Moreover, infection with delNS1 virus stimulates IFN production by activating NF-κB and IFN regulatory factor 3 (IRF-3) transcription factors. DelNS1 virus reacquires virulence and replicates in lungs of PKR −/− mice, also suggesting an important role of NS1 in the inhibition of PKR, an important component of the IFN system. These data underline the importance of NS1-mediated inhibition of IFN activated pathways in the pathogenesis of influenza A virus infection. © 2001 Elsevier Science B.V. All rights reserved.

Keywords: Influenza virus; NS1 protein; α/β Interferon; Interferon-stimulated pathways; IRF-3; PKR; NK-kB

1. Introduction

The interaction between an infectious foreign agent and the host starts a series of attack and counterattack mechanisms that may end with (i) the victory of the host and the

---

* Corresponding author. Tel.: +1-212-241-7769; fax: +1-212-534-1684.
E-mail address: adolfo.garcia-sastre@mssm.edu (A. García-Sastre).

0531-5131/01/$ – see front matter © 2001 Elsevier Science B.V. All rights reserved.
PII: S 0 5 3 1 - 5 1 3 1 (0 1) 0 0 6 3 4 - 3

clearance of the infection, or (ii) the victory of the pathogen, which replicates, induces disease, and/or establish persistent infection, and propagates to new hosts. In this battle, interferon (IFN) plays a critical role. Type I (α/β) IFN and type II (γ) IFN are quickly secreted after infection by all (type I) or specialized immune cells (type II) to defend the organism from a new pathogen. However, viruses have evolved intriguing mechanisms to prevent the IFN-mediated antiviral responses [1]. This review will focus on the role of the NS1 protein of influenza virus as an inhibitor of the type I IFN system during influenza virus infection.

2. Initiation of the IFN response

IFN was discovered in the late 1950s [2] as a cellular released factor that was able to *interfere* with viral replication. However, it took many years to understand its effectors, and only a few out of the many IFN-activated genes/pathways are now fully understood. There are at least 12 subtypes of αIFN and 1 subtype βIFN. Functions of all these different IFN species are still largely unknown but all α/β IFNs act through the same receptor [3].

Upon viral infection, the generation of dsRNA during viral replication stimulates IFN production. This is a very fast event and type I IFN is released only a few hours after the first contact with the pathogen. This rapid response is mediated by constitutively expressed transcriptional regulators, such as the IFN regulatory factor 3 (IRF-3). The importance of IRF-3 in the initiation of the innate antiviral response has only recently been demonstrated [4–7]. After virus infection or exposure to dsRNA, IRF-3 is rapidly activated by phosphorylation of several C-terminal serine and threonine residues. Phosphorylation of IRF-3 results in its nuclear accumulation, where it assembles with other transcription factors and contributes to the induction of the transcription of specific defense genes, including βIFN.

Another critical factor in the regulation of βIFN transcription is NF-κB. Under physiological conditions, NF-κB is retained in the cell cytoplasm by its bound inhibitor IκB. As a response to an external offence (i.e. bacterial or viral infection), IκB kinase (IKK) gets activated, leading to phosphorylation of IκB, which gets released from its complex with NF-κB. Phosphorylated IκB undergoes proteosome-mediated degradation while NFκB is free to migrate into the nucleus where it contributes to the transcriptional stimulation of several genes including βIFN [8].

3. IFN signaling

After production by the infected cells, α/β IFN is released and binds its receptor on the same cells or on neighboring cells. IFN binding induces dimerization of the receptor, resulting in activation of the Janus kinases JAK1 and Tyk2. Activated JAK1 and Tyk2 induce tyrosine phosphorylation of the receptor. The phosphorylated tyrosines now provide a docking site for the STAT proteins. Upon binding, STAT1 and STAT2 become themselves activated by phosphorylation, form heterodimers, recruit IRF-9 protein and translocate to the nucleus. In the nucleus, this protein complex, also called IFN-stimulated gene factor 3 (ISGF3), modulates the expression of target genes by activation of IFN-stimulated response element- (ISRE-) containing promoter(s) [3].

4. PKR

α/β IFN regulates the transcription of many genes, some of which are involved in the establishment of an 'antiviral state' [9]. Among the latter, one of the most extensively studied is the dsRNA activated protein kinase (PKR) gene. PKR is constitutively expressed but its synthesis is increased by IFN. However, PKR is usually in an inactive form and requires activation to display kinase activity. Activation of PKR is triggered by binding to dsRNA which is produced during viral infection. After activation, PKR inactivates by phosphorylation the translation factor eIF-2α stopping protein synthesis [10].

5. The NS1 protein of influenza A virus, an antagonist of the α/β IFN response

The NS1 protein of influenza A virus is expressed from RNA segment 8. This segment also encodes the NEP protein through alternatively splicing. The NS1 protein is produced early during influenza virus infection, can be found in both the nucleus and the cytoplasm and is one of the most abundant proteins in infected cells. While the NEP has been recently characterized as a nuclear export factor for the viral RNA segments [11], the role of the NS1 protein has been linked for many years to the regulation of viral and cellular protein expression. This protein has been implicated in enhancement of translation [12–14], inhibition of splicing [15,16], inhibition of host mRNA polyadenylation [17] and inhibition of nuclear export of host mRNAs [15,18,19]. In addition, early studies demonstrated that the NS1 protein blocks the dsRNA induced activation of PKR [20]. This activity was dependent on the ability of the NS1 protein to bind to dsRNA [21], and then might be mediated by competition between NS1 and PKR for the PKR activator. Nevertheless, direct interactions between these two proteins, rather than competition for binding to dsRNA, might be responsible for the inhibition of PKR by the NS1 protein [22].

In order to understand the biological role of the NS1 protein during influenza virus infection, we compared the phenotypic characteristics of wild type influenza A virus with those of a recombinant influenza virus lacking the NS1 gene [23]. Interestingly, delNS1 virus was unable to efficiently replicate in IFN competent systems such as 10-day-old embryonated eggs or MDCK cells, and showed an attenuated phenotype in immunocompetent mice. However, delNS1 virus was able to replicate nearly as well as the wild-type virus in systems where the IFN pathways were altered, such as Vero cells or 6-day-old eggs [23,24]. Moreover, this mutant influenza virus regained virulence and ability to replicate in lungs of STAT1 $-/-$ mice [23]. These experiments were the first to demonstrate in vivo that the NS1 protein protects influenza A virus from the cellular IFN response.

Evidence that the NS1 protein of influenza A virus inhibits the expression of IFN-stimulated genes came from experiments showing that infection with delNS1 virus, the recombinant influenza virus lacking the NS1 gene, resulted in clear stimulation of an ISRE-containing promoter at conditions in which this activation was not observed in cells infected with wild-type influenza A virus [23]. Moreover, expression of α and β IFN mRNAs was readily detected in MEF or HEC1b cells infected with delNS1 virus but not in the same cells infected with wild-type influenza A virus [25,26]. These data suggest that NS1 protein prevents the synthesis of type I IFN during influenza A virus infection. Interestingly, a recombinant influenza A virus expressing a truncated form of the NS1 protein which retained its RNA-binding domain was still able to prevent the synthesis of type I IFN in infected cells [26].

A potential mechanism by which the NS1 protein might inhibit the α/β IFN system of the host is by binding to and sequestering dsRNA generated during influenza virus infection, therefore preventing dsRNA-activated pathways, including the IFN pathways (Fig. 1). In fact, prevention of the activation of IFN regulatory factor 3 (IRF-3), a key regulator of α/β IFN gene expression which can be stimulated by dsRNA, is one of the mechanisms by which the NS1 protein appears to inhibit the induction of IFN expression in infected cells [25]. Thus, IRF-3 activation is prevented in wild-type influenza virus-infected cells but not in cells infected with delNS1 virus. Inhibition of IRF-3 activation could also be achieved by the expression of wild-type NS1 protein in trans, not only in delNS1 virus-infected cells but also in cells infected with a heterologous RNA virus (Newcastle disease virus). However, expression of a mutant NS1 that lacked a functional RNA binding domain (R38AK41A-NS1) did not block the activation of IRF-3 in delNS1 virus-infected cells [25].

We also investigated whether the NS1 protein was able to prevent the activation of NF-κB, which together with activated IRF and ATF2/c-Jun, cooperates in the induction of βIFN production upon virus infection or dsRNA treatment [27]. We found that during infection with delNS1 virus, there was a strong and maintained activation of NF-κB while this activation is only marginal in wild-type virus infected cells [26]. As expected, expression of dominant negative mutants of the NF-κB pathway, such as IκB and IKKβ mutant proteins, resulted in inhibition of both NF-κB activation and βIFN expression in delNS1 infected cells. NF-κB activation and βIFN expression was also inhibited in response to virus infection or dsRNA treatment when cells were transfected with a plasmid expressing the dsRNA-binding domain of the NS1 protein. To confirm these results, we used a recombinant influenza A virus expressing a truncated NS1 protein of 126 amino acids, containing the dsRNA-binding domain. Consistent with the previous results, NS1-126 virus did behave as wild-type influenza A virus and was able to prevent the activation of NF-κB [26]. These data demonstrate that the RNA binding domain of the NS1 protein is essential and sufficient to mediate the inhibition of NF-κB and consequently βIFN induction during influenza A virus infection of tissue culture cells.

In addition to inhibiting the expression of α/β IFN, the NS1 protein also appears to inhibit the activation of PKR, a dsRNA-activated enzyme which is transcriptionally induced by IFN and which inhibits protein synthesis when activated. Thus, temperature-sensitive influenza A virus mutants with mutations in the NS1 gene exhibited defects in protein synthesis at the nonpermissive temperature that correlated with an increased level

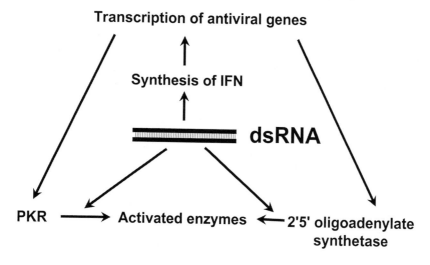

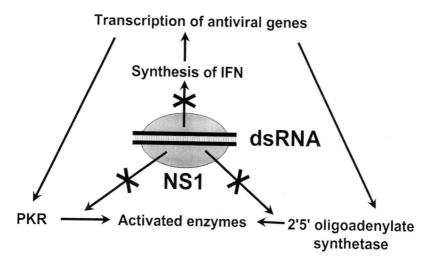

Fig. 1. Antiviral pathways inhibited by the NS1 protein of influenza A virus. dsRNA generated during viral infection triggers the production of IFN, which in turn activates transcription of IFN-stimulated genes, including the dsRNA-activated antiviral enzymes PKR and 2′-5′ oligoadenylate synthetase. The influenza virus NS1 protein, by virtue of its dsRNA-binding properties, inhibits the dsRNA-mediated activation of the host antiviral pathways.

of activated (phosphorylated) PKR and inactivated (phosphorylated) eIF-2α [28]. PKR activation was also readily observed in cells infected with delNS1 virus, in contrast to wild-type influenza A virus [29]. In these experiments, infection of W138 cells with delNS1 virus clearly shifted the balance between phosphorylated and unphosphorylated

PKR towards the activated form of PKR. This shift was almost as pronounced as the one observed upon transfection of cells with dsRNA, the activator of PKR. These results suggested that the NS1 protein inhibits PKR activation in virus-infected cells. We also addressed the relevance of the antiviral effects of PKR in influenza A virus pathogenicity in PKR knockout (PKR −/−) mice [29]. Although wild-type influenza virus efficiently replicates in lungs and cause disease in PKR +/+ and PKR −/− mice, delNS1 virus, which is attenuated in wild-type mice, regained virulence and in PKR −/− infected mice, and replicated in the lungs of these mice to titers comparable to those in mice infected with wild-type virus. These results underscore the biological relevance of the PKR–NS1 interactions during influenza A virus infections.

6. Discussion

Although it has now become clear that the NS1 protein of influenza A virus prevents the activation of the type I IFN system of the host, this critical antiviral system is not completely inhibited during influenza A virus infections. For example, it has been shown that the absence of STAT1 or of PKR is responsible for a broader tissue tropism and higher pathogenicity of wild-type influenza A/WSN/33 virus [30,31]. It will be interesting to determine whether differences in pathogenicity among different influenza virus strains correlate with the ability of their NS1 proteins to function as type I IFN antagonists. In addition, the ability of the NS1 protein to inhibit dsRNA-activated pathways may also result in the inhibition of not only PKR, but of other dsRNA-activated enzymes with antiviral activity, such as the $2'$-$5'$ oligoadenylate synthetases (Fig. 1). Other open questions refer to (i) potential interactions and cooperative effects between the NS1 protein and p58^{IPK}, a cellular inhibitor of PKR which becomes activated during influenza A virus infection [32,33], (ii) the biological role of the carboxy-terminal domain of the NS1 protein in virus pathogenicity and (iii) the role of protein–protein interactions in the NS1 anti-IFN properties. These studies will shed light on the molecular interplay between influenza virus and its host and on the pathogenicity of this medically important virus.

Acknowledgements

This work has been funded in part by National Institutes of Health Grants AI46954 and AI48204 to A.G-S.

References

[1] A. Alcami, U.H. Koszinowski, Viral mechanisms of immune evasion, Immunol. Today 21 (2000) 447–455.
[2] A. Isaacs, J. Lindenmann, Virus interference: 1. The interferon, Proc. R. Soc. London, Ser. B 147 (1957) 258–267.
[3] G.R. Stark, I.M. Kerr, B.R. Williams, R.H. Silverman, R.D. Schreiber, How cells respond to interferons, Annu. Rev. Biochem. 67 (1998) 227–264.
[4] M. Sato, N. Tanaka, N. Hata, E. Oda, T. Taniguchi, Involvement of the IRF family transcription factor IRF-3 in virus-induced activation of the IFN-β gene, FEBS Lett. 425 (1998) 112–116.

[5] S.L. Schafer, R. Lin, P.A. Moore, J. Hiscott, P.M. Pitha, Regulation of type I interferon gene expression by interferon regulatory factor-3, J. Biol. Chem. 273 (1998) 2714–2720.

[6] B.K. Weaver, K.P. Kumar, N.C. Reich, Interferon regulatory factor 3 and CREB-binding protein/p300 are subunits of double-stranded RNA-activated transcription factor DRAF1, Mol. Cell. Biol. 18 (1998) 1359–1368.

[7] M. Yoneyama, W. Suhara, Y. Fukuhara, M. Fukuda, E. Nishida, T. Fujita, Direct triggering of the type I interferon system by virus infection: activation of a transcription factor complex containing IRF-3 and CBP/p300, EMBO J. 17 (1998) 1087–1095.

[8] M. Karin, Y. Ben-Neriah, Phosphorylation meets ubiquitination: the control of NF-kappaB activity, Annu. Rev. Immunol. 18 (2000) 621–663.

[9] S.D. Der, A. Zhou, B.R. Williams, R.H. Silverman, Identification of genes differentially regulated by interferon alpha, beta, or gamma using oligonucleotide arrays, Proc. Natl. Acad. Sci. U. S. A. 95 (1998) 15623–15628.

[10] B.R. Williams, PKR: a sentinel kinase for cellular stress, Oncogene 18 (1999) 6112–6120.

[11] R.E. O'Neill, J. Talon, P. Palese, The influenza virus NEP (NS2 protein) mediates the nuclear export of viral ribonucleoproteins, EMBO J. 17 (1998) 288–296.

[12] S. de la Luna, P. Fortes, A. Beloso, J. Ortín, Influenza virus NS1 protein enhances the rate of translation initiation of viral mRNAs, J. Virol. 69 (1995) 2427–2433.

[13] T. Aragón, S. de La Luna, I. Novoa, L. Carrasco, J. Ortín, A. Nieto, Eukaryotic translation initiation factor 4GI is a cellular target for NS1 protein, a translational activator of influenza virus, Mol. Cell. Biol. 20 (2000) 6259–6268.

[14] K. Enami, T.A. Sato, S. Nakada, M. Enami, Influenza virus NS1 protein stimulates translation of the M1 protein, J. Virol. 68 (1994) 1432–1437.

[15] P. Fortes, A. Beloso, J. Ortín, Influenza virus NS1 protein inhibits pre-mRNA splicing and blocks mRNA nucleocytoplasmic transport, EMBO J. 13 (1994) 704–712.

[16] Y. Lu, X.Y. Qian, R.M. Krug, The influenza virus NS1 protein: a novel inhibitor of pre-mRNA splicing, Genes Dev. 8 (1994) 1817–1828.

[17] M.E. Nemeroff, S.M. Barabino, Y. Li, W. Keller, R.M. Krug, Influenza virus NS1 protein interacts with the cellular 30 kDa subunit of CPSF and inhibits 3'end formation of cellular pre-mRNAs, Mol. Cell 1 (1998) 991–1000.

[18] X.Y. Qian, F. Alonso-Caplen, R.M. Krug, Two functional domains of the influenza virus NS1 protein are required for regulation of nuclear export of mRNA, J. Virol. 68 (1994) 2433–2441.

[19] Z. Chen, Y. Li, R.M. Krug, Influenza A virus NS1 protein targets poly(A)-binding protein II of the cellular 3'-end processing machinery, EMBO J. 18 (1999) 2273–2283.

[20] Y. Lu, M. Wambach, M.G. Katze, R.M. Krug, Binding of the influenza virus NS1 protein to double-stranded RNA inhibits the activation of the protein kinase that phosphorylates the elF-2 translation initiation factor, Virology 214 (1995) 222–228.

[21] E. Hatada, R. Fukuda, Binding of influenza A virus NS1 protein to dsRNA in vitro, J. Gen. Virol. 73 (1992) 3325–3329.

[22] S.L. Tan, M.G. Katze, Biochemical and genetic evidence for complex formation between the influenza A virus NS1 protein and the interferon-induced PKR protein kinase, J. Interferon Cytokine Res. 18 (1998) 757–766.

[23] A. García-Sastre, A. Egorov, D. Matassov, S. Brandt, D.E. Levy, J.E. Durbin, P. Palese, T. Muster, Influenza A virus lacking the NS1 gene replicates in interferon-deficient systems, Virology 252 (1998) 324–330.

[24] J. Talon, M. Salvatore, R.E. O'Neill, Y. Nakaya, H. Zheng, T. Muster, A. García-Sastre, P. Palese, Influenza A and B viruses expressing altered NS1 proteins: a vaccine approach, Proc. Natl. Acad. Sci. U. S. A. 97 (2000) 4309–4314.

[25] J. Talon, C.M. Horvath, R. Polley, C.F. Basler, T. Muster, P. Palese, A. García-Sastre, Activation of interferon regulatory factor 3 is inhibited by the influenza A virus NS1 protein, J. Virol. 74 (2000) 7989–7996.

[26] X. Wang, M. Li, H. Zheng, T. Muster, P. Palese, A.A. Beg, A. García-Sastre, Influenza A virus NS1 protein prevents the activation of NF-κB and induction of type I IFN. J. Virol. 74 (2000) 11566–11573.

[27] M.G. Wathelet, C.H. Lin, B.S. Parekh, L.V. Ronco, P.M. Howley, T. Maniatis, Virus infection induces the

assembly of coordinately activated transcription factors on the IFN-beta enhancer in vivo, Mol. Cell 1 (1998) 507–518.

[28] E. Hatada, S. Saito, R. Fukuda, Mutant influenza viruses with a defective NS1 protein cannot block the activation of PKR in infected cells, J. Virol. 73 (1999) 2425–2433.

[29] M. Bergmann, A. García-Sastre, E. Carnero, H. Pehamberger, K. Wolff, P. Palese, T. Muster, Influenza virus NS1 protein counteracts PKR-mediated inhibition of replication, J. Virol. 74 (2000) 6203–6206.

[30] A. García-Sastre, R.K. Durbin, H. Zheng, P. Palese, R. Gertner, D.E. Levy, J.E. Durbin, The role of interferon in the tropism of influenza virus, J. Virol. 72 (1998) 8550–8558.

[31] S. Balachandran, P.C. Roberts, L.E. Brown, H. Truong, A.K. Pattnaik, D.R. Archer, G.N. Barber, Essential role for the dsRNA-dependent protein kinase PKR in innate immunity to viral infection, Immunity 13 (2000) 129–141.

[32] T.G. Lee, J. Tomita, A.G. Hovanessian, M.G. Katze, Purification and partial characterization of a cellular inhibitor of the interferon-induced protein kinase of Mr 68,000 from influenza virus-infected cells, Proc. Natl. Acad. Sci. U. S. A. 87 (1990) 6208–6212.

[33] M.W. Melville, S.L. Tan, M. Wambach, J. Song, R.I. Morimoto, M.G. Katze, The cellular inhibitor of the PKR protein kinase, P58(IPK), is an influenza virus-activated co-chaperone that modulates heat shock protein 70 activity, J. Biol. Chem. 274 (1999) 3797–3803.

International Congress Series 1219 (2001) 521–525

Sialyl sugar chains as receptors and determinants of host range of influenza A viruses

Yasuo Suzuki[a,*], Toshihiro Ito[b], Takashi Suzuki[a], Daisei Miyamoto[a],
Kazuya I.-P.J. Hidari[a], Chao-Tan Guo[a], Hiroshi Kida[c],
Robert G. Webster[d], Thomas M. Chambers[e], Yoshihiro Kawaoka[f,g]

[a]*Department of Biochemistry, University of Shizuoka School of Pharmaceutical Sciences,
52-1 Yada, Shizuoka 422-8526, Japan*
[b]*Faculty of Agriculture Tottori University, Tottori, Japan*
[c]*Graduate School of Veterinary Medicine, Hokkaido University, Sapporo, Japan*
[d]*St. Jude Children's Research Hospital Memphis, USA*
[e]*Department of Veterinary Science, 108 Gluck Equine Research Center,
University of Kentucky, Lexington, KY, USA*
[f]*School of Veterinary Medicine, University of Wisconsin-Madison, Madison, WI, USA*
[g]*Institute of Medical Science, University of Tokyo, Tokyo, Japan*

Abstract

Sialic acids (SA) in host cell receptors are widely distributed in animals; however, the molecular species and the sialyl linkages vary among animal species. Previous studies have shown that the sialyllacto/sialylneolacto-series sugar chains, SAα2–3(6)Galβ1–3(4)GlcNAcβ1-, in glycoproteins and glycolipids are the functional receptor sugar chains for influenza A and B viruses from humans and animals. Amino acid substitutions in hemagglutinin (HA), the glycoprotein responsible for receptor binding of influenza viruses, have resulted in changing receptor specificity for the molecular species (Neu5Ac, Neu5Gc) as well as sialyl linkage (SA2–3Gal, SA2–6Gal). The host range is influenced by host cell receptors; the Neu5Gc2–3Gal moiety present on crypt epithelial cells of duck colon has been shown to play an important role in the enterotropism of avian influenza viruses. In addition, a virus with an HA recognizing the Neu5Ac2–6Gal but not Neu5Ac2–3Gal or Neu5Gc2–3Gal, failed to replicate in horses, while one with an HA recognizing the Neu5Gc2–3Gal moiety replicated in horses. The abundance of the Neu5Gc2–3Gal moiety in epithelial cells of horse trachea supports that recognition of this moiety is critical for viral replication in horses. Thus, substantial evidence suggests the significance of the molecular species and linkage in the host range of the

---

* Corresponding author. Tel.: +81-54-264-5725; fax: +81-54-264-5721.
E-mail address: suzukiy@ys7.u-shizuoka-ken.ac.jp (Y. Suzuki).

0531-5131/01/$ – see front matter © 2001 Published by Elsevier Science B.V.
PII: S 0 5 3 1 - 5 1 3 1 (0 1) 0 0 6 3 0 - 6

influenza. Here we report the biological role of receptor sialyl sugar chains in host range determination of influenza A viruses. © 2001 Published by Elsevier Science B.V.

Keywords: Hemagglutinin; Sialidase; Sialic acid; Receptor binding specificity; Host range variation

Influenza A viruses have been isolated from a variety of animals, including human, pigs, horses, sea mammals and wild waterfowl, including ducks and poultry [1]. Among these animals, wild waterfowl is the major reservoir of influenza viruses and all influenza viruses in other animal species are thought to be derived from these birds. In fact, the causative viruses of the 1957 Asian and 1968 Hong Kong pandemic influenza A strains are reassortant viruses between human and avian influenza viruses, indicating the introduction of avian virus hemagglutinin genes into the human population. All subtypes of the hemagglutinin, H1 to H15, and sialidase, N1 to N9, are maintained in the avian world. Hemagglutinin subtypes of pig influenza viruses are similar to those of humans.

Influenza viruses bind to sialic acid (SA) receptors containing sugar chains on the host cell membranes. In nature, at least 28 molecular species have been reported, including N-acetylneuraminic acid (Neu5Ac), N-glycolylneuraminic acid (Neu5Gc), and several kinds of O-acetylated Neu5Ac [2]. Among them, two major molecular species, N-acetyl and N-glycolylneuraminic acids, are important for the influenza A and B virus infections.

This report describes the sialyl sugar chains as receptors and as determinants of host range of influenza A viruses.

1. Materials and methods

The viruses were propagated in the allantoic cavities of 11-day-old embryonated chicken eggs or MDCK cells. Molecular species of sialic acid, Neu5Ac and Neu5Gc, were determined fluorometrically by HPLC [3]. Antibody directed against GM3(Neu5Gc) gangliosode was developed in chickens which are known to lack Neu5Gc [4]. Frozen sections of tissues were stained to detect Neu5Gc2–3Gal immunologically by the antibody. Specificities of the virus hemagglutinin were determined by thin layer chromatography/virus binding assays as previously described [5].

2. Results and discussion

After determining the binding specificity of more than 100 native and synthetic sialyl sugar chains we found that the dominant receptors of influenza A and B viruses were sialylglycoproteins and gangliosides containing monosialo-lactosamine type I and II, SAα2–3(6)Galβ1–3(4)GlcNAcβ1-. One terminal sialic acid is necessary, but tandem sequences of sialic acid and also sialic acid linked to an internal galactose in a sugar chain, such as GM1 gangliosides, are not recognized. Influenza viruses specifically recognized selected sialyl sugar chains and molecular species of sialic acid.

We determined the receptor binding specificity of human, swine, avian and equine influenza A viruses and also the sialyl linkage present on the cells of the host target organs, trachea epithelium for humans, pigs, and horse and intestinal mucosa for birds, using lectins which recognize sialyllinkages, 2–3 or 2–6 [6].

Human influenza viruses isolated in MDCK cells bind Neu5Ac2–6Gal sequences; however, equine and avian viruses bind 2–3 predominantly. Interestingly, swine viruses bind both 2–6 and 2–3, equally or with a slight predominance toward 2–6. Human trachea expresses sialyl 2–6Gal significantly, while horse trachea and duck intestinal mucosa express 2–3. By contrast, pig trachea expresses both 2–3 and 2–6 linkages. Thus, according to their ability to support replication of both avian and human influenza viruses, pigs have been implicated as intermediate hosts, serving as mixing vessels for avian and human viruses. As indicated by the previous data, the availability of receptors, such as 2–3 and 2–6 moieties, in host animals correlates with the receptor specificity of influenza viruses from those host animals, suggesting that receptor specificity is an important determinant of the host range restriction of influenza viruses.

We found at least two possible mechanisms for host range variation of influenza A viruses: selection due to the presence of antibody in the host and selection by the host cell receptor based on the type of sialylsugar chains of host cell receptors. A single amino acid substitution in the viral hemagglutinin changes the binding specificity to sialyl linkages Neu5Ac2–3Gal (2–3) and Neu5Ac2–6Gal (2–6). Ser 205 located in the antgenic site D. Although distant from the receptor binding site, this amino acid is proximate to the receptor binding site of the next subunit. By the substitution of the Ser to bulky amino acid Tyr, the receptor binding specificity changes from 2–3 to 2–6. This amino acid substitution can be generated experimentally using antibodies directed against the viral hemagglutinin.

We also found that when amino acid Leu 226, located in the receptor binding pocket, is substituted to Gln, a dramatic change in receptor binding specificity from 2–6 to 2–3 occurred. Experimentally this has been demonstrated by culturing influenza isolates from human trachea with 2–6 specificity in the allantoic membrane of embryonated chicken eggs which have sialyl2–3Gal receptor. These results indicate that the amino acid 205 in antigenic site and 226 in the receptor binding pocket are critical for recognition and regulation of receptor binding specificity, 2–3 and 2–6. If these single amino acid alterations occurred in host animals in nature, the virus would acquire a new receptor binding specificity, allowing the infection to different animal species. This may be an important mechanism for host mediated variation, the transmission of influenza virus between different hosts, as well as the emergence of new subtypes of influenza viruses in the human population. Amino acid 226 is located on the left edge of the receptor binding pocket, which is near the glycosidic linkage of the receptor sialyl linkage. It is, therefore, quite reasonable that alteration of this amino acid alone caused the specificity to change from 2–6 to 2–3 sialyl linkages.

Recently, we also determined the sialic acid species in the target organs for influenza viruses. Humans have no Neu5Gc species in their tissue or cells; however, pig and horse trachea epithelial cells, which are targets for influenza A viruses, contain significant amounts of Neu5Gc. We also found Neu5Gc in duck intestinal epithelial cells. Analysis of the intestinal cells of the duck, chicken, and MDCK cells using anti Gc-GM3 (hematoside) antibody which specifically recognizes Gc2–3Gal but not Ac2–3Gal, confirmed the location of Gc2–3Gal in the target organs and cells. It failed to react with chicken intestine, which lacks Gc, but did react with Gc containing MDCK cells. The crypt cells of duck colon epithelium reacted strongly with the antiserum, demonstrating the presence of Neu5Gc. The epithelial cells of duck jejunum and cecum were also positive, though to a lesser extent, and those of duodenum were not, suggesting that much higher concentrations of Gc are present in the lower intestine of ducks. The molar ratio of Ac and Gc in the sample of epithelial cells obtained by EDTA treatment of duck intestine was 98:2, indicating that the epitherial cells in duck intestine contain Gc2–3Gal, albeit as a minor species.

We examined whether duck viruses universally bind Gc2–3Gal [5]. All four duck viruses, representing a variety of HA subtypes, recognized Gc2–3Gal, except A/duck/Ukraine/1/63(H3N8). Since duck/Ukraine virus has been passaged extensively for many years in chicken eggs, which lack Neu5Gc recognition, this altered specificity may be a result of egg adaptation and may explain why the virus no longer replicates well in ducks. By contrast, other duck viruses with substantial ability to recognize Gc2–3Gal replicated well in duck intestine (with titers of 10^4 EID50/g) and progeny viruses were isolated from their feces. The human isolate Udorn (H3 subtype) preferentially bound Ac2–6Gal, whereas, the isolate Mallard/NY bound to all three sialyl–Gal moieties of gangliosides tested (Gc2–3Gal, Ac2–3Gal, and Ac2–6Gal, in order of preference). To determine the molecular basis for these differences in specificity, we prepared reassortant viruses containing HAs with amino acid substitution at 226, Leu to Gln only at both 226, Leu to Gln and 228, Ser to Gly. The mutation from Leu to Gln at 226 (R3 virus) shifted the specificity of the human Udorn virus HA from Ac2–6Gal to Ac2–3Gal. However, the R3 virus still preferentially recognized Ac2–3, and Gc2–3 only marginally. Surprisingly, an additional mutation from Ser to Gly at 228 (R2) resulted in approximately equal recognition of Ac2–3 and Gc2–3. Thus, amino acids 226 and 228 in the viral hemagglutinin are very important for receptor binding specificity and can be manipulated to change the receptor specificity of human influenza viruses.

In the case of horses, more than 90% of the sialic acid in the epithelial cells of horse trachea is Neu5Gc, while the remaining proportion is Neu5Ac. The anti Gc2–3Gal antiserum bound to epithelial cells lining horse trachea, but not to those of chicken trachea, which lack Neu5Gc. We found that influenza viruses isolated from horses bind to Neu5Gc2–3Gal and Neu5Ac2–3Gal, whereas the human isolate, PR/8/34 did not bind to Neu5Gc GM3, indicating that influenza viruses isolated from Neu5Gc-containing hosts bind to Neu5Gc-containing receptor sugar chains.

Furthermore, we also demonstrated that Gc2–3Gal recognition is essential for viral replication in horses. The human isolate, A/Udorn/307/72 (H3N2) (Udorn), preferentially binds the Ac2–6Gal, but not Ac2–3 or Gc2–3Gal. The following reassortant viruses possessing the Udorn HA, and the remainder of the genes from an equine virus, A/equine/Kentucky/1/91(H3N8)(Eq/Ky) were generated: (1) Udorn-Eq/Ky virus containing the human virus, Udorn HA; (2) Leu226Gln-Eq/Ky virus containing the Udorn Leu226Gln mutant HA; and (3) Leu226Gln/Ser228Gly-Eq/Ky, containing the Udorn HA possessing alterations at both 226 and 228. Ponies were experimentally infected with 10^7 EID50 of aerosolized virus. Viruses were recovered from nasal swabs, taken daily inoculating by the swab suspensions into embryonated eggs. Eq/Ky virus, whose HA recognizes not only Ac2–3Gal but also Gc2–3Gal, replicated for up to 1 week (5 days in three ponies and 8 days in one pony) producing high-titer virus on day 2. By contrast, the Udorn-Eq/Ky virus, whose HA preferentially recognizes Ac2–6Gal over the Gc2–3Gal moiety, did not replicate in ponies at all, demonstrating an essential contribution of the HA to host range restriction. Interestingly, the Leu226Gln-Eq/Ky virus, whose HA preferentially recognizes the SA2–3Gal with Neu5Ac, while binding much less avidly to the Neu5Gc moiety, replicated in one of the three ponies tested, but for only 2 days. However, the Leu226Gln/Ser228Gly-Eq/Ky virus, whose HA recognizes both Ac2–3Gal and Gc2–3Gal, replicated in all three ponies tested for as long as 1 week, with titers ranging from $10^{1.8}$ to $10^{3.8}$ EID50.

These findings demonstrate that recognition of the Gc2–3Gal moiety is critical for the efficient replication of influenza A viruses in horses and also ducks. The above results are the evidence of the biologic effect of different sialic acid species in different animals.

References

[1] E.D. Kilbourne, Influenza, Plenum Medical Book, New York, 1987.
[2] A. Varki, Essentials of Glycobiology, Cold Spring Harber Laboratory Press, New York, 1999.
[3] S. Hara, Y. Taketomi, M. Yamaguchi, M. Nakamura, Y. Ohkuma, Fluorometric high-performance liquid chromatography of N-acetyl- and N-glycolylneuraminic acids and its application to their microdetermination in human and animal sera, glycoproteins, and glycolipids, Anal. Biochem. 164 (1987) 138–145.
[4] Y. Hirabayashi, T. Suzuki, Y. Suzuki, M. Taki, M. Matsumoto, H. Higashi, S. Kato, A new method for purification of anti-glycosphingolipid antibody, Avian anti-hematoside (NeuGc) antibody, J. Biochem. 94 (1983) 327–330.
[5] Y. Suzuki, Y. Nakao, T. Ito, N. Watanabe, Y. Toda, G. Xu, T. Suzuki, T. Kobayashi, Y. Kimura, A. Yamada, K. Sugawara, H. Nishimura, F. Kitame, K. Nakamura, E. Deya, M. Kiso, A. Hasegawa, Structural determination of gangliosides that bind to influenza A, B, and C viruses by an improved binding assay: Strain-specific receptor epitopes in sialo-sugar chains, Virology 189 (1992) 121–131.
[6] T. Ito, J. Nelson, S.S. Couceiro, S. Kelm, L.G. Baum, S. Krauss, M.R. Castrucci, I. Donatelli, H. Kida, J.C. Paulson, R.G. Webster, Y. Kawaoka, Molecular basis for the generation in pigs of influenza A viruses with pandemic potential, J. Virol. (1998) 7367–7373.

International Congress Series 1219 (2001) 527–531

Lectins in innate host defence against influenza virus

E. Margot Anders*, Patrick C. Reading, Joanna L. Miller

Department of Microbiology and Immunology, University of Melbourne, Melbourne, Victoria 3010, Australia

Abstract

Soluble collagenous C-type lectins (collectins) present in plasma and lung fluids display antiviral activity against influenza virus in vitro. Our studies in the mouse model of influenza indicate that the collectin lung surfactant protein D (SP-D) plays an important role in vivo in innate defence of the respiratory tract against the virus. Furthermore, studies with diabetic mice indicated a direct link between their increased susceptibility to influenza virus infection and interference with collectin-mediated host defence of the lung by glucose. Macrophages are another important component of innate immunity to influenza virus, uptake of the virus leading to nonproductive viral replication and secretion of proinflammatory cytokines and type 1 interferons (IFN-α/β). Our recent studies on infection of murine macrophages by influenza virus indicate that uptake is mediated by the macrophage mannose receptor, an integral membrane C-type lectin with carbohydrate specificity similar to that of the collectins. The oligosaccharide present on influenza viral glycoproteins thus appears to act as a target for recognition of the virus by endogenous lectins of the innate immune system. Evasion of such recognition by poorly glycosylated viruses may contribute to their virulence. © 2001 Elsevier Science B.V. All rights reserved.

Keywords: Collectins; Macrophage; Mannose receptor; Glycosylation; Diabetes; Innate immunity

1. Introduction

Effective immunity to influenza depends on innate as well as specific immune mechanisms [1]. Innate defences act early in infection to contain replication and spread of the virus in the period before specific T and B cell responses develop, and may be critical in determining whether the infection remains subclinical or proceeds to clinical disease. Well-studied components of innate immunity include macrophages, natural killer (NK) cells, IFN-α/β and complement. Our work with the mouse model of influenza has

* Corresponding author. Tel.: +61-3-8344-5702; fax: +61-3-9347-1540.
E-mail address: emanders@unimelb.edu.au (E.M. Anders).

0531-5131/01/$ – see front matter © 2001 Elsevier Science B.V. All rights reserved.
PII: S 0 5 3 1 - 5 1 3 1 (0 1) 0 0 3 8 6 - 7

indicated an important role also for endogenous lectins in innate defence against the virus. These molecules include members of the collectin family—soluble collagenous lectins found in plasma and lung fluids—and a membrane lectin, the macrophage mannose receptor, which appears to be important in uptake of the virus into macrophages.

2. Collectins

The collectins are a family of soluble lectins present in plasma and lung fluids and possessing collagenous segments linked to Ca^{2+}-dependent (C-type) lectin domains [2]. Members of this family include serum mannose-binding lectin (MBL, also known as mannose- or mannan-binding protein, MBP), and lung surfactant proteins A (SP-A) and D (SP-D); two additional plasma collectins, conglutinin and CL-43, are found only in cattle and other *Bovidae*. The collectins all bind to mannan and to mannose-containing oligosaccharides and appear to function in innate immunity to microbial infection, binding to a wide range of Gram-positive and Gram-negative bacteria, yeasts and parasites and acting as opsonins for their uptake by phagocytes [3–5].

All of the collectins bind to influenza virus and display antiviral activity in vitro. For SP-A, the interaction involves binding of the virus through its hemagglutinin (HA) to sialic acid on SP-A [6]. The other collectins function as so-called β inhibitors of influenza virus [7], binding in a Ca^{2+}-dependent manner through their lectin domains to glycans on the viral HA and neuraminidase (NA) glycoproteins. The in vitro activities of collectins against influenza virus include hemagglutination inhibition, virus neutralization, virus aggregation, and opsonization of the virus for interaction with neutrophils [6–14], properties which suggested a possible role for these molecules in innate defence in vivo against influenza virus infection.

3. In vivo role of collectins in murine influenza

To investigate the role of collectins in vivo, we examined the relationship between sensitivity of influenza viruses to the collectins SP-D and MBL and their ability to replicate in the mouse lung [13]. Viruses of the H3 subtype differ in the degree of glycosylation of their HA molecules: early strains (1968–1972) carry seven potential glycosylation sites (five on the stalk, two on the globular head of HA), whereas later strains carry an additional one, two or three sites on the head of the molecule. This increase in glycosylation is accompanied by an increase in sensitivity to neutralization by collectins SP-D and MBL. A marked inverse correlation was observed between collectin sensitivity and ability of a virus to replicate in the mouse lung. The later, more heavily glycosylated, strains of virus grew very poorly, whereas earlier strains replicated well to moderately well in the lung. A/PR/8/34 virus (H1N1, Mt. Sinai strain), which is highly virulent for mice and grows to high titre in mouse lung, carries no glycans on the head of its HA molecule and is essentially resistant to neutralization by SP-D and MBL. Together, the data indicated that growth of glycosylated strains of virus in the lung is limited by their sensitivity to collectins. Consistent with this notion, inclusion of a ligand of the collectins (yeast mannan or α-methylmannoside) with the virus inoculum led to marked enhancement of growth of the glycosylated strains of virus but no effect on growth of A/PR/8/34 even from a low inoculum.

SP-D is present in the airways of normal mice [15], and levels in lung lavage fluids were shown to increase rapidly on influenza virus infection [13]. SP-D is thus available to act immediately on the infecting virus and during the early rounds of viral replication. In contrast, MBL is absent from the airways of normal mice but could be detected in lung lavage 3 days after infection; MBL may thus be important in preventing spread of influenza virus into the bloodstream and may contribute directly to defence of the lung later in infection.

4. Compromise of collectin-mediated host defence of the lung in diabetes

Glucose is one of the preferred ligands of SP-D and hence a potential inhibitor of SP-D function in diabetes. Using the RIP-K^b transgenic mouse model of diabetes [16,17], we showed that diabetic mice are indeed more susceptible to influenza virus infection than their nondiabetic littermates. This difference in susceptibility applied to strains of virus that are sensitive to collectins but not to the virulent strain A/PR/8/34, which is collectin-resistant. The susceptibility of the mice correlated directly with their blood glucose levels, and neutralization of influenza virus in vitro by SP-D was shown to be inhibited by levels of glucose commonly found in the blood of diabetic mice. Together, these findings suggest a direct link between increased susceptibility of diabetic mice to influenza virus infection and interference with collectin-mediated innate immune mechanisms by glucose [18].

5. Infection of macrophages by influenza virus and role of the mannose receptor

Macrophages represent an important component of innate immunity to influenza virus: infection of macrophages is abortive and hence a dead end for the virus [19,20]; infection also leads to production of IFN-α/β and proinflammatory cytokines which will further act to limit virus spread [21]. We observed a marked difference among influenza virus strains in their ability to infect macrophages that paralleled their sensitivity to collectins, A/PR/8/34 virus giving particularly low levels of infection [22]. The macrophage mannose receptor (MR) is an integral membrane protein that mediates the uptake of glycoproteins terminating in mannose, fucose or N-acetylglucosamine [23,24]. Since the carbohydrate specificity of the MR overlaps that of the collectins, influenza virus glycoproteins represent potential ligands for this receptor. The possible role of the MR in infectious entry of influenza virus into macrophages was therefore investigated.

Competitive binding experiments with ^{125}I-labelled mannosylated-BSA, a ligand of the MR, indicated a direct interaction of influenza HA/NA glycoproteins with the MR and the avidity of the interaction correlated with the ability of the respective viruses to infect macrophages. Efficiency of infection also correlated with the level of expression of MR on the macrophages. Infection of macrophages, but not Madin–Darby canine kidney cells which lack an MR, was blocked by yeast mannan at a stage subsequent to virus adsorption. Given the known endocytic activity of the MR and the fact that uptake of influenza virus into an endosome following adsorption is an obligatory step in the infectious process, these findings suggested that uptake via the MR represents a major endocytic route for influenza virus into macrophages [22].

6. Conclusions

The studies reported here indicate that the carbohydrate on influenza virus glycoproteins acts as a target for recognition by endogenous lectins of the innate immune system including collectins (SP-D and MBL) and the macrophage mannose receptor. Glycans on the head of the HA molecule appear to be particularly important in conferring sensitivity to these lectins. The virulence of A/PR/8/34 virus for mice is due, at least in part, to its ability to evade these components of innate immunity through its low level of glycosylation. In mice, and perhaps in humans, diabetes predisposes to influenza virus infection through compromise of lectin-mediated host defence by glucose.

Acknowledgements

We gratefully acknowledge the contribution of our collaborators Drs. E.C. Crouch and J. Allison to parts of the work reported here. This work was supported by Project Grants 940742 and 970283 to EMA from the National Health and Medical Research Council of Australia.

References

[1] G.L. Ada, P.D. Jones, The immune response to influenza infection, Curr. Top. Microbiol. Immunol. 128 (1986) 1–54.
[2] S. Thiel, K.B.M. Reid, Structures and functions associated with the group of mammalian lectins containing collagen-like sequences, FEBS Lett. 250 (1989) 78–84.
[3] U. Holmskov, R. Malhotra, R.B. Sim, J. Jensenius, Collectins: collagenous C-type lectins of the innate immune defense system, Immunol. Today 15 (1994) 67–74.
[4] H.-J. Hoppe, K.B.M. Reid, Collectins—soluble proteins containing collagenous regions and lectin domains—and their roles in innate immunity, Protein Sci. 3 (1994) 1143–1158.
[5] R.A.B. Ezekowitz, K. Sastry, K.B.M. Reid (Eds.), Collectins and Innate Immunity, RG Landes, Austin, Texas, 1996.
[6] C.A. Benne, C.A. Kraaijeveld, J.A.G. van Strijp, E. Brouwer, M. Harmsen, J. Verhoef, L.M.G. van Golde, J.F. van Iwaarden, Interactions of surfactant protein A with influenza viruses: binding and neutralization, J. Infect. Dis. 171 (1995) 335–341.
[7] E.M. Anders, C.A. Hartley, D.C. Jackson, Bovine and mouse serum β inhibitors of influenza A viruses are mannose-binding lectins, Proc. Natl. Acad. Sci. U. S. A. 87 (1990) 4485–4489.
[8] C.A. Hartley, D.C. Jackson, E.M. Anders, Two distinct serum mannose-binding lectins function as β inhibitors of influenza virus: identification of bovine serum β inhibitor as conglutinin, J. Virol. 66 (1992) 4358–4363.
[9] K.L. Hartshorn, K. Sastry, M.R. White, E.M. Anders, M. Super, R.A.B. Ezekowitz, A.I. Tauber, Human mannose-binding protein functions as an opsonin for influenza A viruses, J. Clin. Invest. 91 (1993) 1414–1420.

[10] K.L. Hartshorn, K. Sastry, D. Brown, M.R. White, T.B. Okarma, Y.-M. Lee, A.I. Tauber, Conglutinin acts as an opsonin for influenza A viruses, J. Immunol. 151 (1993) 6265–6273.

[11] K.L. Hartshorn, E.C. Crouch, M.R. White, P. Eggleton, A.I. Tauber, D. Chang, K. Sastry, Evidence for a protective role of pulmonary surfactant protein D (SP-D) against influenza A viruses, J. Clin. Invest. 94 (1994) 311–319.

[12] E.M. Anders, C.A. Hartley, P.C. Reading, R.A.B. Ezekowitz, Complement-dependent neutralization of influenza virus by a serum mannose-binding lectin, J. Gen. Virol. 75 (1994) 615–622.

[13] P.C. Reading, L.S. Morey, E.C. Crouch, E.M. Anders, Collectin-mediated antiviral host defense of the lung: evidence from influenza virus infection of mice, J. Virol. 71 (1997) 8204–8212.

[14] K.L. Hartshorn, M.R. White, D.R. Voelker, J. Coburn, K. Zaner, E.C. Crouch, Mechanism of binding of surfactant protein D to influenza viruses: importance of binding to haemagglutinin to antiviral activity, Biochem. J. 351 (2000) 449–458.

[15] C.J. Wong, J. Akiyama, L. Allen, S. Hawgood, Localization and developmental expression of surfactant proteins D and A in the respiratory tract of the mouse, Pediatr. Res. 39 (1996) 930–937.

[16] J. Allison, L. Malcolm, J. Culvenor, R.K. Bartholomeusz, K. Holmberg, J.F.A.P. Miller, Overexpression of β2-microglobulin in transgenic mouse islet β cells results in defective insulin secretion, Proc. Natl. Acad. Sci. U. S. A. 88 (1991) 2070–2074.

[17] J. Allison, I.L. Campbell, G. Morahan, T.E. Mandel, L.C. Harrison, J.F.A.P. Miller, Diabetes in transgenic mice resulting from overexpression of Class I histocompatibility molecules in pancreatic β cells, Nature 333 (1988) 529–533.

[18] P.C. Reading, J. Allison, E.C. Crouch, E.M. Anders, Increased susceptibility of diabetic mice to influenza virus infection: compromise of collectin-mediated host defense of the lung by glucose? J. Virol. 72 (1998) 6884–6887.

[19] M.P. Wells, P. Albrecht, S. Daniel, F.A. Ennis, Host defense mechanisms against influenza virus: interaction of influenza virus with murine macrophages in vitro, Infect. Immun. 22 (1978) 758–762.

[20] B. Rodgers, C.A. Mims, Interaction of influenza virus with mouse macrophages, Infect. Immun. 31 (1981) 751–757.

[21] T. Peschke, A. Bender, M. Nain, D. Gemsa, Role of macrophage cytokines in influenza A virus infections, Immunobiology 189 (1993) 340–355.

[22] P.C. Reading, J.L. Miller, E.M. Anders, Involvement of the mannose receptor in infection of macrophages by influenza virus, J. Virol. 74 (2000) 5190–5197.

[23] S.E. Pontow, V. Kery, P.D. Stahl, Mannose receptor, Int. Rev. Cytol. 137B (1992) 221–244.

[24] P.D. Stahl, R.A.B. Ezekowitz, The mannose receptor is a pattern recognition receptor involved in host defense, Curr. Opin. Immunol. 10 (1998) 50–55.

International Congress Series 1219 (2001) 533–543

Hemagglutinin and neuraminidase as determinants of influenza virus pathogenicity

Ralf Wagner[a], Anke Feldmann[a], Thorsten Wolff[a], Stephan Pleschka[b], Wolfgang Garten[a], Hans-Dieter Klenk[a,*]

[a]*Institut für Virologie, Klinikum der Philipps-Universität Marburg, Robert-Koch-Str. 17, 35037 Marburg, Germany*
[b]*Institut für Virologie, Justus-Liebig-Universität Giessen, Germany*

Keywords: Pathogenicity; Fowl plague virus; Receptor binding specificity; Neurominidase activity

The pathogenicity of influenza viruses is determined by many of its other biological properties, such as efficiency of replication, tissue tropism, host range, spread of infection, as well as response to and modulation of host defense. All of these properties are controlled by the complex interplay of viral and host factors at virtually each stage in the life cycle of the virus. Activation of the hemagglutinin by host cell proteases has been shown in many studies to have a dramatic effect on pathogenesis, and the molecular details of proteolytic activation are well understood [16a]. We will concentrate here on recent studies in which we have analyzed the interplay of hemagglutinin (HA) and neuraminidase (NA) in receptor binding and release and some of the factors that determine spread of infection in the organism.

1. Balance of receptor binding and release regulates virus growth

HA-mediated attachment of influenza viruses to sialic acid containing receptors on the host cell surface is the initial step of infection. Influenza HA contains at the tip a narrow crevice lined with highly conserved amino acids. By its ability to specifically bind sialic acids, this crevice has been identified as the receptor binding site [8,27,38]. The precise structure of this HA domain is known to be of crucial importance for the process of virus

* Corresponding author. Tel.: +49-6421-286-6253; fax: +49-6421-286-8962.
E-mail address: klenk@mailer.uni-marburg.de (H.-D. Klenk).

0531-5131/01/$ – see front matter © 2001 Elsevier Science B.V. All rights reserved.
PII: S 0 5 3 1 - 5 1 3 1 (0 1) 0 0 3 8 1 - 8

binding to its receptor. Accordingly, single amino acid substitutions in the binding pocket can result in altered receptor binding specificity and altered host range of the respective viruses [1,6,36]. Furthermore, employing vector-expressed FPV-HA, we could show that oligosaccharides flanking the binding site modulate receptor affinity [23]. To evaluate the impact of each individual N-glycan at the FPV-HA tip on the growth of intact viruses, we generated recombinant influenza viruses containing the oligosaccharide-deleted HA mutants [37] (Fig. 1). Our studies demonstrate that the glycans flanking the receptor binding pocket are potent regulators of virus growth in cell culture. The oligosaccharide attached to Asn 149 (absent in mutant G2) plays a dominant role in controlling virus spread while that attached to Asn 123 (absent in mutant G1) is less effective. Growth of viruses lacking both N-glycans was found to be reduced in cell culture due to a restricted release of progeny viruses from infected cells (Fig. 2). These findings on the growth of recombinant viruses are an important extension of our previous work investigating the receptor interaction of transiently expressed HA. There is now experimentally based evidence for a distinct regulatory function of individual N-

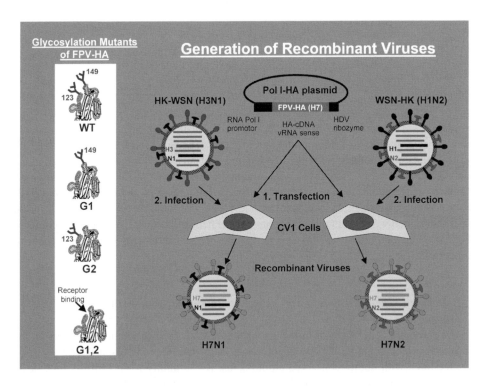

Fig. 1. Inset on the left: the head region of FPV-HA is shown on the top. N-linked oligosaccharides adjacent to the receptor binding pocket are indicated. Mutants G1 and G2 lack the glycosylation sites at Asn 123 and Asn 149, respectively. Both sites are absent in mutant G1,2. The arrow marks the entrance to the receptor binding pocket. Body of figure: recombinant viruses were generated by a RNA-polymerase I-based reverse genetics system. Two reassortants of strain A/WSN/33 were used as helper viruses to obtain two series of HA-mutant viruses only differing in NA.

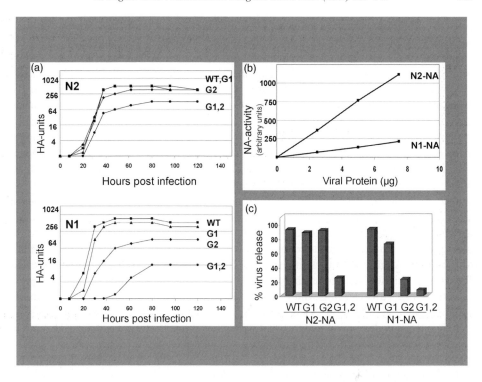

Fig. 2. (a) Growth curves of recombinants in MDCK cells. Cell monolayers were infected at an MOI of 0.001 with recombinant viruses, and supernatants were monitored for HA titers at the time points indicated. The results obtained with viruses of the N2-series and of the N1-series are shown. (■) WT; (▲) G1; (♦) G2; (●) G1,2. (b) Comparison of specific NA-activities of WT/N1 and WT/N2 viruses. Different amounts of purified virus were incubated with 4-methylumbelliferyl *N*-acetylneuraminic acid for 20 min at 37 °C. The reaction was stopped and NA activity was calculated by measuring the fluorescence of the liberated methylumbelliferone. The data are means of three experiments. They indicate that WT/N2 has a higher NA activity than WT/N1. (c) Release of recombinant viruses from MDCK cells. MDCK cells were infected at an MOI of 5 with recombinant viruses and incubated at 37 °C overnight. One hour before virus harvest, VCNA was added to the culture media to one-half of the samples. Titers of progeny viruses released into the media were determined by plaque assay. Levels of virus release in the absence of VCNA are presented as percent values relative to the virus titers released after VCNA treatment (from Ref. [37]).

glycans located at the HA tip on the viral life cycle. By sequentially removing *N*-glycans from the vicinity of the HA receptor binding site, we have also delineated a novel approach to specifically generate influenza viruses with a gradual extension of attenuation in cell culture.

By removing terminal sialic acid residues from oligosaccharide side chains of glycoconjugates, the viral neuraminidase (NA) acts as a receptor-destroying enzyme in influenza viruses [4,18]. When NA activity was blocked by either antibodies [5], inhibitors [12,24], or temperature-sensitive mutations [25], formation of large viral aggregates on the surface of infected cells was observed as was with virus lacking NA either partly [22] or completely [19]. Accordingly, viral NA is regarded an important factor for the release of progeny virus from host cells promoting the efficient progression of an infection. In light of this, it was of special interest to examine how different NA subtypes affect the attenuated phenotype of the recombinant viruses lacking N-glycans at the HA tip. Several N1-NAs have a deletion in the stalk region that is most extensive with FPV-NA [14]. NA enzymatic activity has been reported to vary according to the length of the stalk region of the molecule with NA species containing a deletion in the stalk having a lower activity [2,9,20,21]. By choosing appropriate helper viruses, we generated recombinants in which the HA mutants were combined with either the WSN virus NA (N1 subtype) containing a stalk deletion or the Hong Kong virus NA (N2 subtype) that has no deletion. When assayed for neuraminidase activity, recombinant viruses carrying N2-NA exceeded those with N1-NA at least sixfold (Fig. 2). Thus, our set of recombinants was ideally suited to analyze in depth the impact of different NA activities on the growth of mutant influenza viruses specifically designed to show distinct receptor binding activities. Using this system, we were able to demonstrate that the growth behavior of HA mutant viruses is governed by the nature of the accompanying viral NA. Among the viruses with the high-activity N2-NA, growth restriction was observed only when the G1,2 mutant was present showing the highest receptor affinity, while recombinants containing G1 and G2 grew essentially like virus carrying wild type HA. Yet, the situation was different with viruses containing the low-activity N1-NA. Here, the growth of G1,2 mutant viruses was significantly impeded in cell culture due to a restricted release from host cells. This effect was less pronounced with G2 mutant viruses, but still evident. Obviously, unlike N2-NA, the lower-activity N1-NA is not capable to overcome the high affinity interaction of G1,2 and G2 HA with its receptor (Fig. 2).

Hence, our data clearly point out that, for the establishment of productive infection, influenza viruses are strictly dependent on a highly balanced action of HA and NA. An increase in receptor binding affinity apparently needs to be accompanied by a concomitant increase in the receptor-destroying activity of the viral NA. Otherwise, the enhanced receptor binding is a serious disadvantage in the late stage of infection by preventing the release of progeny viruses from host cells. The need for such a match of HA and NA activities had so far only been deduced from studies analyzing natural virus isolates or laboratory generated reassortants [15,16,21,29]. Taken together, our work represents the first concise study of the functional interrelationship of distinct HA and NA species and provides experimental evidence for the strict requirement of a fine tuning of HA receptor binding and NA receptor destroying activity in order to allow for an efficient influenza virus propagation (Fig. 3).

There is evidence that N-glycans flanking the receptor binding site not only modulate receptor affinity, but also control receptor specificity. Thus, H1 subtype influenza strains with an oligosaccharide in such a position have been shown to bind preferentially to $\alpha2,3$-linked neuraminic acid, whereas mutants lacking this oligosaccharide had a preference for the $\alpha2,6$-linkage [11,13]. Furthermore, it has been shown recently that glycans carrying neuraminic acid in $\alpha2,3$ or $\alpha2,6$ linkages gain access to the receptor binding pocket from opposite sides [8]. Sterical hindrance by a glycan adjacent to the receptor binding site may therefore be a determinant of receptor specificity. Finally, the number and structure of N-glycans neighbouring the receptor binding pocket have been suggested to determine host range and pathogenicity of influenza viruses [7,11,26]. In

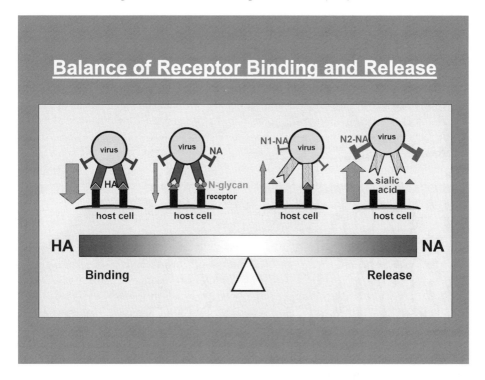

Fig. 3. Regulation of virus binding and release by HA glycosylation and neuraminidase activity. Receptor affinity is controlled by the oligosaccharides adjacent to the receptor binding site on HA. The efficiency of release depends on the activity of NA.

view of these findings, it will now be interesting to employ our panel of recombinant viruses to elucidate the contributions of individual HA tip glycans to tissue tropism and host range.

2. Factors determining endotheliotropism of FPV

Although cleavage of HA is an important determinant of spread of infection in the organism, it is not the only factor involved. This is illustrated by a recent study in which spread of FPV in the chick embryo was investigated [10]. We have found in this study that FPV shows strict endotheliotropism when infecting 11-day-old chick embryos (Fig. 4). Since hemorrhages and edema are major symptoms in FPV-infected chickens, it was not unexpected to see that the vasculature is an important target of infection. However, we were surprised when we could not detect viral replication in other cell types. Besides endothelia, myocytes and lymphatic tissues were found to be sites of virus replication, when hatched chickens were infected with other pathogenic H5 and H7 strains [17,34,35]. These differences in cell tropism may depend on the developmental stage of the host and on the virus strains used.

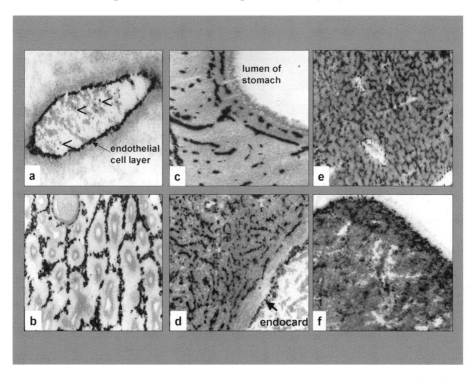

Fig. 4. Localization of FPV-infected cells in embryonic tissues by in situ hybridization. Brightfield photomicrographs showing autoradiograms with black grains representing bound HA-specific riboprobe in organs of the chick embryo. After in situ hybridization, slides were covered by photoemulsion, exposed for 2 days, developed, and counter-stained by hematoxilin-eosin. (a) Blood vessel (arrowheads indicating infected blood cells), (b) lung, (c) stomach, (d) heart, (e) liver, (f) spleen. Magnification × 75 (from Ref. [10]).

The results obtained with reassortants of FPV and virus N clearly indicate that endotheliotropism requires the presence of FPV-HA. This observation is in line with the concept that, because of its susceptibility to ubiquitous proteolytic activation, FPV-HA allows virus entry from the allantoic cavity into the highly vascularized mesenchymal layer of the chorioallantoic membrane, and thus, mediates hematogenic spread of infection. On the other hand, the restricted cleavability of virus N HA confines infection to the inner layer of the membrane and the allantoic cavity [28]. Therefore, reassortants containing virus N HA did not have access to endothelia when infected through the chorioallantoic route.

Whereas cleavage activation of HA proved to be essential for targeting the virus to endothelia, it was not responsible for confining the infection to these cells. Furin and PC5/PC6, the activating proteases of FPV-HA, were identified in all chicken tissues analyzed including endothelial cells. This observation indicates that the lack of spread of infection from endothelia to surrounding tissues cannot be attributed to the absence of activating proteases.

In contrast, tissue-specific expression of virus receptors appears to be an important factor in restricting infection to endothelia. Using lectin binding assays we could detect α-2,3-linked and α-2,6-linked neuraminic acid, which both proved to be able to serve as FPV receptors, only on epithelial cells and on cells of the reticulo-endothelial system. We could not detect, however, receptor determinants on other cells, such as myocytes, fibroblasts, and hepatocytes. Thus, it appears that cells lacking a measurable amount of neuraminic acid receptors cannot be infected by FPV and are therefore a barrier for the spread of infection. This concept is nicely supported by observations made in lung tissue. When this organ is infected via the hematogenic route as is the case in the embryo at day 11, the virus is retained in the endothelial cells of the capillary vessels. Since neuraminic acid is present in α2,6 linkage on these cells, it is clear that this type of neuraminic acid can serve as FPV receptor, although it appears that binding of avian strains is generally determined by the α2,3 linkage. The alveolar epithelia, although expressing virus receptor in large amounts, are not infected because virus access is prevented by the connective tissue lacking neuraminic acid. On the other hand, when embryos are infected through the airways, as can be done by inoculating virus 2 days before hatching into the now almost dry allantoic cavity, virus replication is readily detected in lung epithelia (data not shown).

It has to be pointed out that expression of neuraminic acid in the chick embryo depends on tissue differentiation [3]. This may explain the absence of detectable amounts of neuraminic acid on fibroblasts in situ, whereas cultured fibroblasts readily express receptors as indicated by their ability to allow efficient virus replication. It has also to be assumed that the subendothelial connective tissue is not a very tight barrier in the chorioallantoic membrane where it allows penetration of the virus from the allantoic epithelium into the mesodermal endothelia. In fact, low amounts of virus budding from mesodermal fibroblasts have been observed, indicating that these cells may play a role in mediating spread of infection [28]. Whether the spread through the mesodermal layer is driven by the particularly high virus replication rates in the allantoic epithelium and the presence of neuraminic acid on mesodermal fibroblasts or by some other mechanism remains to be seen.

Our data also show that the polarity of virus budding is another factor contributing to the confinement of infection to endothelial cells. Studies on Sendai virus in a mouse model have shown before that the sidedness of virus maturation has a distinct effect on spread of infection in the organism and on pathogenicity. Wild type Sendai virus released exclusively from the apical surface of lung epithelia is strictly pneumotropic, whereas the mutant F1-R which matures at the apical as well as the basolateral side causes pantropic infection [32,33]. It has long been known that FPV matures preferentially at the luminal side of endothelia [28], and the observations made here on virus budding and HA transport support this concept. The luminal budding polarity of FPV supports therefore the hematogenic spread of the virus and prevents at the same time infection of subendothelial cells.

Taken together, our data indicate that endotheliotropism of FPV in the chick embryo is the result of an interplay of several factors determined by the virus and the host (Fig. 5). These include proteolytic activation of HA by ubiquitous proteases which is responsible for entry of the virus into the vascular system and at least two mechanisms contributing to the confinement of the virus to endothelia: the polarity of virus budding at the luminal side of endothelial cells and cell-specific differences in the expression of neuraminic acid

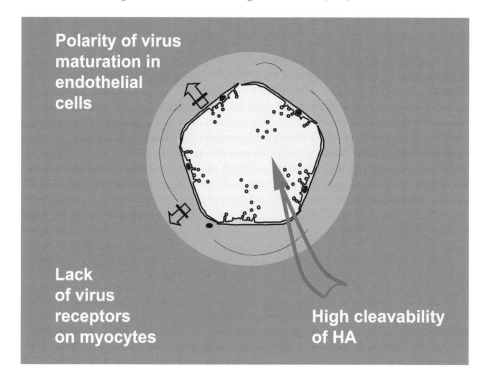

Fig. 5. The factors determining endotheliotropism of FPV. HA cleavage is responsible for virus entry into the vascular system. Polar budding and lack of receptors in adjacent tissues are responsible for restricting infection to endothelia.

receptors. Endotheliotropism without doubt plays an important role in the generalization of FPV infection and in the generation of typical symptoms of the disease, such as hemorrhages and edema. Systemic infection and severe vascular injury are also the central pathogenetic mechanisms of hemorrhagic fevers in primates caused by filoviruses and other agents, and there is evidence that at least some of these viruses replicate also in endothelia [30,31,39]. It will therefore be interesting to see if similar mechanisms as described here for FPV infection play also a role in the pathogenesis of hemorrhagic fevers in other species.

3. Conclusion

The high variability of the influenza virus genome is reflected by a wide spectrum in host tropism, tissue specificity, and pathogenicity, ranging from local infection of the respiratory tract or the gut, as is the case with most mammalian strains and the apathogenic avian viruses, to systemic infection caused by fowl plague virus or other highly pathogenic avian strains. Pathogenicity is determined by the interaction of viral proteins with each other or with host factors. This concept is supported by many studies on the viral envelope proteins. Proteolytic activation of the hemagglutinin as a fusion protein has been known for a long time to be an important determinant of pathogenicity. Receptor specificity is another hemagglutinin trait responsible for host range and tissue tropism. There is a close interdependence between hemagglutinin and neuraminidase in controlling binding and release of virus. The multifactorial character of tissue tropism and pathogenicity is illustrated by recent studies demonstrating that endotheliotropism of fowl plague virus in the chick embryo is determined, on one side, by the high cleavability of the hemagglutinin that mediates virus entry into the vascular system and, on the other hand, by restricted receptor expression and polar budding that prevent spread of infection into tissues surrounding endothelia.

Acknowledgements

We are grateful to R. Rott and C. Scholtissek, Giessen, for helpful discussions and for providing influenza virus reassortants. The electron micrograph was made by B. Agricola. This study was supported by grants from the Deutsche Forschungsgemeinschaft (SFB 286 and KL 238/6-1) and from the Fonds der Chemischen Industrie.

References

[1] S. Aytay, I.T. Schulze, Single amino acid substitutions in the hemagglutinin can alter the host range and receptor binding properties of H1 strains of influenza A virus, J. Virol. 65 (1991) 3022–3028.

[2] M.R. Castrucci, Y. Kawaoka, Biologic importance of neuraminidase stalk length in influenza A virus, J. Virol. 67 (1993) 759–764.

[3] P. Codogno, M. Aubery, Changes in cell-surface sialic acid content during chick embryo development,- Mech. Ageing Dev. 23 (1983) 307–314.

[4] P. Colman, Structure and function of the neuraminidase, in: K.G. Nicholson, R.G. Webster, A.J. Hay (Eds.), Textbook of Influenza, Blackwell, London, England, 1998, pp. 65–73.

[5] R.W. Compans, N.J. Dimmock, H. Meier-Ewert, Effect of antibody to neuraminidase on the maturation and hemagglutinating activity of an influenza A2 virus, J. Virol. 4 (1969) 528–534.

[6] R.J. Connor, Y. Kawaoka, R.G. Webster, J.C. Paulson, Receptor specificity in human, avian, and equine H2 and H3 influenza virus isolates, Virology 205 (1994) 17–23.

[7] C.M. Deom, A.J. Caton, I.T. Schulze, Host cell-mediated selection of a mutant influenza A virus that has lost a complex oligosaccharide from the tip of the hemagglutinin, Proc. Natl. Acad. Sci. U. S. A. 83 (1986) 3771–3775.

[8] M.B. Eisen, S. Sabesan, J.J. Skehel, D.C. Wiley, Binding of the influenza A virus to cell-surface receptors: structures of five hemagglutinin–sialyloligosaccharide complexes determined by X-ray crystallography, Virology 232 (1997) 19–31.

[9] M.C. Els, G.M. Air, K.G. Murti, R.G. Webster, W.G. Laver, An 18-amino acid deletion in an influenza neuraminidase, Virology 142 (1985) 241–247.

[10] A. Feldmann, M.K.-H. Schäfer, W. Garten, H.-D. Klenk, Targeted infection of endothelial cells by the avian influenza virus A/FPV/ROSTOCK/34 (H7N1) in chicken embryos, J. Virol. 74 (2000) 8018–8027.

[11] A.S. Gambaryan, V.P. Marinina, A.B. Tuzikov, N.V. Bovin, I.A. Rudneva, B.V. Sinitsyn, A.A. Shilov, M.N. Matrosovich, Effects of host-dependent glycosylation of hemagglutinin on receptor-binding properties on H1N1 human influenza A virus grown in MDCK cells and in embryonated eggs, Virology 247 (1998) 170–177.

[12] L.V. Gubareva, R. Bethell, G.J. Hart, K.G. Murti, C.R. Penn, R.G. Webster, Characterization of mutants of influenza A virus selected with the neuraminidase inhibitor 4-guanidino-Neu5Ac2en, J. Virol. 70 (1996) 1818–1827.

[13] I. Günther, B. Glatthaar, G. Doller, W. Garten, A H1 hemagglutinin of a human influenza A virus with a carbohydrate-modulated receptor binding site and an unusual cleavage site, Virus Res. 27 (1993) 147–160.

[14] J. Hausmann, E. Kretzschmar, W. Garten, H.D. Klenk, Biosynthesis, intracellular transport and enzymatic activity of an avian influenza A virus neuraminidase: role of unpaired cysteines and individual oligosaccharides, J. Gen. Virol. 78 (1997) 3233–3245.

[15] N.V. Kaverin, A.S. Gambaryan, N.V. Bovin, I.A. Rudneva, A.A. Shilov, O.M. Khodova, N.L. Varich, B.V. Sinitsin, N.V. Makarova, E.A. Kropotkina, Post reassortment changes in influenza A virus hemagglutinin restoring HA-NA functional match, Virology 244 (1998) 315–321.

[16] (a) H.D. Klenk, W. Garten, Activation cleavage of viral spike proteins. In: E. Wimmer (Ed.), Cold Spring Harbor Laboratory Press, 1994, pp. 241–280;
(b) N.V. Kaverin, H.D. Klenk, Strain-specific differences in the effect of influenza A virus neuraminidase on vector-expressed hemagglutinin, Arch. Virol. 144 (1999) 781–786.

[17] Y. Kobayashi, T. Horimoto, Y. Kawaoka, D. Alexander, C. Itakura, Pathological studies of chickens experimentally infected with two highly pathogenic avian influenza viruses, Avian Pathol. 25 (1996) 285–304.

[18] R.A. Lamb, R.M. Krug, Orthomyxoviridae: The viruses and their replication, in: B.N. Fields, D.M. Knipe, P.M. Howley (Eds.), Fields Virology, Lippincott-Raven Publishers, Philadelphia, USA, 1996, pp. 1353–1395.

[19] C. Liu, M.C. Eichelberger, R.W. Compans, G.M. Air, Influenza type A virus neuraminidase does not play a role in viral entry, replication, assembly, or budding, J. Virol. 69 (1995) 1099–1106.

[20] G. Luo, J. Chung, P. Palese, Alterations of the stalk of the influenza virus neuraminidase: deletions and insertions, Virus Res. 29 (1993) 321.

[21] M. Matrosovich, N. Zhou, Y. Kawaoka, R. Webster, The surface glycoproteins of H5 influenza viruses isolated from humans, chickens, and wild aquatic birds have distinguishable properties, J. Virol. 73 (1999) 1146–1155.

[22] L.J. Mitnaul, M.R. Castrucci, K.G. Murti, Y. Kawaoka, The cytoplasmic tail of influenza A virus neuraminidase (NA) affects NA incorporation into virions, virion morphology, and virulence in mice but is not essential for virus replication, J. Virol. 70 (1996) 873–879.

[23] M. Ohuchi, R. Ohuchi, A. Feldmann, H.D. Klenk, Regulation of receptor binding affinity of influenza virus hemagglutinin by its carbohydrate moiety, J. Virol. 71 (1997) 8377–8384.

[24] P. Palese, R.W. Compans, Inhibition of influenza virus replication in tissue culture by 2-deoxy-2,3-dehydro-N-trifluoroacetylneuraminic acid (FANA): mechanism of action, J. Gen. Virol. 33 (1976) 159–163.

[25] P. Palese, K. Tobita, M. Ueda, R.W. Compans, Characterization of temperature sensitive influenza virus mutants defective in neuraminidase, Virology 61 (1974) 397–410.

[26] M.L. Perdue, J.W. Latimer, J.M. Crawford, A novel carbohydrate addition site on the hemagglutinin protein of a highly pathogenic H7 subtype avian influenza virus, Virology 213 (1995) 276–281.

[27] G.N. Rogers, J.C. Paulson, R.S. Daniels, J.J. Skehel, I.A. Wilson, D.C. Wiley, Single amino acid substitutions in influenza haemagglutinin change receptor binding specificity, Nature 304 (1983) 76–78.

[28] R. Rott, M. Reinacher, M. Orlich, H.D. Klenk, Cleavability of hemagglutinin determines spread of avian influenza viruses in the chorioallantoic membrane of chicken embryo, Arch. Virol. 65 (1980) 123–133.

[29] I.A. Rudneva, E.I. Sklyanskaya, O.S. Barulina, S.S. Yamnikova, V.P. Kovaleva, I.V. Tsvetkova, N.V. Kaverin, Phenotypic expression of HA-NA combinations in human-avian influenza A virus reassortants, Arch. Virol. 141 (1996) 1091–1099.

[30] E.J. Ryabchikova, L.V. Kolesnikova, S.V. Netesov, Animal pathology of filoviral infections, Curr. Top. Microbiol. Immunol. 235 (1999) 145–173.

[31] H.J. Schnittler, F. Mahner, D. Drenckhahn, H.-D. Klenk, H. Feldmann, Replication of Marburg virus in human endothelial cells: a possible mechanism for the development of viral hemorrhagic disease, J. Clin. Invest. 91 (1993) 1301–1309.

[32] M. Tashiro, J.T. Seto, S. Choosakul, M. Yamakawa, H.D. Klenk, R. Rott, Budding site of Sendai virus in polarized epithelial cells is one of the determinants for tropism and pathogenicity in mice, Virology 187 (1992) 413–422.

[33] M. Tashiro, M. Yamakawa, K. Tobita, J.T. Seto, H.D. Klenk, R. Rott, Altered budding site of a pantropic mutant of Sendai virus F1-R, in polarized epithelial cells, J. Virol. 64 (1990) 4672–4677.

[34] H. van Campen, B.C. Easterday, V.S. Hinshaw, Destruction of lymphocytes by a virulent avian influenza A virus, J. Gen. Virol. 70 (1989) 467–472.

[35] H. van Campen, B.C. Easterday, V.S. Hinshaw, Virulent avian influenza A viruses: their effect on avian lymphocytes and macrophages in vivo and in vitro, J. Gen. Virol. 70 (1989) 2887–2895.

[36] A. Vines, K. Wells, M. Matrosovich, M.R. Castrucci, T. Ito, Y. Kawaoka, The role of influenza A virus hemagglutinin residues 226 and 228 in receptor specificity and host range restriction, J. Virol. 72 (1998) 7626–7631.

[37] R. Wagner, T. Wolff, A. Herwig, S. Pleschka, H.-D. Klenk, Interdependence of hemagglutinin glycosylation and neuraminidase as regulators of influenza virus growth—a study by reverse genetics, J. Virol. 74 (2000) 6316–6323.

[38] W. Weis, J.H. Brown, S. Cusack, J.C. Paulson, J.J. Skehel, D.C. Wiley, Structure of the influenza virus haemagglutinin complexed with its receptor, sialic acid, Nature 333 (1988) 426–431.

[39] S.R. Zaki, C.S. Goldsmith, Pathologic features of filovirus infections in humans, Curr. Top. Microbiol. Immunol. 235 (1999) 97–116.

International Congress Series 1219 (2001) 545–549

Characterization of the 1918 influenza virus hemagglutinin and neuraminidase genes

Jeffery K. Taubenberger*, Ann H. Reid, Thomas A. Janczewski, Thomas G. Fanning

Division of Molecular Pathology, Department of Cellular Pathology, Armed Forces Institute of Pathology, 14th Street and Alaska Avenue NW, Washington, DC 20306-6000, USA

Abstract

In the fall and winter of 1918–1919, an influenza pandemic of unprecedented virulence swept the globe leaving 40 million or more dead in its wake. The virus responsible for this catastrophe was not isolated at the time, however, it has recently become possible to study the genetic features of the 1918 'Spanish' influenza virus using frozen and fixed autopsy tissue. Gene sequences of the 1918 virus can be used to frame hypotheses about the origin of the 1918 virus, and to look for clues to its virulence. The study of the 1918 virus is not just one of historical curiosity. An understanding of the genetic make-up of the most virulent influenza strain in history may facilitate prediction and prevention of future pandemics. Published by Elsevier Science B.V.

Keywords: 1918 influenza virus; Spanish influenza; HA gene; NA gene

The influenza pandemic of 1918–1919 had several distinct waves. The first wave of influenza in the spring and summer of 1918 was highly contagious but caused few deaths. In late August, a virulent form of the disease emerged and spread throughout the globe in 6 months. The main wave of the global pandemic occurred in September through November of 1918, killing over 10,000 people per week in some US cities [1]. Outbreaks of the disease swept not only North America and Europe but also spread as far as the Alaskan wilderness and the most remote islands of the Pacific. Almost one-third of the US population became ill. The disease was also exceptionally severe, with mortality rates among the infected over 2.5%, compared to less than 0.1% in other influenza epidemics. Incredibly, some isolated populations had mortality rates over 70% [1].

* Corresponding author. Tel.: +1-301-319-0323; fax: +1-301-295-9507.
E-mail address: taubenbe@afip.osd.mil (J.K. Taubenberger).

0531-5131/01/$ – see front matter. Published by Elsevier Science B.V.
PII: S0531-5131(01)00629-X

In the 1918 pandemic, most deaths occurred among young adults, a group that usually has a very low death rate from influenza. Influenza and pneumonia death rates for 15–34 year olds were more than 20 times higher in 1918 than in previous years [2], with 99% of excess deaths among people under 65 years of age [3].

The majority of individuals who died during the pandemic succumbed to secondary bacterial pneumonia. However, a subset died rapidly after the onset of symptoms often with either massive acute pulmonary hemorrhage or pulmonary edema. In the hundreds of autopsies performed in 1918, the primary pathologic findings were confined to the respiratory tree and death was due to pneumonia and respiratory failure [4]. These findings are consistent with infection by a well-adapted influenza virus capable of rapid replication throughout the entire respiratory tree.

The natural reservoir of influenza viruses is thought to be wild waterfowl. Periodically, genetic material from avian strains is transferred to strains infectious to humans by reassortment or antigenic shift. Human influenza strains with recently acquired avian surface proteins were responsible for the pandemic influenza outbreaks in 1957 and 1968 [5].

While reassortment appears to be a critical event for the production of a pandemic virus, a significant amount of data exists to suggest that influenza viruses must acquire specific adaptations to spread and replicate efficiently in a new host. Among other features, there must be functional receptor binding and interaction between viral and host proteins. Defining the minimal adaptive changes needed to allow a reassortant virus to function in humans is essential to understanding how pandemic viruses emerge.

Once a new strain has acquired the changes that allow it to spread in humans, virulence is probably due in large part to the presence of novel surface protein(s) which allow the virus to spread rapidly through an immunologically naive population. This was the case in 1957 and 1968 and was almost certainly the case in 1918 [6]. While immunological novelty may explain much of the virulence of the 1918 influenza, it is likely that additional genetic features contributed to its exceptional lethality. Unfortunately, little is known about how genetic features of influenza viruses affect virulence. Virulence of a particular influenza strain is complex and involves a number of features including host adaptation, transmissibility, tissue tropism, and viral replication efficiency. The genetic basis for each of these features is not yet fully characterized, but is most likely polygenic in nature. Sequence analysis of the 1918 influenza virus allows us to address the genetic basis of virulence.

Frozen and fixed lung tissue from three 1918 influenza victims has been used to examine directly the genetic structure of the 1918 influenza virus [7–9]. Two of the cases analyzed were US Army soldiers who died in September 1918, one in New York and the other in South Carolina. A third sample was obtained from an Alaskan Inuit woman who had been interred in permafrost since November 1918. Amplification and sequencing of small overlapping RNA fragments extracted from these tissues allowed complete viral gene sequences to be determined for the two surface protein-encoding genes, hemagglutinin (HA) and neuraminidase (NA). These sequences confirm that the 1918 strain was an H1N1 subtype influenza A virus. Although these cases were widely separated geographically, there is very little heterogeneity amongst them at the sequence level suggesting the virus was optimally adapted to infect a majority of the human population in 1918. Sequencing the complete coding sequences of the six remaining gene segments is in progress.

The sequence of the 1918 HA is most closely related to the oldest available 'classical' swine flu strain, A/Sw/Iowa/30. However, despite this similarity the sequence has many avian features. Of the 41 amino acids that have been shown to be targets of the immune system and subject to antigenic drift pressure in humans, 37 match the avian sequence consensus, suggesting that there was little immunologic pressure on the HA protein before the fall of 1918. Another mechanism by which influenza viruses evade the human immune system is the acquisition of glycosylation sites to mask antigenic epitopes. Modern human H1N1s have up to five glycosylation sites in addition to the four found in all avian strains. The 1918 virus has only the four conserved avian sites.

Influenza virus infection requires binding of the HA protein to sialic acid receptors on the host cell surface. The HA receptor binding site consists of a subset of amino acids that are invariant in all avian HAs but vary in mammalian-adapted HAs. To shift from the avian receptor-binding site to that of swine H1s requires only one amino acid change, E190D. All three 1918 cases have the E190D change. In fact, the receptor-binding site of one of the 1918 cases (A/New York/1/18) is identical to that of A/Sw/Iowa/30. The other two 1918 cases have an additional change from the avian consensus, G225D. Since swine viruses with the same receptor site as Sw/Iowa/30 bind both avian and mammalian-type receptors, A/New York/1/18 probably also had the capacity to bind both. The change at residue 190 may represent the minimal change necessary to allow an avian H1-subtype HA to bind mammalian-type receptors, a critical step in host adaptation.

The principal biological role of NA is the cleavage of the terminal sialic acid residues that are receptors for the virus' HA protein. The active site of the enzyme consists of 15 invariant amino acids that are conserved in the 1918 NA. The functional NA protein is configured as a homotetramer in which the active sites are found on a terminal knob carried on a thin stalk. Some early human strains have short (11–16 amino acids) deletions in the stalk region, as do many strains isolated from chickens. The 1918 NA has a full-length stalk and has only the glycosylation sites shared by avian N1 strains.

Although the antigenic sites on human-adapted N1 neuraminidases have not been mapped, it is possible to align the N1 sequences with N2 subtype NAs and examine the N2 antigenic sites for evidence of drift in N1. There are 22 amino acids on the N2 protein that may function in antigenic epitopes. The 1918 NA matches the avian consensus at 21 of these sites.

Neither the 1918 HA nor NA genes have obvious genetic features that can be related directly to virulence. Two mutations in surface proteins have been shown to affect the virulence of influenza strains. For viral activation HA must be cleaved into two pieces, HA_1 and HA_2 by a host protease. Some avian H5 and H7 subtype viruses acquire a mutation which involves the addition of one or more basic amino acids to the cleavage site, allowing HA activation by ubiquitous proteases. Infection with such a pantropic strain causes systemic disease in birds with near uniform mortality. This mutation was not observed in the 1918 virus.

The second mutation with a significant effect on virulence through pantropism has been identified in the NA gene of two mouse-adapted influenza strains, A/WSN/33 and A/NWS/33. Mutations at a single codon (N146R or N146Y, leading to the loss of a glycosylation site) appear, like the HA cleavage site mutation, to allow the virus to replicate in many tissues outside the respiratory tract. This mutation was also not observed in the 1918 virus.

Therefore, the 1918 influenza virus does not have either of the mutations known to allow the virus to become pantropic. Since clinical and pathological findings in 1918 showed no evidence of replication outside the respiratory system, mutations allowing the 1918 virus to replicate systemically would not be expected. However, the relationship of other structural features of these proteins (aside from their presumed antigenic novelty) to virulence remains unknown. In their overall structural and functional characteristics, the 1918 HA and NA are avian-like but they also have mammalian-adapted characteristics.

While evidence suggests that the 1918 HA and NA gene segments were new to humans, the source of the 1918 influenza surface proteins and how they became part of a human-adapted influenza virus remain unclear. The absence of information about pre-1918 human influenza strains, the lack of influenza strains from birds and pigs around 1918, the gap between the 1918 strain and human and swine strains from the 1930s, and the lack of pre-1918 human serum samples all conspire to make solution of the question on 1918 influenza's origin exceedingly difficult. However, despite these problems, sequence data from the 1918 influenza virus itself is finally providing a basis for answering these questions.

Since virulence cannot yet be adequately explained by sequence analysis of the 1918 HA and NA genes, what can these sequences tell us about the origin of the 1918 virus? The best approach to analyzing the relationships among influenza viruses is phylogenetics, whereby hypothetical family trees are constructed which uses available sequence data to make assumptions about the ancestral relationships between current and historical flu strains. Since influenza genes are encoded by eight discreet RNA segments that can move independently between strains by the process of reassortment, these evolutionary studies must be performed independently for each gene segment.

A comparison of the complete 1918 HA and NA genes with those of numerous human, swine, and avian sequences demonstrates the following. Phylogenetic analyses based upon HA nucleotide changes (total, synonymous, or nonsynonymous) or HA amino acid changes always place the 1918 HA with the mammalian viruses, not with the avian viruses. Phylogenetic analyses of total or synonymous NA nucleotide changes place the 1918 NA sequence with the mammalian viruses, but analyses of nonsynonymous changes or amino acid changes place 1918 NA with the avian viruses. Most analyses place HA and NA near the root of the mammalian clade, suggesting that both genes emerged from an avian reservoir just prior to 1918. Clearly, by 1918 the virus had acquired enough mammalian-adaptive changes to function as a human pandemic virus.

Identifying the minimal changes necessary to allow a virus with avian surface proteins to replicate and be transmitted efficiently in mammalian hosts is extremely important for our understanding of the emergence of pandemic influenza viruses.

Fragmentary sequences of all the remaining gene segments of the 1918 virus have already been deciphered and full-length segment sequences will be completed for several more 1918 influenza genes in the near future. Such sequences will allow the complete phylogenetic analyses of each segment, and will help elucidate the origin of the 1918 virus. Whether any particular genetic features of the virus can be related directly to its exceptional virulence is yet unclear. Even as the genetic structure of the 'Spanish' flu virus is becoming fully known, other questions, such as the role played by differences in immunity in different age groups in 1918 may prove important. It is hoped that knowledge gained by studying this exceptionally lethal human pathogen can be applied to prevent, or at least predict, the emergence of new influenza viruses with pandemic potential.

Acknowledgements

Supported by grants from the Department of Veteran's Affairs and the American Registry of Pathology, and by the intramural funds of the Armed Forces Institute of Pathology. This is US government work; there are no restrictions on its use.

References

[1] A. Crosby, America's Forgotten Pandemic, Cambridge Univ. Press, Cambridge, 1989.
[2] S.D. Collins, Age and sex incidence of influenza and pneumonia morbidity and mortality in the epidemic of 1928–1929 with comparative data for the epidemic of 1918–1919, Public Health Rep. 46 (1931) 1909–1937.
[3] L. Simonsen, M.J. Clarke, L.B. Schonberger, N.H. Arden, N.J. Cox, K. Fukuda, Pandemic versus epidemic influenza mortality: a pattern of changing age distribution, J. Infect. Dis. 78 (1998) 53–60.
[4] E.R. LeCount, The pathologic anatomy of influenzal bronchopneumonia, JAMA 72 (1919) 650–652.
[5] C. Scholtissek, W. Rohde, R. von Hoyningen, R. Rott, On the origin of the human influenza virus subtypes H2N2 and H3N2, Virology 87 (1978) 13–20.
[6] A.H. Reid, J.K. Taubenberger, The 1918 flu and other influenza pandemics: 'over there' and back again, Lab. Invest. 79 (1999) 95–101.
[7] J.K. Taubenberger, A.H. Reid, A.E. Krafft, K.E. Bijwaard, T.G. Fanning, Initial genetic characterization of the 1918 'Spanish' influenza virus, Science 275 (1997) 1793–1796.
[8] A.H. Reid, T.G. Fanning, J.V. Hultin, J.K. Taubenberger, Origin and evolution of the 1918 "Spanish" influenza virus hemagglutinin, PNAS 96 (1999) 1651–1656.
[9] A.H. Reid, T.G. Fanning, T.A. Janczewski, J.K. Taubenberger, Characterization of the 1918 'Spanish' influenza virus neuraminidase gene, PNAS 97 (2000) 6785–6790.

International Congress Series 1219 (2001) 551–555

Inhibition of influenza virus replication by nitric oxide

G.F. Rimmelzwaan*, M. Baars, R.A.M. Fouchier, A.D.M.E. Osterhaus

Department of Virology, Erasmus University Rotterdam, PO Box 1738, 3000 DR Rotterdam, The Netherlands

Abstract

Background: Upon infection with influenza viruses, patients develop a cytokine response including the induction of IFN-γ, TNF-α and IL-1β. These cytokines are known to induce the expression of the inducible form of nitric oxide (NO) synthase (iNOS) in human airway epithelial cells. NO has been shown to exert antiviral activity against a number of different viruses. It is unknown, however, whether NO has antiviral properties against influenza viruses. *Methods*: The effect of the NO-donor *S*-nitroso-*N*-acetylpenicillamine (SNAP) was studied on the influenza virus replication in Madin Darby Canine Kidney (MDCK) cells. To measure influenza virus replication, IFA, hemagglutination assays, measurement of infectious virus in culture supernatants and RNA hybridization techniques were performed. *Results*: SNAP was found to inhibit influenza virus replication in a dose-dependent manner. NO liberated from SNAP inhibited the synthesis of vRNA and mRNA encoding viral proteins severely. Subsequently, fewer influenza-infected cells were detected by IFA and the titer of infectious virus in culture supernatants of infected SNAP treated MDCK cells were reduced. *Conclusion*: It is concluded that NO inhibits the replication of influenza viruses, probably during the early steps of the virus replication cycle, involving the synthesis of vRNA and mRNA encoding viral proteins. Therefore, it is hypothesized that the production of NO by cytokine-induced iNOS in airway epithelial cells provides an antiviral effect in these cells. © 2001 Elsevier Science B.V. All rights reserved.

Keywords: Cytokines; Antiviral activity; Nitric oxide

1. Introduction

Nitric oxide (NO), a gaseous free radical, has been shown to have multiple biological functions. NO is catalytically generated by one of the three isoforms of NO

* Corresponding author. Tel.: +31-10-4088243; fax: +31-10-4089485.
E-mail address: rimmelzwaan@viro.fgg.eur.nl (G.F. Rimmelzwaan).

0531-5131/01/$ – see front matter © 2001 Elsevier Science B.V. All rights reserved.
PII: S0531-5131(01)00649-5

synthase (NOS) from L-arginin. NO generated by the inducible form of NOS (iNOS) has been shown to play a role in the defense against a variety of microbial pathogens, including bacteria, parasites and viruses. iNOS can be induced in a number of different cell types, including human airway epithelial cells [1,2], the primary target for influenza viruses. In these cells, iNOS is induced after stimulation with interferon-γ, tumor necrosis factor-α and interleukin1-β [1,2]. Interestingly, the production of these cytokines is induced shortly after infection with influenza viruses [3,4]. In mouse models, it has been shown that the release of NO after infection with influenza virus can contribute to the pathogenesis of virus induced pneumonia [5,6]. It is unclear whether influenza virus replication is also sensitive to the action of NO. In that case, the release of NO by airway epithelial cells may also provide a first line defense mechanism against influenza viruses. In the present study the effect of S-nitroso-N-acetylpenicillamine (SNAP), a NO donor, was studied on influenza virus replication in vitro.

2. Materials and methods

2.1. Infection procedures

Madin Darby Canine Kidney (MDCK) cells were cultured in minimal essential medium (MEM) containing 10% FCS, 100 IU/ml penicillin and 100 μg/ml streptomycin. After washing the cells twice with PBS, the cells were infected with influenza virus A/Netherlands/19/94 or A/Netherlands/202/94 for 1 h at 37 °C at various multiplicity of infection (MOI). After washing the cells with infection medium (MEM with 4 μg/ml trypsin and 4% BSA), cells were treated with different concentrations of the NO donor SNAP, or a control molecule, which lack the S-nitroso group, N-acetylpenicillamine (NAP), or were left untreated. SNAP and NAP were added directly after the infection procedure or 3 h before infection.

2.2. Measurement of viral replication

After 24 h post-infection, the infectious virus titers in the culture supernatants of infected MDCK cells were determined as previously described [7]. In brief, 10-fold-serially diluted culture supernatants were inoculated in quadruplicate on MDCK cells as described above. After culturing the cells for 6–7 days, the supernatants were tested for HA activity, which was used as an indicator for infection of the cells in individual wells. The infectious titers were calculated according to the method of Spearman–Karber and expressed as $TCID_{50}$/ml.

2.3. Immunofluorescence assay

In parallel experiments, the number of influenza virus infected MDCK cells was determined by IFA. Twelve hours after infection, the cells were fixed in acetone as previously described [8]. Subsequently, the cells were incubated with a monoclonal antibody specific for the influenza virus A nucleoprotein, which was labeled with FITC (IMAGEN, influenza A + B, DAKO Diagnostics).

2.4. RNA hybridization

For the detection of vRNA and mRNA/cRNA corresponding to the NP and HA encoding sequences, positive strand (+) and negative strand (−) DIG labeled probes were used, respectively. These probes were synthesized as previously described [8]. RNA was isolated from the MDCK cells using the RNAzol method 12 h post-infection, according to the recommendations of the manufacturer. One-micrliter volumes of 3-fold-serial dilution of the RNA samples were transferred to a nylon membrane after denaturation in 50% formamide, 7% formaldehyde and $1 \times$ SSC in DEPC treated water. After baking the nylon membranes, they were incubated with the respective DIG labeled probes and developed according to the manufacturers recommendations (Boehringer Mannheim).

3. Results

SNAP, but not NAP, inhibited the replication of influenza viruses in a dose-dependent fashion as shown by measuring the HA titers in the culture supernatants of MDCK cells infected with A/Netherlands/202/95 or B/Netherlands/22/95. The inhibitory effects correlated with the release of NO_{2-}, an intermediate of NO, in the culture medium. The strongest inhibition of the replication by SNAP was observed at a concentration of 400 μM. At this concentration, SNAP also reduced the release of infectious virus into the culture supernatant of MDCK cells infected with AA/Netherlands/202/95 (Fig. 1).

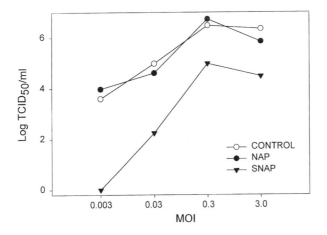

Fig. 1. The addition of the NO donor SNAP inhibits the release of infectious virus into the culture supernatant of MDCK cells infected with influenza virus A/Netherlands/202/95 at the indicated MOI. Directly after infections, the cells were treated with 400 μM SNAP or NAP or left untreated. The infectious virus titers in the culture supernatants were expressed as the Log of 50% tissue culture infectious dose per milliliter (TCID$_{50}$/ml).

Twenty-four hours post-infection of the inhibitory effect of SNAP was most pronounced using a low MOI for the infection of the MDCK cells. SNAP did not affect the viability of the MDCK cells or the neuraminidase and hemagglutination activity of the virus. The inhibitory effect of NO on influenza virus replication was further demonstrated by showing that the addition of 400 μM SNAP 3 h before or directly after infection reduced the number of infected cells in treated cultures as analyzed by IFA performed 12 h after infection [9]. At this time point after infection, RNA hybridization techniques were also performed. Treatment of the MDCK cells with the NO donor 3 h before infection significantly inhibited the synthesis of viral RNA and mRNA. When added 1 h after infection, a reduction of viral RNA was also observed. The levels of β-actin mRNA were not affected by SNAP (data not shown).

4. Conclusion

NO inhibits the replication of influenza viruses, probably during the early steps of the virus replication cycle, involving the synthesis of viral RNA and mRNA encoding viral proteins. Therefore, it can be speculated that the production of NO by iNOS in airway epithelial cells after stimulation with cytokines, which are induced shortly after infection with influenza viruses, provides an antiviral effect in these cells. The release of NO in the airway would reduce the primary replication of influenza viruses before other mechanisms of the immune system are activated to control and clear the infection. Thus, in addition to harmful effects such as cell death and tissue destruction, as has been described in mouse models for influenza, NO also can be beneficial, provided that its production is tightly regulated.

References

[1] F.H. Guo, H.R. De Raeve, T.W. Rice, D.J. Stuehr, F.B.J.M. Thunnissen, S.C. Erzurum, Continuous nitric oxide synthesis by inducible nitric oxide synthase in normal human airway epithelium in vivo, Proc. Natl. Acad. Sci. U. S. A. 92 (1995) 7809–7813.
[2] K. Asano, C.B.E. Chee, B. Gaston, C.M. Lilly, C. Gerard, J.M. Drazen, J.S. Stamler, Constitutive and inducible nitric oxide synthase gene expression, regulation and activity in human lung epithelial cells, Proc. Natl. Acad. Sci. U. S. A. 91 (1994) 10089–10093.
[3] F.G. Hayden, R.S. Fritz, M.C. Lobo, W.G. Alvord, W. Strobe, S.E. Straus, Local and systemic cytokine responses during experimental human influenza A virus infection, J. Clin. Invest. 101 (1998) 643–649.
[4] T. Hennet, H.J. Ziltener, K. Frei, E. Peterans, A kinetic study of immune mediators in the lungs of mice infected with inflluenza A virus, J. Immunol. 149 (1992) 932–939.
[5] T. Akaike, Y. Noguchi, S. Ijiri, K. Setoguchi, M. Suga, Y.M. Zheng, B. Dietzschold, H. Maeda, Pathogenesis of influenza virus induced pneumonia: involvement of both nitric oxide and oxygen radicals, Proc. Natl. Acad. Sci. U. S. A. 93 (1996) 2448–2453.
[6] G. Karupiah, J.-H. Chen, S. Mahalingam, C.F. Nathan, J.D. MacMicking, Rapid interferon-γ dependent clearance of influenza A virus and protection from consolidating pneomonitis in nitric oxide synthase 2-deficient mice, J. Exp. Med. 188 (1998) 1541–1546.
[7] G.F. Rimmelzwaan, M. Baars, R. Van Beek, G. Van Amerongen, K. Lövgren, E.C.J. Claas, A.D.M.E. Osterhaus, Induction of protective immunity against influenza in a macaque model: comparison of conventional and iscom vaccines, J. Gen. Virol. 78 (1997) 757–765.

[8] G.F. Rimmelzwaan, M. Baars, E.C.J. Claas, A.D.M.E. Osterhaus, Comparison of RNA hybridization, hemagglutination assay, titration of infectious virus and immunofluorescence as methods for monitoring influenza virus replication in vitro, J. Virol. Methods 74 (1998) 57–66.
[9] G.F. Rimmelzwaan, M.M.W.J. Baars, P. de Lijster, R.A.M. Fouchier, A.D.M.E. Osterhaus, Inhibition of influenza virus replication by nitric oxide, J. Virol. 73 (1999) 8880–8883.

International Congress Series 1219 (2001) 557–571

Targeted influenza virus infection of endothelial cells and leucocytes

Anke Feldmann, Nikolai Looser, Ralf Wagner, Hans-Dieter Klenk*

Institut für Virologie, Klinikum der Philipps-Universität Marburg, Robert-Koch-Str. 17, 35037 Marburg, Germany

Abstract

The tissue tropism and spread of infection of the highly pathogenic avian influenza virus A/FPV/Rostock/34 (H7N1) were analyzed in 11-day-old chicken embryos by in situ hybridization technique using specific riboprobes directed against the hemagglutinin mRNA. As shown by in situ hybridization, the virus caused generalized infection that was strictly confined to endothelial cells. Studies with reassortants of FPV and the apathogenic avian strain A/chick/Germany/N/49 (H10N1) revealed that endotheliotropism was linked to FPV hemagglutinin (HA). To further analyze the factors determining endotheliotropism, the HA-activating protease furin was cloned from chicken tissue. Ubiquitous expression of furin and other proprotein convertases revealed that proteolytic activation of HA was not responsible for restriction of the infection. Expression of virus receptors in embryonic tissues was analyzed by histochemical analysis of $\alpha2,3$- and $\alpha2,6$-linked neuraminic acid on the cells. Viral receptors were found on endothelial cells, but not on tissues surrounding endothelia. The budding polarity of FPV from the endothelia is strictly at the luminar side of the vessel. Taken together, these observations indicate that endotheliotropism of FPV in the chicken embryo is determined, on one hand, by the high cleavability of HA that mediates virus entry into the vascular system and, on the other hand, by restricted receptor expression and polar budding that prevent spread of infection into tissues surrounding endothelia. Further investigations with H7 and H3 reassortants of the WSN strain also showed endotheliotropism in the chick embryo, whereas wild-type WSN (H1) was observed only in leucocyte infiltration of peripheral tissues. Thus, HA is an important determinant of the tissue tropism of influenza virus. © 2001 Elsevier Science B.V. All rights reserved.

Keywords: Influenza; Pathogenicity; Tissue tropism; Hemagglutinin

* Corresponding author. Tel.: +49-6421-286-6253; fax: +49-6421-286-8962.
E-mail address: klenk@mailer.uni-marburg.de (H.-D. Klenk).

0531-5131/01/$ – see front matter © 2001 Elsevier Science B.V. All rights reserved.
PII: S 0 5 3 1 - 5 1 3 1 (0 1) 0 0 3 9 7 - 1

1. Introduction

Influenza A viruses are found in humans, pigs and several other mammals as well as in many birds. Most influenza A viruses cause local infection that is confined to the respiratory tract or, in the case of some avian strains, to the gut. In contrast, some avian strains belonging to subtypes H5 and H7 cause generalized infection. These viruses are highly pathogenic, killing the birds within a few days. As a result of the systemic infection, virus can be recovered from many organs. Large hemorrhages distributed all over the body, edema, and cutaneous ischemia are major symptoms of the diseases. At the final stage of the infection, neurological signs emerge, such as photophobia and dullness [8,15]. Although hemorrhages and edema indicate an affliction of the vascular system, only few data are available pertaining to cell tropism in the natural host. As one example, the virulent influenza strain A/turkey/Ontario/7732/66 (H5N2) has a pronounced effect on lymphocytes and lymphoid tissue of its avian host [30,31]. In contrast, A/turkey/England/ 50-92/91 (H5N1) strongly attacks the cardiovascular system of the birds [13]. An infection of myocytes and endothelial cells was also observed when chickens were experimentally infected with avian and human isolates obtained during the H5N1 outbreak in Hong Kong in 1997 [25]. These examples already show that conclusions on tissue tropism drawn from investigations using one strain are not necessarily applicable to others. Until recently, it was believed that the highly pathogenic avian strains are not transmitted to humans. However, in the course of an H5N1 outbreak among chickens, several human infections with a high case fatality rate were observed in 1997 in Hong Kong [26]. Furthermore, an H7N7 virus was isolated in 1996 from man with milder disease symptoms that proved to be closely related to the avian isolate A/turkey/Ireland/PV74/95 [1,14]. These observations demonstrate that H5 and H7 strains can be transmitted from birds to humans without an intermediate host and without reassortment and, even more importantly, that the pathogenic potential of these viruses as determined by HA is preserved to some extent in the new host.

We were interested in finding factors determining tissue and cell tropism of influenza virus in the chick embryo. We found that infection with FPV is confined to endothelial cells. Endotheliotropism is determined, on one hand, by the high cleavability of HA that mediates virus entry into the vascular system and, on the other hand, by restricted receptor expression and polar budding that prevent spread of infection into tissues surrounding endothelia. Further investigations with H7 and H3 reassortants of the WSN strain showed also endotheliotropism in the chick embryo, whereas wild-type WSN (H1) was observed only in leucocyte infiltrations of peripheral tissues. Thus, HA is an important determinant of the tissue tropism of influenza virus.

2. Materials and methods

2.1. Viruses

Influenza virus strains A/FPV/Rostock/34 (H7N1), A/chick/Germany/N/49 (H10N7), (virus N) and reassortants of both influenza strains have been used. The generation of the influenza reassortants and the identification of their genotypes have been described before [17,22,23]. Furthermore, we used A/WSN/33 (H1N1) and the recombinant influenza viruses H3-WSN (H3N1) and H7-WSN (H7N1). The generation of these recombinant viruses has been described previously [33]. Seed stocks of influenza virus were grown in the allantoic cavity of 11-day-old embryonated eggs.

2.2. Generation of riboprobes, cloning of chicken furin (gfur)

[^{35}S]UTP-labeled cRNA probes for furin, H7 HA and H10 HA, were generated from cDNA. cDNAs were obtained by RT-PCR or by screening a chicken liver cDNA gene bank (Stratagene Cat. No.: 965402). The complete gene of gfur was cloned and sequenced (GenBank Z68093). A fragment of 331nt (nt533–864) of bovine furin (GenBank X75956) labeled with [^{32}P CTP] served as a screening probe. A fragment [32] of 461nt, corresponding to nt1252–1713 of the HA cDNA of A/FPV/Rostock/34 (H7N1) [6] (GenBank M24457), was subcloned into the transcription vector pBluescript KS+. A fragment corresponding to nt846–1300 of the HA gene of A/chick/Germany/N/49 (H10N7) [4] (GenBank M21646) was cloned by RT-PCR using viral RNA into the transcription vector pBluescript KS+. [^{35}S]UTP-labeled cRNA probes were generated for A/FPV HA (nt1252–1713), A/WSN HA (nt1267–1775), A/PR8 NA (nt1096–1409) and A/Hong Kong NP (nt113–511) by RT-PCR using viral RNA. The gene fragments were subcloned into the transcription vector pBluescript KS+ (Stratagene). In vitro transcription using the in vitro transcription kit (Boehringer-Mannheim, Germany) was carried out in the presence of 150 μCi [^{35}S]UTP. For purification of the labeled RNA, we used Nucleotide push columns (Stratagene).

2.3. Replication of FPV in blood from the chicken embryo

Ten-microliter blood was taken from the neck vessel of 11-day-old chicken embryos and transferred into an eppendorf-cup containing 200 μl DMEM. Cells were infected with FPV at a multiplicity of infection (MOI) of 10. At different time points, aliquots were taken, centrifuged to pellet the leucocytes, and the supernatant was used to perform plaque assay on MDBK cells. Ten-milliliter blood was taken from adult chickens, the leucocytes isolated by ficoll-gradient centrifugation and then infected as described above.

2.4. In situ hybridization

In situ hybridization was performed according to a reported protocol [3,20].

2.5. Lectin characterization

For detection of SAα-2,3Gal and SAα-2,6Gal on the surface of the cells of chicken embryos, a digoxigenin (DIG) glycan differentiation kit (Boehringer-Mannheim) was used. Twenty-micrometer sections of uninfected chicken embryos were fixed for 2 min in ice-cold methanol containing 1 mM levamisole, a specific inhibitor of the endogenous alkaline phosphatase. A blocking solution supplied with the kit was then incubated with the sections for 12 h. The slides were washed twice with TBS buffer (0.05 M Tris–HCl, pH 8.5, 0.15 M NaCl) for 10 min each and once with buffer 1 (TBS, 1 mM $MgCl_2$, 1 mM $CaCl_2$, 1 mM $MnCl_2$). DIG-labeled lectins [*Sambucus nigra* agglutinin (SNA) specific for SAα-2,6Gal and *Maackia amurensis* agglutinin (MAA) specific for SAα-2,3Gal] dissolved in buffer 1 were then incubated with the slides for 2 h. After three washes with TBS, the sections were incubated for 1 h with anti-DIG antibody conjugated to alkaline phosphatase (1:1000 in TBS). After three washes with TBS, the sections were incubated with buffer 2 (0.1 M Tris–HCl, pH 9.5, 0.05 M $MgCl_2$, 0.1 M NaCl), and the substrate solution NBT/X-phosphate (supplied with the kit) dissolved in buffer 2 containing 1 mM levamisole was applied to the sections. After 5–10 min, the reaction was stopped by washing the slides in H_2O. The sections were coverslipped without counterstaining.

2.6. Electronmicroscopy

The organs of infected chicken embryos were prepared at 18 h p.i. and fixed immediately in ITO buffer according to a published protocol [11]. Subsequently, an additional fixation step with OsO_4 was carried out. The tissue was embedded in Epon and ultrathin sections were prepared and contrasted by uranyl acetate and lead citrate prior to microscopic analysis.

3. Results

3.1. Endothelial cells are the target of FPV

When 11-day-old chicken embryos were infected via the allantoic route with 10^3 PFU of FPV, they died 18 h after infection and showed extensive subcutaneous hemorrhages distributed all over the body. In contrast, embryos infected with virus N that was used as an apathogenic control usually died at 30 h p.i. without significant bleeding signs. By in situ hybridization, we detected viral RNA in all organs of the FPV-infected embryo, indicating that the virus causes a generalized infection. In the chicken embryo infected with virus N, HA-specific RNA was only detected in the cloaca (Fig. 1). The hybridized slides were then covered with nuclear emulsion to visualize the radioactive riboprobe on the tissue. It was interesting to see that viral RNA of FPV was found in every organ, but exclusively in endothelial cells, while virus N-specific RNA was strictly confined to the epithelia of the cloaca (Fig. 1). In addition, we performed in situ hybridization with a riboprobe directed against the vascular endothelial growth factor receptor 2 (flk-2) that is exclusively expressed in endothelial cells [5]. In all organs, we saw similar labeling patterns when we used the HA-specific or the flk-2-specific probes (data not shown). Thus, in 11-day-old chicken embryos, only endothelial cells are infected by FPV.

3.2. FPV HA is necessary and sufficient for endotheliotropism

We analyzed tissue tropism and especially endotheliotropism of a set of reassortants of FPV and virus N to determine the influence of the hemagglutinin molecule

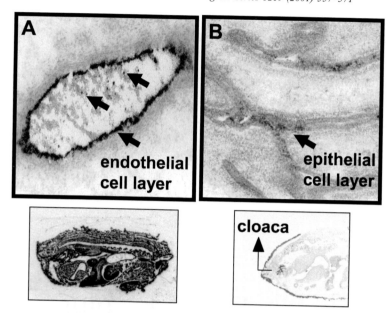

Fig. 1. Spread of FPV and virus N in the chick embryo. Embryonated eggs were infected with 10^3 PFU via the allantoic route. At 17 h (FPV) or 40 h (N), p.i., cryosections were prepared that were subjected to autoradiography after in situ hybridization with $[^{35}S]$UTP-labeled riboprobes directed against mRNA of H7 HA (A) and H10 HA (B). Sections were covered by nuclear photoemulsion and developed after 4 days exposure time. Tissue was counterstained by hematoxilin-eosin staining. Exposure time for autoradiographie was 8 h.

(Table 1). Replication of all reassortants was strictly confined to endothelial cells although, in some cases, even more than half of the viral RNA segments were from virus N. We did not detect viral RNA of the reassortants 108 and 109 in the chicken embryo although they reached high HA titers ($>2^7$) within the allantoic fluid. The

Table 1
Gene constellation and endotheliotropism of the reassortants of FPV and virus N

	PB1	PB2	PA	HA	NP	NA	MS1, MS2	NS1, NS2	Endotheliotropism
106	N	FPV	FPV	FPV	FPV	FPV	FPV	FPV	+
111	FPV	N	FPV	FPV	FPV	FPV	FPV	FPV	+
116	FPV	FPV	N	FPV	FPV	FPV	FPV	FPV	+
114	FPV	FPV	FPV	FPV	N	FPV	FPV	FPV	+
110	FPV	FPV	FPV	FPV	FPV	N	FPV	FPV	+
118	FPV	N	N	FPV	N	N	FPV	FPV	+
119	FPV	N	N	FPV	N	FPV	FPV	N	+
122	FPV	FPV	N	FPV	FPV	N	N	N	+ +
108	FPV	N	N	N	N	FPV	FPV	FPV	−
109	FPV	FPV	N	N	N	FPV	FPV	FPV	−

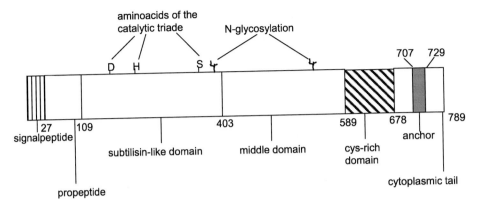

Fig. 2. Protein structure of gfur.

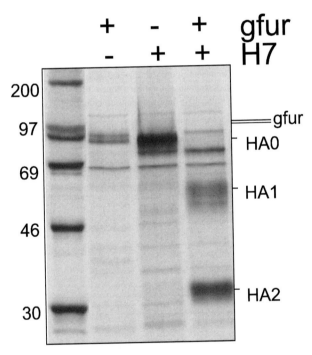

Fig. 3. Cleavage of FPV HA by chicken furin. LoVo cells [27] were infected with VV:gfur and VV:HAwt [16], each at an MOI of 10. Virus inocula were replaced by DMEM without FCS 1 h after infection. At 4 h after infection, LoVo cells were starved for methionine for 1 h and then labeled with 100 μCi of [35S]methionine (1000 Ci/mmol; Amersham, Braunschweig, Germany) for 3 h. The medium was replaced by MEM-containing nonradioactive methionine, and incubation was continued for an additional hour. Immunoprecipitation was carried out using anti-FPV or anti-hfur rabbit serum and proteins were analyzed by SDS-10% PAGE under reducing conditions. Sizes are shown in kilodaltons.

reassortants 108 and 109, in contrast to all other reassortants tested, have the HA of virus N. These experiments show a clear relationship between cleavability of HA and spread of infection. FPV HA is both necessary and sufficient for infection of endothelia.

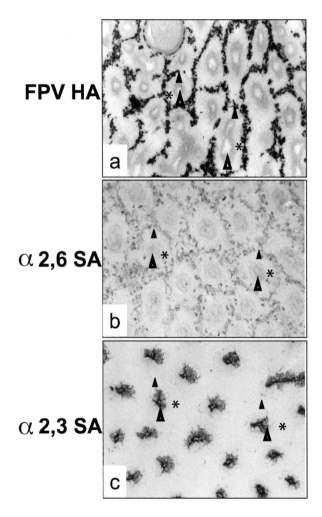

Fig. 4. (a) Localization of FPV-infected cells in embryonic lung tissue by in situ hybridization. Bright-field photomicrographs showing autoradiograms with black grains representing bound HA-specific riboprobe in the endothelial cells of the lung. After in situ hybridization, slides were covered by photoemulsion, exposed for 2 days, developed and counterstained by hematoxylin-eosin. (b, c) Histochemical analysis of NeuAc-α2,6Gal (b) and NeuAc-α2,3Gal (c) in the lung of chicken embryos by lection binding. Cryosections of uninfected chicken embryos were incubated with MAA, specific for NeuAc-α2,3Gal, or SNA, specific for NeuAc-α2,6Gal, as described in Materials and methods. Bound lectins were identified using the DIG-Glycan differentiation kit (Roche). Magnifications × 75. Symbols indicate endothelial cells (solid arrowhead), mesencymal cells (stars), and alveolar epithelia (open arrowheads).

3.3. Proteolytic activation of FPV HA is not responsible for the confinement of infection to endothelial cells

Proteolytic activation of HA by host protein convertases is known to be a strong determinant for spread and severity of influenza virus infection [12]. FPV HA is activated at its multibasic cleavage by furin [24]. To find out if a limited expression of furin is the reason for the restricted infection in chicken embryos, we cloned chicken furin (gfur) from a chicken liver cDNA library (Stratagene). gfur exhibits all structural characteristics of human furin including the propeptide that is autocatalytically removed by cleavage, the subtilisin-like domain, and the cytoplasmic tail (Fig. 2).

We used recombinant vaccinia viruses that expressed FPV HA [16] or gfur to analyze the cleavage of FPV HA by the cloned chicken furin in the furin-deficient LoVo cell line [27]. gfur was expressed in these cells and cleaved FPV HA as does human furin (Fig. 3).

Having found out that in chickens the proprotein convertase furin is expressed and that it can activate FPV HA in expression experiments, we looked for the expression pattern of gfur in 11-day-old chicken embryos by in situ hybridization. As expected, gfur is ubiquitously expressed and is, therefore, not responsible for confinement of infection to endothelia (data not shown).

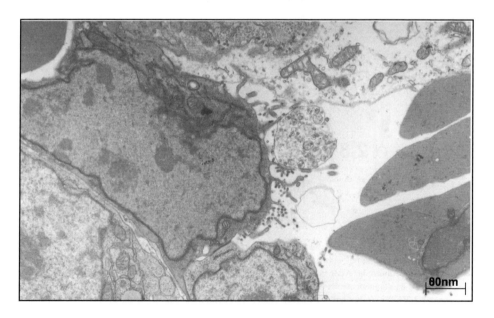

Fig. 5. Electron micrograph of an FPV-infected endothelial cell from a heart capillary. At 18 h p.i., the heart of an infected chicken embryo was prepared for transmission electron microscopy. Numerous virus particles bud from the luminal side of the endothelial cell.

3.4. Neuraminic acid receptors are absent on tissue surrounding endothelial cells

After we had analyzed the expression pattern of HA-activating proteases, we investigated the distribution of viral receptor determinants in the chick embryo. This was done by histochemical analysis using lectins specific for NeuAc-α2,3-Gal, which is preferentially bound by avian influenza virus strains, or NeuAc-α2,6-Gal, which is recognized by mammalian strains. These lectins have also been used by other groups to determine the receptor specificities of different influenza strains [9,10].

By this method, we found that neuraminic acid receptors were not expressed ubiquitously. Fig. 4 shows the results obtained in the lung. Labeling of lung tissue with SNA revealed a characteristic hexagonal endothelial-labeling pattern, identical to that observed after in situ hybridization with the H7-specific probe. The epithelial cells of the lung are only stained by MAA, indicating the presence of NeuAc-α2,3-Gal receptors. By this experiment, we could first show that NeuAc-α2,6-Gal on lung endothelial cells can serve as a viral receptor for FPV-mediating infection of the endothelial cells. Second, the

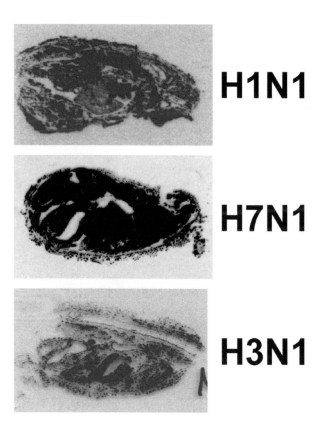

Fig. 6. Spread of WSN (H1N1) and the recombinant viruses H3-WSN (H3N1) and H7-WSN (H7N1) in the chick embryo. Forty hours after infection, cryosections were prepared and subjected to in situ hybridization using riboprobes directed against mRNA of NP. Exposure time for autoradiography was 8 h.

epithelial cells of the lung, although reacting with MAA are not infected by FPV. Third, the mesenchymal cells of the lung between epithelial and endothelial cell layer do not react with either of the two lectins. Therefore, at least with the method employed, no viral receptor determinants can be localized on these cells. These mesenchymal cells, therefore, appear to function as a barrier preventing spread of the infection from endothelial to epithelial cells.

In all organs, we always observed specific labeling of endothelial and epithelial cells; other cells, e.g. hepatocytes, did not react with the lectins used (data not shown). In liver, there is no tight endothelial cell layer; thus, the viruses can easily come into contact with hepatocytes. Also, by in situ hybridization, we did not find viral RNA in hepatocytes, supporting the notion that the absence of viral receptor determinants prevents hepatocytes from being infected.

3.5. FPV shows polar budding from the luminal side of endothelial cells

We analyzed the budding polarity of FPV by electron microscopy of heart tissue. Budding of FPV was seen only at the luminal side of endothelial cells (Fig. 5). We confirmed the data by confocal laser immunofluorescence microscopy and a surface biotinylation assay using FPV-infected primary endothelial cells. Hemagglutinin was found to be strictly transported to the apical part of the cells (data not shown). Taken together, the data show that in chick embryos, FPV buds unidirectionally from endothelial cells into the lumen of the vessels. Therefore, budding prevents the spread of the infection into deeper cell layers and supports the localized infection of endothelial cells.

H1N1   **H3N1**   **H7N1**

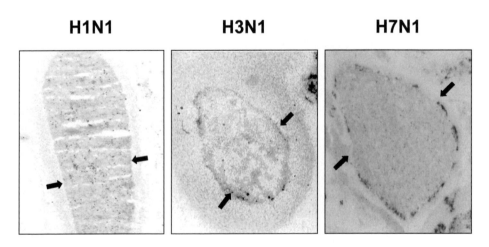

Fig. 7. Localization of influenza-infected cells in blood vessels of embryonic tissue. Bright-field photomicrographs showing autoradiograms with black grains representing bound NP-specific riboprobe in organs of the chick embryo. After in situ hybridization, slides were covered by photoemulsion, exposed for 2 days, developed and counterstained by hematoxylin-eosin. Arrows indicate the endothelial cell layer of the vessel.

WSN from leucocytes

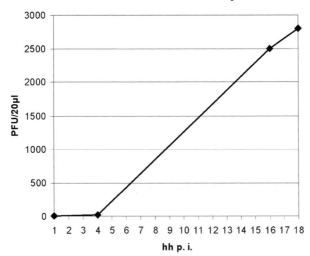

Fig. 8. Leucocytes obtained from the neck vein of 11-day-old chicken embryos were infected with WSN. At different time point, an aliquot was taken and centrifuged to pellet the leucocytes. The supernatant was assayed for viral plaques on MDBK cells.

3.6. Subtype of HA influences tissue tropism in chick embryos

To determine whether the hemagglutinin subtype has an effect on tissue tropism, we investigated the strain A/WSN/33 (H1N1) and the reassortants H3-WSN (H3N1) and H7-WSN (H7N1) that were obtained by classical and recombinant techniques, respectively. The viruses differed only in HA, sharing all other genes. The H7 recombinant and, because of the presence of WSN neuraminidase [7], also the other viruses caused systemic infection in chick embryos (Fig. 6). However, the H3 and H7 viruses replicated in endothelial cells, while WSN virus was only found in the lumen of blood vessels (Fig. 7).

3.7. WSN undergoes productive replication in leucocytes of chick embryos

To exclude the possibility that WSN causes an abortive replication cycle in leucocytes, we infected leucocytes taken from a vein at the neck of the chick embryo as well as leucocytes from adult chickens with WSN virus. At different time points, an aliquot was taken and the presence of progeny viruses was checked by plaque assay on MDBK cells (Fig. 8). WSN produced productive infection in chicken leucocytes; therefore, the inability of the virus to infect endothelial cannot be explained by an abortive infection in leucocytes.

4. Discussion

We have found that FPV shows strict endotheliotropism when infecting 11-day-old chicken embryos. Since hemorrhages are major symptoms in FPV-infected chickens, it was not unexpected to see that the vasculature is an important target of infection. However, we were surprised when we could not detect viral replication in other cell types. The results obtained with the reassortants of FPV and virus N, in agreement with the results obtained with WSN, H3-WSN and H7-WSN, clearly indicate that generalization of the infection requires high cleavability of HA. Cleavability of the hemagglutinin due either to a multibasic cleavage site (H7) or to the presence of WSN neuraminidase (H1; H3) [7] is a prerequisite for the access of the virus to the vascular system. In contrast, the restricted cleavability of virus N HA confines infection to the inner layer of the chorioallantoic membrane and the allantoic cavity [18].

Whereas cleavage activation of HA proved to be essential for targeting the virus to endothelial cells, it was not responsible for confining the infection to these cells. To demonstrate this, we first had to clone chicken furin because this HA-activating proprotein convertase had not been identified in the natural host. The gene shows 84% nucleotide sequence homology to human furin [24]. We showed that gfur is able to cleave FPV HA by coexpression experiments of gfur and FPV HA in furin-deficient LoVo cells. We performed in situ hybridization assays to investigate the expression of gfur in chicken tissue. As known from mammals, we found gfur ubiquitously expressed in chicken tissue. Taken together, these observations indicated that the lack of spread of the infection from endothelial to surrounding tissues cannot be attributed to the absence of activating proteases.

Our data show, however, that the polarity of FPV budding is a factor contributing to the confinement of infection to endothelial cells. Studies on Sendai virus in a mouse model have shown before that the side of virus maturation has a distinct effect on spread of infection in the organism. Wild-type virus is strictly released from the apical surface of lung epithelia causing a strictly pneumotropic infection, whereas the mutant F1-R that matures in a bipolar fashion causes generalized infection in mice [28,29]. It has long been known that FPV preferentially buds on the apical part of endothelial cells [18], and the observations made here on virus budding from endothelial cells of a heart capillary support this concept. The luminal budding, therefore, supports the hematogenic spread of the virus and at the same time prevents infection of subendothelial cells.

Tissue-specific expression of virus receptors was the next topic we were interested in and it appears to be an important factor in restricting infection to endothelia. With the lectin-binding assays employed in this study, we could detect α2,3-linked and α2,6-linked neuraminic acid, both of which proved to be able to serve as influenza receptors on epithelia and cells of the reticuloendothelial system. We could not detect receptor determinants on other cells, such as myocytes and fibroblasts. Thus, it appears that cells lacking a measurable number of neuraminic acid receptors cannot be infected. The results obtained with lung tissue showed that α2,6-linked-neuraminic acid can serve as an FPV receptor because on endothelial cells α2,3-linked neuraminic acid was not detected by the method used. In contrast, epithelial cells of the lung that are not involved in infection were heavily stained with the lectin specific for NeuAc-α2,3-Gal. The access to these cells is prevented by the lack of neuraminic acid receptors on the connective tissue that functions as a barrier to the spread of infection between endothelial and epithelial cells. It has to be pointed out that expression of neuraminic acid in the chick embryo depends on tissue differentiation [2]. This may explain differences in tissue tropism that are seen between infected chicken embryos and infected adult chickens [13].

In the case of WSN, infection is confined to leucocytes. NeuAc-α2,6-Gal that is present on endothelial cells is known to be a receptor determinant of WSN. Therefore, the limited spread of the infection cannot be explained by the absence of viral receptors. Furthermore, WSN causes a productive replication in chicken leucocytes, so the cell-specific infection cannot be explained by a lack of proteolytic activation of WSN HA. Therefore, it is difficult to understand why we did not observe any infection of endothelial cells. To find an explanation for the cell tropism of WSN, we will investigate more recombinant viruses possessing different HA subtypes to generate a common rule for endotheliotropism or replication in leucocytes. In spite of the lack of a complete explanation, the results obtained with the viruses WSN, H3-WSN and H7-WSN clearly show that differences in tissue tropism are directly linked to the HA subtype of the virus.

Taken together, our data indicate that endotheliotropism of influenza virus infection in chick embryos is the interplay between several factors determined by virus and host. These include proteolytic activation of HA, polarity of virus budding at the luminal side of endothelial cells, and cell-specific differences in the expression of neuraminic acid receptors. Endotheliotropism, without doubt, plays an important role in the generalization of FPV infection and in the generation of typical symptoms of the disease, such as hemorrhages. Systemic infection and severe vascular injury are also central pathogenetic mechanisms of hemorrhagic fevers in primates caused by filoviruses and other agents, and there is evidence that at least some of these viruses also replicate in endothelial cells [19,21].

Acknowledgements

We are grateful to R. Rott and C. Scholtissek, Giessen, for helpful discussions and for providing influenza virus reassortants. The electron micrograph was made by B. Agricola.

This study was supported by grants for the Deutsche Forschungsgemeinschaft (SFB 286 and KL 238/6-1) and from the Fonds der Chemischen Industrie.

References

[1] J. Banks, E. Speidel, D.J. Alexander, Characterization of an avian influenza: A virus isolated from a human is an intermediated host necessary for the emergence of pandemic influenza viruses? Arch. Virol. 143 (1998) 781–787.

[2] P. Codogno, M. Aubery, Changes in cell-surface sialic acid content during chick embryo development, Mech. Ageing Dev. 23 (1983) 307–314.

[3] A. Feldmann, M.K.-H. Schafer, W. Garten, H.-D. Klenk, Targeted infection of endothelial cells by avian influenza virus A/FPV/Rostock/34 (H7N1) in chicken embryos, J. Virol. 74 (2000) 8018–8027.

[4] H. Feldmann, E. Kretzschmar, B. Klingeborn, R. Rott, H.D. Klenk, W. Garten, The structure of serotype H10 hemagglutinin of influenza A virus: comparison of an apathogenic avian and a mammalian strain pathogenic for mink, Virology 165 (1988) 428–437.

[5] I. Flamme, G. Breier, W. Risau, Vascular endothelial growth factor (VEGF) and VEGF receptor 2 (flk-1) are expressed during vasculogenesis and vascular differentiation in the quail embryo, Dev. Biol. 169 (1995) 699–712.

[6] W. Garten, D. Linder, R. Rott, H.D. Klenk, The cleavage site of the hemagglutinin of fowl plague virus, Virology 122 (1982) 186–190.

[7] H. Goto, Y. Kawaoka, A novel mechanism for the acquisition of virulence by a human influenza A virus, Proc. Natl. Acad. Sci. U. S. A. 95 (1998) 10224–10228.

[8] E. Gratzl, H. Koehler, Gefluegelpest, Ferdinand Enke Verlag, Stuttgart, 1968.

[9] T. Ito, Y. Suzuki, L. Mitnaul, A. Vines, H. Kida, Y. Kawaoka, Receptor specificity of influenza A viruses correlates with the agglutination of erythrocytes from different animal species, Virology 227 (1997) 493–499.

[10] T. Ito, Y. Suzuki, A. Takada, A. Kawamoto, K. Otsuki, H. Masuda, M. Yamada, T. Suzuki, H. Kida, Y. Kawaoka, Differences in sialic acid-galactose linkages in the chicken egg amnion and allantois influence human influenza virus receptor specificity and variant selection, J. Virol. 71 (1997) 3357–3362.

[11] M.J. Karnovsky, The ultrastructural basis of transcapillary exchanges, J. Gen. Physiol. 52 (Suppl. 95s) (1968) 64.

[12] H.D. Klenk, R. Rott, The molecular biology of influenza virus pathogenicity, Adv. Virus Res. 34 (1988) 247–281.

[13] Y. Kobayashi, T. Horimoto, Y. Kawaoka, D. Alexander, C. Itakura, Pathological studies of chickens experimentally infected with two highly pathogenic avian influenza viruses, Avian Pathol. 25 (1996) 285–304.

[14] I. Kurtz, J. Manvell, J. Banks, Avian influenza virus isolated from a woman with conjunctivitis, Lancet (1996) 348901–348902.

[15] O. Narayan, J. Thorsen, T.J. Hulland, G. Ankeli, P.G. Joseph, Pathogenesis of lethal influenza virus infection in turkeys: I. Extraneural phase of infection, J. Comp. Pathol. 82 (1972) 129–137.

[16] P.C. Roberts, W. Garten, H.D. Klenk, Role of conserved glycosylation sites in maturation and transport of influenza A virus hemagglutinin, J. Virol. 67 (1993) 3048–3060.

[17] R. Rott, M. Orlich, C. Scholtissek, Correlation of pathogenicity and gene constellation of influenza A viruses: III. Non-pathogenic recombinants derived from highly pathogenic parent strains, J. Gen. Virol. 44 (1979) 471–477.

[18] R. Rott, M. Reinacher, M. Orlich, H.D. Klenk, Cleavability of hemagglutinin determines spread of avian influenza viruses in the chorioallantoic membrane of chicken embryo, Arch. Virol. 65 (1980) 123–133.

[19] E.J. Ryabchikova, L.V. Kolesnikova, S.V. Netesov, Animal pathology of filoviral infections, Curr. Top. Microbiol. Immunol. 235 (1999) 145–173.

[20] M.K.H. Schaefer, R. Day, In Situ Hybridization Techniques to Map Processing Enzymes, vol. 23, Academic Press, London, 1992.

[21] H. Schnittler, R.P. Franke, D. Drenckhahn, Role of the endothelial actin filament cytoskeleton in rheology and permeability, Z. Kardiol. 78 (1989) 1–4.

[22] C. Scholtissek, I. Koennecke, R. Rott, Host range recombinants of fowl plague (influenza A) virus, Virology 91 (1978) 79–85.

[23] C. Scholtissek, B.R. Murphy, Host range mutants of an influenza A virus, Arch. Virol. 58 (1978) 323–333.

[24] A. Stieneke-Grober, M. Vey, H. Angliker, E. Shaw, G. Thomas, C. Roberts, H.D. Klenk, W. Garten, Influenza virus hemagglutinin with multibasic cleavage site is activated by furin, a subtilisin-like endoprotease, EMBO J. 11 (1992) 2407–2414.

[25] D.L. Suarez, L.L. Perdue, N. Cox, T. Rowe, J.H. Bender, D.E. Swayne, Comparisons of highly virulent H5N1 influenza A viruses isolated from humans and chickens from Hong Kong, J. Virol. 72 (1998) 6678–6688.

[26] K. Subbarao, A. Klimov, J. Katz, H. Regnery, W. Lim, H. Hall, M. Perdue, D. Swayne, C. Bender, J. Huang, M. Hemphill, T. Rowe, M. Shaw, X. Xu, K. Fukuda, N. Cox, Characterization of an avian influenza A (H5N1) virus isolated from a child with fatal respiratory illness, Science 279 (1998) 393–396.

[27] S. Takahashi, T. Nakagawa, K. Kasai, T. Banno, S.J. Duguay, W.J. Van de Ven, K. Murakami, K. Nakayama, A second mutant allele of furin in the processing-incompetent cell line, LoVo. Evidence for involvement of the homo B domain in autocatalytic activation, J. Biol. Chem. 270 (1995) 26565–26569.

[28] M. Tashiro, J.T. Seto, S. Choosakul, M. Yamakawa, H.D. Klenk, R. Rott, Budding site of Sendai virus in polarized epithelial cells is one of the determinants for tropism and pathogenicity in mice, Virology 187 (1992) 413–422.

[29] M. Tashiro, M. Yamakawa, K. Tobita, J.T. Seto, H.D. Klenk, R. Rott, Altered budding site of a pantropic mutant of Sendai virus, F1-R, in polarized epithelial cells, J. Virol. 64 (1990) 4672–4677.

[30] H. Van Campen, B.C. Easterday, V.S. Hinshaw, Destruction of lymphocytes by a virulent avian influenza A virus, J. Gen. Virol. 70 (1989) 467–472.

[31] H. Van Campen, B.C. Easterday, V.S. Hinshaw, Virulent avian influenza A viruses: their effect on avian lymphocytes and macrophages in vivo and in vitro, J. Gen. Virol. 70 (1989) 2887–2895.

[32] M. Vey, W. Schafer, S. Berghofer, H.D. Klenk, W. Garten, Maturation of the trans-Golgi network protease furin: compartmentalization of propeptide removal, substrate cleavage, and COOH-terminal truncation, J. Cell. Biol. 127 (1994) 1829–1842.

[33] R. Wagner, T. Wolff, A. Herwig, S. Pleschka, H.-D. Klenk, Interdependence of hemagglutinin glycosylation and neuraminidase as regulators of influenza virus growth: a study by reverse genetics, J. Virol. 74 (2000) 6316–6323.

International Congress Series 1219 (2001) 573–579

Mechanisms of differential induction of apoptosis by H3N2 and H1N1 influenza viruses

Clive Sweet[a],[*], Susan J. Morris[a], Mustafa A. Mohsin[a], Harry Smith[b]

[a]School of Biosciences, University of Birmingham, Edgbaston, Birmingham, B15 2TT, UK
[b]Medical School, University of Birmingham, Birmingham, UK

Abstract

Background: The abilities of seven H3N2 and four H1N1 influenza viruses to infect MDCK cells and produce apoptosis were measured and related to their neuraminidase (NA) activity and the role of individual influenza virus proteins in induction of apoptosis was also investigated by transient transfection assays in HeLa cells with expression vectors containing individual virus genes. *Methods*: MDCK cells were inoculated at a high multiplicity of infection (5 EID_{50}/cell) and apoptosis was measured by cytotoxicity and morphology while infection was quantified by fluorescence staining with anti-nucleoprotein (NP) antibody. The Invitrogen Voyager™ vector expressing influenza virus genes as VP22 fusion proteins was transfected into HeLa cells using lipofectamine. *Results and discussion*: H3N2 viruses with high NA activities (1.4–1.8 μmol/l/min) induced high levels of apoptosis (83–94%) and infected 91–98% of cells, while H1N1 viruses with low NA activities (0.22–0.33 μmol/l/min) were poor apoptosis inducers (11–19%) and infected few (15–21%) cells. The differences in % infected cells reflected differences in haemagglutinin (HA) receptor binding affinity. Treatment of viruses with bacterial NA to remove sialyl groups from oligosaccharides on virus HA increased their ability to infect MDCK cells and the increase correlated inversely with the number of potential glycosylation sites around the receptor binding site. Transfection experiments showed that NA (from clone 7a but not A/Fiji) and NS1 (from clone 7a and A/Fiji) induced apoptosis, while NP (clone 7a and A/Fiji) did not. © 2001 Elsevier Science B.V. All rights reserved.

Keywords: NS1; Neuraminidase; Transfection; M1; Nucleoprotein; Haemagglutinin

1. Introduction

Two influenza viruses, A/Fiji/15899/83 (H1N1) and clone 7a (H3N2) of the A/Puerto Rico/8/34 (H1N1) × A/England/939/69 (H3N2) reassortant virus, induced apoptosis in

---

[*] Corresponding author. Tel.: +44-121-414-6554; fax: +44-121-414-5925.
E-mail address: C.Sweet@bham.ac.uk (C. Sweet).

MDCK cells [1], but A/Fiji induced less than clone 7a. Several lines of evidence suggested that the virion neuraminidase (NA) was involved in apoptosis: (i) it activates transforming growth factor (TGF)-β, a known inducer of apoptosis in epithelial cells [2]; (ii) antibody to TGF-β reduced virus-induced apoptosis [2]; (iii) several anti-NA compounds partially blocked apoptosis induction by both clone 7a and A/Fiji when applied during the viral attachment/entry phase but not subsequently [3]. Also, with regard to the differences in apoptotic activity, the NA of clone 7a was more active than that of A/Fiji against several substrates (fetuin, α-2,6 sialyl lactose) [3]. However, other factors connected with virus replication are also involved in the induction of apoptosis as the latter was considerably reduced when UV-irradiated virus, which retained $> 75\%$ of its NA activity, was used, and ammonium chloride (which prevents virus entry) and amantadine (which inhibits virus uncoating) also reduced influenza virus-induced apoptosis [3].

These studies have now been extended to six more N2 and three more N1 viruses to determine whether there was a connection between the ability to infect MDCK cells, the extent of apoptosis and NA activity. In addition, transient transfection assays with expression vectors containing individual influenza virus genes from clone 7a and A/Fiji were performed to investigate the role of virus proteins in apoptosis.

2. Materials and methods

Seven H3N2 and four H1N1 viruses were examined for their ability to cause apoptosis (measured by a combination of lactate dehydrogenase release and acridine orange staining) and to infect (measured by fluorescence staining of nucleoprotein (NP) using an anti-NP monoclonal antibody) MDCK cells [1]. Haemagglutination was quantified using erythrocytes of human, avian and equine origin. Affinity for receptors on human and avian erythrocytes was determined by measuring inhibition of haemagglutination using horse serum containing α-macroglobulin rich in sialic acid-linked α-2,6 to galactose [4]. NA activity was measured against fetuin [3]. The effect of bacterial NA on virus infection was determined by incubating the virus (5×10^6 EID_{50}/ml) with 0.156 units of *Clostridium perfringens* NA for 1 h at 37 °C followed by inoculation of cells with treated virus in the presence of the NA inhibitor DANA. The Invitrogen Voyager$^{\text{™}}$ vector expressing influenza virus genes as VP22 fusion proteins were transfected into HeLa cells using lipofectamine plus reagent (Gibco BRL).

3. Results and discussion

The N2-containing viruses induced greater levels (38–94%) of apoptosis than the N1 viruses (11–35%) (Table 1). NA activities against fetuin paralleled this response (Table 1) and a linear regression analysis showed a good correlation (0.81). Overall, the N2 viruses produced higher cell infection rates than the N1 viruses (Table 1) and again there was a good correlation (0.99) between % infection and % apoptosis and between % infection and NA activity (0.82). This suggested that all three parameters were linked. The differences in infection between the viruses were surprising as all were inoculated at a high moi of 5

Table 1
Comparison of % apoptosis, neuraminidase activity and % cell infection produced by N2 and N1 influenza viruses

Virus	Total mean % apoptosis[a]	NA activity (μmol/l/min)[b]	Total mean % infection[c]
H3N2 viruses			
A/Udorn/307/72	94.1 (5.2)[d]	1.79 (0.13)	97.8 (1.1)
Clone 7a	85.1 (13.3)	1.64 (0.14)	96.4 (1.6)
A/Finland/4/74	83.2 (4.3)	1.40 (0.28)	91.3 (3.6)
A/Victoria/3/75	61.6 (13.9)	0.74 (0.07)	62.8 (1.04)
A/Bangkok/1/79	51.1 (12.5)	0.81 (0.12)	50.2 (3.7)
A/Belgium/2/81	38.2 (12.4)	0.11 (0.01)	40.5 (3.4)
H2N2 virus			
A/Tokyo/3/67	46.6 (14.8)	0.69 (0.03)	45.9 (3.2)
H1N1 viruses			
A/Chile/1/83	19.3 (3.4)	0.33 (0.09)	21.6 (3.0)
A/Fiji/15899/83	11.8 (2.9)	0.22 (0.03)	16.1 (2.5)
A/Firenze/13/83	11.0 (2.3)	0.22 (0.02)	15.4 (1.9)
Hsw1N1 virus			
A/New Jersey/8/76	35.0 (9.1)	1.05 (0.09)	35.9 (1.7)

[a] Total mean % apoptosis was calculated by combining the number of cells which have died (as measured by LDH release) with those remaining but apoptotic (as measured by acridine orange staining).

[b] μmol/l NANA released per minute. The amount of virus used in all assays was 10^7 EID$_{50}$.

[c] Total mean % infection was calculated by combining the number of cells which have died (as measured by LDH release) and hence were infected with those remaining but infected (as measured by staining with monoclonal antibody to nucleoprotein).

[d] Standard deviation of the mean.

EID$_{50}$/cell and replication was limited to a single cycle by omission of trypsin from the medium.

One possible explanation for these differences in infection was variation of receptor affinity/specificity. While the N2 (H3 and H2) and N1 (H1 and Hsw1)-containing viruses utilised only α-2,6-containing receptors (as judged by ability to agglutinate human and avian but not equine erythrocytes), those viruses which induced the highest levels of infection for MDCK cells (i.e. H3N2 viruses) bound more strongly to the α-2,6 receptor-rich α-macroglobulin of horse serum (Table 2). These latter results are interpreted as H3N2 viruses having a greater affinity for α-2,6-containing receptors as they are prevented from agglutinating erythrocytes by lower levels of α-macroglobulin in higher dilutions of horse serum. In accord with this result seen with all viruses, clone 7a (H3N2) attached more rapidly and to higher levels than A/Fiji (H1N1) to MDCK cells (Table 3). Interestingly, the important residues involved in haemagglutinin (HA) specificity are Leu226 and Ser228, which were found in the HAs of all the N2 (H3 and H2) viruses, while the H1N1 viruses had Gln and Gly at these positions, typical of viruses with NeuAcα-2,3 Gal specificity [5] and poor affinity for human cells [6].

Table 2
Haemagglutination-inhibition (HI) titres of influenza virus by horse serum

Virus	HI titre using RBCs from[a]	
	Humans	Chickens
H3N2 viruses		
A/Udorn/307/72	1024	1024
Clone 7a	512	256
A/Finland/4/74	512	512
A/Victoria/3/75	128	64
A/Bangkok/1/79	64	64
A/Belgium/2/81	32	16
H2N2 virus		
A/Tokyo/3/67	32	32
H1N1 viruses		
A/Chile/1/83	32	64
A/Fiji/15899/83	16	32
A/Firenze/13/83	16	16
Hsw1N1 virus		
A/New Jersey/8/76	64	64
Avian H3N8 virus		
A/Duck/Ukraine/63	0	0

[a] Reciprocal of highest dilution of horse serum which caused complete inhibition of haemagglutination using four HAs per well.

Another possible explanation for differences in infectivity is that binding of HA to its receptor is weakened by the presence of oligosaccharides around the receptor binding site (RBS) [7–10]. Comparison of nucleotide sequences showed that all the N2 viruses had HAs (H3, H2) containing six to seven potential glycosylation sites, while the H1N1 viruses had 7–10 such sites; the number of such potential sites adjacent to the RBS varies with the virus (Table 4). Treatment of viruses with bacterial NA increased their ability to

Table 3
% Cells infected following incubation of MDCK cells with virus (5 EID_{50}/cell) for specified times at room temperature

Virus	% Cells infected after incubating for			
	30 min[a]	45 min[a]	60 min[a]	60 + 60 min[b]
Clone 7a	61	70	80	94
A/Fiji	4	6	11	24

[a] Virus incubated with MDCK cells at room temperature for 30, 45 or 60 min followed by incubation at 37 °C for a further 24 h prior to determining the % infected cells.

[b] Virus incubated with MDCK cells at room temperature for 60 min and then for a further 60 min at 37 °C followed by incubation at 37 °C for a further 23 h prior to determining the % infected cells.

Table 4
Effect of bacterial neuraminidase treatment on % infection

Virus	Number of oligosaccharides surrounding RBS of HA	% Increase infection on treatment with bacterial NA
Clone 7a (H3N2)	1	10
A/Belgium/2/81 (H3N2)	2[a]	31
A/New Jersey/8/76 (Hsw1N1)	1[a]	14
A/Fiji/15899/83 (H1N1)	4	84

[a] From sequence database.

infect MDCK cells and the magnitude of the increase correlated inversely with the number of glycosylation sites (Table 4). As an important function of viral NA is to remove sialic acid residues from virion HA [11], and this removal is inefficient for viruses with N1 NAs [11], it seems likely that the poor ability of the H1N1 viruses to infect MDCK cells relates to their lack of ability to remove sialic acid from oligosaccharides on their HAs. It is in this way also that NA could contribute to apoptosis.

The role of individual virus proteins in induction of apoptosis was examined using the Invitrogen Voyager™ vector, which allows the study of viral protein function in cells without the need to create stable cell lines. It takes advantage of the ability of the 32 kDa Herpes simplex type 1 structural protein VP22 to translocate between cells. Any virus VP22 fusion proteins expressed in transfected cells will translocate and localise to the nuclei of virtually 100% of adjacent non-transfected cells [12]. While the process of transfection with vector alone induced some apoptosis (4–5%), this was enhanced when VP22 was fused with clone 7a NA (12–14%) but not A/Fiji NA (Table 5). The NA probably activates latent TGF-β in the medium or on cell surfaces as the former translocates to non-transfected cells via the medium. The apoptosis-inducing activity of NA was blocked by anti-TGF-β antibody present in the medium and was considerably reduced by the anti-NA compound GG167 (Table 5) even though GG167 did not enter

Table 5
% Apoptosis 24 h post-transfection with vectors expressing clone 7a or A/Fiji NA in the presence or absence of anti-TGF-β antibody or the anti-NA compound GG167

Vector	% Apoptosis			
	Anti-TGF-β[a]		GG167[b]	
	−	+	−	+
Control	1.5 (1.0)[c]	1.9 (1.0)	1.2 (0.5)	1.3 (0.5)
VP22	5.4 (0.6)	4.9 (1.0)	3.9 (1.2)	3.8 (1.1)
VP22/Fiji NA	5.8 (0.6)	5.7 (0.9)	5.3 (1.2)	5.2 (1.2)
VP22/7a NA	11.8 (2.5)	6.8 (1.7)*	14.2 (2.5)	9.5 (1.8)*

[a] Anti-TGF-β was added 3 h post-transfection at 33.3 μg/ml and remained in the medium for the subsequent 21 h.

[b] GG167 was added 3 h post-transfection at 500 μg/ml and remained in the medium for the subsequent 21 h.

[c] Standard deviation of the mean.

* Statistically significant from untreated control at $P < 0.01$.

Table 6
% Apoptosis following transfection with vectors expressing clone 7a or A/Fiji NS1 in the presence or absence of poly I:C

Vector	% Apoptosis		
		Poly I:C[a]	
		−	+
C	2.0^b $(0.5)^c$	1.7 (0.4)	30.6 (5.9)
VP22	11.8 (1.3)	8.4 (2.3)	32.3 (4.9)
VP22/Fiji NS1	16.9 (3.0)*	15.1 (4.2)*	16.9 (6.2)**
VP22/Fiji delNS1	17.8 (2.6)*	15.0 (4.5)	19.9 (5.5)**
VP22/7a NS1	21.2 (4.3)*	18.4 (3.2)*	13.5 (3.8)**

[a] Apoptosis determined 24 h post-transfection. Poly I:C was added 3 h post-transfection at 50 μg/ml and remained in the medium for the subsequent 21 h.
[b] Apoptosis determined 48 h post-transfection.
[c] Standard deviation of the mean.
* Statistically significant from VP22 alone at $P < 0.01$.
** Statistically significant from VP22 alone + poly I:C at $P < 0.01$.

cells [3]. NS1 of both clone 7a and A/Fiji induced apoptosis in transfected cells, and for A/Fiji NS1, this occurred with both full-length and a deleted NS1 lacking 107 amino acids of the C-terminal sequence (Table 6). NS1 has been shown to induce apoptosis when expressed constitutively in MDCK cells [13] but recent studies have shown it to be anti-apoptotic in infected cells [14]. Influenza virus can block activation of the dsRNA-dependent protein kinase (PKR), which is known to induce apoptosis [15], but this does not occur with mutant virus defective in NS1 [16]. NS1 is anti-apoptotic in transfected cells in the presence of dsRNA as apoptosis induced by poly I:C in HeLa cells was significantly reduced (>50%) when cells were transfected with either clone 7a or A/Fiji NS1 (Table 6).

Similar studies with vectors expressing NP from either clone 7a or A/Fiji showed that it does not induce apoptosis.

Acknowledgements

S.J. Morris is the recipient of a BBSRC research studentship.

References

[1] G.E. Price, H. Smith, C. Sweet, Differential induction of cytotoxicity and apoptosis by influenza virus strains of differing virulence, J. Gen. Virol. 78 (1997) 2821–2829.
[2] S. Schultz-Cherry, V.S. Hinshaw, Influenza virus neuraminidase activates latent transforming growth-factor β, J. Virol. 70 (1996) 8624–8629.
[3] S.J. Morris, G.E. Price, J.M. Barnett, S.A. Hiscox, H. Smith, C. Sweet, Role of neuraminidase in influenza virus-induced apoptosis, J. Gen. Virol. 80 (1999) 137–146.
[4] K.A. Ryan-Poirer, Y. Kawaoka, α2-Macroglobulin is the major neutralising inhibitor of influenza virus in pig serum, Virology 193 (1993) 974–976.

[5] R.J. Connor, Y. Kawaoka, R.G. Webster, J.C. Paulson, Receptor specificity in human, avian, and equine H2 and H3 influenza virus isolates, Virology 205 (1994) 17–23.

[6] M. Matrosovich, A. Tuzikov, N. Bovin, A. Gambaryan, A. Klimov, M.R. Castrucci, I. Donatelli, Y. Kawaoka, Early alterations of the receptor-binding properties of H1, H2, and H3 avian influenza virus hemagglutinins after their introduction into mammals, Virology 74 (2000) 8502–8512.

[7] R. Ohuchi, M. Ohuchi, W. Garten, H.-D. Klenk, Oligosaccharides in the stem region maintain the influenza virus hemagglutinin in the metastable form required for fusion activity, J. Virol. 71 (1997) 3719–3725.

[8] S. Aytay, I.T. Schulze, Single amino acid substitutions in the hemagglutinin can alter the host range and receptor binding properties of H1 strains of influenza virus, J. Virol. 65 (1999) 3022–3028.

[9] D.M. Crecelius, C.M. Deom, I.T. Schulze, Biological properties of a hemagglutinin mutant of influenza virus selected by host cells, Virology 139 (1984) 164–177.

[10] R. Wagner, T. Wolff, A. Herwig, S. Pleschka, H.-D. Klenk, Interdependence of hemagglutinin glycosylation and neuraminidase as regulators of influenza virus growth: a study by reverse genetics, Virology 74 (2000) 6316–6323.

[11] N.V. Kaverin, A.S. Gambaryan, N.V. Bovin, I.A. Rudneva, A.A. Shilov, O.M. Khodova, N.L. Varich, B.V. Sinitsin, N.V. Makarova, E.A. Kropotkina, Postreassortment changes in influenza A virus hemagglutinin restoring HA–NA functional match, Virology 244 (1998) 315–321.

[12] A. Phelan, G. Elliott, P. O'Hare, Intercellular delivery of functional p53 by the herpesvirus protein VP22, Nat. Biotechnol. 16 (1998) 440–443.

[13] S. Schultz-Cherry, R.M. Krug, V.S. Hinshaw, Induction of apoptosis by influenza virus, Semin. Virol. 8 (1998) 491–495.

[14] O.P. Zhirnov, T. Wolff, T. Konakova, H.-D. Klenk, Host-dependent variations of apoptosis in cells infected with NS1 deficient influenza A virus, 11th International Conference on Negative Strand Viruses, Quebec City, Canada, June 24th–29th, 2000, Abstract number 99.

[15] J. Gil, J. Alcami, M. Esteban, Induction of apoptosis by double-stranded-RNA-dependent protein kinase (PKR) involves the subunit of eukaryotic translation factor 2 and NF-kappaB, Mol. Cell. Biol. 19 (1999) 4653–4663.

[16] E. Hatada, S. Saito, R. Fukuda, Mutant influenza viruses with a defective NS1 protein cannot block the activation of PKR in infected cells, J. Virol. 73 (1999) 2425–2433.

International Congress Series 1219 (2001) 581–585

Influenza-induced bacterial infection: reduced number of airway macrophages

Margaret L. Dunkley*, Robert L. Clancy

*Discipline of Immunology and Microbiology, School of Biomedical Sciences, Faculty of Medicine and
Health Sciences, The University of Newcastle, Newcastle, NSW, Australia*

Abstract

Background: Influenza-induced bacterial superinfection causes morbidity and mortality associated with influenza epidemics. Certain bacterial species are commonly isolated from such infections, but it is unclear why certain bacterial species are preferentially affected. In this study, dual infection of influenza A virus (A/Qld/6/72) with various bacteria (*H. influenzae*, *S. pneumoniae*, *S. aureus* and *P. aeruginosa*) was studied in a mouse model of acute respiratory infection to assess the degree of bacterial superinfection, and effect on airway leukocytes. *Methods*: Mice were infected with A/Qld alone, bacteria alone, or a mixture of virus and bacteria. After 22 h mice were killed and broncho-alveolar lavage (BAL) fluid and lung tissue homogenates were assayed for live bacteria and BAL leukocyte subsets. *Results*: Influenza A/Qld caused a significant increase in *H. influenzae* and *S. pneumoniae* infection. Neutrophil (PMN) numbers were primarily related to the number of bacteria present. Macrophage numbers were reduced during mixed infection of A/Qld with *H. influenzae* or *S. pneumoniae* but were not affected by A/Qld plus *P. aeruginosa* or *S. aureus* infection. *Conclusion*: Differential effects of influenza/bacteria combinations on macrophages may partially account for preferential enhancement of particular bacterial infections during influenza infection. © 2001 Elsevier Science B.V. All rights reserved.

Keywords: Influenza; Bacterial superinfection; Macrophages

1. Introduction

Secondary bacterial pneumonia is the most common pulmonary complication of influenza virus infection and is primarily responsible for influenza-related morbidity

---

* Corresponding author. Discipline of Immunology and Microbiology, Royal Newcastle Hospital, Level 4 David Maddison Building, King St., Newcastle, NSW 2300, Australia. Tel.: +61-249-236581; fax: +61-249-236205.

E-mail address: mdunkley@mail.newcastle.edu.au (M.L. Dunkley).

0531-5131/01/$ – see front matter © 2001 Elsevier Science B.V. All rights reserved.
PII: S0531-5131(01)00383-1

and mortality, particularly in the elderly and those with compromised lung function [1–3]. Certain bacteria such as *S. pneumoniae*, *S. aureus* and *H. influenzae* are commonly isolated following influenza infection in man [1,4,5]. Bacteria have also been shown to enhance influenza infection via cleavage of the haemagglutinin precursor polyprotein by bacterial proteases [6,7].

Several mechanisms have been proposed to explain bacterial superinfection. It has been proposed that influenza infection enhances bacterial adherence to the epithelium [8], and that influenza virus has a deleterious effect on anti-bacteria immunity. Indeed effects of influenza virus on neutrophils have been described [9,10].

This study employs a mouse model of acute respiratory infection to examine airway leukocyte numbers in mixed influenza virus/bacterial infection using influenza A/Qld and the bacteria *H. influenzae*, *S. pneumoniae*, *S. aureus* and *P. aeruginosa*. These bacteria were chosen for study due to the common isolation of *H. influenzae*, *S. pneumoniae* and *S. aureus* in infectious exacerbations in patients with chronic bronchitis, the isolation of these bacteria in post-influenza bacterial infection, and the importance of *P. aeruginosa* in chronic infection in cystic fibrosis.

2. Materials and methods

2.1. Mice

C57BL/6 specific pathogen-free (SPF) mice 8–10 weeks of age were obtained from the University of Newcastle Central Animal House or the Animal Resource Centre, Murdoch, Western Australia. Mice were held in isolator cages for the duration of the experiment. All experiments were approved by the University of Newcastle Animal Care and Ethics Committee and the University of Newcastle Safety Committees.

2.2. Influenza viruses

Influenza virus A/Qld/6/72, H3N2 (AQld) was grown in embryonated chicken eggs for 72 h at 33–34 °C. Virus was harvested and purified by centrifugation on sucrose gradients. The virus titer was determined by plaque assay in confluent cultures of a Madin–Darby canine kidney (MDCK) cell line [11]. Virus was stored at − 70 °C until required.

2.3. Bacteria

Two non-typeable *H. influenzae* strains were used. One was a previously encapsulated strain that had lost its capsule (Hi uncaps). The second was a true nontypeable strain (NTHi). Both strains were biotype I. *H. influenzae* were grown on chocolate agar plates, *S. pneumoniae* on blood–agar plates and *P. aeruginosa* and *S. aureus* on nutrient agar plates. Bacteria were harvested into PBS and the concentration determined by measurement of optical density and comparison with pre-prepared regression curves. Bacteria preparations were washed with PBS once before use and resuspended in PBS.

2.4. Mouse model of acute respiratory infection

Groups of mice were infected intra-tracheally with either bacteria, virus, or a mixture of bacteria and virus. For infection, mice were anaesthetised with pentobarbitone administered by the intra-peritoneal route. The trachea was exposed by cutting the skin and gently pushing aside the salivary glands and soft tissue using a cotton bud. Fifty microliters of the infection dose was injected into the trachea. The skin wound was sutured and the mice

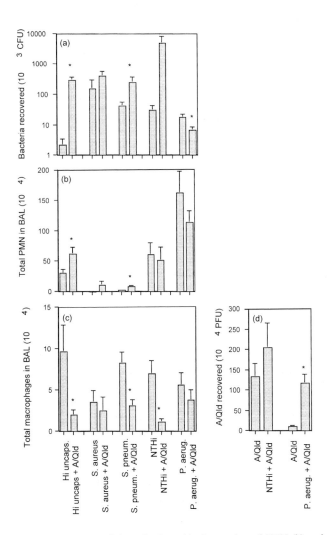

Fig. 1. The number of bacteria recovered from the lung (a), the number of PMN (b) and macrophages (c) recovered from the airways, and the number of influenza virus recovered from the lung (d). The x-axis describes the infection delivered to the mouse group, i.e. bacteria alone or bacteria plus influenza A/Qld. * denotes a significant difference between the group infected with bacteria only and the group infected with the same bacteria plus influenza A/Qld.

kept warm during recovery from anaesthesia. Bacteria were used at a dose of 0.625–1.25×10^6 and influenza virus at 1.25×10^7. Mice were killed 22 h after infection by overdose of sodium pentobarbitone. The lungs were lavaged with 2×1 ml of PBS to obtain pooled bronchoalveolar lavage (BAL) fluid, and the lavaged lungs were homogenised in 10 ml of PBS. A total leukocyte count was performed on the BAL fluid and a cytospin prepared for a differential count. Samples of BAL and lung homogenate (LH) were serially diluted (10-fold dilutions) and 20 µl placed onto nutrient agar plates (*P. aeruginosa* or *S. aureus* infection), chocolate agar plates (*H. influenzae* infection) or blood agar plates (*S. pneumoniae* infection). After overnight culture at 37 °C the colonies were counted and the total colony forming units (CFU) in BAL and LH determined. The total lung bacteria was determined by adding the number for BAL and LH. BAL and LH were also analysed by the MDCK plaque assay to quantitate the number of plaque-forming units (PFU) of influenza virus in the samples [11].

2.5. Statistical analysis

Groups of mice were compared by unpaired *t*-test (Statview 4.0 for Macintosh). Differences between groups were considered significant if $P < 0.05$.

3. Results

3.1. Bacterial superinfection caused by influenza A/Qld in C57Bl/6 mice

Fig. 1a shows the total live bacteria recovered from the lungs of mice infected with either bacteria alone or bacteria plus influenza A/Qld. The presence of influenza A/Qld caused significantly enhanced infection for *S. pneumoniae* and the two *H. influenzae* strains and caused a small non-significant increase in the level of *S. aureus*. In contrast the level of infection of *P. aeruginosa* was significantly decreased by A/Qld.

Fig. 1b shows the number of polymorphonuclear neutrophils (PMN) and Fig. 1c the number of macrophages recovered from the BAL of these mice. The PMN number is only significantly different in the presence of A/Qld (compared to bacterial infection alone) in *S. pneumoniae* infection and infection with *H. influenzae* Hi uncaps. The macrophage number is significantly reduced when A/Qld is present for both *H. influenzae* strains and for the *S. pneumoniae* infection. There is no significant effect on macrophage numbers for either *S. aureus* or *P. aeruginosa* infection.

Fig. 1d shows the influenza A/Qld levels in mice infected with A/Qld alone or with A/Qld plus NTHi or *P. aeruginosa*. Both bacteria caused an increase in A/Qld infection but this was particularly evident for *P. aeruginsosa*.

4. Discussion

This study has demonstrated that in C57Bl mice influenza A/Qld induced enhanced infection of *H. influenzae* and *S. pneumoniae* but not *S. aureus* or *P. aeruginosa*. Where such bacterial superinfection was observed there was a significant decrease in airway macrophage numbers compared to infection with bacteria alone. This suggests that certain influenza virus/bacteria combinations cause a decrease in airway macrophage numbers, which may be contributing to the enhanced bacterial infection observed.

Acknowledgements

This work was supported by a National Health and Medical Research Council of Australia Project Grant number 980355. The research assistance of Ms. Catherine Delahunty is gratefully acknowledged.

References

[1] M. Wiselka, Influenza: diagnosis, management, and prophylaxis, BMJ 308 (1994) 1341–1345.
[2] D.W. Alling, W.C. Black, C.H. Stuart-Harris, A study of excess mortality during influenza epidemics in the United States, 1968–1976, Am. J. Epidemiol. 113 (1981) 30–43.
[3] W.H. Barker, J.P. Mullooly, Pneumonia and influenza deaths during epidemics: implications for prevention, JAMA 142 (1982) 85–89.
[4] R.M. Wadowsky, S.M. Meitzner, D.P. Skoner, W.J. Doyle, P. Fireman, Effect of experimental influenza A virus infection on isolation of *streptococcus pneumoniae* and other aerobic bacteria from the oropharynges of allergic and non-allergic adult subjects, Infect. Immun. 63 (1995) 1153–1157.
[5] C.B. Smith, C. Golden, M.R. Klauber, R. Kanner, A. Renzetti, Interactions between viruses and bacteria in patients with chronic bronchitis, J. Infect. Dis. 134 (1976) 552–561.
[6] M. Tashiro, P. Cibrowski, M. Reinacher, J.D. Klenk, G. Pulverer, R. Rott, Role of staphylococcal protease in the development of influenza pneumonia, Nature 325 (1987) 536–537.
[7] H. Scheiblauer, M. Reinacher, M. Tashiro, R. Rott, Interactions between bacteria and influenza A virus in the development of influenza pneumonia, J. Infect. Dis. 166 (1992) 783–791.
[8] V. Fainstein, D.M. Musher, T.R. Cate, Bacterial adherance to pharangeal cells during viral infection, J. Infect. Dis. 141 (1980) 172–176.
[9] R. Spera, D.H. Shepp, Influenza viruses, in: H. Chmel, M. Bendinelli, H. Friedman (Eds.), Pulmonary Infections and Immunity, Plenum, New York, 1994, pp. 281–308.
[10] G. Pang, R. Clancy, C. Ma, M. Ortega, Z. Ren, G. Reeves, Influenza virus inhibits lysozyme secretion by sputum neutrophils in subjects with chronic bronchial sepsis.
[11] K. Tobita, A. Sugiura, C. Enomoto, M. Furuyama, Plaque assay and primary isolation of influenza A viruses in an established line of canine kidney cells (MDCK) in the presence of trypsin, Med. Microbiol. Immunol. 162 (1975) 9–14.

International Congress Series 1219 (2001) 587–590

Genetic approach to studying influenza pathogenesis

Gabriele Neumann[a], Yoshihiro Kawaoka[a,b,*]

[a]*Department of Pathobiological Sciences, School of Veterinary Medicine, University of Wisconsin, Madison, WI, USA*
[b]*Institute of Medical Science, University of Tokyo, Tokyo, Japan*

Abstract

In 1990, Enami et al. [PNAS 87 (1990) 3802] established a method (reverse genetics) that allowed one to generate influenza virus containing a gene segment derived from cloned cDNA. Although this method contributed tremendously to our understanding of influenza pathogenesis, the requirement of helper viruses limited its use in many experimental settings. Recently, we [PNAS 96 (1999) 9345] and others [J. Virol. 73 (1999) 9679] established systems for the generation of influenza viruses entirely from cloned cDNAs. This system requires only DNA cloning and transfection techniques, and is therefore easily adaptable by laboratories working in the field of molecular biology and virology. Thus, for the first time, a system is now available that allows highly efficient generation of influenza virus without technical limitations. Using this technology, one can now dissect influenza pathogenesis, a complex biologic process, at the molecular level. © 2001 Elsevier Science B.V. All rights reserved.

Keywords: Reverse genetics; Influenza virus; Virulence

1. Introduction

Reverse genetics of negative-sense RNA viruses is defined as the generation of viruses from cloned cDNAs. To artificially generate negative-sense RNA viruses, functional ribonucleoprotein (RNP) complexes have to be provided. This task had been accomplished for nonsegmented, negative-sense RNA viruses of both the Rhabdo- and

* Corresponding author. Department of Pathobiological Sciences, School of Veterinary Medicine, University of Wisconsin-Madison, 2015 Linden Drive West, Madison, WI 53706, USA. Tel.: +1-608-265-4925; fax: +1-608-265-5622.

E-mail address: kawaokay@svm.vetmed.wisc.edu (Y. Kawaoka).

Paramyxoviridae families. In 1994, Schnell et al. [4] reported the generation of infectious rabies virus from cloned DNA. Plasmids encoding the full-length viral genome and the nucleoprotein and polymerase proteins, all under the control of the T7 RNA polymerase promoter, were transfected into cells that had been infected with recombinant vaccinia virus expressing T7 RNA polymerase. Since then, similar systems have been described for viruses of all genera of the Rhabdo- and Paramyxovirus families [5–17]. The genomes of segmented, negative-sense RNA viruses had long been refractory to generation from cloned cDNAs, likely because multiple vRNPs have to be provided. Following the approach outlined by Schnell et al. [4], Bridgen and Elliott [18] reported the generation of Bunyamwera virus, belonging to the family Bunyaviridae whose genome is composed of three segments; however, the efficiency of virus generation was low. The generation of influenza A virus is far more challenging since its genome is composed of eight segments of RNA. To generate influenza A virus from cloned cDNAs, all eight viral RNAs have to be provided in the cell nucleus, together with the three-polymerase proteins and the nucleoprotein. Here, we review influenza reverse genetics and how one can use this system for studying the pathogenesis of this virus.

2. Reconstitution of functional RNP complexes

The first step towards the generation of influenza virus was the reconstitution of functional RNP complexes. RNP complexes can be assembled from purified NP and polymerase proteins [19] or isolated from detergent-treated virus [20]. Parvin et al. [21] and Honda et al. [22] were able to transcribe short synthetic RNAs or full-length vRNAs by RNP complexes reconstituted from purified viral proteins. Because of inherent technical difficulties, the purification of viral proteins and their reassembly with synthetic RNAs to form functional vRNP complexes was not an efficient approach to artificially generate influenza viruses. Nevertheless, these early studies paved the road for the next steps by demonstrating that the three polymerase proteins and NP are sufficient for transcription and replication of viral RNAs.

3. Helper virus-dependent reverse genetics

Enami et al. [1] were the first to generate influenza virus containing an artificially produced gene. The neuraminidase protein of A/WSN/33 virus confers trypsin-independent virus growth in MDBK cells. The authors transfected in vitro generated A/WSN/33 NA vRNPs into cells that had been infected with a virus containing an NA from a trypsin-dependent strain. Thus, in the absence of trypsin, virus containing the A/WSN/33 NA gene segment was selected. Since this success, a number of viruses containing mutations in different gene segments (i.e., PB2, HA, NP, NA, M, and NS) were produced. However, because of the requirement of helper virus, and thus, the difficulty of selecting a virus containing a transfected gene, this method had limitations.

4. Generation of influenza A virus entirely from cloned cDNAs

A decade after the generation of influenza A virus containing a single gene derived from cloned cDNA, we [2], and shortly thereafter, Fodor et al. [3] succeeded in synthesizing influenza A virus entirely from cloned cDNAs. We cloned cDNAs encoding all eight vRNAs of A/WSN/33 virus between the human RNA polymerase I promoter and mouse RNA polymerase I terminator [2]. Transfection of the resulting plasmids into 293T cells yields vRNA synthesized by cellular RNA polymerase I. Cotransfection of protein expression plasmids for all viral structural proteins yielded 8×10^7 infectious viruses per milliliter of supernatant, one of the most efficient among reverse genetics systems. Infection with helper virus is no longer required circumventing the need for cumbersome selection of transfectant viruses. Thus, for the first time, researchers have made available a system for designing influenza virus. The system is simple, since it only requires DNA cloning, purification, and transfection technique-methods that are well established in molecular biology and virology laboratories.

5. Use of reverse genetics for pathogenesis studies

Because of the extremely high efficiency of our helper virus-independent system, we can now generate influenza virus with non-lethal mutations in any gene segment. Traditionally, when there are two influenza viruses that differ in their biologic phenotypes, reassortant viruses between the two viruses are generated. However, generation of a panel of reassortant viruses that would lead to a clear conclusion was difficult. With this technology, such reassortants can easily be made. Thus, reverse genetics technology will likely reveal new viral factors responsible for virulence of influenza virus.

Acknowledgements

We thank the members of our laboratory for the production of data presented in this review article and Krisna Wells for editing the manuscript. Support for this work came from NIAID Public Health Service research grants and from the Japan Health Sciences Foundation and the Ministry of Education and Culture of Japan.

References

[1] M. Enami, W. Luytjes, M. Krystal, P. Palese, Introduction of site-specific mutations into the genome of influenza virus, PNAS 87 (1990) 3802–3805.
[2] G. Neumann, T. Watanabe, H. Ito, S. Watanabe, H. Goto, P. Gao, M. Hughes, D.R. Perez, R. Donis, E. Hoffmann, G. Hobom, Y. Kawaoka, Generation of influenza A viruses entirely from cloned cDNAs, PNAS 96 (1999) 9345–9350.
[3] E. Fodor, L. Devenish, O.G. Engelhardt, P. Palese, G.G. Brownlee, A. Garcia-Sastre, Rescue of influenza A virus from recombinant DNA, J. Virol. 73 (1999) 9679–9682.
[4] M.J. Schnell, T. Mebatsion, K.K. Conzelmann, Infectious rabies viruses from cloned cDNA, EMBO J. 13 (1994) 4195–4203.

[5] M.D. Baron, T. Barnett, Rescue of rinderpest virus from cloned cDNA, J. Virol. 71 (1997) 1265–1271.

[6] U.J. Buchholz, S. Finke, K.K. Conzelmann, Generation of bovine respiratory syncytial virus (BRSV) from cDNA: BRSV NS2 is not essential for virus replication in tissue culture, and the human RSV leader region acts as a functional BRSV genome promoter, J. Virol. 73 (1999) 251–259.

[7] D.K. Clarke, M.S. Sidhu, J.A. Johnson, S.A. Udem, Rescue of mumps virus from cDNA, J. Virol. 74 (2000) 4831–4838.

[8] P.L. Collins, M.G. Hill, E. Camargo, H. Grosfeld, R.M. Chanock, B.R. Murphy, Production of infectious human respiratory syncytial virus from cloned cDNA confirms an essential role for the transcription elongation factor from the 5' proximal open reading frame of the M2 mRNA in gene expression and provides a capability for vaccine development, PNAS 92 (1995) 11563–11567.

[9] A.P. Durbin, S.L. Hall, J.W. Siew, S.S. Whitehead, P.L. Collins, B.R. Murphy, Recovery of infectious human parainfluenza virus type 3 from cDNA, Virology 235 (1997) 323–332.

[10] B. He, R.G. Paterson, C.D. Ward, R.A. Lamb, Recovery of infectious SV5 from cloned DNA and expression of a foreign gene, Virology 237 (1997) 249–260.

[11] M.A. Hoffman, A.K. Banerjee, An infectious clone of human parainfluenza virus type 3, J. Virol. 71 (1997) 4272–4277.

[12] H. Jin, D. Clarke, H.Z. Zhou, X. Cheng, K. Coelingh, M. Bryant, S. Li, Recombinant human respiratory syncytial virus (RSV) from cDNA and construction of subgroup A and B chimeric RSV, Virology 251 (1998) 206–214.

[13] N.D. Lawson, E.A. Stillman, M.A. Whitt, J.K. Rose, Recombinant vesicular stomatitis viruses from DNA, PNAS 92 (1995) 4477–4481.

[14] B.P. Peeters, O.S. de Leeuw, G. Koch, A.L. Gielkens, Rescue of Newcastle disease virus from cloned cDNA: evidence that cleavability of the fusion protein is a major determinant for virulence, J. Virol. 73 (1999) 5001–5009.

[15] F. Radecke, P. Spielhofer, H. Schneider, K. Kaelin, M. Huber, C. Dotsch, G. Christiansen, M.A. Billeter, Rescue of measles virus from cloned DNA, EMBO J. 14 (1995) 5773–5784.

[16] A. Romer-Oberdorfer, E. Mundt, T. Mebatsion, U.J. Buchholz, T.C. Mettenleiter, Generation of recombinant lentogenic Newcastle disease virus from cDNA, J. Gen. Virol. 80 (1999) 2987–2995.

[17] S.P. Whelan, L.A. Ball, J.N. Barr, G.T. Wertz, Efficient recovery of infectious vesicular stomatitis virus entirely from cDNA clones, PNAS 92 (1995) 8388–8392.

[18] A. Bridgen, R.M. Elliott, Rescue of a segmented negative-strand RNA virus entirely from cloned complementary DNAs, PNAS 93 (1996) 15400–15404.

[19] B. Szewczyk, W.G. Laver, D.F. Summers, Purification, thioredoxin renaturation, and reconstituted activity of the three subunits of the influenza A virus RNA polymerase, PNAS 85 (1988) 7907–7911.

[20] A. Honda, K. Ueda, K. Nagata, A. Ishihama, Identification of the RNA polymerase-binding site on genome RNA of influenza virus, J. Biochem. 102 (1987) 1241–1249.

[21] J.D. Parvin, P. Palese, A. Honda, A. Ishihama, M. Krystal, Promoter analysis of influenza virus RNA polymerase, J. Virol. 63 (1989) 5142–5152.

[22] A. Honda, J. Mukaigawa, A. Yokoiyama, A. Kato, S. Ueda, K. Nagato, M. Krystal, Purification and molecular structure of RNA polymerase from influenza virus A/PR8, J. Biochem. 107 (1990) 624–628.

International Congress Series 1219 (2001) 591–594

Role of plasminogen-binding neuraminidase in influenza pathogenicity

Hideo Goto[a], Yoshihiro Kawaoka[a,b,*]

[a]Division of Virology, Department of Microbiology and Immunology, The Institute of Medical Science,
The University of Tokyo, 4-6-1 Shirokanedai, Minato, Tokyo 108-8639, Japan
[b]Department of Pathobiological Sciences, School of Veterinary Medicine,
University of Wisconsin-Madison, Madison, WI, USA

Abstract

Because hemagglutinin (HA) cleavage by proteases is a prerequisite for the infectivity of influenza A virus, it is a major determinant of viral pathogenicity. Although a mechanism by which HA cleavage plays a role in pathogenicity has been well studied in avian influenza viruses, in mammalian viruses it is not well understood. We demonstrated that the neuraminidase (NA) of a human isolate A/WSN/33, which is highly pathogenic in mice, bound and sequestered plasminogen, resulting in increased HA cleavability. To prove that plasminogen-binding activity of the NA determines the pathogenicity of influenza virus in mice, we generated mutant viruses that are deficient in plasminogen-binding activity by reverse genetics. © 2001 Elsevier Science B.V. All rights reserved.

Keywords: Influenza virus; Plasmin; Virulence; Proteolytic processing

1. Introduction

HA cleavability is one of the major determinants of pathogenicity of influenza A virus because HA cleavage is essential for infectivity [1,2]. The HA of highly pathogenic avian influenza viruses is susceptible to cleavage by ubiquitous proteases, furin and PC6 [3]. Thus, these viruses are able to propagate in a variety of organs, resulting in systemic

* Corresponding author. Division of Virology, Department of Microbiology and Immunology, The Institute of Medical Science, The University of Tokyo, 4-6-1 Shirokanedai, Minato, Tokyo 108-8639, Japan. Tel.: +81-3-5449-5310; fax: +81-3-5449-5408.
E-mail address: kawaoka@ims.u-tokyo.ac.jp (Y. Kawaoka).

0531-5131/01/$ – see front matter © 2001 Elsevier Science B.V. All rights reserved.
PII: S 0 5 3 1 - 5 1 3 1 (0 1) 0 0 6 3 3 - 1

infection. However, the molecular mechanisms by which influenza virus causes severe disease in mammals are poorly understood. Among mammalian influenza viruses, a human isolate A/WSN/33 (WSN) shows unique biological properties that are similar to highly pathogenic avian influenza viruses. It can replicate in cultured cells without the addition of trypsin and in a range of murine tissues, including brain [4,5]. The fact that the HA of WSN is not susceptible to furin or PC6 suggests a unique mechanism of HA cleavage for this virus. Genetic studies indicated that the WSN NA is critical for HA cleavage and viral pathogenicity [6]. Furthermore, Li et al. [7] also reported that glycosylation of the NA determined neurovirulence in mice. Lazarowitz et al. [8] showed that serum plasminogen is responsible for WSN HA cleavage in cell cultures when trypsin is not added. Previously, in an in vitro assay, we demonstrated that the WSN NA had plasminogen-binding activity, leading to higher concentrations of plasmin (which is activated from plasminogen by a cellular activator) and thus to increased HA cleavage [9]. Because plasminogen circulates through the blood stream and exists in a variety of organs, we suggested that plasminogen-binding activity of the NA was associated with high pathogenicity in mice. Here, we generated mutant WSN viruses whose NAs lack plasminogen-binding activity by reverse genetics to obtain direct evidence that NA's plasminogen-binding activity determines the pathogenicity of WSN virus.

2. Materials and methods

2.1. Generation of WSN without plasminogen-binding NA

Full-length cDNA encoding the NA gene of WSN was used for site-directed mutagenesis. Because the carboxyl terminal Lys (at 453) of the WSN NA is essential for plasminogen-binding activity, mutations were introduced to convert AAG (453Lys) to CGC (Arg, K453R), CAA (Gln, K453Q), GAA (Glu, K453E) or CTA (Leu, K453L). The mutant NA genes were placed under the control of human RNA polymerase I promoter and the mouse RNA polymerase I terminator in pHH21 to construct pPolIK453R or pPolIK453L [10]. These plasmids were transfected together with other genome RNA transcription plasmids and viral protein expression plasmids into human embryonic kidney 293T cells using Trans IT LT-1 (Panvera, Madison, WI). Forty-eight hours after transfection, virus was isolated from the culture supernatant.

3. Results

3.1. Generation of WSN viruses with mutations at the carboxyl terminus of the NA

To generate WSN viruses whose NAs lack plasminogen-binding activity, we constructed plasmids encoding an altered amino acid at the carboxyl terminus of the NA, Lys to Arg, K453R; Lys to Glu, K453E; or Lys to Leu, K453L. To exclude the possibility that these mutations negatively affected intracellular transport of the NA, we constructed expression plasmids with the mutant NA genes and transfected cultured cells. Mutant

K453R and K453L NAs were detected on the cell surface. Thus, K453R and K453L NA genes were used to construct plasmids for transcription of genome RNA with RNA polymerase I.

To generate mutant WSN viruses, 293T cells were transfected as described in the Materials and Methods. Virus titers of the mutants in MDCK cells in the presence of trypsin were similar to that of the wild-type WSN virus. Neither mutant viruses grew in MDBK cells in the presence of serum.

4. Discussion

Reverse genetics has been previously used to introduce mutations in the NA of influenza A virus [11]. However, since this prior technology requires a selection system that relies on the unique property of the WSN NA to confer growth ability in the absence of trypsin, we could not apply this system to the present study. Here, however, we succeeded in generating mutant WSN viruses without plasminogen-binding NA by reverse genetics using the RNA polymerase I system [10], which does not require a selection system, thereby exploiting the advantage of this system.

Direct evidence of how plasminogen-binding activity of the WSN NA is involved in virus replication was lacking. Here, we demonstrated that WSN K453R and K453L replicated in MDCK cells in the presence of trypsin, indicating that plasminogen-binding activity is not essential for viral viability. However, the mutant viruses could not propagate in the presence of serum, a source of plasminogen, indicating that plasminogen-binding activity of the NA contributes to virus propagation in cell culture in the presence of plasminogen.

Acknowledgements

We thank Krisna Wells and Ryo Kawaoka for excellent technical assistance. Support for this work came from NIAID Public Health Service research grants and from the Japan Health Sciences Foundation and the Ministry of Education and Culture of Japan.

References

[1] H.D. Klenk, R. Rott, M. Orlich, J. Blodorn, Activation of influenza A viruses by trypsin treatment, Virology 68 (1975) 426–439.

[2] S.G. Lazarowitz, P.W. Choppin, Enhancement of the infectivity of influenza A and B viruses by proteolytic cleavage of the hemagglutinin polypeptide, Virology 68 (1975) 440–454.

[3] H.D. Klenk, W. Garten, Host cell proteases controlling virus pathogenicity, Trends Microbiol. 2 (1994) 39–43.

[4] P.W. Choppin, Replication of influenza virus in a continuous cell line: high yield of infective virus from cells inoculated at high multiplicity, Virology 39 (1969) 130–134.

[5] M.R. Castrucci, Y. Kawaoka, Biologic importance of neuraminidase stalk length in influenza A virus, J. Virol. 67 (1993) 759–764.

[6] J.L. Schulman, P. Palese, Virulence factors of influenza A viruses: WSN virus neuraminidase required for plaque production in MDBK cells, J. Virol. 24 (1977) 170–176.

[7] S. Li, J. Schulman, S. Itamura, P. Palese, Glycosylation of neuraminidase determines the neurovirulence of influenza A/WSN/33 virus, J. Virol. 67 (1993) 6667–6673.

[8] S.G. Lazarowitz, A.R. Goldberg, P.W. Choppin, Proteolytic cleavage by plasmin of the HA polypeptide of influenza virus: host cell activation of serum plasminogen, Virology 56 (1973) 172–180.

[9] H. Goto, Y. Kawaoka, A novel mechanism for the acquisition of virulence by a human influenza A virus, Proc. Natl. Acad. Sci. U. S. A. 95 (1998) 10224–10228.

[10] G. Neumann, T. Watanabe, H. Ito, S. Watanabe, H. Goto, P. Gao, M. Hughes, D.R. Perez, R. Donis, E. Hoffmann, G. Hobom, Y. Kawaoka, Generation of influenza A viruses entirely from cloned cDNAs, Proc. Natl. Acad. Sci. U. S. A. 96 (1999) 9345–9350.

[11] M. Enami, W. Luytjes, M. Krystal, P. Palese, Introduction of site-specific mutations into the genome of influenza virus, Proc. Natl. Acad. Sci. U. S. A. 87 (1990) 3802–3805.

International Congress Series 1219 (2001) 595–600

Molecular correlates of influenza A H5N1 virus pathogenesis in mice

K. Subbarao*, X. Lu, T.M. Tumpey[1], C.B. Smith, M.W. Shaw, J.M. Katz

Influenza Branch, Division of Viral and Rickettsial Diseases, National Center for Infectious Diseases, Centers for Disease Control and Prevention, Mailstop G-16, 1600 Clifton Road, Atlanta, GA 30333, USA

Abstract

Background: In 1997, highly pathogenic avian influenza A H5N1 viruses caused 18 human cases of respiratory illness and six deaths in Hong Kong. The genes of the H5N1 viruses isolated from humans were derived from avian influenza viruses, with no evidence of reassortment with human influenza viruses. The molecular determinants of human pathogenesis were not evident. *Methods*: The BALB/c mouse was used as a mammalian model to evaluate the biological and molecular basis of human H5N1 virus pathogenesis. Molecular correlates of H5N1 virus pathogenicity for mice were sought by analyzing the nucleotide sequence of human H5N1 viruses. *Results*: Based on high and low lethality for mice, the pathogenicity phenotype of 15 human H5N1 viruses was characterized; nine viruses displayed a high, five a low, and one an intermediate pathogenicity phenotype. H5N1 viruses with a high pathogenicity phenotype replicated in multiple solid organs and caused depletion of peripheral blood leukocytes. Sequence analysis determined that five specific amino acids in four proteins correlated with pathogenicity in mice. *Conclusions*: Alone or in combination, these specific residues are the likely determinants of virulence of human H5N1 influenza viruses in this mammalian model. Published by Elsevier Science B.V.

Keywords: Molecular pathogenesis; Influenza H5N1; Mouse pathogenicity

1. Introduction

The molecular determinants and related mechanisms that make certain influenza viruses highly pathogenic for mammalian species, including humans, are poorly under-

---

* Corresponding author. Tel.: +1-404-639-3591; fax: +1-404-639-2334.
E-mail address: KSubbarao@cdc.gov (K. Subbarao).
[1] Present address: USDA/ARS/Southeast Poultry Research Laboratories, Athens, GA, USA.

0531-5131/01/$ – see front matter. Published by Elsevier Science B.V.
PII: S 0 5 3 1 - 5 1 3 1 (0 1) 0 0 6 3 5 - 5

stood. Both viral factors and host factors may determine virulence and studies have shown that influenza virus virulence in mammalian species is a polygenic trait that may require a particular constellation of genes [1–4]. In 1997, highly pathogenic avian H5N1 viruses infected poultry in the live-bird markets of Hong Kong and caused an outbreak of 18 human cases of respiratory illness, including six deaths [5–7]. The H5N1 viruses are the only highly pathogenic avian viruses that have caused an outbreak of respiratory disease in humans. The 16 H5N1 viruses isolated from humans during the 1997 outbreak had avian virus genomes [8]. The outbreak created a new awareness that avian influenza viruses could spread directly from poultry to humans and cause severe respiratory disease in humans, but the molecular basis of the H5N1 virus virulence in humans was not evident.

The BALB/c mouse was previously shown to be a useful mammalian model for the evaluation of human H5N1 virus pathogenesis [9–11]. H5N1 viruses replicate efficiently in the respiratory tract of mice without prior adaptation. Viruses exhibiting high lethality (pathogenicity) replicated in extrapulmonary sites, including the brain, while growth of viruses of low lethality was restricted to the respiratory tract of mice [9,11]. All 16 human H5N1 viruses possessed a multiple basic amino acid motif at the cleavage site between HA1 and HA2, and were lethal for experimentally infected chickens [5,6,8,9,12], suggesting that other molecular features are associated with the high pathogenicity of H5N1 viruses in mammalian species. We investigated the molecular determinants that distinguish 15 H5N1 viruses of high and low pathogenicity in mice.

2. Methods

The 15 H5N1 viruses isolated from confirmed cases in Hong Kong in 1997 were grown in Madin Darby Canine Kidney (MDCK) cells and/or in the allantoic cavity of 10-day-old embryonated hens' eggs at 37 °C for 24 h. Fifty percent egg infectious dose (EID_{50}) titers were calculated by the method of Reed and Muench [13]. The 50% lethal dose (LD_{50}) of the viruses for 6- to 8-week-old female BALB/c mice (Charles River Laboratories, Wilmington, MA) was determined as previously described [11] and was used as a marker for pathogenicity. Viruses with an LD_{50} of $> 10^{6.5}$ were considered to be of low pathogenicity, while viruses with LD_{50} of $< 10^{3.0}$ were considered to be of high pathogenicity.

The complete nucleotide sequences for all coding regions of all gene segments of nine of the H5N1 viruses were determined using gene-specific primer sets. This analysis identified five residues that segregated with the mouse pathogenicity phenotype in genes that encoded the NA, matrix (M1) protein, and viral polymerases PB1 and PB2. To confirm this finding, partial sequence analysis was conducted on these four gene segments from the same virus stocks that were used to determine the pathogenicity phenotype in mice.

3. Results

Amino acid residues 223 (I or T) in the NA, 198 (K or R) and 317 (I or M) in PB1, and 355 (K or Q) in PB2 correlated with high or low pathogenicity, respectively, in 15 of the

Table 1
Nucleotide and deduced amino acid residues in the NA, M1, PB1, and PB2 proteins that correlate with mouse pathogenicity phenotype

H5N1 virus	Mouse pathogenicity phenotype	Genotype									
		NA		M1		PB1				PB2	
		nt 668	aa 223	nt 68	aa 15	nt 617	aa 198	nt 975	aa 317	nt 1090	aa 355
HK/481/97	high	T	I	A	I	A	K	A	I	A	K
HK/483/97	high	T	I	A	I	A	K	A	I	A	K
HK/485/97	high	T	I	A(CC)	T	A	K	A	I	A	K
HK/491/97	high	T	I	A	I	A	K	A	I	A	K
HK/503/97	high	T	I	A	I	A	K	A	I	A	K
HK/514/97	high	T	I	A	I	A	K	A	I	A	K
HK/516/97	high	T	I	A	I	A	K	A	I	A	K
HK/532/97	high	T	I	A	I	A	K	A	I	A	K
HK/542/97	high	T	I	A	I	A	K	A	I	A	K
HK/156/97	intermediate	T	I	A	I	A	K	A	I	A	K
HK/486/97	low	C	T	G	V	G	R	G	M	C	Q
HK/488/97	low	C	T	G	V	G	R	G	M	C	Q
HK/507/97	low	C	T	G	V	G	R	G	M	C	Q
HK/538/97	low	C	T	G	V	G	R	G	M	C	Q
HK/97/98	low	C	T	G	V	G	R	G	M	C	Q

16 viruses analyzed (Table 1). Amino acids at position 15 (I or V) in the M1 protein correlated with high and low pathogenicity, respectively, in 14 of the H5N1 viruses. HK/485/97, a virus of high pathogenicity, possessed a unique codon (ACC) relative to all other H5N1 viruses analyzed, encoding a threonine at position 15 in the M1 protein (Table 1), suggesting either that threonine at this position is permissive for the high-pathogenicity phenotype or that substitution of this residue alone is insufficient to alter the mouse pathogenicity phenotype of the virus.

4. Discussion

Because the human H5N1 viruses are a genetically closely related group of viruses [8,14], it was possible to associate the five specific molecular markers in the NA, PB1, PB2 and M1 genes with the two distinct phenotypes of pathogenicity observed in mice.

Amino acid 223 in the N1 NA corresponds to residue 222 of N2 NA, a conserved framework residue in the enzyme active site in the head of the NA molecule [15]. H5N1 viruses of the low-pathogenicity phenotype possess a threonine at this position, creating a potential glycosylation site (N–X–T) in the enzyme active site. Studies have suggested a role for the NA in influenza virus-induced apoptosis, which has been implicated as a mechanism of pathogenicity among influenza viruses [16,17]. Interestingly, the highly pathogenic H5N1 virus HK/483/97 induces peripheral blood lympho-cyte depletion and apoptosis in the spleens and lungs of infected mice, whereas HK/

486/97, a virus of low pathogenicity, does not [18]. Because the specific residues in the PB1, PB2 and M1 proteins that correlated with mouse pathogenicity were not located in any of the defined functional domains of these proteins, their contribution to the mechanism(s) of virulence remains unknown.

The specific amino acid residues identified in the NA, M1, PB1, and PB2 genes in the present study have not been previously associated with pathogenicity. It is possible that additional molecular markers for pathogenicity were not detected because the findings from complete sequence analysis of nine of the human H5N1 viruses were used to direct partial analysis of the remaining viruses. Mutations in the polymerase genes of influenza viruses have previously been reported to determine host range [19,20], temperature sensitivity, and in some instances, attenuation of influenza viruses for mice, ferrets, and humans [21,22]. Mutations in the M protein have been associated with host range, growth, and virulence phenotypes. Growth properties of influenza viruses can be determined by specific mutations in individual gene segments or by the constellation of genes present in the virus.

To investigate the prevalence of these specific residues in other influenza A viruses, nucleotide sequence alignments for the four gene products were performed using available sequence data, including sequences from human, avian, swine, and equine influenza A viruses. No significant distribution of the specific residues associated with high or low pathogenicity for mice in this study was observed, most likely because of the relatively low genetic relatedness of influenza A viruses from different species.

Although HK/156/97 was shown to be of intermediate pathogenicity in this study, the genotype was that of the high-pathogenicity viruses, presumably due to biological and molecular heterogeneity of this virus isolate [9,23]. One other virus, HK/482/97, consistently yielded an indeterminate mouse pathogenicity phenotype and a genotype that consisted of a mixture of the residues associated with high and low pathogenicity in M1, PB1 and PB2. It is possible that the original HK/482/97 isolate, like HK/156/97, was biologically heterogeneous.

While two distinct pathogenicity phenotypes were observed in this inbred mouse model, a broader spectrum of pathogenicity was observed in humans infected with the H5N1 viruses. The mouse pathogenicity phenotype of four viruses failed to correlate with the severity of disease observed in humans. In addition to the general virulence of the H5N1 viruses, age, underlying medical conditions, and other unknown risk factors may have contributed to the severity of disease in humans. Nevertheless, the fact that H5N1 viruses of high-pathogenicity induced symptoms of disease similar to those observed in severe and fatal human cases, including viral pneumonia, multi-organ involvement, leukopenia, and death, suggests that the mouse is an appropriate model to better understand the molecular basis of influenza virus virulence in mammalian species. However, at present, it is not possible to distinguish between the molecular determinants responsible for general virulence in mammals and those responsible for specific virulence in mice. While it is likely that the polygenic nature of pathogenicity differs among influenza viruses and among host species, the molecular determinants of pathogenicity in this mammalian model may provide a framework for the future identification of influenza A viruses with the potential to cause severe disease.

Acknowledgements

We thank the Epidemiology Section of the Influenza Branch, CDC; Paul Saw, K.H. Mak, Wilina Lim, and others from the Hong Kong Department of Health for the acquisition of specimens and isolation of the H5N1 viruses; Xiyan Xu, Sarah Cantrell, Mark Hemphill, and Alexander Klimov for contributing to the sequence analysis.

References

[1] E.G. Brown, J.E. Bailly, Genetic analysis of mouse-adapted influenza A virus identifies roles for the NA, PB1, and PB2 genes in virulence, Virus Res. 61 (1999) 63–76.

[2] C. Scholtissek, A. Vallbracht, B. Flehmig, R. Rott, Correlation of pathogenicity and gene constellation of influenza A viruses: II. Highly neurovirulent recombinants derived from non-neurovirulent or weakly neurovirulent parent virus strains, Virology 95 (1979) 492–500.

[3] A.C. Ward, Neurovirulence of influenza A virus, J. NeuroVirol. 2 (1996) 139–151.

[4] A.C. Ward, Virulence of influenza A virus for mouse lung, Virus Genes 14 (1997) 187–194.

[5] E.C. Claas, A.D. Osterhaus, R. van Beek, J.C. de Jong, G.F. Rimmelzwaan, D.A. Senne, S. Krauss, K.F. Shortridge, R.G. Webster, Human influenza A H5N1 virus related to a highly pathogenic avian influenza virus, Lancet 351 (1998) 472–477.

[6] K. Subbarao, A. Klimov, J. Katz, H. Regnery, W. Lim, H. Hall, M. Perdue, D. Swayne, C. Bender, J. Huang, M. Hemphill, T. Rowe, M. Shaw, X. Xu, K. Fukuda, N.J. Cox, Characterization of an avian influenza A (H5N1) virus isolated from a child with a fatal respiratory illness, Science 279 (1998) 393–396.

[7] K.Y. Yuen, P.K. Chan, M. Peiris, D.N.C. Tsang, T.L. Que, K.F. Shortridge, P.T. Cheung, W.K. To, E.T.F. Ho, R. Sung, A.F.B. Cheng and Members of the H5N1 Study Group, Clinical features and rapid viral diagnosis of human disease associated with avian influenza A H5N1 virus, Lancet 351 (1998) 467–471.

[8] C. Bender, H. Hall, J. Huang, A. Klimov, N. Cox, A. Hay, V. Gregory, W. Lim, K. Subbarao, Characterization of the surface proteins of influenza A (H5N1) viruses isolated from humans in 1997–1998, Virology 254 (1999) 115–123.

[9] P. Gao, S. Watanabe, T. Ito, H. Goto, K. Wells, M. McGregor, A.J. Cooley, Y. Kawaoka, Biological heterogeneity, including systemic replication in mice, of H5N1 influenza A virus isolates from humans in Hong Kong, J. Virol. 73 (1999) 3184–3189.

[10] L.V. Gubareva, J.A. McCullers, R.C. Bethell, R.G. Webster, Characterization of influenza A/HongKong/ 156/97 (H5N1) virus in a mouse model and protective effect of zanamivir on H5N1 infection in mice, J. Infect. Dis. 178 (1998) 1592–1596.

[11] X. Lu, T.M. Tumpey, T. Morken, S.R. Zaki, N.J. Cox, J.M. Katz, A mouse model for the evaluation of pathogenesis and immunity to influenza A (H5N1) viruses isolated from humans, J. Virol. 73 (1999) 5903–5911.

[12] D.L. Suarez, M.L. Perdue, N.J. Cox, T. Rowe, C. Bender, J. Huang, D.E. Swayne, Comparisons of highly virulent H5N1 influenza A viruses isolated from humans and chickens from Hong Kong, J. Virol. 72 (1998) 6678–6688.

[13] L.J. Reed, H. Muench, A simple method of estimating fifty percent endpoints, Am. J. Hyg. 27 (1938) 493–497.

[14] Y. Hiromoto, Y. Yamazaki, T. Fukushima, T. Saito, S.E. Lindstrom, K. Omoe, R. Nerome, W. Lim, S. Sugito, K. Nerome, Evolutionary characterization of the six internal genes of H5N1 human influenza A virus, J. Gen. Virol. 81 (2000) 1293–1303.

[15] P.M. Colman, J.N. Varghese, W.G. Laver, Structure of the catalytic and antigenic sites in influenza virus neuraminidase, Nature 303 (1983) 41–44.

[16] S.J. Morris, G.E. Price, J.M. Barnett, S.A. Hiscox, H. Smith, C. Sweet, Role of neuraminidase in influenza virus-induced apoptosis, J. Gen. Virol. 80 (1999) 137–146.

[17] S. Schultz-Cherry, V.S. Hinshaw, Influenza virus neuraminidase activates latent transforming growth factor β, J. Virol. 70 (1996) 8624–8629.

[18] T.M. Tumpey, X. Lu, T. Morken, S.R. Zaki, J.M. Katz, Depletion of lymphocytes and diminished cytokine production in mice infected with a highly virulent influenza A (H5N1) virus isolated from humans, J. Virol. 74 (2000) 6105–6116.

[19] J.W. Almond, A single gene determines the host range of influenza virus, Nature 270 (1977) 617–618.

[20] E.K. Subbarao, W. London, B.R. Murphy, A single amino acid in the PB2 gene of influenza A virus is a determinant of host range, J. Virol. 67 (1993) 1761–1764.

[21] M.H. Snyder, R.F. Betts, D. DeBorde, E.L. Tierney, M.L. Clements, D. Harrington, S.D. Sears, R. Dolin, H.F. Maassab, B.R. Murphy, Four viral genes independently contribute to attenuation of live A/Ann Arbor/6/60 (H2N2) cold-adapted reassortant virus vaccines, J. Virol. 62 (1988) 488–495.

[22] E.K. Subbarao, Y. Kawaoka, B.R. Murphy, Rescue of an influenza A virus wild-type PB2 gene and a mutant derivative bearing a site-specific temperature-sensitive and attenuating mutation, J. Virol. 67 (1993) 7223–7228.

[23] Y. Hiromoto, T. Saito, S. Lindstrom, K. Nerome, Characterization of low virulent strains of highly pathogenic A/Hong Kong/156/97 (H5N1) virus in mice after passage in embryonated hens' eggs, Virology 272 (2000) 429–437.

International Congress Series 1219 (2001) 601–607

A mouse model of dual infection with influenza virus and *Streptococcus pneumoniae*

Jonathan A. McCullers[a,*], Robert G. Webster[b,c]

[a]*Department of Infectious Diseases, St. Jude Children's Research Hospital,*
332 North Lauderdale Street, Memphis, TN 38105, USA
[b]*Department of Virology and Molecular Biology, St. Jude Children's Research Hospital,*
332 North Lauderdale Street, Memphis, TN 38105, USA
[c]*Department of Pathology, University of Tennessee, Memphis, 8000 Madison Avenue,*
Memphis, TN 38163, USA

Abstract

Background: A lethal synergism exists between influenza virus and *Streptococcus pneumoniae* accounting for excess mortality during influenza epidemics. A small animal model of dual infection with these organisms would be useful for study of pathogenic mechanisms underlying this interaction. *Methods*: Groups of mice were infected with either mouse adapted influenza virus A/ Puerto Rico/8/34 (H1N1), *S. pneumoniae* strain D39, both simultaneously, or pneumococcus following influenza virus. Weight loss, as a measure of morbidity, and mortality were followed. Blood cultures were collected 24 h after infection. *Results*: Mice infected simultaneously with both influenza virus and pneumococcus exhibited gradual weight loss and mortality commensurate with expectations for an additive process. In contrast, mice infected with pneumococcus 7 days following infection with influenza virus uniformly died in less than 24 h and were highly bacteremic. *Discussion*: A mouse model of sequential infection with influenza virus and *S. pneumoniae* has been developed. Mice infected with pneumococcus seven days after infection with influenza virus exhibit a synergistic lethality caused by overwhelming sepsis. This model will be useful for study of the mechanisms involved in pathogenic interactions between influenza virus and pneumococcus. © 2001 Elsevier Science B.V. All rights reserved.

Keywords: Sepsis; Pneumonia; Bacteria; Mortality; Synergism

* Corresponding author. Tel.: +1-901-495-3486; fax: +1-901-495-3099.
E-mail address: jon.mccullers@stjude.org (J.A. McCullers).

1. Introduction

Lower respiratory tract infections from pneumonia and influenza account for excess mortality during influenza epidemics [1,2]. A lethal synergy exists between influenza virus and *Streptococcus pneumoniae*, the most common cause of community acquired pneumonia [3]. Although several mechanisms have been postulated to explain the synergism between these organisms [4], the interaction remains poorly understood. Study of these pathogenic mechanisms would likely provide targets for drugs or vaccines that could impact on the serious worldwide morbidity and mortality from pneumonia and influenza.

Although the contribution of the synergistic interaction between influenza virus and pneumococcus to development of otitis media has been well studied in the chinchilla model [5], no small animal model of pneumonia or sepsis with these two organisms has been described. We describe here a murine model of pneumonia and sepsis demonstrating lethal synergism between influenza virus and pneumococcus and discuss its utility for further study of pathogenic mechanisms underlying this interaction.

2. Materials and methods

2.1. Infectious agents

Mouse adapted influenza virus A/Puerto Rico/8/34 (H1N1), hereafter referred to as PR8, was grown in Madin–Darby canine kidney (MDCK) cells from stock from the influenza virus repository at St. Jude Children's Research Hospital. The dose of PR8 lethal for 50% of infected mice (MLD_{50}) was the equivalent of 3000 $TCID_{50}$ (the dose infectious for 50% of MDCK tissue culture wells) and 140 MID_{50} (the dose infectious for 50% of mice). *S. pneumoniae* D39, a type 2 encapsulated strain, was obtained from the collection of Elaine Tuomanen, St. Jude Children's Research Hospital, Memphis, TN, and grown in Todd Hewitt broth (Difco Laboratories, Detroit, MI, USA). The MLD_{50} for pneumococcus in mice was equivalent to 5×10^5 CFU on tryptic soy agar (Difco Laboratories) supplemented with 3% v/v sheep erythrocytes.

2.2. Mice

Eight- to ten-week-old female Balb/cByJ mice (Jackson Laboratory, Bar Harbor, ME) were maintained in a Biosafety Level 2 facility in the Animal Resource Center at St. Jude Children's Research Hospital. All experimental procedures were approved by the Animal Care and Use Committee prior to study and were done under general anesthesia with methoxyflurane (Pittman-Moore, Mundelein, IL, USA).

2.3. Blood cultures

Approximately 500 μl blood was obtained from mice via retroorbital puncture with polished, sterile, glass Pasteur pipettes 24 h following infection with pneumococcus and transferred into Isolator 1.5 microbial tubes (Wampole Laboratories, Cranbury, NJ, USA).

Quantitation of colony counts by the Isolator 1.5 system was done by tenfold dilutions on tryptic soy agar plates supplemented with 3% v/v sheep erythrocytes. The assay could quantitate colony counts between 100 and 10^7 CFU/ml blood.

2.4. Mean survival day

A mean survival day (MSD) was calculated using the following formula

$$MSD = [f(d-1)]/N$$

where f is the number of mice recorded dead on day d (survivors on day 21 were included in f for that day), and N is the number of mice in a group [6].

3. Results

3.1. Infectious model

Our first goal was to determine whether mice could be infected with each infectious agent and what the effect of dual infection would be on morbidity, manifest as weight loss, and mortality. Three groups of four mice were infected with 100 μl of a suspension (50 μl in each nostril) in phosphate buffered saline (PBS) of either PR8 (0.7 MLD_{50}), pneumo-coccus (0.2 MLD_{50}), both, or PBS alone. Mice infected with PR8 initially showed no disease signs, but after 3–4 days developed clinical infection manifest as ruffled fur, decreased activity, anorexia, huddling, hunched posture, and shivering. Weight loss was noted after 2 days and peaked at 7–10 days with approximately 30% weight loss (Fig. 1) after which time surviving mice gradually recovered. Mice infected with pneumococcus were clinically ill within 24 h as evidenced by decreased movement, shivering, huddling, hunched posture, and closed eyes. Weight loss occurred between days 1 and 3 but mice recovered quickly by 5 days post infection (p.i.). Mice infected with both agents exhibited signs of each infection with rapid onset of clinical illness and gradual recovery after a weight nadir at 7–10 days (Fig. 1), while mock infected animals had no clinical symptoms and no change in weight. Therefore, we determined that mice could be dually infected with influenza virus and pneumococcus and that simultaneous administration resulted in morbidity and mortality similar to what would be expected from an additive process.

3.2. Lethal synergy when pneumococcal infection follows influenza virus infection

In order to determine whether lethal synergy was due to influenza predisposing to pneumococcal infection, we designed an experiment where pneumococcal challenge followed influenza virus infection by 1 week. Groups of eight mice were infected at doses as detailed above at day 0 with either PR8, pneumococcus, both together, or PBS (mock infection) followed by either pneumococcus or PBS (mock infection) at day 7 (Table 1). Mice were followed for mortality for 21 days, and gross mortality and the MSD were calculated. Infection with either infectious agent alone or both together resulted in clinical illness and 25–50% mortality, following a clinical illness of 9–15 days with a

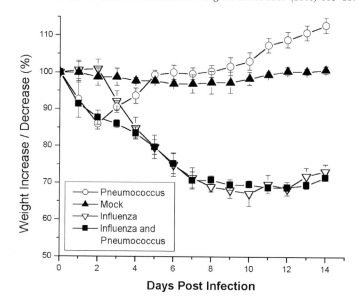

Fig. 1. Groups of mice were weighed daily after infection with either *S. pneumoniae* strain D39, influenza virus A/PR/8/34, both, or diluent as a control at day 0. Error bars represent the standard deviation between groups of four mice.

resulting MSD for these groups between 14 and 16 days. All mock infected mice survived with a maximum attainable MSD of 20. However, mice sequentially infected with PR8 and then pneumococcus at day 7 p.i. uniformly died within 24 h (Table 1). These data indicate that sequential infection with pneumococcus following influenza virus by 7 days results in synergistic lethality in this model.

3.3. Mice sequentially infected with influenza virus then pneumococcus are highly bacteremic

To determine whether the mice dying rapidly following sequential infection with pneumococcus following influenza virus were dying of sepsis, we repeated the experiment and obtained blood cultures in the first 24 h after infection. Groups of eight mice were

Table 1
Infection with pneumococcus following influenza is lethal in mice

Group	Mean survival day	Mortality [no. surviving/total (%)]
Influenza	14.1	4/8 (50)
Pneumococcus	15.6	6/8 (75)
Influenza and Pneumococcus	14.3	4/8 (50)
Influenza then Pneumococcus	0	0/8 (0)
Mock infected	20.0	8/8 (100)

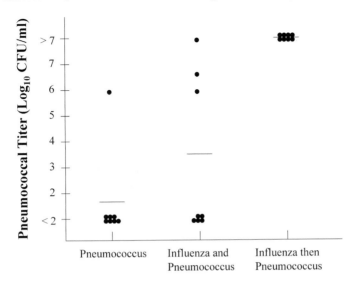

Blood Cultures from Mice 24 Hours After Infection

Fig. 2. Mice were infected with either *S. pneumoniae* strain D39, influenza virus A/PR/8/34 and pneumococcus simultaneously, or influenza virus followed 7 days later by pneumococcus. Blood cultures were collected 24 h after infection with pneumococcus and quantitated. Titers beyond the limits of the assay are expressed as either >7 if greater than 1×10^7 CFU/ml or <2 if less than 100 CFU/ml.

infected with either pneumococcus, PR8 and pneumococcus together, or PR8 followed 7 days later by pneumococcus. Blood cultures were obtained 18–24 h after infection with pneumococcus and quantitated. All mice sequentially infected with pneumococcus 7 days after infection with PR8 were highly bacteremic above the limits of the assay as performed. Only one mouse had bacteremia in the pneumococcus alone group, while the group receiving both simultaneously had intermediate results (Fig. 2). These data suggest that the rapid demise of mice infected sequentially in this model at the given doses is due to overwhelming sepsis.

4. Discussion

The lethal synergism between influenza virus and bacteria such as *S. pneumoniae* has been appreciated since the early part of last century following the influenza pandemic of 1918–1919 [7], and continues to be a major contributor to excess mortality during influenza epidemics worldwide. This is not only a major medical problem but an interesting biological problem deserving of further study. Towards this end, we developed a mouse model of pneumonia and sepsis with influenza virus and pneumococcus. We found that sequential infection with influenza virus followed 1 week later with challenge with pneumococcus resulted in 100% lethality in less than 24 h. These mice were highly bacteremic suggesting that overwhelming sepsis was the cause of death.

In the model as described, infectious doses below the MLD_{50} of influenza virus or pneumococcus resulted in partial mortality, with deaths occurring after a progressive clinical illness. Mice dually infected exhibited clinical courses and mortality as would be expected for an additive process if both infectious agents acted separately on the model. When pneumococcal infection followed influenza virus infection by a period of 1 week, however, synergistic killing occurred with rapid and complete mortality. The fact that lethal synergism occurred only when influenza virus infection preceded pneumococcal infection by one week implies that some alteration in the mouse engendered by influenza virus infection predisposes to sepsis. This may be suppression of the immune system, destruction of the respiratory epithelium exposing basement membrane elements to which pneumococcus can adhere, general debilitation of the mouse, or upregulation of receptors permissive for pneumococcal adherence and invasion through the host cytokine response to influenza virus infection. Although it is likely that multiple factors are responsible for the observed effect, the latter hypothesis is particularly attractive given work demonstrating that PAF receptor can be upregulated in vitro to allow pneumococcal attachment and invasion following exposure to cytokines present during influenza virus infection such as TNF-alpha and IL-1 [8]. The issues of how long must influenza virus infection precede pneumococcal challenge, what infectious doses are necessary to achieve synergistic morbidity and mortality, and what is the relative contribution of each of the proposed mechanisms for synergism are currently being studied.

Further work in this model has demonstrated that reduction of the doses of each infectious agent used can elicit similar results with 100% mortality following sequential infection, but clinico-pathologic disease more consistent with pneumonia than with sepsis (in preparation). Thus, the model should allow study of mechanisms of the synergistic interaction between influenza virus and pneumococcus that are pertinent to the human condition of secondary bacterial pneumonia which accounts for much of the excess mortality seen during influenza epidemics. Identification of specific pathogenic mechanisms should produce targets for intervention with drugs or vaccines that could impact on human disease and mortality.

Acknowledgements

This work was supported by Public Health research grants AI-08831 and AI-29680 from the National Institute of Allergy and Infectious Diseases, Cancer Center Support (CORE) grant CA-21765, and the American Lebanese Syrian Associated Charities (ALSAC).

References

[1] L. Simonsen, The global impact of influenza on morbidity and mortality, Vaccine 17 (1999) S3–S10.

[2] A. Klimov, L. Simonsen, K. Fukuda, N. Cox, Surveillance and impact of influenza in the United States, Vaccine 17 (1999) S42–S46.

[3] G.R. Donowitz, G.L. Mandell, Acute Pneumonia, in: G.L. Mandell, J.E. Bennett, R. Dolin (Eds.), Mandell,

Douglas, and Bennett's Principles and Practices of Infectious Diseases, 4th edn., Churchill Livingstone, New York, 1995, pp. 619–637.

[4] J.M. Hament, J.L. Kimpen, A. Fleer, T.F. Wolfs, Respiratory viral infection predisposing for bacterial disease: a concise review, FEMS Immunol. Med. Microbiol. 26 (1999) 189–195.

[5] S. Giebink, Otitis media: the chinchilla model, Microb. Drug Resist. 5 (1999) 57–72.

[6] R.R. Grunert, J.W. McGahen, W.L. Davies, The in vivo antiviral activity of 1-adamantanamine (amantadine), Virology 26 (1965) 262–269.

[7] A. Abrahams, N. Hallows, H. French, A further investigation into influenzo-pneumococcal and influenzo-streptococcal septicaemia, Lancet (1919) 1–11.

[8] D.R. Cundell, N.P. Gerard, C. Gerard, I. Idanpaan-Heikkila, E.I. Tuomanen, *Streptococcus pneumoniae* anchors to activated human cells by the receptor for platelet-activating factor, Nature 377 (1995) 435–438.

International Congress Series 1219 (2001) 609–613

Acute encephalitis–encephalopathy during influenza epidemics in Japanese children

Takehiro Togashi[a,*], Yoshihiro Matsuzono[b],
Tsuneo Morishima[c], Mitsuo Narita[d]

[a]*Department of Pediatrics, Sapporo City General Hospital, N 11 W 13, Chuo-ku, Sapporo 060-8604, Japan*
[b]*Department of Pediatrics, Abashiri Kousei Hospital, Abashiri, Japan*
[c]*Department of Health Science, Nagoya University, Nagoya, Japan*
[d]*Department of Pediatrics, Sapporo Tetsudo (JR) Hospital, Sapporo, Japan*

Abstract

Background: We previously reported an epidemiological aspect of influenza-associated encephalitis/encephalopathy in Japan. *Patients*: Case 1 is a 7-year-old boy who survived, and case 2 is a 5-year-old boy who died with a fulminant course. *Results*: Both patients showed remarkably high levels of IL-6 in cerebrospinal fluid and a postmortem examination of case 2 revealed generalized vasculopathy. *Conclusion*: The generalized impairment of vascular endothelial cells caused by highly activated cytokines must play a central role in the pathophysiology of this disease. © 2001 Elsevier Science B.V. All rights reserved.

Keywords: Brain stem; IL-6; Cytokine; Thrombus; Vasculopathy; Pathophysiology

1. Introduction

We have reported an epidemiology of influenza-associated encephalitis/encephalopathy (infl-enc) in Japan [1] as well as in Hokkaido, the northernmost island of Japan [2]. Two representative cases are reported here to present clinicopathological findings concerning the etiology of infl-enc.

* Corresponding author. Tel.: +81-11-726-2211; fax: +81-11-726-9541.
E-mail address: ttogashi@pop07.odn.ne.jp (T. Togashi).

2. Patients/results

Case 1, a 7-year-old boy. The child developed a fever of 37.9 °C on January 30, 1998. The fever rose to 39.4 °C by the next morning and he was found unconscious by his elder sister at 1:30 p.m., January 31. A generalized convulsion occurred at 7:00 p.m. and he was intubated. Laboratory findings are shown in Table 1. Prothrombin time was 21 s (40% of a reference), fibrinogen 2.62 g/l, FDP 15.6 mg/l. A brain CT taken at 10:00 p.m. on January 31 showed a low density area in the brain stem (Fig. 1A) and this extended to the bilateral thalami by February 2 (Fig. 1B). With supportive therapy on mechanical ventilation, he gradually regained normal consciousness on February 11. He was extubated on February 20, when the brain lesions still remained (Fig. 1C,D). Influenza virus A (H3N2) was isolated from a bronchial washing fluid taken on January 31 and an anti-H3N2 HI titer was 1:4096 on February 15. He was discharged from the hospital on June 23, by which time he could ride a bicycle.

Case 2, a 5-year-old boy. The child suddenly developed a fever of 40.6 °C with a generalized convulsion at 9:30 p.m. on February 6, 1998. He was in a comatose state on arrival at the hospital and the convulsion was controlled by the intravenous use of diazepam. A brain CT only revealed a mild, generalized edema of the brain. Laboratory findings are shown in Table 1. He again had a generalized convulsion at 0:30 a.m. on

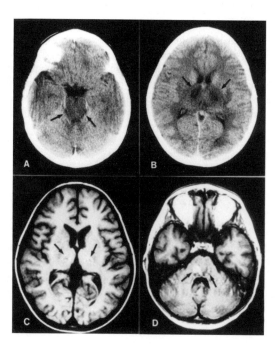

Fig. 1. Brain CT and MRI findings of case 1. (A) CT taken at 10:00 p.m. on January 31. A low density area was observed in the brain stem. (B) CT taken on February 2. The low density area extended symmetrically to the bilateral thalami. (C,D) T2-weighted image (C) and gadolinium-enhanced image (D) of MRI taken on February 19. The brain stem and thalamic lesions still remained.

February 7, which resisted medication. He died at 3:40 a.m. despite intensive care. Postmortem findings are shown in Fig. 2.

IL-6 (Fujirebio, Tokyo, Japan) and TNF-α (Amersham International, Amersham, UK) were measured by the ELISA kits according to the supplier's recommendation. The results

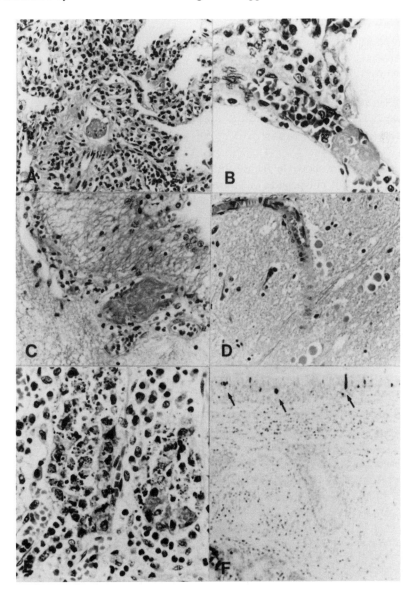

Fig. 2. Postmortem histological findings of case 2. (A,B) Lung tissue showing interstitial pneumonia and microvascular thrombi, (C,D) Medulla tissue showing hydropic degeneration, hyalinization of vessels, and extravasation of plasma proteins. (E) Small intestine tissue showing cryptic necrosis. (F) NP antigen of influenza virus A in the epithelial cells of the lung.

Table 1
Laboratory findings and cytokine test results of cases 1 and 2

		Case 1	Case 2
WBC (cells/mm^3)		9200	5800
AST (IU/L)		607	93
ALT (IU/L)		354	51
CPK (IU/L)		235	160
Glucose (mg/100ml)		155	253
CRP (mg/100ml)		1.32	0
IL-6 (pg/ml)	CSF	855.2	62,250
	Serum	NT	>700,000
TNF-α (pg/ml)	CSF	<7.5	159
	Serum	NT	1059

CSF: cerebrospinal fluid; NT: not tested.

of cytokine assays are shown in Table 1. Influenza virus was detected using a monoclonal antibody against NP polypeptide of influenza virus A, by the courtesy of Dr. Takuya Iwasaki of the National Institute of Infectious Diseases of Japan. The result is shown in Fig. 2F.

3. Discussion

In Japan, infl-enc has now acquired a distinct disease entity, which is characterized by affecting mainly younger children, rapid onset, and poor prognosis. We estimate that the disease occurrence is 260 patients (range, 100–400) per year [1,2]. This disease must not be unique to the Japanese, evidenced by the fact that some cases described in other

Table 2
Differential diagnosis of influenza-associated encephalopathy[a]

	Influenza encephalopathy	Reye's syndrome	Hemorrhagic shock encephalopathy	Acute necrotizing encephalopathy
Age distribution	0-12 years	0-8 years	<1 year	0-10 years
(Median)	(3.8 years)	(6.0 years)	(5.3 months)	(2.5 years)
Male/female	32/22	7/14	8/2	15/19
(Ratio)	(1.9:1)	(0.5:1)	(4.0:1)	(0.8:1)
Mortality rate	28/64	17/21	7/10	4/12
(%)	(43.8)	(81.0)	(70.0)	(33.3)
Influenza virus in throat	+	+/ −	−	+/ −
Clotting disorder	+/ −	−	+	+/ −
Hepatic dysfunction	+/ −	+	+	+
Blood sugar	↑ or →	↓	→	→
Serum ammonia	→	↑	→	→

[a] +: positive, − : negative, +/ − : variable, ↑: elevated, ↓: decreased, → : no change. Referred from: Influenza encephalopathy [2], Reye's syndrome [10], hemorrhagic shock encephalopathy [11], acute necrotizing encephalopathy [12].

countries [3–5] closely resembled what we call infl-enc. Moreover, the histological findings of case 2 closely resembled those described earlier [6]. Differential diagnosis of influenza-associated encephalopathy is shown in Table 2.

Concerning etiology, PCR evidence of direct invasion of the central nervous system by this virus is controversial [2,7,8]. The very rapid onset and the extraordinarily high cytokine levels in cerebrospinal fluid in comparison with encephalitis of other viral or mycoplasmal infections [9], along with the histological findings, suggest that the generalized impairment of vascular endothelial cells caused by highly activated cytokines plays a central role in the pathophysiology of infl-enc.

References

[1] T. Kasai, T. Togashi, T. Morishima, Encephalopathy associated with influenza epidemics, Lancet 355 (2000) 1558–1559.

[2] T. Togashi, Y. Matsuzono, M. Narita, Epidemiology of influenza-associated encephalitis/encephalopathy in Hokkaido, the northernmost island of Japan, Pediatr. Int. 42 (2000) 192–196.

[3] J.A. McCullers, S. Facchini, P.J. Chesney, R.G. Webster, Influenza B virus encephalitis, Clin. Infect. Dis. 28 (1999) 898–900.

[4] M.M. Ryan, P.G. Procopis, R.A. Ouvrier, Influenza A encephalitis with movement disorder, Pediatr. Neurol. 21 (1999) 669–673.

[5] D.B. Neilson, Sudden death due to fulminating influenza, Br. Med. J. 1 (1958) 420–422.

[6] R. Oseasohn, L. Adelson, M. Kaji, Clinicopathologic study of thirty-three fatal cases of Asian influenza, N. Engl. J. Med. 260 (1959) 509–518.

[7] S. Fujimoto, M. Kobayashi, O. Uemura, et al., PCR on cerebrospinal fluid to show influenza-associated acute encephalopathy or encephalitis, Lancet 352 (1998) 873–875.

[8] Y. Ito, T. Ichiyama, H. Kimura, et al., Detection of influenza virus RNA by reverse transcription-PCR and proinflammatory cytokines in influenza-virus-associated encephalopathy, J. Med. Virol. 58 (1999) 420–425.

[9] Y. Matsuzono, N. Narita, Y. Akutsu, T. Togashi, Interleukin-6 in cerebrospinal fluid of patients with central nervous system infections, Acta Paediatr. 84 (1995) 879–883.

[10] R.D.K. Reye, G. Morgan, J. Baral, Encephalopathy and fatty degeneration of the viscera: a disease entity in childhood, Lancet II (1963) 749–752.

[11] M. Levin, M. Hjelm, J.D.S. Kay, et al., Haemorrhagic shock and encephalopathy: a new syndrome with a high mortality in young children, Lancet II (1983) 64–67.

[12] M. Mizuguchi, Acute encephalopathy with necrosis of bilateral thalami: clinical aspects, Neuropathology 13 (1993) 327–331.

International Congress Series 1219 (2001) 615–622

Detection of viral antigens in the encephalopathy brain by influenza A virus

Mitsuo Takahashi[a,*], Tatsuo Yamada[b], Tetsuya Toyoda[c]

[a]Department of Clinical Pharmacology, Faculty of Pharmaceutical Sciences, Fukuoka University,
1-19-8 Nanakuma, Jonan, Fukuoka 814-0180, Japan
[b]Fifth Department of Internal Medicine, School of Medicine, Fukuoka University,
1-45-7 Nanakuma, Jonan, Fukuoka 814-0180, Japan
[c]Department of Virology, School of Medicine, Kurume University, Kurume, Fukuoka, Japan

Abstract

Rapid progressive encephalopathy showing a high fever, consciousness loss and recurrent convulsions has been occasionally reported in childhood during influenza epidemics in Japan since 1995. A clinicopathological study of a 2-year-old female diagnosed with hemorrhagic shock and encephalopathy syndrome associated with influenza A virus (A/Nagasaki/76/98; H3N2) infection showed that the virus antigens are present in CD8-positive T lymphocytes from the lung and spleen, suggesting the possible route of the virus spread. The virus antigens are confined to a very limited part of the brain, especially Purkinje cells in the cerebellum and many neurons in the pons, without inducing an overt immunological reaction of the host. RT-PCR for detecting the hemagglutinin gene demonstrated definite positive bands in all frozen tissues and cerebrospinal fluids taken at autopsy but not in samples on admission. The pathological change induced by the direct viral invasion cannot be sufficient for the rapid and severe clinical course of the disease within 24–48 h after the initial respiratory symptoms. The rapid production of several inflammatory cytokines together with the breakdown of the blood–brain barrier, which will induce severe brain edema, may be the major pathological processes. Any therapeutic strategy to control this multi-step progression could be effective. © 2001 Elsevier Science B.V. All rights reserved.

Keywords: Influenza A virus; Encephalopathy; Autopsy; RT-PCR; Immunohistochemistry

* Corresponding author. Tel.: +81-92-871-6631x6645; fax: +81-92-863-0389.
E-mail address: takahasi@fukuoka-u.ac.jp (M. Takahashi).

0531-5131/01/$ – see front matter © 2001 Elsevier Science B.V. All rights reserved.
PII: S0531-5131(01)00374-0

1. Introduction

Influenza virus is one of the most common causes of respiratory tract infection during the winter season. A wide spectrum of central nervous system (CNS) involvement has been observed during influenza A virus infection [1].

Rapid progressive encephalopathy cases with a high fever, consciousness disturbances and recurrent convulsions have been occasionally reported in children during influenza epidemics in Japan since 1995. Isolation of viruses or viral genomes from throat swabs or other clinical specimens strongly suggests that the encephalitic condition could be associated with influenza virus infection. After reviewing the severe or fatal cases reported previously, we conclude that the clinical signs and symptoms following influenza infection are superimposed by three suggested entities: Rye's syndrome [2], acute necrotizing encephalopathy [3], and hemorrhagic shock and encephalopathy (HSE) syndrome [4].

In this paper, we examined a 2-year-old girl with HSE syndrome, trying to answer several questions for which no histological or virological data exist.

2. Patient and methods

2.1. Case report

A previously healthy 2.5-year-old girl, who had no history of immunization for influenza virus, became pyrexial at 38–39 °C and had a cough 1 day before admission despite having been treated with a cold remedy. She managed to speak a few words and felt uneasy. She looked uncomfortable and sometimes trembled. She could hardly sleep during the following night owing to a continuous feeling of discomfort. She could stand and walk at night. On the following morning, when she asked her mother to take her to the lavatory, her mother noticed that her locomotion was quite unstable and that she could not walk straight. She fell down after voiding and stopped breathing. Her heart beat recovered 30 min after cardiopulmonary resuscitation and she was then transferred to Sasebo Municipal General Hospital. On admission, she was comatose without spontaneous respiration. As shown in Table 1, her clinical course was characterized by coma, DIC, subsequent hemorrhagic diathesis, shock and severe rhabdomyolysis. She died 7 days after admission.

2.2. Nested RT-PCR and Southern blot analysis

One microgram of total RNA was reverse-transcribed using H3 specific primer H3F-7 (ACTATCATTGCTTTGAGC) and avian myeloblastosis virus reverse transcriptase. PCR of the H3 specific HA gene was carried out for 30 cycles with the primer pair of H3F-7 (ACTATCATTGCTTTGAGC) and H3R-1184 (ATGGCTGCTTGAGTGCTT); the expected product size was 1178 base pairs (bp). PCR cycling conditions included denaturation at 95 °C for 5 min, annealing for 2 min at 42 °C, extension for 3 min at 72 °C, and additional extension for 10 min at 72 °C. One microliter of the RT-PCR

Table 1

Variable	On admission	Third day	Sixth day
Body temperature (°C)	30.5	31.5	30.5
Blood pressure (mm Hg)	65/40	100/80	60/50
Urine volume (ml)	640	1110	190
Platelet count/mm^3	297,000	33,000	16,000
Prothrombin time (s)	20.7	65.4	97.0
Aspartate aminotransferase (U/l)	1019	1988	645
Alanine aminotransferase (U/l)	243	552	387
Lactate dehydrogenase (U/l)	2053	17,630	7466
Creatine kinase (U/l)	2127	197,850	9066
Ammonia (μl/dl)	38	22	

products was further PCR-amplified for 30 cycles with the primer pairs of H3-HA5′n (GCACACTGATAGATGCTCTATTGGG) and H3-HA3′n (GGTGCATCTGACCTCAT-TATTGAG) using a Ready-to-Go PCR kit (Pharmacia Biotech); the expected size of the nested PCR product was 629 bp. The conditions of the nested PCR included denaturation at 94 °C for 1 min, annealing for 2 min at 55 °C, and extension for 1 min at 72 °C. As a control, PCR was performed exactly as above but without reverse-transcription. RT-PCR of β-actin was also performed with the primer pairs of β-actin 5′ (ATCATGTTTGA-GACCTTCAA) and β-actin 3′ (CATCTCTTGCTCGAAGTCCA). RT-PCR cycling included reverse transcription at 42 °C for 30 min, followed by denaturation at 95 °C for 1 min, annealing for 1 min at 44 °C, and extension for 1 min at 72 °C using a Ready-to-Go RT-PCR kit (Pharmacia); the expected product size was 308 bp. Digoxygenin-11-dUTP (Boehringer Mannheim Biochemica)-labeled H3 HA of influenza virus A/Nagasaki/93/98 (H3N2) was used as a Southern hybridization probe.

2.3. Viral inoculation of cynomolgus monkey brain

Each monkey received an inoculation into the bilateral frontal lobes of 1.0 ml PBS containing 25 plaque forming units of A/Nagasaki/76/98 (H3N2) with a 22-gauge needle. On days 3 and 7 after inoculation, monkeys were anesthetized and were killed by bilateral common carotid perfusion with 4% PFA and brains were removed. All experimental procedures were approved by the ethical committee for animal experiments at National Institute of Infectious Disease, Tokyo, Japan.

2.4. Immunohistochemistry

Sections were pretreated with 0.2% Triton X-100 (Sigma) in TBS (50 mmol/l Tris–HCl; 150 mmol/l NaCl; pH 7.5) for 20 min to increase permeability to primary antibodies. Peroxidase-like activity in tissue samples was blocked by incubating with 3% hydrogen peroxide in TBS for 10 min. They were then incubated with a primary antibody for 48 h at 4 °C, with 1:1000 biotinylated horse anti-mouse IgG (Vector) preabsorbed by 10% normal human or monkey serum for 2 h, and with 1:1000 avidin-

Table 2
Primary antibodies

Specificity	Species and dilution	Source
Human glial fibrillary acidic protein	Mouse monoclonal, 1:1000	DAKO
Microtubule associated protein-2	Mouse monoclonal, 1:1000	Boehringer
A/Kumamoto/22/76 (H3N2)	Chicken polyclonal, 1:2000	Kida
A/Memphis/96 (H3N2)	Chicken polyclonal, 1:2000	Kida
CD3, CD4, CD8, CD20	Mouse monoclonal, 1:1000	DAKO
Human insulin	Guinea pig polyclonal, 1:100	Lipshaw
Human glucagon	Rabbit polyclonal, 1:100	Lipshaw
Human somatostatin	Rabbit polyclonal, 1:100	Lipshaw

biotinylated horse-radish peroxidase complex (Vector) for 2 h at room temperature. Color development of peroxidase-labeled areas was performed for 15 min in a freshly prepared solution consisting of 20 ml TBS, 1 ml of 10 mg/ml 3,3′-diaminobenzidine (DAB; Dojindo), 3 ml 1% nickel ammonium sulfate and 3.5 µl hydrogen peroxide (30% stock solution). For double immunostaining, the second cycle was carried out in a manner similar to the first after treating sections for 30 min with 0.5% H_2O_2 solution, except that the nickel ammonium sulfate was omitted from the DAB solution, yielding a brown precipitate. The primary antibodies tried in this study and the dilutions used are shown in Table 2. Several negative controls were simultaneously performed: normal sera corresponding to the applied primary antibody as a primary antibody, intrinsic peroxidase detection by DAB solution without any further process, and the procedure without a primary antibody.

3. Results

3.1. Viral isolation and detection of the HA gene by nested RT-PCR

Influenza A virus was isolated in MDCK cells from a throat swab sample taken on admission, and its serotype was identified as influenza A virus (H3N2). Throat swab and cerebrospinal fluid samples were tested for antibody titer to anti-A/Wuhan/ 359/95 (H3N2). The hemagglutinin inhibition (HI) titer of the throat swab sample was 1280.

In nested RT-PCR of HA, positive bands of corresponding sizes, 629 bp for the HA gene segment and 308 bp for β-actin, were obtained in all samples taken at autopsy, and not in CSF and PBMC taken on admission. Specificity of the nested PCR products was confirmed in all samples by Southern blot analysis (Fig. 1).

3.2. Immunohistochemical study of the autopsied samples

Immunohistochemistry of the lung with anti-A/Kumamoto/22/76 (H3N2) showed linear dense staining, probably corresponding to type I alveolar epithelial cells, as well

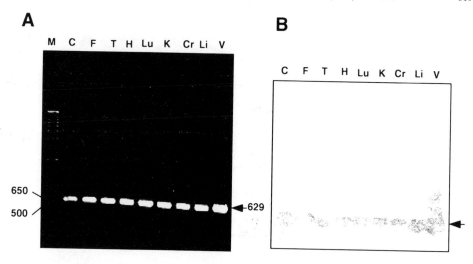

Fig. 1. RNAs from tissues and CSF taken at autopsy were subjected to RT-PCR. The outer and inner pairs of PCR primers were designed to detect the HA gene segment. Positive bands can be seen in all tissues and CSF (A), and the specificity of the amplified PCR products was confirmed by Southern blot (B). The band in lane V is from a positive control using a template of HA cDNA transcribed from RNA of influenza virus A/Nagasaki/76/98 isolated from this case. M: marker; C: CSF; F: frontal lobe; T: temporal lobe; H: hippocampus; Lu: lung; K: kidney; Cr: cerebellum; Li: liver.

as positively stained round cells in alveoli and vessels. Double immunostaining with anti-A/Kumamoto and anti-CD3 showed that there were some double positive cells. In the pancreas, although there was relatively high background staining, islets of Langerhans were positively stained compared to negative controls.

In immunohistochemistry of the spleen with anti-A/Memphis/96 (H3N2) and some lymphocyte markers, anti-A/Memphis/96-positive cells are located in the marginal area of the white pulp, where T cells are ordinarily abundant. In the center of the white pulp, there is no germinal center formation. Residual round, mononuclear cells are stained with anti-A/Memphis/96 and anti-CD4. Doubly stained cells are hardly observed. In contrast, the majority of the virus antigen-positive cells are also positive with anti-CD8. No fatty degeneration or virus antigen was observed in liver tissues.

The brain hemisphere was softened and edematous after 1 week of mechanical respiratory assist. There was no obvious hemorrhage. We could not obtain any parts of the thalamus and basal ganglia due to massive morphological destruction at autopsy. Immunohistochemical studies were shown in Fig. 2. No pathological alterations were seen in the vessels and perivascular spaces.

3.3. Immunohistochemical study of the infected cynomolgus monkey brain

Immunoreactivity with anti-A/Memphis/96 was seen only in the vicinity of injection site of the virus. Adjacent neurons in the pyramidal layer were focally virus antigen

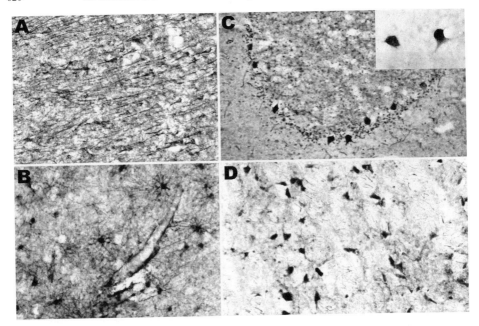

Fig. 2. Immunohistochemistry of the brain tissues. Antigenicity in the fixed brain tissues was checked by staining with anti-MAP-2 (A) and with anti-GFAP (B). Fairly good preservation of the antigenicity was confirmed in each area of the brain examined. Astrocytes seen in the vicinity of blood vessels had the morphology of activated ones (B). However, clear astrocytosis or diffusely activated astrocytes were not observed in all examined areas. (C) Many Purkinje cells in the cerebellum were strongly stained with anti-A/Memphis/96 (H3N2) (inset). Unstained Purkinje cells were sometimes seen even in areas very close to the positively stained cells, reflecting focal invasion of the virus. (D) Various neurons in the pons were positive for virus antigen.

positive. Astrocytic activation and proliferation were seen in the injection site and were positive with anti-A/Memphis/96.

4. Discussion

In the autopsied brain, Purkinje cells in the cerebellum and various neurons in the pons were positive for influenza virus antigen. There was no positive staining in the hippocampus, midbrain, and neocortex. When we consider this parenchymal tissue involvement, the characteristic clinical course of influenza virus-induced encephalopathy is very important. The syndrome is diagnosed clinically by a sudden onset of fever followed by disturbances of consciousness ranging from somnolence to deep coma and convulsions to some degree within a very short period, mostly 24–48 h after the onset of respiratory symptoms during an influenza epidemic [5]. RT-PCR demonstrated that the influenza A virus genome RNA was present in brain tissues as well as other organs and CSF. In contrast, CSF had little or no characteristics corresponding to meningoencephalitic conditions (pleocytosis and protein level elevation) in most reported cases. Immunohistochemical study of the infected cynomolgus monkey brain showed that over 1 week, the infection was restricted to the injection site. The time between the onset of respiratory tract symptoms and CNS involvement is not long enough for the virus to replicate and spread to parts of the brain, which we previously observed in mice showing neurological symptoms due to encephalitis. Therefore, we can assume that the syndrome may occur mainly not by the direct invasion of the brain parenchymal tissues by the virus.

Reports measuring proinflammatory cytokine levels in CSF from children with acute encephalitis showed that soluble TNF receptor 1 (sTNF-R1) and IL-6 levels were significantly higher in those who died or were left with sequelae than in those who survived without neurological deficits. The level of sTNF-R1 during the acute stage of encephalitis is an important index for predicting the neurological outcome. The serum level of IL-6 is also higher in patients with acute influenza virus-induced encephalopathy [6]. Furthermore, hyperactivated coagulation factors associated with DIC would participate in the pathogenesis [7,8].

Some residual mononuclear blood cells in the splenic vessels were double-positive for anti-virus and CD8 corresponding to suppressor T lymphocytes [9,10]. The barrier between the blood and susceptible extra-respiratory tissues is very strong under physiological condition because of the integrity and the insusceptibility of the endothelial cells lining blood vessels. In this study, we observed vascular endothelial cells under light microscopy and found no clear pathological alterations. Future studies are needed to look for ultrastructural changes of the endothelial cells as well as for the measurement of the humoral factors capable of acting on these cells [11].

Acknowledgements

Drs. A. Matsuo and K. Iwasaki at Sasebo Municipal General Hospital kindly provided us a clinical record and autopsied samples. We thank Drs. K. Ito, K. Yamada and K. Yamada at Kurume University for generous gifts of the antibodies shown in Table 2. We also thank Drs. H. Noguchi and T. Ueda at Nagasaki Prefectural Institute on Public Health and Environmental Science for virus isolation. We are grateful to Dr. K. Ami at National Institute of Infectious Disease for animal experiments.

References

[1] Y. Hayase, K. Tobita, Influenza virus and neurological disease, Psychiatry Clin. Neurosci. 51 (1997) 181–184.
[2] R.D.K. Rye, G. Morgan, J. Baral, Encephalopathy and fatty degeneration of the viscera-a disease entity in childhood, Lancet II (1963) 749–752.
[3] M. Mizuguchi, J. Abe, K. Mikkaichi, S. Noma, K. Yoshida, T. Yamanaka, S. Kamoshita, Acute necrotising encephalopathy of childhood: a new syndrome presenting with multifocal, symmetric brain lesions, J. Neurol., Neurosurg. Psychiatry 58 (1995) 555–561.
[4] M. Levin, M. Hjelm, J.D.S. Kay, J.R. Pincott, J.D. Gould, R. Dinwiddie, D.J. Matthew, Haemorrhagic shock and encephalopathy: a new syndrome with a high mortality in young children, Lancet II (1983) 64–67.
[5] S. Kimura, N. Ohtuki, A. Nezu, M. Tanaka, S. Takeshita, Clinical and radiological variability of influenza-related encephalopathy or encephalitis, Acta Paediatr. Jpn. 40 (1998) 264–270.

[6] H. Tsuruoka, H. Xu, K. Kuroda, K. Hayashi, O. Yasui, A. Yamada, T. Ishizaki, Y. Yamada, T. Watanabe, Y. Hosaka, Detection of influenza virus RNA in peripheral blood mononuclear cells of influenza patients, Jpn. J. Med. Sci. Biol. 50 (1997) 27–34.

[7] Y. Nagai, Protease-dependent virus tropism and pathogenicity, Trends Microbiol. 1 (1993) 81–87.

[8] A. Nishino, M. Suzuki, T. Yoshimoto, H. Otani, H. Nagura, A novel aspect of thrombin in the tissue reaction following central nervous system injury, Acta Neurochir. (Suppl.) 60 (1994) 86–88.

[9] I. Mori, T. Komatsu, K. Takeuchi, K. Nakakuki, M. Sudo, Y. Kimura, Viremia induced by influenza virus, Microb. Pathog. 19 (1995) 237–244.

[10] P.G. Stevenson, S. Hawke, C.R.M. Bangham, Protection against lethal influenza virus encephalitis by intranasally primed CD8[+] memory T cells, J. Immunol. 157 (1996) 3065–3073.

[11] I. Joris, G. Majno, E.J. Corey, R.A. Lewis, The mechanism of vascular leakage induced by leukotriene E_4, Am. J. Pathol. 126 (1987) 19–24.

International Congress Series 1219 (2001) 623–629

Hemorrhagic pneumonia by influenza virus: deaths in a low-risk group during the epidemic of dengue in Cuba

Suset Oropesa*, A. Valdivia, I. Abreu, B. Hernandez, L. Morier, Z. Gonzalez, L. Perez

Department of Virology, Instituto de Medicina Tropical Pedro Kouri, Havana, Cuba

Abstract

Background: In Cuba, flu is the first cause of infectious diseases and the fifth general cause of death associated with pneumonia. Lung necropsies were carried out on 15 fatal cases, between 20–54 years old, and dengue was presumptively diagnosed during an epidemic outbreak in 1997. According to virological evaluation, it was demonstrated that the causative agent in nine of these cases was influenza virus. *Techniques and Methods*: Indirect Immunofluorescence (IFI); immunoperoxidase staining (IPS); RT-PCR; nucleotide sequence. Culture was in MDCK cells and chicken eggs and hemagglutination inhibition was used for antigenic characterization. *Results*: With the IFA technique, nine cases (60%) were positive and with IPS, seven cases were positive (46.7%). In MDCK and chicken eggs, six hemagglutinating agents characterized by hemagglutination inhibition were similar to the reference strain A/Johannesburg/33/94 (H3N2). Type and subtype A(H3N2) were demonstrated by RT-PCR, too. Nucleotide sequences were determined and compared. Serological studies showed that the isolated A/Santiago de Cuba/193/97 strain was circulating in the population studied. Morbidity reports during January to May showed an average of 19 600 cases per month; however, morbidity during June and July rose to 39 800 per month. *Conclusion*: This is the first report about the co-circulation of influenza and dengue viruses in Cuba. It also reinforces the necessity of developing prophylactic, clinical and epidemiological actions against flu during dengue virus epidemics. © 2001 Elsevier Science B.V. All rights reserved.

Keywords: Hemorrhagic pneumonia; Influenza viruses; Diagnosis

* Corresponding author. National Reference Laboratory of Influenza, Tropical Medicine Institute Pedro Kouri, Novia del Mediodía Km. 6, La Lisa, Marianao 13, P.O. Box 601, Havana, Cuba. Fax: +53-7246051.
E-mail address: s.oro@ipk.sld.cu (S. Oropesa).

0531-5131/01/$ – see front matter © 2001 Elsevier Science B.V. All rights reserved.
PII: S 0 5 3 1 - 5 1 3 1 (0 1) 0 0 6 6 4 - 1

1. Introduction

In Cuba, acute respiratory infections (ARI) constitute a major health problem and among infectious diseases, they constitute the leading cause of morbidity in all age groups. Influenza virus is well recognized as the most important pathogen accounting for acute viral infections of the upper respiratory tract. This viral infection can give rise to severe complications, pneumonia being the most frequent, mainly in infants under 1 year, and older persons over 65. These two age groups have been considered as high-risk groups. Severity of this infection is shown in our country by the high mortality rates associated with influenza and pneumonia, ranking fifth among the general death and first among infectious diseases. More than 85% of these deaths occur in people aged above 65 years [1,2].

However, the behaviour of these viruses may present exceptional situations. During the month of June and the beginning of July 1997, a dengue epidemic occurred in the city of Santiago de Cuba, in the Eastern part of Cuba. During this epidemic, 15 persons, aged between 20 and 55 years, were presumptively diagnosed with dengue, requiring hospitalization, but died after a rapid evolution of the disease. Further investigations proved that these deaths were not caused by dengue virus, nor were they caused by enterovirus or herpesvirus. Samples were investigated for influenza virus as the possible causative agent of some of these deaths and the results obtained are described in this paper.

2. Material and method

2.1. Group I samples

Samples are 32 cases of necropsies from 15 fatal cases in Santiago de Cuba between June and July 1997, presumptively due to dengue. Ages of the cases were between 20 and 54 years. At the outset, these cases had a fever, which quickly evolved to hemorrhagic pneumonia and death. Only one case was presented with asthma as a chronic condition.

Samples were taken from lungs of all cases and in certain cases from the liver, brain and heart.

The 32 samples of necropsies were macerated and suspended in Dulbecco modified medium containing antibiotics, and centrifuged at 3500 rpm and decanted. All samples were divided into two parts. One part was tested immediately for the presence of influenza viruses by a rapid assay and the other part was frozen at − 70 °C.

2.2. Group II samples

Samples are 27 human sera from both acute and convalescent phases from two outbreaks, and 167 single sera collected from persons of the same region and period of time, were incorporated in this study, after obtaining a positive virological diagnosis of the necropsy samples, in order to assess the circulation of this virus strain in the population.

3. Methods

3.1. Immunofluorescence (IFA)

Group I samples were tested by indirect immunofluorescence (IFA), as previously described by Gadner and McQuilliam [3], using a commercial kit of monoclonal antibodies for respiratory viruses (Chemicon International, Temécula, CA, USA).

3.2. Immunoperoxidase (IPS)

These samples were also inoculated into 96-well cell culture plates (Costar Cambridge, MA), using two pools of Mabs, pool A (1:1000) and pool B (1:500). In addition, the Mabs HA1-71 and HA2-76 were used for subtyping of influenza A virus (1:400), according to the methodology described by Ziegler et al. [4].

Reagents for IFA and IPS development were kindly supplied by the Centers for Disease Control (CDC), Atlanta, GA, USA.

3.3. Isolates

The centrifuged product of the group I samples were grown in embryonated chicken eggs and MDCK, obtained from the American type culture collection (ATCC, Bethesda, MD) and culture was carried out according to the recommended protocol [5].

3.4. Polymerase chain reaction (PCR)

This technique was applied to three of the isolates obtained from lung samples; influenza A and B strains were incorporated as positive controls, RNA of noninoculated MDCK cells, and distilled water (as negative controls). RNA extraction was made with Trizol LS reagent (BRL Life Technologies), according to the manufacturer's instructions.

DNA molecular weight marker used: X174 DNA/Hinf I.

Primers:

Code	Sequence	
AB-41	5′ ATGGCCATCGGATCCTCAAC 3′	Influenza B1 (forward)
AB-42	5′ TGTCAGCTATTATGGAGCTG 3′	Influenza B2 (retro)
AB-43	5′ AAGGGCTTTCACCGAAGAGG 3′	Influenza A1 (forward)
AB-44	5′ CCCATTTCTACTTACTGCTTC 3′	Influenza A2 (retro)

The reaction was run for 30 cycles: 92 °C for 5 min, 50 °C for 2 min, and 72 °C for 3 min. A 10-μl aliquot was analyzed by agarose gel electrophoresis and stained with ethidium bromide. The reaction was carried out according to the protocol described by Class and the CDC, and adapted to our conditions [6].

3.5. Antigenic characterization

The viruses isolated were studied by HI with sheep hyperimmune sera against the A(H3N2) reference strains: A/Beijing/352/89, A/Shangdong/9/93, A/Johannesburg/33/94, A/Wuhan/359/95, A/Sydney/5/97, the A(H1N1) reference strains; A/Singapore/6/86, A/Taiwan/1/86, A/Texas/36/91, A/Beijing/262/95, A/Johannesburg/82/96, influenza B reference strains; B/Panama/45/90, B/Guangdong/08/93, B/Harbing/7/94, B/Beijing/184/93 and 7 influenza A(H3N2) isolates from the season 1985–1986 in Cuba: A/Cuba 820/85, A/Cuba/822/85, A/Cuba/828/85, A/Cuba/833/85, A/Cuba/895/85, A/Cuba/929/85, A/Cuba/933/85 and A/Santiago de Cuba/193/97(H3N2) [7].

3.6. Nucleic acid sequencing of the HA1 portion of the HA gene

From the RT-PCR product, sequencing of the A/Santiago de Cuba/193/97(H3N2) strain was performed following the dideoxy method described by Sanger et al. [8], using the Thermo'Sequenase Radiolabeled Terminator Cycle Sequencing kit, according to the manufacturer instructions and the following primers from data provided by the Centers for Diseases Control and Prevention (CDC).

Position	Sequence
Primer 7	+5′ ACTATCATTGCTTTGAGC 3′
Primer 362	+5′ TAAGGGTAACAGTTGCTG 3′
Primer 570	+5′ TGGCATAGTCACGTTCAG 3′

For analysis and comparison of the results, PC/Gene software was used.

Group II samples were tested by Hemagglutination Inhibition with A(H3N2) antigens A/Shangdong/9/93, A/Johannesburg/33/94, A/Wuhan/359/95, A/Sydney/5/97, A(H1N1) antigens; A/Texas/36/91, A/Beijing/262/95, A/Johannesburg/82/96, and influenza B antigens; B/Panama/45/90, B/Guangdong/08/93, B/Harbing/7/94, B/Beijing/184/93 and A/Santiago de Cuba/193/97.

4. Results

All the samples that are positive by the different techniques were obtained from lungs and the presence of influenza virus was not detected in samples from liver, brain, and heart.

Identification of the specimens from necropsies with monoclonal antibodies by IFA: Nine positive specimens (60%) were characterized as type A [3].

Type and specific subtype by immunoperoxidase staining: An intense cytoplasmic staining was observed in cells infected with influenza A and B reference strains, in using the A and B antiserum pools, respectively. The absence of staining in the cell controls indicated the specificity of the method. Viruses of the A(H3N2) subtype showed similar staining with the monoclonal antibodies HA1-71 and HA2-76 and the A(H1N1) subtype with the monoclonal HA2-76 (positive and negative controls) [9].

Of the 32 inoculated samples, seven samples reacted with the monoclonal antibodies HA1-71 and HA2-76, and were classified within the AH3N2 subtype (46.7%). In the rest of the samples, no cell staining was detected [10].

By observation of the cytopathic effect in monolayer cell samples that produced a clear positive hemadsorption and confirmed positive by IFA, six were confirmed as positive (40%) [7].

Polymerase chain reaction: It was confirmed that the isolates belonged to the influenza A type. Primers from conserved regions were used, which allowed the amplification of a nucleotide sequence of a single size for each type of influenza virus; type A generating amplification products of 190 bp, and type B, 241 bp [11,12].

Viral isolation in embryonated chicken eggs was positive in six samples. In the antigenic characterization by HI, none of these six hemagglutinating agents reacted with A(H1N1) subtype or the B type antisera. Furthermore, no antibody levels were detected with sera produced against strains isolated in Cuba during the years 1985–1986.

Different antihemagglutinin antibody levels were observed with A(H3N2) reference sera (from <20 to 1/160). Titres of the reference strains with homologous sera oscillated between 1:320 and 1:640. The isolates reacted to highest titre with sera to A/Johannesburg/33/94 (H3N2) and A/Santiago de Cuba/193/97 strains (1:1280).

Sequence: In the A/Santiago de Cuba/193/97 strain, a change of C by G, at nucleotide position 163 was observed.

Serologic study: Of the 27 paired sera, the majority of the subjects showed an increase in antibody titre (37.5%) and seroconvertion (60%) with A/Johannesburg/33/94 and A/Santiago de Cuba/193/97 strains. For the 167 unpaired single sera, HI antibody to the A/Johannesburg/33/94 and A/Santiago de Cuba/193/97 strains was found in 38% of sera.

5. Discussion

Results of the IFI, the IPS and the PCR techniques were all valued in this investigation, accurately indicating that the causative agent in these cases was the A(H3N2) influenza virus.

The techniques of IFA and IPS were specific and sensitive, providing rapid detection of the specific viral antigen, and the opportunity to utilise this in the management of the patient. The PCR was also demonstrated to be specific, yielding products of the current size for the strains of types A and B of influenza, as reported in the literature [13,14].

Antigenic characterization demonstrated that the isolates were closely related or were very similar to the A/Johannesburg/33/94 (H3N2) international reference strain. The circulation of this strain was widely reported as responsible for epidemic influenza outbreaks, and in 1995, of the 407 isolates characterized by CDC, 41% were antigenically related to this virus [7].

From the analysis of the serological results of the paired sera obtained and of the 167 unpaired control sera [15], it was concluded that the influenza strains similar to A/Johannesburg/33/94 and A/Santiago de Cuba/193/99 were circulating throughout the

Eastern region of our country, within all age groups. However, no similar cases were observed in other Eastern provinces.

From an epidemiological viewpoint, these deaths coincide with the summer influenza outbreak that sometimes occurs in Cuba, during the months of June and July. During that time, medical care given due to ARI in Santiago de Cuba increased from 19 800 (from January to May) to 39 000 consultations in a population of scarcely 1 million inhabitants.

The HA1 sequence of the A/Santiago de Cuba/193/97 strain, one of the isolates, was compared with the nucleotide sequence of the homologous segments of the A/Johannesburg/33/94 (H3N2) reference strain. Only one change was observed in the position 163 (C to G), i.e. a homology of 99.56%. The presence of changes in other regions of the genome should be further explored, with the objective of explaining the unusual behaviour of this influenza strain, the causative agent of at least nine of the deaths among the cases studied and whose clinical picture was basically characterized by hemorrhagic pneumonia, with rapid progress in low-risk persons (age group between 20 and 55 years) [16,17]. Chronic asthma was observed as a possible risk factor in only one individual.

A situation of this nature had not been reported previously in Cuba, either virologically or clinically. Furthermore, a similar situation has not been found in the international literature, except those referring to the great pandemics of the century. These observations confirm that the behaviour of the influenza strains and their pathogenicity may vary unpredictably.

The circumstances of this finding, in necropsies of fatal cases with a preliminary diagnosis of dengue, confirm the need of individualized diagnosis in clinical practice and the possible difficulties when dengue and influenza occur together [18].

Acknowledgements

The authors are grateful to Dr. Nancy Cox, Helen Regnery and Dr. A. Klimov (CDC, Atlanta, USA), to Dr. Hay (NIMR, UK) and Dr. Wood (NIBSC, UK) for the support of this investigation. The authors especially thank Lic Armando Martinez and Orquidea Biart for their dedication and help.

References

[1] C. Weissenbasher, W. Avila, Los virus como causa de IRA alta y baja en ninos: Características generales y diagnostico, in: Y. Benguigui, F. Antunano, G. Schmunis, J. Yunes (Eds.), Infecciones Respiratorias en Ninos. EEUU:OPS/OMS, Lippincott-Raven Publishers, New York, 1997.

[2] B. Murphy, G. Robert, Orthomixoviruses: influenza, in: B.N. Fields, D.M. Knipe, H.P. Fields (Eds.), Virology, vol. I, Lippincott-Raven, New York, 1996.

[3] P.S. Gardner, J. McQuillin, Rapid Virus Diagnosis in Application of Immunofluorescence, 2nd edn., Butterworth and Co., London, 1980.

[4] T. Ziegler, H. Hall, A. Sánchez-Fauquier, W.C. Gamble, N. Cox, Type and subtype-specific detection of influenza viruses in clinical specimens by rapid culture assay, J. Clin. Microbiol. 33 (2) (1995) 318–321.

[5] H. Meguro, J.D. Bryant, A.E. Torrence, P.F. Wright, Canine kidney cells line for isolation of respiratory viruses, J. Clin. Microbiol. 9 (1979) 175–179.

[6] E.C. Class, M.J. Sprenger, G.E. Kleter, R. van Beek, Type-specific identification of influenza viruses A, B and C by the polymerase chain reaction, J. Virol. Methods 39 (1992) 1–13.

[7] D. Palmer, W. Dowdle, M. Coleman, G. Schild, Advanced laboratory techniques for influenza diagnosis, Part 2: Procedural guide US Department of Health Educat. and Public Health Service, Immunology Series 6 (1975) 25–62.

[8] F. Sanger, S. Nicklen, A.R. Coulsen, DNA sequencing with chain-terminating inhibitors, Proc. Natl. Acad. Sci. U. S. A. 74 (1987) 5463–5467.

[9] Caracterización de influenza virus por el método de inmunoperoxidasa utilizando anticuerpos monoclonales: montaje y validación, Rev. Cubana Med. Trop. 48 (3) (1996), En imprenta, Cuba.

[10] Detección y caracterización rápida de virus influenza A y B en secreciones nasofaríngeas utilizando el método de la inmunoperoxidasa, Rev. Cub. de Med. Trop. 49 (2) (1997), En imprenta, Cuba.

[11] D.A. Buonagurio, S. Nakada, J.D. Parvin, M. Krystal, P. Palese, W.M. Fitch, Evolution of human influenza A viruses over 50 years: rapid uniform rate of change in NS gene, Science 232 (1986) 980–982.

[12] P. Chomeznski, N. Sacchi, Single-step method of RNA isolation by acid guanidinium thioajanate–phenol–chloroform extraction, Anal. Biochem. 162 (1987) 156–159.

[13] N.J. Deacon, M. Lah, The potential of the polymerase chain reaction in research and diagnosis, Aust. Vet. J. 66 (1989) 442–444.

[14] E.C.J. Claas, M.J.N. Spienger, G.E.M. Kleter, R. van Beek, W.G. Quint, N. Masurel, Type specific identification of influenza viruses A, B and C by the polymerase chain reaction, J. Virol. Methods 39 (1992) 1–3.

[15] World Health Organization, Influenza: Antigenic activity of recent influenza virus isolates and influenza activity in the Southern hemisphere, WER 70 (39) (1995) 277–280.

[16] N.J. Cox, T.L. Brammer, H.L. Regnery, Influenza: global surveillance for epidemic and pandemic variants, Eur. J. Epidemiol. 10 (4) (1994) 467–470.

[17] J. Ellis, P. Chakraverthy, J. Clewley, Genetic and antigenic variation in the hemagglutinin of recently circulating human influenza A(H3N2) virus in the United Kingdom, Arch. Virol. 140 (11) (1995) 1889–1904.

[18] C. Lasalle, P. Grizeau, H. Isautier, O. Bagnis, et al., Sourveillance epidemiologique de la grippe et de la dengue, Bull. Soc. Pathol. Exot. 91 (1) (1998) 61–63.

International Congress Series 1219 (2001) 631–635

Impact of influenza on the functional status of frail older persons

William Barker*, Hannah Borisute, Christopher Cox, Ann Falsey

Departments of Preventive Medicine, Medicine and Biostatistics, University of Rochester Medical Center, Rochester, NY, USA

Abstract

Background: Little is known regarding the impact of influenza on functional status. We report an ongoing body of work to assess functional decline following influenza among older patients in nursing home and hospital settings. *Methods*: In nursing homes, a case-comparison design was used. One hundred and sixteen residents who developed influenza-like illness (ILI) during laboratory confirmed outbreaks of influenza A/H3N2 served as cases; 127 residents without ILI served as the comparison subjects. Measures of functional status before outbreak and 4 months after outbreak were collected from medical records. Matched pairs analyses were conducted to ascertain changes in measures of functional status. *Results*: Among case and comparison subjects, 25% and 16%, respectively, experienced decline in at least one major function ($p = 0.04$) including bathing, dressing and mobility for a net 9% or 1 patient in 10 with decline attributable to influenza. *Conclusion*: Decline in major physical functions constitutes an important new and costly measure of impact of influenza on the frail elderly. A comparison study of functional decline among elders hospitalized with pneumonia during influenza season, involving 300 cases and 300 controls, is in the planning stages. © 2001 Elsevier Science B.V. All rights reserved.

Keywords: Influenza; Functional status; Frail older persons

1. Introduction

In spite of extensive literature on the impact of influenza on mortality, hospitalization, sickness days and cost of care, there are virtually no published data on impact of acute

* Corresponding author. Department of Community and Preventive Medicine, University of Rochester, 601 Elmwood Avenue, Box 644, Rochester, NY 14642, USA. Tel.: +1-716-275-3357; fax: +1-716-461-4532.
E-mail address: William_Barker@urmc.rochester.edu (W. Barker).

0531-5131/01/$ – see front matter © 2001 Elsevier Science B.V. All rights reserved.
PII: S 0 5 3 1 - 5 1 3 1 (0 1) 0 0 4 1 2 - 5

influenza on functional status [1–3]. To begin to redress this gap in knowledge, this paper reports on the following body of observational research designed to measure the frequency and pattern of changes in physical status among frail older persons following acute influenza-like illness (ILI).

1. First and primarily we present selected findings from a completed study among elderly nursing home residents experiencing influenza.
2. Secondly, we briefly present a planned companion study among community dwelling elderly persons hospitalized with pneumonia during the influenza season.

2. Nursing home study

2.1. Setting and methods

The nursing home (NH) study, conducted in cooperation with the Medicare Influenza Vaccine Demonstration [4], is based on six homes, all which experienced laboratory documented influenza A/H3N2 outbreaks with 10 or more cases in the winter of 1991–1992. We conducted a retrospective medical record review of 131 NH residents who developed influenza-like illness during the outbreaks and 132 randomly selected comparison subjects from the same NHs who did not develop influenza-like illnesses.

Data collected on baseline characteristics include age, sex, flu vaccination status, presence of major chronic conditions (cardio-pulmonary, other) and selected measures of functional status. Outcome measures include deaths, functional status changes, and intercurrent deterioration in general health during the 4 months following the outbreak. Functional status data were obtained from standardized Patient Review Instruments routinely used to document the functional status on all NH residents at approximately 2-month intervals.

We used the Wilcoxan Signed Rank Test to test for significant changes in functional status using paired observations made pre-outbreak and at 3 to 4 months post-outbreak. These tests for change over time were run separately for case and comparison pairs.

2.2. Results

Clinical manifestations recorded among the 131 laboratory diagnosed influenza cases were typical of acute flu and included cough (90%), congestion (76%), and malaise or myalgia (25%). Mean duration of recorded symptoms was 6.2 days and mean highest recorded temperature was 101.5 °F. Pneumonia was diagnosed in 6% of cases.

Among the original 131 influenza cases and the 132 comparison subjects there were 15 and 5 deaths, respectively, during the 4-month period following the influenza outbreak with pneumonia and cardiovascular disease the predominant causes of death. Our study focuses on the 116 cases and 127 comparisons that survived at least 4 months.

Baseline characteristics of the 116 cases and 127 comparison subjects were essentially similar for age, sex, presence of major underlying chronic conditions, and percent who had received influenza vaccine — over 80% in both groups. The two groups were also similarly distributed with respect to levels of functioning for bathing, dressing, and mobility, as well as other physical and mental activities. Measures of functional status are expressed in terms of the individual's ability to perform an activity (e.g. bathing) independently or with partial or complete assistance of caregivers [5].

2.3. Functional status change

No significant changes in functional status were observed among case or comparison subjects at 1 to 2 months; however, at 3 to 4 months post-outbreak, we did observe significant net decline in functional status or independence in bathing, dressing and mobility among cases but not among comparison subjects. These findings are shown in Table 1.

For each section of Table 1, dealing respectively with bathing, dressing and mobility, assessment of changes among the 116 cases is shown first, followed by assessment of changes among the 127 comparison subjects. For each activity studied, the number of persons classified by each level of function–independent, partial, or complete assist at pre-outbreak baseline is shown in the left-hand column. The respective changes, if any, in levels of function from baseline are shown as numbers and percents in the rows in the tables. For bathing, of 34 cases who were independent as baseline, 27 (79%) were still independent, 15% had become partially dependent and 6% had become completely dependent 3 to 4 months following a bout of influenza. Similarly, among 26 partially dependent at baseline, 18 or 69% were unchanged while 27% had become completely dependent at 3 to 4 months. The net changes were highly significant at a p-value of 0.008. Among 51 comparison subjects who were independent in bathing at baseline and 22 who were partially dependent, 94% and 91% respectively remained unchanged at 3 to 4 months, representing essentially no significant change. Analysis for change in level of dependency for dressing and mobility at 3 to 4 months post-outbreak again showed in both instances a statistically significant pattern of functional decline among influenza cases but not among comparisons.

In aggregating the observations for each group of study subjects, 25% of the 116 influenza cases experienced worsening in one or more functions as opposed to 16% of the 127 comparison subjects, a statistically significant difference. This in essence represents a

Table 1
Clinical characteristics of 131 cases of influenza-like illness

	N	(%)
Cough	118	(90)
Congestion	100	(76)
Headache	6	(5)
Malaise	33	(25)
Pneumonia	8	(6)
Mean Temperature (SD) (°F)	101.5	(1.3)
Mean Days (SD)	6.2	(3.2)
Rx Antibiotics	29	(25)
Rx Amantadine	23	(18)
Vaccinated	108	(82)

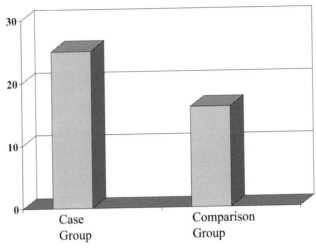

Chi² test for differences, p=0.037

Fig. 1. Percent of cases and comparison subjects with decline in one or more measures of physical functions at 4 months post-outbreak.

net residual negative effect on function and quality of life among 9% or 1 in 10 of those with influenza who survived (Fig. 1).

As a further measure of impact of acute influenza, we reviewed medical records for evidence of intercurrent deterioration of general health among case and comparison subjects during the 2-month period following the influenza outbreak including worsening of underlying medical conditions, mental status changes, and other. These were all more common among former influenza cases than among comparison subjects.

3. Planned pneumonia study

A planned companion study, which goes beyond the experience of NH residents, will assess impact on functional status of pneumonia hospitalizations caused by influenza and other common pathogens among community dwelling older persons. In pilot observations during the 1999–2000 influenza season, among approximately 120 pneumonia patients, 33% required partial or complete assistance in one or more physical functions; influenza, respiratory syncytial virus and pneumococcus were the most common etiologies. We plan to enroll and follow-up 300 pneumonia cases and 300 well-matched comparisons in the months of November–April during the years 2000–2002.

3.1. Summary and conclusion

Among a series of nursing home residents with acute influenza, 9% experienced significant long-term decline in independence in one or more major physical functions attributable to the influenza illness, which translates to 10 of every 100 cases. While data are limited due to retrospective nature of the study, our findings appear valid and document for the first time the significant impact of acute influenza on functional status of frail older persons. The observed functional decline is non-specific (bathing, dressing, mobility), likely due to "deconditioning" from bed rest, and may be reduced by reconditioning following acute illness [6,7]. A planned companion study will measure decline in function among community dwelling older persons following pneumonia hospitalization during the influenza season.

In conclusion, we submit that the impact of acute influenza on functional status is a very real and under-appreciated burden among the elderly population most vulnerable to the effects of influenza and that this is an important outcome to be measured in future studies of effectiveness of vaccines as well as the new anti-viral drugs which are receiving much attention among scientists participating in this Congress.

References

[1] K.J. Lui, A.P. Kendal, Impact of influenza epidemics on mortality in the United States from October 1972 to May 1985, Am. J. Public Health 77 (1987) 712–716.
[2] W.H. Barker, Excess pneumonia and influenza hospitalization in the U.S. due to influenza epidemics 1970–78, Am. J. Public Health 76 (1986) 761–765.
[3] A.S. Monto, Influenza: quantifying morbidity and mortality, Am. J. Med. 82 (1987) 20–25.
[4] W. Barker, N. Bennett, M. LaForce, et al., "McFlu." The Monroe County, New York, medicare vaccine demonstration, Am. J. Prev. Med. 16 (35) (1999) 118–127.
[5] W. Applegate, J. Blass, T.F. Williams, Instruments for functional assessments of older patients, NEJM 332 (1990) 1207–1214.
[6] C.M. Harper, Y.M. Lyles, Physiology and complications of bed rest, J. Am. Geriatr. Soc. 36 (1988) 1047–1054.
[7] W. Bortz, Disuse and aging, JAMA 250 (1982) 1203–1208.

International Congress Series 1219 (2001) 637–643

Indicators and significance of severity in influenza patients

D.M. Fleming[a],*, A.B. Moult[b], O. Keene[b]

[a]*Northfield Health Centre, 15 St. Heliers Road, Northfield, Birmingham, B31 1QT, UK*
[b]*Glaxo Wellcome, Greenford, UK*

Abstract

Background: In routine practice, influenza is diagnosed on clinical grounds. When influenza is known to be circulating locally, this is usually accurate, but awareness of the markers of influenza severity could be used by physicians to aid diagnosis and begin appropriate treatment early. This analysis compared baseline symptom profiles of subjects with severe and non-severe influenza. *Methods*: Symptoms of influenza-like illness (ILI) were recorded from 2235 subjects in six clinical trials of inhaled zanamivir 10 mg bd. ILI was defined as fever (37.8 °C) or feverishness plus at least two of the following: headache, myalgia, cough, sore throat, weakness, nasal congestion, loss of appetite. *Results*: Thirty percent (474/1572) of influenza-positive subjects were classified as having severe influenza and had a higher mean baseline temperature of 38.5 vs. 38.1 °C ($P < 0.001$). Symptom profiles were similar in severe and non-severe groups; severe subjects had higher symptom scores but did not consult their physician earlier than non-severe. Zanamivir reduced the time to alleviation by 3 days (8 vs. 5 days, $P < 0.001$) in severe subjects and by 1 day (5.5 vs. 4.5 days, $P < 0.001$) in non-severe subjects. In severe subjects ≥ 50 years old, zanamivir reduced the time to alleviation by 7 days (11.5 vs. 4.5 days, $P = 0.004$) compared with 2 days in severe subjects < 50 years (7.5 vs. 5.5 days, $P < 0.001$). *Conclusions*: Symptom profiles of subjects with severe and non-severe influenza were broadly similar; baseline temperature and total symptom scores were markers of severity. Time to alleviation was variable in untreated patients, but was reduced with zanamivir to between 4.5 and 5.5 days regardless of age or severity of illness. © 2001 Elsevier Science B.V. All rights reserved.

Keywords: Zanamivir; Symptom; Alleviation; Temperature; Age

---

* Corresponding author.

0531-5131/01/$ – see front matter © 2001 Elsevier Science B.V. All rights reserved.
PII: S 0 5 3 1 - 5 1 3 1 (0 1) 0 0 3 7 3 - 9

1. Introduction

Clinical features of influenza range from asymptomatic infection, through a respiratory illness with systemic features, multi-system complications, to death, usually from viral or bacterial pneumonia. Individuals over 65 years old and those with chronic heart or lung disease, diabetes, renal failure or immune suppression are at increased risk for complications and may have a more severe illness. The severity of illness may be influenced by previous infection with an antigenically related strain, smoking or pregnancy, and some viral antigenic types such as H3N2 appear to be associated with more severe diseases than others. Vaccination is efficacious and cost effective, but immunological senescence in the frail elderly reduces its effectiveness.

Patients with a classic "flu-like" illness present after a short incubation period of 2–3 days typically with an abrupt onset of symptoms, which may include myalgia, headache, fever (often 38–40 °C), chills, malaise, and anorexia, dry cough, and sore throat. Fever, if untreated, usually lasts between 3 and 8 days, at which time other systemic symptoms also begin to improve. Clinical diagnosis is usually accurate when influenza is known to be circulating locally [1], and accurate diagnosis is particularly important in subjects with severe symptoms of influenza or at high risk of complications. Markers of influenza severity could be used by physicians to aid diagnosis and commence treatment early.

This analysis compares the baseline symptom profile of subjects with severe influenza to that of those with non-severe influenza and investigates if any of the symptoms were predictive markers of influenza severity. Subject's age, high-risk status, vaccine status and infecting virus type (influenza A or B) were also investigated with a view to developing an understanding of the factors that might be associated with influenza severity.

2. Patients and methods

Data regarding the severity of patients' symptoms were collected and pooled from six phase II and III double blind, placebo-controlled studies designed to evaluate the use of the antiviral agent zanamivir (Table 1) [2]. Study participants were required to have fever (≥ 37.8 or ≥ 37.2 °C for subjects ≥ 65 years old in NAIA/B3002) or a symptom of 'feverishness', plus at least two influenza-like symptoms such as headache, myalgia, cough, or sore throat. The maximum duration of symptoms prior to study entry was 2 days or 48 h for all, except for one of the studies where it was 36 h [2]. Patients were supplied with relief medication in the form of paracetamol/acetaminophen and a cough suppressant in all, except one study (where only paracetamol was given), and instructed to use these medication only as dictated by the severity of their symptoms.

Confirmation of the clinical diagnosis of influenza was made on the basis of a positive result from viral antigen detection, virus isolation, polymerase chain reaction (PCR) assay or a four-fold rise in anti-haemagglutinin antibody (HAI) titre from baseline to day 21 or 28. High-risk subjects (aged ≥ 65 years and any subject with underlying cardiovascular, respiratory, metabolic or endocrine conditions, or those who were immunocompromised) were included in all studies except NAIA2005 and NAIB2005. Patients with chronic, unstable illness were excluded.

Table 1
Zanamivir phase II and III studies

Protocol number	Location/year	Placebo (n)	Zanamivir 10 mg inhaled (n)
NAIA2005[a]	NH/1995–1996	81	68
NAIB2005[a]	NH/1995–1996	63	64
NAIB2007[a]	SH/1995 and 1996	183	188
NAIB3001	SH/1997	228	227
NAIA3002	NH/1997–1998	365	412
NAIB3002	NH/1997–1998	182	174

[a] These trials also included a treatment arm of inhaled and intranasal zanamivir.

Physicians recruiting patients made an overall assessment of illness severity, which was rated as mild, moderate or severe. Patients recorded severity of individual symptom scores on a four-point scale (none $= 0$, mild $= 1$, moderate $= 2$, severe $= 3$). For this analysis, data from severe and non-severe (mild or moderate) groups (physician assessment) were compared on the basis of baseline temperature and total symptom score for the five main symptoms of influenza (headache, myalgia, feverishness, sore throat and cough). Scores were expressed as a percentage of the maximum achievable. Baseline temperature was compared between severe and non-severe patients using analysis of variance allowing for study differences. Symptom score was compared between these groups using a Wilcoxon test, stratified by study. These tests were also used to compare these measurements between patients aged < 50 and ≥ 50 years and between patients with type A and type B influenza. The proportion of severe patients was compared between type A and type B influenza using a Mantel–Haenszel test, stratified by study. Time to consultation from onset of symptoms was compared using an extended Mantel–Haenszel test, stratified by study.

The effect of zanamivir treatment in severe and non-severe subjects was also assessed based on the time to alleviation of symptoms used as the primary end-point in zanamivir treatment studies. Alleviation was defined as no fever (temperature < 37.8 °C and feverishness score of 'none') and no other main symptom recorded as more than 'mild' on the diary card. All these criteria had to be maintained further for 24 h. Time to alleviation was compared between zanamivir and placebo using the Generalized Wilcoxon test, stratified by study. Patients with no evidence of alleviation were included as censored at their last diary card entry. Corresponding median times to alleviation were calculated from Kaplan–Meier estimates of success rates.

3. Results

In the six studies evaluated for this analysis (Table 1), 1133 subjects received zanamivir and 1102 received placebo. In all, 1572/2235 subjects (70%) were influenza-positive with 474 (30%) of these being in the severe group. Subjects classified as severe on recruitment had a significantly higher median temperature (38.5 °C) than those who were non-severe (38.1 °C, $P < 0.001$) and 84% of those in the severe group were febrile at baseline

Table 2
Baseline characteristics and time to consultation in influenza-positive subjects

Time to consultation (h)	Severe ($n = 474$, %)	Non-severe ($n = 1098$, %)
≤ 24	35	38
24–36	46	45
>36	20	17

(temperature $\geq 37.8\ °C$) compared to 75% in the non-severe group. There were no substantial differences in the symptom profile of subjects classified as severe or non-severe, but overall symptom scores were higher for those in the severe (73) than the non-severe category (60, $P < 0.001$). Subjects with severe symptoms did not consult earlier than those without (Table 2).

The median baseline symptom scores for the five main symptoms for those aged < 50 ($n = 1309$) and ≥ 50 years ($n = 263$) were 67 and 60, respectively ($P = 0.012$). The baseline temperature in the older group was 38.3 °C compared with 38.2 °C in the younger group ($P = 0.916$), with similar numbers being febrile (80%) compared to the younger group (78%). Subjects with influenza A had a higher median baseline symptom score (67, $n = 1342$) than those with influenza B (53, $n = 220$, $P = 0.004$) and a higher baseline temperature (38.3 vs. 37.9 °C, $P = 0.071$). Overall, 82% of influenza A subjects were febrile at baseline, compared with 59% of those with influenza B. Forty-six patients (21%) with influenza B and 425 (32%) with influenza A were classified as severe on recruitment ($P = 0.001$).

When placebo recipients in these studies were investigated, the time to alleviation of symptoms was 2.5 days longer in subjects considered severe at recruitment (8 days) than

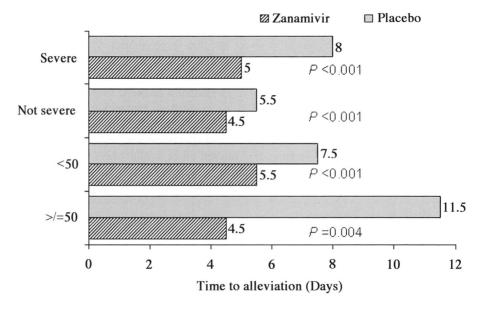

Fig. 1. Time to alleviation of clinically significant symptoms in subjects assessed as severe.

those who were not severe (5.5 days), and 1.5 days longer in subjects who were ≥ 50 years old (7.5 days) compared to those < 50 (6 days). Moreover, older placebo recipients (≥ 50 years) considered severely ill at recruitment had an even longer course of disease (11.5 days).

In the population classified as severe on recruitment, zanamivir treatment ($n = 222$) significantly reduced the time to alleviation by 3 days compared to placebo ($n = 252$) (8 vs. 5 days, $P < 0.001$). In subjects categorised as non-severe, the time to alleviation was reduced from 5.5 days in the placebo group ($n = 543$) to 4.5 days in the zanamivir group

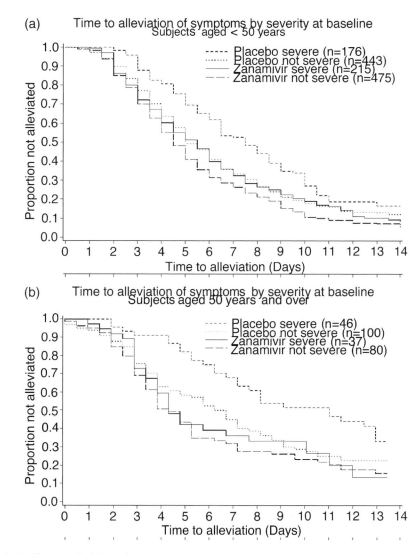

Fig. 2. (a) Time to alleviation of symptoms by severity at baseline; subjects aged < 50 years. (b) Time to alleviation of symptoms by severity at baseline; subjects aged 50 years and above.

($n = 555$, $P < 0.001$). In those ≥ 50 rears old with severe illness, the time to alleviation was reduced by 7 days (from 11.5 to 4.5 days, $P = 0.004$), and in those < 50 years by 2 days (from 7.5 to 5.5 days, $P < 0.001$) (Fig. 1).

Treatment with zanamivir reduced the time to alleviation regardless of vaccination status, with a reduction of 3.0 days for unvaccinated subjects and 2.5 days for vaccinated subjects (Fig. 1).

In untreated subjects, the length of disease was longer in subjects ≥ 50 years old and in those considered severe on recruitment. In zanamivir-treated patients, the time to alleviation of symptoms was similar in these populations, regardless of the time to alleviation in untreated subjects, where it varied substantially with age and severity (Fig. 2).

4. Discussion

The data generated from this large cohort of subjects indicate that increasing severity of influenza and increasing age are both independently associated with increased length of disease as measured by time to alleviation of symptoms. Subjects ≥ 50 years old with severe influenza reported an even longer time to alleviation of symptoms. Subjects with severe illness did not consult earlier than the non-severe. Baseline temperature, total and individual symptom scores were markers of severity. Subjects aged ≥ 65 years were not analysed as a separate sub-group. However, a longer course of disease has been demonstrated in unvaccinated subjects over 65 [4].

The baseline symptom scores reported by subjects and the proportion febrile was higher in subjects who had influenza A than those with influenza B, but subjects infected with either virus type reported a similar symptom profile. A larger proportion of influenza A than influenza B subjects was considered severe on recruitment. Nevertheless, 21% of subjects with influenza B were in the severe group, reinforcing the importance of an effective treatment for influenza B infection. Zanamivir has been shown to be effective in the treatment of influenza B, reducing the time to alleviation by 2 days ($P < 0.001$) [3]. Overall, 115 subjects received prior vaccination, with only 29 of these being assessed as severe at recruitment indicating that vaccination does not always prevent subjects from acquiring a severe infection.

The time to alleviation of symptoms in subjects who received placebo varied between 5 and 11.5 days in the different sub-groups analysed here. There was much less variability in time to alleviation in the zanamivir treatment groups. The time to alleviation in zanamivir treatment groups varied only between 4.5 and 5.5 days and was similar regardless of age or severity.

5. Conclusions

Subjects aged ≥ 50 years old and those considered severely ill at recruitment experience a longer duration of illness than those who are aged < 50 years old or non-severe. Zanamivir reduced the time to alleviation by up to 7 days compared to placebo, to between 4.5 and 5.5 days regardless of age or severity of illness at presentation.

Acknowledgements

Financial support was provided by Glaxo Wellcome.

References

[1] A.S. Monto, S. Gravenstein, M. Elliott, M. Colopy, J. Schweinle, Clinical signs and symptoms predicting influenza infection, Arch. Intern. Med., in press.

[2] A.S. Monto, A. Webster, O. Keene, Randomized, placebo controlled studies of inhaled zanamivir in the treatment of influenza A and B: pooled efficacy analysis, J. Antimicrob. Chemother. 44 (Topic B) (1999) 23–29.

[3] A. Osterhaus, J. Hedrick, K. Henrickson, M. Mäkelä, A. Webster, O. Keene, Clinical efficacy of inhaled zanamivir for the treatment of influenza B: a pooled analysis of randomized, placebo-controlled studies, Clin. Drug Invest., in press.

[4] S. Gravenstein, B. Freund, J. McElhaney, M. Schilling, et al., Greater effectiveness from zanamivir treatment of influenza with antecedent influenza vaccination in older adults, World Organisation of National Colleges, Academies and Academic Associations of General Practitioners/Family Physicians (WONCA), Vienna, Austria, July 2nd–6th 2000, Abstract 114.

Current strategies for
improved control by vaccination

International Congress Series 1219 (2001) 647–653

Measuring the effect of influenza vaccination programs—the Japanese schoolchildren experience revisited

T.A. Reichert[a,*], N. Sugaya[b], D.S. Fedson[c], W.P. Glezen[d], L. Simonsen[e], M. Tashiro[f]

[a]*Becton Dickinson & Co/Entropy Limited, 262 W. Saddle River Road, Upper Saddle River, NJ 07458, USA*
[b]*Nippon Kokan Hospital, Kawasaki, Japan*
[c]*Aventis-Pasteur-MSD, Lyon, France*
[d]*Baylor College of Medicine, Houston, TX, USA*
[e]*National Institute of Allergy and Infectious Disease, Washington, DC, USA*
[f]*National Institute of Infectious Disease, Tokyo, Japan*

Abstract

Background: An important consequence of influenza epidemics is increased mortality in elderly persons and those with high-risk conditions. Most developed countries have focused on vaccination of this group. In Japan, the control of influenza centered on the vaccination of schoolchildren. From 1962 to 1987, most Japanese schoolchildren received influenza vaccine. With the level of coverage achieved, it is possible that herd immunity was achieved. If this were the case, the impact of disease should have been reduced in older persons, and a reduction in winter excess mortality should have occurred. *Methods*: All-cause and pneumonia and influenza (P&I) excess mortality for both Japan and the US were estimated for 50 winters, 1949–1998. *Results*: Estimates of P&I and all-cause excess mortality were highly correlated. The winter excess of mortality in Japan was sharply reduced from ~1963 to about 1990, after which it again rose. The timing of these changes matches that of the Japanese Schoolchildren Vaccination Program. *Conclusions*: All-cause and P&I mortality represent the impact of influenza about equally well. That impact is three to four times greater in Japan than in the US. Schoolchildren vaccination appears to have averted ~37,000 deaths/year, or one for each ~420 vaccinations; and must be included in comprehensive pandemic planning. © 2001 Elsevier Science B.V. All rights reserved.

Keywords: Herd immunity; Excess mortality; Schoolchildren vaccination

* Corresponding author. Tel.: +1-201-934-9365; fax: +1-201-934-1467.
E-mail address: doctom_us@yahoo.com (T.A. Reichert).

1. Introduction

Today, in virtually all developed countries, influenza vaccination is recommended for elderly persons and high-risk patients. While, in all such countries except Japan, vaccine distribution has steadily increased [1], few countries have achieved vaccine coverage rates >50%, even in targeted populations. In Japan, however, the use of influenza vaccine has markedly decreased [2]. Japan based its policy for controlling influenza on a strategy of vaccinating schoolchildren [3]. During the Asian influenza pandemic of 1957, the importance of schools and schoolchildren as an amplifier of epidemics was clearly recognized. In 1962, a mass immunization program was begun in Japan. From that year to the late 1980s, vaccine coverage levels among Japanese schoolchildren ranged from 50% to 85%. Vaccination was mandatory beginning in 1977. In 1987, however, new legislation allowed parents to refuse influenza vaccination for their children. The use of influenza vaccine in Japan fell to very low levels; and in 1994, the government discontinued the mass immunization of schoolchildren, entirely [4].

Indirect protective effects of influenza vaccination were first reported by Monto et al. [5] who noted that vaccination of 85% of the schoolchildren in Tecumseh, MI reduced, three-fold, influenza-like illness among adults, compared with a neighboring community in which schoolchildren were not vaccinated. Mathematical models also suggested that high vaccine coverage rates in schoolchildren might substantially reduce the community-wide impact of influenza [6–8]. Because vaccination coverage levels over 50% were regularly achieved among Japanese schoolchildren during the 1970s and 1980s, it is possible that a degree of herd immunity in the population may have been achieved. If this was so, the impact of epidemic influenza, as measured by a change in mortality, principally in elderly people, might have been reduced. The purpose of our study was to determine whether or not this had occurred.

2. Methods

We examined excess mortality in Japan, before, during, and after the mass immunization of schoolchildren, contrasted with that of the US, for the same time period. From monthly mortality and population data from both countries [9–11], all-cause and pneumonia and influenza (P&I) excess mortality were estimated using an adaptation of the method of Simonsen et al. [12] In this adaptation, a baseline was defined as the 3-year moving average of the monthly mortality in November. This baseline was subtracted from the mortality for each winter month, November through May, and the algebraic sum was taken as the estimate of the excess deaths. The estimates produced by our method were very highly correlated with those of Simonsen et al. [12], for both all-cause and P&I excess mortality, differing only by a constant. Note that since the estimates produced by various methods differ either by a constant or exhibit a linear relationship with a slope on the order of one, differences between estimates made for two time points, using any method, will be very similar.

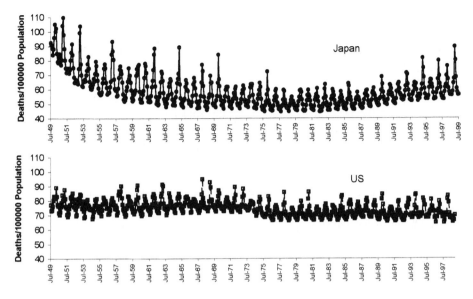

Fig. 1. All-cause monthly mortality in Japan and the US, 1949–1999.

Data on the amount of influenza vaccine produced and distributed in Japan and the US were obtained from the records of the Association of Biological Manufacturers of Japan and the US Center for Disease Control and Prevention, respectively [13].

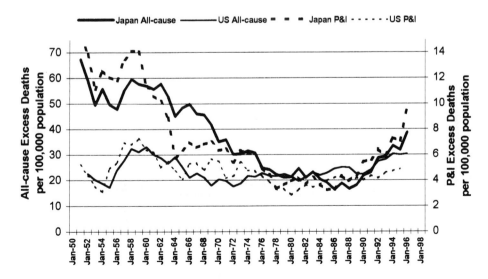

Fig. 2. The 5-year moving average of excess deaths for both P&I and all-cause mortality for Japan and the US.

3. Results

   The population of both Japan and the US increased linearly, from 1950 to 1980, each growing 18%. Japan's population was about 1/2 that of the US, throughout; but there was a greater increase in elderly in Japan (7–12% vs. 10–12% for the US). The all-cause mortality experience for Japan and the US is shown in Fig. 1, as rates adjusted for population. The taller peaks mark years of locally epidemic influenza activity, and these are much larger in Japan. In Japan, the large spikes in winter season mortality are attenuated beginning about 1971. From 1972 through the late 1980s, there is only one large peak, in 1975–1976, the year of the emergence of the variant strain, A/Victoria (H3N2). Very large peaks occur again in Japan, after 1994.

   Fig. 2 displays all-cause and P&I excess death rates for both Japan and the US as 5-year moving averages. A distinct notch in excess mortality rates occurred in Japan, coincident with the timing of the Japanese schoolchildren vaccination program. The three- to four-fold drop in excess mortality rates during the years of the Japanese schoolchildren vaccination program corresponds to reductions of ~9000 deaths/year in P&I mortality; and about 37,000 deaths/year in all-cause mortality, using 1960 population figures.

   In Fig. 3, we show P&I excess deaths rates, adjusted for population. The 5-year moving average is again displayed. We have also superimposed the vaccine usage in each country.

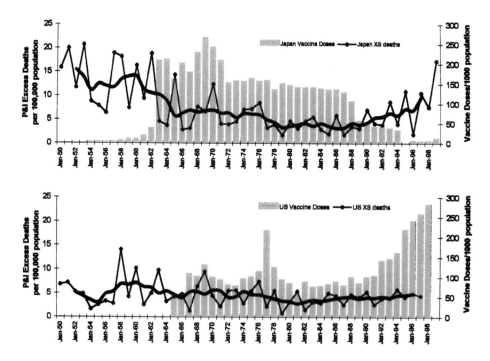

Fig. 3. Excess deaths attributable to pneumonia and influenza over 50 years in Japan (upper panel) and the US (lower panel). The 5-year moving average (centered) is included. The vaccine usage history for each country is superimposed.

Very soon after the wide scale introduction of influenza vaccine, Japanese excess death rates abruptly dropped about one-half in level. For the 10-year period of mandatory vaccination, 1977–1987, excess death rates declined still further, again, dropping nearly one-half. At these lowest levels, Japanese rates were comparable to those in the US. After 1990, Japanese excess deaths returned to values similar to those seen in Japan prior to 1962. In the US, year-to-year variation has diminished steadily since 1970. The association of the changes in excess death rates with vaccine usage, in both countries, is clear.

4. Discussion

In Japan, the mass immunization of schoolchildren began in 1962 and ended, practically in 1987, and officially in 1994. The official purpose of the Japanese Influenza Vaccination Program was to protect schoolchildren and reduce community transmission of infection, particularly to the elderly and those with chronic, high-risk conditions. Very few of the elderly and high-risk patients directly received influenza vaccine in that country [14]. Unfortunately, assessments of program effectiveness were also not focused on older or other high-risk individuals. Only discontinuation of the program has allowed its effects to become clear.

The most likely explanation for the large changes seen in excess mortality in Japan is protection of the elderly by herd immunity generated by the mass immunization of schoolchildren. Could these large changes in excess mortality be attributed to other factors? Certainly, in the same time period, Japan experienced exceptional economic development, with accompanying improvements in social infrastructure and technical advances. These factors may all have contributed to the observed decrease in excess death. However, it is the rapid increase of excess death after 1994, which most strongly supports the notion that the observed effect was due to herd immunity induced by the mass immunization program. If anything, social factors may have amplified the effects of the program. For example, the proportion of Japanese elderly living with their children is high compared with other developed countries. Thus, the high vaccination coverage levels achieved amongst schoolchildren could have directly prevented the transmission of influenza virus to their grandparents.

Figs. 2 and 3 show that, from 1955 to 1970, rates of excess mortality were two to three times higher in Japan than in the US, whereas during the 1970s and 1980s, rates in the two countries were comparable. Using the 1960 census population for Japan, we estimate that at least 37,000 all-cause excess deaths were averted, annually, during the period when the National Influenza Vaccination Program for Japanese Schoolchildren was in effect. Since the population of Japan is now about 25% larger, the number of excess deaths to which the observed difference in rates would now correspond is proportionately larger, about 48,000 all-cause deaths/year. Dowdle et al. [3] reported that, in 1977, about 20 million persons were vaccinated in Japan, including 17 million schoolchildren. Oya and Nerome [4] suggested that the number of schoolchildren vaccinated may have been somewhat lower (~14 million). Therefore, it appears, that for each 380–460 schoolchildren vaccinated, one death was prevented. In a study of direct vaccination amongst the enrollees of a US managed care group, age-restricted to 65–74, Nichol and Goodman [15] estimated that

270 vaccinations averted one death. Given the special characteristics of the population studied by these authors, we can say that only the effect of directly vaccinating the at-risk population appears to be of similar order as protection from herd immunity, as attained in Japan.

In 1997, Japan issued recommendations for influenza vaccination of elderly persons and those with chronic medical conditions. Rapid implementation of these recommendations to high levels of vaccine coverage should produce easily discernible reductions in all-cause and P&I excess mortality, permitting a straight-forward assessment of the benefit of administering vaccine directly to the population at greatest risk. Since many older persons have a reduced ability to develop protective immunity in response to vaccination, these two vaccination strategies could be overlapping, additive or synergistic. Rapid implementation of the 1997 guidelines, within Japan, could help elucidate the relationship between these two approaches.

Recent studies in the US have shown that giving preschool children live attenuated, cold-adapted influenza vaccine provides a high level of protection against influenza-induced illness [16,17]. Still other recent studies have demonstrated a regular association of influenza outbreaks with increases in hospitalizations for cardiopulmonary conditions, in children [18–20]. Our findings, together with the results of ongoing studies, should prompt a reconsideration of current recommendations for the use of influenza vaccines in both children and adults. This reconsideration will be especially important in planning for an influenza pandemic [21].

References

[1] F. Ambrosch, D.S. Fedson, Influenza vaccination in 29 countries: an update to 1997, PharmacoEconomics 16 (Suppl. 1) (1999) 47–54.

[2] Y. Hirota, D.S. Fedson, M. Kaji, Japan lagging in influenza jabs, Nature 380 (1996) 18.

[3] W.R. Dowdle, J.D. Millar, L.B. Schonberger, F.A. Ennis, J.R. LaMontagne, Influenza immunization policies and practices in Japan, J. Infect. Dis. 141 (1980) 258–264.

[4] A. Oya, K. Nerome, Experiences with mass vaccination of young age groups with inactivated vaccines, in: A.P. Kendal, P.A. Patriarca (Eds.), Options for the Control of Influenza, Alan R. Liss, New York, 1986, pp. 183–192.

[5] A.S. Monto, F.M. Davenport, J.A. Napier, et al., Modification of an outbreak of influenza in Tecumseh, Michigan by vaccination of schoolchildren, J. Infect. Dis. 122 (1970) 16–25.

[6] L.R. Elveback, J.P. Fox, E. Ackerman, A. Langworthy, et al., An influenza simulation model for immunization studies, Am. J. Epidemiol. 103 (1976) 152–165.

[7] I.M. Longini, E. Ackerman, L.R. Elveback, An optimization model for influenza A epidemics, Math. Biosci. 38 (1978) 141–157.

[8] I.M. Longini Jr., J.S. Koopman, M. Haber, G.A. Cotsonis, Statistical inference for infectious diseases, Risk-specific household and community transmission parameters, Am. J. Epidemiol. 128 (1988) 845–859.

[9] Vital Statistics of Japan, Statistics and Information Department, Minister's Secretariat, Ministry of Health and Welfare, Tokyo, 1949–1998.

[10] National Center for Health Statistics, Vital Statistics of the United States, 1949–1992, vol. II, Public Health Service, Washington, 1951–1994, mortality, part A.

[11] Advance report of final mortality statistics, 1993–1998, Monthly Vital Statistics Report, National Center for Health Statistics, Hyattsville, MD, 1994–1998.

[12] L. Simonsen, M.J. Clarke, L.B. Schonberger, et al., Pandemic versus epidemic influenza mortality: a pattern of changing age distribution, J. Infect. Dis. 178 (1998) 53–60.

[13] Centers for Disease Control and Prevention, Biologics Surveillance, Reports No. 1–94, Published series of intermittent reports from the US National Immunization Program, CDC, covering the period 1963 to the present.

[14] N. Sugaya, Influenza vaccination for children and adults in Japan (Japanese), Jpn. J. School Health 35 (1993) 537–542.

[15] K.L. Nichol, M. Goodman, The health and economic benefits of influenza vaccination for healthy and at-risk persons aged 65 to 74 years, PharmacoEconomics 16 (Suppl. 1) (1999) 63–71.

[16] R.B. Belshe, W.C. Gruber, J. Treanor, et al., The efficacy of live attenuated, cold-adapted, trivalent, intra-nasal influenza virus vaccine in children, N. Engl. J. Med. 20 (1998) 1405–1412.

[17] R.B. Belshe, W.C. Gruber, P.M. Mendelman, et al., Efficacy of vaccination with live attenuated, cold-adapted, trivalent influenza virus vaccine against a variant (A/Sydney) not contained in the vaccine, J. Pediatr. 136 (2000) 168–175.

[18] K.M. Neuzil, B.G. Mellen, P.F. Wright, E.F. Mitchel Jr., M.R. Griffin, The effect of influenza on hospitalizations, outpatient visits and courses of antibiotics in children, N. Engl. J. Med. 342 (2000) 225–231.

[19] H.S. Izuretta, W.W. Thompson, P. Kramarz, et al., Influenza and the rates of hospitalization for respiratory disease among infants and young children, N. Engl. J. Med. 342 (2000) 232–239.

[20] N. Sugaya, K. Mitamura, M. Nirasawa, K. Takahashi, The impact of winter epidemics of influenza and respiratory syncytial virus on paediatric admissions to an urban general hospital, J. Med. Virol. 60 (2000) 102–106.

[21] World Health Organization, Influenza pandemic preparedness plan, The role of WHO and guidelines for national and regional planning, World Health Organization, Geneva, Switzerland, April 1999.

International Congress Series 1219 (2001) 655–660

Modeling the effects of updating the influenza vaccine on the efficacy of repeated vaccination

Derek J. Smith[a,b,*], Alan S. Lapedes[b,c], Stephanie Forrest[b,d],
Jan C. de Jong[a], Albert D.M.E. Osterhaus[a], Ron A.M. Fouchier[a],
Nancy J. Cox[e], Alan S. Perelson[b,c]

[a]*Department of Virology and WHO National Influenza Centre, Erasmus University,
Dr. Molewaterplein 50, 3015 GE Rotterdam, Netherlands*
[b]*Santa Fe Institute, Santa Fe, NM, USA*
[c]*Los Alamos National, Laboratory, Los Alamos, NM, USA*
[d]*Department of Computer Science, University of New Mexico, Albuquerque, NM, USA*
[e]*Influenza Branch, Centers for Disease Control and Prevention, Atlanta, GA, USA*

Abstract

Background: The accumulated wisdom is to update the vaccine strain to the expected epidemic strain only when there is at least a 4-fold difference [measured by the hemagglutination inhibition (HI) assay] between the current vaccine strain and the expected epidemic strain. In this study we investigate the effect, on repeat vaccinees, of updating the vaccine when there is a less than 4-fold difference. *Methods*: Using a computer model of the immune response to repeated vaccination, we simulated updating the vaccine on a 2-fold difference and compared this to not updating the vaccine, in each case predicting the vaccine efficacy in first-time and repeat vaccinees for a variety of possible epidemic strains. *Results*: Updating the vaccine strain on a 2-fold difference resulted in increased vaccine efficacy in repeat vaccinees compared to leaving the vaccine unchanged. *Conclusions*: These results suggest that updating the vaccine strain on a 2-fold difference between the existing vaccine strain and the expected epidemic strain will increase vaccine efficacy in repeat vaccinees compared to leaving the vaccine unchanged. © 2001 Elsevier Science B.V. All rights reserved.

Keywords: Original antigenic sin; Vaccine efficacy; Antigenic distance

* Corresponding author. Tel.: +31-10-408-8066; fax: +31-10-408-9485.
E-mail address: dsmith@santafe.edu (D.J. Smith).

0531-5131/01/$ – see front matter © 2001 Elsevier Science B.V. All rights reserved.
PII: S 0 5 3 1 - 5 1 3 1 (0 1) 0 0 4 0 1 - 0

1. Introduction

Generally, the influenza vaccine strain is updated when there is at least a 4-fold difference in HI titer between the existing vaccine strain and the expected epidemic strain. Public health recommendations are for individuals in high-risk groups to be revaccinated annually [1]; thus, vaccine efficacy in repeat vaccinees is particularly important. However, the efficacy of repeated vaccination has been difficult to determine definitively: meta-analysis has shown a statistically significant heterogeneity in the efficacy of repeated vaccination in serology-based field trials [2], and different studies have draw different conclusions as to the effectiveness of repeated vaccination [3,4]. To explain this heterogeneity, we introduced the "antigenic distance" hypothesis [5], which states that prior exposure to influenza virus or vaccine can influence the subsequent response depending upon the degree of cross-reactivity among the antigens used in the vaccines

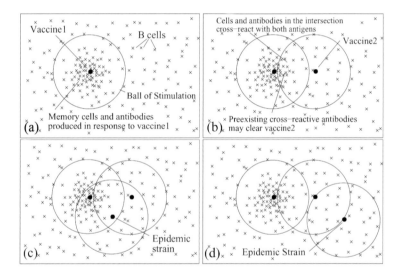

Fig. 1. An illustration of the antigenic distance hypothesis. These *Shape space* diagrams are a way to illustrate both the affinities of multiple B cells/antibodies to multiple antigens, and also the antigenic distances among multiple antigens [10]. In these diagrams, the affinity between a B cell or antibody (×) and an antigen (•) is represented by the distance between them. Similarly, the distance between antigens is a measure of how similar they are antigenically. (a) B cells with sufficient affinity to be stimulated by an antigen lie within a *ball of stimulation* centered on the antigen. Thus, a first vaccine (vaccine1) creates a population of memory B cells and antibodies within its ball of stimulation. (b) Cross-reactive antigens have intersecting balls of stimulation, and antibodies and B cells in the intersection of their balls—those with affinity for both antigens—are the cross-reactive antibodies and B cells. The antigen in a second vaccine (vaccine2) will be partially eliminated by pre-existing cross-reactive antibodies (depending on the amount of antibody in the intersection), and thus the immune response to vaccine2 will be reduced [6,7]. (c) If a subsequent epidemic strain is close to vaccine1, it will be cleared by pre-existing antibodies. (d) However, if there is no intersection between vaccine1 and the epidemic strain, there will be few pre-existing cross-reactive antibodies to clear the epidemic strain quickly, despite two vaccinations. Note, in the absence of vaccine1, vaccine2 would have produced a memory population and antibodies that would have been protective against both the epidemic strains in panels c and d. For an antigen with multiple epitopes (such as influenza), there would be a ball of stimulation for each epitope. Figure taken from Ref. [5], copyright (1999) National Academy of Sciences, USA, used with permission.

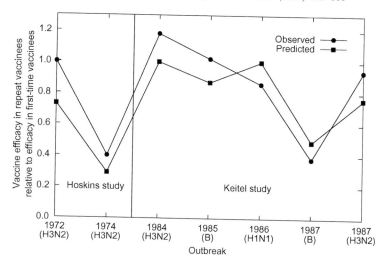

Fig. 2. The observed and predicted vaccine efficacy in repeat vaccinees relative to the efficacy in first-time vaccinees. The prediction of relative efficacy had good correlation with the observed data ($r = 0.87$, $p = 0.01$); however, the model did not accurately predict absolute vaccine efficacies, suggesting additional variation in each vaccine not accounted for in the model (discussed further in Ref. [5]). Figure taken from Ref. [5], copyright (1999) National Academy of Sciences, USA, used with permission.

and the epidemic influenza strains in each study year (Fig. 1). Using a computer model, we showed that this hypothesis offered a parsimonious explanation for the observed variation in repeated vaccination within and between the Hoskins et al. [3] and Keitel et al. [4] repeated vaccination studies (Fig. 2). Here we use the antigenic distance hypothesis, and the same computer model, to reason quantitatively about the effects, on repeat vaccinees, of updating the vaccine strain on a less than 4-fold difference.

2. Methods

The computer model consists of B cells, plasma cells, memory B cells, antibodies, and antigens. The model captures the essence of the primary and secondary humoral immune response, and the cross-reactive immune response. More details of the model can be found in Ref. [5], full details can be found in the supplemental material of Ref. [5] at http://www.pnas.org/, and the software for the simulator is available from http://www.santafe.edu/~dsmith/software/PNAS-model.html.

The computer experiment simulated two influenza seasons. A control group of 200 simulated individuals received no vaccinations and was challenged with replicating virus 2 months into the second influenza season. Four first-time vaccination groups, each of 200 simulated individuals, were vaccinated at the start of the second influenza season, and were challenged 2 months into the second influenza season with either homologous virus, or virus 2-, 4- or 8-fold different from the vaccine strain. Sixteen repeated vaccination groups, each of 200 simulated individuals, all received the same "vaccine1" (v1) strain at

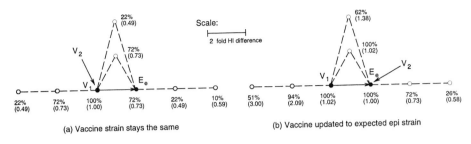

Fig. 3. Predictions from the model for vaccine efficacy in repeat vaccinees (given V_1 and V_2), and in parenthesis, relative efficacy compared to that in first-time vaccinees (given V_2 only), for two vaccine2 strain choices given a variety of actual epidemic strains (hollow circles) up to 4-fold from both vaccine strains. There was a 2-fold difference between the existing vaccine (V_1) and the expected epidemic strain (E_e) in both panels a and b.

the start of the first influenza season. At the start of the second influenza season, 8 of the 16 groups were vaccinated with the same strain as used for the first vaccination, and the other eight groups received a "vaccine2" (v2) strain that was 2-fold different[1] from the vaccine1 strain. All 16 repeat vaccination groups were challenged 2 months into the second influenza season with replicating virus up to 4-fold different from each of the vaccine strains (Fig. 3). In all cases, the vaccine dose was 1000 "units" of nonreplicating virus, and the epidemic dose was 500 units of replicating virus.

If the viral load exceeded 1500 units it was deemed to have passed a "disease threshold" and the simulated individual was considered symptomatic. The attack rate within a group was defined as the proportion of the group in which the viral load exceeded the disease threshold. Vaccine efficacy was defined as $1 - (ar_{vac}/ar_{nonvac})$, where ar_{vac} is the attack rate in a vaccinated group and ar_{nonvac} is the attack rate in the nonvaccinated control. Two sample z-tests were used to compare proportions. Two-tailed testing was used for p values.

3. Results

The attack rate in the nonvaccinated control was 1.0.[2] Attack rates in first-time vaccinees were 0.0, 0.02, 0.55, and 0.83 for homologous, 2-fold, 4-fold, and 8-fold differences, respectively, between the vaccine strain and the actual epidemic strain. Efficacies in repeat vaccinees when the vaccine was updated, and when it was not updated, and for various actual epidemic strains, are shown in Fig. 3. Ratios of efficacy in repeat vaccinees to efficacy in first-time vaccinees ranged from 0.49 to 3.00 (Fig. 3).

Updating the vaccine on a 2-fold difference between the existing epidemic strain and the expected epidemic strain resulted in higher predicted vaccine efficacy in repeat vaccinees in all cases compared to when the vaccine was not updated ($p < 0.01$ in all

---

[1] 2- 4- and 8-fold differences corresponds to "antigenic distances" 1, 2, and 3, respectively in Ref. [5].

[2] Each simulated individual was challenged with a large dose of virus, resulting in higher attack rates than in influenza vaccine field trials.

cases other than in the case when the actual epidemic strain was the same as the vaccine1 strain). Efficacies when the vaccine was not updated were dependent only on the antigenic distance between the vaccine strain and the actual epidemic strain. When the vaccine was updated to the expected epidemic strain, efficacies in repeat vaccinees depended on the antigenic distances between the actual epidemic strain and both vaccine1 and vaccine2 strains. Repeat vaccine efficacy was higher when there was a triangular configuration between the three strains (for example, when the actual epidemic strain was 4-fold different from both the vaccine1 and vaccine2 strains, and vaccine1 and vaccine2 strains were 2-fold different from each other). Vaccine efficacy in repeat vaccinees exceeded that in first-time vaccinees in some groups ($p < 0.01$) when the vaccine was updated to the expected epidemic strain, and not at all when the vaccine was not updated.

Somewhat surprisingly, for actual epidemic strains closer to vaccine1 than to the expected epidemic strain (strains to the left of vaccine1 in Fig. 3), the predicted efficacy in repeat vaccinees was higher ($p < 0.01$) when the vaccine was updated than when it remained unchanged—even though leaving the vaccine unchanged would result in a vaccine strain closer to those actual epidemic strains.

4. Discussion

Updating the vaccine when there is a 2-fold difference between the existing vaccine strain and the expected epidemic strain gave a higher vaccine efficacy in repeat vaccinees than leaving the vaccine unchanged (Fig. 3). It is similarly advantageous to update the vaccine on a 4-fold or more difference (data not shown). These results support the current strategy to update the vaccine strain on a 4-fold or more difference between the existing vaccine strain and the expected epidemic strain. Moreover, these results suggest that also updating the vaccine on a 2-fold difference will increase vaccine efficacy in repeat vaccinees compared to leaving the vaccine unchanged.

Influenza epidemics occur in most years, and public health recommendations are for at-risk individuals to be revaccinated annually. Thus, optimizing the vaccine efficacy for a single year by updating the vaccine strain to an expected epidemic strain 2-fold from the existing vaccine is not necessarily the best strategy over multiple years. For example, an advantage of only updating the vaccine when there is at least a 4-fold difference is that there will be less "negative interference" (antigenic sin effect [6,7]) from prior vaccinations. Thus, keeping the vaccine unchanged trades off reduced efficacy in repeat vaccinees in the year when the vaccine did not change, for increased efficacy in the subsequent year. To fully assess the tradeoffs for repeat vaccinees in updating the vaccine or not requires examining the effects over multiple years (manuscript in preparation).

A difficulty of updating the vaccine strain on a 2-fold difference in HI titer is that the resolution and reliability of the HI assay are such that only at least a 4-fold difference between strains has typically been considered significant. Beyer and Masurel [8], and Lapedes and Farber [9] have used mathematical techniques to address some of the inherent difficulties in obtaining accurate measurements of antigenic distance from HI data. These techniques are investigated further in a manuscript in preparation.

Acknowledgements

We thank David Ackley, Walter Beyer, Henrietta Hall, Jacqueline Katz, Alexander Klimov, and Guus Rimmelzwaan. This work was supported by the National Science Foundation (grants IRI-9711199, CDA-9503064, and ANIR-9986555), the Office of Naval Research (grant N00014-99-1-0417), Defense Advanced Projects Agency (grant AGR F30602-00-2-0584), the Intel Corporation, the Joseph P. and Jeanne M. Sullivan Foundation, and the Los Alamos National Laboratory LDRD program. The research of ASL was supported by the Department of Energy under contract W-7405-ENG-36. Portions of this work were performed under the auspices of the US Department of Energy. The hospitality of the Santa Fe Institute, where part of this work was performed, is gratefully acknowledged. Computational resources were donated by Popular Power.

References

[1] CDC, Prevention and control of influenza: recommendations of the advisory committee on immunization practices (ACIP), Morb. Mortal. Wkly. Rep. 45 (RR5) (1996) 1–24

[2] W.E.P. Beyer, I.A. DeBruijn, A.M. Palache, R.G.J. Westendorp, A.D.M.E. Osterhaus, Protection against influenza after annually repeated vaccination: a meta-analysis of serologic and field studies, Arch. Intern. Med. 159 (1999) 182–188.

[3] T.W. Hoskins, J.R. Davis, A.J. Smith, C.L. Miller, A. Allchin, Assessment of inactivated influenza-A vaccine after three outbreaks of influenza A at Christ's Hospital, Lancet i (1979) 33–35.

[4] W.A. Keitel, T.R. Cate, R.B. Couch, L.L. Huggins, K.R. Hess, Efficacy of repeated annual immunization with inactivated influenza virus vaccines over a five-year period, Vaccine 15 (1997) 1114–1122.

[5] D.J. Smith, S. Forrest, D.H. Ackley, A.S. Perelson, Variable efficacy of repeated annual influenza vaccination, Proc. Natl. Acad. Sci. 96 (1999) 14001–14006.

[6] S.F. de St. Groth, R.G. Webster, Disquisitions of original antigenic sin: II. Proof in lower creatures, J. Exp. Med. 124 (1966) 347–361.

[7] R.G. Webster, J.A. Kasel, R.B. Couch, W.G. Laver, Influenza virus subunit vaccines. II. Immunogenicity and original antigenic sin in humans, J. Infect. Dis. 134 (1976) 48–58.

[8] W.E.P. Beyer, N. Masurel, Antigenic heterogeneity among influenza A(H3N2) field isolates during an outbreak in 1982/83, estimated by methods of numerical taxonomy, J. Hyg. Camb. 94 (1985) 97–109.

[9] A.S. Lapedes, R. Farber, The geometry of shape space: Application to influenza, J. Theoret. Biol., in press.

[10] A.S. Perelson, G.F. Oster, Theoretical studies of clonal selection: Minimal antibody repertoire size and reliability of self- non-self discrimination, J. Theor. Biol. 81 (1979) 645–670.

International Congress Series 1219 (2001) 661–664

Recommendations for the use of inactivated influenza vaccines and other preventive measures

D. Lavanchy[a,*], A. Monto[b], J. Wood[c]

[a]Division of Emerging and Other Communicable Disease Surveillance and Control,
Communicable Disease Surveillance and Response (CSR),
World Health Organization (WHO), 20, Avenue Appia, CH-1211, Geneva 27, Switzerland
[b]School of Public Health, University of Michigan, 109 Observatory Road, Ann Arbor, MI 48109, USA
[c]NIBSC, Blanche Lane, South Mimms, Potters Bar, Hertfordshire, EN6 3QG, UK

WHO formulated recommendations for national health authorities on measures for the prevention of influenza by vaccination and other means. These were published in the Weekly Epidemiological Record (WER), 2000, 75, 281–288 and Vaccine 2001. The recommendations are not intended to replace current national prevention measures or to preclude individual countries, health providers or individuals from undertaking additional measures consistent with local priorities and resources. There is increasing awareness among WHO member states of the disease burden of influenza and its social and economic impact, which has been enhanced by longer life expectancy in many countries. It was noted that experience in the use and benefits of influenza vaccination has increased and that a number of anti-influenza drugs has been developed and evaluated.

About 50 countries have government funded national influenza immunization programmes and the vaccine is available in many others. Specific recommendations for the use of the vaccine vary, but generally involve annual immunization for individuals of advanced age and those over 6 months at increased risk of severe illness because of a pre-existing chronic medical condition. In some countries, vaccine is used to reduce spread of influenza to those at increased medical risk. Member states need to consider the benefit of influenza prevention activities in the context of their overall public health priorities.

These recommendations addressed mainly the use of inactivated vaccines and the following topics were reviewed:

Vaccine types
Composition of the vaccines (annual recommendations by WHO)

* Corresponding author. Tel.: +41-22-791-2656; fax: +41-22-791-4878.

Standardization of vaccine
Efficacy
Safety
Economic aspects
Timing and administration of vaccination
Logistics of vaccine supply
Resources

The following recommendations for use of inactivated vaccine were made:
Many national programmes for control of priority diseases, are based upon reliable data on the seasonal occurrence of influenza, and its impact and knowledge about the effectiveness of influenza control measures.

In such countries each of the following groups are usually targeted for vaccination:

Individuals who are
• residents of institutions for the elderly or the disabled;
• elderly non-institutionalized individuals with one or more of the following chronic conditions: chronic cardiovascular, pulmonary, metabolic or renal disease, or who are immunocompromized;
• other individuals (adults and children >6 months) in the community who have chronic cardiovascular, pulmonary, metabolic or renal disease, or are immuno-compromized;
• are above a nationally defined age limit irrespective of their medical risk status (most countries define the limit of age >65 years);
• other groups defined on the basis of national data.

Those with regular, frequent contact with high-risk persons such as
• health care workers in contact with high risk persons;
• household contacts of high risk persons.

It was recognized that not all countries have extensive knowledge about influenza, or the resources to implement the same level of Public Health prevention. In such cases, it is recommended the first priority be given to residents of institutions for the elderly and disabled. As resources become available, countries should sequentially add additional groups as listed above, modified as appropriate by national priorities.

From time to time countries may decide that it is important to immunize vulnerable groups such as, refugees or disaster victims housed in long-term camps or shelters, large groups of pilgrims gathering in one area for several weeks, orphans living in long-term residential institutions, and their attendants. These decisions should be made at the local level. Many of these countries also recommend that individuals, who wish to avoid influenza by being immunized at their own expense, should have access to the vaccine.

In some countries, due to limited data on the occurrence of influenza and chronic diseases in the population, as well as limited health care facilities, resources, and existence of other unmet health needs, vaccination against influenza in medical high-risk groups may not at present be a current priority.

Implementation of vaccine programmes will involve different combinations of efforts by public and private components of the health care system in different countries. In some cases, vaccine will be purchased and distributed mainly by national authorities, whereas under other circumstances, vaccines are largely provided through the private sector. In determining priorities for the use of vaccine, National Health authorities should take into account information from countries in their region with similar climate, populations, and health infrastructure.

Other preventive measures were also considered, but not generally recommended.

Live attenuated vaccines
Antiviral agents

The main conclusions for the use of inactivated influenza vaccines and other preventive measures were:

• The primary objective of influenza prevention is to reduce the incidence of severe disease and influenza related mortality in persons at high risk of developing severe consequences of influenza infection.

• Vaccination with inactivated vaccines is the single most effective measure available; many member states have successfully implemented regular annual immunization programmes with considerable tangible benefits to public health.

• Inactivated influenza vaccines, which comply with WHO guidelines on quality and are consistent with WHO annual recommendation on vaccine composition have a long history of safety and efficacy.

• Member states should consider the implementation or expansion of influenza prevention programmes in the context of other public health priorities. Careful long-term planning for availability of resources, supplies of vaccine and a clear vaccination strategy based on sound epidemiological information were regarded as essential for countries contemplating introduction or extension of vaccination.

• The consultation identified population groups who were a high priority for vaccination; these included residents of institutions for the elderly and disabled, those with chronic medical conditions and the elderly. However, it was agreed that high-risk groups might vary from country to country, and even within a country.

• Accurate epidemiological surveillance and characterization of prevalent viruses will enhance the preventive effects of influenza vaccination. Wherever possible member states should collaborate with WHO to intensify its surveillance programmes. Local information is regarded as an important prerequisite to the design of influenza vaccine programmes.

• There are promising developments in the field of live influenza vaccines and additional antiviral drugs are becoming more available for prevention of influenza. Antiviral drugs should not be used as an alternative to vaccination, which remains the preventive measure of first choice.

It was emphasized that these recommendations are not intended to cover pandemics, which occur occasionally following the emergence of a virus subtype against which large sections of the population around the world lack immunity. Separate national recommendations for response to pandemics of influenza are needed. The current recommendations for annual prevention will provide a foundation for such national pandemic planning efforts and in addition improve coordination of responses to a pandemic.

Acknowledgements

These recommendations were developed by a WHO group of international experts at a consultation held in Tokyo, Japan, in June 2000 in collaboration with the WHO Collaborating Centres for Influenza Reference and Research, located at the Centers for Disease Control and Prevention, Atlanta, USA; the National Institute for Medical Research, London, UK; the WHO Collaborating Centre, Melbourne, Australia; the National Institute of Infectious Diseases, Tokyo, Japan; the Therapeutic Goods Administration Laboratories, Canberra, Australia; the National Institute for Biological Standards and Control, Potters Bar, UK; and the Center for Biologics Evaluation and Research, Food and Drug Administration, Rockville, USA; The School of Public Health, University of Michigan, Ann Arbor; Department of Microbiology and Immunology, University of Melbourne; The National Immunization Program, CDC. WHO was assisted in organizing the consultation by the Biomedical Sciences Association, Tokyo, Japan, the European Scientific Working Group on Influenza (ESWI) and by the Rollins School of Public Health, Emory University, Atlanta, USA.

International Congress Series 1219 (2001) 665–669

Influenza vaccination recommended for all adults aged 50 years and older, United States

Raymond A. Strikas [a,*], Carolyn B. Bridges[b], James A. Singleton[a]

[a]National Immunization Program, MS E-52, Centers for Disease Control and Prevention, Atlanta, GA 30333, USA
[b]Influenza Branch, Division of Viral and Rickettsial Diseases, National Center for Infectious Diseases, Centers for Disease Control and Prevention, Atlanta, GA, USA

Abstract

The U.S. Public Health Services' Advisory Committee on Immunization Practices added the 41 million U.S. adults aged 50–64 years to its recommended primary target group for universal annual influenza vaccination, beginning with the 2000–2001 influenza season. Several reasons prompted lowering the recommended age from ≥ 65 years. (1) Between 10 and 13 million (24–32%) of persons aged 50–64 years are at high risk for influenza-related hospitalizations (80–400 hospitalizations per 100,000 persons aged 45–64 years) and death because of chronic medical conditions. (2) Strategies to increase vaccination based on age-specific recommendations have been more successful than those based on medical conditions (e.g., in 1997, 63% of all persons aged ≥ 65 years reported influenza vaccination compared to 40% of persons aged 50–64 years reporting one or more high-risk medical conditions). (3) Increased vaccination would reduce disease transmission from the substantial number in this age group who are contacts of persons at risk for influenza-related complications, such as the elderly and other high-risk adults. (4) Past data show that vaccination of healthy adults < 65 years who are at low risk for serious illness reduced the number of illnesses, physician visits, workdays missed, and antibiotic use. (5) Fifty years is an age when other preventive services begin and when routine assessment of vaccination and other preventive services has been recommended. © 2001 Elsevier Science B.V. All rights reserved.

Keywords: Influenza vaccine; Adults 50 years and older; United States

* Corresponding author. Tel.: +1-404-639-8813; fax: +1-404-639-8828.
E-mail address: rstrikas@cdc.gov (R.A. Strikas).

0531-5131/01/$ – see front matter © 2001 Elsevier Science B.V. All rights reserved.
PII: S0531-5131(01)00670-7

1. Introduction

Influenza vaccine has been recommended for certain persons at increased risk of complications of influenza by the United States (U.S.) Public Health Service's Advisory Committee on Immunization Practices (ACIP) since 1964 [1]. The 1964 recommendations recommended influenza vaccination for older persons, and identified those > 45 years as at moderately increased risk of influenza complications, and those > 65 years as at higher risk of complications [1]. Beginning in 1974, the ACIP specifically identified persons >65 years of age as at increased risk, and recommended annual vaccination for persons in this age group [2]. In 1999, the ACIP voted to lower the age to 50 years and older for recommended annual influenza vaccination for the 2000–2001 influenza vaccination season [3]. As of 1999, no other countries recommend influenza vaccination for persons beginning at age 50 years; Belgium, Germany, and Iceland recommend vaccination beginning at age 60 years ([4], D.S. Fedson, personal communication).

This report will describe the rationale and data supporting the new ACIP recommendation for routine vaccination of persons aged 50–64 years as follows. (1) There is a large proportion of persons at high risk for influenza complications among those 50–64 years of age in the United States [3]. (2) Strategies to increase vaccination based on age-specific recommendations have been more successful than those based on medical conditions [5]. (3) Increased vaccination of persons in this age group would reduce disease transmission from the substantial number in the 50–64-year age group who are contacts of persons who are at risk for influenza-related complications, such as the elderly and other high-risk adults [3]. (4) Previous data show vaccination of healthy adults at low risk for serious illness reduces the number of illnesses, physician visits, workdays missed, and antibiotic use [6–10]. (5) There are existing recommendations for other preventive services to begin at age 50 years [11,12]. In addition to the technical recommendations, recently recommended strategies to improve vaccination coverage will be discussed [13], as well as the impact influenza vaccine supply in the United States may have on these new recommendations [4].

2. Rationale and data

There are an estimated 41 million persons aged 50–64 years in the United States, and 10–13 million of them have chronic underlying medical conditions [3]. The burden of influenza-related morbidity and mortality among persons 45–64 years is significant. Hospitalization rates for persons in this age group have varied between 80/100,000 and 400/100,000 for those with high-risk conditions, and from approximately 20/100,000 to 40/100,000 in those without such conditions [15,16]. In contrast, among persons ≥ 65 years, the hospitalization rate ranges from 200/100,000 to >1000/100,000 [15–17]. Nearly 90% of influenza-associated excess deaths occur among those ≥ 65 years of age [3]. About 9% of influenza-associated deaths occur among persons 50–64 years of age (United States Centers for Disease Control and Prevention [CDC], unpublished data).

Influenza vaccine use has markedly increased in the United States since 1989, particularly among persons > 65 years, for whom annual influenza vaccination has been specifically recommended by the ACIP since 1974. The total number of net doses distributed has increased from approximately 24 million doses in 1989 to 74 million doses in 1999 (CDC, unpublished data). Data from CDC's National Health Interview Survey indicate that self-reported use of vaccine increased between 1989 and 1997 from 33% to 63% in those ≥ 65 years, while it only increased from 10% to 28% in all persons 50–64 years of age, and from 16–24% to 41% in high-risk persons in this age group (Table 1) ([18], CDC, unpublished data, 2000), suggesting that the age based recommendation for persons ≥ 65 years was more successfully implemented than the risk condition-based recommendation for younger persons. Among persons 18–49 years overall and among those with high-risk conditions, the vaccination rate in 1997 was even lower (Table 1: 13% and 21%, respectively; CDC, unpublished data, 2000). Lowering the age for routine influenza vaccination to 50 years may increase vaccination levels in persons 50–64 years of age more than would occur in the absence of such a recommendation, although at the cost of recommending vaccination to low-risk healthy adults for whom influenza vaccination is less of a priority.

The ACIP recommends that persons who have household or occupational contact with persons at high risk of influenza complications also receive annual influenza vaccination. Estimates of the number of persons age 50–64 years who do not have other vaccine indications in the United States, but who have such household contact range from 6.8 to 8.6 million. While the vaccination level in this group in the United States is unknown, it is likely no higher than that for health care workers in this age group, or 48% [19]. The recommendation to vaccinate all persons beginning at age 50 years is expected to increase the vaccination rate among person with household or occupational high-risk contacts

Several studies have documented reductions in illness, work absenteeism and health care resource utilization following influenza vaccination of healthy working adults [6–10]. It is anticipated that broader use of influenza vaccine in persons 50–64 years of age may further increase health and economic benefits to persons 50–64 years of age.

The United States Preventive Services Task Force has recommended that several preventive services begin at or about age 50 years [11]. These include breast cancer screening with mammography, colorectal cancer screening and counseling postmeno-

Table 1
Percentage of selected adult populations reporting influenza vaccination in the previous year, National Health Interview Survey, United States, 1989, 1997

Age/risk group	1989	1997
18–49 years, healthy[a]	3.5	13
18–49 years, high risk[b]	4–12	21
50–64 years, healthy[a]	10	28
50–64 years, high risk[b]	16–24	41
≥ 65 years, all	33	63

[a] For 1989, includes all persons in the age group. For 1997, includes persons reporting no high-risk medical conditions putting them at increased risk of complications from influenza.

[b] Includes persons reporting one or more high-risk conditions as identified by the U.S. Advisory Committee on Immunization Practices [3]. The 1989 survey did not allow identification of person with multiple risk conditions; the range represents independent estimates for persons with heart disease, lung disease and diabetes.

pausal women about hormone replacement therapy. In 1995, the ACIP recommended that age 50 also be a time for health-care providers to (1) review adult vaccination status, (2) administer tetanus and diphtheria toxoids as indicated, and (3) determine whether a patient has one or more risk factors that indicate a need to receive one dose of pneumococcal vaccine and begin annual influenza vaccination [12]. Therefore, moving to a routine influenza vaccination recommendation beginning at age 50 years is a logical progression from the earlier recommendation.

3. Strategies for improving vaccination coverage

Recently, an evidence-based review of the literature suggested that certain strategies will raise vaccination levels among children, adolescents and adults. The United States Task Force on Community Preventive Services, an independent advisory committee to the U.S. Department of Health and Human Services [13], has been recommending these strategies. These include health care provider and patient reminder and recall systems, standing orders for vaccination, assessment and feedback of vaccination levels, expanding access to vaccination, use of home medical visits for vaccination, multicomponent interventions that include education and reducing out-of-pocket costs [13]. Implementing these recommended strategies in concert with publicizing age 50 years as the new beginning age for routine influenza vaccination should enhance influenza vaccination levels in these adults.

4. Vaccine supply

During the 2000/2001 influenza season, there will be a substantial delay and possible shortage of influenza vaccine supply in the U.S. due to the lower than expected yields of the A/Panama (H3N2) vaccine virus strain earlier in the production period and other manu-facturing problems [14]. The availability of a significant number of doses will be delayed about a month. Preparedness strategies will attempt to ensure that vaccine is administered to those at highest risk for serious influenza-related complications. In the context of a possible vaccine shortage, it will be appropriate for contingency plans covering the 50–64-year age group to focus primarily on vaccinating persons with high-risk conditions rather than this entire age group. The CDC is working with state and local health departments and other organizations to develop and implement strategies that maximize provision of vaccine to those at high risk and encourage vaccination into late December 2000 and January 2001. CDC is also conducting studies to evaluate the impact of a delay and shortage on vaccine utilization and disease, including persons in the 50–64-year age group.

5. Summary

The United States Public Health Service has adopted a unique recommendation for routine annual influenza vaccination beginning at age 50 years, lowering the age for routine vaccination from 65 years. The recommendation was adopted because among persons 50–64 years of age, (1) there is a significant burden of influenza-related disease; (2) there are low vaccination levels and high rates of medical conditions and household and occupational contacts for whom influenza vaccination was already recommended; (3) low vaccination levels will likely improve with an age-based recommendation; (4) economic benefits may be realized; and (5) other preventive services are recommended beginning at age 50 years.

References

[1] CDC, Influenza Surveillance Report No. 80, U.S. Department of Health Education, and Welfare, Public Health Service, Atlanta, GA, 1964, pp. 8–11.

[2] CDC, Recommendations of the public health service advisory committee on immunization practices: Influenza, MMWR 23 (1974) 215.

[3] CDC, Prevention and control of influenza: Recommendations of the advisory committee on immunization practices, MMWR 49 (No. RR-3) (2000) 1–38.

[4] F. Ambrosch, D.S. Fedson, Influenza vaccination in 29 countries, An update to 1997, Pharmacoeconomics 16 (Suppl. 1) (1999) 47–54.

[5] D.S. Fedson, Adult immunization: summary of the national vaccine advisory committee report, JAMA, J. Am. Med. Assoc. 272 (1994) 1133–1137.

[6] K.L. Nichol, A. Lind, K.L. Margolis, et al., The effectiveness of vaccination against influenza in healthy, working adults, N. Engl. J. Med. 333 (1995) 889–893.

[7] J.A. Wilde, J.A. McMillan, J. Serwint, J. Butta, M.A. O'Riordan, M.C. Steinhoff, Effectiveness of influenza vaccine in health care professionals: a randomized trial, JAMA, J. Am. Med. Assoc. 281 (1999) 908–913.

[8] D.S. Campbell, M.H. Rumley, Cost-effectiveness of the influenza vaccine in a healthy, working-age population, J. Occup. Environ. Med. 39 (1997) 408–414.

[9] J.W.G. Smith, R. Pollard, Vaccination against influenza: a five-year study in the post office, J. Hyg. 83 (1979) 157–170.

[10] C.B. Bridges, W.W. Thompson, M.I. Meltzer, et al., Effectiveness and cost-benefit of influenza vaccination of healthy working adults: a randomized placebo controlled study, JAMA, J. Am. Med. Assoc. 284 (2000) 1655–1663.

[11] U.S. Preventive Services Task Force, Guide to Clinical Preventive Services, 2nd edn., Williams & Wilkins, Baltimore, 1996.

[12] CDC, Notice to readers: assessing adult vaccination status at age 50 years, MMWR 44 (1995) 561–563.

[13] Task Force on Community Preventive Services, Recommendations regarding interventions to improve vaccination coverage in children, adolescents, and adults, Am. J. Prev. Med. 18 (1) (2000) 92–96 (Supplement 1).

[14] CDC, Notice to readers: Delayed supply of influenza vaccine and adjunct ACIP influenza vaccine recommendations for the 2000–01 influenza season, MMWR 49 (2000) 619–622.

[15] Wh. Barker, J.P. Mullooly, Impact of epidemic type A influenza in a defined adult population, Am. J. Epidemiol. 112 (1980) 798–811.

[16] W.P. Glezen, M. Decker, D.M. Perrotta, Survey of underlying conditions of persons hospitalized with acute respiratory disease during influenza epidemics in Houston, 1978–1981, Am. Rev. Respir. Dis. 136 (1987) 550–555.

[17] W.P. Glezen, Influenza surveillance in an urban area, Can. J. Infect. Dis. 4 (1993) 272–274.

[18] CDC, Influenza and pneumococcal vaccination coverage levels among persons ≥ 65 years-United States, 1973–1993, MMWR 44 (1995) 506–507, 513–515.

[19] F.J. Walker, J.A. Singleton, P.J. Lu, R.A. Strikas, Influenza vaccination of healthcare workers in the United States, 1989–97, Infect. Control Hosp. Epidemiol. 21 (2000) 113.

International Congress Series 1219 (2001) 671–675

Impact of influenza vaccination policies on staff coverage in long-term care facilities

B. Henry[a,b,c], M. Naus[b,c,*], R. Stirling[a,b,c]

[a]*Field Epidemiology Training Program, Population and Public Health Branch, Health Canada*
[b]*Faculty of Medicine, University of Toronto, Toronto, Canada*
[c]*Disease Control Service, Public Health Branch, Ontario Ministry of Health and Long-Term Care,
Toronto, Canada*

Abstract

Background: Influenza vaccine has been provided to staff of long-term care facilities (LTCFs) in Ontario through the public health program since 1993. To promote high levels of coverage, in 1999 the Ministry issued an influenza prevention and control protocol for LTCFs emphasizing staff vaccination. The protocol requires reporting of coverage by the facility, which facilitated an examination of factors associated with high and low rates. *Methods*: Coverage reports were collected and compared with reports of LTCF outbreaks. LTCFs from high and low coverage groups were selected for a survey of factors that contributed to higher immunization levels. *Results*: The majority of LTCFs had staff coverage rates greater than 70% and 38% had rates greater than 90%. 100 of these facilities were randomly selected and compared with 97 facilities with rates lower than 70%. A 77% response was achieved in both groups. Educational sessions, individual counseling and on-site immunization clinics were associated with higher coverage rates. The development of facility specific policies, particularly those with a policy that excluded unimmunized workers from the facility without pay during an outbreak, were associated with higher staff coverage rates. *Conclusion*: Influenza vaccination policies are an effective measure to increase staff influenza vaccination rates in LTCFs. © 2001 Elsevier Science B.V. All rights reserved.

Keywords: Influenza vaccination; Health care workers; Elderly; Influenza control policies

* Corresponding author. Disease Control Service, Public Health Branch, 5700 Yonge Street, 8th Floor, Toronto, Ontario, Canada M2M 4K5. Tel.: +1-114163277412; fax: +1-114163277439.
E-mail address: monika.naus@moh.gov.on.ca (M. Naus).

0531-5131/01/$ – see front matter © 2001 Elsevier Science B.V. All rights reserved.
PII: S 0 5 3 1 - 5 1 3 1 (0 1) 0 0 6 7 1 - 9

1. Introduction

In Canada, health care is a provincial responsibility, funded partially by federal transfer payments. The province of Ontario, with a population of 11.5 million people, is home to approximately one third of Canadians. Vaccines for public health programs are purchased by the province and given mainly by the 13 thousand physicians in the province.

Prior to 1988, the influenza vaccine was available through the Ontario drug benefit program, targeting mainly seniors, with limited uptake and promotion. In 1988, a public health program was established to target persons >65 years of age, all residents of nursing homes and homes for the aged (henceforth called long-term care facilities (LTCFs), and those persons <65 years of age with high risk medical conditions. In 1993, the program was expanded to include patient care staff of LTCFs. In 1999, the program was further expanded to include all staff of LTCFs and rest and retirement homes, as well as all members of the regulated health professions (including physicians, nurses, occupational therapists, physiotherapists, pharmacists, and dentists) and emergency services workers (fire, police and ambulance). Most recently, for the 2000/2001 season the influenza vaccine program was expanded to include all Ontario residents.

To reduce morbidity and mortality caused by influenza in LTCFs, public health departments have developed a strong liaison with local facilities and provide instruction about outbreak recognition and control. Amantadine prophylaxis has increasingly been used in Ontario for outbreak control. There is interest in use of neuraminidase inhibitors for this purpose but these have been licensed for treatment only and rimantidine has not been licensed for any indications. In conjunction with the expanded immunization program in 1999, the Ministry introduced a policy for influenza prevention and control for all 508 LTCFs, which house about 55,000 residents. The policy was not issued under regulatory provisions. It emphasizes annual influenza vaccination for both residents and staff. In addition, vaccination coverage levels in residents and staff are to be reported to the local medical officer of health by December 1 of each year. Finally, the policy advises that unimmunized staff should be excluded from work in a facility during an outbreak unless they become immunized or take antiviral prophylaxis.

Several factors led to the issuance of this policy. The number of outbreaks in health care institutions, including LTCFs, increased eightfold in the 2 years of A/Sydney (1997/1998 and 1998/1999) compared to the previous 7 years. In December 1998, a large nursing home outbreak in a facility with fewer than half of the staff immunized, resulted in 25 deaths among 240 residents, and led to a coroner's inquest. The jury's key recommendation was that staff vaccination should be mandatory. A third factor was mounting evidence from studies showing reduced resident morbidity and mortality with higher levels of health care worker immunization [1–3] coupled with an increasing frailty index among Ontario residents in LTCFs.

To evaluate the policy components and their influence on coverage, we examined the relationship between coverage and reported outbreaks in the 1999/2000 season. We also conducted a survey of facilities about factors that contributed to increased staff coverage.

2. Methods

Facility coverage rates were collected for the 1999/2000 season through local health departments. Each facility was asked to report numbers of residents and staff immunized, and the number eligible for vaccine. Reports of outbreaks of laboratory confirmed influenza were received through the routine influenza surveillance program. Facilities in the two resultant databases were matched using the facility unique number. Attack rates, rates of hospitalization and rates of pneumonia in high staff coverage facilities were compared with those in low coverage facilities.

In the second part of this study, a self-administered questionnaire about factors influencing staff vaccination was administered to the person responsible for infection control in each of 197 nursing homes and homes for the aged. One hundred facilities with high coverage rates (>70%) were randomly selected and compared with all 97 facilities which reported coverage rates less than 70%. Information was collected about facility demographics, promotional strategies used, the level of institutional support, the existence and components of a facility-specific influenza prevention and control policy, and the facility's prior influenza outbreak experience. Data were analyzed using SPSS (Version 10, Chicago, IL).

3. Results

Overall staff immunization in LTCFs in Ontario in 1999/2000 was reported to be 86.3%. Of 508 facilities, 88.5% had staff coverage rates >70% and 38% of facilities had coverage rates >90%.

No association was found between staff immunization rates and the occurrence of an influenza outbreak in the 1999/2000 season. There were 338 confirmed institutional outbreaks from 318 institutions. The overall attack rate in LTCF outbreaks was 14.7%. The overall case fatality due to influenza was 5.3%, 4.8% of cases had radiologically confirmed pneumonia, and 7.2% of cases were hospitalized. All of these indicators showed decreases from the 1998/1999 season when the attack rate was 47% higher at 27.8% for all outbreaks, case fatality was 5.9%, and among cases, hospitalization occurred in 8.8% and pneumonia in 5.9%.

Seventy-seven percent of facilities responded to the questionnaire (Fig. 1). High and low coverage facilities were compared. There were no differences by type of facility (nursing home vs. home for the aged), size of facility and percent of staff belonging to a union. In the low coverage group, rates of staff immunization ranged from 10% to 69% with 50% of these facilities reporting rates from 30% to 60%.

Strategies associated with increased staff immunization levels included holding educational sessions for staff, providing individual counseling sessions for staff who had concerns about vaccination, and holding on-site immunization clinics on day, evening and night shifts. Facilities with high staff immunization coverage were significantly more likely to have a written facility policy for influenza prevention and control. In addition, this policy was more likely to contain a clause that excluded unimmunized staff from working in the facility during an outbreak if they refused to take anti-viral medication.

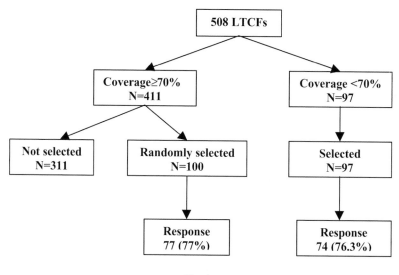

Fig. 1.

Policies that excluded workers without pay were also significantly associated with higher staff immunization coverage.

Preliminary analysis of the data did not show any association between staff immunization rates and prior influenza outbreak experience in the facility during the preceding three seasons. Almost one quarter of survey respondents expressed concern that community based physicians who provided primary care services to staff did not provide immunization to these staff when requested as they "did not fit into the high risk categories." Finally, active involvement of the local health department with the facility was associated with higher staff coverage rates. Analysis of this study is ongoing and we intend to publish a complete report in the future.

4. Discussion

With the introduction of the *Influenza Prevention and Surveillance Protocol for Ontario Long-Term Care Facilities*, staff coverage rates in LTCFs in the 1999/2000 season were much higher than in past years. This important increase was not associated with decreased numbers of influenza outbreaks in the 1999/2000 season, however, attack rates, rates of pneumonia and rates of hospitalization were lower than in the 1998/1999 season. These findings are consistent with those found in studies of LTCFs in the UK [1,2].

Influenza prevention and control policies at a provincial and facility level are effective measures to increase staff influenza immunization rates in LTCFs. Policies that include exclusion of workers without pay during an outbreak appear to have the greatest effect. A group union grievance challenging the exclusion of unimmunized staff was recently reviewed by an appeals board. The board determined that facility administration may reasonably expect staff to be immunized each fall, and exclude unimmunized staff during outbreaks in order to protect residents. The Ontario Nurses Association and public opinion, as reflected by the coroner's jury recommendations, are also supportive of these policy directions. With the expanded immunization program in 2000/1, efforts are being made at all levels to encourage any person who visits a LTCF or has contact with elderly or at risk persons to be immunized.

Acknowledgements

The authors would like to acknowledge the sage advice provided by the Ontario Influenza Study Working Group and the assistance of Kerri Watkins and Gina Pohani in the development of the database.

References

[1] J. Potter, D.J. Stott, M.A. Roberts, et al., Influenza vaccination of health care workers in long-term care hospitals reduces the mortality of elderly patients, JID 175 (1997) 1–6.
[2] W.F. Carman, A. Elder, L. Wallace, et al., Effects of influenza vaccination of health-care workers on mortality of elderly people in long-term care: a randomized controlled trial, Lancet 355 (2000) 93–97.
[3] J.A. Wilde, J.A. McMillan, J. Serwint, et al., Effectiveness of influenza vaccine in health care professionals, JAMA, J. Am. Med. Assoc. 281 (1999) 908–913.

International Congress Series 1219 (2001) 677–679

Informing consumers about influenza increases vaccine acceptance—the Denver experience

Steven R. Mostow*

Department of Medicine, University of Colorado Health Sciences Center, 4200 East Ninth Avenue, Box A-020 Denver, CO 80262, USA

Abstract

Influenza remains an important disease worldwide and vaccine acceptance by high-risk patients has not been optimal. Most campaigns have emphasized the role of the physician and enthusiasm has varied from exuberant to negative. By going directly to the public with television, radio, and electronic print information about the risks of influenza and the ability to reduce this risk with vaccine, Colorado has been able to improve vaccine acceptance rates in all age and risk categories. In fact, Colorado has the highest percentage of immunized elderly in the USA. Flu-like illness reports to the Health Department have decreased and mortality has decreased as well. Thus, when patients themselves are informed about the risks of a disease as well as the best means to obviate that risk, they respond by accepting influenza vaccine in record numbers. © 2001 Elsevier Science B.V. All rights reserved.

Keywords: Influenza; Vaccine; Public education

Approximately 20 years ago, several colleagues were concerned about the meager acceptance of influenza vaccine amongst high-risk patients in the USA. Even though our population of at-risk Americans was becoming rapidly larger, less than 20% of these patients received vaccine. The absolute number of Americans receiving vaccine was about 13 million. Since our plea to physicians had not been effective over a number of years, it was decided to approach the American Thoracic Society and the American Lung Association with a novel idea–informing the public directly about the importance of influenza [1]. We also had obtained initial financial support from Dupont Laboratories, the producer of amantadine, an antiviral for the treatment of influenza Type A. With that

---

* Tel.: +1-303-372-9190; fax: +1-303-372-9246.
E-mail address: Steven.Mostow@UHColorado.edu (S.R. Mostow).

0531-5131/01/$ – see front matter © 2001 Elsevier Science B.V. All rights reserved.
PII: S0531-5131(01)00353-3

support, a movie was made which was shown to the public on national television. Subsequently, interviews about influenza were carried out on radio, television, and in newspapers. This aroused interest in the disease and there was a modest gain in vaccine usage because at-risk patients asked their physicians for vaccine rather than waiting for the physician to offer vaccine.

Sixteen years ago, the American Lung Association of Colorado (an affiliate of the national organization) was convinced to become interested in influenza and its control. Further, they were asked to add the control of influenza to their traditional list, which included chronic lung disease, smoking cessation, and childhood asthma. A large group of nurses, known as the Visiting Nurses Association of Colorado, was recruited to participate. This nursing group historically makes home visits to care for patients. They were asked to participate in a small coalition to inform the public about influenza and to provide vaccine at alternative sites, such as local health clinics. An owner of a large grocery store chain was also convinced to permit the nurses to administer influenza vaccine in the grocery store during normal business hours. On the first day of this unique program, sales receipts for groceries and other items exceeded expectations by US$10,000. After that, more and more grocery store managers requested that the program be provided in their stores [2]. In the second year of this program, the first major press conference was held. This inaugural press conference informed the public about the importance of influenza in terms of disease and costs, as well as disease prevention with vaccine and treatment with antiviral medication. The press coverage was phenomenal, and coverage has remained exceptional for the past 16 years, expanding far beyond the borders of the state of Colorado. It rapidly became clear that financial support was needed to expand the program and in fact, the three major grocery companies in Colorado now donate money. Private medical insurance companies also support these efforts with posters for pharmacies and grocery stores, and free telephone messaging services for individuals to call for information on vaccine sites. Each grocery store usually has one clinic per influenza vaccine season; there are approximately 375 such stores participating in the program.

The coalition has now grown to more than 80 members representing the various supporters. These include the federal health system (Medicare and related departments), State Health Department, numerous county health departments, television and radio organizations, private health insurance companies, and pharmaceutical companies.

With financial donations, in-kind contributions and gifts it has been possible to print grocery bags, milk cartons and cashier receipts with a flu message and/or phone numbers for information about vaccine. Posters and educational brochures are printed and distributed as well [3]. We even have an automobile (a Volkswagen Bug) with flu messages and logos, which is parked at major sporting and public events.

What has been the impact? In the first year of operation, about 30,000 persons were immunized in alternative sites. The traditional sites immunized another 100,000 persons in a state with a population then of 3 million. In the past vaccine season almost 300,000 persons were immunized in alternative sites and more than 1 million were immunized in physician offices [4]. Therefore, not only have new options been provided for persons to receive vaccine in unusual sites such as supermarkets, pharmacies, and office buildings [5], the public now is intensely aware of the complications of influenza and that has resulted in the public going to their primary care physician and asking or even demanding influenza vaccine. Further, this has resulted in a diminution of cases and deaths for the state of Colorado. The federal government has announced that Colorado has the highest rates per capita of vaccine acceptance and data supports that the number of deaths, hospitalizations and cost of this preventable disease has been a direct result of this program.

Acknowledgements

The author wishes to acknowledge Catherine O'Grady, R.N., of the Visiting Nurses Association for 16 years of constant work, encouragement, and support.

References

[1] S.R. Mostow, Influenza—a preventable disease not being prevented, Am. Rev. Respir. Dis. 134 (1986) 1.
[2] S.R. Mostow, Influenza: a preventable disease finally being prevented in Colorado, Colo. Med., (November 1990) 332.
[3] S.R. Mostow, Prevention of influenza in Colorado, Am. J. Respir. Crit. Care Med. 149 (4) (1994) A807.
[4] Prevention and control of influenza: recommendations of the Advisory Committee of Immunization Practices (ACIP). MMWR 2000;49(RR-3).
[5] Adult immunization programs in nontraditional settings: quality standards and guidance for program evaluation. MMWR 2000;49(RR-1).

An update on the use of influenza vaccination in Wales and the impact of changes in government policy

John Watkins*

*Department of Epidemiology and Public Health, University of Wales College of Medicine,
Heath Park, Cardiff, Wales, UK*

Abstract

Background: Influenza vaccine uptake in the United Kingdom has been improving steadily during the 1990s. In late 1998 the government announced that it was revising its guidelines for vaccine use to include all those 75 years and above as well as those in the previous high-risk categories. The author and others have shown that these changes would increase the high-risk pool of individuals, in Wales (population 2.9 million), recommended for vaccination to 15%. This present study builds on previous work on vaccine usage by Welsh general medical practitioners and quantifies the response to the policy change at both a national and practice level. *Methods*: Using information from the prescription pricing authority for Wales and computerised medical practices, vaccine uptake rates were calculated nationally for Wales, by administrative health regions, with a population of 550,000 on average, and by individual practices in southeast Wales. This data has been available from the early 1990s to the present day and covers the winter of 1998/1999, when policy was changed. *Results*: Since the 1980s, the uptake of vaccine has risen marginally in Wales from 8.7% of the population being vaccinated in 1993 to 9% in 1998/1999. Despite the change in government policy, no significant increase in response to this was seen at any population level. Less than 50% of those recommended for vaccination received it, with a 10-fold variation in the percentage of the population vaccinated by individual general medical practices. *Conclusions*: This study demonstrates that changes in government vaccination policy have made little difference to the vaccination practices of individual doctors. There still exists a shortfall between 2% and 6% (assuming that all vaccine doses are given to those who require it) between the vaccine delivered and the pool of the population at risk. In the United Kingdom, a vaccination policy left to individual practices to organise, with little central

* Department of Epidemiology and Public Health, University of Wales College of Medicine, c/o Gwent Health Authority, Mamhilad, Pontypool, Gwent NP4 0YP, UK. Tel.: +44-1495-765126.
  E-mail address: john.watkins@gwent-ha.wales.nhs.uk (J. Watkins).

0531-5131/01/$ – see front matter © 2001 Elsevier Science B.V. All rights reserved.
PII: S0531-5131(01)00376-4

coordination or funding, leads to wide-scale variation and a large percentage of the population left unprotected. © 2001 Elsevier Science B.V. All rights reserved.

Keywords: High-risk groups; Medical practice variation; Primary care

1. Introduction

Over 80% of the deaths from influenza occur in those aged 65 years and older and vaccination has been shown to be both effective and cost saving in the elderly [1–6] reducing the clinical symptoms of influenza by 40–60%, hospitalisations by 40–80% and deaths by up to 45%. Recipients, recommended for vaccine, are deemed to be at special risk of developing complications from clinical influenza and are more likely to be hospitalised or die if not protected [7–13]. Despite this evidence of effectiveness, Nguyen-Van-Tam and Nicholson [14] showed that in the 1991/1992 winter, only 41% of the population recommended for vaccination in over 600 medical practices in England were immunised. A similar conclusion was reached by Watkins [15] in 1994/1995 when he showed that less than half of all vaccine used by practices in southeast Wales went to people in high-risk categories, while less than half of those recommended for vaccination received it. In 1998, using the General Practice Morbidity Database for Wales (GPMD) [16], Watkins et al. [17] estimated the impact on healthcare systems of the introduction of an age-based policy in the UK for influenza vaccination, targeting all those aged 75 and older, in addition to those of all ages with chronic disease. The policy change meant that in the United Kingdom and similar western countries, between 12% and 15% of the population were recommended for vaccination. Against this backdrop presented here is a review of influenza vaccination use in Wales, a region of the United Kingdom with a population of 2.9 million, using data obtained from prescriptions for vaccines dispensed by general medical practitioners in Wales. In addition, for the first time, the uptake figures of influenza vaccine by high-risk groups following the 1998 policy change [18] in those practices involved in the GPMD, and a comparison of this uptake with the population coverage for Wales using prescription pricing information will be shown. This work will further the debate on the shortfall between policy and practice in relation to preventative health care.

2. Methods

In Wales, the primary vehicle for delivering influenza vaccine is through general medical practices and family physicians, with little or no vaccination being carried out by other agencies. Data used in this study came from two sources. The first being the computerised information held by the Prescription Pricing Authority for Wales, which holds complete information on all doses of vaccine administered by Welsh medical practitioners for the study period 1993–1999. The second source of data used in this study came from the General Practice Morbidity Database for Wales (GPMD) with a total population of 297,086 patient records, some 10% of the Welsh total, collected from the computer systems in 32 general medical practices in Wales for the 1998/1999 winter. Practices that contribute data to the GPMD have been recruited since 1993 and each one has needed to demonstrate a high level of data entry and quality before they contribute to the project. GPMD records an average of 2 million consultations per annum the details of which are pooled to form the core data. Patient and practice confidentiality is maintained by GPMD. The present study utilised aggregated data extracted by age, sex and the presence or absence of factors that would entitle patients to receive influenza vaccine under the Department of Health guidance. We were able to identify individuals with single or multiple morbidity that places them at special risk from the complications of influenza. These included diseases of the cardiovascular, respiratory and renal systems as well as those suffering with diabetes. We were not able to identify those who were immuno-compromised, from disease or therapy, or those living in a residential or nursing home setting. From previous work [15], these latter two categories are likely to be small, particularly in the younger population who are recommended for vaccination on the basis of health status and where respiratory and cardiovascular disease are orders of magnitude more common. From the GPMD, we were able to estimate the percentage of the population that fall into the high-risk pool recommended for vaccination in Wales. Also, we were able to calculate the recorded uptake of vaccine in the age bands 65–74 years, 75 years and older and high risk below aged 65. In addition, we were able to examine the use of vaccine outside of recommendations in both males and females.

Using the prescription pricing information, uptake rates of influenza vaccine were calculated per 1000 of the population, for each administrative health region in Wales, each with a population of around 550,000 and for each of the 112 general practices in southeast Wales, for the winters between 1993 and 1999. In addition, presented here are the findings from the GPMD vaccine usage at the individual patient level. This approach allowed the completeness of the data in the GPMD, to be assessed for the year 1998/1999 when vaccination policy changes were introduced.

The present study has limitations in that even though 10% of the Welsh population is covered by GPMD, the sample population of general medical practices is biased towards those larger practices who use their computer systems effectively with protocols for the recording of clinical information. As such, they are likely to be more organised than other practices in their use of information technology to aid patient care.

3. Results

3.1. Population uptake

From prescription pricing information, the overall influenza vaccine uptake by the Welsh population registered with all practices in Wales, between 1993 and 1999 is shown in Table 1.

Between 1993 and 1999, the number of vaccine doses given rose over this period from 87 doses per 1000 to a maximum of 94 doses in 1996/1997. In subsequent years, this figure declined and in 1998/1999, the year that the government announced an expansion to the vaccination programme, we saw levels decline still further. In southeast Wales, the

Table 1
Influenza vaccine usage by region of Wales and by general medical practice in southeast Wales

Year	Vaccine uptake for Welsh administrative regions per 1000 population (range in brackets)	Vaccine uptake for general medical practices in southeast Wales per 1000 population (range in brackets)
1993–1994	87 (81–94)	89 (25–251)
1994–1995	82 (80–86)	83 (18–256)
1995–1996	92 (88–96)	88 (21–219)
1996–1997	94 (90–98)	91 (20–250)
1997–1998	92 (90–93)	96 (27–401)
1998–1999	90 (86–92)	94 (21–178)

uptake of vaccine each year was overall slightly higher than the regional average, but again showed a decrease in the year 1998/1999. In addition from Table 1, it can be seen that whereas at a population level, the vaccine uptake figures appear comparable across the principality, when we examine individual medical practice we see a 10-fold variation with many practices vaccinating less than 1% of their practice population.

3.2. Uptake of vaccine in 1998/1999 winter by high-risk groups

For the population of 297,086 patients registered with the 32 general medical practices in the GPMD, we found that 18% were aged 65 years or older, with a further 5.6% below this age with high-risk conditions (Table 2).

Table 2
Summary results and population characteristics for individuals registered with general medical practitioners participating in the General Practice Morbidity Database for Wales for the winter 1998–1999

(a) Population base used in the analysis from 32 practices	297,086
(b) Population aged 65 years and older; percentage of total population in brackets	53,747 (18.1%)
(c) Population aged less than 65 years with high-risk conditions; percentage of total population in brackets	16,728 (5.6%)
(d) Percentage population recommended for vaccination in 2000/2001 winter (%sum of (b)+(c))	23.7%
Current uptake in over 65 age group; percentage of total 65 and over population vaccinated in brackets (includes all 75 and older)	14,648 (27.25%)
Uptake of influenza vaccine in over 75 age group; percentage of total 75 and over population vaccinated in brackets	7515 (17.54%)
Uptake of vaccine by high risk under 65; percentage of high risk in brackets	2316 (13.8%)

Table 3

Female high-risk population for 2000/2001 winter recommended for influenza vaccination by chief medical officer England and uptake of influenza vaccination during the 1998/1999 winter following introduction of vaccination to all aged 75 years and older

Age bands	Total population in age band	Number in age band receiving vaccination; percentage of age band population in brackets	Number in age band with high-risk conditions[a]; percentage of age band population in brackets	Number of high-risk vaccinated; percentage of high-risk population vaccinated in brackets
0–14	26,012	100 (0.38)	1412 (5.42)	50 (3.54)
15–34	39,239	428 (1.1)	1808 (4.61)	140 (7.74)
35–64	54,711	3477 (6.36)	5218 (9.54)	1022 (19.58)
65–74	14,142	3715 (26.27)	2968 (21.0)	1032 (34.77)
75–84	11,246	3358 (29.86)	2266 (20.15)	854 (37.69)
85+	5836	1284 (22.0)	643 (11.0)	185 (28.77)
Total	151,186	12,362 (8.2)	14,315 (9.46)	3283 (22.93)

[a] Those with chronic medical conditions recommended for vaccination including diseases of the heart, chest and kidneys and diabetes mellitus but excluding those in residential homes and the immuno-suppressed.

During the winter of 1998/1999, the first winter that a 75 and over, aged-based policy, was introduced, 7515 individuals in this age group were vaccinated with an uptake rate of 17.5% of the age group. In addition 14,648 (27.25%) of those aged 65 years and over received vaccine. In both these age groups, there was a slightly higher uptake in men than women (Tables 3 and 4).

Table 4

Male high-risk population for 2000/2001 winter recommended for influenza vaccination by chief medical officer England and uptake of influenza vaccination during the 1998/1999 winter following introduction of vaccination to all aged 75 years and older

Age bands	Total population in age band	Number in age band receiving vaccination; percentage of age band population in brackets	Number in age band with high risk conditions[a]; percentage of age band population in brackets	Number of high-risk vaccinated; percentage of high-risk population vaccinated in brackets
0–14	27,674	138 (0.5)	1964 (7.1)	69 (3.51)
15–34	40,455	300 (0.74)	1503 (3.7)	96 (6.39)
35–64	55,248	2896 (5.24)	4823 (8.7)	939 (19.47)
65–74	12,583	3418 (27.16)	2571 (20.4)	957 (37.22)
75–84	7291	2369 (32.5)	1537 (21.1)	601 (39.1)
85+	2649	504 (19.03)	295 (11.1)	93 (31.53)
Total	145,900	9625 (6.6)	12,693 (8.7)	2755 (21.7)

[a] Those with chronic medical conditions recommended for vaccination including diseases of the heart, chest and kidneys and diabetes mellitus but excluding those in residential homes and the immuno-suppressed.

3.3. Vaccine uptake outside of recommended groups

Both Tables 3 and 4 demonstrate that at all ages below age 65, a half to two thirds of influenza vaccine is given to individuals who are outside of the high-risk groups recommended for vaccination. This may reflect the broader use by general practitioners of vaccine to include others with chronic conditions, not clearly defined as fitting into the current guidelines, or it may be lack of computer classification by practices. The majority of patients with high-risk chronic conditions failed to receive vaccine.

3.4. Validity

The overall population coverage of influenza vaccine for individuals registered with practices in the GPMD was 74 doses of vaccine per 1000 of the population. This figure is less than the uptake for the population of Wales in total, calculated from general practice prescription pricing information (Table 1).

The discrepancy between the population coverage information from these two sources could be interpreted in a number of ways; firstly, it could represent a real difference between the practices within the study in their behaviour towards influenza vaccine compared with all practices in Wales. This explanation seems unlikely since the practices themselves differ from the larger pool of Welsh practices, a difference arising from the selection bias of the GPMD towards larger, better organised practices, attributes one could argue are more likely to enhance vaccine uptake rather than the converse.

The other more obvious explanation would be that not all the vaccine information about patients is stored on the GP computer systems and it is this missing data that accounts for the discrepancy seen. If we take this discrepancy into account and assume that all the additional vaccine doses not recorded were given to patients with high-risk conditions, or aged 75 years or over, we would still achieve a coverage rate far short of 50%. This finding is consistent with other studies [14,15].

4. Discussion

It is clear from the results presented here that over the past decade, a period when the percentage of the UK population recommended for vaccination has risen from at least 12% to 23% in 2000, we have seen a less significant rise in population coverage and a 10-fold variation in vaccination practices among individual doctors. The introduction of an aged-based policy in 1998, from the findings presented here, seems to have had no real impact on doctors who appear to use the majority of vaccine for uses outside of government policy.

The United Kingdom influenza policy has a mixture of age- and disease-based inclusion criteria. The targeting of influenza vaccine at individuals, in order to offer personal protection to that individual on the basis of risk related to their own health status, makes estimates of the recipient population prevalence difficult for those under age 65 years. The high-risk population are difficult to quantify on the basis of chronic disease category alone, since many have overlapping comorbidities, particularly in the older age group where people have multiple chronic diseases. We addressed the question of comorbidities the last time the United Kingdom influenza vaccination policy was changed [17]. This present study estimates that 23% of the United Kingdom population, an increase of nearly 10%, will be eligible for vaccination against influenza during the autumn of 2000, 18% of the population being 65 years and older, while the remaining 5% are in the younger age group with chronic health problems.

Vaccine uptake findings, derived using our methodology, seem to underestimate the total population uptake for influenza vaccine found from other methods, such as prescription pricing information. However, it agrees with uptake estimates derived by others from similar sources using other research databases.

5. Implications

Introduction of an age-based vaccination policy makes the use of a computerised patient register an effective tool to improve uptake for the majority of those recommended for vaccination in many western countries [21]. Computerised patient registers allow an easily defined cohort of the population to be identified, from which uptake rates can be calculated. However, this study reinforces the need for judicial use of influenza vaccine by targeting effectively those most at risk. It also emphasizes that while financial systems, such as those introduced in the United Kingdom to pay incentives to doctors to inoculate the elderly [19,20], may ensure greater uptake in this older age group, it is important that such policies do not result in a detrimental impact on uptake in younger patients with chronic high-risk conditions.

It has been shown here that at least 23% of the population of most developed countries would benefit from protection against influenza; yet, over the past 10 years in one region of the United Kingdom, under half this amount of vaccine has been delivered to its citizens with perhaps only 20% of the entire eligible population appropriately receiving cover. This has major implications for policy makers.

References

[1] D.S. Fedson, A. Wajda, P. Nicol, G.W. Hammond, D.L. Kaiser, L.L. Roos, Clinical effectiveness of influenza vaccination in Manitoba, JAMA 270 (1993) 1956–1961.

[2] R. Schmitz, D. Kidder, A. Schwarz, P. Cook, Final results: medicare influenza vaccine demonstration in selected states, 1988–1992, MMWR 42 (1993) 601–604.

[3] K.L. Nichol, K.L. Margolis, J. Wuorenma, T. Von Steinberg, The efficacy and cost effectiveness of vaccination against influenza among elderly persons living in the community, N. Engl. J. Med. 331 (1994) 778–784.

[4] J.P. Mullooly, M.D. Bennett, M.C. Hornbrook, W.H. Barker, W.W. Williams, P.A. Patriarca, et al., Influenza vaccination programs for elderly persons: cost-effectiveness in a health maintenance organization, Ann. Intern. Med. 121 (1994) 947–952.

[5] J. Perez-Tirse, P.A. Gross, Review of cost-benefit analyses of influenza vaccine, PharmacoEconomics 2 (1992) 198–206.

[6] T.M. Govaert, C.T. Thijs, N. Masurel, M. Sprenger, C. Dinant, J.A. Knott Nerus, The efficacy of influenza vaccination in elderly individuals, A randomized double-blind placebo-controlled trial, JAMA 272 (1994) 1661–1665.

J. Watkins / International Congress Series 1219 (2001) 681–688

[7] K.G. Nicholson, Impact of influenza and respiratory syncytial virus on mortality in England and Wales from January 1975 to December 1990, Epidemiol. Infect. 116 (1996) 51–63.

[8] I. Ashley, T. Smith, K. Dunnell, Deaths in Great Britain associated with the influenza epidemic of 1989/90, Popul. Trends 65 (1991) 16–20.

[9] K.J. Lui, A.P. Kendal, Impact of influenza epidemics on mortality in the United States from October 1972 to May 1985, Am. J. Public Health 77 (7) (1987) 2–6.

[10] G.O. Williams, Vaccines in older patients: combating the risk of mortality, Geriatrics 35 (1980) 55–64.

[11] W.P. Glezen, Serious morbidity and mortality associated with influenza epidemics, Epidemiol. Rev. 4 (1982) 25–44.

[12] T.C. Eickhoff, I.L. Sherman, R.E. Serfling, Observations on excess mortality associated with epidemic influenza, JAMA 176 (1961) 776–782.

[13] D.W. Ailing, W.C. Blackwelder, C.W. Stuart-Harris, A study of excess mortality during influenza epidemics in the United States, 1968–1976, Am. J. Epidemiol. 113 (1981) 30–43.

[14] J.S. Nguyen-Van-Tam, K.G. Nicholson, Influenza immunization; vaccine offer, request and uptake in high risk patients during the 1991/2 season, Epidemiol. Infect. 111 (1993) 347–355.

[15] J. Watkins, Effectiveness of influenza vaccination policy at targeting patients at high risk of complications during 1995–696: cross sectional survey, BMJ 317 (1997) 1069–1070.

[16] General Practice Morbidity Database Wales, The GPMD Website is located at http://www.cymruweb.wales.nhs.uk/whcsa/phmis/gpmd/gpmdmenu.html.

[17] J. Watkins, C. Rogers, J. Evans, Implications of age based policies for influenza immunisation, Lancet 353 (1999) 208–209.

[18] Department of Health, Influenza immunisation: extension of current policy to include all those aged 75 years and over, CMO letter PL/CMO/98/4.

[19] Department of Health, Major Changes to the policy on Influenza vaccination, CMO's Update 26; May 2000: 1–2.

[20] Department of Health, Influenza Immunisation, CMO Letter PL/CMO/2000/3.

[21] F. Ambrosch, D.S. Fedson, Influenza vaccination in 29 countries: an update to 1997. PharmacoEconomics 16 (Suppl. 1) (1999) 47–54.

International Congress Series 1219 (2001) 689–695

Influenza vaccination in the Netherlands: a successful system approach

G.A. van Essen[a,*], M.M. Kuyvenhoven[a], N. Masurel[b],
R.J.A. Diepersloot[c], M. van der Graaf[d,1], Th.J.M. Verheij[a]

[a]*Julius Center for General Practice and Patient-oriented Research, University Medical Center Utrecht,
P.O. Box 85060, 3508 AB Utrecht, The Netherlands*
[b]*Erasmus University Rotterdam, Rotterdam, The Netherlands*
[c]*Diakonessen Hospital, Utrecht, The Netherlands*
[d]*Pleiade Management & Consultancy, Amsterdam, The Netherlands*

Abstract

Background: In the Netherlands, the influenza vaccination rate increased from 6% in the eighties up to 16% in the late nineties. The Dutch Influenza Council, founded in the early nineties, started a series of activities in a multitargeted intervention strategy. The increase in vaccination rate is related to the activities in this intervention. *Methods*: In the yearly reports of the Dutch Influenza Council, all data on government policy, vaccination rate, patient and doctor behavior were assembled, together with data from other sources (Dutch Bureau for Statistics, Prevention project of the Dutch College of General Practitioners). *Results*: In a timetable, all activities are presented. Patient knowledge on high-risk groups improved. The rise in vaccination rate shows two tops: in 1992 at the start of the Dutch Influenza Council, and in 1996 at the start of the national GP-prevention project. In 1999, the vaccination rate in high-risk groups was 76%. *Conclusions*: This multitargeted system approach was successful in increasing vaccination rates, especially in high-risk groups. This combined effort of government, private enterprise and national GP organizations sets an example for other national preventive actions. © 2001 Elsevier Science B.V. All rights reserved.

Keywords: Vaccination rate; Patient knowledge; Age criterion; Dutch Influenza Council; Selection software

* Corresponding author. Tel.: +31-30-2538188; fax: +31-30-2539028.
E-mail address: GAvEssen@knmg.nl (G.A. van Essen).
1 Formerly with Dutch Influenza Council.

0531-5131/01/$ – see front matter © 2001 Elsevier Science B.V. All rights reserved.
PII: S 0 5 3 1 - 5 1 3 1 (0 1) 0 0 3 9 3 - 4

1. Introduction

Since the nineties, influenza vaccination rates have risen in many countries, such as the United Kingdom and Belgium. In other countries, as Germany, Denmark, Sweden, Norway, hardly any change has occurred [1]. In the Netherlands, after decades of a constant annual vaccination rate of about 60 per 1000 inhabitants, there was a big increase in the nineties to 160 per 1000. Several groups played a roll in this increase as members of a 'task force': health authorities, patients and patient organizations, medical professionals and their organizations, and the vaccine manufacturers.

In 1991, the Dutch national health authorities concluded that the influenza vaccination rate of less than 30% of the high-risk groups remained far too low, in spite of the yearly letter to all healthcare providers to inform them about the influenza vaccine for that season and the valid high-risk groups. Vaccination was stimulated by means of joint activities by the health administration and the vaccine manufacturers. The Dutch Influenza Council (NIS) was set up by several influenza researchers as a typical Dutch private-enterprise institution, funded by both parties, in order to start a campaign for both the general population and the medical profession. This council was the center of a series of activities.

This paper firstly aims to describe the structure and the organization of influenza vaccination in the Netherlands in the early nineties. The increase in vaccination rate is described and related to the increased activities of the NIS. The goal of this study is to give an example for future activities in the field of preventive medicine in the Netherlands and possibly in other countries.

2. Material and methods

In summary, the Dutch Influenza Council had the following goals.

(1) To provide information to convince the patients at risk (an estimated 3.2 million) and the general public (as the environment of the patients at risk) about the benefits of influenza vaccination. This was mainly achieved by television and radio commercials and by providing posters and flyers in the waiting rooms of general practices, hospitals and at pharmacies. The impact of the campaign was also increased by free publicity around the start of the campaign (interviews, photo opportunities, etc.).

(2) To inform and convince the participients who were directly involved in the execution of the vaccination process—the GPs, the assistants of the GPs and (till 1996) the pharmacists—in order to implement an effective vaccination strategy. The advised strategy focussed on three points: registration of the patients at risk, annual postal notice and a fixed and widely advertised vaccination hour. This was achieved in cooperation with their national organizations, by putting the topic on the agenda and by assisting with establishing and communicating the best strategy. The NIS also targeted the GPs directly by mailing and publishing articles in various professional journals.

(3) To inform participants so that they used their influence to increase the vaccination rate: health insurance companies, societies of medical specialists, the regional health authorities, hospital staff and other related organizations.

Each year, the NIS presented the results of the campaign for evaluation and feedback in evaluation reports using several methods:

- a random telephone interview of 400 persons (200 at risk);
- a personal interview of 200 GPs spread over the country about their specific activities in this field: the way they registered the high-risk patients in their information system, the sending of a mail cue to the patients at risk, the presence of a special vaccination hour in their office and the way of monitoring of the vaccinations.

The results of these interviews were available and published within a few months after the campaign [2]. For this study, the data of the NIS are analyzed again and compared with data from other sources.

The influenza vaccination rate is assessed in several ways.

- The vaccine producers presented their figures about vaccine sales each year in the yearly report of the NIS;
- The Dutch Central Bureau of Statistics (CBS) carried out a continuing health survey in about 5000 persons each year [3]. The results have proved to be valid and reliable, but their publication is some years behind and could not be used for evaluation of the vaccination campaign each year.
- The NIS telephone interviews gave a less accurate, but faster indication of the vaccination rate, both in the high-risk population, and in the general population.
- Since 1997, GP organizations evaluated the vaccination rate each year.

3. Results

3.1. The process: activities of all actors in the field

In Fig. 1, the specific activities of all the actors in the field in influenza vaccination are presented. The annual letter to all healthcare providers started in the seventies and was continued to 1997. The Dutch Influenza Council started its activities in 1992 and continued until 1996. The Dutch College of General Practitioners (DCGP) guidelines on influenza vaccination were published in 1993. In 1995, the Dutch GP prevention Project started. In 1996, one month before the campaign started, the age-criterion was added to the guidelines and a fee for vaccination of high-risk patients agreed on (about ECU 7 for the injection, ECU 3 for the vaccine). All costs for influenza vaccination of patients in the high-risk groups and persons 65 years and over are covered by national health insurance. In 1997, vaccine was delivered directly to the GPs, eliminating the role of the pharmacists.

The information campaigns for the public were conducted via mass media (radio and television, national and local newspapers) and through magazines of patient organizations of the high-risk groups. Press conferences were held, free publicity was asked for in news programs, interviews of specialists in the field of influenza were promoted, and articles for

Annual letter health authorities

Dutch Influenza Council

DCGP guideline on influenza

GP Prevention Project

Over-65-criterion

Renumeration for GP

Vaccine in surgery

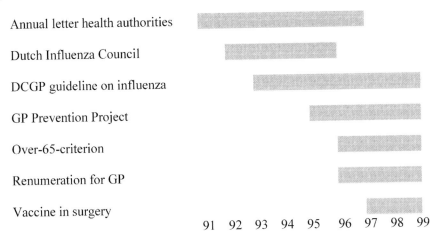

```
91   92   93   94   95    96   97   98   99
```

Fig. 1. Activities of all actors in the field of influenza vaccination in The Netherlands 1991–1999.

advertising in local newspapers were written. As a result of NIS activities, each year, an average of 213 articles and 30 TV and radio messages were published (Table 1). Each year many radio and TV spots were broadcasted.

The NIS activated the DCGP to write guidelines for influenza and influenza vaccination. These guidelines were published in September 1993 [4]. All Dutch GPs were offered information booklets for their patients and a poster for the waiting room. Invitation postcards were also offered for free to send to eligible patients. For all these activities, close contact was maintained with the responsible GP officials. The message to the GPs was also positive: be a good doctor and be active in inviting your patients to be vaccinated.

The activities of GPs show a gradual improvement from 1992 until 1996 (Table 2). Flagging the risk for influenza in the computer, sending a postal cue, organizing special vaccination hours and controlling the compliance of patients, all increased, as did the use of the special NIS invitation postcard. In 1998, more than 90% of the GPs used an information system which could support the special influenza module. In the Dutch Health Survey, it was found that the initiative for vaccination usually came from the

Table 1
Press releases in 1992–1996 (numbers) and percentage of high-risk groups reached

Public messages	1992	1993	1994	1995	1996
Patient magazines	23	32	39	34	45
Doctors journals	20	15	26	19	24
Newspapers	34	39	155	285	271
Radio programs[a]	15	17	39	44	11
TV programs[a]	–	7	7	7	3
% High-risk groups reached	68%	75%	62%	74%	64%

[a] Excluding radio and TV spots.

Table 2
Activities of general practitioners around influenza vaccination from 1992–1996

GP activities	1992	1993	1994	1995	1996
Flagging risk	71%	75%	82%	77%	87%
Personal call	53%	55%	59%	60%	76%
Vaccination hour	63%	68%	73%	78%	83%
Monitoring	59%	60%	63%	64%	76%
NIS Postcard	–	27%	35%	43%	58%

GP; the percentage increased from 57% of the responding patients in 1991 to 74% in 1996.

After the Council stopped its activities in 1996, the information to the general public was provided by the National Sick Fund. Since 1996, information to the general practitioners has been provided by the National Association and the Dutch College of General Practitioners. In 1995, a nationwide prevention project for general practice started, in which influenza vaccination was the first activity. The GP organizations carried out their own evaluation of the results of the prevention program [5].

3.2. The outcome: the change in vaccination rate

Fig. 2 shows the vaccination rate in sold doses of influenza vaccine per 1000 inhabitants since 1980, supplied by the vaccine producers. There is a slight increase in the eighties, from 44 to 66 doses per 1000. In the nineties, the rate increased to 166 per 1000 inhabitants in 1998. The strongest relative increase was in 1992, the start of the first NIS campaign, and in 1996, the first year the age criterion was advised.

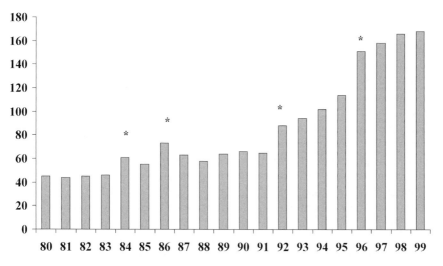

Fig. 2. Influenza vaccination rate in The Netherlands in high-risk patients 1991–1999.

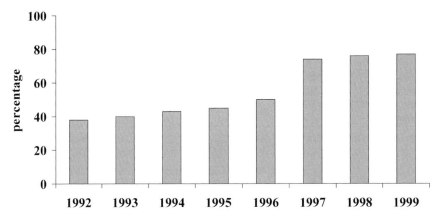

Fig. 3. Influenza vaccination rates in The Netherlands 1980–1999 (number of doses per 1000 inhabitants).

In the eighties, there were only two small peaks in the vaccination rate. After the double epidemic with influenza H1N1 and B in the beginning of 1984, there was a small peak in vaccination rate [6]. In 1986, there was another peak, perhaps caused by publicity about the late change of the composition of the vaccine (a fourth component was added) [7].

In Fig. 3, the vaccination rate in high-risk groups is presented, as measured by the CBS, by the NIS and the GP-prevention project from 1991 through 1999.

4. Discussion

Vaccination rates improved considerably in the nineties in the Netherlands from 28% of the high-risk population in 1991 to 77% in 1999. The strongest relative increase was in 1992, the start of the first NIS campaign, and in 1996, the first year the age criterion was advised. The expansion of the high-risk groups, only one month before the vaccination period, did not lead to a lowering of the relative vaccination rate.

In this complex, social field of government, health officials, vaccine manufacturers, interested scientists, general practitioners, medical specialists, pharmacists and, most of all, patients, it is hard to single out one cause for this improvement. Sending an annual letter to healthcare professionals did not alter their behavior in the eighties. Starting publicity for the general public gave an improvement, but changing GPs behavior proved to be more influential. The guidelines on influenza vaccination were adopted in 1993. Although most general practitioners are well acquainted with guidelines, knowledge does not, unfortu- nately, invariably lead to application [8]. The last big raise came when the fee for the GP was bargained. The extension with the healthy over-65s was easily absorbed.

Single interventions give temporary results at best. A 'shotgun' of interventions, aimed at all players in the field, has resulted in a change of behavior [9]. Gyorkos et al. [10] demonstrated in a meta-analysis of 36 publications that the pooled effect of influenza immunization strategies differed quite a lot according to the sort of strategy. Client-oriented strategies gave an improvement of 12%, provider-oriented 17%, system-oriented 39% and a mixed intervention 17%. Litt and Lake [11] concluded that a combined approach could lead to a greater coverage of influenza vaccine, including appropriate information to high-risk groups and greater use of registers and doctor and patient reminder systems. It is likely that a combination of interventions at different levels in the community during a number of years has the opportunity of changing patients' and doctor's behavior.

Acknowledgements

For this study, a grant was received from the Dutch Influenza Council.

References

[1] D.S. Fedson, C. Hannoun, J. Leese, et al., Influenza vaccination in 18 developed countries, 1980–1992, Vaccine 7 (1995) 623–627.

[2] M. van der Graaf, G.A. van Essen, R.J.A. Diepersloot, M.J.W. Sprenger, N. Masurel, Influenzavaccinatie in de huisartspraktijk, De effecten van de voorlichtingscampagne 1992, Med. Contact 48 (1993) 115–117.

[3] Statistics Netherlands, Ministry of Health, Welfare and Sports, Vademecum of Health Statistics of The Netherlands 1997, SDU, The Hague, 1997.

[4] G.A. van Essen, Y.C.G. Sorgedrager, G.W. Salemink, Th.M.E. Govaert, J.P.H. van den Hoogen, J.R. van der Laan, NHG-Standaard Influenza and Influenzavaccinatie, Huisarts Wet 36 (1993) 342–346.

[5] M. Tacken, H. van den Hoogen, W. Tiersma, D. de Bakker, J. Braspenning, LINH, De Influenzavaccinatie-Campagne 1997, WOK/Nivel, Nijmegen/Utrecht, 1998.

[6] N. Masurel, W.E.P. Beyer, Gelijktijdig optreden van influenza B-en influenza A-(H1N1)virus in de winter 1983/'84, Ned. Tijdschr. Geneeskd. 128 (1984) 2050–2051.

[7] N. Masurel, W.E.P. Beyer, Drift van het influenza A (H1N1)-virus; wijziging van het influenzavaccin voor het seizoen 1986/'87, Ned. Tijdschr. Geneeskd. 130 (1986) 1929–1930.

[8] R. Grol, National standard setting for quality of care in general practice: attitudes of general practitioners and response to a set of standards, Br. J. Gen. Pract. 40 (1990) 361–364.

[9] G.A. van Essen, M.M. Kuyvenhoven, R.A. de Melker, Implementing the Dutch College of General Practitioners' guidelines for influenza vaccination: an intervention study, Br. J. Gen. Pract. 47 (1997) 25–29.

[10] T.W. Gyorkos, T.N. Tannenbaum, M. Abrahamowicz, et al., Evaluation of the effectiveness of immunization delivery methods, Can. J. Public Health 85 (1994) S14–S30 (supplement).

[11] J.C.B. Litt, P.B. Lake, Improving influenza vaccine coverage in at-risk groups, Good intentions are not enough, Med. J. Aust. 44 (1993) 542–547.

International Congress Series 1219 (2001) 697–702

Government policy change in 1997 was essential for the implementation of an influenza vaccination strategy for New Zealand

Lance C. Jennings[a,*], Simon Baker[b]

[a]*Virology Section, Canterbury Health Laboratories, P.O. Box 151, Christchurch, New Zealand*
[b]*Health Funding Authority, Auckland, New Zealand*

Abstract

In 1997, the New Zealand Government introduced a policy to provide influenza vaccination free to all New Zealanders aged 65 years and older, and a target of 75% coverage for the year 2000 was set. In 1999, the policy of free vaccination was extended to include all individuals aged 6 months or over with a chronic medical condition. Prior to 1997, vaccine distributors had been the main promoters of influenza vaccination. Only 68 vaccine doses per 1000 population were distributed in 1996. In 1997, the first year of the new policy, vaccine coverage among those aged 65 and over rose from an estimated 28% to 38%, and to 44% in 1998. With the extension of the policy of free influenza vaccination in 1999, the number of vaccine doses distributed increased to 137 per 1000 population and coverage among those aged 65 and over rose to 55%. Coverage for those aged 65 and over varied by health locality from 40% to 68%. Localities with higher coverage had active local "influenza awareness" strategies in place to co-ordinate healthcare provider efforts. Coordinated National influenza immunisation promotion was introduced as a strategy for the year 2000, with objectives of both public and healthcare provider education. © 2001 Elsevier Science B.V. All rights reserved.

Keywords: Influenza immunisation; Policy; Coverage

1. Background

Both the seriousness of influenza as a public health threat, and the benefits of influenza immunisation in protecting those at high risk from influenza, are well recognised.

* Corresponding author.
E-mail address: Lance.Jennings@chmeds.ac.nz (L.C. Jennings).

0531-5131/01/$ – see front matter © 2001 Elsevier Science B.V. All rights reserved.
PII: S0531-5131(01)00387-9

Nonetheless, influenza vaccine remains under-utilised worldwide. Among the factors increasing vaccine usage is the degree of endorsement by public health and Governmental authorities.

New Zealand recommendations for influenza immunisation are typical of those of many countries, and target those at greatest risk of developing complications or dying following infection with influenza, rather than attempting to control the spread of influenza. Individuals may be at higher risk because of their age, or the presence of a chronic medical condition [1]. Although these recommendations have been in place for many years, prior to 1997 there had been no Government policy to encourage medical practitioners to immunise their at-risk patients against influenza, and promotion had been carried out largely by vaccine distributors. As a result, coverage rates were well below that of our nearest Pacific neighbour, Australia, and below that of other developed countries [2].

The cornerstone of influenza immunisation strategy is influenza surveillance. The maintenance of optimal vaccine efficacy is dependent on achieving a close antigenic match between the vaccine and circulating strains. The early detection of changes that may occur in the influenza virus is the primary goal of influenza surveillance. An influenza surveillance network was established by the World Health Organisation (WHO) in 1947 [3]. New Zealand joined this network in 1953 and has remained an active participant. The composition of influenza vaccines and guidance for public health measures in the event of an influenza epidemic or pandemic are both reliant on surveillance. However, apart from contributing data to the WHO and the Australian Influenza Immunisation Advisory Committee to assist with the annual determination of the vaccine composition for the coming Southern Hemisphere season, little additional use has been made of the extensive surveillance data available [4].

In 1996, recommendations were made to the New Zealand Government that influenza vaccine should be made available free to those at high risk of complications from influenza. The outcome was the implementation of new policy for the 1997 influenza season, making influenza vaccine available free to individuals aged 65 years and older, with a future extension to those under 65 years once the risk groups had been determined. A target of 75% coverage of those aged 65 and over for the year 2000 was set. Coverage monitoring was introduced, and a health promotion budget established.

This paper reviews the influence of this policy on influenza vaccine coverage rates in New Zealanders.

2. Methods

Prior to 1997, influenza vaccine coverage could only be estimated by combining the number of units of vaccine distributed in New Zealand with national census data. Vaccine distribution unit numbers were accessed directly from the commercial vaccine distributors. No estimates were available for vaccine wastage. Since February 1997, coverage data from reimbursement claims for individuals aged 65 years and older have been available. Medical practitioners purchase the vaccine, then once administered, claim reimbursement from the Government's Health Funding Authority via Health Benefits

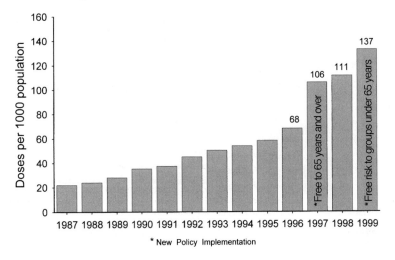

Fig. 1. New Zealand influenza vaccine distribution, 1987–1999.

Limited. A random auditing process checks the validity of claims. The policy extension in 1999 (to include risk groups under 65 years) has also extended the coverage data available.

3. Results

The number of doses of influenza vaccine distributed in New Zealand per 1000 population since 1987 is shown in Fig. 1. Following the availability of national claims data in 1997, influenza immunisation coverage rates for New Zealanders aged 65 and over could be more clearly defined (Table 1). National coverage for this high-risk group increased from 38% in 1997 to 44% in 1998 and 55% in 1999. Vaccine coverage data by

Table 1
Influenza vaccine coverage rates for persons aged 65 years and over, 1997–1999

Health region	Year					
	1997		1998		1999	
	No. at Risk	% Cover	No. at Risk	% Cover	No. at Risk	% Cover
Northern	132,780	30	134,980	24	137,445	48
Midland	84,190	40	85,935	50	87,270	57
Central	97,670	37	98,530	48	99,170	52
Southern	122,160	48	123,380	58	124,390	64
National	436,800	38	442,825	44	448,275	55
Increase over previous year (%)		Est 10		6		11

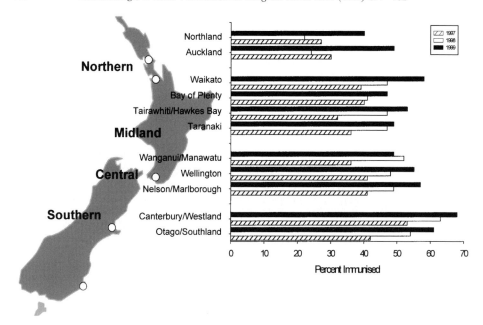

Fig. 2. Influenza immunisation coverage ≥ 65 years, 1997–1999.

locality are shown in Fig. 2. Coverage among those under 65 years with a chronic medical condition is estimated at 19% for 1999.

4. Discussion

Government endorsement of influenza immunisation has been the single most important contributing factor to the increased influenza vaccine use among New Zealand's 3.8 million people. Up until 1996, when 68 doses of vaccine/1000 population were distributed, there had been little Government intervention, and a slow increase in influenza vaccine sales. This was despite the presence of public health recommendations for influenza immunisation in line with other countries. During this period, promotion of the vaccine nationally was largely carried out by the commercial vaccine suppliers. This included television advertising from 1995. In 1996, enterprising medical practitioners established influenza vaccination clinics in public areas such as shopping malls and supermarkets. These strategies contributed to community influenza awareness and may have resulted in the increase in vaccine sales in 1996.

Government endorsement of influenza vaccination in 1997, through the provision of free vaccine to those aged 65 years and older, then extension of this policy to those under 65 years in defined risk groups, has resulted in a substantial increase in vaccine usage. Vaccine distribution increased from 68 doses per 1000 in 1996 to 106 doses per 1000 in 1997 (a 56% increase), reaching 137 doses/1000 population in 1999 (a further

29% increase). This represents a more than 100% increase over 3 years. However, comparison of the per capita distribution of influenza vaccine with Australia (170 doses/1000 population in 1999) suggests that although endorsement has been essential for the accelerated increase in vaccine uptake in New Zealand, other strategies are also needed.

Between 1996 and 1997, coverage increased by 10%, from an estimated 28% to 38%. The introduction of free vaccine to those aged 65 and over, Ministry of Health circulars to medical practitioners, provision of posters and pamphlets about influenza vaccination, and promotion by the vaccine distributor all occurred just prior to the 1997 influenza season. From 1997, reimbursement claims have provided coverage data, which previously could only be estimated. Coverage nationally has increased from 38% in 1997, to 44% in 1998 and 55% in 1999. The smaller 6% increase in coverage between 1997 and 1998 may have been related to the lack of new initiatives in vaccine promotion for the 1998 influenza season. In 1999, an 11% increase in coverage was observed. No new Ministry of Health promotion initiative had been introduced; however, an influenza kit had been developed by the vaccine supplier and distributed nationally to all general practitioners.

Coverage data from individual health localities shows considerable variation. Due to the unavailability of influenza vaccination data by geographical area prior to 1997, the impact of the availability of free vaccine in 1997 cannot be estimated for individual health localities. However, from 1997 to 1999, increases in coverage among persons 65 years and over ranged from 7% in the Bay of Plenty to 28% in Waikato. The locality with the highest level of coverage (53%) in 1997 was Canterbury/West Coast. This locality is likely to have benefited from the establishment of a coordinated influenza awareness program prior to the 1997 influenza season. In addition, influenza awareness was heightened by a severe A/Wuhan/353/95 (H3N2) epidemic in 1996, and health authorities were keen to reduce the impact on the health care system through excessive admissions to hospital.

For high-risk individuals under 65 years, reimbursement claims data is also available for 1999. The extension of the free vaccine policy to include this group followed an analysis of published data on the benefits of influenza immunisation in a range of chronic disease categories [5]. Health Benefits Limited claims data suggests that 19% of this group received vaccine in 1999. This is likely to be an underestimate, since a large number of those under 65 will have received vaccination privately, or through employer subsidised schemes, and will therefore not appear in claims data.

Along with the implementation of the 1997 free vaccine policy, a budget for promotion was also established. Limited promotion was carried out over this period. However, the need for an influenza awareness programme for the promotion of the benefits of influenza immunisation was recognised in some localities. The Elder Care Canterbury programme, a collaborative effort between 17 health care providers, was initiated in 1997, and has seen the Canterbury coverage rate for those 65 years and older increase to 68% in 1999. The success in Canterbury has provided the model for the formation of the National Influenza Immunisation Strategy Group. This group has the twin aims of educating the public on the seriousness of influenza, and informing health care professionals of the benefits of immunisation to those at risk for influenza. Through this approach, the 75% target will be achieved in some health localities.

References

[1] Ministry of Health, Immunisation Handbook, Ministry of Health, Wellington, 1996.
[2] F. Ambrose, D.S. Fedson, Influenza vaccination in 29 developed countries: an update to 1997, Pharmacoeconomics 16 (suppl. 1) (1999) 47–54.
[3] WHO, Standardization and improvement of influenza surveillance: memorandum from a WHO/GEIG meeting, Bull. WHO 70 (1992) 23–25.
[4] L.C. Jennings, Influenza surveillance in New Zealand, Vaccine 17 (1999) S115–S117.
[5] N. Wilson, A. Hampson, L.C. Jennings, The evidence for benefit from influenza immunisation for specific populations aged under 65 years (Unpublished report for the Transitional Health Authority), Wellington, 1997.

International Congress Series 1219 (2001) 703–706

Use of alternative sites to administer influenza vaccine improves acceptance by both physicians and patients

Steven R. Mostow*

Department of Medicine, University of Colorado Hospital, 4200 East Ninth Avenue, Box A-020, Denver, CO 80262, USA

Abstract

Influenza remains an important and largely uncontrolled disease. In the USA, estimated direct and indirect costs exceed US$14 billion, reported annual deaths are in excess of 20,000/year, and the impact on the health care system is dramatic. In the state of Colorado, a volunteer coalition of health professionals, electronic and print consultants, health departments, nursing groups, and pharmaceutical companies have worked to improve vaccination rates. Advertising on radio, TV, newspapers and on electronic billboards at public sporting events has increased awareness. Messages about flu shots are also displayed on a donated automobile. Vaccines can be obtained through standard channels such as physician offices and health departments, but also can be obtained in alternative sites such as grocery stores, pharmacies, and office sites. At the inception of this program 15 years ago, only 32,000 doses of vaccine were delivered at alternative sites and less than 100,000 doses were dispensed in the entire state in physician offices and health departments. In the 1998–1999 season, more than 249,000 doses were dispensed in alternative sites and more than 800,000 in physician offices. This year, an automobile named the "Flubug" displaying positive influenza vaccine messages was strategically placed at sporting and cultural events. A toll-free "hotline" was also established so potential vaccine candidates could phone and obtain information on where vaccine was available on a daily basis. Vaccine delivered at alternative sites will exceed 300,000 this year in the state of Colorado alone. Influenza-like illness reported to the state health department has declined each year as the number of doses administered increases. Alternative site administration of influenza vaccine is a cost effective and successful strategy to improve immunization rates. © 2001 Elsevier Science B.V. All rights reserved.

Keywords: Influenza; Vaccine; Alternative sites

* Tel.: +1-303-372-9190; fax: +1-303-372-5385.
  E-mail address: Steven.Mostow@UHColorado.edu (S.R. Mostow).

0531-5131/01/$ – see front matter © 2001 Elsevier Science B.V. All rights reserved.
PII: S 0 5 3 1 - 5 1 3 1 (0 1) 0 0 6 5 8 - 6

Influenza is an important, preventable, treatable disease, and now with rapid diagnostic technology, easy to recognize and confirm in the clinic. In the USA, influenza outbreaks and epidemics occur annually and are responsible for approximately 114,000 hospitalizations and between 20,000 and 40,000 deaths/year [1]. Since the early 1970s, there have been six seasons where more than 40,000 persons died due to this preventable disease [2]. Historically, each year individuals interested in the control of influenza would approach physicians in an attempt to encourage the doctors and their office staff to make special efforts to immunize high-risk patients in the practice to prevent the ravages of this disease. These efforts did not substantially impact the number of citizens receiving vaccine (about 13 million/year) [3]. In Colorado, to address this issue locally, a coalition was formed to try a new idea to improve immunization rates. The coalition consisted of physicians, nurses, and public health officials as one might expect, but also included persons from the advertising industry, pharmaceutical industry, and medical insurance industry. The coalition decided that a physician should lead the efforts and promote the benefits of influenza vaccine publicly, and that an effort should be made to make influenza vaccine available to high-risk patients and others requesting the vaccine in alternative sites (such as grocery stores, pharmacies, banks, places of work, local public health clinics, as well as other more traditional sites). The coalition was based at the American Lung Association of Colorado (ALAC), a nonprofit organization, which traditionally was interested in informing the public of the risks of chronic lung disease and asthma as well as the risks of smoking cigarettes. The coalition was able to convince the ALAC to add the control of influenza as a fourth objective. Furthermore, the coalition was able to convince the president of the largest grocery store chain in Colorado to permit the administration of influenza immunizations in one of the grocery stores for a 4-h period on a single day. Recipients had to pay for the vaccine and its administration (US$5). On that day, because so many people appeared for vaccine, cash receipts of that particular grocery store were US$10,000 higher than average; soon all other store managers within that grocery store chain wanted clinics in their individual stores. During the first year of the program, we immunized 32,332 persons at alternative sites. Physicians in traditional office practices and sites immunized only an additional 100,000 during that season (1985–1986). The population of Colorado in the early 1980s was approximately 3 million inhabitants. In the most recent season (1999–2000), nearly 300,000 persons were immunized in alternative sites and physicians in traditional sites immunized more than 1 million persons. As seen in Table 1, as the number of persons immunized in alternative sites increased, the number of cases and number of deaths reported to and by the Colorado Department of Health decreased. This, in spite of the fact that our total population has grown during this period from just under 3 million to approximately 4.5 million (US Census data). In other words, by having an intense publicity campaign, patients were informed about influenza, its complications and costs, and were encouraged to talk to their physician about their candidacy for vaccine. From our earlier research, we learned that patients in general wait for a physician to offer vaccine [4]. When it is not offered it is often not accepted. Our strategy was to encourage patients to ask their physician about vaccine and actually ask to receive it. Although early in our campaign physicians were very

Table 1
Impact of alternative vaccination sites in Colorado

Year	1985–1986	1988–1989	1993–1994	1996–1997	1999–2000
Vaccinated	33,322	64,337	197,033	213,567	280,482
Cases reported	16,300	15,369	4951	1798	1200
Deaths	1750	1300	972	980	803
Rate/100,000[a]	>15.0	>14.5	13.9	12.5	<12.0

[a] Rates are estimates due to data processing in progress.

skeptical about our motives and were in general nonsupportive, they feared the coalition was competing for their patients, they are now very enthusiastic as documented by an increase of more than 900,000 persons receiving vaccines in physician offices in a single year (1999–2000). The excess number of patients receiving vaccines in a private practice setting over the 16 years is likely to be several million.

There were other impacts as well. As more persons received the vaccine, the absolute number of cases reported to the Colorado Department of Health decreased from more than 30,000 to less than 2000. Furthermore, the number of deaths the Colorado Department of Health reports to the Centers for Disease Control in Atlanta decreased substantially (Table 1) in spite of a population growth of more than 25%.

In summary, by forming a coalition of concerned health providers, business persons, media representatives, insurance executives, and by having physicians willing to be visible and vocal on television, radio, and electronic print media, we have been able to convince an entire US state to become concerned with and sensitive to the issues concerning influenza. Children were encouraged to talk with their parents and grand-parents about receiving vaccine. Vaccine was made available in alternative sites. Nurses administered vaccine and a physician prescription was not required. We were even able to convince the federal government to permit electronic billing for persons covered by Medicare. Financial support to provide brochures, posters, telephone lines, newspaper advertisements, television reminders during prime time, and even a Volkswagen (with influenza messages all over its surface) were obtained from individual contributors, government grants, and donations from the pharmaceutical industry. In-kind contributions from volunteers, television stations broadcasting flu messages, brewing companies, and others helped us accomplish our goals. Coalition members were not paid, but their respective employers permitted them to work for the coalition and for the project.

Acknowledgements

The author wishes to acknowledge the 80-member coalition (Colorado Influenza and Pneumonia Alert Committee — CIPAC), but in particular Catherine O'Grady, RN, of the Visiting Nurses Association for her tireless efforts, encouragement, and support.

References

[1] Prevention and control of influenza: recommendations of the Advisory Committee on Immunization Practices (ACIP), MMWR, 49 (RR-3) (2000).
[2] Surveillance for influenza — United States, 1994–1995, 1995–1996, and 1996–1997 seasons, MMWR, 49 (SS-3) (2000).
[3] S.R. Mostow, Influenza: a preventable disease not being prevented, Am. Rev. Respir. Dis. 134 (1986) 1.
[4] S.R. Mostow, Community prevention of influenza in Colorado, Colo. Med. 89 (1992) 376.

International Congress Series 1219 (2001) 707–711

Antibody responses in elderly to influenza vaccination in case of an antigenic mismatch

J.C. de Jong[a,*], W.E.P. Beyer[a], A.M. Palache[b], G.F. Rimmelzwaan[a], A.D.M.E. Osterhaus[a]

[a]Department of Virology and WHO National Influenza Centre, Erasmus University, Dr. Molewaterplein 50, 3015 GE Rotterdam, The Netherlands
[b]Solvay Pharmaceuticals, Weesp, The Netherlands

Abstract

Background: The vigour of immune responses declines at higher ages. The present study examined sera from influenza vaccinees to assess the magnitude of this effect in case of an antigenic mismatch. *Methods*: Sera taken in mid-1997 from influenza vaccinees of various ages, including residents of nursing homes, were used in haemagglutination inhibition (HI) tests. In the following influenza season of 1997/1998, a major antigenic mismatch of the H3N2 vaccine component occurred. *Results*: At advanced age, the homologous antibody response was lowered, starting above 60 years. Also, the cross-reactivity of the formed antibodies to the drifted field virus decreased with age, starting above 70 years. *Conclusion*: The effect of ageing on the induction of "protective" titres (≥ 40) of HI antibodies against an emerging deviant strain can be severe: in the 1997/1998 season, above 80 years, the percentage of vaccinees acquiring such titres against the major epidemic H3N2 virus was only about 15%. © 2001 Elsevier Science B.V. All rights reserved.

Keywords: Influenza vaccine efficacy; Cross-reactive antibodies

1. Introduction

The efficiency of antiviral immunity decreases with rising age. The present study investigated the possible consequences of this phenomenon for the protection provided by influenza vaccination against homologous and drifted viruses. A preliminary report has been published [1].

* Corresponding author. Tel.: +31-10-408-8066; fax: +31-10-408-9484.
E-mail address: jc.de.jong@wxs.nl (J.C. de Jong).

0531-5131/01/$ – see front matter © 2001 Elsevier Science B.V. All rights reserved.
PII: S0531-5131(01)00392-2

2. Materials and methods

During influenza vaccination studies performed in mid-1997, sera were obtained from vaccinees of various ages, including residents of nursing homes over 60 years of age. As a surrogate marker for induction of protection by influenza vaccination, we studied the haemagglutination inhibition (HI) antibody response of the vaccinees to vaccine and epidemic strains of the three (sub)types A(H3N2), A(H1N1), and B. Statistical methods included the paired t-test, the McNemar χ^2-test, the one-way ANOVA, the Pearson χ^2-test, and a "minimum-maximum" analysis, newly developed by Dr G. Lüchters from Bonn. In accordance with usual practice, the "50% protective threshold" of HI antibodies was set at ≥ 40.

3. Results

In mid-1997 in Australia and in 1997/1998 in the northern hemisphere, unexpectedly, an H3N2 variant, A/Sydney/5/97 ("Syd"), emerged, which deviated considerably from the H3N2 vaccine virus RESVIR-9, a reassortant of A/Wuhan/359/95 ("Wu") [2]. We examined the vaccination responses in 1997 against the homologous vaccine strain ("Wuhan-vaccine") two 1997/1998 H3N2 virus isolates from Netherlands, one like the old A/Wuhan/359/95 strain ("Wu-field/97+") and the other like the new A/Sydney/5/97 strain ("Syd-field/97+") (Table 1). As expected, homologous antibody responses proved to decrease with increasing age of the vaccinees (Table 2 and Fig. 1). Antibody titres against Syd-field/97+ were on an average 7.6-fold lower than those against Wuhan-vaccine. This cross-reactivity ratio proved to be age-dependent. Below 80 years of age, the ratio Wuhan-vaccine/Sydney-field was on an average about 6.8, at higher ages 11.9 (Table 2). The newly developed "minimum–maximum analysis" revealed a turning-point at 67 years of age (95% CI: 47 to 87). It indicated a plateau of 6.6-fold for the ratio W/F below this age, whereas above 67 years, the ratio progressively deteriorated to 15.2-fold (Fig. 2).

The impact of the antigenic mismatch on the proportions of subjects with "protective" postvaccination HI titres ≥ 40 against the H3N2 vaccine strain and

Table 1

Cross-reactivities of vaccine and field influenza A(H3N2) virus strains in the 1997/1998 season as assessed using ferret antisera

Influenza virus strain	HI titres of postinfection ferret antisera to:		
	Wuhan-vaccine (RESVIR-9)	Wu-field/97+[a] (N/005/98 –)	Syd-field/97+ (N/300/97+)
Wuhan-vaccine	1280[b]	1280	40
Wu-field/97+	320	1280	80
Syd-field/97+	80	320	2560

[a] "97+" as well as "98 –" designates the 1997/1998 season.
[b] Homologous titres are underlined and in bold type.

Table 2
Postvaccination geometric mean titres (95% CI) and Wu-v/Syd-f quotient (post-GMT against Wuhan-vaccine/post-GMT against Sydney-field)

Age class years	N	Antigens used in the HI titrations			
		Wuhan-vaccine	Wuhan-field	Sydney-field	Wu-v/Syd-f
19–59	48	794 (592–1066)	731 (540–990)	111 (78–156)	7.2 (5.9–8.8)
60–79	66	261 (194–352)	450 (321–631)	40 (29–56)	6.5 (5.0–8.4)
80–99	30	171 (118–248)	155 (111–218)	14 (11–19)	11.9 (8.5–16.6)
All ages	144	346 (282–426)	424 (342–525)	45 (36–57)	7.6 (6.5–8.9)
P*		<0.001	<0.001	<0.001	0.010

* P-values were calculated by one-way ANOVA.

the major H3N2 field strain is given in Fig. 3. The rate for the field strain appeared significantly lower in the age group 60 to 79 years and deteriorated even further in the age group of 80 to 99 years, resulting in a seriously impaired protection of the

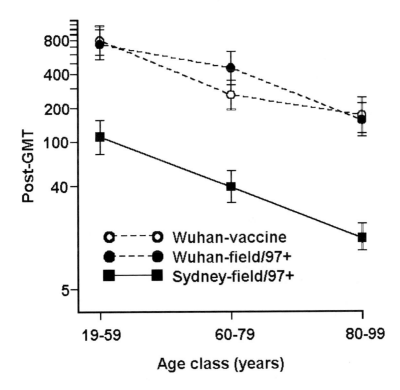

Fig. 1. Postvaccination geometric mean HI titres to H3N2 vaccine and the major H3N2-epidemic ("field") influenza virus strain in the 1997/1998 season according to three age classes. The vertical bars indicate the 95% confidence intervals.

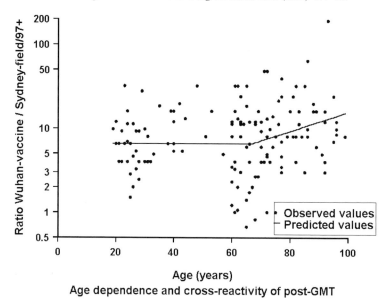

Age dependence and cross-reactivity of post-GMT

Fig. 2. Ratios of the HI titres of individual postvaccination sera against the H3N2 vaccine strain and the major H3N2 field strain in the 1997/1998 season (dots), and the corresponding values calculated by the statistical minimum–maximum method (lines).

latter individuals against the field strain, namely about 13% on an average (95% confidence interval 4–31%).

4. Discussion

In 1997, the influenza H3N2 vaccination antibody response to the deviant H3N2 field strain of 1997/1998 was found to be impaired in the elderly in three ways:

1. Antigenic distance between vaccine and field strain;
2. Reduction of homologous antibody response, starting above 60 years;
3. Reduction of cross-reactivity of vaccine-induced antibodies to the deviant strain, starting above 70 years.

The mechanism of the decline of cross-reactivity may have been the deteriorating ability of the immune system of older individuals to mount effective antibody levels to new antigens [3,4]. It should be noted that the reductions mentioned do not invariably occur. We also titrated the vaccinee sera used for the present study against the H1N1 and B components of the administered influenza vaccine and against H1N1 and B field viruses, which emerged in the 1999/2000 and 1998/1999 seasons, respectively. In these

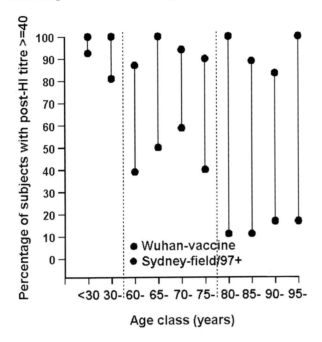

Fig. 3. Proportions of subjects with postvaccination HI titres ≥ 40 in the 1997/1998 season according to 10 age classes. Circles at the upper ends of the vertical bars refer to the H3N2 vaccine strain and circles at the bottom ends to the major H3N2 field strain.

two cases, no decline of the homologous responses, nor decline of the cross-reactivity with increasing age, was observed (data not shown).

Acknowledgements

The authors thank R. van Beek, M. Baars, and L.J. van der Kemp for their excellent technical assistance.

References

[1] J.C. De Jong, W.E.P. Beyer, A.M. Palache, G.F. Rimmelzwaan, A.D.M.E. Osterhaus, Mismatch between the 1997/1998 influenza vaccine and the major epidemic A(H3N2) virus strain as the cause of an inadequate vaccine-induced antibody response to this strain in the elderly, J. Med. Virol. 61 (2000) 94–99.
[2] Anonymous, Recommended composition of influenza virus vaccines for use in the 1998–1999 season, Wkly. Epidemiol. Rec. 73 (1998) 56–61.
[3] W.E.P. Beyer, A.M. Palanche, M. Baljet, N. Masurel, Antibody induction by influenza vaccines in the elderly: a review of the literature, Vaccine 7 (1989) 385–394.
[4] J.E. McElhaney, G.S. Meneilly, K.E. Lechelt, B.L. Beattie, R.C. Bleackley, Antibody response to whole-virus and split-virus influenza vaccines in successful ageing, Vaccine 11 (1993) 1055–1060.

International Congress Series 1219 (2001) 713–721

Influenza vaccination is less effective for stimulating a Granzyme B response in older adults

Caroline R. Letter, Stefan Gravenstein, Janet E. McElhaney*

Glennan Center for Geriatrics and Gerontology, Eastern Virginia Medical School, 825 Fairfax Avenue, Suite 201, Norfolk, VA 23507, USA

Abstract

Cytotoxic T lymphocyte (CTL) activity against influenza declines with age and is only partially improved with influenza vaccination. Granzyme B (Grz B) is a key enzyme in CTL-mediated killing of virus-infected cells. The purpose of this study was to determine age-related differences in the number of virus-specific precursor CTL (pCTL) and Grz B levels after influenza vaccination. Our hypothesis was that Grz B is less effectively stimulated by killed-virus vaccines in older compared to young adults. We measured pCTL frequency by enzyme-linked immunospot (ELISPOT) and Grz B levels in lysates of peripheral blood mononuclear cells (PBMC) stimulated with live influenza virus under ex vivo and in vitro conditions. Prior to influenza vaccination, healthy young and older adults had similar levels of Grz B in A/Sydney-stimulated PBMC. Four weeks after vaccination, the Grz B levels in PBMC from young adults were significantly higher than PBMC from older adults (young, 6.35 U/mg protein; older, 2.94 U/mg protein; $p < 0.0001$). Young adults had a higher proportion of pCTL compared to older adults ($p < 0.001$), but the two groups had a similar increase in the number of pCTL in response to vaccination (pre to post: young, 0.44–0.50%; older, 0.36–0.44% of PBMC). The level of Grz B per pCTL in young adults showed a 3.4-fold rise compared to a 1.7-fold rise in older adults in response to vaccination. We conclude that vaccination with killed virus is more effective in young compared to older adults for restimulating a previously primed response to influenza, but only weakly stimulates virus-specific pCTL. © 2001 Elsevier Science B.V. All rights reserved.

Keywords: Granzyme B; Cytotoxic T lymphocytes; Influenza vaccination; Aging

* Corresponding author. Tel.: +1-757-446-7040; fax: +1-757-446-7049.
E-mail address: mcelhaje@evms.edu (J.E. McElhaney).

0531-5131/01/$ – see front matter © 2001 Elsevier Science B.V. All rights reserved.
PII: S 0 5 3 1 - 5 1 3 1 (0 1) 0 0 3 4 0 - 5

1. Introduction

Influenza vaccination is recommended for all persons age 50 years and above and is a cost-saving medical intervention in older adults due to the prevention of serious complications of influenza illness [1]. However, the current parenteral, inactivated vaccines are only 50–60% effective in preventing illness and may offer little protection for institutionalized older adults [2]. The increased susceptibility to complications of influenza infections and the decline in vaccine efficacy in older adults has been attributed to diminished T-cell responses, rather than a primary B-cell defect.

The effect of aging on the cytotoxic T lymphocyte (CTL) response to influenza vaccination results in decreased peak CTL activity in older people, while the duration of the CTL response appears similar to the young adult population [3]. While inactivated influenza vaccines stimulate CTL responses in adults who have been previously primed by exposure to influenza virus, this response is not as robust in older adults and may be related to changes in CTL function.

Granzyme B (Grz B) is a key enzyme in CTL-mediated killing of virus-infected host cells and is contained in granules within CTL [4,5]. Upon activation of CTL, granules are transported to the point of contact with the target cell and the contents are released into the intercellular space. Grz B is ultimately transported to the nucleus of the target cell as part of the catalytic cascade that leads to DNA fragmentation and apoptotic cell death [6]. The unique substrate specificity of Grz B is used in an enzymatic assay of its activity [7] where cleavage of the substrate, N-t-butyloxycar-bonyl-L-alanyl-L-alanyl-L-aspartyl-paranitroanilide, results in colorimetric change in the assay. We have correlated Grz B levels in influenza virus-stimulated peripheral blood mononuclear cell (PBMC) cultures with cytolytic activity in a chromium (^{51}Cr) release assay [8].

Traditional assays of the CTL response to influenza vaccination in people require restimulation of CTL, such that proliferation and differentiation under in vitro conditions may not reflect the in vivo response to vaccination. Using in vitro restimulation, both Grz B assays and the labor-intensive technique of ^{51}Cr-release assays for measuring cytolytic activity have shown an age-related decline in the CTL response to influenza vaccination [3]. Studies of CTL responses using ex vivo cultures have been limited and have not included older adults. The purpose of this study was to measure the age-related changes in the number of virus-specific precursor CTL (pCTL), and Grz B levels in ex vivo cultures as measures of the CTL response to influenza vaccination.

2. Methods

2.1. Subjects

PBMC were obtained from 10 healthy young (median age, 37.5 years; range, 19–46 years; three males, seven females) and older (median age, 73 years; range, 63–83 years, four males, six females) adults prior to and 4 weeks after vaccination. Subjects were screened and excluded from the study for the following: acute illness occurring within 72 h before enrollment; any known or suspected allergy to eggs, thimerosal or formaldehyde; pregnancy; or immunosuppressant medication. All subjects received the 1999–2000 influenza vaccine that contained 15-μg each of A/Beijing/262/95 (H_1N_1), A/Sydney/5/97 (H_3N_2), and B/Beijing/184/93 (Pasteur Merieux Connaught, Swiftwater, PA). Blood samples (30 cc) were collected prevaccination and 4 weeks postvaccination.

2.2. Ex vivo and in vitro stimulation

PBMC were isolated from venous blood samples using ficoll-hypaque gradient purification and resuspended in AIM V medium (Gibco, Grand Island, NY). Cell cultures were prepared at a concentration of 1.5×10^6 PBMC/ml and stimulated with each of three live H_3N_2 strains of influenza virus (A/Sydney/5/97, A/Nanchang/933/95, A/Johannesburg/33/94) at 10^5 $TCID_{50}$/ml. Recombinant human interleukin-7 (IL-7) was also added to ex vivo cultures at 25 ng/ml to shorten the period over which activation occurs and thus increase peak CTL activity [9]. PBMC cultures were incubated at 37 °C, 5% CO_2 and harvested after 17 h (ex vivo cultures) or 6 days (in vitro cultures). PBMC were pelleted from the cultures and lysed with 100 μl of lysis buffer (1% Triton X-100/150 mM NaCl/15 mM Tris–HCl, pH 8.0). Three freeze–thaw cycles were used to ensure complete lysis. Cell lysates were frozen at -80 °C until the time of assay for Grz B activity. Cell nuclei were pelleted from the lysate by centrifugation at $250 \times g$ for 10 min at 4 °C before removing aliquots of lysate for the Grz B assay.

2.3. Granzyme B assay

The assay was modified from our previously published method [8]. Triplicate samples containing 10 μl of cell lysate were prepared in a 200-μl reaction volume (0.1 M Hepes pH 7.5, 10 mM $CaCl_2$) containing 4 mM of the substrate, *t*-butyloxycarbonyl-Ala-Ala-Asp-paranitroanilide (BAADpna; BACHEM, Torrance, CA) and incubated for 20 h at room temperature. Cleavage of the substrate by Grz B at the aspartate residue (ASPase activity) releases the paranitroaniline that forms a colored product detected at 405 nm using a microtiter plate reader (PowerWave X, Bio-Tek Instruments) using KC4 (Kinetcalc for Windows). The amount of protein in each PBMC lysate was determined using the BCA (bicinchoninic acid) assay (Pierce, Rockford, IL). ASPase activity was calculated as A_{405}/mg protein in the PBMC lysate. Unstimulated PMBC (17 h and day 6) were included as negative controls and gave a reading equivalent to the background. PBMC stimulated with 10 μg/ml concanavalin A (Con A) were included as positive controls.

2.4. Interferon-γ ELIspot assay

Enzyme-linked immunospot (ELIspot) assays were performed pre- and postvaccination on 6 of 10 study participants [10]. PBMC were prepared at concentrations of 1×10^6 cells/ml and incubated with anti-CD4 Dynabeads (Dynal, Lake Success, NY) and anti-CD56 coated Pan Mouse IgG Dynabeads (PharMingen International, San

Diego, CA) (Dynal) to remove helper T cells (CD4+) and natural killer (NK) cells from PBMC to yield CD8+, CD56-, CD4-PBMC for the ELIspot assay. Ninety-six well nitrocellulose plates (Millititer, Millipore, Bedford, MA) were coated with 50 μl mouse anti-human interferon-γ (INF-γ) monoclonal antibody (Mabtech, Stockholm, Sweden) overnight at 4 °C, washed with phosphate buffered saline (PBS) supplemented with 0.25% Tween 20 (Sigma, St. Louis, MO) and blocked with PBS supplemented with 5% fetal bovine serum for 30 min at 37 °C. One hundred microliters of RPMI 1640 (Gibco) supplemented with 10% human AB serum, 2 mM L-glutamine, 50 μM β-mercaptoethanol, 100 units/ml penicillin and 100 μg/ml streptomycin sulfate were added to the plates and incubated for 10 min, diluting any remains of Tween 20. Serial 1:2 dilutions of the CD8+, CD4-, CD56-PBMC starting with 5×10^5/ml, were stimulated with influenza A/Sydney (H$_3$N$_2$), A/Nanchang (H$_3$N$_2$), and A/Johannesburg (H$_3$N$_2$) at 10^5 TCID$_{50}$/ml and 25 ng/ml IL-7 and incubated for 17 h (37 °C, 5% CO$_2$) in antibody-coated plates. Serial dilutions of unstimulated PMBC- and Con A-stimulated PBMC were similarly prepared as negative and positive controls. Plates were washed 13 times with the PBS/Tween 20 solution and incubated with 50 μl/well of biotinylated polyclonal mouse anti-human IFN-γ antibody (Mabtech) for 2 h at 22 °C. The assay was completed with six washes of PBS/Tween 20, a 2-h incubation at 22 °C in 100 μl/well of avidin-horseradish peroxidase (Sigma) (1 μg/ml), six washes with PBS/Tween 20, a 30-min incubation at 22 °C in 25 μl/well of aminoethyl carbazole solution (Sigma) incubated for 30 min at 22 °C, and three washes with distilled water to stop color development. The colored spots on air-dried plates were counted using a stereomicroscope.

2.5. Statistical analysis

Comparisons between the young and older adult groups used the Mann–Whitney U-test. Comparisons of pre- to postvaccination changes and the difference between virus strains were analyzed by an analysis of variance (ANOVA) within each of the age groups. The statistical package used was Statview 5.1 (Abacus concepts).

2.6. Ethics approval

This protocol and consent form were reviewed and approved by the Institutional Review Board at Eastern Virginia Medical School, Norfolk, VA.

3. Results

The ex vivo CTL response to influenza vaccination was measured according to changes in virus-specific CTL frequency and Grz B levels in virus-activated PBMC from healthy young and older adults. For the determination of virus-specific pCTL frequency by the ELISPOT assay, other potential IFN-γ-producing PBMC (Th and NK cells) were removed from the cultures by negative selection so that only remaining IFN-γ-producing cells were virus-activated CTL. Our previous experiments using negative selection to remove CD56+

and CD4+ cells, or CD8+ cells, showed that Grz B activity in ex vivo cultures resides in measurable amounts only in the CD8+ subset of PBMC (data not shown). Thus, the measurement of the CTL response using an assay of Grz B activity in virus-activated PBMC did not require cell separation.

Virus-specific pCTL frequency was signifcantly higher in the young compared to the older adult group for each of the three strains of virus at both the pre- and postvaccination time points ($p < 0.001$ for all comparisons, Mann–Whitney U-test) (Fig. 1). There was a statistically significant, albeit limited response to vaccination ($p < 0.0001$, ANOVA) with a similar absolute increase in the number of virus-specific CTL in the two age groups for each of the three influenza A/H_3N_2 strains. Three different H_3N_2 strains of influenza with presumed cross-reactivity for the CTL epitopes were used activate (ex vivo) or stimulate (in vitro) CTL. However, a comparison of the response to the three H_3N_2 strains showed incomplete cross-reactivity; lower pCTL frequencies were observed in cultures stimulated with the older compared to more recently circulating A/H_3N_2 strains of virus (A/Sydney > A/Nanchang > A/Johannesburg; $p < 0.0001$, ANOVA with Bonnferoni–Dunn correction).

Grz B activity measured in ex vivo PBMC from the young and older adult groups showed similar prevaccination levels for each of the three strains of virus (Fig. 2). Postvaccination, Grz B levels increased significantly in both age groups for all three strains of virus ($p < 0.0001$ for all comparisons, ANOVA). However, the amount of increase in Grz B levels was dependent on age and virus strain. The young compared to the older adult group had significantly higher levels of Grz B at 4 weeks postvaccination

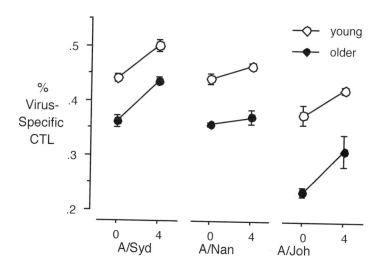

Fig. 1. The percent of IFN-γ-producing CD8+ cells in ex vivo (17 h), influenza virus-activated PBMC are shown as the mean % virus-specific pCTL from six young and six older adults. Results for the three different H_3N_2 strains at pre (0 weeks) and post (4 weeks) vaccination time points are shown. CD56+ and CD4+ cells were removed from the culture. Error bars represent 95% confidence intervals. The effects of age, vaccination and virus strain were all statistically significant in the analysis.

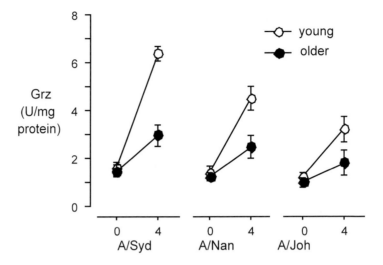

Fig. 2. Grz B activity in ex vivo (17 h), influenza virus-activated PBMC are shown as the mean U/mg protein from 10 young and 10 older adults. Results for the three different H_3N_2 strains at pre- (0 weeks) and post- (4 weeks) vaccination time points are shown. Error bars represent 95% confidence intervals. Postvaccination results were statistically different between the two age groups and the three strains of virus.

for each of the stimulating strains of virus ($p < 0.0001$ for A/Sydney, $p = 0.0006$ for A/Nanchang, and $p = 0.003$ for A/Johannesburg; Mann–Whitney U-test). A comparison between the three strains of virus showed the greatest increase in Grz B in cultures

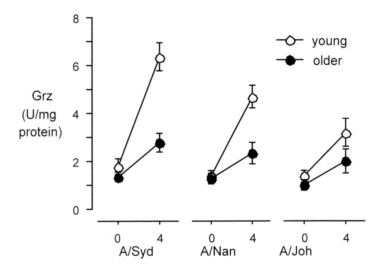

Fig. 3. In vitro Grz B activity (6 days), influenza virus-stimulated PBMC are shown as the mean U/mg protein from 10 young and 10 older adults. Results for the three different H_3N_2 strains at pre (0 weeks) and post (4 weeks) vaccination time points are shown. Error bars represent 95% confidence intervals. Postvaccination results were statistically different between the two age groups and the three strains of virus.

stimulated with the vaccinating strain of virus, A/Sydney. By comparison, there was a significantly weaker response and older A/H$_3$N$_2$ strains stimulated lower postvaccination levels of Grz B, again demonstrating incomplete cross-reactivity between the strains ($p < 0.0001$ for all comparisons, ANOVA).

Grz B levels of in vitro cultures were similar to those measured ex vivo for both age groups and the three stimulating strains of virus (Fig. 3) and the statistical significance of the results were similar to those for the ex vivo data. Earlier experiments showing that in vitro Grz B levels correlate with cytotoxicity, suggest that the ex vivo data would also be correlated with ^{51}Cr-release assays in virus-activated PBMC. Using negative selection, we have previously shown that a small portion of the Grz B activity of in vitro cultures may be derived from other cell populations, such as CD4+ and NK, in addition to CD8+ cells in these proliferating virus-stimulated cultures. These observations contrast with the ex vivo experiments, in which all of the measurable Grz B activity in virus-activated PBMC is within the CD8+ population.

The amount of Grz B activity per virus-specific pCTL was calculated to examine the potential qualitative effect of vaccination on CTL function. In the young adult population, there was a 3.4-fold increase in the amount of Grz B activity produced on a per pCTL basis, while the level increased only 1.7-fold in the older adult population (Fig. 4) for stimulation with the A/Sydney strain ($p = 0.004$, Mann–Whitney U-test). Grz B activity per pCTL after vaccination showed the greatest degree of stimulation with the vaccinating strain of virus and decreased with the older strains (A/Sydney>A/Nanchang = A/Johannesburg) again reflecting incomplete cross-reactivity of the Grz B response to vaccination across the three H$_3$N$_2$ strains.

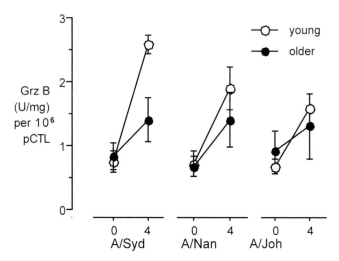

Fig. 4. Grz B activity calculated according to the number of virus-specific pCTL in ex vivo (17 h) cultures in influenza virus-activated PBMC, are shown for six young and older adults. Results for the three different H$_3$N$_2$ strains at pre (0 weeks) and post (4 weeks) vaccination time points are shown. Error bars represent 95% confidence intervals. Only the postvaccination results for A/Sydney were significantly different between the two age groups ($p = 0.004$).

4. Discussion

Prior to vaccination, young compared to older adults had higher pCTL frequencies for all H_3N_2 strains with similar levels of Grz B production. Lower pCTL frequencies and Grz B levels were observed with the older circulating strains of virus compared to more recently circulating strains of influenza, suggesting that there is a gradual strain-specific decline in pCTL frequency over a period of at least 5 years. This data is consistent with previously published estimates of the duration of CTL memory in young adults [11]. This decline may be more rapid in older compared to young adults. The lack of a cross-reactive response to vaccination in both age groups is inconsistent with the known cross-reactivity CTL epitopes between different virus strains within influenza A or B [12].

Vaccination with a split-virus (killed) vaccine stimulated a limited CTL response with respect to the increase in pCTL frequency in both young and older adults. This result is predicted from the theoretical requirement for viral peptides to be derived from replicating virus for presentation on the class I major histocompatibility complex (MHC I) to stimulate CTL. More recently, it has been recognized that antigen presentation of peptides derived from killed virus may occur through nonclassical pathways and is presumed to be the mechanism by which killed vaccines stimulate CTL [13]. The nonclassical pathway may be the mechanism by which the vaccine stimulates a significant Grz B response in primed individuals. These results suggest two different mechanisms for stimulating the CTL response to vaccination, one for stimulating the limited increase in pCTL frequency and another for increasing Grz B levels within activated CTL, the latter being less effectively stimulated in older compared to young adults. Also, the mechanism for stimulating Grz B appears to be more strain-specific than the mechanism for increasing in pCTL frequency.

The difference in the Grz B response to vaccination between young and older adults in this study parallels clinical observations of age-related changes in influenza vaccine efficacy where, in both cases, there is $\sim 50\%$ reduction with age. We have also shown in a larger parallel study that there was no significant difference between young and older adults in the postvaccination antibody titers to A/Sydney with the same preparation of influenza vaccine (unpublished results) suggesting that antibody titers may not be a useful surrogate of vaccine efficacy. Because ex vivo activation of CTL provides a model for the initial in vivo response to influenza challenge, and is the least affected by the function of other cells in PBMC cultures, ex vivo Grz B levels may be preferable to in vitro cultures for measuring a cellular response to influenza vaccination.

In summary, an ex vivo assay of Grz B activity provides a relatively simple assay of the CTL response to influenza vaccination and is a likely candidate as a surrogate for vaccine efficacy that could be used to test new vaccines in older adults.

References

[1] Centers for Disease Control Prevention and Control of Influenza, Update: Influenza activity—United States, and worldwide, 1999–2000 season and composition of the 2000–2001 influenza vaccine. Practices Advisory Committee, JAMA, J. Am. Med. Assoc. 283 (2000) 2781–2783.

[2] P.A. Gross, A.W. Hermogenes, H.C. Sacks, J. Lau, R.A. Levandowski, The efficacy of influenza vaccine in the elderly persons, Ann. Intern. Med. 123 (1995) 518–527.

[3] D.C. Powers, R.B. Belshe, Effect of age on cytotoxic T lymphocte memory as well as serum and local antibody responses elicited by inactivated influenza virus vaccine, J. Infect. Dis. 167 (1993) 584–592.

[4] M.M. Simon, M. Hausmann, T. Tran, et al., In vitro- and ex vivo-derived cytolytic leukocytes from granzyme A × B double knockout mice are defective in granule-mediated apoptosis but not lysis of target cells, J. Exp. Med. 186 (1997) 1781–1786.

[5] P.C. Doherty, D.J. Topham, R.A. Tripp, R.D. Cardin, J.W. Brooks, P.G. Stevenson, Effector CD4+ and CD8+ T-cell mechanisms in the control of respiratory virus infections, Immunol. Rev. 159 (1997) 105–117.

[6] A.J. Darmon, D.W. Nicholson, R.C. Bleackley, Activation of the apoptotic protease CPP32 by cytotoxic T-cell-derived granzyme B, Nature 377 (1995) 446–448.

[7] S. Odake, C.M. Kam, L. Narasimhan, M. Poe, J.T. Blake, O. Krahenbuhl, J. Tschopp, J.C. Powers, Human and murine cytotoxic T lymphocyte serine proteases: subsite mapping with peptide thioester substrates and inhibition of enzyme activity and cytolysis by isocoumarins, Biochemistry 30 (1991) 2217–2227.

[8] J.E. McElhaney, M.J. Pinkoski, C.M. Upshaw, R.C. Bleackley, The cell mediated cytotoxic response to influenza vaccination using an assay for granzyme B activity, J. Immunol. Methods 190 (1996) 11–20.

[9] A. Lalvani, T. Dong, G. Ogg, A.A. Pathan, H. Newell, A.V. Hill, A.J. McMicheal, S. Rowland-Jones, Optimization of a peptide-based protocol employing IL-7 for in vitro restimulation of human cytotoxic T lymphocyte precursors, J. Immunol. Methods 210 (1997) 65–77.

[10] C. Czerkinsky, Z. Moldoveanu, J. Mestecky, L.-A. Nilsson, O. Ouchterlony, A novel two colour ELISPOT assay: I. Simultaneous detection of distinct types of antibody-secreting cells, J. Immunol. Methods 155 (1988) 31–37.

[11] A.J. McMichael, F.M. Gotch, G.R. Noble, P.A. Beare, Cytotoxic T-cell immunity to influenza, N. Engl. J. Med. 309 (1983) 13–37.

[12] J.W. Yewdell, J.R. Bennink, G.L. Smith, B. Moss, Influenza virus nucleoprotein is a major target antigen for cross-reactive anti-influenza A virus cytotoxic T lymphocytes, Proc. Natl. Acad. Sci. U. S. A. 82 (1985) 1785–1789.

[13] A. Bender, L.K. Bui, M.A. Feldman, M. Larsson, N. Bhardwaj, Inactivated influenza virus, when presented on dendritic cells, elicits human CD8+ cytolytic T cell responses, J. Exp. Med. 182 (1995) 1663–1671.

International Congress Series 1219 (2001) 723–731

The epidemiology of influenza vaccination: implications for global vaccine supply for an influenza pandemic

David S. Fedson*

Aventis Pasteur MSD, 8, rue Jonas Salk, 69367 Lyon Cedex 07, France

Keywords: Influenza; Vaccination; Pandemic

The societal benefits of influenza vaccination are firmly established [1]. Among elderly persons, vaccination reduces both hospitalization for influenza-associated respiratory conditions and all-cause mortality. Among healthy working adults, schoolchildren and pre-schoolchildren, vaccination prevents influenza-related respiratory illness and work and school absence. In pre-schoolchildren it also reduces the occurrence of otitis media. For people of all ages, influenza vaccination is highly cost-effective. Nonetheless, the full benefits of influenza vaccination have not been achieved. If this is to occur, one requirement will be a better understanding of the epidemiology of influenza vaccination.

Other reports in this volume address issues related to influenza vaccination by individual practitioners or within regions of individual countries. This article focuses on the comparative use of influenza vaccine in different countries. Three earlier publications document vaccine use for the period 1980 to 1997 [2–4]. Information on vaccination in 1998 has also been presented [5]. Understanding the changing patterns of vaccine use in interpandemic years has been useful. It is likely to be even more helpful in planning for vaccine use in the event of an influenza pandemic.

1. Influenza vaccine use in individual countries, 1999–2000

Fig. 1 shows the use of influenza vaccine in Western Europe, the United States, Canada and Australia during the period July 1, 1999 to June 30, 2000. Although all of these

---

* Tel.: +33-4-37-28-40-60; fax: +33-4-37-28-44-11.

E-mail address: dfedson@fr.aventis-pasteur-msd.com (D.S. Fedson).

PII: S0531-5131(01)00657-4

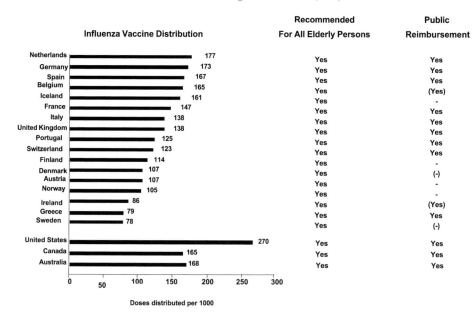

Influenza Vaccine Distribution	Recommended For All Elderly Persons	Public Reimbursement
Netherlands 177	Yes	Yes
Germany 173	Yes	Yes
Spain 167	Yes	Yes
Belgium 165	Yes	(Yes)
Iceland 161	Yes	-
France 147	Yes	Yes
Italy 138	Yes	Yes
United Kingdom 138	Yes	Yes
Portugal 125	Yes	Yes
Switzerland 123	Yes	Yes
Finland 114	Yes	-
Denmark 107	Yes	(-)
Austria 107	Yes	-
Norway 105	Yes	-
Ireland 86	Yes	(Yes)
Greece 79	Yes	Yes
Sweden 78	Yes	(-)
United States 270	Yes	Yes
Canada 165	Yes	Yes
Australia 168	Yes	Yes

Doses distributed per 1000

Fig. 1. Influenza vaccine use in Western Europe, the United States, Canada and Australia in 1999–2000. Vaccine use is shown as the estimated number of doses distributed per 1000 total population. Vaccine data were provided by Aventis Pasteur MSD and by Marika Iwane, Centers for Disease Control and Prevention, Atlanta, GA. For Canada, data for 1998 are shown because 1999 data were not available. Elderly persons were those ≥ 65 years in age except for Belgium, Germany and Iceland (≥ 60), France (≥ 70) and the United Kingdom (≥ 75). In Denmark and Sweden, publicly supported programs for influenza vaccination were conducted in Copenhagen and Stockholm.

countries had age-based recommendations for older adults, those without some form of public reimbursement tended to use less vaccine. For calendar year 1999, substantial vaccine use was also reported for several other countries: in South America—Argentina, Uruguay, Brazil, Chile and Mexico; in Central and Eastern Europe—Russia, Poland, Latvia, Slovakia, the Czech Republic and Estonia; in the Middle East—Tunisia and Lebanon; in East Asia—the Republic of Korea, Japan, Taiwan and Hong Kong; and in South Africa. In all other countries for which data are available, little if any influenza vaccine was used.

It is important to recognize that influenza vaccine is produced in only a few countries [6]. In the United States, three companies produce influenza vaccine and in Canada there is one producer. In Western Europe, Italy has three producers, Germany has two and Austria, Belgium, France, the United Kingdom, the Netherlands and Switzerland have one each. There are no vaccine producers in Ireland, Spain or Scandinavia. In Central and Eastern European, Russia is the main producer, and apparently there are small production facilities in Romania (2), Slovakia and the former Republic of Yugoslavia. In East Asia, there are at least six producers in Japan (1999) and one each in the Republic of Korea and Australia.

Not only are there few influenza vaccine producers, the production capacities of many producers are limited. To illustrate this, if it is assumed that each country with one or more vaccine producers obtained all of the doses it used in 1999–2000 from domestic

Table 1
Influenza vaccination outside Western Europe, North America and Australia, 1999

Region	Estimated number of doses distributed (000s)[a]	Source of vaccine supply (%)	
		Within region	Western Europe, North America or Australia
Central Europe, Eastern Europe and Russia[b]	12,581	59.1	40.9
East Asia	22,258	38.7	61.3
Latin America	19,115	1.1	98.9
Middle East and Africa	4495	–	100.0
Total	58,449	28.2	71.8

[a] Vaccine distribution data were provided by Aventis Pasteur.

[b] Includes Israel. No data were available on vaccine use in Belarus, Bulgaria, Moldova and the countries of Southeast Europe.

producers, only 10 countries could be considered self-sufficient: the United States, Belgium, France, Italy, the Netherlands, Switzerland, Australia, Russia, Japan and the Republic of Korea. For this reason, there is substantial international trade in influenza vaccines. Table 1 shows for 1999 the source of supply of the influenza vaccine used in countries outside Western Europe, North America and Australia. In Central and Eastern Europe and in Russia, almost all of the doses produced were used in Russia. Countries outside Russia had to import their vaccine. In East Asia, vaccine companies in Japan and Korea supplied their own domestic needs, yet almost two-thirds of the 22 million doses used in the region had to be imported. In Latin America, the Middle-East and Africa, virtually all of the vaccine used was imported.

2. Two lessons for vaccine supply for an influenza pandemic

In recent years, many countries have developed national plans for managing a future influenza pandemic [7]. The World Health Organization (WHO) has issued an important set of guidelines for national and regional pandemic preparedness planning [6]. Included in these guidelines are a set of points to consider regarding vaccine production and distribution. Unfortunately, there is little historical experience to tell us how the WHO guidelines for pandemic vaccine supply might be implemented. Experience in the United States in 1976, however, gives some indication of what to expect. In that year, the isolation of a Swine influenza virus from a military recruit who died of influenza eventually led to the national program to produce and administer a Swine influenza vaccine to a large proportion of the U.S. population [8]. Many problems arose as the program unfolded, including concerns among the vaccine producers about legal liability. The occurrence of Guillain Barré syndrome in vaccine recipients six weeks after the vaccination program began led to its abrupt cessation. Although only 45 million doses had been given, this decision was considered reasonable because by then there was no indication a pandemic would occur.

The 1976 Swine influenza experience provided at least two important lessons for the future supply of vaccine for a pandemic; one hopeful, the other disturbing. First, because American vaccine companies had been able to produce approximately 25 million doses of a trivalent, full-strength (45 μg HA antigen) vaccine in 1975, they were able to produce approximately 150 million doses of a monovalent, half-strength (7.5 μg HA) Swine influenza vaccine [8]. Second, because 150 million doses were insufficient to provide one dose for every person in the United States, the vaccine producers were not allowed to export Swine influenza vaccine to other countries.

3. Increasing influenza vaccine use in interpandemic years and its importance for vaccine supply in a pandemic

All health officials concerned with influenza pandemic preparedness planning acknowledge the importance of increasing the levels of vaccine use in interpandemic years before a pandemic actually arrives. Increasing the levels of interpandemic vaccine use leads vaccine companies to expand their production capacities. Furthermore, by increasing vaccine coverage, healthcare systems gain valuable experience in dealing with practical issues of vaccine delivery. For a pandemic, it is almost certain that a monovalent vaccine will be produced. If a dose of 15 μg HA is sufficient, the supply of a pandemic vaccine could be three times the number of doses of trivalent vaccine used in the most recent interpandemic year, a "3-for-1" scenario. If a half-strength pandemic vaccine is sufficient, the supply could increase sixfold, a "6-for-1" scenario.

The epidemiology of influenza vaccine use in 1999 provides useful insight into why increasing the level of interpandemic vaccine use will be important for the future supply of a pandemic vaccine. Under the optimistic "6-for-1" scenario, any country that continues to use ≥ 167 doses of trivalent vaccine per 1000 population will theoretically have one dose

Table 2
Vaccine supply for an influenza pandemic

Countries	Population, 1999 (millions)	Estimated number of doses of vaccine distributed, 1999 (millions)[a]	Additional doses of trivalent–equivalent vaccine needed (millions)[b]
United States, Canada, Australia	323	82.0	(28.2)
Western Europe	386	56.4	8.1
Argentina, Brazil, Chile, Mexico and Uruguay	328	18.7	34.6
Central Europe, Eastern Europe and Russia[c]	298	12.8	40.0
Japan, Republic of Korea	176	6.4	13.1
Total	1511	176.3	67.6
29 other countries	3148	7.5	?

[a] Vaccine distribution data were provided by Aventis Pasteur MSD and Aventis Pasteur. The estimates refer to the number of doses distributed by all vaccine producers.

[b] Additional doses of trivalent vaccine needed to reach a level of 167 doses per 1000 population. Achieving this level will ensure that one dose of monovalent pandemic vaccine (7.5 μg HA) is available for each person.

[c] Includes Israel, but excludes Belarus, Bulgaria, Moldova and the countries of Southeast Europe.

of pandemic vaccine for each of its citizens ($1000 \div 6 = 167$). Fig. 1 and Table 2 show that in 1999–2000, only eight countries met or exceeded this cut off level (≥ 160 doses). Western Europe as a whole fell short by 8.1 million doses. In Latin America, the five countries that used influenza vaccine (very little vaccine was used in the other Latin American countries) fell short of the cut off by 35 million doses. Central Europe, Eastern Europe and Russia fell short by 40 millions doses, and Japan and the Republic of Korea also failed to reach the cut off level. Under the "6-for-1" scenario, only the United States would have had the ability to export a pandemic vaccine. If this vaccine were sent only to the countries shown in Table 2, they would still have needed to increase their collective use of trivalent influenza vaccine by 67.6 million doses (27%) to reach the cut off level of 167 doses per 1000 population. Under the less optimistic "3-for-1" scenario, they would have had to increase their level of trivalent vaccine use by 326.8 million doses (185%). The countries shown in Table 2 accounted for almost all of the influenza vaccine used in 1999, yet they contained only one-fourth of the world's population. Very little vaccine was used in the rest of the world.

4. Distributing the global supply of pandemic influenza vaccine: the limitations of the market

The WHO Influenza Pandemic Preparedness Plan identifies several issues that will affect the production and distribution of a pandemic vaccine [6]. Scientific and technical issues include the possibility of preparing a number of potential pandemic virus "vaccine seeds". In the event of a pandemic, the appropriate seed will be provided to all vaccine producers. New testing reagents, new production procedures (especially cell culture) and centralized registration will be critically important if production times are to be reduced and vaccine supplies increased.

In addition to vaccine production, the WHO guidelines suggest that countries should plan for emergencies when negotiating vaccine procurement contracts, stating, "each vaccine manufacturer *should discuss* (italics added) with the country(ies) where. . . vaccine is usually produced or distributed,. . . what can be the expected rate of production. . . It *may be desirable* to build flexibility into procurement procedures to allow for different vaccination strategies . . .Each government and vaccine supplier *will need to consider* how much vaccine they will guarantee to purchase or sell in an emergency situation. The cost per dose may be different if vaccine is being purchased by governments. . . (or) at the user's expense. Without a "clearing house", . . .cost considerations rather than public health *may drive* vaccine distribution (and). . .non-industrialized countries. . .*may be completely overlooked* . . .A central clearing house, operated and funded by a number of co-operating countries, *might allow* for vaccine purchases to be "pooled" and distributed more equitably. . . (and could ensure that some). . .vaccine is purchased as a humanitarian donation for. . . (those). . . in non-industrialized countries. . . who play essential long-term roles in society" [6].

The WHO guidelines identify many of the key issues for global supply of a pandemic influenza vaccine. However, in outlining what should be done, the guidelines do not say how it could be accomplished. Instead, the guidelines implicitly rely on the continued use of market mechanisms. Currently, individual countries either negotiate with one or more vaccine producers to provide a one-year supply of vaccine or, more commonly, several vaccine companies either bid for public contracts or sell their vaccines privately to distributors, pharmacies and individual physicians. This market mechanism allows vaccine producers to prudently expand their production capacity to meet next year's market forecast. However, because this mechanism functions on a year-to-year basis, it provides companies with little guidance for making decisions on long-term investments that would increase production capacity. Given the current situation, one can easily imagine that when a pandemic threat appears, scores of governmental health agencies will simultaneously attempt to negotiate vaccine supply contracts with a limited number of producers, in effect leaving decisions on who will or will not be vaccinated in the hands of company executives. Alternatively, the U.S. experience in 1976 might be repeated, and the governments of the few countries which have their own influenza vaccine producers could in one way or another "nationalize" their companies in order to guarantee an adequate domestic supply of vaccine. Such a long-term arrangement has already been negotiated with the one vaccine producer in Canada (G. Ball, personal communication). Once domestic needs have been met, any excess production could be exported to other countries. If this happens, country presidents and prime ministers will have the power to decide who will or will not be vaccinated.

5. The rationale for developing a global approach for pandemic vaccine supply

The solutions to several of mankind's most important problems can be achieved only by efforts that are transnational in nature [9–11]. Whenever a solution is achieved, it is called a global public "good" [12,13]. Public goods are essential resources or services that, by their very nature, cannot be provided solely by the "invisible hand" of the market and require some form of governmental intervention [13]. Within nations, effective policing, a sound currency and widespread literacy are recognized as public goods, and their provision is ensured through a variety of laws and regulations. At the international level, different approaches must be taken to ensure global public goods. For example, the global consequences of environmental change have been addressed through legally binding international agreements and institutions, including the Vienna Convention for the Protection of the Ozone Layer, the Montreal Ozone Protocol and the London Amendments enacted in the 1980s, and more recently by the Framework Convention on Climate Change [14].

For global public health there may be no greater challenge than developing effective approaches to meet the threat of emerging and re-emergent infectious diseases. WHO can and should be expected to play a leading role in meeting this challenge. For decades, WHO has administered a set of international health regulations which apply to plague, yellow fever and cholera [9]. Although WHO established a unit for emerging infections in the mid-1990s, its activities have been largely concerned with strengthening the international public health infrastructure in order to improve research, training, and surveillance activities needed to deal with threats posed by emerging infectious diseases [9]. Public health institutions in individual countries have been encouraged to improve their capacities and to coordinate their activities with those of other countries and WHO. None of these efforts has relied on international health law.

WHO began to use a new approach to confronting a global threat to public health when in 1999 the World Health Assembly authorized multilateral negotiations for a Framework Convention on Tobacco Control (FCTC) [14]. Scientific evidence for the devastating health and economic consequences of tobacco use was well known. What was new was a recognition that the global nature of the tobacco industry and the international trade in tobacco products required a public health response that transcended that of individual national governments. Under the FCTC, a Technical Working Group was charged with developing protocols to cover issues such as tobacco pricing, taxation, advertising, sponsorship, package design and labelling, smuggling, agriculture, information sharing and the Internet. The first meeting of the FCTC's Intergovernmental Negotiating Body was held in October 2000. This group will negotiate and draft the proposed FCTC and related protocols which will be presented to the World Health Assembly for adoption in May 2003. In authorizing the FCTC, the World Health Assembly has firmly committed WHO to using international health law to address a problem of enormous importance for global public health.

6. A proposal to implement the WHO Influenza Pandemic Preparedness Plan and ensure vaccine supply

The fundamental weakness of WHO's Influenza Pandemic Preparedness Plan regarding vaccine production is self-evident; it offers no solution to the problem of maximizing the global supply of a pandemic vaccine and ensuring its equitable distribution. It is highly unlikely that market mechanisms can be counted on to effectively deal with this problem because they force company executives or national political leaders to make decisions on who will and will not be vaccinated. It also seems self-evident that the only way health authorities and vaccine producers will be able to optimise the production and distribution of a pandemic vaccine will be to work out the necessary conditions well before a pandemic threat appears. Failure to do so could have serious political as well as health and economic consequences worldwide [9,15,16].

Because the issues of pandemic vaccine supply will require negotiations between health officials representing a large number of countries and company officials representing a small number of vaccine producers, they are likely to succeed only if the negotiations are legally binding and conducted on a global basis. One possible mechanism to accomplish this would be a Framework Convention for Pandemic Influenza Vaccine Supply. If authorized by a resolution of the World Health Assembly, a Framework Convention would establish Technical Working Groups (TWGs) that would meet a least once a year. The TWGs would include representatives of the health ministries of all national governments that wish to participate in the process. These health officials would be invited to present five-year forecasts of the annual number of doses of trivalent influenza vaccine they will commit to purchase and how the vaccine will be paid for. The TWGs would also include representatives of each company that produces influenza vaccine as well as representatives of regulatory authorities, international agencies and nongovernmental organizations. Through a process that is consistent with the international competition policies and trade regulations and yet also recognizes the primacy of global public health, the vaccine producers would determine the extent to which they will be able to meet the vaccine supply needs that health officials have forecasted and how the needs of public and private markets can be accommodated. If additional production capacity is required, the negotiators might need to explore tax credits or other financial incentives to ensure that companies are able to make the necessary capital investments. The TWGs would also need to anticipate and propose solutions to regulatory problems, especially if new production techniques such as cell culture are involved.

The rolling five-year forecasts of trivalent vaccine supply would serve as the basis for determining, according to several plausible scenarios, how vaccine companies would produce, finance and distribute a pandemic vaccine. Once the TWGs have prepared their protocols, an Intergovernmental Negotiating Body should draft and negotiate a Framework Convention for Pandemic Influenza Vaccine Supply. It could serve as a forerunner to the recently proposed Framework Convention on Global Infectious Disease Prevention and Control [17].

7. Conclusion

The health benefits of annual influenza vaccination are evident [1] and may be greater than currently understood [18,19]. The importance of annual influenza vaccination in interpandemic years has been acknowledged in a recent WHO statement [20]. Moreover, the urgent need for an effective mechanism for pandemic vaccine supply has been emphasized by the H5N1 experience in Hong Kong [21].

A Framework Convention for Pandemic Influenza Vaccine Supply would provide a legally binding mechanism for optimizing the production and distribution of a pandemic vaccine. It would accelerate the already increasing use of trivalent influenza vaccine in developed and developing countries. It could also provide useful experience for forecasting the needs for other vaccines for children and adults [22] and for anticipating global mechanisms that could be used to introduce vaccines against HIV, tuberculosis and malaria, a goal that leaders of the G8 countries are committed to achieving [23]. Unlike the Framework Convention on Tobacco Control, which pits the needs of global public health against the interests of international tobacco companies, a Framework Convention for Pandemic Influenza Vaccine Supply would benefit both individual countries and vaccine producers. Ensuring that such a process is actually established, however, will require the active support of health officials, physicians and scientists throughout the world.

Acknowledgements

The author thanks Isabelle Berthaut, Vincent Demenil, Salah Eddine Mahyaoui and Karim Kashi for information on influenza vaccine distribution; Paula Soper for information on the World Health Organization's Tobacco Free Initiative; and David P. Fidler for comments on the manuscript.

References

[1] A.S. Monto, Individual and community impact of influenza, Pharmacoeconomics 16 (Suppl. 1) (1999) 1–6.
[2] D.S. Fedson, C. Hannoun, J. Leese, et al., Influenza vaccination in 18 developed countries, 1981–1992, Vaccine 13 (1995) 623–627.
[3] D.S. Fedson, Y. Hirota, H.K. Shin, et al., Influenza vaccination in 22 developed countries; an update to 1995, Vaccine 15 (1997) 1506–1511.
[4] F. Ambrosch, D.S. Fedson, Influenza vaccination in 29 countries, An update to 1997, Pharmacoeconomics 16 (Suppl. 1) (1999) 47–54.
[5] F. Ambrosch, D.S. Fedson, Epidemiology of influenza vaccine distribution (abstract), Options for the Control of Influenza IV, (September 23–28, 2000) 126.
[6] World Health Organization, Influenza Pandemic Preparedness Plan, World Health Organization, Geneva, April 1999.
[7] A.S. Monto (Ed.), Pandemic Influenza: Confronting A Re-Emergent Threat, J. Infect. Dis. 176 (Suppl. 1) (1997) S1–S90.
[8] W.R. Dowdle, The 1976 experience, J. Infect. Dis. 176 (Suppl. 1) (1997) S69–S72.
[9] D.P. Fidler, Globalization, international law, and emerging infectious diseases, Emerging Infect. Dis. 2 (1996) 77–84.
[10] D. Yach, D. Bettcher, The globalization of public health: I. Threats and opportunities, Am. J. Public Health 88 (1998) 735–738.
[11] D. Yach, D. Bettcher, The globalization of public health: II. The convergence of self-interest and altruism, Am. J. Public Health 88 (1998) 738–741.
[12] L.C. Chen, T.G. Evans, R.A. Cash, Health as a global public good, in: I. Kaul, M.A. Grunberg (Eds.), Global Public Goods, Oxford University Press, New York, 1999, pp. 284–304.
[13] I. Kaul, I. Grundberg, M.A. Stern, Defining global public goods, in: I. Kaul, M.A. Grunberg (Eds.), Global Public Goods, Oxford University Press, New York, 1999, pp. 2–19.
[14] A.L. Taylor, D.W. Bettcher, WHO Framework Convention on Tobacco Control: a global "good" for public health, Bull. W.H.O. 78 (2000) 920–929.
[15] E. O'Brien, The diplomatic implications of emerging diseases, in: K.M. Cahill (Ed.), Preventive Diplomacy, Basic Books, New York, 1996, pp. 244–268.
[16] G. Alleyne, Health and national security, Bull. Pan. Am. Health Org. 30 (1996) 158–163.
[17] D.P. Fidler, International Law and Infectious Diseases, Oxford University Press, New York, 1999.
[18] T.A. Reichert, D.S. Fedson, W.P. Glezen, N. Sugaya, M. Tashiro, Measuring the effect of influenza vaccination programs, The Japanese experience revisited (abstract), Options Control Influenza IV, (September 23–28, 2000) 60.
[19] D.S Siscovick, T.E. Raghunathan, D. Lin, et al., Influenza vaccination and the risk of primary cardiac arrest, Am. J. Epidemiol. 152 (2000) 674–677.
[20] World Health Organization, Influenza vaccine, Wkly. Epidemiol. Rec. 35 (2000) 281–288.
[21] R. Snaken, A.P. Kendal, L. Haaheim, J.M. Wood, The next influenza pandemic: lessons from Hong Kong, 1997, Emerging Infect. Dis. 5 (1999) 195–203.
[22] World Health Organization, Guidelines for the International Procurement of Vaccines and Sera, World Health Organization, Geneva, 1998.
[23] J. Watts, G8 countries set priorities for infectious diseases but fail to make progress on debt relief, Bull. W.H.O. 78 (2000) 1168.

International Congress Series 1219 (2001) 733–736

Influenza pandemic planning: review of a collaborative state and national process

K.F. Gensheimer[a,*], R.A. Strikas[b], K. Fukuda[b], N.J. Cox[b],
C.M. Sewell[c], Z.F. Dembek[d], M. Myers[b]

[a]*Maine Department of Human Services, Augusta, ME, USA*
[b]*National Immunization Program, Centers for Disease Control and Prevention,
MS E-52, Atlanta, GA 30333, USA*
[c]*New Mexico Department of Health, Santa Fe, NM, USA*
[d]*Connecticut Department of Public Health, Hartford, CT, USA*

Abstract

In the United States, planning for the next influenza pandemic is occurring in parallel at national, state and local levels. Certain issues, such as conducting surveillance and purchasing pandemic vaccine, require coordination at the national level. However, most prevention and control actions will be implemented at the state and local level, which vary widely in terms of population demographics, culture (e.g., rural versus urban), and available resources. In 1995, a survey by the Council of State and Territorial Epidemiologists (CSTE) found that only 29 (59%) states perceived a need to develop a specific influenza pandemic plan for their jurisdiction. Since then, the process of developing state and local plans has gained considerable momentum. Integration of these efforts with the national planning process has been facilitated by: (1) the mutual involvement of state and federal staff in both processes; (2) the sharing of draft documents; (3) the ongoing occurrence of local and national coordinating meetings; and (4) the provision of financial resources by the federal government. So far, approximately 12 states either have drafted or begun drafting a state and local influenza pandemic plan. One of the benefits of the collaborative planning process has been the development of new working relationships and partnerships among several agencies at the state, local and national levels. Such efforts will improve our collective ability to rapidly investigate and control other emerging or re-emerging public health threats in the 21st century, be it a bioterrorist event, an influenza pandemic, or any other catastrophic health event. © 2001 Elsevier Science B.V. All rights reserved.

Keywords: Influenza pandemic planning; Vaccine; Public health threats

* Corresponding author. Tel./fax: +1-207-287-5183.
E-mail address: Kathleen_F.Gensheimer@state.me.us (K.F. Gensheimer).

0531-5131/01/$ – see front matter © 2001 Elsevier Science B.V. All rights reserved.
PII: S 0 5 3 1 - 5 1 3 1 (0 1) 0 0 3 8 9 - 2

The United States approach to pandemic planning is national in scope in that the federal government has involved multiple partners from the state and local level throughout the process. Since 1993, the Council of State and Territorial Epidemiologists (CSTE) has been one of the many partners involved in these efforts and has worked actively with the national working group on Influenza Pandemic Preparedness and Emergency Response (GRIPPE). Together, these partners have created a comprehensive conceptual "Influenza Pandemic Preparedness Plan" outlining critical areas needed on a national level to limit the burden of disease; to minimize social disruption and to reduce economic loss. National planners also recognized the need for states to formalize their own influenza pandemic response initiatives, acknowledging that a parallel planning effort at the state and local level would be a critical component to the national efforts. Certain issues, such as conducting surveillance and purchasing vaccine, would require coordination at the national level during an influenza pandemic. However, most prevention and control actions will be implemented at the state and local level, where a diversity of population demographics, governmental infrastructure, culture, and financial resources will dictate unique responses by states and localities to such a crisis.

Until recently, most state and local public health agencies did not have a plan for the management of an influenza pandemic, nor for any other rapidly emerging infectious disease threat that has the potential to affect the entire population within a short period of time. In 1995, a survey by the CSTE found that only 29 (59%) states perceived a need to develop a specific influenza pandemic plan for their jurisdiction. As a result of the recognition of this gap in preparedness, a formal mechanism with limited funding support provided by the Centers for Disease Control and Prevention (CDC) was established in 1995 to address state specific influenza pandemic planning issues. One of the first projects under this CSTE/CDC cooperation agreement was convening a meeting of 40 state and local representatives in 1996 to develop critical elements of a pandemic response plan. The outcome of these discussions was drafted into the document, "Pandemic Influenza, a Planning Guide for State and Local Officials." The model guidelines were intended to orient state and local health officials regarding the need for planning during both the interpandemic and the pandemic time periods; to identify persons within the public and private sector organizations and agencies who would be involved in the planning process; to provide assurances that appropriate state and local statutes were in place for dealing with the pandemic; to promote strategies for marketing the plan to appropriate partners to obtain the necessary support for implementing the plan and to develop strategies to implement or expand specific components of the plan, including surveillance, biologicals/delivery, communications, and emergency preparedness.

A CDC/CSTE steering committee has worked together since 1995 to guide the CSTE/CDC cooperative agreement process to collaborate on the state and local guidelines as well as to further promote influenza pandemic planning efforts at the state and local level. The steering committee has worked to support states who were interested in initiating pandemic planning by providing limited funding support as "seed money" through the cooperative agreement to begin the planning process; by providing technical and moral support to states involved in pandemic planning and by working together to resolve issues felt to be critical to influenza pandemic planning efforts. In 1998, six sites: Connecticut, Maine, Missouri, New Mexico, New York and Mercer County, New

Jersey pilot tested the draft guidelines, receiving limited funding support for this effort through the cooperative agreement. As a result of feedback received from these sites, this document became the framework for promoting and enhancing pandemic preparedness efforts at the state level. California, Maryland, Minnesota, and South Carolina were selected to receive funding in 1999 through the CDC/CSTE cooperative agreement to produce their own state specific influenza pandemic plans. In January 2000, Florida, Indiana, New Hampshire, New Jersey, and Massachusetts became the second group of states selected to develop state specific plans through the cooperative agreement process. Other states have initiated the process of pandemic planning as part of other emerging infections, bioterrorism preparedness or catastrophic health planning initiatives. Integration of State planning efforts with the national planning process has been facilitated by the mutual involvement of state and federal staff in both processes; the sharing of draft documents; the ongoing occurrence of local and national coordinating meetings; the provision of financial resources through the CDC/CSTE cooperative agreement and the promotion and the marketing of the need for influenza pandemic planning through national teleconferences and other national meetings.

The process of developing state and local plans has gained considerable momentum. A second follow-up national influenza pandemic meeting, convened by the CSTE/CDC steering committee in September 2000 was attended by 140 participants, representing 42 states, Puerto Rico and the District of Columbia. The meeting provided the opportunity to share state influenza pandemic plans and lessons learned, as well as allowing the CSTE/CDC steering committee to obtain objective input on specific issues requiring state and federal cooperation including: surveillance issues; vaccine priority groups and use of antivirals. Reflections from the 1976 and the 1997 pandemic warning provided a sobering reality to conference deliberations. A recent year 2000 survey of the CSTE membership was also shared with program participants. Of note, 49 (98%) states perceived a need to develop a specific influenza pandemic plan for their jurisdiction, with 39 (78%) states actually involved in the process of developing a plan. Other competing demands, lack of personnel resources, and lack of financial resources were cited as the three most important impediments faced in initiating the development of an influenza pandemic plan. Respondents noted that the two most important resources needed by states to complete each work were provision of funding support and completion of a national plan. Six states indicated that they had completed influenza pandemic plans with an additional 25 states indicating that plans are to be completed by the end of 2001. Clearly, the above efforts have been fruitful in promoting and enhancing influenza pandemic planning efforts nationally.

Pandemic influenza planning offers an exciting opportunity to work together proactively with various partners and stakeholders at the national, state and local level to plan comprehensively for this potential catastrophic health event. The national influenza pandemic planning process has offered a unique approach to planning for an infectious disease crisis, requiring broad cooperation and collaboration across national, state and local agencies which until this time, had minimal knowledge of each other's function or existence. New relationships with the private medical community and other outside agencies and organizations have also been established. Although these hurdles have posed unique challenges; the effort has been strengthened by the partnerships established and will ultimately improve our ability to rapidly investigate and control whatever public health threats emerge or reemerge in the 21st century. Coordination of such efforts not only makes sense, but also will in the end assure a more viable national approach to a potential public health threat with implementation of a comprehensive response taking place at the state and local level.

International Congress Series 1219 (2001) 737–744

Pandemic planning in a temperate country with no vaccine producer

Lance C. Jennings[a,*], N. Wilson[b], D. Lush[b]

[a]*Virology Unit, Canterbury Health Laboratories, P.O. Box 151, Christchurch, New Zealand*
[b]*Ministry of Health, Wellington, New Zealand*

Abstract

Influenza is an ongoing threat to public health in New Zealand with yearly winter epidemics causing considerable morbidity and mortality. In line with the global concern of the emergence of novel influenza strains, a national pandemic plan has been prepared to assist government and non-government agencies prepare their contingency arrangements. The primary objectives are to reduce the morbidity and mortality from influenza illness. The key elements of this plan require activity during interpandemic periods. This includes the further development of surveillance networks for early warning, the development of an influenza awareness program along with the promotion of influenza immunisation, and modelling to assist the development of influenza management strategies including guidelines for antiviral use. New Zealand does not have the ability to manufacture vaccine and this highlights the need for national health intervention planning. © 2001 Elsevier Science B.V. All rights reserved.

Keywords: Influenza; Pandemic plan; Vaccine

1. Introduction

The New Zealand National Influenza Pandemic Plan (NZIPP) has been prepared to facilitate a national response to minimise the morbidity and mortality of future pandemics of influenza. It follows the World Health Organisation's (WHO) definitions of levels of alertness and preparedness and pandemic planning guidelines [1].

The purpose of the plan is to assist hospital and health services, public health services and other agencies with the preparation of their contingency arrangements in the event of a

---

* Corresponding author.
E-mail address: lance.jennings@chmeds.ac.nz (L.C. Jennings).

0531-5131/01/$ – see front matter © 2001 Elsevier Science B.V. All rights reserved.
PII: S 0 5 3 1 - 5 1 3 1 (0 1) 0 0 3 5 4 - 5

pandemic of influenza. The objectives of these contingency arrangements are to reduce the morbidity and mortality from influenza infection through:

1. optimising the preventive options available,
2. effective management of the cases,
3. ensuring essential services are maintained,
4. minimising social disruption and economic losses associated with an influenza pandemic, and
5. providing timely information and advice to health professionals, the media and the public.

This paper focuses on aspects of the development of a pandemic plan for New Zealand, a country of 3.8 million people that has no vaccine manufacturing capability and is likely to face scarcity of vaccine and other resources during a pandemic threat. By the ongoing optimisation of surveillance and preventative measures during the interpandemic period, mechanisms for the delivery of appropriate control measures during a pandemic can be developed.

2. Kinetics of viral spread

The probability of a future global influenza pandemic is high and it is unlikely that New Zealand will be unaffected. Three pandemics have affected New Zealand during the 20th century (Fig. 1). A review of the entry times of these novel viruses into New Zealand suggests that a 3–7-month delay could be expected for a future novel virus, with a

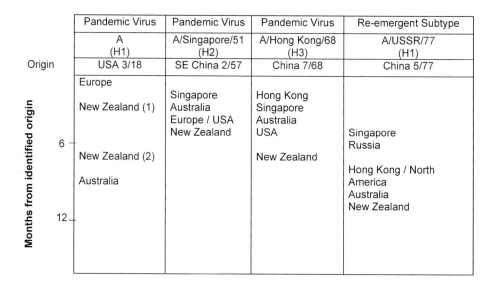

Fig. 1. Origin and rate of spread of influenza A viruses.

possible further delay to the first epidemic peak in illness. If the Asian subcontinent is the most likely source of the next pandemic virus, the substantial increases in tourism and trade and students from this region are likely to enhance the speed of virus arrival in New Zealand.

3. Worldwide vaccine production capacity:

Worldwide vaccine production capacity is not clear. There are 26 major manufacturers worldwide in 18 countries; however, only three countries may have sufficient capacity to be self-sufficient [2]. During a pandemic, embargoes on vaccine must be anticipated, as countries are likely to see a pandemic as a national health emergency. New Zealand's initial response planning is based on the probability that vaccine will not be available. This is for two reasons: firstly, there is no influenza vaccine manufacturing capacity, and secondly, it is unlikely that current technology will be able to produce substantial quantities of vaccine within the expected 3–7-month time period for virus entry. Obtaining vaccine might be plausible if New Zealand was late in encountering the first wave of the pandemic and during subsequent waves of disease in the following years. We believe influenza vaccination should not be excluded in the planning process despite potential supply issues.

4. The impact of influenza

The development of a national plan for a future pandemic needs to be based on as accurate as possible understanding of the impact of influenza on the community. There are two approaches to identifying and quantifying the potential impact. The first is simply by reviewing the national information that is already available; in New Zealand, extensive interpandemic data exists. The second approach is by projection through the application of modelling.

4.1. Community disease surveillance

Although New Zealand exhibits a temperate climate epidemiologic pattern for influenza, virological surveillance is carried out year round by five regional Virus Diagnostic laboratories. All respiratory virus diagnoses made from hospital in-patients and outpatients are reported centrally, and data are then publicised nationally in a Weekly Virus Report. During the 'influenza season' months of May through September, national voluntary sentinel surveillance (both disease and virological) is run [3]. Sentinel sites are distributed on a population basis (approximately 1 per 50,000) throughout the country's Health Districts. Each sentinel practice records the daily number of consultations that fit a case definition for an influenza-like illness (ILI), and these data are collected each Friday. Sentinel practices also provide respiratory samples from patients seen with an ILI each week. A weekly Influenza Report is produced and distributed nationally the following Wednesday. Surveillance data suggest that between 2% (36 000) and 5% (95 000) of New

Zealand's population consult a general practitioner annually with an influenza-like illness, placing a considerable burden of the counties primary health care system.

4.2. Hospital-based morbidity and mortality

All influenza-related hospitalisations and mortality in New Zealand are included in the ICD-9CM 487-diagnosis classification. In 10 years, from 1990 to July 1999, a total of 4113 influenza-related hospitalisations were recorded. Of these, 23% of admissions were in the 65 years and above age group, and 77% were under 65 years. Severe epidemics in New Zealand, as occurred in 1996, resulted in 767 first hospitalisations being recorded as due to influenza and 1670 first hospitalisations for pneumonia and influenza. Overall, hospitalisation rates are highest for infants under 5 years of age, and increasing with age from 55 years. Admission rates for Maori have exceeded the rates for Europeans in most years. Influenza mortality data from 1990 to 1997 show the majority of deaths (94.7%) was reported in the 65 and over age group, the largest number being reported in 1996 during the A(H3N2) epidemic year. Influenza deaths in the 0–64 years age group contributed 5.3% to the total mortality. Influenza has a substantial impact on the secondary health care system in most years.

4.3. Modelling

Modelling can be carried out to estimate the differential effects of influenza on morbidity, mortality and social disruption. The model by Boyce [4] for pandemic influenza has been widely used as a basis for these calculations. Using this model for New Zealand suggests that the number of expected influenza cases for incidence rates in the 15% to 35% range are 0.6 to 1.3 million cases, with 286 000 to 673 000 cases being unable to work. The model also suggests that there would be 258 000 to 602 000 medical consultations and 4500 to 10 500 people hospitalised. There would also be 1300 to 3000 deaths (90% CI = 800–4100), with half of these occurring in the under 65 years age group. Maori, Pacific peoples and low-income New Zealanders are likely to be at increased risk both of contracting pandemic influenza and of adverse health outcomes associated with it. Urban dwellers are also likely to be at increased risk of infection relative to rural dwellers. Pandemic modelling and planning can determine the priority groups and logistics for immunisation when pandemic-strain vaccine becomes available.

5. Interpandemic contingency planning

Contingency arrangements can be initiated during the interpandemic period. These initiatives can include the following.

5.1. Strengthening surveillance

A timely, representative and efficient surveillance system is the cornerstone of influenza detection. During the interpandemic period, surveillance should be strengthened. This should include a review of the voluntary sentinel general practice network to ensure that the network is as representative as possible of the population. Further, the quality of the data collected can be improved by use of standardised computerised patient-record systems, with electronic transfer to the surveillance centre. Motivation of participating health professionals through possible incentive systems or at least with the provision of regular feedback via electronic newsletters should be established.

Influenza hospitalisation data are not readily available. Improving both the quality and timeliness of these data can contribute to influenza monitoring. The quality of the routine virology diagnostic system can be improved, especially the detection and reporting of out-of-season cases. Laboratories also need to improve the turn-around-time for virus detection and typing and the forwarding of isolates to the Regional WHO Collaborating Centre can also be improved.

When a pandemic alert is established, intensified surveillance may be required to provide data about the initial occurrence, spread and impact of a novel influenza virus. This will need to be focused on travellers returning to New Zealand, hospitalised patients with severe viral pneumonia and contacts of these groups. The speed of influenza spread and rapid human movements may make this approach impractical, reinforcing the need for a high-quality nationally standardised system.

5.2. Improving vaccine coverage

Increasing the interpandemic use of vaccine is an important and cost-effective health care strategy. In New Zealand, recommendations for immunisation of at risk groups are in line with other countries and have been in place for many years. However, since 1997 when government endorsement through the provision of free vaccine to those 65 years and over, then extension of this policy to include those under 65 years with high risk conditions, vaccine usage has increased. However, coverage of the 65 and older group is currently 55%. Further active promotion of influenza immunisation is required to increase coverage levels.

During a pandemic alert situation, cost-effectiveness of preventing hospitalisation and death are the most likely health outcomes to be used to drive decision making on immunisation policy. In an attempt to assist this decision making, modelling has been carried out to estimate the potential benefit of immunisation [1]. The uncertainties in the effectiveness of any new vaccine created in response to the pandemic strain and the wide range of plausible gross incidence rates are difficult to take into consideration. The findings (Table 1) indicate that the most cost-effective intervention to prevent death is likely to be immunising those in high-risk groups' aged less than 65 years. Following this would be vaccinating the population 65 years and over. Vaccinating smokers aged 45–64 who were not in any risk groups would also be fairly cost-effective, but less so the adult population aged 20–64 years who were not in a high-risk group. Nevertheless, immunising the latter group may still be reasonably cost-effective compared to other health sector interventions when considered in terms of the cost per years of life saved. It is hard to calculate the benefit of preventing influenza among the population of essential service providers. This is because these workers might be able to save the lives and protect the welfare of others by providing appropriate medical care and social services.

Table 1
Cost effectiveness of various influenza immunisation strategies during a pandemic in New Zealand (for a gross incidence rate of 35% and a 50% vaccine effectiveness in preventing death) [5]

Populations	Estimated population in NZ	Deaths expected (if no immunisation)	Assumed vaccine uptake rate during a pandemic	Deaths prevented	Total cost ($NZ million)	Cost per death prevented ($NZ)
(A) High-risk groups under 65 years	388000	1500	50%	375	6.1–10.2	16000–27000
(B) Population aged 65 and over	460000	1440	70%	504	10.2–17.0	20000–34000
(C) Smokers aged 45–64 who are not in any risk groups	120000	290	40%	58	1.5–2.5	26000–44000
(D) Adult population aged 20–64 (excluding those covered in group A)	1660000	40	30%	6	15.8–26.2	2.6 M–4.4 M
(E) Population aged 0–19 (excluding those at risk, i.e., in A)	1100000	20	20%	2	7.0–11.6	3.5 M–5.8 M
(F) Selected essential service providers (health professionals, police, fire fighters, army personnel)	82300	Not assessed	60%	Not assessed	1.6–2.6	Benefit is in terms of social stability and providing services

Given the evidence for the cost-effectiveness of influenza immunisation during interpandemic periods, it is possible that immunisation would be even more cost-effective when a pandemic did occur. This is because of the higher incidence rate of infection and the increased risk of serious health outcomes and death in the younger age groups, typically seen during pandemics. However, the priority groups will need to be scrutinised at the time of a pandemic based on what is known about the novel virus.

Additional vaccine strategies include the use of pneumococcal vaccine; however, the cost-effectiveness of pneumococcal immunisation is still not entirely clear even though this intervention could in theory significantly reduce mortality during an influenza pandemic.

5.3. Antivirals

Antiviral drugs may be the only specific intervention available for treatment and prophylaxis; however, like vaccines, supply is unlikely to meet demand. There is less clarity than vaccines about their use in a pandemic situation; nevertheless, the assessment of antiviral requirements, establishment of guidelines for use and stockpiling issues need to be addressed. The objectives of antiviral drug use would be to control outbreaks in closed populations, to treat seriously ill patients in hospital, and to provide prophylaxis until vaccine is available. No cost-effectiveness studies have been carried out in New Zealand. However, in terms of the development of a prophylaxis strategy, it would make sense to follow the existing recommendations for use of influenza vaccine, with appropriate adjustment once the epidemiological characteristics of a novel virus are know in a pandemic threat.

5.4. Public health interventions to reduce spread

New Zealand has in place a public health network, which is closely associated with most communities. Strategies to close schools and control other public meetings may be the main public health strategies available following the entry of a novel virus. There may be scope for limiting population movements to small isolated rural communities and to small islands, but the benefits and costs of these strategies need further consideration and consultation with the communities involved. Such measures are included in the Health Act 1956 and will be included in new public health legislation, which is being drafted.

5.5. Communication and influenza awareness

The imminent threat of a pandemic will require a communication strategy to minimise panic and uncertainty. During the interpandemic period, strategies can be put in place to increase influenza awareness. Along with the implementation of the 1997 free vaccine policy in New Zealand, a budget for influenza awareness was also established. The success of local promotions has provided the model for the formation of the National Influenza Immunisation Strategy Group. This group has the twin aims of educating the public of the seriousness of influenza, and informing health care professionals of the benefits of immunisation to those at risk for influenza. This has allowed the development of lines of communication involving the national media, professional medical organisations, health authorities and other parties, which will be essential during a pandemic threat.

The pharmaceutical industry also plays a role in promoting immunisation via television advertising and other promotions, and their involvement in this process is essential. However, with the licensing of the new antivirals, the role of the pharmaceutical industry in influenza awareness has become more prominent. An important aspect of the commercial strategy is the wide dissemination of influenza surveillance data, particularly within the primary health care sector for the targeted use of these drugs. Partnerships are essential to ensure the maximum public health benefit from the collection and use of these data.

5.6. Linkages

Both national and international linkages are required for emergency preparedness. A National Civil Defence Plan exists in New Zealand, and while a threat of pandemic influenza will require a unique response, in comparison with a natural disaster, the linkages with emergency planning plans and processes already in place are important.

New Zealand's response to a pandemic alert, or response related to influenza activity during interpandemic periods, will necessitate co-ordination with Australia. The establishment of the Australian IPPC under the auspices of the Communicable Diseases Network Australia New Zealand (CDNANZ) provides this linkage.

6. Conclusions

Pandemic planning is an ongoing and evolving process. By focusing on contingency initiatives in the interpandemic period, annual influenza hospitalisations and deaths are minimised, and the awareness of the seriousness of influenza improved in the community and in the primary and secondary health care sectors. The process of pandemic planning enables public health authorities to improve the efficiency of current influenza control strategies.

References

[1] World Health Organisation, Influenza Pandemic Preparedness Plan, WHO, Geneva, 1999.
[2] M.I. Meltzer, N.J. Cox, K. Fukuda, Modeling the economic impact of pandemic influenza in the United States: priorities for intervention, Emerg. Infect. Dis. 5 (1999) 659–671.
[3] L.C. Jennings, Influenza surveillance in New Zealand, Vaccine 17 (1999) S115–S117.
[4] N. Boyce, "Ready or not...", New Sci. 166 (2000) 16–17.
[5] N. Wilson, A preliminary examination of the impact of an influenza pandemic on New Zealand (unpublished report for the New Zealand Ministry of Health), 2000.

International Congress Series 1219 (2001) 745–749

Influenza pandemic planning in the tropics (Singapore)

A.E. Ling*

Department of Pathology, Pathology Building, Singapore General Hospital, Singapore, Singapore

Certain features unique to the region influence planning for influenza pandemics in the tropics. In the tropics and sub-tropic regions, influenza occurs throughout the year, with one or, more commonly, two seasonal peaks of varying intensity, roughly corresponding to the winter periods of the north and south [1] (Figs. 1 and 2). Large outbreaks, however, may occur "out of season". Surveillance data from Singapore show very little time lag between appearances of new strains seen in other parts of the world. Indeed, first isolations of epidemic and pandemic strains have occurred in Singapore, as in the Asian flu pandemic in 1957 caused by A/Singapore/1/57 (H2N2) and that caused by B/Singapore222/79, in 1979.

A look at the outpatient clinic attendance for acute respiratory tract infections shows that attendance goes up in conjunction with the influenza seasons, but also may be high during inter-seasonal periods (Fig. 1). Attendance in these periods may coincide with other respiratory infections, in particular, respiratory syncytial virus, which usually presents after the influenza seasons.

In the absence of specific studies, and low figures for mortality, it is felt that influenza does not cause significant morbidity or mortality in Singapore in inter-epidemic periods. This, coupled with the need for twice yearly immunisation to enable year round protection, the possibility of "out of season" outbreaks and the probability of having to face a new strain not covered by a vaccine are reasons that regular mass immunisation is not implemented.

However, despite its apparent low mortality and morbidity in the inter-epidemic years, it is a fact that morbidity and mortality are severe during large epidemics, as experienced in the major epidemic in Singapore due to the A/Victoria/3/75 strain which occurred from mid-April to mid-June, 1976 [2]. Hence, in Singapore, the contingency plan to deal with an influenza pandemic takes into consideration that it may not be possible to halt the initial

---

* Fax: +65-222-6826.

0531-5131/01/$ – see front matter © 2001 Elsevier Science B.V. All rights reserved.
PII: S0531-5131(01)00355-7

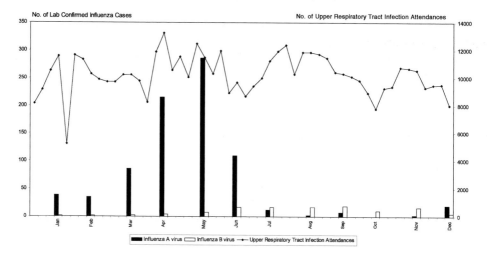

Fig. 1. Monthly distribution of lab-confirmed influenza cases and weekly upper respiratory tract infection attendance at Polyclinics, 1998.

spread of a new strain of influenza. The plan is based on maintenance of good surveillance systems and measures to minimise the consequences of a pandemic.

The following summarises the Singapore Ministry of Health's contingency plan, which has as its objectives:

1. Reduction of morbidity and mortality from influenza
2. Ensuring the adequate capacity of the health services to rapidly cope with increased numbers of infected persons

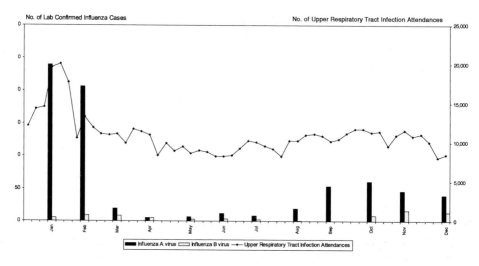

Fig. 2. Monthly distribution of lab-confirmed influenza cases and weekly upper respiratory tract infection attendance at Polyclinics, 1999.

3. Ensuring that health facilities have the means to vaccinate and administer chemo-prophylaxis to large numbers of persons
4. Make provision for adequate stocks of vaccines and anti-influenza drugs
5. Disseminate timely and accurate information for health professionals, the public and media at all stages to prevent panic and provide useful information.

The operation of the contingency plan and its direction and co-ordination will be handled by the Influenza Pandemic Task Force. This comprises the Deputy Director of Medical Services, Public Health Division, Ministry of Health (MOH), the Head of the Quarantine and Epidemiology Department (QED), the Director of the Agro Veterinary Agency (AVA), Clinical Director, Communicable Disease Centre, Laboratory Director of the National Influenza Centre, the Director of the National Pharmaceutical Administration (NPA), the Director of the Family Health Service (FHS) and the Director of Epidemiology and Disease Control (EDC).

The Task Force co-ordinates efforts among those involved in the treatment of patients, procurement of drug and vaccine stocks, animal health, the laboratory as well as public relations officers. The task force will also advise on steps to be taken during an epidemic or pandemic, e.g., mass vaccination, closure of public swimming pools, kindergartens, nurseries and childcare centres, etc.

This committee is to be convened in times of impending epidemics to confirm and implement control measures for influenza.

One important aspect of influenza control is the administration of the surveillance system for influenza in Singapore. This is based on

(a) Routine monitoring of attendance at government polyclinics for acute respiratory infections (ARIs) coupled with notification of an unusual increase in the daily number of cases.

(b) An alert system of selected sentinel private general practitioners that inform the Ministry of Health whenever unusual numbers of patients with acute respiratory tract infections are seen.

(c) Active laboratory surveillance by the National Influenza Centre that carries out a year round active laboratory surveillance of influenza viruses. This is based on

(I) The number of positive tests for influenza immunofluorescence and serology for influenza
(II) The number and types of virus isolates from:
18 weekly random throat swabs taken from patients presenting with ARI at specified government polyclinics and submitted to the National Influenza Centre.
Ad hoc samples from patients with ARI sent by doctors from public and private hospitals/clinics

(d) Reports from animal surveillance. The Agro Veterinary Agency actively and systematically tests a random representative number of samples from domestic and imported birds and animals.

The contingency plan is divided into six phases:

Phase 0	Inter-epidemic/pandemic period
Phase 1	Influenza epidemic/pandemic outside Singapore
Phase 2	Increased incidence of influenza in Singapore
Phase 3	Influenza epidemic/pandemic in Singapore
Phase 4	Influenza epidemic/pandemic with complications
Phase 5	End of epidemic/pandemic

The main activity in phase 0 — interpandemic/epidemic period is surveillance. This involves monitoring the weekly attendance at government polyclinics, fortnightly returns from the National Influenza Centre on positive laboratory tests for influenza, notification of abnormal or new strains of influenza virus isolates and notification from the AVA of any new strains or highly pathogenic avian influenza virus isolated from animals or an abnormal mortality among animals from influenza.

The Ministry of Health updates the National Pharmaceutical Administration (NPA) on the current WHO recommended vaccine formulation to allow rapid licensing of such vaccines for use. The NPA's task is to ensure availability of vaccines and anti-influenza drugs for the Travel Clinics and polyclinics. Polyclinics will administer vaccines to the target population as part of the influenza epidemic control programme.

Phase 1 is activated when there is an influenza epidemic or pandemic reported in another country. Activities in phase 1 are meant to take steps necessary to deal with an impending epidemic. In addition to measures already mentioned, co-operation with the Ministry of the Environment, National Influenza Centre and AVA is implemented. If animals and birds are implicated, increased influenza surveillance on livestock is implemented. The Ministry will issue a press statement to advise travellers to the affected country to take appropriate precautionary measures, and alert all medical practitioners of the outbreak and the strain of influenza virus.

Phase 2 is activated if outpatient attendance at government polyclinics for ARI increase over the "warning" threshold, and/or the number of positive tests for influenza increases. The number of cases of ARIs and the laboratory returns will be monitored weekly instead of fortnightly, and press releases sent out to advise on appropriate precautionary measures to be taken by the public. Immediate notification of deaths or complications resulting from influenza is implemented. The National Influenza Centre will in addition to its usual surveillance, update the Ministry of Health on strains isolated, or any abnormal or new strains and seek the assistance of the WHO Collaborating Centres for Influenza where necessary. Arrangements will be made with authorised distributors of influenza vaccines and antivirals to ensure sufficient stocks.

Phase 3 is activated if there is an increase in OPD attendance for ARIs to above the epidemic threshold and there is a corresponding increase in the number of positive immunofluorescence influenza tests (i.e., there is an influenza epidemic/pandemic in Singapore). The network of information will be expanded, and a decision made as to whether or not to administer mass immunisation. The deployment of a larger number of staff to man clinics may have to be implemented. Vaccination and prophylactics will be made available to the nursing homes and homes for the aged. Medical personnel will also be offered vaccination or prophylactics.

If the epidemic is caused by a new strain of influenza virus, which may be imported, the AVA will be informed so that surveillance of implicated animals is stepped up, or imports are stopped.

In addition to all other steps taken for phase 2, isolation facilities will be set up, and monitoring of all cases, and number of deaths from influenza will be recorded.

Phase 4:

This is activated if there are more than three cases of death arising from complications of influenza (in particular, influenza–pneumonia). For this, full reports of death cases are monitored, the press kept informed of the situation, adequate beds in hospitals, drug supplies and equipment and additional staff deployed, and a decision made as to whether to administer mass vaccination. Closing down of schools/kindergartens/nurseries may be necessary.

Phase 5:

End of epidemic/pandemic is declared when outpatient attendance for ARI, and the number of positive immunofluorescence influenza tests have gone back to base line (interepidemic) levels. At this time, the Ministry of Health will prepare a report, reviewing the effectiveness of the contingency plan and the lessons learnt from the outbreak, and modify the plan accordingly.

Acknowledgements

Figs. 1 and 2 were reproduced with permission from the Quarantine and Epidemiology Department, Epidemiology and Disease Control Division, Ministry of the Environment, Ministry of Health, Singapore and the National Influenza Centre, Department of Pathology, Singapore General Hospital.

References

[1] S. Doraisingham, K.T. Goh, A.E. Ling, M. Yu, Influenza surveillance in Singapore: 1972–86, Bulletin of the World Health Organisation 66 (1) (1988) 57–63.
[2] K. Vellayappan, S. Doraisingham, Clinical Features in Children of Infection Caused by the Influenza A_2 Variant A/Victoria/3/75, 18: No. 2, (1976) 125–130.

International Congress Series 1219 (2001) 751–759

Developing vaccines against potential pandemic influenza viruses

J.M. Wood[a,*], K.G. Nicholson[b], M. Zambon[c], R. Hinton[d],
D.L. Major[a], R.W. Newman[a], U. Dunleavy[a], D. Melzack[a],
J.S. Robertson[a], G.C. Schild[a]

[a]*National Institute for Biological Standards and Control, Blanche Lane, South Mimms,
Potters Bar, Hertfordshire EN6 3QG, UK*
[b]*Leicester Royal Infirmary, Leicester, UK*
[c]*Central Public Health Laboratory, Colindale, UK*
[d]*Centre for Applied Microbiology and Research, Porton Down, UK*

Abstract

In the event of an influenza pandemic, there will be an urgent need for a vaccine. The human infections with influenza A (H5N1) and A (H9N2) viruses served as pandemic warnings and initiated worldwide efforts to develop suitable vaccines. This was not straightforward however, due to safety considerations and many practical problems that were encountered. This is primarily on account of the three main strategies for H5 vaccine development: attenuation of the pathogenic A/Hong Kong/97 (H5N1) virus; expression of H5 haemagglutinin in baculovirus vectors; use of avirulent H5 avian viruses. Progress with H9 vaccine development is also reviewed. Over the past $2\frac{1}{2}$ years, we have learnt a great deal about our ability to respond to an influenza pandemic. Some of the improvements that could be made for the future, are summarised. © 2001 Elsevier Science B.V. All rights reserved.

Keywords: H5N1 vaccines; H9N2 vaccines

1. Introduction

During the period May–December 1997, an outbreak of human influenza A (H5N1) infections in Hong Kong S.A.R. gave serious cause for concern [1]. At the time there was no indication whether human infection would remain linked to poultry infections, or

---
* Corresponding address. Tel.: +44-1707-654753; fax: +44-1707-646730.
E-mail address: jwood@nibsc.ac.uk (J.M. Wood).

0531-5131/01/$ – see front matter © 2001 Elsevier Science B.V. All rights reserved.
PII: S 0 5 3 1 - 5 1 3 1 (0 1) 0 0 3 8 5 - 5

whether the H5N1 virus would acquire the ability to transmit from person-to-person. A few months later, human infections caused by a further avian influenza virus subtype, H9N2 were detected in China and Hong Kong S.A.R. [2,3]. In response to these events, there was an urgent need to develop H5N1 and H9N2 vaccines, which could be used to combat possible pandemic activity. Several laboratories throughout the world were involved with vaccine development and at the time of writing, two such vaccines have been clinically evaluated and a third is under test. Although neither an H5N1 nor an H9N2 pandemic actually materialised, the process of vaccine development was extremely useful nonetheless. Different development strategies were adopted, some more successful than others and most laboratories encountered problems at some stage of vaccine development. There are important lessons to be learned from our experiences, which should help us to respond more effectively in future. The following is an account of vaccine development.

2. Safety issues

Ideally, an influenza vaccine should be safe for man and the environment both during vaccine development and also during clinical use. The H5N1 virus was highly pathogenic for man and several species of animals [4] and the H9N2 virus caused clinical illness in man, was capable of infecting chickens and ducks without symptoms, but was pathogenic in mice [5]. It was important therefore to review safety procedures, before vaccine development could begin. By common consent among WHO influenza laboratories, a high level of containment (e.g., BSL 3 or 4) was necessary for the H5N1 virus, whereas the H9N2 virus was less of a hazard and could be handled at lower levels of containment (BSL 2+ or BSL3). There were also important public health and veterinary regulations to observe and permits to be obtained before work could begin. The first stages of H5N1 vaccine development were directed at producing a safe vaccine virus and this work together with initial preparation for safe handling of the pathogenic H5N1 virus, meant that some delays were experienced.

One of the general safety issues that emerged was the safe handling of novel viruses within vaccine production areas. Most production areas are designed to protect the product from extraneous agents, but not to protect staff. Thus, in order to avoid accelerating a possible pandemic by infecting staff, a containment facility would be needed for vaccine production. This is an important consideration during the time when a novel virus is not circulating widely (e.g., WHO pandemic plan phases 0 and possibly 1 [6]). It may be considered appropriate, however, to relax such precautions if vaccine production is based on an attenuated virus or indeed if a pandemic is imminent.

3. Vaccine production

Three main strategies were adopted for H5N1 vaccine production:

- Attenuate the pathogenic A/Hong Kong/97 virus so that it was no longer lethal for poultry and other animal species.

- Produce purified H5 haemagglutinin (HA) by recombinant technology using genetically modified baculovirus vectors.
- Produce a conventional inactivated virus vaccine from an apathogenic H5N1.

3.1. Attenuation of A/Hong Kong/97 virus

Three laboratories pursued this approach. In the USA [7], the HA gene of A/Hong Kong/97 virus was genetically modified by deleting the stretch of basic amino acids at the cleavage site. Then by reverse genetics, the modified H5 HA gene and the NI NA gene from HK/97 virus were rescued into the attenuated cold-adapted A/Ann Arbor/60 virus background. The resulting 6:2 reassortant had trypsin-dependant replication in mammalian cells, was apathogenic in chickens and ferrets, possessed the cold-adapted phenotype and grew well in eggs. A second laboratory in the USA attempted to rescue a modified H5 HA gene and the N1 gene into either A/PR/8/34 (H1N1) or A/Mal/New York/78 (H2N2) viruses, but this approach appeared to be less successful (K. Subbarao, personal communication). In Japan, similar modifications to A/HK/97 HA were made and a reassortant was prepared using an avirulent strain A/Duck/Hong Kong/836/80 (H3N1) [8]. The reassortant was avirulent in a variety of animal species and grew well in eggs (M. Tashiro, personal communication).

As yet, safety for man for such genetically attenuated viruses is unknown, but there is clearly considerable potential for this approach to quickly develop safe and productive seed viruses for use in inactivated vaccines. Furthermore, the use of cold-adapted parental strains, provides a basis for development of live attenuated vaccines for use in a pandemic.

3.2. Recombinant proteins

The first H5 vaccine to be available anywhere in the world was a recombinant HA protein expressed in recombinant baculovirus-infected *S. frugiperda* cells. At present only small amounts of vaccine can be produced using this technology, but there is potential for scale-up to meet future demands.

3.3. Vaccines derived from apathogenic avian H5 viruses

An avirulent H5N3 strain, A/Duck/Singapore–Q/F119-2/97 was selected for vaccine development due to the antigenic and genetic similarity of the HA with that of the HK/97 HA. Furthermore, the DK/Sing virus did not have the polybasic amino acids at the HA cleavage site and it was not pathogenic in poultry (D. Alexander, personal communication). Unfortunately the virus grew poorly in hens' eggs and had an N3, not an N1 NA. Attempts were made to improve the situation by producing high growth reassortants. However, despite repeated attempts in several laboratories to produce reassortants by conventional means in eggs, there has been only limited success. Virus growth has been improved by selecting variants of DK/Sing, NIB-40 and ARIV-1, but it was not possible to substitute the NA. It is significant, that the only complete success to produce a high growth H5N1 virus from DK/Sing virus was in MDCK cells using plaquing techniques [9]. An avirulent H5N1 vaccine virus has also been developed in Japan [8], by producing an H5N1 reassortant, R513 between A/Duck/Hokkaido/67/96 (H5N4) and A/Duck/Hong Kong/301/78 (H7N1). The HA of DK/Hok virus was antigenically related to that of A/HK/97 virus. Experimental lots of NIB-40 and R513 have been produced for animal studies, but only NIB-40 has been used on a larger scale to produce clinical trial lots of purified surface antigen vaccine [10]. Here the greatest problem was that of poor virus growth, which created difficulties in downstream processing (A. Colegate, personal communication). Another significant issue was the availability of eggs. It was fortunate that only small amounts of vaccine were needed for clinical trial and this could be accommodated during a normal vaccine production season. If an H5N1 pandemic had materialised, it would have been difficult to mass-produce an egg-grown NIB-40 vaccine.

3.4. H9N2 vaccines

In Europe, clinical trial lots of conventional whole virus and surface antigen vaccines have been made from the A/Hong Kong/99 (H9N2) virus. The virus grew well in eggs and vaccine processing was not a problem. Again the availability of eggs was an issue and, as mentioned earlier, containment facilities were needed for the early stages of vaccine production.

A recombinant H9 HA protein has also been produced for experimental use (L. Lambert, personal communication).

3.5. General production issues

In 1998, plans were developed in the UK to produce pilot lots (approximately 1000 doses) of an inactivated vaccine from the pathogenic HK/97 virus, for subsequent clinical comparison with NIB-40 vaccines. The first stages of vaccine production took place at BSL4 containment and this was very successful. However, during downstream processing at another site, there were severe problems, which led to complete loss of the vaccine. Such losses were due to processing small amounts of experimental vaccine in a normal vaccine production facility. It is likely that if a small-scale production facility had been available, the losses would have been avoided. This was extremely unfortunate but the experience does illustrate that it should be possible to produce pilot lots of vaccine from unmodified novel viruses and this could be a first response while attempts are being made to seek safer alternatives.

4. Immunogenicity and efficacy

4.1. Attenuated A/Hong Kong/97 vaccines

Pre-clinical assessment of the attenuated viruses was performed in the USA and Japan. Cold-adapted reassortants were administered to chickens by the intravenous route and they stimulated serum haemagglutination-inhibition (HI) responses against wild-type HK/97 virus, When the chickens were challenged with lethal HK/97 viruses, 11 out of 16 chickens survived [7]. Studies with inactivated vaccines prepared from attenuated HK/97 virus were performed in Japan. Mice were immunised by the intraperitoneal route and one dose stimulated HI and virus neutralising (VN) antibody responses. When vaccine was administered by the intranasal route, mucosal and systemic antibody was produced and approximately 90% of mice survived a lethal HK/97 challenge [8].

These experiments illustrate the potential of vaccines prepared from attenuated influenza viruses and plans are in place to assess their safety and immunogenicity in man.

4.2. Recombinant proteins

Immunogenicity and protective efficacy of baculovirus-expressed avian H5 and H7 HAs in animals has been demonstrated [11] and there are ample results to show immunogenicity of human influenza HAs in man. The first lots of recombinant H5 HA were available for clinical use early in 1998 and they were administered as two 10- or 20-μg doses to 56 subjects in a phase-I trial. Somewhat surprisingly, only 2 of 28 subjects receiving the 10-μg dose and only 6 of 28 subjects receiving the 20-μg dose, developed significant VN antibody titres (≥ 80). [12]. This was a weaker immune response than expected, in view of earlier trials of HA derived from conventional human influenza viruses. In a subsequent phase II dose escalating study even two 90-μg doses could only stimulate significant VN antibody in 40% of recipients [13]. Thus, although the recombinant H5 protein was well tolerated, it was only modestly immunogenic.

4.3. Vaccines derived from apathogenic avian H5 viruses

In order to assess the protective efficacy of DK/Sing vaccines, mouse challenge studies were performed. For comparative purposes, four experimental inactivated whole-virus vaccine were prepared: (1) DK/Sing virus, (2) A/Hong Kong/156/97 virus, (3) A/Hong Kong/489/97 virus, (4) A human H3N2 virus, A/Shanghai/24/90. Balb/C mice were immunised with two intramuscular doses of 15 μg HA, given 21 days apart. High levels of HI antibody to HK/156 virus HA were induced by HK/156 and HK/489 vaccines, whereas the HI titres induced by DK/Sing vaccine were somewhat lower. This reflected the small antigenic differences between the DK/Sing vaccine and the HK/156 virus used for serological tests. The Shg/90 vaccine was as immunogenic as the H5 vaccines (high H3 antibody titres). The mice were subsequently challenged in a BSL4 laboratory with a lethal infection of HK/156 virus. All the mice died within a 7-day period in an unvaccinated control group and in the H3N2 vaccine group, but there was complete survival of mice in all three H5 vaccine groups [14].

Similar results have been obtained in other laboratories using inactivated vaccine prepared from DK/Sing virus [15] or from A/Hokkaido/67/96 (H5N4) or an H5N1 reassortant R513 described earlier [8]. In each case, the avirulent H5 avian virus provided an effective inactivated vaccine against lethal HK/97 virus challenge.

As was described earlier, pilot lots of NIB-40 vaccine have been produced for clinical evaluation. In a phase-I dose escalating trial, a conventional surface antigen vaccine was compared with an MF59-adjuvanted surface antigen vaccine. Subjects received one or two doses of 7.5, 15 or 30 μg HA. Although both types of vaccine were well tolerated, there were significant differences in immunogenicity. Two doses of the non-adjuvanted vaccine produced seroconversion in only 22% of individuals (VN data), whereas 94% of individuals seroconverted after receiving two doses of the adjuvanted vaccine (Nicholson et al, unpublished data). The conclusion from this study is that a conventional surface antigen vaccine prepared from DK/Sing is poorly immunogenic and normal doses are unlikely to protect against the pathogenic HK/97 viruses.

4.4. H9N2 vaccines

Pre-clinical evaluation of inactivated vaccines prepared from HK/99 virus have been performed in mice. A whole virus vaccine stimulated good HI responses in all mice and gave complete protection against challenge with HK/99 virus, whereas a surface antigen vaccine was poorly immunogenic even after two doses and gave incomplete protection [16]. This is further evidence that surface antigen vaccines may not make good pandemic vaccines. Clinical trial evaluation of the H9N2 vaccines is currently underway.

4.5. Other H5N1 vaccines

H5 DNA vaccines have been shown to protect mice against the lethal effects of HK/ 97 virus challenge (J. Robertson, unpublished data), even when the encoded H5 DNA (A/Turkey/Ireland/1/83) differed by 12% in the HA1 region from the HK/156 challenge virus [17]. However, neither the H5 nor an H9 DNA vaccine appeared to be capable of preventing virus replication after challenge. Thus, a DNA vaccine may offer adequate protection, even if a homologous vaccine is not available. At present the most likely use of a DNA vaccine in the context of a pandemic is to protect chickens and to prevent an initial focus of infection. The safety and efficacy of DNA vaccines in man is as yet, unproven.

The efficacy of ISCOMs as adjuvants for H5N1 vaccines has been investigated in chickens. Purified surface antigens of HK/97 virus induced no antibody responses and no protection against lethal H5N1 challenge, whereas the same surface antigens prepared as ISCOMs were highly immunogenic and gave complete protection [18]. ISCOMs are, at present, undergoing evaluation for use in normal human influenza vaccines and they offer potential to augment immune responses to pandemic vaccines.

4.6. Vaccine serology

It was extremely difficult to detect antibody to H5N1 human infections in Hong Kong, using the conventional HI test and it was necessary to use alternative tests such as VN [19]. The inadequacies of the HI test were further revealed when immune responses to baculovirus HA vaccines [12] and NIB-40 inactivated vaccines (K. Nicholson, unpublished data) were examined. It was only by the use of VN, ELISA or single-radial haemolysis techniques that vaccine immunogenicity could be evaluated. If HI insensitivity is a general phenomenon among avian subtypes, it is important that alternative safe and reliable techniques are developed.

5. Reagents for vaccine potency testing

The internationally accepted test for measurement of influenza vaccine potency is single-radial diffusion (SRD). It was therefore important to develop SRD reagents (calibrated antigen and specific anti-HA sera) for H5 and H9 vaccines prior to evaluation of their immunogenicity. Normally it takes about 2 months to develop SRD reagents, but much longer was needed for H5 (4 months) and H9 (10 months) reagents. The delays were due to a variety of reasons such as poor virus growth; need for containment facilities; difficulties in purifying H9 HA; availability of recombinant HA. Although the reagents were available in time for the animal and human vaccine studies there may have been problems if the H5N1 or H9N2 viruses had become pandemic.

6. Conclusions

Over the past $2^1/_2$ years, we have learnt a great deal about our ability to respond to an influenza pandemic. We cannot ignore the fact that it took 8 months (dating from the second human H5N1 case) to produce the first lots of H5 vaccine by conventional means, that the vaccine virus grew so poorly that mass vaccination would have been virtually impossible and that conventional surface antigen vaccines probably would not have afforded adequate protection. The H5N1 and H9N2 outbreaks have served as warnings that improvements are needed, before we can effectively combat an influenza pandemic by vaccination.

The following are some lessons that can be learnt:

- Develop and maintain dialogue between veterinary and public health authorities to reduce administrative barriers and to obtain appropriate permits and containment facilities.
- Develop and rehearse contingency plans for production of pandemic vaccines. Such plans should involve the use of containment laboratories.
- Develop methods to attenuate pathogenic viruses by reverse genetics.
- Develop alternative technologies (e.g., plaquing in cell cultures; reverse genetics) for production of high growth reassortants.
- Produce libraries of vaccine viruses from a range of avian subtypes, beginning with those considered most likely to transmit to mammals (e.g., H2, H5, H7, H9).
- Develop new vaccine technologies that do not depend upon the availability of hens' eggs; produce vaccine quicker than conventional methods; and/or present vaccine more efficiently to the immune system (e.g., mammalian cell culture vaccine, recombinant proteins, DNA vaccines, adjuvants).
- Reach a consensus on the role of live attenuated vaccines in a pandemic.
- Prepare contingency plans for fast-track licensing and official testing of pandemic vaccines. Such plans should allow novel vaccines to be used.
- Evaluate dose requirements and immunogenicity for conventional vaccines, adjuvanted vaccines and novel vaccines prepared from novel subtypes.

- Develop antiserum reagents to standardise the potency of vaccines made from novel subtypes.
- Strengthen and maintain pandemic response teams to develop vaccines. The teams could include Directors of WHO Influenza Centres, public health officials, national control authorities, clinicians, academic institutions and vaccine manufacturers.

Acknowledgements

We are grateful for helpful discussion and permission to use unpublished information from Drs. J. Katz, A. Klimov and K. Subbarao, CDC, USA; L. Lambert NIAID, USA; R. Levandowski, CBER, USA; M. Tashiro, NIID, Japan; A. Osterhaus, Erasmus University, The Netherlands; and A. Colegate, Chiron Vaccines, Italy.

References

[1] C. Bender, H. Hall, J. Huang, A. Klimov, N. Cox, A. Hay, V. Gregory, K. Cameron, W. Lim, K. Subbarao, Characterisation of the surface proteins of influenza A (H5N1) viruses isolated from humans in 1997–1998, Virology 254 (1999) 115–123.

[2] M. Peiris, K.Y. Yuen, C.W. Leung, K.H. Chan, P.L.S. Ip, R.W.M. Lai, W.K. Orr, K.F. Shortridge, Human infection with influenza H9N2, Lancet 354 (1999) 916–917.

[3] Y. Guo, J.W. Li, I. Cheng, Discovery of humans infected by avian influenza A (H9N2) virus, Chin. J. Exp. Clin. Virol. 15 (1999) 105–108.

[4] K.F. Shortride, N.N. Zhou, Y. Guan, P. Gao, T. Ito, Y. Kawaoka, S. Kodihalli, S. Krauss, D. Markwell, K.G. Murti, M. Norwood, D. Senne, L. Sims, A. Takada, R.G. Webster, Characterisation of avian H5N1 influenza viruses from poultry in Hong Kong, Virology 252 (1998) 331–342.

[5] Y.J. Guo, S. Krauss, D.A. Senne, I.P. Mo, K.S. Lo, X.P. Xiong, M. Norwood, K.F. Shortridge, R.G. Webster, Y. Guan, Characterisation of the pathogenicity of members of the newly established H9N2 influenza virus lineages in Asia, Virology 267 (2000) 279–288.

[6] Influenza Pandemic Preparedness Plan, WHO, Geneva, Switzerland, 1999.

[7] S. Li, C. Liu, A. Klimov, K. Subbarao, M. Perdue, D. Mo, Y. Ji, L. Woods, S. Hietala, M. Bryant, Recombinant influenza A virus vaccines for the pathogenic human A/Hong Kong/97 (H5N1) viruses, J. Infect. Dis. 179 (1999) 1132–1138.

[8] A. Takada, N. Kuboki, K. Okazaki, A. Ninomiya, H. Tanaka, H. Ozaki, S. Itamura, H. Nishimura, M. Enami, M. Tashiro, K.F. Shortridge, H. Kida, Avirulent avian influenza virus as a vaccine strain against a potential human pandemic, J. Virol. 73 (1999) 8303–8307.

[9] T. Mabrouk, Vaccines and related biological products advisory committee meeting regarding influenza vaccine formulation for 1999–2000. 1999. www.fda.gov/ohrms/dockets/ac/99/transcpt/3494t1.

[10] J.M. Wood, Vaccines and related biological products advisory committee meeting regarding influenza vaccine formulation for 1999–2000. 1999. www.fda.gov/ohrms/dockets/ac/99/transcpt/3494t1.

[11] J. Crawford, B. Wilkinson, A. Vosnesensky, G. Smith, M. Garcia, H. Stone, M.L. Perdue, Baculovirus-derived haemagglutinin vaccines protect against lethal influenza infections by avian H5 and H7 subtypes, Vaccine 17 (1999) 2265–2274.

[12] J. Katz, J. Treanor, Vaccines and related biological products advisory committee meeting regarding influenza vaccine formulation for 1999–2000. 1999. www.fda.gov/ohrms/dockets/ac/99/transcpt/3494t1.

[13] J.J. Treanor, B. Wilkinson, W. Blackwelder, J.M. Katz, Evaluation of the haemagglutinin (HA) of the H5N1 influenza A/Hong Kong/156/97 virus expressed in insect cells by recombinant baculovirus (rH5) as an influenza vaccine in healthy adults [Abstract No. 682], 39th International Conference on Antimicrobial Agents and Chemotherapy, San Francisco, 1999.

[14] J.M. Wood, D. Major, J. Daly, R.W. Newman, U. Dunleavy, C. Nicholson, J.S. Robertson, G.C. Schild, Vaccines against H5N1 influenza, Lett. Vaccine 19 (2000) 579–580.

[15] X. Lu, T.M. Tumpey, T. Morken, S.R. Zaki, N.J. Cox, J.M. Katz, A mouse model for the evaluation of pathogenesis and immunity to influenza A (H5N1) viruses isolated from humans, J. Virol. 73 (1999) 5903–5911.

[16] D. Major, R.W. Newman, U. Dunleavy, A. Heath, K. Ploss, J.M. Wood, Evaluation of candidate H9N2 influenza vaccine strains in Balb C mice, in: A.D.M.E. Osterhaus, et al. (Eds.), Options for the Control of Influenza IV, Exerpta Med. Int. Congr. Ser., Elsevier, 2001, pp. 789–794.

[17] S. Kodihalli, H. Goto, D.L. Kobasa, S. Krauss, Y. Kawaoka, R.G. Webster, DNA vaccine encoding haemagglutinin provides protective immunity against H5N1 influenza virus infection in mice, J. Virol. 73 (1999) 2094–2098.

[18] G.F. Rimmelzwaan, E.C.J. Claas, G. Van Amerongen, J.C. de Jong, A.D.M.E. Osterhaus, ISCOM vaccine induced protection against a lethal challenge with a human H5N1 influenza virus, Vaccine 17 (1999) 1355–1358.

[19] T. Rowe, R.A. Abernathy, J. Hu-Primmer, W.W. Thompson, X. Lu, W. Lin, K. Fukuda, N.J. Cox, J.M. Katz, Detection of antibody to avian influenza A (H5N1) virus in human serum by using a combination of serological assays, J. Clin. Microbiol. 37 (1999) 937–943.

International Congress Series 1219 (2001) 761–766

A single radial haemolysis assay for antibody to H5 haemagglutinin

J.M. Wood[a,*], D. Melzack[a], R.W. Newman[a], D.L. Major[a],
M. Zambon[b], K.G. Nicholson[c], A. Podda[d]

[a]National Institute for Biological Standards and Control, Blanche Lane, South Mimms, Potters Bar,
Herts EN6 3QG, UK
[b]Control Public Health Laboratory, Colindale, UK
[c]Leicester Royal Infirmary, Leicester, UK
[d]Chiron Vaccines, Siena, Italy

Abstract

Background: It has been recognised that the haemagglutination–inhibition (HI) test is not sufficiently sensitive to detect human antibody to H5N1 influenza virus and alternative serological tests are needed. A modified single radial haemolysis (SRH) test is described. *Methods*: Sera from H5N1 human cases in Hong Kong SAR and from H5 vaccine trials were tested by an H5 SRH test which included a virus adsorption step to remove cross-reactive antibody. Test specificity was examined using reference animal antisera. *Results*: The SRH test recognised antibody in a specific antiserum to A/Hong Kong/489/97 (H5N1) virus, yet rabbit antibody to an A (H10N7) avian virus and human antibody to A (H1N1) or A (H3N2) viruses did not react. H5 SRH antibody induced by human H5N1 virus infection and A/Duck/Singapore/97 (H5N3) vaccination, correlated with antibody detected by microneutralisation techniques. *Conclusion*: The modified SRH test offers an alternative serological technique for detecting antibody to H5 haemagglutinins, which does not depend on use of live pathogenic H5N1 virus. © 2001 Elsevier Science B.V. All rights reserved.

Keywords: SRH; Influenza; HA; H5 antibody

1. Introduction

Although haemagglutination–inhibition (HI) is considered to be the standard technique for measurement of antibody to influenza virus, it is insufficiently sensitive for detecting

* Corresponding author. Tel.: +44-1707-654753; fax: +44-1707-646730.
E-mail address: jwood@nibsc.ac.uk (J.M. Wood).

0531-5131/01/$ – see front matter © 2001 Elsevier Science B.V. All rights reserved.
PII: S0531-5131(01)00410-1

antibody responses to avian viruses in mammalian sera [1,2]. This view was reinforced during the 1997 outbreak of H5N1 virus in Hong Kong SAR, when H5 HI titres were either very low or negative in patients with confirmed H5N1 infections [3]. Similarly, during serological investigation of Phase I trials of recombinant H5 HA vaccine, HI was found to be insensitive [4].

Alternative serological techniques to be developed for H5 HAs include microneutralization (MN), ELISA and Western blots [3]. A combination of MN or ELISA and confirmation by Western blot gave a high degree of sensitivity and specificity for subjects aged ≤ 60 years and this approach was used for seroepidemiological studies in Hong Kong SAR [5,6]. However, one drawback with the MN test was the need for infectious virus and hence, a high level of containment.

Single radial haemolysis (SRH) was developed in 1975 [7] and has gradually gained acceptance, particularly in Europe for evaluation of the antibody response to vaccination [8]. Studies in the 1980s [9] have suggested that SRH could be used to detect human antibody to avian influenza viruses, although there is concern about the lack of specificity in such tests [3]. We have developed an SRH test, which appears to have adequate sensitivity and specificity for detection of H5 antibody.

2. Materials and methods

2.1. Viruses

The influenza viruses used in this study were A/Hong Kong/489/97 (H5N1) (HK/489), A/Duck/Singapore–Q/F119-3/97 (H5N3) (DK/Sing), A/Chicken/Germany/49 (H10N7) (CK/Ger), A/Beijing/262/95 (H1N1) (Bj/95) and RESVIR-13 reassortant with surface antigens of A/Sydney/5/97 (H3N2). Viruses were propagated in embryonated hens' eggs and purified by rate zonal centrifugation on sucrose gradients. The HK/97 virus was cultivated in BSL-4 containment and inactivated by β-propiolactone before purification.

2.2. Serum samples

Sera from five H5N1 patients in Hong Kong were kindly provided by Drs J. Katz, CDC, USA, M. Peiris, University of Hong Kong SAR and W.L. Lim, Queen Mary Hospital, Hong Kong, SAR. Human sera were also obtained from a Phase I clinical trial of a DK/Sing subunit vaccine (Nicholson et al. unpublished data), from a 1998 clinical trial of a licensed influenza vaccine (kindly supplied by Dr H. Engelmann, SKB, Germany) and from UK blood donations (kindly supplied by Dr M. Ferguson, NIBS-C,UK).

Ferret antiserum to HK/489 virus was obtained by intranasal infection, followed by an intranasal boost after 2 weeks and blood taken 2 weeks later. Rabbit antiserum to CK/Ger HA was obtained by intramuscular injection of purified CK/Ger HA followed by three boosts with HA at weekly intervals and blood taken 7 weeks after the initial injection.

2.3. Single radial haemolysis

The SRH immunoplates were prepared as described by Schild et al. [7] using turkey erythrocytes. The amount of influenza virus (either DK/Sing or inactivated HK/489) used to sensitise the erythrocytes was 100 μg virus protein per 1 ml of a 15% erythrocyte suspension. All sera were heated at 56 °C for 30 min and 5 μl volumes were added to wells in the SRH plates. After incubation for 18 h at 37 °C, zones of haemolysis were measured and zone annulus areas were calculated. In experiments to remove non-specific (i.e. non-HA or NA) antibody, heat-treated sera (6 μl) were absorbed with a 6 μl mixture of Bj/95 and RESVIR-13 viruses (10 mg virus protein/1 ml).

3. Results

3.1. Test specificity

Normal human sera and sera from trials of a licensed 1998 influenza vaccine were tested in SRH plates containing DK/Sing virus. Ten out of 31 (32%) sera gave small non-specific zones, which could be removed by adsorption with influenza A (H1N1) and A (H3N2) viruses (serum 3 in Fig. 1). A large number (61%) of the sera also had SRH antibody to influenza A (H1N1) or A (H3N2) viruses and all sera showing non-specific responses also had antibody to other influenza A strains. Thus, without the adsorption step, the SRH test was too cross-reactive to reliably measure anti-H5 HA antibody. A rabbit antiserum to the HA of an H10N7 virus CK/Ger gave no SRH zones before or after adsorption (serum 6 in Fig. 1).

Tests of human sera from a Phase I trial of a DK/Sing vaccine (sera 1 and 2 in Fig. 1) and a ferret serum to HK/489 (serum 5 in Fig. 1) revealed clear SRH zones and the zone size was unaffected by adsorption.

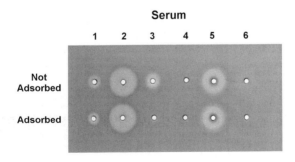

Fig. 1. Single radial haemolysis test of antisera to H5 haemagglutinins. Two human sera from a DK/Sing vaccine trial (sera 1 and 2), a human serum from a 1998 trial of a licensed vaccine (serum 3), a normal human serum (serum 4), a ferret antiserum to HK/489 virus (serum 5), and a rabbit antiserum to CK/Ger virus (serum 6) were tested for SRH antibody to DK/Sing virus. Sera were tested before and after adsorption with a mixture of an H1N1 and H3N2 viruses.

In further tests for cross-reactivity (not illustrated), none of the positive H5 sera gave zones on SRH plates containing CK/Ger virus, whereas the rabbit antiserum to CK/Ger gave clear zones. Thus, a DK/Sing SRH test with the addition of a virus adsorption step, was considered sufficiently specific for further evaluation.

3.2. Comparison of SRH, HI and MN for detection of H5 antibody induced by DK/Sing vaccine

Sera from the DK/Sing vaccine trial were also tested by HI and MN (M. Zambon, unpublished data). In comparison of SRH and HI tests (data not shown), SRH detected 51 positive responses (SRH area ≥ 4 mm^2) from 128 sera tested (40%), whereas HI detected only 26 positives (HI ≥ 10) (20%). There were 27 sera which had SRH antibody but no HI antibody.

In MN tests of the same sera, 63 were positive (MN ≥ 20) (49%) and there was an equivalent number of sera that were SRH positive/MN negative (9) or were SRH negative/MN positive (11). Thus, the H5 SRH test appeared to have similar sensitivity to the MN test and both were approximately twice as sensitive as the HI test.

3.3. SRH tests of post-infection sera from H5N1 cases

Sera from five cases of H5N1 infection from Hong Kong were tested in SRH plates containing inactivated HK/489 virus. Only one serum sample was available for four of the cases (sera 1–4 in Fig. 2). These were equivalent to the S2 sera described by Katz et al. [5]. For one case, acute and convalescent sera were available (sera 5 and 6 in Fig. 2). H5 SRH zones were produced by sera from all five H5N1 cases tested and seroconversion was clearly detected. Serum adsorption did not reduce the size of the SRH zones. Positive H5 SRH zones were again obtained with ferret antiserum to HK/489 (serum 7, Fig. 2) and no zones were obtained with rabbit antiserum to CK/Ger HA (serum 8, Fig. 2). However, in

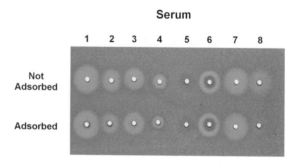

Fig. 2. Detection of H5 SRH antibody in sera from H5N1 cases. Sera from the following H5N1 cases: case 7 (serum 1), case 4 (serum 2); case 16 (serum 3), case 8 (serum 4), case 5 acute phase (serum 5), case 5 convalescent phase (serum 6), were tested for SRH antibody to HK/489 virus. Control sera tested were ferret antisera to HK/489 virus (serum 7) and rabbit antiserum to CK/Ger virus (serum 8). Sera were tested before and after adsorption as in Fig. 1.

this SRH test, the CK/Ger serum appeared to possess some non-specific activity before adsorption. All the sera from H5N1 cases were also screened for antibody to the 1997 H3N2 strain RESVIR-13 and only one serum was positive (serum 4, data not illustrated). The H5 SRH titres were compared with MN titres (J. Katz, unpublished data) and there was a good correlation ($r = 0.83$) between the two tests.

4. Discussion

A modified SRH test has been developed for detection of antibody to avian H5 HAs. From limited data available, the H5 SRH test appears to be as sensitive as VN tests and much more sensitive than HI tests. There is thus potential for use of SRH in seroepidemiology and in serology of vaccine trials.

The main advantage of SRH over MN is one of safety. The VN test requires live influenza virus and thus a high level of containment is needed for H5N1 tests. The SRH test works well with inactivated viruses so that H5N1 serology can be safely performed at BSL2 containment.

This study has also demonstrated that caution must be exercised in planning and interpreting SRH tests. The H5 SRH test could detect non-specific antibody in human and rabbit sera, but the antibody could be removed by adsorption with other influenza A viruses. It is likely that the cross-reactivity is due to antibody induced by influenza A internal proteins. Therefore, for SRH detection of antibody to influenza A viruses, a preliminary screen for cross-reactivity, a confirmatory test with an alternative serological technique or a virus adsorption step are recommended.

We have demonstrated the potential of SRH for detecting antibody to H5 HAs and there is a need to extend the studies to other avian influenza subtypes.

Acknowledgements

We are grateful to Dr Jackie Katz, CDC for permission to use unpublished MN data.

References

[1] V.S. Hinshaw, R.G. Webster, B.C. Easterday, W.J. Bean, Replication of avian influenza A viruses in mammals, Infect. Immun. 34 (1981) 354–361.

[2] M.L. Profeta, G. Palladino, Serological evidence of human infections with avian influenza viruses, Arch. Virol. 90 (1986) 355–360.

[3] T. Rowe, R.A. Abernathy, J. Hu-Primmer, W.W. Thompson, X. Lu, W. Lim, K. Kukuda, N.J. Cox, J.M. Katz, Detection of antibody to avian influenza A (H5N1) virus in human serum by using a combination of serologic assays, J. Clin. Microbiol. 37 (1999) 937–943.

[4] J. Katz, Vaccines and related biological products advisory committee meeting regarding influenza vaccine formulation for 1999–2000, 1999, http://www.fda.gov/ohrms/dockets/ac/99/transcpt/3494tl.

[5] J.M. Katz, W. Lim, C.B. Bridges, T. Rowe, J. Hu-Primmer, X. Lu, Antibody response in individuals infected with avian influenza A (H5N1) viruses and detection of anti-H5 antibody among household and social contacts, J. Infect. Dis. 180 (1999) 1763–1770.

[6] C.B. Bridges, J.M. Katz, W.H. Seto, P.K.S. Chan, D. Tsang, W. Ho, K.H. Mak, W. Lim, J.S. Tam, M. Clarke, S.G. Williams, A.W. Mounts, J.S. Bresee, L.A. Conn, T. Rowe, J. Hu-Primmer, R.A. Abernathy, X. Lu, N.J. Cox, K. Fukuda, Risk of influenza A (H5N1) infection among health care workers exposed to patients with influenza A (H5N1), Hong Kong, J. Infect. Dis. 181 (2000) 344–348.

[7] G.C. Schild, M.S. Pereira, P. Chakraverty, Single-radial-haemolysis: a new method for the assay of antibody to influenza haemagglutinin, Bull. WHO 52 (1975) 43–50.

[8] CPMP, Note for guidance on harmonisation of requirements for influenza vaccines, http://www.eudra.org/humandocs/PDFs/BWP/021496en.

[9] K.F. Shortridge, Pandemic influenza—a blueprint for control at source, Chin. J. Clin. Virol. 2 (1988) 75–89.

International Congress Series 1219 (2001) 767–773

Cross-protection studies with H5 influenza viruses

Yuri A. Smirnov[a,*], Nikolai V. Kaverin[a], Elena A. Govorkova[a],
Alexander S. Lipatov[a], Eric C.J. Claas[b], Natalia V. Makarova[a],
Asya K. Gitelman[a], Robert G. Webster[c], Dmitri K. Lvov[a]

[a]The D.I. Ivanovsky Institute of Virology RAMS, 16 Gamaleya, 123098, Moscow, Russia
[b]Department of Virology, CKVL, Leiden University Medical Center, Leiden, Netherlands
[c]Department of Virology and Molecular Biology, St. Jude Children's Research Hospital, Memphis, TN, USA

Abstract

Background: The direct transmission of avian influenza H5N1 virus from infected poultry into humans raised questions about the level of protection induced by different strains within the H5 subtype. *Methods*: In this study, the hemagglutinins (HA) of four avian H5 viruses and the human A/ Hong Kong/156/97 (H5N1) strain were analyzed antigenically and their phylogenetic relationships were established. These viruses were further characterized in cross-protection studies in mice. Mice were immunized with β-propiolactone-inactivated viruses, and three weeks later challenged with 10 MLD_{50} of the mouse-adapted A/Mallard Duck/Pennsylvania/10218/84. *Results*: The HI test with a panel of HA-specific monoclonal antibodies showed different reactivity patterns for the five H5 influenza viruses studied. Phylogenetic analysis revealed genetic diversity among these H5 viruses as well. Cross-protection experiments indicated that mice immunized with American viruses exhibited a high level of protection (94.4–100.0%) against challenge with the virus from the same phylogenetic lineage. Immunization with Eurasian viruses induced lower levels of protection in mice (50.0– 55.5%). *Conclusions*: Due to the heterogeneity of the H5 viruses, no single broad reactive strain is available as an appropriate vaccine candidate for a potential H5 influenza pandemic. © 2001 Elsevier Science B.V. All rights reserved.

Keywords: Influenza A viruses; Hemagglutinin; Immunization; Cross-protection

* Corresponding author. Tel.: +7-95-190-3056; fax: +7-95-190-2867.
E-mail address: yusmirnov@hotmail.com (Y.A. Smirnov).

0531-5131/01/$ – see front matter © 2001 Elsevier Science B.V. All rights reserved.
PII: S 0 5 3 1 - 5 1 3 1 (0 1) 0 0 3 5 6 - 9

1. Introduction

Phylogenetic studies have established that the previous pandemic human influenza A viruses have been partly of avian origin, with three antigenic variants (H1N1, H2N2 and H3N2) [1,2]. Avian influenza viruses do not replicate efficiently in humans [3], and before the outbreak of influenza in 1997 in Hong Kong caused by avian-like H5N1 strains [4,5] it was considered that an intermediate mammalian host was required for the transmission of an avian influenza viruses to humans. The Hong Kong H5N1 influenza viruses were shown to replicate in mice and to cause lethal disease without prior adaptation [6,7]. The highly pathogenic avian influenza viruses encoding the HA gene associated with the H5N1 outbreak are still circulating in poultry in Asia [8]. In the present study, we characterized antigenic specificity of the HA and phylogenetic relationships among five H5 influenza viruses. Cross-protection experiments were carried out to determine the protective efficacy of these viruses in a mouse model.

2. Material and methods

2.1. Viruses

The H5 avian influenza viruses were used in this study included: A/Tern/South Africa/61(H5N3), A/Duck/Ho Chi Minh/014/78 (H5N3) (A/DK/Ho Chi Minh/78), A/Ruddy Turnstown/Delaware/244/91 (H5N2) (A/RT/Delaware/ 244/91), A/Mallard Duck/Pennsylvania/10218/84 (H5N2) (A/Ml/Pennsylvania /10218/84), and human A/Hong Kong/156/97 (H5N1) virus. A highly pathogenic mouse-adapted (MA) variant of A/Ml/Pennsylvania/10218/84 strain was obtained by 23 serial lung-to-lung passages in mice [9]. Purified virus preparations were collected from infected allantoic fluid by centrifugation through 20% (w/v) sucrose cushion and inactivated by treatment with β-propiolactone [10].

Antigenic characterization of the viruses was performed in hemagglutination-inhibition (HI) test with the panel of HA-specific monoclonal antibodies (MAbs) raised against A/Chicken/Pennsylvania/1370/83 (H5N2) [11].

2.2. Sequencing of the HA genes

RNA was extracted from virus-containing allantoic fluids and amplified by RT-PCR as described previously [12]. PCR products were purified and subsequently subjected to sequence analysis using a Dye-Terminator Cycle Sequencing ready reactions kit (Perkin-Elmer, Applied Biosystems, Foster City, CA).

Phylogenetic analysis of the nucleotide sequences of the HA1 subunit of the HA gene was performed for the viruses used in cross-protection studies, together with sequences from the GenBank. Analysis was done using a combination of the Neighbour-Joining method for the detection of distance and the Maximum-Parsimony method for the generation of phylogenetic tree using PHYLIP (the PHYLogeny Interface Package) version 3.57C software.

2.3. Immunization and experimental infection

Outbred albino mice (10–12 g) were immunized intramuscularly and into the base of the tail with inactivated whole virus preparations mixed with an equal volume of complete Freund's adjuvant (20 μg total virus protein per mouse) [13]. Control mice were injected with PBS/adjuvant (1:1) mixture. Twenty-one days after immunization, ether anaesthetized mice were infected intranasally with 50 μl of PBS-diluted allantoic fluid containing 10 MLD_{50} of A/Ml/Pennsylvania/10218/84-MA. The survival rates of mice were assessed after an observation period of 10 days.

3. Results

3.1. Antigenic reactivity of H5 influenza viruses in the HI test

The results of the HI test established that two American strains, A/RT/Delaware/244/91 and A/Ml/Pennsylvania/10218/84-MA, were closely related and showed similar reactivity patterns with five out of seven MAbs used (Table 1). Eurasian viruses were antigenically heterogeneous and demonstrated detectable antigenic drift. All MAbs reacted with influenza A/Hong Kong/156/97 virus, while only three MAbs reacted with influenza A/Tern/South Africa/61 virus, which was antigenically distinguishable from all other H5 viruses tested (Table 1).

3.2. Phylogenetic analysis of the HA genes

We analyzed the nucleotide sequences of the HA1 portion of the HA gene of the above five influenza H5 viruses together with previously published sequences (Fig. 1). The analysis revealed that influenza A/RT/Delaware/244/91 and A/Ml/Pennsylvania/10218/84-MA viruses belong to the American lineage and are located on distinct branches of the phylogenetic tree. Three other influenza viruses tested belong to the Eurasian lineage, and influenza A/Tern/South Africa/61 virus formed a separate branch.

Table 1
Antigenic reactivity of the HA of H5 influenza viruses with monoclonal antibodies

Virus	HI titer[a] with MAbs[b]						
	22	28	34	46	55	58	79
A/Tern/South Africa/61	<[c]	<	100	25,600	<	800	<
A/DK/Ho Chi Minh/014/78	800	200	800	<	800	6400	6400
A/Hong Kong/156/97	1600	800	1600	1600	3200	6400	6400
A/RT/Delaware/244/91	200	<	6400	25,600	51,200	51,200	102,400
A/Ml/Pennsylvania/10218/84-MA	12,800	400	3200	51,200	102,400	102,400	102,400

[a] HI titer is expressed as the reciprocal of the highest antibody dilution inhibiting 4 HA units of virus.
[b] MAbs were prepared to the HA of influenza A/CK/Pennsylvania/1370/83 (H5N2) virus.
[c] HI titer less than 100.

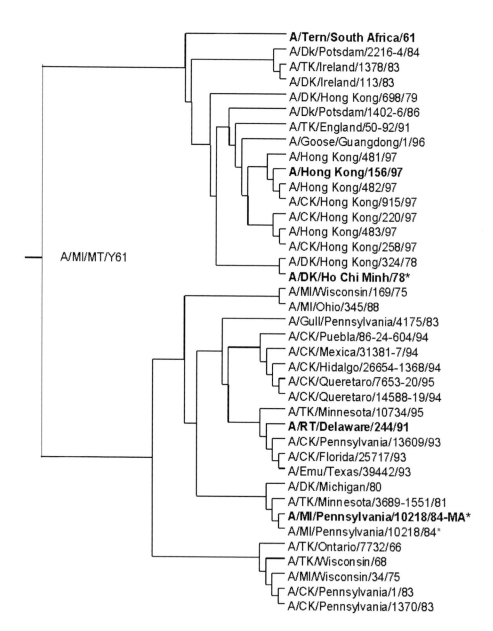

Fig. 1. Phylogenetic tree for H5 influenza A viruses HA genes. The tree is rooted to the nucleotide sequence from A/Mallard/MT/Y61 (H2N2), (L11136). Horizontal distances are proportional to the number of nucleotide changes in the HA1. The viruses studied in cross-protection experiments are typed in bold letters. * — New sequences: A/DK/Ho Chi Minh/014/78 (accession number AF290443); A/Ml/Pennsylvania/10218/84-MA (accession number AF100179) and A/Ml/Pennsylvania/10218/84 (accession number AF100180).

Table 2
Protection of mice immunized with influenza H5 viruses against lethal challenge with A/Ml/Pennsylvania/10218/84-MA

Virus used for immunization	Survivals/t total	Survival rate (%)	P-value[a]	P-value[b]
A/Tern/South Africa/61	10/20	50.0	0.0003	0.02
A/DK/Ho Chi Minh/ 014/78	10/18	55.5	0.0005	0.015
A/Hong Kong/156/97	10/18	55.5	0.0005	0.015
A/RT/Delaware/244/91	17/18	94.4	0.16	<0.00001
A/Ml/Pennsylvania/10218/84-MA	18/18	100.0	–	<0.00001
Control	3/21	14.3	<0.00001	–

P-values were calculated using two-sided Fisher's Exact test.

[a] Comparison of the survival rates between the mice immunized with heterologous strain and homologous virus A/Ml/Pennsylvania/10218/84-MA.

[b] Comparison of the survival rates between the immunized and control groups of mice.

3.3. Cross-protection experiments in mice

To determine if the observed antigenic and genetic differences among five H5 influenza viruses can influence their protective properties, cross-protection experiments were done in mice (Table 2). The viruses studied could be divided in two groups. The first group included influenza A/Tern/South Africa/61, A/DK/Ho Chi Minh/78 and A/Hong Kong/156/97 viruses; the survival rates in mice immunized with these viruses were in the range from 50.0% to 55.5%. The second group included influenza A/RT/Delaware/244/91 virus and A/Ml/Pennsylvania/10218/84-MA. Mice immunized with these viruses achieved a high level of protection (respectively, 94.4% and 100%) after challenge with A/Ml/Pennsylvania/10218/84-MA. The survival rates of animals immunized with different viruses were statistically significant as compared with those of the controls. The number of survivals was greater among mice immunized with influenza A/RT/Delaware/244/91 virus and A/Ml/Pennsylvania/10218/84-MA ($P<0.00001$), while the other experimental groups were protected from lethal infection at a lower level of significance ($P<0.1$).

4. Discussion

Protective immunity towards influenza is based mainly on the presence of virus neutralising antibodies against the surface glycoprotein HA, which is considered to be a major antigenic determinant of the influenza viruses. Previously, we have shown that mice immunized with different H2 influenza viruses exhibited different levels of protection against lethal challenge with the virus of the same HA subtype [13,14]. The grouping of the strains in accordance with their cross-protection efficiency does not coincide with H2 phylogenetic branches [14].

In the present study, we determined the protective efficacy for the H5 influenza viruses, which showed antigenic differences and belong to different phylogenetic lineages of the HA. Immunization of mice with the strains belonging to the American lineage completely protected animals against the lethal challenge with the virus of same lineage, whereas only half of the animals were protected when Eurasian strains were used for immunization. The extent of amino acid homology in the HA1 regions among the viruses used for immunization and challenge strain was relatively high (96% for American virus and 87–92% for Eurasian viruses). Avian-like A/Hong Kong/156/97 virus demonstrated a similar level of protection as the other Eurasian viruses, in spite of the lowest percentage of homology to the challenge virus (87%). Previous studies have shown that HA-based DNA vaccines conferred protection in chickens and ferrets against challenge with antigenic variants that differed from the primary antigen by 11% to 13% in the HA1 region [15]. However, in a mouse model a DNA vaccine made with a heterologous H5 strain did not prevent infection by H5N1 avian influenza viruses [16]. These data made it possible to suggest that the level of homology of the HA between the challenge virus and the virus used for immunization is important but is not the sole determinant of protective immunity. It can be concluded that none of the H5 viruses can be used as broad reactive vaccine strain as both the Eurasian and the American lineage will have to be represented in such a vaccine. Obviously, rapid identification and use of the emerging influenza strain with pandemic potential itself will provide a vaccine with optimal protective properties.

Acknowledgements

This work was supported by NATO Linkage Grant OUTR LG 971250, Awards RN1-412 and RB1-2023 of the U.S. Civilian Research and Development Foundation for the Independent States of the Former Soviet Union (CRDF), and Award 00-04-48000 of the Russian Foundation for Basic Research (RFBR).

References

[1] R.G. Webster, W.J. Bean, O.T. Gorman, T.M. Chambers, Y. Kawaoka, Evolution and ecology of influenza A viruses, Microbiol. Rev. 56 (1992) 152–179.

[2] R.G. Webster, Influenza virus transmission between species and relevance to emergence of the next human pandemic, Arch. Virol. 13 (1997) 105–113 (suppl).

[3] A.S. Beare, R.G. Webster, Replications of avian influenza viruses in humans, Arch. Virol. 119 (1991) 37–42.

[4] J.C. De Jong, E.C.J. Claas, A.D.M.E. Osterhaus, R.G. Webster, W.L. Lim, A pandemic warning? Nature 389 (1997) 554.

[5] E.C.J. Claas, A.D.M.E. Osterhaus, R. Van Beek, J.C. De Jong, G.F. Rimmelzwaan, D.A. Senne, S. Krauss, K.F. Shortridge, R.G. Webster, Human influenza A(H5N1) virus related to a highly pathogenic avian influenza virus, Lancet 351 (1998) 472–477.

[6] P. Gao, S. Watanabe, T. Ito, H. Goto, K. Wells, M. McGregor, A.J. Cooley, Y. Kawaoka, Biological heterogeneity, including systemic replication in mice, of H5N1 influenza A virus isolates from humans in Hong Kong, J. Virol. 73 (1999) 3184–3189.

[7] X. Lu, T.M. Tumpey, T. Morken, S.R. Zaki, N.J. Cox, J.M. Katz, A mouse model for the evaluation of pathogenesis and immunity to influenza A (H5N1) viruses isolated from humans, J. Virol. 73 (1999) 5903–5911.

[8] A.N. Cauthen, D.E. Swayne, S. Schultz-Cherry, M.L. Perdue, D.L. Suarez, Continued circulation in China of highly pathogenic avian influenza viruses encoding the hemagglutinin gene associated with the 1997 H5N1 outbreak in poultry and humans, J. Virol. 74 (2000) 6592–6599.

[9] Y.A. Smirnov, A.S. Lipatov, R. Van Beek, A.K. Gitelman, A.D.M.E. Osterhaus, E.C.J. Claas, Characterization of adaptation of an avian influenza A (H5N2) virus to a mammalian host, Acta Virol. 44 (2000) 1–8.

[10] E.I. Budowsky, Y.A. Smirnov, S.F. Shenderovich, Principles of selective inactivation of viral genome: VIII.

The influence of β-propiolactone on immunogenic and protective activities of influenza virus, Vaccine 11 (1993) 343–348.

[11] Y. Kawaoka, A. Nestorowicz, D.J. Alexander, R.G. Webster, Molecular analysis of the hemagglutinin genes of H5 influenza viruses. Origin of a virulent turkey strain, Virology 158 (1987) 218–227.

[12] L.L. Shu, W.J. Bean, R.G. Webster, Analysis of the evolution and variation of the human influenza A virus nucleoprotein gene from 1933 to 1990, J. Virol. 67 (1993) 2723–2729.

[13] E.A. Govorkova, Y.A. Smirnov, Cross-protection of mice immunized with different influenza A (H2) strains and challenged with viruses of the same HA subtype, Acta Virol. 41 (1997) 251–257.

[14] N.V. Kaverin, Y.A. Smirnov, E.A. Govorkova, I.A. Rudneva, A.K. Gitelman, A.S. Lipatov, N.L. Varich, S.S. Yamnikova, N.V. Makarova, R.G. Webster, D.K. Lvov, Cross-protection and reassortment studies with avian H2 influenza viruses, Arch. Virol. 145 (2000) 1059–1066.

[15] S. Kodihalli, J.R. Haynes, H.L. Robinson, R.G. Webster, Cross-protection among lethal H5N2 influenza viruses induced by DNA vaccine to the hemagglutinin, J. Virol. 71 (1997) 3391–3396.

[16] S. Kodihalli, H. Goto, D.L. Kobasa, S. Krauss, Y. Kawaoka, R.G. Webster, DNA vaccine encoding hemagglutinin provides protective immunity against H5N1 influenza virus infection in mice, J. Virol. 73 (1999) 2094–2098.

International Congress Series 1219 (2001) 775–781

Infection with H9N2 influenza viruses confers immunity against lethal H5N1 infection

Eduardo O'Neill[a], Sang H. Seo[a], David L. Woodland[b,1],
Kennedy F. Shortridge[c], Robert G. Webster[a,*]

[a]Department of Virology and Molecular Biology, St. Jude Children's Research Hospital,
332 North Lauderdale, Memphis, TN 38105-2794, USA
[b]Department of Immunology, St. Jude Children's Research Hospital, Memphis, TN 38105-2794, USA
[c]Department of Microbiology, The University of Hong Kong, University Pathology Building,
Queen Mary Hospital, Hong Kong SAR, China

Abstract

Background: The bird flu incident in Hong Kong in 1997 was caused by a highly pathogenic H5N1 influenza virus. Influenza viruses of the H9N2 and H5N1 serotypes were cocirculating in the poultry markets during the 1997 Hong Kong outbreak, but mortality was only marginally above background. *Methods*: Chickens and mice were immunized with an H9N2 virus and subsequently challenged with a lethal H5N1 virus. *Results*: Both chickens and mice survived a lethal H5N1 challenge if previously immunized with an H9N2 containing internal proteins that are homologous in both types of viruses. *Conclusions*: Previous immunization of chickens with an H9N2 virus establishes cellular immunity and protects against lethal H5N1 infection. H9N2-immunized mice also survive a lethal H5N1 challenge, suggesting that mammals can be effectively immunized using a similar strategy. © 2001 Elsevier Science B.V. All rights reserved.

Keywords: Hong Kong outbreak; Heterosubtypic immunization; Cytotoxic T cells

1. Introduction

Influenza viruses of the H9N2 serotype were cocirculating with H5N1 viruses in the poultry markets during the 1997 outbreak in Hong Kong [1]. In fact, both serotypes

---

* Corresponding author. Tel.: +1-901-495-3400; fax: +1-901-523-2622.
E-mail address: robert.webster@stjude.org (R.G. Webster).
[1] Present address: The Trudeau Institute, 100 Algonquin Avenue, P.O. Box 59, Saranac Lake, NY 12983-0059, USA.

0531-5131/01/$ – see front matter © 2001 Elsevier Science B.V. All rights reserved.
PII: S0531-5131(01)00396-X

continue to be isolated from the poultry markets, and H9N2 infection was recently detected in humans [2–4]. The potential for genetic reassortment of these viruses and for human disease is a continuous threat.

The pathogenicity of the H5N1 viruses isolated from the poultry markets during the 1997 incident is different from that seen in chickens and mice infected with H5N1 in a laboratory setting [5–8]. Interestingly, chickens seemed healthy despite harboring H5N1 viruses that were lethal to laboratory animals [1]. A likely explanation for this phenomenon is that the genes encoding the internal proteins of the H9N2 virus are homologous to those of H5N1; this finding suggests that previous infection with an H9N2 virus results in cellular immunity that would be protective against lethal H5N1 infection. Cellular immunity against cross-reactive epitopes has been shown to provide protection against serologically distinct viruses. The effectiveness of this type of immunity against highly virulent strains of influenza remains to be elucidated.

In the current report, we demonstrate that infection with an H9N2 virus in a laboratory setting generates a cytotoxic T lymphocyte (CTL) response in chickens and mice. We confirmed that this response is T cell- and not B cell-mediated in both systems. Chickens that were primed with H9N2 before an H5N1 challenge were protected and shed the H5N1 virus in their feces, a finding that suggested that this shedding was a mechanism of transmission to humans during the Hong Kong outbreak of 1997. The fact that mice can also be protected in the same manner suggests that mammals may also benefit from heterosubtypic immunization against H5N1. Moreover, this mouse model could be a very useful system for examining specific aspects of immunity against highly lethal viruses such as H5N1.

2. Methods

2.1. Viruses, chickens, mice, and infection

All viruses used were grown in the allantoic cavities of 10-day-old embryonated chicken eggs. A/Hong Kong/156/97 (HK156), A/Silkie Chicken/HK/P21/97 (CHKP21), and A/Chicken/HK/728/97 (CHK728) are H5N1 viruses, and A/Quail/HK/G1/97 (QHKG1) and A/Chicken/HK/G9/97 (CHKG9) are H9N2 viruses. The viruses were used at St. Jude Children's Research Hospital in the biosafety level three containment facility.

Outbred 3- to 4-week-old SPF White Leghorn (WL) chickens were purchased from SPAFAS (Norwich, CT). C57BL/6 and BALB/c mice were purchased from the Jackson Laboratory (Bar Harbor, ME). Inbred chickens (B^2/B^2) were obtained from the University of Michigan, East Lansing. All animals were maintained in specific pathogen-free conditions before infection.

All immunizations were done with live preparations of virus. Briefly, chickens were immunized with 3 $\log_{10}$ chicken infectious doses (CID_{50}) of CHKG9 and challenged with 10 chicken lethal doses (CLD_{50}) of CHK728. Mice were immunized with 4.5 $\log_{10}$ egg infectious doses (EID_{50}) of QHKG1 and challenged with 2.8 $\log_{10}$ EID_{50} of HK156. All viruses were administered intranasally, and the survival of the animals was monitored daily.

2.2. Cytotoxic assay

Cytotoxic activity was analyzed by using the CytoTox96 Non-Radioactive Cytotoxicity Assay (Promega, Madison, WI) which measures the release of endogenous lactate dehydrogenase. The percent cytotoxicity was calculated by using the following formula: %cytotoxicity=[(experimental − spontaneous)/(maximal − spontaneous)] × 100.

3. Results

3.1. Heterologous protection against lethal H5N1 in WL chickens

Previous studies have shown that the H5N1 virus isolates from the 1997 Hong Kong outbreak are lethal to chickens in a laboratory setting [6,11,12]. To determine whether an H9N2 virus provides protection against lethal H5N1 infection in chickens, we infected WL chickens with CHKG9 (H9N2) and then challenged them 30 days later with CHK728 (H5N1); 90% of the chickens survived (Table 1). Among the surviving chickens, 33% shed H5N1 virus from their cloacae, and 100% shed the virus from their tracheae (data not shown). These results support the hypothesis that H9N2 viruses cocirculating at the time of the H5N1 outbreak [1,13] provided poultry with protection against lethal H5N1 infection. Also, our finding that protected chickens in our study shed H5NI in their feces concurs with Shortridge's observation that healthy birds in the Hong Kong markets do the same [1].

Hemagglutinin inhibition assays revealed that experimental infection of WL chickens with H9N2 did not provide serologic cross-reactivity against the H5N1 serotype (data not shown); therefore, we set out to determine whether cellular immunity was established. A CTL response was generated in H9N2-infected birds: 74% cytotoxicity was detected in their spleens (Fig. 1). The specific cytotoxic activity was equally effective against target cells infected with H9N2 and those infected with H5N1 (Fig. 1). Adoptive transfer of T cells (specifically CD8$^+$ cells) from H9N2-infected chickens into naive inbred chickens provided protective immunity (data not shown); however, adoptive transfer of B cells did not.

Table 1
Survival of H9N2-immunized chickens

Days after H9N2 infection[a]	Survivors/total challenged
0[b]	0/5
10	4/5
30	9/10

[a] Chickens were infected with 3 $\log_{10}$ chicken infectious dose (CID_{50}) of A/Chicken/HK/G9/97 (H9N2) before they were challenged at the indicated times with 10 chicken lethal doses (CLD_{50}) of A/Chicken/HK/728/97 (H5N1). Infected animals were monitored daily for 15 days.

[b] Uninfected chickens.

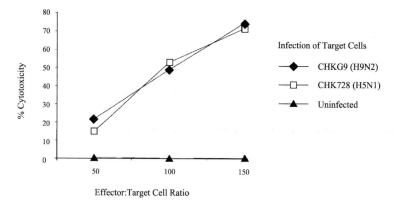

Fig. 1. Cytotoxic activity of splenic T cells from chickens previously infected with an H9N2 virus. The effector cells used were splenocytes collected from inbred chickens (B^2/B^2) infected with CHKG9 (H9N2) 7 days earlier. Lung target cells infected with H9N2 or H5N1 viruses served as the target cells.

3.2. Heterologous protection against lethal H5N1 infection in C57BL/6 mice

Avian-to-human transmission of influenza had not been reported before the 1997 Hong Kong outbreak [12]. Since then, H9N2 has been found to be transmitted to humans in a similar manner [3,4]. To determine whether H9N2 viruses can protect

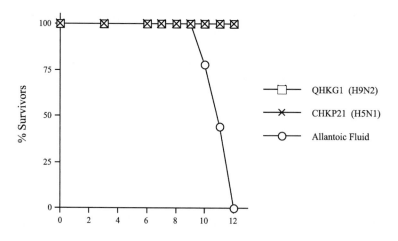

Fig. 2. Heterologous protection against a lethal dose of HK156. C57BL/6 mice were immunized with 4.5 $\log_{10}$ EID_{50} of QHKG1 (H9N2), 3.2 $\log_{10}$ EID_{50} of CHKP21 (H5N1), or 100 µl of allantoic fluid. Four weeks after immunization, mice were challenged with 2.8 $\log_{10}$ EID_{50} of HK156, and their weight and survival monitored daily. Data are representative of three independent experiments and are presented as the percent of mice which survived the challenge.

against lethal H5N1 infection in a mammalian system, we immunized C57BL/6 mice with QHKG1 (H9N2) and then subjected the mice to a lethal challenge of HK156 (H5N1). The HK156 virus requires no adaptation in mice [6,8,14] and killed 100% of the non-immunized animals (Fig. 2). However, 100% of the mice that were immunized with QHKG1 (H9N2) survived the challenge (Fig. 2). It should be noted that QHKG1 (H9N2)-infected animals did exhibit a temporary weight loss (as much as 15% of initial weight) that was not observed in the CHKP21 (a non-lethal H5N1 virus)-primed mice, presumably caused by homotypic antibodies against H5N1 that prevent infection by HK156 [15,10]. A temporary loss of weight is typical of heterosubtypic immunity, which is unable to block the initial infection of the animals; therefore, we investigated whether the HK156 and QHKG1 viruses induced CTL responses. C57BL/6 mice were infected with QHKG1, and bronchoalveolar lavage (BAL) was performed at 10 days after infection. BAL specimens from QHKG1-infected mice showed 30% cytotoxicity against QHKG1-infected target cells (Table 2). Similarly, BAL specimens from HK156-infected mice were cytotoxic against HK156-infected targets, albeit at lower levels. Tumpey et al. [17] found that a reduction in the number of lymphocytes and a decrease in cytokine production follows influenza infection, a finding that may explain our observation in the primary response against HK156 infection. BAL specimens from control mice infected with HKx31 (H3N2) showed a level of cytotoxicity against HKx31-infected target cells that was similar to that seen in BAL specimens from QHKG1-infected mice against QHKG1-infected target cells. These results indicated that a CTL response was readily generated in the mammalian system.

No serologic cross-reactivity was seen in hemagglutination inhibition experiments; thus, in agreement with those studies done in WL chickens, our study showed that protective immunity against H5N1 in mice did not appear to be humoral in origin (data not shown). QHKG1 immunization partially protected B-cell-deficient mice against HK156 challenge because there was a significant delay in the death of most of the mice (data not shown). These findings support the hypothesis that H9N2 protects mice against H5N1 via heterosubtypic immunity.

Table 2
Cytotoxic activity of cells from infected mice

Target cells	Infection[1]	Effectors[2]	Effector: target ratio[3]	
			20:1	5:1
L929-D[2]	HKx31[4]	HKx31	30	19
L929-K[2]	HKx31	HKx31	9	1
L929-D[2]	HK156	HK156	13	14
L929-K[2]	HK156	HK156	2	0
L929-D[2]	QHKG1	QHKG1	30	0

[1] Target cells were infected with the indicated virus previous to incubation with effector cells.

[2] Effector cells were obtained from bronchoalveolar lavages of mice 10 days after infection with the indicated virus.

[3] Data are expressed as percent cytotoxicity.

[4] HKx31 is an H3N2 laboratory reassortant that contains the surface molecules of A/Aichi/68 and the internal components of A/Puerto Rico/8/34.

4. Discussion

H9N2 viruses continue to circulate in the poultry markets in Hong Kong [2] and the presumed precursor of the H5N1 hemagglutinin, A/Goose/Guangdong/1/96 (H5N1), is still circulating in geese in southern China [18]. The fact that the majority of market birds in 1997 did not succumb to infection with H5N1 viruses, which are lethal to chickens in an experimental setting [1], and the fact that there is no humoral cross-reactivity between these serotypes, emphasize the value of heterosubtypic immunity in influenza infection. We demonstrated that previous infection with an H9N2 virus that contains genes encoding internal proteins that are homologous to those of the lethal H5N1 virus is protective in chickens and that some of these birds shed H5N1 virus. Thus, the pathogenic potential that these viruses posed to the human population during the 1997 outbreak was masked by the fact that the chickens carrying lethal isolates of H5N1 appeared healthy.

We also demonstrated that the same model of protective immunity can be achieved in mice. This finding suggests that mammals can be immunized against lethal H5N1 viruses with a strategy that emphasizes cellular immunity. Although Jameson et al. [19] found a degree of cross-protection against HK156-infected target cells in humans that had been previously infected with circulating influenza strains, Tumpey et al. [17] showed that lethal H5N1 virus infection depleted lymphocytes and decreased cytokine production in mice. In agreement with Tumpey et al. [17] we find that the cytotoxic response against a primary H5N1 infection is lower than that exhibited against H9N2 in mice. Thus, this system can be used as a model to study specific aspects of heterosubtypic immunity achieved against H5N1. It is imperative that research efforts continue to focus on highly pathogenic strains of virus so that we can understand the ability of cellular immunity to control this type of infection.

Acknowledgements

This work was supported by National Institutes of Health grants AI07372 (EO), AI29680 (SS), AI95357 (RGW), and AI37597 (DLW); by Cancer Center Support CORE grant P30 CA21765 from the National Cancer Institute; by the American Lebanese Syrian Associated Charities (ALSAC); and by the Trudeau Institute.

References

[1] K.F. Shortridge, Poultry and the influenza H5N1 outbreak in Hong Kong, 1997: abridged chronology and virus isolation, Vaccine 17 (1999) S26–29.
[2] Y. Guan, K.F. Shortridge, S. Krauss, P.S. Chin, K.C. Dyrting, T.M. Ellis, R.G. Webster, M. Peiris, H9N2 influenza viruses possessing H5N1-like internal genomes continue to circulate in poultry in southeastern China, J. Virol. 74 (2000) 9372–9380.
[3] Y.P. Lin, M. Shaw, V. Gregory, K. Cameron, W. Lim, A. Klimov, K. Subbarao, Y. Guan, S. Krauss, K. Shortridge, R. Webster, N. Cox, A. Hay, Avian-to-human transmission of H9N2 subtype influenza A viruses: relationship between H9N2 and H5N1 human isolates, Proc. Natl. Acad. Sci. U. S. A. 97 (2000) 9654–9658.
[4] M. Peiris, K.Y. Yuen, C.W. Leung, K.H. Chan, P.L. Ip, R.W. Lai, W.K. Orr, K.F. Shortridge, Human infection with influenza H9N2 [letter], Lancet 354 (1999) 916–917.

[5] J.K. Dybing, S. Schultz-Cherry, D.E. Swayne, D.L. Suarez, M.L. Perdue, Distinct pathogenesis of Hong Kong-origin H5N1 viruses in mice compared to that of other highly pathogenic H5 avian influenza viruses, J. Virol. 74 (2000) 1443–1450.

[6] K.F. Shortridge, N.N. Zhou, Y. Guan, P. Gao, T. Ito, Y. Kawaoka, S. Kodihalli, S. Krauss, D. Markwell, K.G. Murti, M. Norwood, D. Senne, L. Sims, A. Takada, R.G. Webster, Characterization of avian H5N1 influenza viruses from poultry in Hong Kong, Virology 252 (1998) 331–342.

[7] P. Gao, S. Watanabe, T. Ito, H. Goto, K. Wells, M. McGregor, A.J. Cooley, Y. Kawaoka, Biological heterogeneity, including systemic replication in mice, of H5N1 influenza A virus isolates from humans in Hong Kong, J. Virol. 73 (1999) 3184–3189.

[8] X. Lu, T.M. Tumpey, T. Morken, S.R. Zaki, N.J. Cox, J.M. Katz, A mouse model for the evaluation of pathogenesis and immunity to influenza A (H5N1) viruses isolated from humans, J. Virol. 73 (1999) 5903–5911.

[10] J.W. Yewdell, J.R. Bennink, G.L. Smith, B. Moss, Influenza A virus nucleoprotein is a major target antigen for cross-reactive anti-influenza A virus cytotoxic T lymphocytes, Proc. Natl. Acad. Sci. U. S. A. 82 (1985) 1785–1789.

[11] D.L. Suarez, M.L. Perdue, N. Cox, T. Rowe, C. Bender, J. Huang, D.E. Swayne, Comparisons of highly virulent H5N1 influenza A viruses isolated from humans and chickens from Hong Kong, J. Virol. 72 (1998) 6678–6688.

[12] K.Y. Yuen, P.K. Chan, M. Peiris, D.N. Tsang, T.L. Que, K.F. Shortridge, P.T. Cheung, W.K. To, E.T. Ho, R. Sung, A.F. Cheng, Clinical features and rapid viral diagnosis of human disease associated with avian influenza A H5N1 virus [see comments], Lancet 351 (1998) 467–471.

[13] Y. Guan, K.F. Shortridge, S. Krauss, R.G. Webster, Molecular characterization of H9N2 influenza viruses: were they the donors of the "internal" genes of H5N1 viruses in Hong Kong? Proc. Natl. Acad. Sci. U. S. A. 96 (1999) 9363–9367.

[14] L.V. Gubareva, J.A. McCullers, R.C. Bethell, R.G. Webster, Characterization of influenza A/HongKong/156/97 (H5N1) virus in a mouse model and protective effect of zanamivir on H5N1 infection in mice, J. Infect. Dis. 178 (1998) 1592–1596.

[15] S. Kodihalli, J.R. Haynes, H.L. Robinson, R.G. Webster, Cross-protection among lethal H5N2 influenza viruses induced by DNA vaccine to the hemagglutinin, J. Virol. 71 (1997) 3391–3396.

[17] T.M. Tumpey, X. Lu, T. Morken, S.R. Zaki, J.M. Katz, Depletion of lymphocytes and diminished cytokine production in mice infected with a highly virulent influenza A (H5N1) virus isolated from humans, J. Virol. 74 (2000) 6105–6116.

[18] A.N. Cauthen, D.E. Swayne, S. Schultz-Cherry, M.L. Perdue, D.L. Suarez, Continued circulation in China of highly pathogenic avian influenza viruses encoding the hemagglutinin gene associated with the 1997 H5N1 outbreak in poultry and humans, J. Virol. 74 (2000) 6592–6599.

[19] J. Jameson, J. Cruz, M. Terajima, F.A. Ennis, Human CD8+ and CD4+ T lymphocyte memory to influenza A viruses of swine and avian species, J. Immunol. 162 (1999) 7578–7583.

International Congress Series 1219 (2001) 783–788

Vaccines against avian influenza A H9N2 viruses

J.M. Katz*, X. Lu, M. Renshaw, T.M. Tumpey[1], N.J. Cox

Influenza Branch, Division of Viral and Rickettsial Diseases, National Center for Infectious Diseases, Centers for Disease Control and Prevention, MS G-16, 1600 Clifton Road, Atlanta, GA 30333, USA

Abstract

Background: Avian influenza A H9N2 viruses are now widespread in poultry and were recently isolated from children with influenza-like illness in Hong Kong. The development and evaluation of vaccines against H9N2 viruses is a priority for pandemic preparedness. *Methods*: The immunogenicity and protective efficacy of live and inactivated H9N2 viruses that represented two antigenically and genetically distinct sublineages of Eurasian H9N2 viruses, G1 and G9, were evaluated in BALB/c mice. Mice were either infected intranasally with live virus or vaccinated intramuscularly with formalin-inactivated purified virus and challenged with G1-like and G9 viruses. *Results*: Infection or vaccination of mice with a G1-like virus induced substantially lower serum antibody responses against homologous virus, compared with mice infected or vaccinated with a G9 virus. The G1-like inactivated vaccine, but not the G9 vaccine, induced modest levels of antibody that cross-reacted with the heterologous H9 virus. Mice infected with either G1-like or G9 viruses or vaccinated with inactivated G1-like vaccine were protected from challenge with either virus. However, mice immunized with G9 vaccine, although completely protected from homologous challenge, were only partially protected against challenge with the G1-like virus. *Conclusions*: This study has identified differences in immunogenicity between the G1 and G9 H9N2 virus sublineages that have consequences for the design of optimal vaccines against circulating H9 viruses. Published by Elsevier Science B.V.

Keywords: Vaccines; Influenza H9N2; Mouse model

1. Introduction

In 1997 in Hong Kong, highly pathogenic avian influenza A H5N1 viruses were transmitted directly from poultry to humans, resulting in 18 human cases, 6 of them fatal [1–5]. Prior to the depopulation of poultry in Hong Kong, H5N1 viruses were isolated from 19.5% of chickens [6]. Other avian influenza subtypes, most notably the H9

---

* Corresponding author. Tel.: +1-404-639-3591; fax: +1-404-639-2334.
E-mail address: jkatz@cdc.gov (J.M. Katz).
[1] Present address: USDA/ARS/Southeast Poultry Research Laboratories, Athens, GA, USA.

0531-5131/01/$ – see front matter. Published by Elsevier Science B.V.
PII: S 0 5 3 1 - 5 1 3 1 (0 1) 0 0 3 9 4 - 6

subtype, were also isolated during this study. H9 viruses were isolated from 4.4% of chickens and from 36.6% of environmental samples collected at one retail market [6]. Three genetically distinct Eurasian sublineages, represented by A/Quail/Hong Kong/G1/97 (G1), A/Chicken/Hong Kong/G9/97 (Ck/G9) and A/Duck/Hong Kong/Y439/97 (Korean lineage) viruses have been identified [7]. In 1998, avian H9N2 viruses were isolated from domestic pigs [8], while in March 1999, H9N2 viruses were isolated from two children in Hong Kong [9,10]. Both children had uncomplicated febrile respiratory illnesses and recovered completely. Additional reports of H9N2 infections in humans in southern China have recently been reported [11].

G1-like and G9-like H9N2 viruses are currently widespread in domestic poultry in southern China [6,7,12] and, thus, remain a potential source of further human infections and, possibly, a new pandemic strain. Vaccine development is complicated by the co-circulation of the two antigenically and genetically distinct H9 sublineages [7]. G1 and G9 viruses differ by 8% in HA amino acid sequence [7,13]. Although the human Hong Kong isolates are G1-like, the H9N2 viruses that infected pigs are G9-like [13]. To provide a rational basis for H9N2 vaccine design, we have compared the human virus A/Hong Kong/1073/99 (HK/1073), a G1-like virus with the avian Ck/G9 virus, for immunogenicity and cross-protective efficacy in the BALB/c mouse model.

2. Material and methods

Six- to 8-week-old female BALB/c mice (Charles River Laboratories, Wilmington, MA. USA) were infected intranasally (i.n.) with 10^6 to 10^7 50% egg infectious doses (EID_{50}) of HK/1073 or Ck/G9 viruses or were vaccinated intramuscularly (i.m.) with 10 μg of formalin-inactivated purified whole virus H9N2 vaccines. The HA content of the vaccines was estimated to be 35–39% of the total viral proteins. Inactivated H9N2 vaccines were administered to mice in the presence or absence of 1% alum (Alhydrogel; Superfos Biosectors, Kvistgaard, Denmark). For the protection studies, mice were challenged i.n. with one hundred 50% mouse infectious doses (MID_{50}) of HK/1073 ($=10^{5.5}EID_{50}$) or Ck/G9 ($=10^{6.3}EID_{50}$) virus. Mice were lightly anesthetized with CO_2, and 50 μl of infectious virus diluted in PBS was inoculated i.n. Three days post-challenge, lungs were collected from euthanized mice. Clarified lung homogenates were titrated for virus infectivity in eggs from initial dilutions of 1:10. The limit of virus detection was $10^{1.2}$ EID_{50} /ml. Virus titers were calculated using the method of Reed and Muench [14]. Sera were collected from mice prior to challenge and were tested for the presence of hemagglutination-inhibition (HI) antibody or neutralizing (neut) antibody by standard methods [15,16].

3. Results

3.1. Cross-reactive immunity induced by intranasal infection with H9N2 viruses

The G1 and G9 viruses replicate efficiently in the lungs of BALB/c mice without prior adaptation to this host [12]. In the present study, peak titers ($10^{6.1}$ to $10^{8.8}$ EID_{50} /ml) were observed on day 3 post-infection. The human G1-like virus HK/1073 replicated in the lungs of mice to substantially higher titers than Ck/G9 virus. Extrapulmonary replication of these H9N2 viruses was not observed and infection of mice with either virus did not result in weight loss or fatal disease (data not shown). Sera from mice infected 1 month previously were tested for the presence of HI and neut antibody (Table 1). Infection of mice with HK/1073 induced modest titers of homologous HI and neut antibody. Homologous antibody titers induced by infection with Ck/G9 virus were ≥fourfold higher than those induced by the G1-like virus. Infection of mice with either HK/1073 or Ck/G9 virus failed to induce cross-reactive antibody to the heterologous H9N2 virus detected by HI or neutralization assays. Mice were then challenged i.n. with 100 MID_{50} of either HK/1073 (G1-like) or Ck/G9 virus. Despite the lack of detectable cross-reactive antibody, mice infected with HK/1073 virus were completely protected from infection with either HK/1073 or Ck/G9 virus. Likewise, mice previously infected with the Ck/G9 virus were essentially protected from challenge with virus of either sublineage. In contrast, all control mice, infected with PBS alone, had high titers of viruses in the lung tissues. These results indicate that infection of mice with live HK/1073 or Ck/G9 viruses results in protection from challenge with the heterologous H9N2 virus in the absence of detectable cross-reactive serum HI or neut antibody responses.

3.2. Immunogenicity and cross-protective efficacy of inactivated H9N2 virus vaccines

Mice were immunized once with 10 μg of purified formalin-inactivated HK/1073 or Ck/G9 vaccine, with or without alum, an adjuvant licensed for use in humans. Table 2 shows the serum HI and neutralizing antibody responses of mice vaccinated 3 months previously. The administration of one dose of either of the H9N2 vaccines without alum resulted in 100% of mice achieving an HI titer of ≥40 to the homologous virus. Addition of alum resulted in homologous antibody titers that were two- to eightfold higher than titers achieved without adjuvant. The HK/1073 vaccines induced detectable but modest antibody titers against Ck/G9 virus. In contrast, the Ck/G9 vaccine induced only G9-specific HI and neut antibody,

Table 1

Serum antibody responses and cross-protective efficacy in mice following primary infection with H9N2 viruses[a]

Virus used to infect	Antibody titer against[b]				Protection against challenge[c]			
	HK/1073		Ck/G9		HK/1073		Ck/G9	
	HI	Neut	HI	Neut	Mean lung titer (log_{10})	No. protected/ Total no.	Mean lung titer (log_{10})	No. protected/ Total no.
HK/1073	40	106	5	20	<1.2	7/7	<1.2	8/8
Ck/G9	5	20	160	485	1.7±0.1	4/5	<1.2	5/5
None	5	20	5	20	8.8±0.3	0/5	6.1±0.3	0/5

[a] Mice were infected with 10^6 to 10^7 EID_{50} of virus.

[b] Antibody was measured in sera collected 1 month post-infection. HI titers were obtained using a pool of sera from all animals in a group and neutralizing antibody (neut) titers are expressed as the geometric mean of individual sera.

[c] Mice were challenged with 100 MID_{50} of virus 2 months after primary infection. Lungs were collected on day 3 post-infection. Virus titers are expressed as log_{10} EID_{50}/ml. The limit of virus detection was $10^{1.2}$ EID_{50}/ml. Mice were considered to be protected from challenge virus if no virus was detected in the lungs.

Table 2
Serum antibody responses and cross-protective efficacy in mice immunized with inactivated H9N2 vaccines[a]

Vaccine group	Antibody titer against[b]				Protection against challenge[c]			
	HK/1073		Ck/G9		HK/1073		Ck/G9	
	HI	Neut	HI	Neut	Mean lung titer ($\log_{10}$)	No. protected/ Total no.	Mean lung titer ($\log_{10}$)	No. protected/ Total no.
HK/1073	40	1600	10	400	<1.2	7/7	1.8±1.6	7/8
HK/1073+alum	160	3200	40	800	<1.2	7/7	<1.2	8/8
Ck/G9	5	100	160	12,800	3.5±1.5[d]	1/7	<1.2	8/8
Ck/G9+alum	5	100	1280	25,600	1.5±0.5	5/7	<1.2	8/8
Alum	5	100	5	100	7.5±0.7	0/7	5.9±1.1	0/8

[a] Mice were vaccinated with a single dose of 10 μg of purified formalin-inactivated whole H9N2 virus with or without 1% alum, or with alum alone.

[b] Antibody was measured in sera collected 3 month post-vaccination. HI and neutralizing (neut) antibody titers were obtained using a pool of sera from all animals in a group.

[c] Mice were challenged with 100 MID_{50} of virus 2 months after vaccination. Lungs were collected on day 3 post-infection. Virus titers are expressed as $\log_{10}$ EID_{50}/ml. The limit of virus detection was $10^{1.2}$ EID_{50}/ml. Mice were considered to be protected from challenge virus if no virus was detected in the lungs.

[d] Lung virus titers in mice administered Ck/G9 vaccine without alum were significantly higher than those in mice administered HK/1073 vaccine alone following challenge with HK/1073 virus ($P<0.01$) but were significantly lower than those of mice that received alum alone ($P<0.01$).

even following co-administration of Ck/G9 vaccine with alum. Next, the cross-protective efficacy of the H9N2 vaccines was investigated. Mice administered inactivated HK/1073 vaccine, with or without alum, were completely protected from infection of the lungs with homologous HK/1073. The HK/1073 vaccine also substantially protected mice from challenge with the heterologous Ck/G9 virus, and when formulated with alum the vaccine was 100% cross-protective. While mice vaccinated with Ck/G9 were protected from homologous virus challenge, only partial protection from heterologous challenge with HK/1073 virus was demonstrated. Virus was detected in the lungs of six of seven mice that received the Ck/G9 vaccine alone. The mean virus titers were significantly ($P<0.01$) lower than those in mice that received alum alone, but significantly higher than those that received the HK/1073 vaccine ($P<0.01$). Addition of alum to the Ck/G9 vaccine resulted in further reduction of virus titers, protection from HK/1073 virus infection was again incomplete.

4. Discussion

H9N2 viruses continue to circulate widely in domestic poultry in Asia [6,7,11,12]. Although no significant human-to-human spread of these viruses has been documented [17], a virus with the ability to efficiently transmit among humans may arise either by mutation of the avian H9N2 virus genome and/or by reassortant between an avian and human influenza A virus. Therefore, the development of a human influenza vaccine for H9N2 viruses is considered a high priority in pandemic preparedness.

We evaluated the relative immunogenicity and protective efficacy of immunization of mice with live or formalin-inactivated H9N2 viruses of the G1 and G9 sublineage.

Differences in relative immunogenicity between the HK/1073 G1-like virus and Ck/G9 virus were observed, either following infection or i.m. administration of inactivated vaccine. Although the HK/1073 inactivated vaccine induced substantially lower homologous antibody titers compared with the G9 vaccine, the antibody response was more cross-reactive since modest antibody titers against the Ck/G9 virus were detected. Infection of mice with either live G1-like or Ck/G9 viruses resulted in essentially complete cross-protection against subsequent re-infection with the heterologous virus, despite a lack of detectable HI or neutralizing cross-reactive serum anti-H9 antibody. Although infection with H9N2 virus may have also induced anti-NA antibody and memory cytotoxic T lymphocyte response that may contribute to enhanced viral clearance, it is unlikely that either of these immune mechanisms alone would result in complete lack of virus 3 days after re-infection with the heterologous virus. Mice infected with Ck/G9 virus had substantial titers of anti-HK/1073 HA (G1-like) serum IgG, IgA and IgM and mucosal IgG and IgA antibody (data not shown). These non-neut anti-HA antibodies may play a role in cross-protection. The Ck/G9 inactivated vaccine also provided partial protection against challenge with the HK/1073 virus in the absence of any detectable HI or neut antibody. However, serum IgG reactive with HK/1073 HA was detected in mice vaccinated with Ck/G9 (data not shown).

Our results suggest that the G1-like vaccine induced antibody that was more broadly cross-reactive, as well as more cross-protective against the heterologous H9 virus compared with the Ck/G9 inactivated vaccine. The G1-like viruses also have the advantage of growing to high titers in embryonated eggs, a property that may eliminate the need for preparation of a high-growth reassortant. It was noteworthy that administration of a single dose of either of the H9N2 vaccines without alum resulted in 100% of mice achieving homologous HI titers comparable to the response of animals following i.n. infection with live HK/1073 virus. Nevertheless, the cross-protective efficacy of both G1-like and Ck/G9 vaccines was improved by the co-administration of alum. It will be important to determine whether H9 vaccine candidates are similarly immunogenic in humans and whether inactivated vaccines prepared from a G1-like virus can induce titers of cross-reactive HI antibody that may be considered adequate for protection in humans.

Acknowledgements

We thank Wilina Lim, the Government Virus Unit of the Department of Health, Hong Kong for providing the human H9N2 virus and Robert Webster, Department of Virology and Molecular Biology, St. Jude Children's Research Hospital, Memphis, TN, for providing the avian H9N2 virus.

References

[1] J.C. de Jong, E.C.J. Claas, A.D.M.E. Osterhaus, R.G. Webster, W.L. Lim, A pandemic warning? Nature 389 (1997) 554.

[2] K. Subbarao, A. Klimov, J. Katz, H. Regnery, W. Lim, H. Hall, M. Perdue, D. Swayne, C. Bender, J. Huang, M. Hemphill, T. Rowe, M. Shaw, X. Xu, K. Fukuda, N. Cox, Characterization of an avian influenza A (H5N1) virus isolated from a child with a fatal respiratory illness, Science 279 (1998) 393–396.

[3] E.C. Claas, A.D. Osterhaus, R. van Beek, J.C. de Jong, G.F. Rimmelzwaan, D.A. Senne, S. Krauss, K.F. Shortridge, R.G. Webster, Human influenza A H5N1 virus related to a highly pathogenic avian influenza virus, Lancet 351 (1998) 472–477.

[4] K.Y. Yuen, P.K. Chan, M. Peiris, D.N.C. Tsang, T.L. Que, K.F. Shortridge, P.T. Cheung, W.K. To, E.T.F. Ho, R. Sung, A.F.B. Cheng, Members of the H5N1 study group. Clinical features and rapid viral diagnosis of human disease associated with avian influenza A H5N1 virus, Lancet 351 (1998) 467–471.

[5] J.M. Katz, W. Lim, C.B. Bridges, T. Rowe, J. Hu-Primmer, X. Lu, R.A. Abernathy, M. Clarke, L. Conn, H. Kwong, M. Lee, G. Au, Y.Y. Ho, K.H. Mak, N.J. Cox, F. Fukuda, Antibody response in individuals infected with avian influenza A (H5N1) viruses and detection of anti-H5 antibody among household and social contacts, J. Infect. Dis. 180 (1999) 1763–1770.

[6] K.F. Shortridge, Poultry and the influenza H5N1 outbreak in Hong Kong 1997: abridged chronology and virus isolation, Vaccine 17 (1999) 26–29.

[7] Y. Guan, K.F. Shortridge, S. Krauss, R.G. Webster, Molecular characterization of H9N2 influenza viruses: were they the donors of the "internal" gene of H5N1 viruses in Hong Kong? Proc. Natl. Acad. Sci. U. S. A. 96 (1999) 9363–9367.

[8] M. Peiris, W.C. Yam, K.H. Chan, P. Ghose, K.F. Shortridge, Influenza A H9N2: aspects of laboratory diagnosis, J. Clin. Microbiol. 37 (1999) 3426–3427.

[9] Anonymous, Influenza: Hong Kong special administrative region of China, WHO Wkly. Epidemiol. Rec. 14 (1999) 111.

[10] M. Peiris, K.Y. Yuen, C.W. Leung, K.H. Chan, P.L.S. Ip, R.W.M. Lai, W.K. Orr, K.F. Shortridge, Human infection with influenza H9N2, Lancet 354 (1999) 916–917.

[11] Y.J. Guo, J.G. Li, X.W. Cheng, M. Wang, Y. Zhou, X.H. Li, F. Cai, H.L. Miao, H. Zhang, F. Guo, Discovery of men infected by avian influenza A (H9N2) virus, Chin. J. Exp. Clin. Virol. 13 (1999) 105–108.

[12] Y.J. Guo, S. Krauss, D.A. Senne, P. Mo, K.S. Lo, X.P. Xiong, M. Norwood, K.F. Shortridge, R.G. Webster, Y. Guan, Characterization of the pathogenicity of members of the newly established H9N2 influenza virus lineages in Asia, Virology 267 (1999) 279–288.

[13] Y.P. Lin, M. Shaw, V. Gregory, K. Cameron, W. Lim, A. Klimov, K. Subbarao, Y. Guan, S. Krauss, K. Shortridge, R. Webster, N. Cox, A. Hay, Avian-to-human transmission of H9N2 subtype influenza A viruses: relationship between H9N2 and H5N1 human isolates, Proc. Natl. Acad. Sci. U. S. A. 97 (2000) 9654–9658.

[14] L.J. Reed, H. Muench, A simple method of estimating fifty per cent endpoints, Am. J. Hyg. 27 (1938) 493–497.

[15] A.P. Kendal, J.J. Skehel, M.S. Pereira, Concepts and procedures for laboratory-based influenza surveillance, CDC, Atlanta, 1982, pp. B17–B35.

[16] T. Rowe, R.A. Abernathy, J. Hu-Primmer, W.W. Thompson, X.H. Lu, W. Lim, K. Fukuda, N.J. Cox, J.M. Katz, Detection of antibody to avian influenza A (H5N1) virus in human serum by using a combination of serologic assays, J. Clin. Microbiol. 37 (1999) 937–943.

[17] T.M. Uyeki, Y. Chong, J.M. Katz, W. Lim, Y. Ho, S.S. Wang, T.H.F. Tsang, W.W. Au, S. Chan, T. Rowe, J. Hu-Primmer, J.C. Bell, W.W. Thompson, C.B. Bridges, N.J. Cox, K.H. Mak, K. Fukuda, Lack of evidence for human-to-human transmission of avian influenza A (H9N2) viruses in Hong Kong, China 1999, Emerging Infect. Dis., in press.

International Congress Series 1219 (2001) 789–794

Evaluation of H9N2 influenza vaccines in Balb/c mice

D.L. Major*, R.W. Newman, U. Dunleavy, A.B. Heath, K. Ploss, J.M. Wood

National Institute for Biological Standards and Control, Blanche Lane, South Mimms, Potters Bar, Herts EN6 3QG, UK

Abstract

Background: Following the emergence of H9N2 influenza virus in humans it was important to develop vaccines. Protection studies were performed in mice to assess influenza virus strains for their potential as vaccine strains and to evaluate H9N2 influenza vaccines prepared for use in human clinical trials. *Methods*: Groups of Balb/c mice were immunised intramuscularly with one or two doses of whole virus or subunit influenza vaccines. Antibody responses were measured by virus neutralisation assay (VN), haemagglutination inhibition assay (HI) and neuraminidase inhibition assay (NI). Fourteen days after the second immunisation animals were challenged with a live human H9N2 influenza virus. Virus excretion in nasal washes was monitored daily for 10 days following challenge. *Results*: Good HI responses to all but the subunit vaccine were detected. VN titres correlated well with the HI data. NI responses were detectable in all groups of mice except those that had received a single dose of subunit vaccine. Following challenge virus was not recovered from any animal immunised with two doses of whole virus vaccine prepared from human H9N2 virus. Virus excretion in the single dose group and groups immunised with whole virus vaccine prepared from swine H9N2 virus was significantly reduced. Virus excretion in the groups immunised with subunit H9N2 vaccine or H3N2 vaccine was similar to that in the controls. *Conclusions*: Whole virus H9N2 vaccine is more immunogenic and protective in mice than subunit vaccine. The mouse model is useful for preclinical evaluation of candidate pandemic influenza vaccines although it requires clinical validation. © 2001 Elsevier Science B.V. All rights reserved.

Keywords: Challenge; Protection; Animal model; Neuraminidase

* Corresponding author. Tel.: +44-1707-654753; fax: +44-1707-646730.
E-mail address: dmajor@nibsc.ac.uk (D.L. Major).

0531-5131/01/$ – see front matter © 2001 Elsevier Science B.V. All rights reserved.
PII: S0531-5131(01)00357-0

1. Introduction

In March 1999, an influenza A (H9N2) virus infected two children in Hong Kong. The human viruses were antigenically similar to an avian H9N2 virus isolated in Hong Kong at the time of the H5N1 outbreak in humans, A/Quail/Hong Kong/G1/97 (Qu/HK) [1]. These viruses could be distinguished antigenically from a second group of H9N2 viruses that comprised viruses isolated from pigs and poultry in Hong Kong in the late1990s. The antigenic relationship between the neuraminidases of these viruses is less clear, however they appear to be more closely related to that of human H2N2 viruses than that of recently circulating H3N2 strains. In view of concern about an impending H9N2 pandemic, we evaluated candidate vaccines in mice. The mouse protection studies assessed vaccines prepared from representative strains of the two H9N2 groups, a recent H3N2 vaccine strain and an H2N2 virus isolated in 1957. We also evaluated two H9N2 vaccines prepared for use in a clinical trial.

2. Materials and methods

2.1. Viruses and vaccines

Experimental whole virus vaccines were prepared from the H9N2 human influenza strain A/HK/1073/99 (HK/1073), an H9N2 virus from a pig A/swine/Hong Kong/10/98 (Sw/HK), RESVIR-13 reassortant virus with surface antigens of A/Sydney/5/97 (H3N2) and A/Singapore/1/57 (H2N2) (Sing/57). Virus was propagated in embryonated hen eggs, inactivated using β-propiolactone and purified by centrifugation on sucrose gradients. Whole virus vaccine (HK/1073 WV) and subunit vaccine (HK/1073 SU) prepared for use in human clinical trial were gifts from Berna (Switzerland) and Solvay Pharmaceuticals (the Netherlands), respectively. The haemagglutinin (HA) content of Sw/HK vaccine was determined by protein and polyacrylamide gel electrophoresis analysis. HA content of all other vaccines was determined by single radial immunodiffusion using the relevant standard reagents [2].

2.2. Antibody analysis

HI and NI were performed by standard methods [3]. Turkey erythrocytes were used in HI. X-15 (H7N2) a reassortant virus with neuraminidase (NA) derived from A/Japan/1/57 (H2N2) and HA from A/equine/Prague/56 (H7N7) was used in NI to eliminate problems arising from potential interference by antibody to HA. VN was performed on MDCK cells using Qu/HK infectious virus and turkey erythrocytes to detect residual virus infectivity [4].

2.3. Challenge studies

Groups of 10 female Balb/c mice were immunised intramuscularly with whole virus experimental vaccines prepared from the strains HK/1073, Sw/HK, and RESVIR-13. Two doses containing 15 μg HA were given, 14 days apart. Animals were bled from a superficial vein 14 days after each immunisation. Fourteen days after the second immunisation animals were challenged with HK/1073 virus ($50MID_{50}$/mouse). On days 1–10, the virus present in nasal washings was determined by titration on MDCK cells.

In a separate study, animals were immunised with the clinical trial vaccines HK/1073 WV, HK/1073 SU and an experimental whole virus vaccine prepared from the strain Sing/57. Groups of animals received one or two doses of vaccine and immune responses and resistance to challenge were assessed as above.

3. Results

After a single immunisation all experimental whole virus vaccines induced good HI responses to the vaccine viruses, (data not shown) which rose slightly following a second dose (Table 1a).

Sw/HK vaccine failed to induce an HI response to the challenge strain HK/1073. Conversely, HK/1073 vaccines did not induce HI responses to Sw/HK virus (data not shown). Post-immunisation mouse sera clearly distinguished between the two groups of H9N2 viruses in HI tests. In tests of clinical trial vaccines (Table 1b) HI responses to HK/1073 SU were significantly lower than responses to HK/1073 WV vaccine after one and two doses.

Antibody was tested by VN using Qu/HK virus which showed a similar pattern of reactivity in HI to that of HK/1073 virus (data not shown).VN titres correlated well with HI data showing a similar pattern of reactivity and similar relative levels of response.

All vaccines but one dose of HK/1073 SU and RESVIR-13 gave antibody responses to N2 NA. The cross-reactivity of the post-vaccination antibody indicated the antigenic

Table 1

Post-immunisation antibody responses to influenza vaccines in Balb/c mice

Vaccine	No. doses	HI GMT		VN[a] vs. Qu/HK	NI[a] vs. X-15
		vs.HK/1073	vs. vaccine virus		
(a)					
HK/1073	2	744	744	1280	100
Sw/HK	2	<20	3458	<60	35
RESVIR-13	2	<20	3062	<60	<20
None	NA	<20	NA	<60	<20
(b)					
HK/1073WV	1	123	123	201	35
HK/1073WV	2	383	383	805	50
HK/1073SU	1	21	21	<60	<20
HK/1073SU	2	81	81	113	20
Sing/57	1	<20	294	<60	320
Sing/57	2	<20	1641	<60	80
None	NA	<20	NA	<60	<20

[a] Sera pooled from 10 mice.

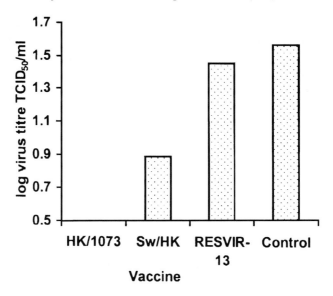

Fig. 1. Virus shedding in mice immunised with experimental vaccines. Bars represent mean virus shedding in each of the vaccine groups indicated over a 10-day period.

similarities of the NAs from the two groups of H9N2 viruses and Sing/57 virus. Higher NA antibody responses were induced by HK/1073 whole virus vaccines than HK/1073 subunit vaccine.

Following challenge no virus was recovered from animals immunised with experimental HK/1073 vaccine (Fig. 1). Virus excretion in the Sw/HK group was significantly reduced and in the RESVIR-13 group was similar to that in unimmunised controls.

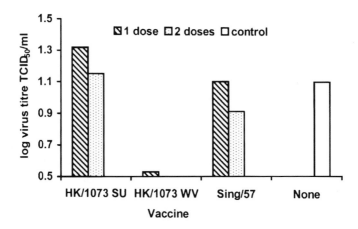

Fig. 2. Virus shedding in mice immunised with clinical trial vaccines. Bars represent mean virus shedding in each of the vaccine groups indicated over a 7-day period.

In tests of the clinical trial vaccines virus recovery from mice immunised with one dose of HK/1073 WV vaccine was significantly reduced compared with control mice (Fig. 2) and no virus was recovered from animals that received two doses of the vaccine. Virus excretion in animals that received one or two doses of subunit vaccine was similar to that in control animals. The moderate reduction in virus excretion in mice immunised with two doses of Sing/57 vaccine was not significant.

4. Discussion

Inactivated influenza vaccines used for interpandemic control are immunogenic and protective [5] and a single dose is sufficient for protection. However, clinical trials have provided some evidence that whole virus vaccines elicit better HI responses than subunit vaccines in unprimed individuals and it is possible that whole virus vaccines may be more appropriate for control of pandemic viruses.

Our studies were designed to examine the efficacy of candidate H9N2 vaccine strains in mice, which may indicate their potential for use in man.

We have demonstrated that two doses of HK/1073 WV vaccine give complete protection, whereas HK/1073 SU was ineffective. The relative efficacy of HK/1073 WV and HK/1073 SU vaccines were in good agreement with the observed post-immunisation antibody responses, but the partial protection provided by Sw/HK and Sing/57 vaccines could not be explained by the observed immune responses. The Sw/HK vaccine induced significant protection in the absence of HI or VN responses to the challenge strain. Conversely, HK/1073SU vaccine induced HI and VN responses to the challenge strain but failed to protect against infection.

Amerding et al. [6] reported enhanced survival following lethal challenge in mice immunised with heterologous inactivated whole virus vaccine. It is therefore possible that immune responses to the antigenically conserved internal proteins may have some protective effect, although this is unlikely in our studies because the H3N2 and H2N2 vaccines differed in protective efficacy, despite possessing antigenically similar internal proteins.

It is more likely that responses to NA contributed to protective immunity in this study. Mice immunised with Sw/HK or Sing/57 vaccine developed antibody to N2 NA and it has been shown previously that the N2s of Sw/HK, Sing/57 and HK/1073 are antigenically related [1]. The reduction in virus replication in these animals is similar to an effect reported by Johansson et al. [7] in challenged mice immunised with purified NA protein.

It is well established that antibody to HA is the major determinant of protection against influenza virus infection, therefore the primary goal of vaccine development for pandemic control must be to produce vaccines that induce demonstrable antibody response to the HA protein. We have confirmed this general concept, as the vaccine that induced the highest levels of antibody to HA afforded the best protection. However, our study has also demonstrated that immune responses to other viral proteins can induce partial protection in mice and that protection can be induced in the absence of significant antibody to HA. The effect of immune responses to influenza virus proteins other than HA should therefore be considered during development of pandemic vaccines.

Although the subunit H9N2 vaccine was ineffective in mice, it is premature to speculate about its use in man before the results of H9N2 vaccine clinical trials are available. It should also be borne in mind that our results have no relevance for interpandemic use of subunit vaccines, where they are as effective as other forms of inactivated vaccines.

References

[1] Y.P. Lin, M. Shaw, V. Gregory, K. Cameron, W. Lim, A. Klimov, K. Subbarao, Y. Guan, S. Krauss, K. Shortridge, R. Webster, N. Cox, A. Hay, Avian-to-human transmission of H9N2 subtype influenza A viruses: relationship between H9N2 and H5N1 human isolates, Proc. Natl. Acad. Sci. U. S. A. 96 (2000) 9654–9658.

[2] J.M. Wood, G.C. Schild, R.W. Newman, V. Seagroatt, An improved single radial immunodiffusion technique for the assay of influenza haemagglutinin antigen: application for potency determinations of inactivated whole virus and subunit vaccines, J. Biol. Stand. 5 (1977) 237–247.

[3] A.P. Kendal, M.S. Pereira, J.J. Skehel, 1982. Concepts and Procedures for Laboratory-Based Influenza Surveillance. U.S. Department of Health and Human Services, (Centers Dis. Control, Atlanta).

[4] A.B. Brokstad, R.J. Cox, D. Major, J.M. Wood, L.R. Haaheim, Cross-reaction but no avidity change of the serum antibody response after influenza vaccination, Vaccine 13 (1995) 1522–1528.

[5] K.L. Nichol, Efficacy/clinical effectiveness of inactivated influenza virus vaccines in adults, in: K.G. Nicholson, R.G. Webster, A.J. Hay (Eds.), Textbook of Influenza, Blackwell, Oxford, 1998, pp. 358–372.

[6] D. Amerding, H. Rossiter, I. Ghazzouli, E. Liehl, Evaluation of live and inactivated influenza A virus vaccines in a mouse model, J. Infect. Dis. 145 (1982) 320–330.

[7] B.E. Johansson, D.J. Bucher, E.D. Kilbourne, Purified influenza virus haemagglutinin and neuraminidase are equivalent in stimulation of antibody response but induce contrasting types of immunity to infection, J. Virol. 63 (1988) 1239–1246.

Current strategies for
improved control by antivirals

International Congress Series 1219 (2001) 797–806

Influenza virus neuraminidase inhibitors: clinical aspects

Frederick G. Hayden[*]

Department of Internal Medicine, University of Virginia School of Medicine, Box 800473, Charlottesville, VA 22901, USA

Keywords: Zanamivir; Oseltamivir; Treatment; Prophylaxis; Antiviral

1. Introduction

Because of the essential role of neuraminidase (NA) in influenza virus replication and the highly conserved enzyme active site in influenza A and B viruses, interest has focused on the development of selective inhibitors of this enzyme. In recent years tremendous progress has been made in the clinical development of this new class of anti-influenza agents. Inhaled zanamivir entered clinical trials in 1994 and is now approved for treatment of influenza infection in many countries. The first orally active NA inhibitor, oseltamivir, entered clinical trials in 1997 and was approved initially for treatment of influenza in adults in Switzerland and the United States in 1999. Oseltamivir was subsequently approved for treatment in children and for prevention of influenza in teenagers and adults in 2000 in the United States. A second oral NA inhibitor, RWJ-270201 (BCX-1812), entered clinical trials in 1999. This article provides an overview of the pharmacologic properties, tolerability, and clinical efficacy of the currently approved NA inhibitors (reviewed by Gubareva et al. [1]).

2. Antiviral activity

Each of these molecules interacts in a different manner within the enzyme active site, which may influence antiviral activity and emergence of resistant variants. However, all three agents are potent selective inhibitors, active at nanomolar to subnanomolor concentrations for influenza A and B virus NAs . They inhibit the NA activity of a wide range of

---

[*] Tel.: +1-804-924-5059; fax: +1-804-924-9065.
E-mail address: fgh@virginia.edu (F.G. Hayden).

strains, including clinical isolates and all nine influenza A NA subtypes present in birds, and are inhibitory for amantadine- and rimantadine-resistant influenza A viruses. Although these agents tend to be less active against influenza B than influenza A enzymes, the clinical importance of differences in inhibitory concentrations is currently uncertain. Inhibition of human and other non-influenza sialidases requires much higher concentrations (generally $\geq 10^6$-fold), and consequently, these agents are not effective for other respiratory viral infections.

These agents show dose-dependent activity in animal models of influenza A and B virus infection. Of note, intranasal zanamivir and oral oseltamivir protected against the highly virulent avian influenza H5N1 strain that caused a human outbreak in Hong Kong in 1997. Intranasal zanamivir and oral oseltamivir are effective for prevention and early treatment of experimental influenza A virus infections in volunteers [2,3]. Both have significant antiviral effects in experimental human influenza B infections [4]. In addition, oral RWJ-270201 shows dose-related antiviral activity after oral administration in experimental influenza A and B infection [5].

3. Pharmacokinetics

Zanamivir and oseltamivir have important differences in their pharmacokinetic properties and associated routes of administration. However, both drugs have prolonged durations of antiviral activity, so that dosing can be infrequent (twice daily for treatment, once daily for prophylaxis).

3.1. Zanamivir

The oral bioavailability of zanamivir is very low (<5% in humans), and most clinical studies have administered it topically to the respiratory tract as a dry powder aerosol by oral inhalation. The aerosol contains a lactose powder carrier (5 mg zanamivir per 20 mg lactose) and is self-administered by a proprietary Diskhaler® device (Glaxo Wellcome). Scintigraphic studies indicate that an average of 13–15% of inhaled zanamivir is deposited in the tracheobronchial tree and lungs and 78% in the oropharynx [6]. No comparable studies have been reported in influenza-infected persons or those with underlying chronic airways diseases. Zanamivir levels are high (> 1000 ng/ml) in induced sputum at 6 h post-inhalation and remain detectable to 24 h [15,26]. Following inhalation, low plasma levels are detectable (30–50 ng/ml), and overall systemic exposure, based on urinary recovery, is estimated to be 15% of dose. The plasma elimination half-life after inhalation averages about 2.5–5 h, and zanamivir is rapidly cleared by the kidney without metabolism [7]. Zanamivir does not inhibit or induce cytochrome $P450$ isoenzymes, or affect expression of liver microsomal isoenzymes in animals [8]. Plasma protein binding is low, and no adverse drug interactions have been recognized.

3.2. Oseltamivir

Oseltamivir (GS4104) is an ethyl ester prodrug that is well absorbed and quickly metabolized, primarily by esterases in the liver, to the antivirally active oseltamivir carboxylate (GS4071) [9,10]. The bioavailability of the carboxylate is estimated to be about 80% following oral oseltamivir. Systemic exposure to the prodrug is low, approximately 3–5% relative to oseltamivir carboxylate based on plasma AUC measurements. Oseltamivir carboxylate levels usually peak at 3–4 h after dosing with levels of approximately 350 ng/ml after doses of 75 mg in adults. The carboxylate distributes well to middle ear and sinus secretions in uninfected persons [11] and to bronchoalveolar lavages in animals. Plasma levels decline slowly with a half-life of 6–10 h. Systemic exposure to oseltamivir carboxylate at steady-state is about 25% higher in elderly persons, but dose adjustments are not necessary. Food reduces the risk of gastrointestinal side effects and slows absorption but does not significantly reduce peak plasma levels or overall bioavailability. The carboxylate is eliminated through the kidney by filtration and tubular secretion via the anionic pathway without further metabolism. Plasma protein binding is low, and no significant drug interactions have been recognized to date. Dose adjustments are indicated for advanced renal insufficiency (creatinine clearance <30 ml/min).

4. Safety and tolerability

Most persons enrolled in clinical studies to date have been previously healthy adults or those with stable underlying medical conditions of mild–moderate severity. Safety has not been established in hospitalized patients and those with unstable medical problems. Surveillance for infrequently occurring events will be important as the drugs gain wider clinical use.

4.1. Zanamivir

In published treatment studies, the frequency and types of adverse events have been no different in zanamivir and placebo (lactose vehicle) recipients, and the most reported adverse effects appear to relate to the underlying influenza illness [12]. The lactose dose (80 mg per dose) is insufficient to cause symptoms in lactose-deficient persons.

The major safety concern with inhaled zanamivir is possible exacerbation of reactive airways disease. No acute bronchospasm or respiratory tract irritation was recognized in controlled clinical trials with inhaled zanamivir, but wider scale use has been associated with uncommon reports of wheezing and sometimes severe bronchospasm, including death, following inhaled zanamivir [13]. In uninfected patients with mild–moderate asthma, no overall changes in methacholine-induced airway reactivity were found during 14 days of zanamivir exposure [14]. A recently completed treatment study of asthma and COPD patients with influenza, found no differences in adverse events, respiratory exacerbations, spirometric changes, or clinical asthma exacerbations (14% each for placebo and zanamivir) compared to placebo. Although inhaled zanamivir appears to be well tolerated in mild to moderate asthmatics, its tolerability remains to be established in those with serious bronchopulmonary disease and hospitalized patients. Although influenza itself causes acute deteriorations in airflow, zanamivir treatment should be used only under carefully monitored conditions in patients with underlying airway disease.

The breath-activated proprietary Diskhaler® device for delivery of inhaled zanamivir requires a cooperative patient who can effectively inspire. Compliance has generally been excellent but certain groups (children <5 years, dementia, very frail elderly) are not able to use it. Nursing home studies have found that most elderly residents are ably to comply with administration [15,16].

4.2. Oseltamivir

Oral oseltamivir is associated with dose-related adverse upper gastrointestinal effects, specifically nausea of mild to moderate intensity and less often vomiting. These symptoms usually are transient, occurring most often after first dose, and resolve within 1–2 days despite continued drug administration. In adults with influenza illness, the excess frequencies of nausea alone and emesis are each about 8–10% compared to placebo. The frequencies of gastrointestinal adverse effects appear no higher in treating elderly and high-risk patients and lower when used for prophylaxis [17]. Gastrointestinal upset appears likely due to local irritation, and ingestion with food reduces the risk of such complaints [3]. A small increase in headache frequency was observed in one elderly prophylaxis study [18], but oseltamivir appears to avoid the central nervous system intolerance associated with M2 inhibitors, especially amantadine.

Administration of NA inhibitors would not be anticipated to affect the humoral immune inactivated influenza vaccine, a point which has been established with zanamivir [19]. Consequently, NA inhibitors could be used for immediate protection in conjunction with late season immunization. Oral oseltamivir and possibly inhaled zanamivir might reduce the replication and immunogenicity of intranasal, live-attenuated influenza vaccines.

5. Clinical efficacy

5.1. Experimental influenza

Studies of experimental influenza with the NA inhibitors have provided valuable information regarding both drug efficacy and the pathogenesis of human influenza. Intravenous zanamivir was highly protective against experimental influenza A and the associated elaboration of nasal cytokines and chemokines [20,21]. Early treatment with oral oseltamivir also reduced proinflammatory cytokine levels (IL-6, TNF-alpha, IFN-gamma) in the upper respiratory tract [3]. These observations indicate that the sequence of influenza virus replication, cytokine elaboration, and symptom production can be inhibited by specific antiviral therapy. Early treatment with inhaled zanamivir or oral oseltamivir significantly reduced the otologic manifestations, including middle ear pressure abnormalities, of experimental influenza [22], whereas oral rimantadine did not. The beneficial effects of NI therapy on middle ear pressures in experimentally infected adults suggest that reductions in otitis media would be possible in treating influenza in children.

5.2. Treatment of natural influenza

A substantial number of treatment studies have been conducted with zanamivir and oseltamivir to assess the effects of treatment on the duration and severity of influenza symptoms, functional status and quality of life measures, and occurrence of complications. Because these studies have been conducted largely in previously healthy ambulatory persons with acute influenza and because of their size, these trials have not addressed whether treatment can reduce influenza-related hospitalizations or mortality. In addition, there have been no direct comparisons of therapeutic efficacy between NA inhibitors and M2 inhibitors or between zanamivir and oseltamivir. The NA inhibitors have received limited study in patients at increased risk for influenza complications because of age or underlying conditions, and no controlled trials have been published from patients hospitalized with influenza. The safety and possible therapeutic value of these agents in treating viral pneumonia or other lower respiratory tract disease due to influenza are uncertain. Studies to assess the pharmacokinetics and antiviral activity of oral oseltamivir and aerosolized or intravenous zanamivir in patients hospitalized with pneumonia or severe lower respiratory tract disease are needed. An alternative delivery system for zanamivir, such as nebulization, needs to be developed for younger children and infants at increased risk of pulmonary complications.

The first phase 2 trial in previously healthy adults with acute influenza found that twice daily inhaled zanamivir reduced the time to alleviation of influenza illness by 1 day (20% reduction) overall and by 3 days (40% reduction) in those with febrile illness or those treated within 30 h of symptom onset [23]. The addition of intranasal zanamivir reduced nasal symptoms and possibly the risk of upper respiratory tract complications without affecting overall recovery. Increasing the dose frequency for combined intranasal and inhaled zanamivir from twice to four times daily provided no additional benefit [24]. Subsequent phase 3 studies showed that inhaled zanamivir 10 mg twice daily for 5 days provided 1–2.5 day reductions in time to alleviation of illness compared to placebo in adults and teenagers ≥12 years old treated within 2 days of symptom onset [25,26]. Recently, similar therapeutic benefits were found with zanamivir treatment of acute influenza in children aged 5–12 years old [27]. These studies found comparable clinical benefits in influenza A and B virus illness. Those aged 50 years or older and those judged to have more severe influenza by their physicians had greater symptom relief benefits [26]. Zanamivir recipients also experienced more rapid functional recovery and required 40% fewer antibiotic prescriptions for lower respiratory complications [28]. Among elderly (≥65 years) adults developing influenza despite immunization [29a], zanamivir treatment appeared to have similar therapeutic effects and tolerance as in younger adults. In higher-risk adults, mostly mild asthma patients, zanamivir appeared to provide symptom benefit and reduced complications leading to antibiotics compared to placebo [29b]. Intranasal but not inhaled zanamivir reduced nasal virus recovery [23,30]. Inhaled zanamivir reduced pharyngeal virus replication in one study [31], but data regarding effects on lower respiratory tract viral replication are not published.

Phase 3 trials of oral oseltamivir found similar therapeutic benefits in previously healthy adults with febrile influenza treated within 11/2 days of illness onset. Oseltamivir 75 mg twice daily for 5 days reduced the time to illness alleviation by approximately 1.2–

1.4 days, illness severity (30–40% reduction in scores), and time to resumption of usual activities by several days [32,33]. The frequency of secondary complications leading to antibiotic prescriptions was reduced by approximately 50% compared to placebo. In general, no greater clinical effects were found at twofold higher doses. Reductions in fever duration, cough, ancillary medication use, and viral titers were also found in these studies. In children aged 1–12 years old, oseltamivir 2 mg/kg twice daily for 5 days reduced illness duration by 1.5 days, time to resuming usual activities, upper respiratory viral titers, and the risk of secondary complications, particularly otitis media, leading to antibiotic use [34]. Treatment in elderly ambulatory adults (≥65 years) indicates that illness reduction and tolerance are similar to those observed in younger adults with acute influenza. Data on oseltamivir treatment of natural influenza B illness are limited.

Studies of zanamivir and oseltamivir have both shown that early antiviral treatment (within 1 day of symptom onset) provides greater clinical benefits. It remains uncertain whether later onset of therapy (after 2 days) is useful, particularly in patient groups that have more protracted virus replication and illness. Whether treatment of ill persons might reduce transmission of virus to contacts has not been rigorously studied, although such a benefit was found in one study with amantadine and rimantadine. NA inhibitor treatment does not interfere with the serum antibody response to acute influenza.

5.3. Prevention of natural influenza

Both inhaled zanamivir and oral oseltamivir are effective for prevention of influenza illness. One 4-week seasonal prophylaxis study in largely nonimmunized adults found that inhaled zanamivir 10 mg once daily reduced the risk of laboratory documented influenza infection by 31%, of influenza illness by 67%, and of febrile influenza illness (≥37.8 °C) by 84% [35]. A post-contact prevention study in families employed both treatments of the ill index case and 10-day prophylaxis of healthy family members. Compared to placebo, once daily inhaled zanamivir reduced the likelihood of influenza illness in contacts by 79%, and no zanamivir-resistant viruses were recovered [13]. In contrast, an earlier similarly designed study of oral rimantadine failed in part due to the rapid emergence and transmission of drug-resistant influenza viruses. Prophylaxis with intranasal zanamivir alone is ineffective against natural influenza [36a]. A recent study compared the efficacy of 2-week courses of inhaled zanamivir or oral rimantadine in preventing influenza in immunized nursing home residents during recognized outbreaks [36b]. Zanamivir prophylaxis resulted in an additional protective efficacy of 61% compared to rimantadine, largely because of rimantadine prophylaxis failures due to acquisition of drug-resistant variants. An open trial found that inhaled zanamivir (10 mg daily for 14 days) appeared to terminate an outbreak of influenza continuing despite amantadine use [16]. Such findings suggest that the protection provided by inhaled zanamivir is additive to that of vaccine.

In nonimmunized working adults, a 6-week seasonal prophylaxis trial found that oral oseltamivir 75 mg once daily reduced the risk of influenza infection by 50%, of influenza illness by 76%, and of influenza illness with fever by 90% [17]. No greater protection was seen with twice daily administration. In elderly nursing home residents, over 80% of whom had been immunized, 6 weeks of daily oseltamivir prophylaxis reduced the risk of influenza illness by 92% in homes experiencing outbreaks [18]. It appeared to provide additive protection to immunization and also reduced the risk of influenza-related complications. When used for post-contact prophylaxis in households, once daily oseltamivir reduced the risk of illness by 89% in household contacts of an influenza-infected index case [37].

6. Resistance to neuraminidase inhibitors

Because of the experience with resistance to the M2 protein inhibitors, amantadine and rimantadine, the potential for development of antiviral resistance with associated loss of clinical efficacy is an important issue for the NA inhibitors. In vitro passage of influenza virus in the presence of zanamivir or oseltamivir carboxylate leads to in vitro resistance, and resistant variants have now been identified during clinical use. Both NA-independent and NA-dependent mechanisms of resistance have been recognized (reviewed by Tisdale [38] and McKimm-Breschkin [39]). Mutations in or close to the HA receptor-binding site reduced efficiency of virus binding to cellular receptors, which results in decreased dependence on NA function and lack of inhibition by all NA inhibitors in cell culture. Such variants usually remain susceptible to NA inhibitors in animal models of influenza, and their clinical significance is uncertain.

Resistance also results from amino acid substitutions at the conserved residues in the NA enzyme active site. Differences in degree of cross-resistance result from differences in drug interactions within the active enzyme site. NA mutations typically compromise enzyme activity and/or stability. These variants usually show reduced infectivity and virulence in animal models. Because replication of influenza virus in the respiratory tract imposes higher requirements on HA and NA functions, changes in these surface glycoproteins are likely to decrease influenza virus virulence and transmissibility in vivo, unlike the experience with M2 inhibitors.

No reliable cell culture method for resistance surveillance is currently available [38]. Current screening is based on determining NA enzyme inhibition phenotype complemented by NA and HA sequence analyses. The frequency of resistance emergence has been low in clinical trials to date. In post-treatment isolates recovered during clinical trials of inhaled zanamivir, no reduced NA susceptibility or changes in the receptor-binding site of the HA were observed following zanamivir therapy [30,31]. One infant with a bone marrow transplantation complicated by influenza B virus pneumonia did not clear virus despite treatment with aerosolized ribavirin followed by 2 weeks of nebulized zanamivir [40]. A zanamivir-resistant isolate had point mutations in both the HA, which altered both receptor binding and antigenicity, and the NA catalytic site at Arg152, which reduced susceptibility to zanamivir but also compromised NA function and reduced infectivity in animals. In immunocompetent adults treated with oral oseltamivir, resistant variants have been recovered very uncommonly (~1.5%) [32]. In children aged 1–12 years treated with oseltamivir, the frequency of resistant variants is about threefold higher. These variants possessed amino acid substitutions (primarily Arg292Lys) in the active site of the NA that are associated with markedly impaired replication in animals. No drug-induced HA variants have been recognized to date in oseltamivir studies.

The available data suggest that resistance to this class of anti-influenza drugs is infrequent and impairs viral fitness, such that resistance emergence is unlikely to limit clinical usefulness in most settings. However, the potential for resistance development requires further study, particularly in those who may have prolonged viral replication, including children, frail elderly, and immunocompromised hosts. A global NA Inhibitor Susceptibility Network (NISN) with participation from the World Health Organization reference laboratories, Centers for Disease Control, and academia, has been established to select appropriate assays for resistance monitoring, collect data regarding baseline susceptibility of influenza subtypes (before widescale use of the NA inhibitors), and prospectively monitor for changes in susceptibility patterns over an extended period of use (≥ 5 years) [41].

7. Summary

The NA inhibitors represent a significant advance in anti-influenza chemotherapy. Compared to the M2 inhibitors amantadine and rimantadine, the NA inhibitors have the advantages of broader spectrum of antiviral activity including both influenza A and B viruses; lesser potential for emergence of clinically important drug-resistant viruses; better tolerability without the central nervous system adverse effects associated with amantadine and less often rimantadine; and documented efficacy in reducing respiratory events leading to antibiotic use following influenza.

Inhaled zanamivir and oral oseltamivir are effective for treatment of acute influenza in ambulatory persons. Early treatment reduces illness severity and duration, speeds functional recovery, and reduces the likelihood of antibiotic use for respiratory events following influenza. Efficacy has been established in febrile illness of short duration in adults and more recently in children. Large databases should prove useful in determining whether early treatment will reduce hospitalization and mortality particularly in elderly or high-risk patients. More information is needed regarding the efficacy and tolerability of treatment with these agents in persons with severe influenza, underlying airways disease, immunocompromise and/or unstable underlying conditions.

Although not currently approved for prevention in most countries, available evidence indicates that the NA inhibitors are effective for chemoprophylaxis and could be used for long-term protection of those unable to receive vaccine or not responding to it, or when the vaccine is unavailable or ineffective due to the appearance of antigenically novel viruses. Short-term prevention (10–14 days) could be considered for outbreak control in institutions, for immediate protection in conjunction with late season immunization, post-exposure prevention in households, and in travelers likely to be exposed out of season.

References

[1] L.V. Gubareva, L. Kaiser, F.G. Hayden, Influenza virus neuraminidase inhibitors, Lancet 355 (2000) 827–835.
[2] F.G. Hayden, J.J. Treanor, R.F. Betts, M. Lobo, J.D. Esinhart, E.K. Hussey, Safety and efficacy of the neuraminidase inhibitor GG167 in experimental human influenza, JAMA 275 (4) (1996) 295–299.

[3] F.G. Hayden, J.J. Treanor, R.S. Fritz, M. Lobo, R. Betts, M. Miller, et al., Use of the oral neuraminidase inhibitor oseltamivir in experimental human influenza, JAMA 282 (13) (1999) 1240–1246.

[4] F.G. Hayden, L. Jennings, R. Robson, G. Schiff, H. Jackson, B. Rana, et al., Oral oseltamivir in human experimental influenza B infection, Antiviral Ther. 5 (2000) 205–213.

[5] F.G. Hayden, J.J. Treanor, R. Qu, C.L. Fowler, Safety and efficacy of an oral neuraminidase inhibitor RWJ-270201 in treating experimental influenza A and B in healthy adult volunteers, Abstracts of the 40th Interscience Conference on Antimicrobial Agents and Chemotherapy, Toronto, Canada, September 17–20, 2000, p. 270, Abst #1156.

[6] L. Cass, J. Brown, M. Pickford, S. Fayinka, S. Newman, C.J. Johansson, et al., Pharmacoscintigraphic evaluation of lung deposition of inhaled zanamivir in healthy volunteers, Clin. Pharmacokinet. 36 (Suppl. 1) (1999) 21–31.

[7] L. Cass, C. Efthymiopoulos, A. Bye, Pharmacokinetics of zanamivir after intravenous, oral, inhaled or intranasal administration to healthy volunteers, Clin. Pharmacokinet. 36 (Suppl. 1) (1999) 1–11.

[8] M.J. Daniel, J.M. Barnett, B.A. Pearson, The low potential for drug interactions with zanamivir, Clin. Pharmacokinet. 36 (Suppl. 1) (1999) 41–50.

[9] G. He, J. Massarella, P. Ward, Clinical pharmacokinetics of the prodrug oseltamivir and its active metabolite Ro 64-0802, Clin. Pharmacokinet. 37 (6) (1999) 471–484.

[10] A. Bardsley-Elliot, S. Noble, Oseltamivir, Drugs 58 (5) (2000) 851–860.

[11] M. Kurowski, J. Barrett, E. Waalberg, H. Wiltshire, Oral oseltamivir rapidly delivers active drug levels to middle ear and sinuses in humans, Abstracts of the 40th Interscience Conference on Antimicrobial Agents and Chemotherapy, Toronto, Canada, September 17–20, 2000, p. 19, Abst #509.

[12] B. Freund, S. Gravenstein, M. Elliott, I. Miller, Zanamivir—a review of clinical safety, Drug Saf. 21 (4) (1999) 267–281.

[13] US Food and Drug Administration, Public Health Advisory: Safe and Appropriate Use of Influenza Drugs, 1-12-2000.

[14] L. Cass, K. Gunawardena, M. MacMahon, A. Bye, Pulmonary function and airway responsiveness in mild to moderate asthmatics given repeated inhaled doses of zanamivir, Respir. Med. 94 (2000) 166–173.

[15] M. Schilling, L. Povinelli, P. Krause, M. Gravenstein, A. Ambrozaitis, H.H. Jones, et al., Efficacy of zanamivir for chemoprophylaxis of nursing home influenza outbreaks, Vaccine 16 (18) (1998) 1771–1774.

[16] C. Lee, M. Loeb, A. Phillips, J. Nesbitt, K. Smith, M. Feaon, et al., Use of zanamivir (AZ) to control an outbreak of influenza A (FluA), Abstracts of the 39th Interscience Conference on Antimicrobial Agents and Chemotherapy, San Francisco, CA, Sept 26–69, 1999, p. 421 (Abst #283).

[17] F.G. Hayden, R.L. Atmar, M. Schilling, C. Johnson, D. Poretz, D. Parr, et al., Use of the selective oral neuraminidase inhibitor oseltamivir to prevent influenza, N. Engl. J. Med. 341 (1999) 1336–1343.

[18] P.H. Peters, P. Norwood, V. DeBock, T. VanCouter, M. Gibbens, T. VonPlanta, et al., Oseltamivir is effective in the longterm prophylaxis of influenza in vaccinated frail elderly, Abstracts of the II International Symposium on Influenza and other Respiratory Viruses, December 10–12, Grand Cayman, Cayman Islands, British West Indies, 1999.

[19] A. Webster, M. Boyce, S. Edmundson, I. Miller, Coadministration of orally inhaled zanamivir with inactivated trivalent influenza vaccine does not adversely affect the production of antihaemagglutinin antibodies in the serum of healthy volunteers, Clin. Pharmacokinet. 36 (Suppl. 1) (1999) 51–58.

[20] D.P. Calfee, A.W. Peng, L. Cass, M. Lobo, F.G. Hayden, Safety and efficacy of intravenous zanamivir in preventing experimental human influenza A virus infection, Antimicrob. Agents Chemother. 43 (7) (1999) 1616–1620.

[21] R.S. Fritz, F.G. Hayden, D.P. Calfee, L. Cass, A.W. Peng, G. Alvord, et al., Nasal cytokine and chemokine responses in experimental influenza A virus infection: results of a placebo-controlled trial of intravenous zanamivir treatment, J. Infect. Dis. 180 (1999) 586–593.

[22] J.B. Walker, E.K. Hussey, J.J. Treanor, A. Montalvo, F.G. Hayden, Effects of the neuraminidase inhibitor zanamivir on otologic manifestations of experimental human influenza, J. Infect. Dis. 176 (1997) 1417–1422.

[23] F.G. Hayden, A.D.M.E. Osterhaus, J.J. Treanor, D.M. Fleming, F.Y. Aoki, K.G. Nicholson, et al., Efficacy and safety of the neuraminidase inhibitor zanamivir in the treatment of influenza virus infections, N. Engl. J. Med. 337 (13) (1997) 874–879.

[24] A.S. Monto, D.M. Fleming, D. Henry, R. DeGroot, M. Makela, T. Klein, et al., Efficacy and safety of the

neuraminidase inhibitor zanamivir in the treatment of indluenza A and B virus infections, J. Infect. Dis. 180 (2) (1999) 254–261.

[25] MIST Study Group, Randomized trial of efficacy and safety of inhaled zanamivir in treatment of influenza A and B virus infections, Lancet 352 (1998) 1877–1881.

[26] A.S. Monto, A. Webster, O. Keene, Randomized, placebo-controlled studies of inhaled zanamivir in the treatment of influenza A and B: pooled efficacy analysis, J. Antimicrob. Chemother. 44 (1999) 23–29.

[27] J.A. Hedrick, A. Barzilai, U. Behre, F.W. Henderson, J. Hammond, L. Reilly, et al., Zanamivir for treatment of symptomatic influenza A and B infection in children five to twelve years of age: a randomized controlled trial, Pediatr. Infect. Dis. J. 2000 19 (5) (2000 May) 410–417.

[28] L. Kaiser, O.N. Keene, J. Hammond, M. Elliott, F.G. Hayden, Impact of zanamivir on antibiotics use for respiratory events following acute influenza in adolescents and adults, Arch. Int. Med. 160 (2000) 3234–3240.

[29] (a) S. Gravenstein, B. Freund, J.E. McElhaney, M. Schilling, O. Keene, Greater effectiveness from zanamivir treatment of influenza with antecedent influenza vaccination in older adults, Abstracts of the 39th Interscience Conference on Antimicrobial Agents and Chemotherapy, San Francisco, CA, Sept 26–69, 1999, p. 436 (Abst #1902).

(b) K.R. Murphy, A. Eivindson, K. Pauksen, W.J. Stein, G. Tellier, R. Watts, P. Leophonte, S.J. Sharp, E. Leoschel, Efficacy and safety of inhaled zanamivir for the treatment of influenza in patients with asthma or chronic obstructive pulmonary disease, Clin. Drug Invest. 20 (5) (2000) 337–349.

[30] J. Barnett, A. Cadman, D. Gor, M. Dempsey, M. Walters, A. Candlin, et al., Zanamivir susceptibility monitoring and characterization of influenza virus clinical isolates obtained during phase II clinical efficacy studies, Antimicrob. Agents Chemother. 44 (1) (2000) 78–87.

[31] G. Boivin, N. Goyette, I. Hardy, F.Y. Aoki, A. Wagner, S. Trottier, Rapid antiviral effect of inhaled zanamivir in the treatment of naturally occurring influenza in otherwise healthy adults, J. Infect. Dis. 181 (2000) 1471–1474.

[32] J.J. Treanor, F.G. Hayden, P.S. Vrooman, R.A. Barbarash, R. Bettis, D. Riff, et al., Efficacy and safety of the oral neuraminidase inhibitor oseltamivir in treating acute influenza, JAMA 283 (8) (2000) 1016–1024.

[33] K.G. Nicholson, F.Y. Aoki, A.D. Osterhaus, S. Trottier, O. Carewicz, C.H. Mercier, et al., Efficacy and safety of oseltamivir in treatment of acute influenza; a randomized controlled trial, Lancet 335 (2000) 1845–1850.

[34] R.J. Whitley, F.G. Hayden, K.S. Reisinger, N. Young, R. Dutkowski, D. Ipe, et al., Oral oseltamivir treatment of influenza in children, Pediatric Infectious Disease Journal 20 (2) (2001) 127–133 (Feb.).

[35] A.S. Monto, D.P. Robinson, L. Herlocher, J.M. Hinson, M. Elliott, A. Crisp, Zanamivir in the prevention of influenza among healthy adults, JAMA 282 (1) (1999) 31–36.

[36] (a) L. Kaiser, D. Henry, N. Flack, O. Keene, F.G. Hayden, Short-term zanamivir to prevent influenza:results of a placebo controlled study, Clin. Infect. Dis. 30 (2000) 587–589.

(b) S. Gravenstein, P. Drinka, D. Osterweil, M. Schilling, J.E. McElhaney, M. Elliot, J. Hammond, O. Keene, P. Krause, N. A. Flack, Multicenter prospective double-blind randomized controlled trial comparing the relative safety and efficacy of ranamivir to rimantadine for nursing home influenza outbreak control. Abstracts of the 40th Interscience Conference on Antimicrobial Agents and Chemotheraphy, Toronto, Canada, September 17–20, 2000, p. 270, Abst #1155.

[37] R. Welliver, A.S. Monto, O. Carewicz, E. Schatteman, M. Hassman, J. Hedrick, H.C. Jackson, et al., Effectiveness of Oseltamivir in preventing influenza in household contacts: A randomized controlled trial, JAMA 285 (6) (2001) 748–754.

[38] M. Tisdale, Monitoring of viral susceptibility: new challenges with the development of influenza NA inhibitors, Rev. Med. Virol. 10 (2000) 45–55.

[39] J.L. McKimm-Breschkin, Resistance of influenza viruses to neuraminidase inhibitors—a review, Antiviral Res. 47 (2000) 1–17.

[40] L.V. Gubareva, M.N. Matrosovich, M.K. Brenner, R. Bethell, R.G. Webster, Evidence for zanamivir resistance in an immunocompromised child infected with influenza B virus, J. Infect. Dis. 178 (5) (1998) 1257–1262.

[41] M. Zambon, F.G. Hayden, Position statement: global neuraminidase inhibitor susceptibility network, Antiviral Res. 49 (2001) 147–156.

International Congress Series 1219 (2001) 807–811

Oral oseltamivir reduces febrile illness in patients considered at high risk of influenza complications

C. Martin[a,*], P. Mahoney[b], P. Ward[b]

[a]Roche Global Development, Basel, CH, Switzerland
[b]Roche Global Development, Welwyn, UK

Abstract

Background: Influenza poses a serious burden to patients at high risk of influenza complications and vaccination against the disease may be inadequate due to poor uptake rates or impaired immune response. We investigated the efficacy and safety of oral oseltamivir treatment in two studies of elderly patients or those with underlying cardiac/pulmonary disease (at-risk). *Methods*: 1138 high-risk patients (13–97 years) presenting within 36 h of onset of influenza symptoms were randomized to oseltamivir 75 mg or placebo bid for 5 days. Endpoints included duration of febrile illness, fever and other symptoms, viral shedding and complications. *Results*: 727 (64%) patients were influenza-infected (ITTI) (at-risk: placebo 133, oseltamivir 118; elderly: placebo 254, oseltamivir 222). In the ITTI population, oseltamivir reduced median duration of fever by 37% in at-risk patients and by 25% in elderly patients compared with placebo. Acute febrile illness and respiratory complications were reduced with oseltamivir treatment by approximately 30% in both patient populations. Viral shedding was reduced by 70% in oseltamivir-treated at-risk patients. Oseltamivir was well tolerated, with similar incidence of gastrointestinal events reported in placebo and oseltamivir recipients. *Conclusions*: Oseltamivir reduces the duration of fever, febrile illness, individual influenza symptoms and complications in high-risk patients. © 2001 Elsevier Science B.V. All rights reserved.

Keywords: Treatment; Prevention; Neuraminidase inhibitor

* Corresponding author. F. Hoffmann-La Roche AG, PDC2, Bldg. 52, 1013, CH-4070, Basel, Switzerland. Tel.: +41-61-688-1456; fax: +41-61-688-7085.
   E-mail address: corine.martin@roche.com (C. Martin).

1. Introduction

Influenza infection poses a serious burden to elderly patients and those with chronic pulmonary or cardiac diseases. This high-risk population can be affected by a number of serious influenza-related complications such as bronchitis, asthma, pneumonia and myocarditis, which may lead to hospitalization and death [1]. Further, influenza infection can lead to exacerbation of an underlying chronic conditions [2].

Although such high-risk patients are recommended to receive the influenza vaccine [3], protection against the disease may be inadequate because of low vaccination uptake rates or a poor immune response [1,3]. Oral oseltamivir, the prodrug of the neuraminidase inhibitor oseltamivir carboxylate, is an effective and safe treatment for acute influenza infection in otherwise healthy adults [4,5]. Thus, oral oseltamivir provides an additional management option in these high-risk patients.

We investigated the efficacy and safety of oral oseltamivir in the treatment of an influenza-infected high-risk population of elderly patients and patients with chronic cardiac and/or respiratory disease (at-risk).

2. Material and methods/patients

Patients with chronic cardiac and/or respiratory disease (13–88 years) and elderly patients (65–97 years) were enrolled into two multi-centre, randomized, placebo-controlled, double-blind, parallel-group studies. Patients presenting within 36 h of onset of influenza symptoms [fever ≥ 38.0 °C (≥ 37.5 °C if subject aged ≥ 65 years) plus one systemic (headache, malaise, myalgia, sweats/chills or prostration] and one respiratory (cough, sore throat, nasal symptoms) symptom received oseltamivir 75 mg or placebo twice daily for 5 days. Influenza was confirmed by positive virus culture or ≥ 4-fold rise in influenza-specific HAI antibody titres. At-risk patients were stratified for the absence/presence of COAD or cardiac disease. Patients made diary entries of symptoms until day 21. Measured variables included temperature (twice daily) and influenza virus titres (from nasal and throat swabs) in the influenza-infected (ITTI) population. Twelve lead ECGs and the forced expiratory volume in 1 s (FEV1) were obtained at baseline, on day 21 and during the study if required. Adverse events were recorded throughout the study.

Table 1
Patient demographics for 402 at-risk and 736 elderly patients treated with oseltamivir 75 mg or placebo bid for 5 days

	At-risk ($n=402$)		Elderly ($n=736$)	
	Placebo ($n=203$)	Oseltamivir ($n=199$)	Placebo ($n=376$)	Oseltamivir ($n=360$)
Mean age (range), year	50 (13–88)	53.7 (13–86)	73 (65–97)	73 (65–96)
Number of males (%)	91 (45)	86 (43)	166 (44)	150 (42)
Number with COAD (%)	150 (74)	155 (78)	38 (10)	24 (7)
Number of vaccinated (%)	55 (27)	56 (28)	172 (46)	143 (40)
Number of influenza-infected (%)	133 (66)	118 (59)	254 (68)	222 (62)

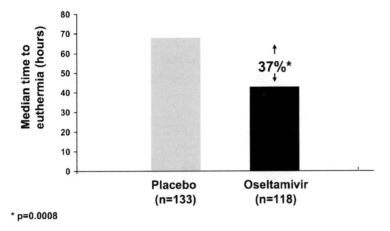

Fig. 1. Median duration of fever in (a) at-risk and (b) elderly patients treated with oseltamivir 75 mg or placebo bid for 5 days.

The studies were performed in accordance with the Declaration of Helsinki (amended) and written informed consent was obtained from each patient before inclusion within the trial.

3. Results

Four-hundred and two at-risk (203 placebo, 199 oseltamivir) and 736 elderly (376 placebo, 360 oseltamivir) patients were randomized and received at least one dose of study drug. Of the at-risk patients 76% had COAD and less than 30% of this group were vaccinated. Overall, 64% of patients were influenza-infected and comprised the ITTI population. Patient demographics for both patient populations are shown in Table 1.

Oral oseltamivir significantly reduced the median duration of fever (temperature ≥ 37.2 °C) by 37% compared with placebo in at-risk patients (placebo 67.9 h, oseltamivir 42.8 h; $p = 0.0008$) and by 25% in elderly patients (placebo 89.5 h, oseltamivir 66.9 h) (Fig. 1a and b). Time to alleviation of acute febrile illness (defined both as fever/chills/

Table 2

Alleviation of acute febrile illness in 251 at-risk and 476 elderly influenza-infected patients treated with oseltamivir 75 mg or placebo bid for 5 days

	Median time to alleviation (h)		Reduction (%)
	Placebo	Oseltamivir	
At-risk	$n = 133$	$n = 118$	
Fever/chills/myalgia	57.9	40.8 ($p = 0.0005$)	30
Fever/cough/coryza	117.3	96.0	18
Elderly	$n = 254$	$n = 222$	
Fever/chills/myalgia	50.5	36.0 ($p = 0.005$)	29
Fever/cough/coryza	132.3	115.0	13

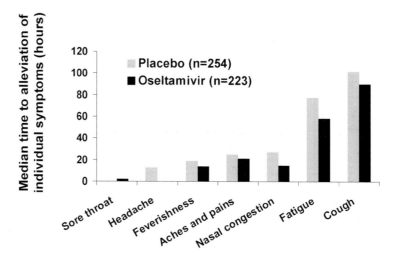

Fig. 2. Median duration of individual influenza symptoms in (a) at-risk and (b) elderly patients treated with oseltamivir 75 mg or placebo bid for 5 days.

myalgia and fever/cough/coryza) was also reduced by approximately 30% in both patient populations with oseltamivir treatment (Table 2). Furthermore, individual influenza symptoms were reduced by oseltamivir treatment (Fig. 2a and b). The beneficial effects of oseltamivir on influenza illness was underlined by a potent antiviral effect, with at-risk oseltamivir recipients experiencing a 70% reduction in the proportion of patients shedding virus on day 4 compared with placebo [placebo 11/98 (11%), oseltamivir 3/90 (3%); $p = 0.05$]. The treatment benefits associated with oseltamivir translated into a 25% reduction in the number of days that this population was restricted to bed (placebo 4 days, oseltamivir 3 days). Moreover, as could be anticipated, there was an overall 28% reduction in the incidence of lower respiratory tract complications (bronchitis, pneumonia and other respiratory infections) in the pooled population [placebo 69/387 (18%), oseltamivir 44/341 (13%)], and a 50% reduction in exacerbation of asthma in at-risk

Table 3

Adverse events and discontinuations in the at-risk and elderly population treated with oseltamivir 75 mg or placebo bid for 5 days (safety population)

	Placebo, n (%)	Oseltamivir, n (%)
At-risk	$n = 202$	$n = 199$
Nausea	13 (6)	19 (10)
Vomiting	6 (3)	9 (5)
Diarrhoea	23 (11)	8 (4)
Discontinuations	7 (3)	3 (1)
Elderly	$n = 373$	$n = 362$
Nausea	27 (7)	21 (6)
Vomiting	11 (3)	17 (5)
Diarrhoea	19 (5)	9 (2)
Discontinuations	11 (3)	9 (2)

patients [placebo 12/202 (6%), oseltamivir 6/199 (3%)]. Oral oseltamivir was well tolerated in both populations and discontinuations due to adverse events were low (<2% placebo, <1% oseltamivir). Gastrointestinal effects occurred with similar frequency in placebo and oseltamivir-treated patients (Table 3).

4. Discussion

Oral oseltamivir, 75 mg twice daily for 5 days, was highly effective in reducing the duration and symptoms of febrile illness in elderly patients or patients with underlying chronic cardiac and/or respiratory disease. As anticipated, the antiviral effect of oseltamivir translated into a reduction in respiratory complications in this patient population and fewer exacerbations of underlying disease in at-risk patients. These results confirm results from studies in otherwise healthy adults [4,5]. Oseltamivir was well tolerated by both patient populations in patients up to 97 years of age. In conclusion, oseltamivir treatment is highly beneficial in patients at high risk from influenza complications.

References

[1] K.L. Nichol, L. Baken, A. Nelson, Relation between influenza vaccination and outpatient visits, hospitalization, and mortality in elderly persons with chronic lung disease, Ann. Intern. Med. 130 (1999) 397–403.
[2] K.G. Nicolson, Human influenza, in: K.G. Nicholson, R.G. Webster, A.J. Hay (Eds.), Textbook of Influenza, Blackwell, London, 1998, pp. 219–264.
[3] Centers for Disease Control and Prevention. Prevention and control of influenza: recommendations of the Advisory Committee on Immunization Practices (ACIP) MMWR 48 (RR-04) (1999) 1–28.
[4] J.J. Treanor, F.G. Hayden, P.S. Vrooman, et al., Efficacy and safety of the oral neuraminidase inhibitor oseltamivir in treating acute influenza, JAMA 283 (2000) 1016–1024.
[5] K.G. Nicholson, F.Y. Aoki, A.D.M.E. Osterhaus, et al., Efficacy and safety of oseltamivir in treatment of acute influenza: a randomised controlled trial, Lancet 355 (2000) 1845–1850.

International Congress Series 1219 (2001) 813–816

Effective treatment of influenza with oral oseltamivir in a vaccinated population of high-risk patients

M. Zaug[a,*], P. Mahoney[b], P. Ward[b]

[a]F. Hoffman-La Roche Ltd., PDC2 Bldg. 52/1115, CH-4070, Basel, Switzerland
[b]Roche Global Development, Welwyn, UK

Abstract

Background: Annual vaccination is recommended for patient groups considered at risk from significant morbidity and mortality from influenza, however, vaccination does not provide complete protection against influenza. Oral oseltamivir is effective for the treatment of influenza in healthy unvaccinated patients. We evaluated oseltamivir for the treatment of influenza in vaccinated 'at-risk' patients, including the elderly and patients with pre-existing cardiac and/or pulmonary disease. *Methods*: 226 vaccinated patients (>13 years) from a pooled dataset of 613 at-risk patients with acute febrile influenza (≤ 36 h duration) were randomized to receive oral oseltamivir 75 mg or placebo twice daily for 5 days. Influenza symptoms were recorded (0 = absent, 1 = mild, 2 = moderate, 3 = severe) in a diary twice daily. The primary endpoint was duration of illness (symptoms score ≤ 1 for ≥ 24 h). *Results*: 62% of vaccinated patients had confirmed influenza (placebo: $n = 76$, oseltamivir: $n = 64$). The median duration of illness was reduced by 1.8 days by oseltamivir compared with placebo (placebo: 8.2 days, oseltamivir: 6.4 days). Oseltamivir reduced individual influenza symptoms, secondary complications and viral shedding compared with placebo. Oseltamivir was well tolerated. *Conclusions*: Oral oseltamivir provides additional clinical benefit to vaccination for influenza-infected at-risk patients who develop the disease. © 2001 Elsevier Science B.V. All rights reserved.

Keywords: Neuraminidase inhibitor; At-risk patients; Antiviral

* Corresponding author. Tel. +41-61-688-7117; fax: +41-61-688-2790.
E-mail address: michel.zaug@roche.com (M. Zaug).

0531-5131/01/$ – see front matter © 2001 Elsevier Science B.V. All rights reserved.
PII: S0531-5131(01)00360-0

1. Introduction

Vaccination against influenza infection is recommended for the elderly population and those considered at risk from the substantial morbidity and mortality associated with influenza infection (e.g. subjects with chronic cardiac and/or pulmonary disease) [1]. Death rates from influenza have not changed over the last 60 years, despite the increased use of influenza vaccination [2]. As vaccination does not provide complete protection against influenza infection [1], a substantial proportion of previously vaccinated patients still develop influenza illness.

Oral oseltamivir, the prodrug of the potent and specific neuraminidase inhibitor oseltamivir carboxylate, is an effective and safe treatment for influenza infection in unvaccinated otherwise healthy patients [3,4]. We studied the benefits of oseltamivir treatment of influenza in a vaccinated population, using data pooled from three studies that included elderly patients and those with chronic cardiac/pulmonary disease.

2. Methods

Patients (>13 years) who had been vaccinated in the study season and who presented within 36 h of the onset of symptoms of influenza were eligible for inclusion into the analysis population. Influenza symptoms were defined as fever (≥ 38 °C/≥ 100 °F for patients <65 years, ≥ 37.5 °C/99.5 °F for patients ≥ 65 years) plus one respiratory symptom (cough, sore throat or nasal congestion) and one constitutional symptom (feverishness/chills, headache, myalgia or fatigue).

Influenza infection was confirmed by either positive virus culture or ≥ 4-fold rise in influenza specific antibody titres. Influenza symptoms were self-reported and graded for severity using a four-point categorical scale twice daily on a diary card (0 = absent, 1 = mild, 2 = moderate, 3 = severe) throughout the study period (21 days).

The primary endpoint was the duration of illness, defined as the length of time from initiation of study drug until all symptoms were alleviated (i.e. symptom scores remained at 0 or 1 for at least 24 h). Efficacy analyses were performed on vaccinated patients with confirmed influenza (ITTI population: placebo $n = 76$, oseltamivir $n = 64$). Safety data was based on all patients who received at least one dose of trial medication (placebo $n = 117$, oseltamivir $n = 109$).

3. Results

Influenza infection was confirmed in 62% (140/226) of vaccinated patients (ITTI population). Most (131/140, 94%) infected patients had nose/throat swabs taken at baseline and 64 (46%) patients (35 placebo, 29 oseltamivir) at both baseline and day 3 of therapy. In the ITTI population, the median duration of illness was reduced by almost 2 days (42.5 h) in oseltamivir recipients (placebo, P, 196.3 h [8.2 days]; oseltamivir, O, 153.8 h [6.4 days]) (Fig. 1). In addition, the median time to alleviation of each individual

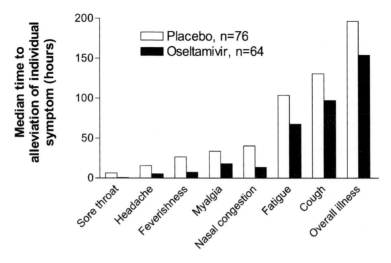

Fig. 1. Oseltamivir 75 mg bid for 5 days reduces the median time to alleviation of individual symptoms in vaccinated patients compared with placebo.

symptom was shorter in oseltamivir recipients compared with placebo, most notably feverishness, myalgia, fatigue and cough (Fig. 1).

The mean baseline titres were similar in both treatment groups (3.5 for placebo and 3.3 $\log_{10}$ TCID$_{50}$/ml with oseltamivir). By day 3 of treatment, the viral titre was reduced 10-fold in the oseltamivir group compared with placebo (placebo: 2.3 $\log_{10}$ TCID$_{50}$/ml, oseltamivir: 1.2 $\log_{10}$ TCID$_{50}$/ml) (Fig. 2). In addition to alleviating influenza symptoms and reducing virus titre, oseltamivir reduced the incidence of influenza-related secondary respiratory complications (mainly bronchitis) compared with placebo (Table 1).

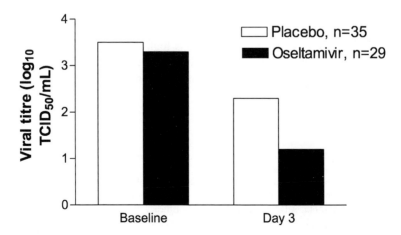

Fig. 2. Oseltamivir 75 mg bid for 5 days reduces the quantity of virus shed in vaccinated patients compared with placebo.

Table 1
Oseltamivir 75 mg bid for 5 days reduces the incidence of secondary respiratory complications (bronchitis, LRTI[a], pneumonia) in vaccinated patients compared with placebo

	Placebo (n = 76)	Oseltamivir (n = 64)
Bronchitis (%)	11 (14)	5 (8)
LRTI[a] (%)	1 (1)	1 (2)
Pneumonia (%)	2 (3)	2 (3)
All respiratory complications (%)	13 (17)	8 (12.5)

[a] LRTI: Lower respiratory tract infection.

Oseltamivir was well tolerated in this at-risk population. Adverse events were reported with similar frequency in the placebo and oseltamivir-treated groups (placebo: 55%, oseltamivir: 46%). Diarrhoea and vomiting were more common in the placebo group than oseltamivir (diarrhoea: placebo 12 [10%], oseltamivir 5 [5%]; vomiting: placebo 6 [5%], oseltamivir 2 [2%]). Nausea was reported more often by oseltamivir recipients (placebo 5 [4%], oseltamivir 8 [7%]). Consistent with the reduced frequency of influenza-related secondary complications, fewer oseltamivir recipients reported respiratory or cardiac events compared with placebo (respiratory: placebo 14 [12%], oseltamivir 10 [9%]; cardiac: placebo 4 [3%], oseltamivir 2 [2%]).

4. Discussion

Our analysis showed that treatment with oral oseltamivir provides additional, clinically significant benefits for patients who develop influenza despite having received an annual vaccination. These data confirm previous results from studies in otherwise healthy unvaccinated adults [3,4].

The quantity of virus shed by oseltamivir recipients was reduced by more than 10-fold compared with placebo. This antiviral effect translated into faster resolution of illness (by almost 2 days) and individual symptoms compared with placebo and a reduced incidence of secondary complications.

Finally, oseltamivir was well tolerated by this high-risk population: the incidence of adverse events was similar in both groups. Oseltamivir-treated patients with cardiac and/or pulmonary conditions reported fewer exacerbations of underlying disease compared with placebo.

References

[1] Prevention and control of influenza: recommendations of the Advisory Committee on Immunization Practices (ACIP) MMWR 49 (RR-03) (2000) 1–38.
[2] K.G. Nicholson, Human influenza, in: K.G. Nicholson, R.G. Webster, A.J. Hay (Eds.), Textbook of Influenza, Blackwell Science, Oxford, 1998, pp. 219–264.
[3] K.G. Nicholson, F.Y. Aoki, A.D.M.E. Osterhaus, et al., Efficacy and safety of oseltamivir in treatment of acute influenza: a randomised controlled trial, Lancet 355 (2000) 1845–1850.
[4] J.J. Treanor, F.G. Hayden, P.S. Vrooman, et al., Efficacy and safety of the oral neuraminidase inhibitor oseltamivir in treating acute influenza: a randomized, controlled trial, JAMA, J. Am. Med. Assoc. 283 (2000) 1016–1024.

International Congress Series 1219 (2001) 817–822

Antiviral use during influenza outbreaks in long-term care facilities

Susan E. Tamblyn*

Perth District Health Unit, 653 West Gore Street, Stratford, Ontario, Canada N5A 1L4

Abstract

Background: Influenza outbreaks (OBs) are common in long-term care facilities (LTCF) and can cause high morbidity and mortality. Outbreak control with antivirals is successful but problematic. I reviewed the Perth County experience with antivirals in LTCF OBs including the introduction of neuraminidase inhibitors (NI). *Methods*: Health department and facility records of all LTCF influenza OBs were reviewed including line listings, epidemic curves, laboratory studies, control measures, and antiviral dosing and side effects. *Results*: Amantadine prophylaxis was used in 29 LTCF influenza A OBs between 1989 and 2000. In 22 (76%) transmission stopped within 48–72 h but seven OBs (24%) were not controlled. Amantadine susceptibility testing in six OBs with amantadine failure showed emergence of resistant organisms in three and ongoing transmission of susceptible organisms in three. Amantadine failure was associated with simultaneous prophylaxis and treatment in the facility. Side effects were reported in 1.7% of residents and drug stopped in 0.7%. Attempts to limit amantadine use to only part of a facility were not successful. Logistical problems including delay in starting prophylaxis, inappropriate schedules, low staff uptake, knowing when to start or stop amantadine and treatment issues. In the 99/00 season, NI were used for persons with contraindications to amantadine, and for treating ill residents when amantadine prophylaxis was initiated for OB control (to prevent resistance). Switching residents to oseltamivir successfully stopped one OB that amantadine failed to control. *Conclusions*: Amantadine prophylaxis successfully controls most LTCF influenza A OBs but failures occur due to both resistant and sensitive viruses. NI have considerable potential in LTCF OBs. © 2001 Elsevier Science B.V. All rights reserved.

Keywords: Influenza outbreaks; Long-term care facilities; Amantadine; Neuraminidase inhibitors

* Tel: +1-519-271-7600x255; fax: +1-519-271-2195.
E-mail address: tamblyn@pdhu.on.ca (S.E. Tamblyn).

0531-5131/01/$ – see front matter © 2001 Elsevier Science B.V. All rights reserved.
PII: S0531-5131(01)00361-2

1. Introduction

Influenza outbreaks are common in long-term care facilities (LTCF) and can cause high morbidity and mortality. Their occurrence and severity has been reduced, but not eliminated, by vaccination programs for residents and staff [1]. Antiviral prophylaxis for outbreak control provides additional benefit and is now widely used in Canada. Many problems with its use have been recognized and personally experienced. These include difficulties in rapid initiation of prophylaxis, complexity of prophylaxis and treatment regimes, troublesome side effects and emergence of drug resistance leading to failed prophylaxis [1–3]. The approval of two neuraminidase inhibitors in Canada in fall 1999, albeit for treatment not prophylaxis, provided opportunities to explore their use in the LTCF setting and see if the problems occurring with amantadine can be overcome.

In Ontario public health staff provide consultation to LTCF regarding outbreak control and collect information on each respiratory outbreak. I reviewed our Perth County experience with antivirals in LTCF outbreaks from the 1989/1990 to the 1999/2000 season. There are 11 licensed LTCF in the county, many with attached retirement home beds, and four free-standing retirement homes. During this period influenza vaccination levels increased from 93% to 96% for residents and from 21% to 88% for staff.

2. Methods

Health department records of all LTCF influenza outbreaks were reviewed and supplemented if necessary with additional information from the LTCF. These included line listings of cases, epidemic curves, outbreak control measures and laboratory studies. Antiviral issues studied included use for prophylaxis and/or treatment in residents and staff, dosing, reported side effects, degree of outbreak control and results of amantadine susceptibility testing of isolates in outbreaks not brought under control. Outbreaks not controlled by amantadine were compared with successfully controlled outbreaks in terms of percentage of residents prophylaxed or treated, duration and dosage of amantadine, simultaneous treatment and prophylaxis in the facility, and isolation of treated patients.

Testing for amantadine resistance of 1999 and 2000 isolates was carried out at the Canadian Science Centre for Human and Animal Health using a method based on RT-PCR restriction analysis. Testing of earlier isolates was performed by the Influenza Virus Laboratory, Centres for Disease Control and Prevention using biological and molecular assays.

3. Results

Amantadine prophylaxis was used for outbreak control in 29 of the 33 confirmed influenza A outbreaks that occurred over the 11 influenza seasons studied. The amantadine protocol used for outbreak control consisted of amantadine prophylaxis for all well residents and for unvaccinated staff until the outbreak was declared over [4]. Ill residents

(< 48 h from onset) were treated with amantadine for a maximum of five days at physician option, and were to be isolated from those on prophylaxis.

Amantadine doses for residents were individually tailored according to recommendations of the National Advisory Committee on Immunization that are based on calculated creatinine clearance [4]. For staff prophylaxis, the recommendation was 200 mg/day; last season this was reduced to 100 mg/day.

Few side effects were reported for residents on amantadine, probably because with individually tailored doses most received less than 100 mg/day. Side effects were reported in only 1.7% of 2176 treated residents and amantadine was discontinued in 0.7%. Reported side effects included dizziness and confusion, mild gastrointestinal symptoms and four falls. In contrast, side effects were reported by 12.8% of staff, mainly dizziness, agitation or gastrointestinal symptoms.

Five facilities whose outbreak began in an isolated cottage or wing attempted to limit their use of amantadine to that area. In all cases, however, influenza quickly spread to other parts of the facility, probably because of shared staff.

Facilities that were inexperienced with amantadine often faced problems in implementing its use for outbreak control. Most of these were successfully overcome as the facilities gained experience and the Health Unit provided more specific recommendations and in-service (Table 1).

Outbreak control was defined as cessation of transmission of influenza A to residents within 72 h of starting amantadine. Amantadine prophylaxis was successful in 22/29 (76%) outbreaks where it was used. However, seven (24%) outbreaks were not controlled. In these uncontrolled outbreaks, testing of the influenza isolates showed emergence of amantadine-resistant organisms in three outbreaks and ongoing transmission of susceptible organisms in three. Fig. 1 provides an example of the former. The seventh outbreak had only pre-amantadine isolates available for testing, which were susceptible.

The comparison of LTCF outbreaks that were not controlled by amantadine with those where it worked found only two significant factors associated with failure—amantadine

Table 1
Problems experienced with amantadine use for outbreak control

Problem	Solution
Delay in starting amantadine prophylaxis	Advance orders and consents
	Keep stock on hand
Inappropriate schedules	In-service, advance orders
	Simpler regimen
Low staff uptake	Provide free, dispense on-site
	Policy requiring use for unvaccinated staff or face exclusion
When to start/stop	Nasopharyngeal swabs and rapid tests
	Provincial guidelines
Treatment dilemma	Guidelines for use—3–5 days duration, within 48 h of onset, isolation
	Use neuraminidase inhibitors
Failure to control outbreak	More appropriate use of amantadine
	Search for other organism
	Switch to neuraminidase inhibitors

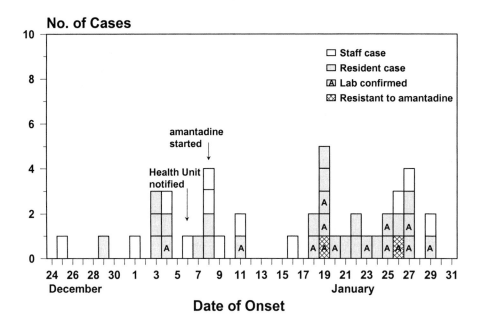

Fig. 1. LTCF A, Perth County, influenza A outbreak—1996/97.

treatment of ill residents in the facility while others were being prophylaxed (100% vs. 45%, $p = 0.04$), and treatment of a higher proportion of cases (48% vs. 27%, $p = <0.001$). The only difference found between the failed outbreaks due to resistant vs. sensitive virus was a higher proportion of cases in shared rooms in the resistant virus outbreaks (83% vs. 60%, $p = 0.003$). Observed problems in some failed outbreaks included prolonged treatment and inability to segregate residents on treatment.

Increasing recognition of amantadine failure and other problems in outbreak control in Ontario LTCF led to updated guidelines for the 1999/2000 season [5]. These emphasized discontinuing amantadine in persons who became ill while on prophylaxis and de-emphasized treatment unless the resident could be properly isolated. A new protocol required unvaccinated staff to be excluded during outbreaks unless on amantadine [6]. Timely licensure of zanamivir and oseltamivir provided a treatment alternative during amantadine prophylaxis, though these drugs were not yet government funded for LTCFs.

In the 1999/2000 season, outbreaks were shorter and smaller than in previous seasons but one facility experienced three separate outbreaks due to virus reintroduction. Zanamivir or oseltamivir was used to treat ill residents in 5/8 confirmed influenza A outbreaks using amantadine prophylaxis. One outbreak with amantadine failure was successfully controlled by switching residents to oseltamivir (Fig. 2). No side effects were reported from this use of neuraminidase inhibitors. Provincially neuraminidase inhibitor prophylaxis was used successfully in 14 LTCF outbreaks, eight as initial prophylaxis and six after amantadine failure (Dr. Allison McGeer, personal communica-

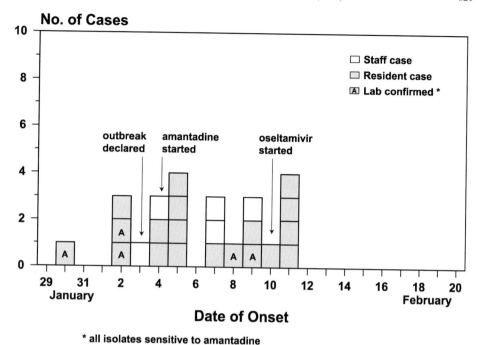

Fig. 2. LTCF B, Perth County, influenza A outbreak—2000.

tion). Neuraminidase inhibitors were also substituted for amantadine in individuals at risk of serious side effects from amantadine.

4. Discussion

Our experience through the years with amantadine prophylaxis in LTCF outbreaks has shown that its use is safe and usually effective. Our success rate of 76% is comparable to the 60–80% reported by Ontario LTCF in the past two seasons [7,8]. Our findings confirm previous observations that combining amantadine treatment and prophylaxis in the same facility seems to set the stage for transmission of amantadine-resistant virus [9,10]. However, amantadine failure with sensitive virus is less easily understood. Concerns that tailored dosing leads to safe but less effective regimes because of underdosing of many individuals could not be tested. Logistical problems in dealing with amantadine were largely overcome through guidelines and education.

Neuraminidase inhibitors have considerable promise in the LTCF setting for outbreak control, either as initial prophylaxis or after amantadine failure, and for treatment of ill residents especially while amantadine is being used for prophylaxis. Ease of adminis-tration, effectiveness against both influenza A and B, low risk of side effects and reduced selection of resistance suggest they will become drugs of choice. However, it will be important to monitor their effectiveness and the potential for resistance in the combined prophylaxis-treatment situation.

Acknowledgements

I wish to thank the following for contributing information used in this report: Jennifer Duffin, PHN and July deGrosbois, PHI at Perth District Health Unit for outbreak investigations; influenza labs at CDC (US) and LCDC (Canada) for amantadine sensitivity testing; and Lewinda Knowles, University of Toronto MHSc practicum student, for analyses of amantadine failure (with grant support from Roche).

References

[1] S.F. Bradley, The Long-Term-Care Committee of the Society for Healthcare Epidemiology of America, Prevention of influenza in long-term-care facilities, Infect. Control Hosp. Epidemiol. 20 (1999) 629–637.

[2] S.E. Tamblyn, Amantadine use in influenza outbreaks in long-term care facilities, Can. Med. Assoc. J. 157 (1997) 1573–1574.

[3] A. McGeer, D.S. Sitar, S.E. Tamblyn, F. Kolbe, P. Orr, F.Y. Aoki, Use of antiviral prophylaxis in influenza outbreaks in long term care facilities, Can. J. Infect. Dis. 11 (2000) 187–192.

[4] National Advisory Committee on Immunization (NACI), Statement on influenza vaccination for the 1999–2000 season, Can. Commun. Dis. Rep. 25 (AC-2,3,4) (1999) 1–16.

[5] Ontario Ministry of Health and Long-Term Care, Recommendations of the Ontario Working Group on Influenza, September 1999.

[6] Ontario Ministry of Health and Long-Term Care, Influenza Prevention and Surveillance Protocol for Ontario Long-Term Care Facilities, November 1, 1999.

[7] B. Henry, Summary report of the Ontario influenza 1998/99 season, Public Health Epidemiol. Rep. Ont. 10 (1999) 144–159.

[8] B. Henry, J. Nsubuga, Summary report of the 1999/00 Ontario influenza season, Public Health Epidemiol. Rep. Ont. 11 (2000) 137–156.

[9] E.E. Mast, M.W. Harmon, S. Gravenstein, S.P. Wu, N.H. Arden, R. Circo, et al., Emergence and possible transmission of amantadine-resistant viruses during nursing home outbreaks of influenza A (H3N2), Am. J. Epidemiol. 134 (1991) 988–997.

[10] J. Degelau, S.K. Somani, S.L. Cooper, D.R.P. Guay, R.B. Crossley, Amantadine-resistant influenza A in a nursing facility, Arch. Intern. Med. 152 (1992) 390–392.

International Congress Series 1219 (2001) 823–828

Zanamivir use during transmission of amantadine-resistant influenza A in a nursing home

Yan Li[a], Christine Lee[b], Mark Loeb[c], Anne Phillips[d],
Judy Nesbitt[e], Karen Smith[e], Margaret Fearon[f],
Margaret M. McArthur[b], Tony Mazzulli[b], Allison McGeer[b,*]

[a]National Microbiology Laboratory, Health Canada, Winnipeg, Manitoba, Canada
[b]Department of Microbiology, Mount Sinai and Princess Margaret Hospitals, University of Toronto,
Toronto, Ontario, Canada
[c]Department of Pathology and Molecular Medicine, McMaster University, , Hamilton, Ontario, Canada
[d]Glaxo-Wellcome, Inc., Toronto, Ontario, Canada
[e]Aurora Resthaven Nursing Home, Newmarket, Ontario, Canada
[f]Ministry of Health and Long Term Care, Laboratory Branch, Ontario, Canada

Abstract

Background: Nursing home influenza outbreaks are common. Amantadine is effective for prophylaxis, but fails to control all outbreaks. We describe an outbreak of influenza A which continued due to amantadine resistance. Zanamivir use was associated with termination of the outbreak. *Outbreak*: The outbreak occurred in a 176-bed residential home for the elderly. Cases of respiratory illness started on March 5, and three of four nasopharyngeal swabs tested positive for influenza A. Amantadine was given to residents from 9 to 19 March; however, new cases continued to occur. The number of new cases increased to 11 on March 25, and five of six nasopharyngeal swabs tested were positive for influenza A. Despite re-initiation of amantadine, new cases continued. Nine nasopharyngeal swabs yielded amantadine-resistant influenza A. *Intervention*: Prophylactic zanamivir inhalations were initiated on April 2. Despite the level of dementia, 95% of residents cooperated, 74% had no difficulty with inhalations. *Results*: In the 2 weeks after the initiation of zanamivir, two new cases of respiratory illness occurred, neither confirmed as influenza A. No side effects were associated with zanamivir. *Conclusion*: Zanamivir use was associated with termination of an outbreak which amantandine had failed to control. Zanamivir was well tolerated and effective in the control of influenza A. © 2001 Elsevier Science B.V. All rights reserved.

Keywords: Zanamivir; Nursing home; Influenza A

---

* Corresponding author. Department of Microbiology, Mount Sinai Hospital, Room 1460, 600 University Avenue, Toronto, Ontario, Canada M5G 1X5. Tel.: +1-416-586-3118.
E-mail address: amcgeer@mtsinai.on.ca (A. McGeer).

0531-5131/01/$ – see front matter © 2001 Elsevier Science B.V. All rights reserved.
PII: S 0 5 3 1 - 5 1 3 1 (0 1) 0 0 3 6 2 - 4

1. Introduction

Despite vaccination of residents and staff, as many as 40% of nursing homes in Canada report at least one influenza outbreak in any given year [1,2]. Both the US and Canadian expert bodies recommend antiviral prophylaxis for the control of nursing home outbreaks of influenza A [3,4]. Only amantadine is licensed in Canada. Amantadine is now used to control more than 80% of influenza A outbreaks in Ontario long-term care facilities [1,2]. However, use of amantadine may be limited by side effects, and by the emergence of resistance [5–8].

Zanamivir is a new antiviral agent shown to be effective for treatment [9] and prophylaxis [10,11] of influenza. In the winter of 1999, the continuation of a nursing home outbreak of influenza A despite amantadine prophylaxis led us to study the feasibility of using zanamivir as prophylaxis in this setting.

2. Background

Aurora Resthaven is a 176-bed residential long-term care facility for the elderly (median age 84 years). Seventy percent of staff and 90% of residents received the 1998–1999 influenza vaccine in the fall of 1998.

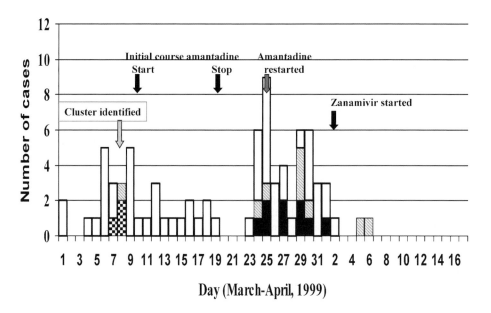

Fig. 1. Epidemic curve of influenza A outbreak in a long-term care facility. Closed bars represent those cases from whom amantadine-resistant influenza A was isolated; dotted bars, those from whom amantadine susceptible virus was isolated; hatched bars, those from whom no virus was isolated; and open bars, those for whom no nasopharyngeal swab was tested.

On March 8/9, rapid antigen testing of nasopharyngeal swabs identified influenza as the cause of a cluster of respiratory illness. Outbreak control measures included case finding, recommending vaccine to unimmunized residents and staff, droplet isolation precautions for ill residents, restriction of ill staff and visitors, and cancellation of communal activities. In addition, a 10-day course of amantadine hydrochloride was offered to all residents and unimmunized staff.

Five days after the completion of this course of amantadine, in response to an increasing number of cases and rapid antigen testing indicating continuing influenza A transmission (Fig. 1), a second course of amantadine prophylaxis was offered to asymptomatic residents. Cases of influenza continued to occur, and on April 2, zanamivir prophylaxis was recommended.

3. Methods

A case was defined as an episode of acute respiratory illness (at least two of: temperature >37.4 °C, cough, sore throat, myalgia, coryza, new wheezes or crackles on chest exam) occurring between March 1 and April 16. Cases were classified as confirmed if influenza A was identified from a nasopharyngeal swab by culture or antigen detection, and probable if viral culture and antigen detection were not done or negative.

Residents were assessed daily for respiratory symptoms from March 9–April 16. Nasopharyngeal swabs were obtained from four new cases on March 25, six new cases on March 30, and all new cases from March 31 onward. Resident charts were reviewed for medical and demographic information.

Zanamivir prophylaxis (10 mg once daily) was offered to asymptomatic residents, and treatment (10 mg twice daily) to case residents ill for <48 h. Nursing staff categorized each resident's ability to comply with instructions for zanamivir inhalations (sealing lips around the device and taking a deep breath) as able to comply without difficulty, able to comply but with difficulty, and not able to comply. Investigators (CL and AM) assessed compliance ability in a sample of residents.

Rapid antigen detection for influenza A was performed on nasopharyngeal swabs from residents using a membrane ELISA (Directigen, Becton-Dickinson, Cockeysville, MD), or an in-house direct fluorescent antigen detection method. Specimens were inoculated into monolayer rhesus monkey kidney and Hep2 cells, and incubated for 2 weeks. Viral isolates were subtyped by hemagglutination inhibition, and tested for amantadine susceptibility testing by RT-PCR restriction and sequence analysis of the M2 gene [12].

4. Results

Thirteen definite and 66 probable cases occurred (Fig. 1). Twelve (15%) developed pneumonia, seven (9%) were hospitalized and two (2.6%) died. Vaccine efficacy was estimated to be 14% (95% confidence limits, − 39%, 53%) for prevention of respiratory illness, 71% (95% CL, − 38%, 94%) for prevention of hospitalization, and 88% (95% CL, 1%, 100%) for prevention of death. All of the 12 influenza A isolates were similar to

A/Sydney/05/97, the H3N2 component of the 1998–1999 vaccine. Three isolates obtained from residents before amantadine use were susceptible to amantadine. In contrast, all nine isolates obtained between March 25th and 30th were resistant to amantadine, and had the same point mutation resulting in a change from leucine to phenylalaline at amino acid position 26 in the transmembrane region of the M2 protein. One of these isolates was from a case-resident who did not receive amantadine during the initial phase of the outbreak.

On April 2, 10 residents were eligible for treatment with zanamivir, and 130 for prophylaxis. Eleven of these (8%) were unwilling or unable to attempt inhalations ($P = 0.11$ compared to amantadine). Of the remaining 129 residents, 100 (78%) were considered by staff to have no difficulty complying with instructions regarding inhalations. Twenty-nine (22%) residents attempted inhalations but had some difficulty (e.g. weak inhalation, incomplete seal of lips on device). Study staff agreed with the nursing home staff assessment in all residents assessed. Difficulty complying with inhalations was associated with poor functional status, and increasing dementia (Table 1).

In the 2 weeks after the initiation of zanamivir, only two new cases of respiratory illness occurred. No residents required hospitalization, and none died. Nasopharyngeal swabs taken the day of onset in both cases were negative for all respiratory viruses by direct immunofluorescence and culture. None of the 128 residents had side effects associated with zanamivir inhalation.

Table 1
Relationship between long-term care facility resident characteristics and observational assessment of difficulty complying with instructions for zanamivir inhalations

Characteristic	No. (%) of residents with difficulty inhaling zanamivir	P value*
Age group		
< 70 years	1/7 (14%)	
70–79 years	3/25 (12%)	
80–89 years	19/64 (30%)	
≥ 90 years	6/32 (19%)	0.25
Functional status[a]		
Dependent in 0–3 ADL	2/24 (8%)	
Dependent in 4–5 ADL	6/38 (16%)	
Dependent in 6 ADL	6/38 (16%)	
Dependent in all 7 ADL	15/26 (58%)	< 0.001
Orientation to person/place/time[b]		
All three	1/33 (3%)	
Two of three	2/19 (11%)	
One of three	4/25 (16%)	
Not oriented	22/49 (45%)	< 0.001

* Analysis of variance.
[a] Functional status assessed by Katz score [13]; ADL = activities of daily living.
[b] Orientation to person, place, and time as assessed by facility staff at most recent three monthly assessment.

5. Discussion

This outbreak demonstrates that, although vaccination of residents and staff in long-term care facilities reduces mortality in residents and the risk of influenza outbreaks [1,14], the poor efficacy of vaccine in nursing home residents means that outbreaks will continue to occur, and outbreak management continues to be important [2,15].

The reported efficacy of amantadine and rimantadine is 75–90% in influenza A prophylaxis in individuals [16], and several outbreak investigation reports provide convincing evidence of their efficacy in controlling outbreaks [6,17–20]. However, amantadine resistance emerges readily during therapy [21], and several previous reports document the emergence and transmission of amantadine-resistant viruses during nursing home influenza outbreaks [6–8]. The isolation of an amantadine-resistant virus from a resident who had not previously received amantadine confirms transmission of resistant virus in this nursing home. Difficulty in isolating case-residents effectively and the treatment of case residents likely increased selective pressure in this facility.

Several studies have shown that neuraminidase inhibitors, including zanamivir, are effective in treatment and prevention of influenza [9–11]. Zanamivir is delivered topically to the respiratory tract by inhalation. Although minimal respiratory pressure is required to deliver the medication, some nursing home residents may not be able to fully cooperate with use of the Diskhaler®. In this facility, the majority (78%) of residents attempting inhalations complied without difficulty. Difficulty with inhalations was greatest in residents who were not oriented and were totally dependent in activities of daily living. As expected, zanamivir was well tolerated and no side effects were observed.

Because zanamivir was introduced late in the outbreak, it is not possible to be sure that zanamivir was responsible for the termination of transmission of influenza A. Nonetheless, the use of zanamivir was temporally associated with control of transmission of amantadine-resistant influenza A, and has been associated with protection against influenza and termination of outbreaks in other reports [11,22]. Neuraminidase inhibitors may be useful adjuncts to the management of influenza in long-term care facilities.

References

[1] C. Stevenson, M.A. McArthur, M. Naus, E. Abraham, A. McGeer, Respiratory disease prevention in Canadian long term care facilities: can we do better? CMAJ 64 (2001) 1413–1419.

[2] B. Henry, Summary report of the Ontario influenza 1998/9 season, Public Health Epidemiol. Rep., Ont. 10 (1999) 144–159.

[3] Advisory Committee on Immunization Practices, Prevention and control of influenza, MMWR 48 (1999) RR-4.

[4] National Advisory Committee on Immunization. Statement on influenza vaccination for the 1999–2000 season, CCDR 25:ACS-2.

[5] W.L. Atkinson, N.H. Arden, P.A. Patriarca, et al., Amantadine prophylaxis during an institutional outbreak of type A (H1N1) influenza, Arch. Intern. Med. 146 (1986) 1751–1756.

[6] E.E. Mast, M.W. Harmon, S. Gravenstein, S.P. Wu, N.H. Arden, et al., Emergence and possible transmission of amantadine-resistant viruses during nursing home outbreaks of influenza A (H3N2), Am. J. Epidemiol. 134 (1991) 988–997.

[7] J. Degelau, S. Somani, S. Cooper, D. Guay, K. Crossley, Amantadine-resistant influenza A in a nursing facility, Arch. Intern. Med. 152 (1992) 390–392.

[8] P. Houck, M. Hemphill, S. LaCroix, D. Hirsh, N. Cox, Amantadine-resistant influenza A in a nursing homes, Arch. Intern. Med. 155 (1995) 533–537.

[9] F.G. Hayden, A.D.M.E. Osterhaus, J.J. Treanor, Efficacy and safety of the neuraminidase inhibitor zanamivir in the treatment of influenza virus infections, N. Engl. J. Med. 337 (1997) 874–880.

[10] A.S. Monto, D.P. Robinson, M.L. Herlocher, et al., Zanamivir in the prevention of influenza among healthy adults, JAMA 282 (1999) 31–35.

[11] M. Schilling, L. Povinelli, P. Krause, et al., Efficacy of zanamivir for chemoprophylaxis of nursing home outbreaks, Vaccine 16 (1998) 1771–1774.

[12] A.I. Klimov, E. Rocha, F.G. Hayden, R.A. Schult, L.F. Roumillat, N.J. Cox, Prolonged shedding of amantadine-resistant influenza A viruses by immunodeficient patients: detection by polymerase chain reaction-restriction analysis, J. Infect. Dis. 172 (1995) 1352–1355.

[13] S. Katz, T.D. Downs, H.R. Cash, R.D. Frotz, Progress in the development of the index of ADL, Gerontologist 10 (1970) 20–30.

[14] W.F. Carman, A.G. Elder, L.A. Wallace, K. McAulay, et al., Effects of influenza vaccination of health-care workers on mortality of elderly people in long-term care: a randomized controlled trial, Lancet 355 (2000) 93–97.

[15] P.A. Gross, A.W. Hermogenes, H.S. Sacks, J. Lau, R.A. Lenadowski, The efficacy of influenza vaccine in elderly persons. A meta-analysis and review of the literature, Ann. Intern. Med. 123 (1995) 518–527.

[16] R. Dolin, R.C. Reichman, H.P. Madore, et al., A controlled trial of amantadine and rimantadine in the prophylaxis of influenza A in humans, N. Engl. J. Med. 307 (1982) 580–584.

[17] K. Staynor, G. Foster, M. McArthur, A. McGeer, M. Petric, A.E. Simor, Influenza A outbreak in a nursing home: value of early diagnosis and the use of amantadine hydrochloride, Can. J. Infect. Control 9 (1994) 109–111.

[18] N.H. Arden, P.A. Patriarca, M.B. Fasano, et al., The roles of vaccination and amantadine prophylaxis in controlling an outbreak of influenza A (H3N2) in a nursing home, Arch. Intern. Med. 148 (1988) 865–868.

[19] N.L. Peters, S. Oboler, C. Hair, L. Laxson, J. Kost, G. Meiklejohn, Treatment of an influenza A outbreak in a teaching nursing home. Effectiveness of a protocol for prevention and control, J. Am. Geriatr. Soc. 37 (1989) 210–218.

[20] Anonymous, Control of influenza A outbreaks in nursing homes: amantadine as an adjunct to vaccine—Washington, 1989–90, MMWR 40 (1991) 841–844.

[21] H.G. Hayden, R.B. Belshe, R.D. Clover, et al., Emergence and apparent transmission of rimantadine-resistant influenza A virus in families, N. Engl. J. Med. 321 (1989) 1696–1702.

[22] W. Lee, M. McArthur, A. Kam, P. Friedman, A. Phillips, A. Simor, M. Loeb, A. McGeer, Use of Zanamivir to Control an Outbreak of Influenza A in a Nursing Home, Abstract presented at: Community and Hospital Infection Control Association of Canada 2000, Toronto, Ontario, May 29–31 2000.

International Congress Series 1219 (2001) 829–834

The effect of Relenza treatment on the early immune response induced after influenza vaccination

Rebecca J. Cox[a,*], Eva Mykkeltvedt[a], Håkon Sjursen[b],
Lars R. Haaheim[a]

[a]Department of Molecular Biology, University of Bergen, N-5020, Bergen, Norway
[b]Department of Infectious Diseases, Haukeland Hospital, University of Bergen, N-5020, Bergen, Norway

Abstract

Background: Although the new anti-influenza drugs are licensed for therapeutic use, it is anticipated that they will also play a role in prophylaxis in combination with vaccine. It is thus imperative to know the minimal time necessary for antiviral prophylaxis before a vaccine-induced protective immune response can be anticipated. *Methods*: We have conducted a double blind placebo controlled trial with 40 young healthy volunteers (18 males, 22 females; age range 21–32 years old) who were vaccinated intramuscularly with licensed split virus vaccine and received 20-mg Relenza (24 subjects) or placebo (16 subjects) daily for a period of 14 days. Heparinised blood was collected prevaccination and up to 42 days postvaccination and analysed using the ELISPOT and HI assays. *Results*: No significant differences were observed in the magnitude or time course of the antibody response between the Relenza and placebo groups for the influenza A/H3N2 and B strains. However, the placebo group responded better to the A/H1N1 strain than the Relenza group at 7 and 9 days postvaccination. *Conclusions*: Relenza treatment was necessary for a minimum of 1 week and by day 12 the majority of volunteers (>80%) had a protective HI titre to all three strains. © 2001 Published by Elsevier Science B.V.

Keywords: Relenza treatment; Immune response; Influenza vaccination

1. Introduction

Currently, the main method of influenza prophylaxis is the use of parenterally administered inactivated influenza vaccine. However, a new anti-influenza drug, Relenza,

* Corresponding author. Tel.: +47-55584385; fax: +47-55589683.
E-mail address: Rebecca.Cox@mbi.uib.no (R.J. Cox).

0531-5131/01/$ – see front matter © 2001 Published by Elsevier Science B.V.
PII: S 0 5 3 1 - 5 1 3 1 (0 1) 0 0 3 7 2 - 7

has recently been licensed for the treatment of influenza A and B viruses, and functions by inhibiting the activity of the influenza neuraminidase. Relenza is effective at reducing the severity of illness in infected individuals as well as preventing influenza in uninfected individuals [1,2]. During an epidemic and particularly in a pandemic scenario, administration of vaccine to unvaccinated risk groups could be combined with antiviral drug to provide protection whilst the antibody response develops. We have shown in a number of studies that by 7–9 days postvaccination most subjects produce protective serum antibody levels [3,4], demonstrating the possibility of immunising in periods of high influenza activity. This raises the question of how long chemoprophylaxis is required before vaccination provides protective immunity. The only available study of co-administration of Relenza and vaccine found that Relenza treatment did not affect the development of HI antibody responses after vaccination, and that similar HI antibody titres were observed at both 2 and 4 weeks postvaccination [5]. In this study, we have examined the effect of Relenza treatment on the early kinetics of the humoral immune response induced after influenza vaccination.

2. Materials and methods

2.1. Study design

Forty healthy human volunteers (age range 21–32 years old, 18 males and 22 females) enrolled in this study, of whom only one subject had been previously vaccinated with influenza vaccine in the preceding season. Volunteers were vaccinated intramuscularly with 0.5-ml licensed trivalent inactivated split virus vaccine (Pasteur-Merieux MSD, France) containing 15 µg HA of each of the following viruses, A/Sydney/5/97 (H3N2), A/Beijing/262/95 (H1N1) and B/Yamanashi/166/98. Volunteers were randomly assigned 20-mg inhaled Relenza or placebo (40-mg inhaled lactose) daily for a period of 14 days. Twenty-four volunteers received Relenza (mean age 25 years and 2 months; 14 females and 10 males) and 16 volunteers received placebo (mean age 25 years and 2 months; 8 females and 8 males). All volunteers completed a side-reactions form to identify any adverse reactions. The study was approved by the Regional Ethics Committee and was carried out in a period of no recorded influenza virus activity in the local community.

2.2. Samples and immunological assays

Heparinised blood samples were collected from all subjects prior to and up to 42 days postvaccination. The ELISPOT assay was used to investigate the number and class (IgG, IgA and IgM) of influenza specific antibody secreting cells (ASC) as previously described [4]. The serum antibody response was analysed by the haemagglutination inhibition test (HI).

2.3. Statistics

The Mann–Whitney U test was performed using SPSS version 10.0 for windows.

3. Results

All participants took Relenza or placebo for the complete 14 days, and of the 280 planned blood samples only 4 were not collected. Fifty percent of the volunteers had local symptoms for the first 3 days after vaccination, which commonly were pain, redness and induration at the injection site. None of the volunteers had symptoms that could be attributed to Relenza or placebo inhalation.

3.1. The influenza specific ASC response

No or low numbers of influenza specific ASC were detected prior to vaccination to all strains (Table 1), which increased in numbers by 5 days postvaccination. The peak in numbers of ASC was observed in all groups on day 7 and the numbers of ASC declined by day 9 and reached baseline numbers by day 15. IgG was the predominant antibody class detected with lower numbers of IgA and IgM ASC found to all strains in all groups (results not shown). The highest response was observed to the H1N1 virus, and higher numbers of influenza-specific ASC were detected in the placebo group on the peak day than in the group which received Relenza treatment ($p < 0.095$). The lowest response was observed to the H3N2 strain, and the placebo group had higher numbers of ASC on the peak day. However, the Relenza group had higher numbers of ASC on the peak day to the B strain than the placebo group.

3.2. HI antibody response

Low HI antibody titres were detected prior to vaccination in most individuals and the titres remained low at 5 days postvaccination (Fig. 1). The HI titres increased at 7 days postvaccination and generally continued to increase until day 12 and then remained constant in the majority of individuals for the remainder of the study. The HI response to the H3N2 and B viruses followed a similar time course in the Relenza and placebo groups, and there were similar percentages of subjects in both groups with protective HI titres and/

Table 1
The influenza-specific ASC response after influenza vaccination in subjects treated with Relenza or placebo

Viral Strain	Treatment	Days postvaccination						
		0	5	7	9	12	15	21–42
A/Sydney/5/97 (H3N2)	Relenza	0*	90 ± 7	225 ± 15	94 ± 10	20 ± 3	1 ± 0	1 ± 0
	Placebo	0*	64 ± 4	372 ± 31	75 ± 8	8 ± 1	1 ± 0	1 ± 0
A/Beijing/262/95 (H1N1)	Relenza	0*	92 ± 8	609 ± 64	485 ± 45	61 ± 5	2 ± 0	2 ± 0
	Placebo	0*	80 ± 7	934 ± 97	491 ± 52	55 ± 9	1 ± 0	1 ± 0
B/Beijing/184/93	Relenza	0*	60 ± 5	780 ± 64	249 ± 18	38 ± 5	3 ± 0	1 ± 0
	Placebo	0*	70 ± 6	620 ± 59	202 ± 23	12 ± 2	1 ± 0	1 ± 0

The data are presented as the mean number of influenza-specific ASC per 500 000 ± standard error of the mean (SEM). 0* refers to < 0.4 specific ASC detected.

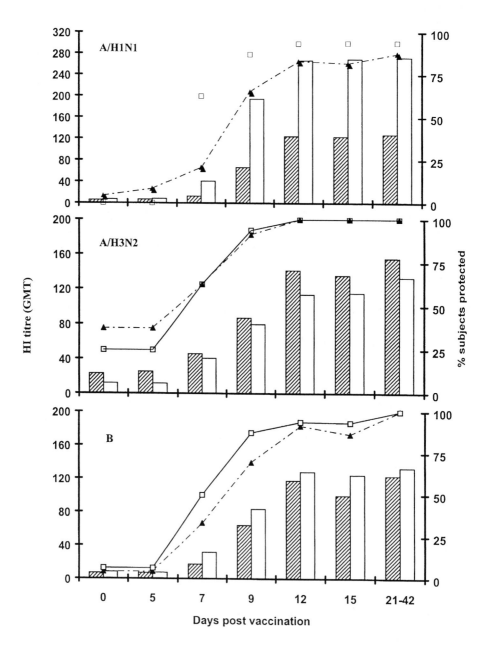

Fig. 1. The effect of Relenza treatment on the HI response after influenza vaccination. The bars represent the geometric meantitre (GmT) for Relenza (shaded)- or placebo (clear)-treated subjects. The lines represent the number of subjects protected after Relenza-treated (dashed line) or placebo (solid line)-treated subjects. HI titres of ≥ 40 were considered protective antibody levels [6] and for calculation purposes, HI antibody titres < 10 were assigned a value of 5.

or exhibiting a ≥ 4-fold rise. However, the HI response to H1N1 was lower in the Relenza group than in the placebo group at days 7 and 9. But by day 12, 83% of volunteers had a protective antibody titre to H1N1 in the Relenza group compared to 94% in the placebo group. The difference in the two groups was influenced in part by three nonresponders and generally lower HI titres to the H1N1 in the Relenza group. Whereas in the placebo group, there were four subjects who had very strong HI responses (≥ 1920) to the H1N1 strain and only 1 nonresponder.

4. Discussion

Relenza has been found to be effective when used both therapeutically and prophylactically. Treatment results in a more rapid resolution of illness and resumption of normal activities [1]. Currently, influenza vaccines are under-utilised in high-risk groups and Relenza may therefore provide a useful adjunct to vaccine in unvaccinated individuals in times of high influenza activity. The only study to date of the combined use of vaccine and Relenza found that 10-mg Relenza administered once daily for a period of 28 days did not affect the serum HI antibody response induced after influenza vaccination [5]. This study also found no increase in HI antibody titres between 2 and 4 weeks postvaccination in the Relenza and placebo groups [5]. We have previously shown in a number of studies that the majority of subjects have a protective antibody response by 7–9 days after vaccination [3,4]. It is thus important to define the necessary period of time for drug prophylaxis, before a protective vaccine immune response is induced. In this study, we found that Relenza treatment was necessary for a minimum of 1 week and by 12 days postvaccination >80% of volunteers were protected.

In our study, Relenza was well tolerated with most side reactions reported as minor and almost exclusively vaccine related. No serious adverse events were observed and similar numbers of side reactions were reported in the two groups, in agreement with other studies [1,2]. The bell-shaped curve of appearance of specific ASC in the blood peaking on day 7 after influenza vaccination is concurrent with the increase in serum antibody, which agrees with our previously published results [3,4,7]. Generally, the antibody response increased reaching maximum titres at 12–15 days postvaccination. Similarly to our previous observations of the time course of the response, there was individual variation in the magnitude of the response, but not in the time course [3,4,7].

We found no significant differences in the response to influenza A/H3N2 and B strains after vaccination between the Relenza and the placebo groups. The antibody response followed a similar time course and was of similar magnitude in the two groups to each of the vaccine strains. Generally, the antibody response to A/H1N1 developed earlier in the placebo group and remained at a higher level than in the Relenza group throughout this study. Previous priming with H1N1 virus results in memory cells, which are probably more effectively re-stimulated by the H1N1 vaccine component because the H1N1 viruses have drifted slowly since their reappearance in 1977 [8]. The history of previous priming is important in determining the response to inactivated influenza vaccine [7], and therefore a larger study is needed to observe if Relenza effects the time course and magnitude of antibody response to the priming virus. If differences are found in a larger study, this may not represent a real problem as all individuals would be unprimed in times of pandemic activity. However, Relenza treatment of 10 mg daily for 28 days was not found to effect the HI response in a larger number of volunteers who had a higher mean age [5]. In our young healthy volunteers an increase in the number of protected subjects was observed 7 days after vaccination (21–63%) and continued to increase with more than 80% of the volunteers protected by 12 days postvaccination. These results and those of our previous studies [3,4,7,9] suggest that it would be necessary to continue Relenza therapy for a minimum of 1 week after vaccination and could lead to better utilisation of a limited supply of Relenza in times of high influenza activity. In conclusion, administration of 20-mg Relenza for a 14-day period did not effect the immune response to A/H3N2 or B strains, however, a better antibody response was initially observed in the placebo group to A/H1N1.

Acknowledgements

We would like to thank the following people at the University of Bergen who helped with this study: Steinar Sørnes, Wenche Trovik, Einar Aaland, Steinar Skrede, Karl Brokstad and also Diane Major from NIBSC, UK. Glaxo Wellcome Norway is thanked for financial support, and for providing and coding the medicines; thanks to Solvay Pharmaceuticals, Holland, for supplying the surface antigens.

References

[1] A.S. Monto, D.M. Fleming, D. Henry, R. de Groot, M. Makela, T. Klein, M. Elliott, O.N. Keene, C.Y. Man, Efficacy and safety of the neuraminidase inhibitor zanamivir in the treatment of influenza A and B virus infections, J. Infect. Dis. 180 (2) (1999) 254–261.

[2] A.S. Monto, D.P. Robinson, M.L. Herlocher, J.M. Hinson Jr., M.J. Elliott, Crisp A Zanamivir in the prevention of influenza among healthy adults: a randomized controlled trial, JAMA 282 (1) (1999 Jul. 7) 31–35.

[3] R.J. Cox, K.A. Brokstad, M.A. Zuckerman, J.M. Wood, L.R. Haaheim, J.S. Oxford, An early humoral immune response in peripheral blood following parenteral inactivated influenza vaccination, Vaccine 12 (11) (1994) 993–999.

[4] K.A. Brokstad, R.J. Cox, J. Olofsson, R. Jonsson, L.R. Haaheim, Parenteral influenza vaccination induces a rapid systemic and local immune response, J. Infect. Dis. 171 (1) (1995) 198–203.

[5] A. Webster, M. Boyce, S. Edmundson, I. Miller, Coadministration of orally inhaled zanamivir with inactivated trivalent influenza vaccine does not adversely affect the production of antihaemagglutinin antibodies in the serum of healthy volunteers, Clin. Pharmacokinet. 36 (Suppl. 1) (1999) 51–58.

[6] D. Hobson, R.L. Curry, A.S. Beare, A. Ward-Gardner, The role of serum haemagglutination-inhibiting antibody in protection against challenge infection with influenza A2 and B viruses, J. Hyg. (London) 70 (4) (1972) 767–777.

[7] A. El-Madhun, R.J. Cox, A. Søreide, J. Olofsson, L.R. Haaheim, Systemic and mucosal immune responses in young children and adults after parenteral influenza vaccination, J. Infect. Dis. 178 (1998) 933–939.

[8] A.M. Iorio, T. Zei, M. Neri, A. Alatri, Possible correlation between low antigenic drift of A(H1N1) influenza viruses and induction of HI antibodies, Eur. J. Epidemiol. 12 (6) (1996) 589–594.

[9] K.A. Brokstad, R.J. Cox, D. Major, J.M. Wood, L.R. Haaheim, Cross-reaction but no avidity change of the serum antibody response after influenza vaccination, Vaccine 13 (16) (1995) 1522–1528.

International Congress Series 1219 (2001) 835–838

A consideration of animal models used for study of influenza virus inhibitors

Robert W. Sidwell*

Institute for Antiviral Research, Utah State University, 5600 Old Main Hill, Logan, UT 84322-5600 USA

Abstract

When an animal model is sought for the study of potential anti-influenza virus agents, investigators commonly turn to the mouse or ferret, which can be experimentally infected by the virus. The ferret will develop febrile illness when infected with influenza A viruses and has successfully been used for study of influenza virus inhibitors. Evaluation parameters commonly include temperature elevation, virus recovery from respiratory tissues and nasal washes and pneumonia-associated mortality. The mouse is often chosen because of its lower cost, ready availability, and ease of handling. Disease parameters using this model include pneumonia-associated mortality, decline in arterial oxygen saturation, lung consolidation, lung virus titers, host weight loss, and increase in serum (α_1-acid glycoprotein. Antiviral data using both animal models are usually comparable; based on studies with amantadine, rimantadine, zanamivir, and oseltamivir, they are predictive for efficacy in the clinic. Rapid development of viral resistance to amantadine and rimantadine and a failure to observe resistance development to the influenza neuraminidase inhibitors has been demonstrated in the murine model. Immunocompromised mice have been used in studies with the latter compounds to demonstrate that their disease-inhibitory effect is not dependent upon the host's immune system. The concepts in the utilization of animal models for study of antiviral drugs will be reviewed. © 2001 Published by Elsevier Science B.V.

Keywords: Mice; Ferrets; Neuraminidase inhibitors; Antiviral

1. Introduction

Influenza continues to be of great public health importance. Much research has, therefore, been expended in the design and development of drugs for the treatment of this significant viral disease. The utilization of appropriate *in vivo* test systems that will

---

* Tel.: +1-435-797-1902; fax: +1-435-797-3959.
E-mail address: Rsidwell@cc.usu.edu (R.W. Sidwell).

0531-5131/01/$ – see front matter © 2001 Published by Elsevier Science B.V.
PII: S 0 5 3 1 - 5 1 3 1 (0 1) 0 0 3 8 8 - 0

clearly establish the efficacy of new drugs as therapies for influenza is, therefore, a primary concern. This review will consider the animal models used.

2. Overview of animal models

The animal models utilized in the study of influenza virus inhibitors are summarized in Table 1. These include the mouse, ferret, chicken, duck, swine, and squirrel monkey. While each species has been used in antiviral studies and offer interesting disease parameters for use in evaluating antiviral drugs, the mouse and ferret have been primarily used, because of their smaller size, lower cost, and ability to predict antiviral efficacy that can translate to the clinic. This review will focus on these latter species for study of influenza virus inhibitors.

3. The ferret

The ferret exhibits many of the typical signs of human influenza infection, such as nasal discharge, fever, loss of appetite, congested eyes, and otologic manifestations [1–3]. High titers of virus can be recovered from the respiratory tract. The animal appears to be a permissive host for non-animal-adapted human influenza viruses [4]. For these reasons, the ferret has often been used for *in vivo* anti-influenza evaluations. A potential problem with the use of ferrets, however, is the indication that they appear more sensitive to infections induced by influenza A than to influenza B viruses [5].

A number of compounds found effective against influenza in the clinic have been demonstrated to be inhibitory to infections in ferrets. Ribavirin, which has exhibited variable effects in the clinic, has reduced the virus-induced febrile response, nasal wash protein, and nasal antibody and virus titers in ferrets [3,6,7]. Zanamivir and oseltamivir, which have been approved for clinical influenza, markedly reduce febrile response, nasal wash influenza virus titers, and nasal inflammatory cell counts of infected ferrets [7,8]. In contrast are reports that the clinically active drug, amantadine, appeared to enhance the

Table 1
Available *in vivo* influenza virus models

Animal	Disease parameters
Mouse	Death, pneumonia-associated lung consolidation, arterial oxygen decline, lung virus titers, host weight loss, rales, water intake decrease, immunosuppressive acidic protein increase.
Ferret	Nasal discharge, appetite loss, congested eyes, ruffled fur, rise in body temperature, virus in nasal washings, turbinates, trachea, lungs. Pneumonia, death if heavily infected. Less sensitive to influenza B virus.
Chicken, duck	Death, temperature elevation, fecal virus shedding, sneezing, rales, viral recovery from multiple organs, leg and foot hemorrhage, hock swelling.
Swine	Pneumonia-associated mortality, coughing, diaphragm spasms (thumps), lung consolidation, virus in nasal washes, resp. tissue.
Squirrel monkey	Fever, cough, sneezing, coryza, increased respiratory rate, virus in nasal washings, lessened food intake.

infection in ferrets as indicated by increased mortality, lung damage, and higher rectal temperatures [9,10].

The ferret has been useful in the determination of infectivity and virulence of influenza virus mutants resistant to the neuraminidase inhibitors [11,12]. A zanamivir-resistant influenza virus having a neuraminidase and hemagglutinin mutation has been shown to be sensitive to the drug when assayed in ferrets, but to exhibit a mild decrease in zanamivir sensitivity in mice [13].

4. The mouse

Influenza viruses, in order to induce acceptable infections in mice, generally require some adaptation to the mouse by multiple passage through their lungs. The mouse-adapted viruses develop an ability to infect alveolar cells [14] and are associated with changes in surface hemagglutinin antigenicity [15]. Clinical isolates, which are not adapted to mice, may induce a toxic pneumonitis at high concentrations without significant viral replication in the lung [15].

The mouse infected with murine-adapted influenza virus offers a spectrum of disease parameters [16]. These include death of the animal, lung consolidation shown by excessive plum coloration and increased lung weights, decline in arterial oxygen saturation (SaO_2), host weight loss, high lung virus titers, pulmonary gas exchange, rales, and, as we have recently reported, increase in serum (α_1-acid glycoprotein [17].

Clinically active drugs have shown efficacy against the mouse influenza infection. Ribavirin, administered orally, has prevented deaths, inhibited lung consolidation, reduced SaO_2 decline, and lessened titers of virus in the lungs, but only at relatively high dosages approaching those which are maximally tolerated, indicating a low therapeutic index (TI) [18]. Amantadine and rimantadine have also proven efficacious using these same parameters [19], even using a non-mouse-adapted virus [20]. Zanamivir and oseltamivir have exhibited remarkable influenza-inhibitory effects in the mouse at low doses, indicative of a high TI [8,21,22]. Surprisingly, zanamivir was also effective in mice when administered orally [22].

The mouse has been used to illustrate the rapid development of amantadine-resistant influenza virus [23] which also occurs in the clinic. The animal has been widely used to determine infectivity and virulence of drug-resistant influenza virus mutants [11,12].

Since the immune system of the mouse has been well studied, aided by the assortment of commercial kits available for assay of immune factors, the animal has been used extensively in studying immunomodulating agents and to ascertain if clinically effective anti-influenza drugs would affect the immune system [24].

References

[1] W. Smith, C.H. Andrewes, P.P. Laidlow, A virus obtained from influenza patients, Lancet 1 (1933) 66–68.

[2] H. Smith, C. Sweet, Lessons for human influenza from pathogenicity studies with ferrets, Rev. Infect. Dis. 10 (1988) 56–65.

[3] C.W. Potter, J.P. Phair, L. Vodinelich, R. Fenton, R. Jennings, Antiviral, immunosuppressive, and antitumor effects of ribavirin, Nature 259 (1976) 496–497.

[4] B.R. Murphy, R.G. Webster, Orthomyxoviruses, in: B.N. Fields, B.N. Knipe, P.M. Howley, et al. (Eds.), Fields Virology, Lippincott-Raven, Philadelphia, 1996, pp. 1397–1445.

[5] C.A. Pinto, R.F. Haff, R.C. Stewart, Pathogenesis and recovery from respiratory syncytial and influenza infections in ferrets, Arch. Gesamte Virusforsch. 26 (1969) 225–237.

[6] K.P. Schofield, C.W. Potter, D. Edey, et al., Antiviral activity of ribavirin on influenza infection in ferrets, J. Antimicrob. Chemother. 1 (Suppl. 4) (1975) 63–69.

[7] D.M. Ryan, J. Ticehurst, M.H. Dempsey, GG167 (4-guanidino-2,4-dideoxy-2,3-dehydro-N-acetylneuraminic acid) is a potent inhibitor of influenza virus in ferrets, Antimicrob. Agents Chemother. 39 (1995) 2583–2584.

[8] D.B. Mendell, C.Y. Tai, P.A. Escarpe, W. Li, et al., Oral administration of a prodrug of the influenza virus neuraminidase inhibitor GS4071 protects mice and ferrets against influenza infection, Antimicrob. Agents Chemother. 42 (1998) 640–646.

[9] K.W. Cochran, H.F. Massab, A. Tsunoda, B.S. Berlin, Studies on the antiviral activity of amantadine hydrochloride, Ann. N. Y. Acad. Sci. 130 (1965) 432–439.

[10] S.L. Squires, The evaluation of compounds against influenza virus, Ann. N. Y. Acad. Sci. 173 (1970) 239–248.

[11] L.V. Gubareva, L. Kaiser, F.G. Hayden, Influenza virus neuraminidase inhibitors, Lancet 355 (2000) 827–835.

[12] J.L. McKimm-Breshkin, Resistance of influenza viruses to neuraminidase inhibitors–a review, Antiviral Res. 47 (2000) 1–17.

[13] T.J. Blick, A. Sahasradudhe, A. McDonald, et al., The interaction of neuraminidase and hemagglutinin mutations in influenza virus in resistance to 4-guanidino-Neu4Ac2en, Virology 246 (1998) 95–103.

[14] J. Mulder, J.F.P. Hers, Influenza, Walters-Noordhoff, Groningen, 1972, pp. 214–238.

[15] A.K. Gitelman, N.V. Kaverin, I.G. Kharitonenkov, et al., Antigenic changes in mouse-adapted influenza virus strains, Lancet 1 (1983) 1229.

[16] R.W. Sidwell, The mouse model of influenza virus infection, in: O. Zak, M. Sande (Eds.), Handbook of Animal Models of Infection, Academic Press, London, 1999, pp. 981–987.

[17] M.H. Wong, D.L. Barnard, M.K. Jackson, et al., Utilization of alpha$_1$-acid glycoprotein levels in the serum as a parameter for in vivo assay of influenza virus inhibitors, Antiviral Res. 46 (2000) A61(Abst. 85).

[18] R.W. Sidwell, Ribavirin: a review of antiviral efficacy, in: G. Pandalai (Ed.), Recent Res. Dev. Antimicrob. Agents Chemother., vol. 1. Research Signpost, Kerala, 1996, pp. 219–256.

[19] C.E. Hoffman, Amantadine HCl and related compounds, in: W.A. Carter (Ed.), Selective Inhibitors of Virus Functions, CRC Press, Cleveland, 1973, pp. 199–211.

[20] R.W. Sidwell, K.W. Bailey, M.H. Wong, J. Huffman, In vitro and in vivo sensitivity of a non-mouse-adapted influenza A (Beijing) virus infection to amantadine and ribavirin, Chemotherapy 41 (1995) 455–461.

[21] D.M. Ryan, J. Ticehurst, M.H. Dempsey, C.R. Penn, Inhibition of influenza virus replication in mice by GG167 (4-guanidino-2,4-dideoxy-2,3-dehydro-N-acetylneuraminic acid) is consistent with extracellular activity of viral neuraminidase (sialidase), Antimicrob. Agents Chemother. 38 (1994) 2270–2275.

[22] R.W. Sidwell, J.H. Huffman, D.L. Barnard, et al., Inhibition of influenza virus infections in mice by GS4104, an orally effective influenza virus neuraminidase inhibitor, Antiviral Res. 37 (1998) 107–120.

[23] J.S. Oxford, I.S. Logan, C.W. Potter, In vivo selection of an influenza A2 strain resistance to amantadine, Nature 226 (1970) 82–83.

[24] R.A. Burger, J.L. Billingsley, J.H. Huffman, et al., Immunological effects of the orally administered neuraminidase inhibitor GS4104 in influenza virus-infected and uninfected mice, Immunopharmacology 47 (1999) 45–52.

International Congress Series 1219 (2001) 839–843

Evaluation of neuraminidase inhibitors in the human experimental infection model

John Treanor*

Infectious Diseases Unit, University of Rochester, 601 Elmwood Avenue, Rochester, NY 14642, USA

Abstract

Determining the effect of antiviral agents against influenza in the field is made more difficult by the need to find infected individuals early in the course of illness and by the seasonal nature of influenza epidemics. One method that can be used to generate preliminary data in humans quickly is the experimental infection model. In these studies, healthy adults are selected for relative susceptibility by serum antibody levels and infected intranasally or by aerosol with a well-characterized pool of wild-type influenza virus. Under these conditions, the majority of subjects will be infected and develop a mild, influenza-like illness, accompanied by recovery of virus from the nasopharynx. This model has been used to evaluate antiviral agents, including neuraminidase inhibitors, for both prophylaxis and treatment. In general, the results of experimental infection studies have been predictive of subsequent results in the field, making this a useful system for initial testing of potential antivirals. © 2001 Elsevier Science B.V. All rights reserved.

Keywords: Experimental infection; Influenza; Human

Intentional inoculation of susceptible human volunteers with live influenza virus has been used as a tool for the study of the pathogenesis and potential control of influenza for many years [1]. In fact, the first such inoculations took place shortly after the discovery of influenza virus, and studies utilizing experimental infection have played an important role in the development of both vaccines and antiviral agents for this disease.

Several significant advantages of these experimental infection studies (Table 1) are responsible for the great enthusiasm with which this model has been embraced,

---

* Tel.: +1-716-275-5871; fax: +1-716-442-9328.

E-mail address: john_treanor@urmc.rochester.edu (J. Treanor).

0531-5131/01/$ – see front matter © 2001 Elsevier Science B.V. All rights reserved.
PII: S0531-5131(01)00363-6

Table 1
Advantages and disadvantages of experimental infection of humans for evaluation of antivirals

Advantages
- Most inoculated subjects will become infected, so that the study design can be very efficient.
- Intense (multiple times daily) monitoring of viral shedding and other responses to infection and treatment is possible.
- The timing of exposure to virus and onset of therapy is under the control of the investigator.
- Studies can be done at any time of the year and do not depend on the timing and intensity of any particular influenza epidemic season for success.

Disadvantages
- Viruses used in the experiment may have decreased virulence because of extensive laboratory passage prior to use.
- Pathogenesis of illness may differ slightly from that of naturally acquired infection because of the mode of administration of virus.
- Symptoms are generally not as severe as seen in naturally acquired flu, and upper respiratory symptoms are more common than systemic symptoms in some experiments.
- Subjects available for use (i.e., adults) are not immunologically naïve, even if screened for low levels of antibody prior to inoculation.

particularly in recent studies of neuraminidase inhibitors. Perhaps the most significant advantages is that all components of the interaction between the virus, the host, and the experimental agent are under the control of the investigator, including the specific viral strain to which the subjects will be exposed, the health and baseline immunity of the subjects, and the exact timing of drug administration with relationship to viral exposure. In addition, the close monitoring of subjects which is possible in this type of study facilitates determination of drug effects on viral replication and intense evaluation of immunologic responses. On the other hand, it is important to recognize that these studies represent a highly artificial situation compared to naturally acquired influenza virus infection with some inherent disadvantages (Table 1). Despite these imperfections, experimental infection studies have proven to be very useful in the initial evaluation of many antiviral drugs.

The features of the model that have emerged over time as critical to success are summarized in Table 2. Chief among these is the selection of a uniformly susceptible population of subjects so that differences between treatment groups are not confounded by differences in the baseline level of immunity. The general features of the study design used to evaluate an antiviral drug in the model are shown in Fig. 1. After subjects are determined to be relatively susceptible based on low levels of serum hemagglutination-inhibiting (HI) antibody to the specific strain of virus to be used and to be in good general health, they are admitted to a facility where they can be isolated from each other and from

Table 2
Critical features of the experimental challenge model

Subjects must be screened for susceptibility, and the level of susceptibility to infection be made uniform among all treatment groups.
A suitable, appropriately prepared live viral preparation must be available for use.
Facilities must be available for appropriate isolation and clinical monitoring of subjects.
Ideally, there should be a significant relationship between the extent of viral replication and the severity of symptoms.

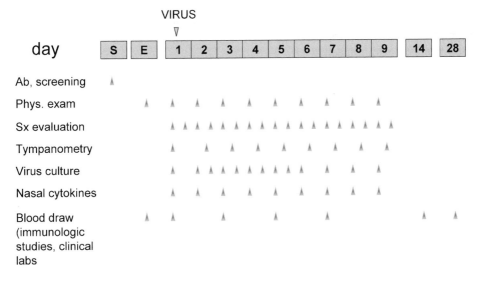

Fig. 1. Schematic diagram showing the typical design of a trial using experimental infection of humans to assess antiviral activity.

the outside world. Following a brief acclimatization period, the influenza virus preparation to be used is administered usually by intranasal drops, and the response to infection is monitored. The antiviral agent may be administered either before or after viral inoculation, depending on the purposes of the study. Clinical outcomes are generally subjective since experimental influenza rarely produces objective clinical signs. For this reason, daily monitoring of viral shedding is usually the primary outcome measurement, with other features, such as digital typanometry and nasal cytokine production used as secondary outcomes.

The first neuraminidase inhibitor (NI) to be evaluated in this setting was zanamivir [2]. Subjects were inoculated with the influenza A/Texas/36/91 (H1N1) virus at a dose of approximately 10^5 TCID$_{50}$ by intranasal drops, and zanamivir was administered by either intranasal drops or spray at various doses either prophylactically (beginning 4 h before virus inoculation) or therapeutically (beginning either 24 or 36 h after virus inoculation). This study was the first study to demonstrate that NIs could be effective antivirals in humans. Administered as either spray or drops, prophylactic zanamivir was associated with an 82% reduction in infection following challenge. When zamamivir was administered by nasal drops 24 h after virus inoculation, significant antiviral effects were seen, with a reduction in the duration of virus shedding by 3 days and an 87% reduction in viral AUC. This was accompanied by significant reductions in fever, total symptom scores, cough, and nasal mucus weight. In contrast, more delayed treatment, while also resulting in reductions in virus shedding, were not associated with significant clinical benefit because symptoms were already at their peak before therapy was initiated. This finding, that earlier therapy is of significantly greater benefit, has been consistent throughout the clinical trials of neuraminidase inhibitors. The effect of zanamivir treatment on the development of middle ear over- and underpressures as assessed with digital tympanometry was also evaluated as a secondary outcome measurement in this study. The frequency of middle ear abnormalities among infected subjects was also decreased significantly by early treatment with zamamivir [3].

Subsequent studies evaluated the orally administered neuraminidase inhibitor oseltamivir in similar fashion [4]. In these studies, also conducted with the A/Texas/36/91 virus, oseltamivir was administered either beginning 26 h prior to virus inoculation, or 28 h after virus inoculation, at a variety of doses. Prophylactic administration of oseltamivir resulted in 100% protection against virus shedding following challenge, while therapeutic administration was resulted in significant reductions in the level and duration of nasopharyngeal shedding, reduced clinical symptoms, and reduced nasal mucus weights. Because induction of cytokines has been implicated in the pathogenesis of acute influenza [5], the levels of nasal cytokines were also assessed in a subset of subjects in this study. Among infected individuals, treatment with oseltamivir resulted in complete abolition of the nasal IL-6, TNF-alpha, and IFN-gamma response to infection [4].

More recently, preliminary evaluation of the cyclopentane NI RWJ270201 has been performed in the model. This agent is also orally bioavailable, and has a relatively prolonged plasma half-life allowing once daily administration. Therapeutic administration of RWJ270201 beginning 24 h after nasal inoculation with the A/Texas/36/91 virus resulted in a dose-dependent antiviral effect and significant reductions in clinical symptoms [6].

There is relatively less experience with evaluation of NIs in adults experimentally infected with influenza B viruses [7]. It has been well recognized that determination of the pre-infection level of susceptibility of potential subjects to influenza B virus is considerably more difficult than for influenza A virus because of the relative insensitivity of the

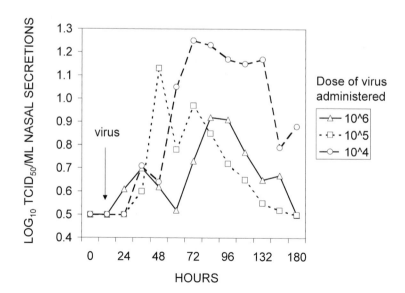

Fig. 2. Nasopharyngeal viral shedding following inoculation of susceptible volunteers intranasally with doses of 10^4, 10^5, or 10^6 TCID$_{50}$ of the influenza B/Yamagata/88 virus.

HI assay of antibody to the B viruses. Perhaps for this reason, or possibly due to intrinsically lower levels of virulence of influenza B viruses, challenge with these agents has generally resulted in lower rates of infectivity and clinical symptoms than seen in similar studies with influenza A viruses. An example of the pattern of viral shedding seen in a recent study of the influenza B/Yamagata/88 virus is shown in Fig. 2. However, evaluation of neuraminidase inhibitors in the B challenge model has been needed since the recent influenza epidemics have not featured influenza B viruses very prominently, thereby limiting the opportunities to evaluate the efficacy of these drugs against naturally acquired influenza B virus infection.

Ultimately, the utility of the experimental model is reflected in the degree to which the results predict the behavior of these drugs in the real world. In this regard, the challenge model has proven to be highly reliable. Both zanamivir [8] and oseltamivir [9] have proven to have significant antiviral and clinical effect when administered early in the course of acute influenza in otherwise healthy adults. In addition, as predicted by the effects of neuraminidase inhibitors on such features as cytokine production and middle ear abnormalities, treatment of natural disease is associated with decreased systemic symptoms and fever, and with a reduction in complications including otitis media in children [10]. Both drugs are also effective for prevention of influenza, as predicted by the results of experimental infection studies. Given the success of these studies in establishing potential clinical efficacy early in the drug development process, the experimental infection model is likely to play an important role in the further development of NIs and other antiviral approaches.

References

[1] J.J. Treanor, F.G. Hayden, Volunteer virus challenge studies, Textbood of Influenza, Nicholson, Webster, Hay, 1999.

[2] F.G. Hayden, J.J. Treanor, R.F. Betts, et al., Safety and efficacy of the neuraminidase inhibitor GG167 in experimental human influenza, JAMA 275 (1996) 295–299.

[3] J.B. Walker, E.K. Hussey, J.J. Treanor, et al., Effects of the neuraminidase inhibitor zanamivir on otologic manifestations of experimental human influenza, J. Infect. Dis. 176 (1997) 1417–1422.

[4] F.G. Hayden, J.J. Treanor, R.S. Fritz, et al., Use of the oral neuraminidase inhibitor oseltamivir in experimental human influenza, JAMA 282 (1999) 1240–1246.

[5] F.G. Hayden, R.S. Fritz, M. Lobo, et al., Local and systemic cytokine responses during experimental human influenza A virus infection, J. Clin. Invest. 101 (1998) 643–649.

[6] F.G. Hayden, J. Treanor, R. Qu, C. Fowler, Safety and efficacy of an oral neuraminidase inhibitor RWJ-270201 in treating experimental influenza A and B in healthy adult volunteers, 40th Interscience Conference on Antimicrobial Agents and Chemotherapy, Toronto CA. A1154.

[7] F.G. Hayden, R. Robson, L.C. Jennings, et al., Efficacy of oral oseltamivir in experimental influenza B virus infection, [Abstract] Clin. Infect. Dis. 29 (1999) 1879.

[8] F.G. Hayden, A.D.M.E. Osterhaus, J.J. Treanor, et al., Efficacy and safety of the neuraminidase inhibitor zanamivir in the treatment of influenzavirus infections, N. Engl. J. Med. 337 (1997) 874–880.

[9] J.J. Treanor, F.G. Hayden, P.S. Vrooman, et al., Efficacy and safety of the oral neuraminidase inhibitor oseltamivir in treating acute influenza: a randomized, controlled trial, JAMA 283 (2000) 1016–1024.

[10] F.G. Hayden, K.S. Reisinger, R. Whitly, et al., Oral oseltamivir is effective and safe in children for the treatment of acute influenza A and B, Options for the Control of Influenza IV, Hersonissos, Crete, September 2000.

International Congress Series 1219 (2001) 845–853

Accumulation of segment 6 sgRNAs of influenza A viruses in the presence of neuraminidase inhibitors

Marina S. Nedyalkova[a,b], Frederick G. Hayden[a,c],
Robert G. Webster[d,e], Larisa V. Gubareva[a,b,*]

[a]*Department of Internal Medicine, University of Virginia School of Medicine, PO Box 800473,
Charlottesville, VA, USA*
[b]*D.I. Ivanovsky Institute of Virology, Moscow, Russia*
[c]*Department of Pathology, University of Virginia, Charlottesville, VA, USA*
[d]*Department of Virology and Molecular Biology, St. Jude Children's Research Hospital, USA*
[e]*Department of Pathology, University of Memphis, Memphis, TN, USA*

Abstract

Background: RNA segment 6 of influenza A viruses only encodes neuraminidase (NA), whereas the same segment of influenza B viruses encodes an additional protein, NB. The NA activity is not required for virus replication but is necessary for virus release from infected cells. In contrast, the NB is an essential influenza B viral membrane protein with an ion channel function. *Methods*: Influenza A and B viruses were passaged in Madine–Darby canine kidney (MDCK) cells in the presence of NA inhibitors. The segment 6 sequences of the selected viruses were analyzed. *Results*: Accumulation of subgenomic (sg) RNAs of segment 6 in influenza A, but not influenza B viruses, was observed as a result of passage in the presence of NA inhibitors. Sequencing of sgRNAs revealed that there were internal deletions of the NA gene both in-frame and with a shift in reading frame. Additional passage of the virus without NA inhibitor resulted in a reduction in the amount of sgRNAs, suggesting that it is a reversible phenomenon. *Conclusions*: Accumulations of sgRNAs could serve as an indicator of reduced viral dependence on NA function during the release of influenza A virus from infected cells. We speculate that the coding capacity of RNA segment 6 of influenza B viruses is preserved because of the essential role of the NB protein and possibly NA in influenza B virus replication. © 2001 Elsevier Science B.V. All rights reserved.

Keywords: Zanamivir; Oseltamivir; RWJ-270201; Deletion mutant; Subgenomic RNA; Antiviral

---

* Corresponding author. Department of Internal Medicine, University of Virginia School of Medicine, PO Box 800473, Charlottesville, VA 22908-0473, USA. Tel.: +1-4343-243-2705; fax: +1-434-982-0384.
E-mail address: lvg9b@virginia.edu (L.V. Gubareva).

0531-5131/01/$ – see front matter © 2001 Elsevier Science B.V. All rights reserved.
PII: S 0 5 3 1 - 5 1 3 1 (0 1) 0 0 3 9 8 - 3

1. Introduction

Influenza A and B viruses are the cause of annual epidemics in humans. Influenza virus is an enveloped virus in which eight sets of viral nucleocapsids are coated with the plasma membrane of infected cells. The envelope contains two major glycoproteins, the hemagglutinin (HA) and neuraminidase (NA). The segment 6 of influenza A viruses encodes the NA, whereas the same segment of influenza B viruses encodes two proteins NA and NB [1].

Recently, a new class of antiinfluenza virus drugs that are specific inhibitors of viral NA has been developed. Two NA inhibitors zanamivir and oseltamivir have been approved for treatment of influenza A and B infections. RWJ-270201 is a novel NA inhibitor that is currently undergoing clinical trials [2]. Inhibition of the receptor-destroying activity of influenza NA by these compounds results in the aggregation of progeny virions on the surface of the infected cell and limiting virus spread to neighboring cells [3,4].

It has been shown that multiple passages of influenza A and B viruses in MDCK cells in the presence of the NA inhibitors result in selection of resistant mutants with amino acid substitutions in the HA and/or NA [4–8]. Substitutions in the enzyme active site resulted in its resistance to the inhibitor and were accompanied by impairment of NA structural integrity and function [7,9,10]. Mutants of influenza A virus with substitutions in the NA active site have been recovered from the patients treated with oseltamivir [11]. A zanamivir-resistant mutant of influenza B strain was isolated from one immunocompromised patient after a prolonged treatment [12]. The role of HA in the development of virus resistance to NA inhibitors is more difficult to evaluate because of heterogeneity of the HA sequences due to antigenic drift and a host cell variation, as well as a low predictability of the sequence data for assessment of virus susceptibility to the drugs.

Here we report that passage of influenza A viruses, but not influenza B viruses in Madine–Darby canine kidney (MDCK) cells in the presence of NA inhibitors (zanamivir, oseltamivir or RWJ-270201), was accompanied by accumulation of sub-genomic (sg) RNAs of segment 6 which encodes the NA. We also present evidence that such viruses demonstrated reduced susceptibility to three NA inhibitors in cell culture, despite the absence of the mutations in their NA enzyme active site or the HA receptor-binding site.

2. Methods

2.1. Viruses and cells

Influenza viruses A/turkey/Minnesota/833/80 (H4N2), B/Memphis/20/96 and B/Memphis/15/85 were from the repository in St. Jude Children's Research Hospital. Clinical isolates A/Charlottesville/28/95 (H1N1), A/Charlottesville/31/95 (H1N1), A/Charlottesville/34/96 (H3N2) were provided by Dr. F.G. Hayden.

Confluent monolayers of Madin–Darby canine kidney (MDCK) cells were infected with viruses as previously described [4]. The NA inhibitors were added to the monolayers simultaneously with the virus. Control viruses were passaged in parallel in MDCK cells without the NA inhibitors. Viruses were harvested on day 3 p.i. and propagated once in MDCK cells without the drug before analysis.

Plaque reduction assay was performed as described previously [4]. The NA inhibitors were added to the agar-containing media following virus adsorption.

2.2. NA inhibition assay

The neuraminidase inhibition (NI) assay was performed according to Potier et al. [13] with modifications in a fluorometric assay with 4-methyl-umbelliferyl-N-acetyl neuraminic acid (MUNANA) as a substrate. Reactions were done in the buffer containing 32.5 mM MES (2-[N-Morpholino] ethanesulfonic acid), 4 mM $CaCl_2$, 2.5% DMSO, pH 6.5. The IC_{50} values for each virus (concentrations of inhibitor required to inhibit neuraminidase activity by 50%) were determined by serial dilutions of the inhibitor against a standard amount of NA activity. Virus dilutions were preincubated with the inhibitor for 30 min at 37 °C followed by addition of MUNANA (final concentration 100 μM). After incubation for 1 h at 37 °C, reactions were stopped by the addition of 0.1 M glycine buffer (pH 10.7) containing 25% ethanol. The fluorescence of released 4-methylumbelliferone was determined with an HTS-7000 BioAssay Reader (Perkin-Elmer) with an excitation wavelength of 365 nm and an emission wavelength of 460 nm. The data were plotted as log inhibitor concentration against fluorescence inhibition, and the IC_{50} read-out from the graph.

2.3. RT-PCR amplification of the HA and NA viral genes

Viral RNA was extracted from cell culture supernatants with the kit (RNeasy, Qiagen). The synthetic oligonucleotide 5′-AGCAAAAGCAGG-3′ was used as a primer to generate cDNA by using reverse transcriptase, followed by PCR amplification of the NA and the HA genes as described previously [4] with minor modifications. We utilized additional primers designed to be complementary to the 3′ and 5′-noncoding ends of the NA gene, which allowed us to amplify both the full-sized NA gene and the NA gene with internal deletions. After purification with PCR purification kit (QIAquick, Qiagen), the PCR products were analyzed in 1–2% agarose gel and subjected to sequencing. The sequencing reactions were performed by the Center of Biotechnology at the University of Virginia. The Sequencher 4.0 software (Gene Codes) was used for the analysis and translation of nucleotide data.

3. Results and discussion

3.1. Selection of influenza A virus mutants with reduced susceptibility to NA inhibitors

We investigated molecular changes acquired by influenza A viruses in response to growth in the presence of NA inhibitors. Viruses were passaged in MDCK cells in the presence of increasing concentrations of zanamivir, oseltamivir or RWJ-270201. In parallel, viruses passaged in the absence of the NA inhibitors were used as a control. The drug-susceptibility of the viruses passaged in the presence of the NA inhibitor was substantially reduced based on the results of a plaque reduction assay in comparison to the viruses passaged without the inhibitor (Fig. 1A,B). The RWJ-270201-selected virus was also resistant to the other two inhibitors, zanamivir and oseltamivir (Fig. 1C). Despite the reduced drug-susceptibility of the RWJ-270201-selected virus, its enzymes were fully susceptible to the inhibitors in the NA inhibition assay (results not shown). To confirm that the NA active site was unaltered, we performed the sequence analysis of the NA gene of the selected virus (Table 1). It revealed that the mutant of A/Charlottesville/31/95 (H1N1) had two mutations in the NA gene, which resulted in abolishing (58 N→D) or creating (211 Ile→Thr) a potential glycosylation site on the NA molecule. As we reported previously, the clones of the zanamivir-resistant virus A/turkey/MN/833/80 (H4N2) had a single amino acid substitution at residue 249 (R→K) of the NA after seven passages in the presence of the NA inhibitor [4]. Thus in our studies, viruses with reduced

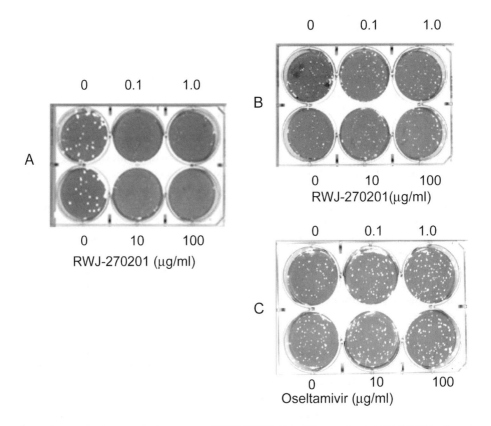

Fig. 1. Plaque reduction assay in the presence of RWJ-270201 (A and B) or oseltamivir (C). MDCK cells were infected with the virus variants of A/Charlottesville/31/95 (H1N1) strain, which have been passaged 18 times in MDCK cells before the assay in the absence of the NA inhibitor (A) or in the presence of RWJ-270201 (B and C).

Table 1
The sequence analysis of the HA and NA genes of influenza A viruses selected in MDCK cells in the presence of the NA inhibitors

NA inhibitor	Virus	Passages with the drug	Predicted amino acid changes in NA	Predicted amino acid changes in HA	Detection of sgRNA of NA gene
Zanamivir	A/turkey/Minnesota/ 833/80 (H4N2)	8	249 R→K	HA2 75 G→E	
	Clone 1				+
	Clone 2				+
RWJ-270201	A/Charlottesville/ 31/95 (H1N1)	18	58 N→D, 211 I→T	None	+
	A/Charlottesville/ 34/96/ (H3N2)	18	ND[a]	None	+
Oseltamivir	A/Charlottesville/ 28/95 (H1N1)	5	None	None	+

[a] ND—sequence analysis is incomplete.

susceptibility to NA inhibitors in cell culture did not necessarily contain amino acid substitutions at the conserved residues of the NA active site [14].

Previous studies showed that changes in the HA could lead to reduced virus susceptibility to NA inhibitors [15,16] by facilitating virus release in the absence of NA activity. Indeed, Sahasrabudhe et al. [17] demonstrated a reduced binding of zanamivir-selected mutants to MDCK cell monolayers where such selection took place. We also demonstrated that zanamivir-selected mutant recovered from an immunocompromised patient contained an amino acid substitution in the receptor-binding site of the HA [12], which reduced the virus affinity for receptors on human cells. Because the HA is a multifunctional glycoprotein with a high sequence heterogeneity, it is difficult to predict the effect of a certain amino acid substitution on the receptor-binding properties of the molecule. Thus in our previous study in MDCK cells [4,18], we described the acquisition of the mutations in the HA2 subunit of the HA in the zanamivir-resistant variant of A/turkey/MN/833/80 (Table 1). The localization of the mutations in the HA2 subunit suggests that the HA's fusogenic properties could be altered by destabilization of the HA1–HA2 interactions in the native state of the molecule. However, the observation that growth in MDCK cells readily select mutants of avian viruses with the changes in the pH optimum of fusion (or human isolates grown in embryonated chicken eggs) [4,19] confounds designation of the mutations in HA2 subunit as zanamivir-related.

In the present study, we have not detected amino acid substitutions in the HA genes of viruses selected in the presence of either oseltamivir or RWJ-270201. The viruses used in the present study were not propagated in chicken eggs at any time. Our results are in accord with the report by Tai et al. [8] where no amino acid changes were detected in the HA of the oseltamivir-selected mutants. Therefore, our data and others [4,8] suggest the existence of a third mechanism leading to reduced virus susceptibility to NA inhibitors, besides the changes in the receptor-binding site of HA or in the enzyme active site of NA.

3.2. Detection of sgRNAs accumulating in the presence of the NA inhibitors

To obtain a full sequence of gene segment 6 of the zanamivir-selected mutants (clones 1 and 2), we performed PCR amplification of two overlapping segments of cDNA encoding the NA gene. The obtained PCR products were purified and sequenced and then their sequences were aligned to produce a sequence of a full-sized NA gene. However, when PCR amplification was done with a pair of primers complementary to the ends of the NA gene, only a very faint band corresponding to the full-sized NA gene was detected. At the same time, an extensive band of a smaller size was seen on the gel. The sequence analysis of this smaller PCR product revealed that it was an NA gene that underwent a massive internal deletion (Table 2). A similar procedure with a second clone of the zanamivir-selected mutant revealed the presence of another internal deletion in the NA gene. Both deletions were in-frame and therefore the defective NA genes encoded the peptides of 111 (clone 1) or 126 (clone 2) amino acid residues in length.

The mutants selected in the presence of RWJ-270201 or oseltamivir also contained defective NA genes with internal deletions (Tables 1 and 2). However, the deletions were not in-frame and peptides encoded by them were predicted to be shorter than those of zanamivir-resistant mutants. In addition, the defective NA gene of the mutant A/Charlottesville/34/96 (H3N2) had an insertion of two nucleotides, which resulted in the formation of a premature stop codon and therefore it encoded the shortest peptide (50 amino acid residues). It is unknown at present whether these peptides are expressed in the infected cells. Nevertheless, it is not likely that these peptides are essential for virus propagation since they do not contain the enzyme active site.

The properties of selected mutants were analyzed after 5–17 passages in the presence of the NA inhibitors. The next question was how early the defective NA genes could be detected. The yields of the virus A/Charlottesville/28/95 (H1N1) were harvested at five subsequent passages in the presence of oseltamivir and subjected to RT-PCR amplification and analysis. The defective NA gene was detected after a single passage (72 h p.i.) in the

Table 2
Sequence analysis of the NA genes with internal deletions

NA inhibitor	Virus	Internal deletion (nt)	In-frame	Length of predicted product (aa)
Zanamivir	A/turkey/Minnesota/833/80 (H4N2)			
	Clone 1	1–79...1220–1466	+	111
	Clone 2	1–145...1166–1466	+	126
RWJ-270201	A/Charlottesville/31/95 (H1N1)	1–292...1173–1461	–	95
	A/Charlottesville/34/96/ (H3N2)	1–389...1121–1466	–	50
			2 nt insertion	
Oseltamivir	A/Charlottesville/28/95 (H1N1)	1–218...1009–1461	–	74

The native NA of N1 subtype has 470 amino acid residues and NA of N2 subtype 469 amino acid residues.

presence of the NA inhibitor, whereas no defective NA genes could be detected in the virus before passage or after five passages in the absence of oseltamivir (Fig. 2). The accumulation of the defective NA gene copies became prominent after four passages when the PCR product of a full-sized gene became undetectable with the use of the primer pairs designed to the gene ends (Fig. 2). The full-sized NA gene in those virus preparations could be easily detected when the gene-end primer was used in a combination with the primer designed to detect the deleted sequence (not shown).

The virus containing the defective NA gene was passaged additionally (five passages) in the absence of the NA inhibitor and then analyzed. Now the presence of the full-sized NA gene copies became apparent (not shown), which indicates that the reduction of the full NA gene copies in the virus preparation and the accumulation of defective NA gene copies was reversible and likely to be drug-related.

If multiplicity of infection was high during virus replication in the presence of the NA inhibitor, it could lead to accumulation of sgRNAs as a result of von Magnus effect; however, in our experiments we used a low multiplicity of infection [20].

It is known that inhibition of NA activity leads to the formation of virus aggregates attached to the cell surface [3,4]. Virus aggregates are infectious in cell culture [4,21]; and a coinfection of virions carrying a complete genome and virions carrying a defective genome could allow replication of the defective genes in the infected cell. If a defective gene is small, it would replicate faster than the full-sized gene and therefore coinfection could lead to accumulation of the progeny virions carrying the defective genes. Thus, virus aggregation in the presence of the NA inhibitor could explain the accumulation of defective NA genes. However, it is important to emphasize that we did not detect the sgRNAs of the HA genes (as well as M and NS genes) in the same virus preparations

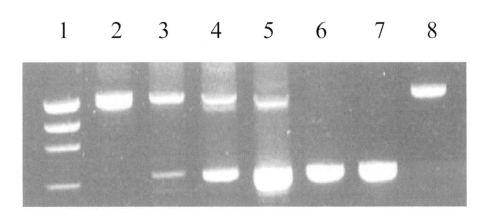

Fig. 2. Detection of the defective NA genes. A/Charlottesville/28/95 (H1N1) was passaged five times in MDCK cells in the presence of increasing concentrations of oseltamivir (10, 100, 500, 1000, and 2000 μM). RNA was extracted from virus yields after each passage, RT-PCR amplification of the NA genes was performed and PCR products were analyzed in 1% agarose gel. Lane 1: molecular weight marker; lane 2: wild type virus; lanes 3–7: virus after one to five passages in MDCK cells in the presence of oseltamivir; lane 8: control virus passaged five times in MDCK cells without oseltamivir.

which contained the sgRNA of the NA gene (data not shown). We believe that accumulation of sgRNAs of the HA gene did not occur because it would not be advantageous for the virus, whereas the accumulation of the sgRNAs of the NA gene could have a lesser impact on virus propagation in vitro. In addition, we did not detect accumulation of defective NA genes in influenza B viruses passaged in the presence of the NA inhibitors. Because the segment 6 of influenza B viruses encodes an additional gene product, the NB protein, we hypothesize that the necessity to preserve a coding capacity for this protein had prevented accumulation of the sgRNAs for the segment 6 of influenza B viruses.

The detection of sgRNAs of NA genes of influenza A viruses was described previously, when viruses were passaged in the presence of exogenous NA from bacterial [22] or viral [23] sources. The reduced virus dependence on its own enzyme was an underlying factor for accumulation of defective NA genes.

In our study, the accumulation of sgRNAs of NA gene coincided with the virus passage in the presence of the NA inhibitors. It is reasonable to assume that during the passage, the virus acquired compensatory changes in the other genes that allowed its spread to the neighboring cells under condition of the inhibited NA enzyme activity. Importantly, we did not detect amino acid substitutions in the HA, a second viral surface glycoprotein which interacts with cellular receptors. Further studies are warranted to elucidate further the molecular changes in the influenza viruses selected in the presence of the NA inhibitors.

Acknowledgements

We thank Douglas Schallon and Yee Soo-Hoo for their excellent technical assistance. This study was supported by Grant AI 45782 from the National Institutes of Health and by R.W. Johnson Pharmaceutical Research Institute.

References

[1] R.A. Lamb, R.M. Krug, Replication of orthomyxoviruses, in: B.N. Fields, D.M. Knipe, et al., (Eds.), Field's Virology, Raven Press, Philadelphia, 1996, pp. 1353–1395.
[2] L.V. Gubareva, L. Kaiser, F.G. Hayden, Influenza virus neuraminidase inhibitors, Lancet 355 (2000) 827–835.
[3] P. Palese, R.W. Compans, Inhibition of influenza virus replication in tissue culture by 2-deoxy-2,3-dehydro-*N*-trifluoro-acetyl-neuraminic acid (FANA): mechanism of action, Journal of General Virology 33 (1976) 159–163.
[4] L.V. Gubareva, R. Bethell, G.J. Hart, K.G. Murti, C.R. Penn, R.G. Webster, Characterization of mutants of influenza A virus selected with the neuraminidase inhibitor 4-guanidino-Neu5Ac2en, Journal of Virology 70 (1996) 1818–1827.
[5] S. Bantia, A.A. Ghate, S.L. Ananth, et al., Generation and characterization of a mutant of influenza A virus selected with the neuraminidase inhibitor BCX-140, Antimicrobial Agents and Chemotherapy 42 (1998) 801–807.
[6] T.J. Blick, T. Tiong, A. Sahasrabudhe, et al., Generation and characterization of an influenza virus neuraminidase variant with decreased sensitivity to the neuraminidase-specific inhibitor 4-guanidino-Neu5A-c2en, Virology 214 (1995) 475–484.

[7] J.M. Colacino, N.Y. Chirgadze, E. Garman, et al., A single sequence change destabilizes the influenza virus neuraminidase tetramer, Virology 236 (1997) 66–75.

[8] C.Y. Tai, P.A. Escarpe, R.W. Sidwell, et al., Characterization of human influenza virus variants selected in vitro in the presence of the neuraminidase inhibitor GS 4071, Antimicrobial Agents and Chemotherapy 42 (1998) 3234–3241.

[9] L.V. Gubareva, M.J. Robinson, R.C. Bethell, R.G. Webster, Catalytic and framework mutations in the neuraminidase active site of influenza viruses that are resistant to 4-guanidino-Neu5Ac2en, Journal of Virology 71 (1997) 3385–3390.

[10] J.L. McKimm-Breschkin, M. McDonald, T.J. Blick, P.M. Colman, Mutation in the influenza virus neura-minidase gene resulting in decreased sensitivity to the neuraminidase inhibitor 4-guanidino-Neu5Ac2en leads to instability of the enzyme, Virology 225 (1996) 240–242.

[11] E. Covington, D.B. Mendel, P.A. Escarpe, C.Y. Tai, K. Soberbarg, N.A. Roberts, Phenotypic and gen-otypic assay of influenza virus neuraminidase indicates a low incidence of viral drug resistance during treatment with oseltamivir, II International Symposium on Influenza and Other Respiratory Viruses, December 10–12, 1999, Grand Cayman, (Abstract).

[12] L.V. Gubareva, M.N. Matrosovich, M.K. Brenner, R.C. Bethell, R.G. Webster, Evidence for zanamivir resistance in an immunocompromised child infected with influenza B virus, Journal of Infectious Diseases 178 (1998) 1257–1262.

[13] M. Potier, L. Mameli, M. Belisle, L. Dallaire, S.B. Melancon, Fluorometric assay of neuraminidase with a sodium (4-methylumbelliferyl-alpha-D-*N*-acetylneuraminate) substrate, Analytical Biochemistry 94 (1979) 287–296.

[14] P.M. Colman, Influenza virus neuraminidase: structure, antibodies, and inhibitors, Protein Science 3 (1994) 1687–1696 [Review].

[15] J.L. McKimm-Breschkin, T.J. Blick, A. Sahasrabudhe, et al., Generation and characterization of variants of NWS/G70c influenza virus after in vitro passage in 4-amino-Neu5Ac2en and 4-guanidino-Neu5Ac2en, Antimicrobial Agents and Chemotherapy 40 (1996) 40–46.

[16] C.R. Penn, J.M. Barnett, R.C. Ethell, R. Enton, K.L. Earing, A.J. Owett, Selection of influenza virus with reduced sensitivity in vitro to the neuraminidase inhibitor GG167 (4-guanidino-Neu5Ac2en): changes in the haemagglutinin may compensate for loss of neuraminidase activity, in: L.E. Brown, A.W. Hampson, R.G. Webster (Eds.), Options for the Control of Influenza III, Elsevier, Amsterdam, The Netherlands, 1996, pp. 735–740.

[17] A. Sahasrabudhe, T.J. Black, J.L. McKimm-Breschkin, Influenza virus variants resistant to GG167 with mutations in the haemagglutinin, in: L.E. Brown, A.W. Hampson, R.G. Webster (Eds.), Options for the Control of Influenza III, Elsevier, Amsterdam, The Netherlands, 2000, pp. 748–752.

[18] L.V. Gubareva, R.C. Bethell, C.R. Penn, R.G. Webster, In vitro characterization of 4-guanidino-Neu5Ac2en-resistant mutants of influenza A virus, in: L.E. Brown, A.W. Hampson, R.G. Webster (Eds.), Options for the Control of Influenza III, Elsevier, Amsterdam, The Netherlands, 1996, pp. 753–760.

[19] Y.P. Lin, S.A. Wharton, J. Martin, J.J. Skehel, D.C. Wiley, D.A. Steinhauer, Adaptation of egg-grown and transfectant influenza viruses for growth in mammalian cells: selection of hemagglutinin mutants with elevated pH of membrane fusion, Virology 233 (1997) 402–410.

[20] D.P. Nayak, T.M. Chambers, R.K. Akkina, Defective-interfering (DI) RNAs of influenza viruses: origin, structure, expression, and interference, Current Topics in Microbiology and Immunology 114 (1985) 103–151 [Review].

[21] M.V. Lakshmi, I.T. Schulze, Effects of sialylation of influenza virions on their interactions with host cells and erythrocytes, Virology 88 (1978) 314–324.

[22] C. Liu, M.C. Eichelberger, R.W. Compans, G.M. Air, Influenza type A virus neuraminidase does not play a role in viral entry, replication, assembly, or budding, Journal of Virology 69 (1995) 1099–1106.

[23] M.T. Hughes, M.N. Matrosovich, M.E. Rodgers, M. McGregor, Y. Kawaoka, Influenza A viruses lacking sialidase activity can undergo multiple cycles of replication in cell culture, eggs, or mice, Journal of Virology 74 (2000) 5206–5212.

International Congress Series 1219 (2001) 855–861

Mechanisms of resistance of influenza virus to neuraminidase inhibitors

Jennifer McKimm-Breschkin*, Anjali Sahasrabudhe, Tony Blick, Mandy McDonald

The Biomolecular Research Institute, 343 Royal Parade, Parkville, 3052, Australia

Abstract

Structure-based inhibitor design has resulted in the development of highly selective inhibitors of the influenza virus neuraminidase (NA). So far, two compounds have been approved for therapeutic use, zanamivir and oseltamivir, but others are under development. However, it is important to establish whether resistance arises readily to these new inhibitors. Unlike amantadine, it takes several passages in culture before resistant variants are isolated. Mutants have also been isolated from oseltamivir-treated patients and from an immunocompromised zanamivir-treated child. Mutations are found in both the NA and the hemagglutinin (HA). In vitro two HA or an HA and NA mutation can act synergistically to increase resistance. The NA mutations are in previously conserved catalytic and structural residues, Glu 119, Arg 152, Arg 292, and His 274. The NA mutations have an adverse effect on NA activity or stability. There are significant quantitative differences observed between the inhibitors upon binding to these mutant NAs. The HA mutations tend to map to regions associated with receptor binding of the HA. The effect of the HA mutations appears to be to reduce the affinity of the HA for the cellular receptor. Their role in vivo is not yet known. © 2001 Elsevier Science B.V. All rights reserved.

Keywords: Resistance; Influenza virus; Neuraminidase

1. Introduction

The influenza virus contains two surface glycoproteins, the haemagglutinin (HA) and neuraminidase (NA). The HA binds to cellular receptors containing terminal sialic acid residues to initiate infection of the target cell. The role of the NA is to remove these

---

* Corresponding author. Fax: +61-3-9662-7101.
E-mail address: jennifer.mckimm@hsn.csiro.au (J. McKimm-Breschkin).

receptors from the cell to enable newly synthesized progeny virions to elute from the surface of the infected cell and from each other. Structural analysis of the influenza virus NA [6,29] revealed there were several highly conserved residues that are both structural and catalytic residues in the NA active site. The first of the NA inhibitors, zanamivir, 4-guanidino-Neu5Ac2en, which has a guanidinium group at the 4-position on the hexose ring, was designed based on the structure of the NA in complex with sialic acid [30]. Zanamivir is around 100-fold more effective than 4-amino-Neu5Ac2en, and 10,000-fold more effective than NeuAc2en or 2-deoxy-2,3-didehydro-D-N-acetyl neuraminic acid (DANA), which was shown to be a weak inhibitor of NA enzyme activity and demonstrated weak antiviral activity in vitro, but not in vivo [24]. Other NA inhibitors have also been developed, GS4071, oseltamivir carboxylate, the active form of the ethyl ester pro-drug, oseltamivir phosphate, GS4104, is a potent carbocyclic inhibitor with a cyclohexene scaffolding [17]. This inhibitor contains a bulky hydrophobic group, a pentyl ether, at the 6-position, replacing the glycerol side chain, and an amino group at the 4-position. More recently a cyclopentane inhibitor, BCX-1812/RWJ-270201, which has a pentyl group at the position corresponding to the 6-position, and a guanidinium group at the 4-position, is being developed [1]. However effective these inhibitors may be, it is critical to determine whether resistance to these new inhibitors arises readily.

2. Generation of mutants

Assays for screening for resistance to the NA inhibitors include an enzyme inhibition assay using either methyl umbelliferone-N-acetyl neuraminic acid (MUNANA) or fetuin as the substrate [3,22,27]. A plaque reduction assay in MDCK cells is also used for screening laboratory-generated mutants [22]. Since the inhibitor prevents release of progeny virions, the initial effect is to reduce the size of the plaque, then at higher concentrations the number of plaques decreases. Mutants with altered drug sensitivity have been selected using either a decrease in plaque size [19] or plaque number [13,25,27]. However, many clinical isolates do not plaque well, in which case sensitivity in a cytopathic effect (cpe) inhibition assay may have to be used [22]. However, the sensitivity in a plaque assay is also complicated if there is a concomitant HA mutation, since HA and NA mutations can act synergistically [4]. The contribution of the NA to resistance can be determined by generating a reassortant that has the NA mutation alone. It is critical to compare sensitivity of the mutant reassortant to the homologous wild type pairing of the reassortant HA and NA since altered pairing of the HA and NA in wild type viruses can lead to decreased drug sensitivity, without the introduction of any mutations [16]. This appears to be a result of generating a virus in which the NA cleaves the new HA receptor more efficiently. The NA can still be inhibited, but retains sufficient activity for virus elution [18].

It takes several passages to generate mutants in MDCK cells by either plaque selection or by limiting dilution passaging under increasing concentrations of drug [22]. Mutations have been found in previously conserved catalytic and structural residues in the NA [7] (reviewed in Ref. [18]). However, the majority of mutations in vitro map to regions in or adjacent to the receptor binding site of the HA [18]. Resistance appears to result from a decrease in affinity of the HA for the cellular receptor, so that the virus is less dependent upon NA activity for elution.

3. Properties of E119 mutants

E119 mutants have been isolated in both influenza A [5,13,14,16,27] and influenza B [2,27] after passaging in zanamivir or oseltamivir in vitro, and in vivo from a patient in an oseltamivir treatment study [8]. The E119G mutants demonstrate a $2-3$ $\log_{10}$ decrease in sensitivity to zanamivir in an enzyme inhibition assay, with around a 10-fold decrease in sensitivity to DANA (Table 1), but no resistance to oseltamivir, or RWJ-270201. The magnitude of resistance in a plaque assay is less, around 1 $\log_{10}$. Three other E119 mutations have been reported, an E119A and E119D in an A/Turkey/Minnesota virus [13,14,16] and an E119V in A/Wuhan/95 from a patient treated with oseltamivir [8]. The E119D is the most resistant, also demonstrating cross-resistance to 4-amino-Neu5Ac2en and oseltamivir [12] (Table 1).

The E119 mutations render the NA more unstable [9,20,26]. This means that a conformational antibody should be used to determine the amount of native protein for specific activity quantification. Using this method, the E119G specific activity is comparable to that of the wild type enzyme [20,22].

Growth of the E119 mutants is compromised in cell culture, producing smaller plaques than the wild type virus [4] and showing a slight delay in growth kinetics [27]. The addition of exogenous *Clostridium* NA in the overlay rescues the plaque size [4], suggesting that the unstable NA does contribute to the growth defect.

Table 1
Enzyme activity and sensitivity to inhibitors of influenza virus neuraminidase mutants

Virus	Mutation	Specific activity (%)	Fold decrease in enzyme sensitivity				
			DANA	4-Amino-Neu5Ac2en	Zanamivir	Oseltamivir	RWJ-270201
NWS/G70C	E119G	100	10	0	250	0	
Recombinant G70C	E119G	30			1000		
	E119A				340		
A/Turkey/Minnesota	E119G	46	10	3	700	0	0
	E119A	23	7	35	600		0
	E119D	3	20	200	2500	3–30	
A/Wuhan/95	E119V					20	
B/HK/Lee	E119G	0.6	resist		500		
B/Beijing/87	E119G				33		
B/Beijing/184/93	R152K	3			1000	25–3000	25–3000
NWS/G70C	R292K	20	20	33	55	6,500	
A/Turkey/Minnesota	R292K		2	4	10	10,000	20
A/Vic/75	R292K			30	24	30,000	
A/Singapore/1/57	R292K				10–20	5000	10–20
A/Texas/36/91	H274Y					400	
A/WS/33	H274Y	50			low	high	

Structural analysis shows that the loss in affinity of the E119G mutant enzyme for zanamivir derives in part from the loss of the stabilizing interactions between the guanidino moiety and the carboxylate residue at 119, and in part from the alterations in solvent structure of the active site [5]. A water molecule occupies the position previously occupied by the carboxylate of the glutamate in the wild type NA. Since the E119G is not resistant to RWJ-270201 it suggests that its guanidinium group may be oriented differently to zanamivir. Although the E119 does not interact directly with the 4-amino group, it is assumed altered solvent structure contributes to the decrease in binding of some mutants to the 4-amino-Neu5Ac2en and oseltamivir.

4. Properties of R292K mutants

R292K mutants have been isolated from influenza A isolates passaged in vitro in zanamivir [16], its 6-carboxamide derivative [23], oseltamivir [28], RWJ-270201 [1] and from patients treated with oseltamivir [10]. The mutant enzymes exhibit a small decrease in binding to substrate, DANA, 4-aminoNeu5Ac2en, zanamivir and RWJ-270201 and a much larger decrease to oseltamivir (Table 1). The same pattern of resistance is seen in cell culture [23]. Virus carrying only the R292K mutation is compromised in its growth. Poor growth can be rescued by either exogenous *Clostridium* NA, or by a concomitant HA mutation [23] which by lowering the affinity would enable a virus with low NA activity to elute.

R292 is one of three highly conserved arginines that form part of the catalytic triad of the NA active site [30]. A small change in the NA active site occurs to enable inhibitors with bulky side chains at the 6-position, such as oseltamivir to be accommodated. E276 changes its position to form a salt link with R224, creating a hydrophobic pocket for the binding of the bulkier substituents. The differences in resistance can be correlated with structural data [31]. There is altered binding of both the triol group and the carboxylate group in sialic acid and all analogues. This results in reduced substrate binding and reduced enzyme activity, as well as altered binding of the inhibitors. The K292 stabilises the E276 from moving, hence the energy penalty is too great for the movement to occur to accommodate oseltamivir, resulting in weak binding, and high resistance. The low resistance seen to the RWJ-270201 suggests that the E276 does not have to move to accommodate its side chain, or that a relatively small energy penalty is involved for the movement to occur.

5. H274Y mutation

This mutant has been isolated from both A/WS/33 and A/Texas/36/91 viruses passaged in oseltamivir in vitro and from oseltamivir challenge studies in vivo [7,32,33]. The virus has a lower specific activity and is around 400-fold less sensitive to oseltamivir, but demonstrates only minor resistance to zanamivir. Growth of the A/Texas/36/91 mutant was said to be reduced both in vitro and in vivo [11], but the A/WS/33 mutant replicated as well as wild type [32]. The mechanism of resistance is probably similar to the R292K mutants, with the Y274 stabilising the E276, so that there is a high-energy penalty for the movement of the E276 to occur.

6. R152K mutation

No resistant variants have yet been isolated from normal patients treated with zanamivir; however, one resistant virus has been isolated from an immunocompromised child [15] infected with an influenza B virus. R152 is conserved in all influenza A and B viruses, and forms a hydrogen bond to the acetamide of sialic acid bound in the active site [6], thus it would be expected to affect binding of substrate and all inhibitors. The enzyme has low activity, and is less sensitive to zanamivir, oseltamivir and RWJ-270201 (Table 1). Sensitivity in cell culture was masked due to the presence of a concomitant HA mutation. While it appears that the T198I decreased binding to terminal $\alpha2,6$ sialic acids, found in humans, it increased binding to the $\alpha2,3$ linked sialic acids found in MDCK cells. The combination of a stronger binding HA and a weak NA masked resistance due to the NA mutation in these cells.

7. HA mutations

The majority of mutants isolated after passaging in NA inhibitors in vitro have had mutations in the HA [18]. One of the characteristics of HA mutations is the cross-resistance to all classes of NA inhibitors. Sequence analysis reveals changes in residues in the vicinity of the receptor binding site. Such mutations could decrease the affinity of the HA for the receptor so that the virus is less dependent on the NA for elution from the infected cells. Some mutants have such a low HA affinity that they adsorb poorly, demonstrating a drug-dependent phenotype [2,13,19,21]. HA mutations can rescue the growth of a mutant virus with low NA activity [4,23] masking the growth defect, but increasing resistance. However, if the HA mutation is generated in a heterologous system, it may increase binding in a different system, and mask an NA mutation [15].

Various assays have been used to evaluate HA binding (reviewed in Ref. [18]). The biggest challenge remains in finding a suitable assay system to reflect the $\alpha2,6$ terminally linked sialic acid receptors found in humans. HA mutations have been found in clinical isolates from an immunocompromised child treated with zanamivir [15] and from patients treated with oseltamivir [10]. The latter has not as yet been shown to play a role in altered drug sensitivity. However, it is clear that the HA and NA cannot be viewed in isolation. The net sensitivity of influenza viruses to NA inhibitors is determined by the affinity of the HA for its cellular receptor, and the efficiency with which the NA cleaves this receptor.

References

[1] S. Bantia, S. Ananth, L. Horn, C. Parker, U. Gulati, P. Chand, Y. Babu, G. Air, Generation and characterization of a mutant of influenza A virus selected with neuraminidase inhibitor RWJ-270201, The 13th International Congress on Antiviral Research, Baltimore, MD, USA, Apr 16–21, 2000. Antiviral. Res. 46 (2000) A60.

[2] J.M. Barnett, A. Cadman, F.M. Burrell, S.H. Madar, A.P. Lewis, M. Tisdale, R. Bethell, In vitro selection and characterisation of influenza B/Beijing/1/87 isolates with altered susceptibility to zanamivir, Virology 265 (1999) 286–295.

[3] R.C. Bethell, G.J. Hart, T.J. Blick, A. Sahasrabudhe, J.L. McKimm-Breschkin, Biochemical methods for the characterization of influenza viruses with reduced sensitivity to 4-guanidino-Neu5Ac2en, in: D. Kinchington, R.F. Schinazi (Eds.), Methods in Molecular Medicine, Humana Press, Totowa, NJ, 1999, pp. 367–374.

[4] T.J. Blick, A. Sahasrabudhe, M. McDonald, I.J. Owens, P.J. Morley, R.J. Fenton, J.L. McKimm-Breschkin, The interaction of neuraminidase and hemagglutinin mutations in influenza virus in resistance to 4-guani-dino-Neu5Ac2en, Virology 246 (1998) 95–103.

[5] T.J. Blick, T. Tiong, A. Sahasrabudhe, J.N. Varghese, P.M. Colman, G.J. Hart, R.C. Bethell, J.L. McKimm-Breschkin, Generation and characterization of an influenza virus neuraminidase variant with decreased sensitivity to the neuraminidase-specific inhibitor 4-guanidino-Neu5Ac2en, Virology 214 (1995) 475–484.

[6] W.P. Burmeister, R.W. Ruigrok, S. Cusack, The 2.2 A resolution crystal structure of influenza B neurami-nidase and its complex with sialic acid, EMBO J. 11 (1992) 49–56.

[7] J. Carr, J. Ives, N. Roberts, L. Kelly, R. Lambkin, J. Oxford, C.Y. Tai, D. Mendel, F. Hayden, Virological assessment in vitro and in vivo of an influenza H1N1 virus with a H274Y mutation in the neuraminidase gene, The 13th International Congress on Antiviral Research, Baltimore, MD, USA, Apr 16–21, 2000. Antiviral Res. 46 (2000) A59.

[8] J. Carr, J. Ives, N.A. Roberts, C.Y. Tai, D.B. Mendel, L. Kelly, R. Lambkin, J. Oxford, An oseltamivir treatment-selected influenza A/Wuhan/359/95 virus with an E119V mutation in the neuraminidase gene has reduced infectivity in vivo, II International Symposium on Influenza and other Respiratory viruses. Grand Cayman, Cayman Islands, Dec 10–12.

[9] J.M. Colacino, N.Y. Chirgadze, E. Garman, K.G. Murti, R.J. Loncharich, A.J. Baxter, K.A. Staschke, W.G. Laver, A single sequence change destabilizes the influenza virus neuraminidase tetramer, Virology 236 (1997) 66–75.

[10] E. Covington, D.B. Mendel, P. Escarpe, C.Y. Tai, K. Soderbarg, N.A. Roberts, Phenotypic and genotypic assay of influenza neuraminidase indicates a low incidence of viral drug resistance during treatment with oseltamivir, II International Symposium on Influenza and other Respiratory viruses. Grand Cayman, Cayman Islands, Dec 10–12.

[11] L. Gubareva, C.Y. Tai, D.B. Mendel, J. Ives, J. Carr, N.A. Roberts, F.G. Hayden, Oseltamivir treatment of experimental influenza A/Texas/36/91 (H1N1) virus infection in humans: selection of a novel neuraminidase variant, The 13th International Congress on Antiviral Research, Baltimore, MD, USA, Apr 16–21, 2000. Antiviral. Res. 46 (2000) A59.

[12] L. Gubareva, R.G. Webster, F.G. Hayden, Cross-resistance of influenza mutants to NA inhibitors: zanamivir, GS4071 and RWJ-270201, The 13th International Congress on Antiviral Research, Baltimore, MD, USA, Apr 16–21, 2000. Antiviral. Res. 46 (2000) A54.

[13] L.V. Gubareva, R. Bethell, G.J. Hart, K.G. Murti, C.R. Penn, R.G. Webster, Characterization of mutants of influenza A virus selected with the neuraminidase inhibitor 4-guanidino-Neu5Ac2en, J. Virol. 70 (1996) 1818–1827.

[14] L.V. Gubareva, R.C. Bethell, C.R. Penn, R.G. Webster, In vitro characterization of 4-guanidino-Neu5Ac2en-resistant mutants of influenza A virus, in: L.E. Brown, A.W. Hampson, R.G. Webster (Eds.), Options for the Control of Influenza III, Elsevier, Amsterdam, 1996, pp. 753–760.

[15] L.V. Gubareva, M.N. Matrosovich, M.K. Brenner, R.C. Bethell, R.G. Webster, Evidence for zanamivir resistance in an immunocompromised child infected with influenza B virus, J. Infect. Dis. 178 (1998) 1257–1262.

[16] L.V. Gubareva, M.J. Robinson, R.C. Bethell, R.G. Webster, Catalytic and framework mutations in the neuraminidase active site of influenza viruses that are resistant to 4-guanidino-Neu5Ac2en, J. Virol. 71 (1997) 3385–3390.

[17] W. Li, P.A. Escarpe, E.J. Eisenberg, K.C. Cundy, C. Sweet, K.J. Jakeman, J. Merson, W. Lew, M. Williams, L. Zhang, C.U. Kim, N. Bischofberger, M.S. Chen, D.B. Mendel, Identification of GS 4104 as an orally bioavailable prodrug of the influenza virus neuraminidase inhibitor GS 4071, Antimicrob. Agents Chemo-ther. 42 (1998) 647–653.

[18] J.L. McKimm-Breschkin, Resistance of influenza viruses to neuraminidase inhibitors—a review, Antiviral Res. 47 (2000) 1–17.

[19] J.L. McKimm-Breschkin, T.J. Blick, A. Sahasrabudhe, T. Tiong, D. Marshall, G.J. Hart, R.C. Bethell, C.R. Penn, Generation and characterization of variants of NWS/G70C influenza virus after in vitro passage in 4-amino-Neu5Ac2en and 4-guanidino-Neu5Ac2en, Antimicrob. Agents Chemother. 40 (1996) 40–46.

[20] J.L. McKimm-Breschkin, M. McDonald, T.J. Blick, P.M. Colman, Mutation in the influenza virus neuraminidase gene resulting in decreased sensitivity to the neuraminidase inhibitor 4-guanidino-Neu5Ac2en leads to instability of the enzyme, Virology 225 (1996) 240–242.

[21] J.L. McKimm-Breschkin, M. McDonald, A. Sahasrabudhe, T. Blick, Infectivity and drug sensitivity studies in the mouse model of zanamivir resistant HA variants of influenza virus, XIth International Congress of Virology. Sydney, Australia, Aug 9–13, VW27.03. (1999) 97.

[22] J.L. McKimm-Breschkin, A. Sahasrabudhe, T. Blick, A.J. Jpwett, R.C. Bethell, Virological methods for the generation and characterization of influenza viruses with reduced sensitivity to 4-guanidino-Neu5Ac2en, in: D. Kinchington, R.F. Schinazi (Eds.), Methods in Molecular Medicine, Humana Press, Totowa, NJ, 1999, pp. 375–381.

[23] J.L. McKimm-Breschkin, A. Sahasrabudhe, T.J. Blick, M. McDonald, P.M. Colman, G.J. Hart, R.C. Bethell, J.N. Varghese, Mutations in a conserved residue in the influenza virus neuraminidase active site decreases sensitivity to Neu5Ac2en-derived inhibitors, J. Virol. 72 (1998) 2456–2462.

[24] P. Palese, J.L. Schulman, Inhibitors of viral neuraminidase as potential antiviral drugs, in: J.S. Osford (Ed.), Chemoprophylaxis and Virus infections of the Upper Respiratory Tract 1, CRC, Cleveland, 1977, pp. 189–205.

[25] C.R. Penn, J.M. Barnett, R.C. Bethell, R. Fenton, K.L. Gearing, N. Healy, A.J. Jowett, Selection of influenza virus with reduced sensitivity in vitro to the neuraminidase inhibitor GG167 (4-guanidino-Neu5-Ac2en): changes in haemagglutinin may compensate for loss of neuraminidase activity, in: L.E. Brown, A.W. Hampson, R.G. Webster (Eds.), Options for Control of Influenza III, Elsevier, Amsterdam, 1996, pp. 735–740.

[26] A. Sahasrabudhe, L. Lawrence, V.C. Epa, J.N. Varghese, P.M. Colman, J.L. McKimm-Breschkin, Substrate, inhibitor, or antibody stabilizes the Glu 119 Gly mutant influenza virus neuraminidase, Virology 247 (1998) 14–21.

[27] K.A. Staschke, J.M. Colacino, A.J. Baxter, G.M. Air, A. Bansal, W.J. Hornback, J.E. Munroe, W.G. Laver, Molecular basis for the resistance of influenza viruses to 4-guanidino-Neu5Ac2en, Virology 214 (1995) 642–646.

[28] C.Y. Tai, P.A. Escarpe, R.W. Sidwell, M.A. Williams, W. Lew, H. Wu, C.U. Kim, D.B. Mendel, Characterization of human influenza virus variants selected in vitro in the presence of the neuraminidase inhibitor GS 4071, Antimicrob. Agents Chemother. 42 (1998) 3234–3241.

[29] J.N. Varghese, W.G. Laver, P.M. Colman, Structure of the influenza virus glycoprotein antigen neuraminidase at 2.9 A resolution, Nature 303 (1983) 35–40.

[30] J.N. Varghese, J.L. McKimm-Breschkin, J.B. Caldwell, A.A. Kortt, P.M. Colman, The structure of the complex between influenza virus neuraminidase and sialic acid, the viral receptor, Proteins 14 (1992) 327–332.

[31] J.N. Varghese, P.W. Smith, S.L. Sollis, T.J. Blick, A. Sahasrabudhe, J.L. McKimm-Breschkin, P.M. Colman, Drug design against a shifting target: a structural basis for resistance to inhibitors in a variant of influenza virus neuraminidase, Structure 6 (1998) 735–746.

[32] Z.M. Wang, C.Y. Tai, D.B. Mendel, Characterization of an influenza A virus variant selected in vitro in the presence of the neuraminidase inhibitor, GS4071, The 13th International Congress on Antiviral Research, Baltimore MD, USA, Apr 16–21, 2000. Antiviral Res. 46 (2000) A60.

[33] Z.M. Wang, C.Y. Tai, D.B. Mendel, Studies on the mechanism by which mutations at His 274 alter sensitivity of influenza A virus neuraminidase type 1 to GS4071 and zanamivir, The 13th International Congress on Antiviral Research, Baltimore, MD, USA, Apr 16–21, 2000. Antiviral Res. 46 (2000) A60.

International Congress Series 1219 (2001) 863–877

Influenza resistance to zanamivir generated in ferrets

M. Louise Herlocher [a,*], Rob Fenton[b], Andrew Merry[c], Stephanie Elias[a], Arnold S. Monto[a]

[a]*Department of Epidemiology, School of Public Health, University of Michigan, 109 Observatory Street, Ann Arbor, MI 48109-2029, USA*
[b]*Medicines Research Centre, Glaxo Wellcome, Stevenage, UK*
[c]*Pathology, University of Michigan, Ann Arbor, MI, USA*

Abstract

Zanamivir (4-Guanidino-2,4-dideoxy-2,3-dehydro-*N*-acetylneuraminic acid), an anti-neuraminidase drug, is highly effective in the treatment of influenza. Influenza resistance to zanamivir has proved difficult to raise. Two neuraminidase mutations leading to resistance in vitro have been identified in several viruses—glu 119 gly and arg 292 lys. Only one resistant virus (an influenza B clone) has been observed in vivo in an immunocompromised child. This series of experiments sought to develop A/LA/1/87 (H3N2) influenza clones resistant to zanamivir in a ferret model. Using this model resistance to amantadine was easily developed within 6 days of treatment. Although most ferrets treated with zanamivir shed virus in the nasal wash, all ferrets were protected from fever and illness when treated with zanamivir. When ferrets were infected with nasal wash from ferrets previously infected with A/LA/1/87 (H3N2) and treated with zanamivir, 20 clones from their nasal wash grew on MDCK cells in the presence of 1 μM zanamivir. Sequencing of the NA genes of these clones revealed no mutations at positions 119 or 292. However, a nucleotide mutation at position 685 was observed in five of the clones. Sequencing of HA1 and HA2 for all genes is underway. Although characterization of the 20 clones is not complete, we can say that resistance to zanamivir will not arise as quickly or with the same frequency as does resistance to amantadine. © 2001 Elsevier Science B.V. All rights reserved.

Keywords: Zanavir; Ferret; Influenza resistance

1. Introduction

Influenza is an acute respiratory infection which causes numerous deaths each year. While this infection is usually a benign self-limiting condition, in children, the elderly and

---

* Corresponding author. Tel.: +1-734-764-5465; fax: +1-734-763-4192.
E-mail address: louise@umich.edu (M.L. Herlocher).

the immunocompromised, influenza infection can be associated with significant mortality [1]. Vaccination is available against circulating antigens; however, the choice of antigens is made based on identification of strain types observed in virus isolates in the preceding year. Since the genes coding for the hemagglutinin and neuraminidase are subject to a high mutation rate, only partial protection may be offered by vaccines against new strains of virus arising in the subsequent influenza season [1].

The antivirals, amantadine and rimantadine, are efficacious in the prophylaxis and treatment of influenza A [2–6]. Both antivirals act by blocking the acid activated ion channel formed by the virion associated M2 protein [7]. M2 protein is not produced by influenza B and so these products have no effect on disease caused by Type B strains. The usefulness of these drugs is further limited by the rapid development of resistance and gastrointestinal and central nervous system side effects [6].

Influenza neuraminidase is considered important for sustained viral replication in humans and is thought to play a role in movement of the virus through mucus in the respiratory tract [8,9]. The highly conserved nature of the influenza neuraminidase active site has led to the expectation that inhibitors of this enzyme would be active against all strains of influenza A and B viruses. Zanamivir (4-guanidino-2,4-dideoxy-2,3-dehydro-N-acetylneuraminic acid), or GG167, has been synthesized based on the crystallographic structure of influenza neuraminidase [10]. It has been shown to be a potent and specific inhibitor of both influenza A and B neuraminidase activity in enzymatic and tissue culture assays [11,12] and has shown efficacy in animal models of influenza [10,13,14]. It has also been proven effective as treatment and prophylaxis in human clinical trials [15,16].

Demonstration of influenza resistance to zanamivir has been difficult to achieve. Two mutations in the neuraminidase of influenza A viruses have been observed independently in vitro by several groups [17–24]: glu 119 gly in an H1N9 virus [17,19,22–24] and arg 292 lys in an H1N9 virus [18]. In an H4N2 virus, both arg 292 lys and glu 119 ala mutations in the NA gene have been created in vitro [20]. The glu 119 gly mutation in the H1N9 virus was accompanied by a mutation in the HA gene at ser 186 phe (which actually appeared following the first passage). Subsequent passages yielded additional HA mutations at either ser 165 asn or lys 222 thr [17,23]. In the H4N2 virus the glu 119 ala mutation was accompanied by a mutation in HA2 of gly 75 glu [21]. One mutation, glu 119 gly, in the neuraminidase of influenza B/HK/8/73 was observed in vitro [19] accompanied by 2 mutations in the HA gene, asn 145 ser and asn 150 ser. It is suggested that the glu 119 gly mutation in the NA gene leads to the abrogation of a salt link between 119 and 156 thus resulting in instability of the NA tetramer [24]. An H2N2 virus resistant to GG167 was generated in vitro with no mutation in the neuraminidase gene but a gly 135 asp mutation in the hemagglutination gene [25]. The H1N9 virus also became 1000-fold less sensitive in plaque assay following passage in tissue culture in the presence of zanamivir. No NA mutation was present; however, mutations in or near the HA binding site were involved; i.e., thr 155 ala, val 223 ile or arg 229 ile/ser [26].

The only in vivo mutant resistant to GG167 recovered was from an immunocompromised patient infected with influenza B [27]. The virus had a neuraminidase mutation at arg 152 lys accompanied by an HA mutation of the 198 ile.

Influenza resistance to oseltamivir (GS 4071) has been observed twice in vivo in an H3N2 virus and once in vivo in an H1N1 virus. In the H3N2 virus, mutants were isolated with mutations in the neuraminidase at arg 292 lys [28] and glu 119 val [29]. His 274 tyr in the neuraminidase was the mutant isolated from the HINI virus [30]. In vitro an H3N2 virus resistant mutant was generated with a mutation in the neuraminidase arg 292 lys accompanied by HA mutations ala 28 thr in HA1 and arg 124 met in HA2 [31].

Mutations in the neuraminidase gene against the anti-neuraminidase drugs have been observed in H3N2, H1N1, H1N9, H3N2, and B influenza viruses at positions 119, 292, 152, and 274. All observed positions are conserved in all known subtypes of neuraminidase [32]. Position 119 is a framework mutation and 152 and 292 are functional mutations in that they make contact with the sialic acid product [33]. Given the preceding resistance history against the anti-neuraminidase drugs, we attempted to generate H3N2 clones resistant to zanamivir (GG167) in vivo.

The ferret as an animal model has been established for 25 years in our laboratories for studying the value of vaccines and antivirals in preventing and treating influenza. We proposed to use the ferret as an animal model for studying the development of influenza resistance to zanamivir because: (1) ferrets respond to influenza similarly to humans (they shed virus, sneeze, cough, and suffer fever and malaise just as humans do when suffering from influenza illness); (2) ferrets are susceptible to human influenza; (3) influenza attaches via an alpha-1,6-glycosidic linkage to the sialic acid of both ferret and human respiratory epithelial cells whereas influenza attaches via the alpha-1,3 linkage of sialic acid in avian and equine epithelial cells [34]; and (4) ferrets respond to zanamivir treatment when infected with influenza [10]. Although a mouse model was used in the past [35,36] to study the epidemic course of influenza, its application to human influenza was limited because the mouse is not a natural host. Ferrets are the only small animal that regularly develops febrile illness when infected with naturally occurring human influenza viruses. The ferret's illness may be monitored by febrile response; shedding of virus may be titered from nasal washes; resistant clones may be plaqued from nasal wash. Since ferrets respond to influenza infection by shedding virus and treatment with zanamivir alleviates illness, mutants arising which are resistant to zanamivir should be detected in virus shed in the nasal wash if the drug indeed induces in vivo resistance.

2. Methods

2.1. Virus

The A/LA/1/87 (H3N2) virus used was obtained from the laboratory of John Maassab. It was isolated in 1987 from a throat swab obtained from the Centers for Disease Control in SPAFAS chicken kidney cells. The passages used in these experiments were A/LA/1/87 CK1 SE1 39 °C SE3-6 35 °C.

2.2. Ferrets

Five- to six-week-old castrated male ferrets were obtained from Marshall Farms. Sera titer against A/LA/1/87 (H3N2) were tested by hemagglutinin inhibition before delivery to ensure seronegativity of animals. After arrival ferrets were treated for 3 days with 0.1 ml

Durapen (300,000 units combined Penicillin). Groups were made up of three or four ferrets with one group consisting of infected controls.

2.3. Amantadine treatment

Ferrets were treated with 50 mg/kg amantadine [37] intraperitoneally (i.p.). They were treated 24 h before infection, 2 h before infection, 5 h after infection, and once daily for 5 or 9 days. One group of animals was not pretreated but was treated for 9 days.

2.4. Zanamivir treatment

Ferrets were treated with 1, 0.3, 0.1, or 0.05 mg/kg zanamivir intranasally (i.n.). Before treatment, they were anesthetized with a combination of 10 mg/kg i.m. Ketamine and 0.2 mg/kg i.m. Rompun. They were treated 24 h before infection, 2 h before infection, 5 h after infection, and twice daily for 9 days.

2.5. Infection

Ferrets were lightly anesthetized with ether and infected i.n. with 1 ml virus (0.5 ml per nares). In Experiments I, II, and III virus used to infect was A/Los Angeles/1/87 (H3N2) grown in eggs and titered at 5×10^5 PFU/ml. In Experiment IV, ferrets were infected with nasal wash from Experiment III—either from control infected ferrets or ferrets infected and treated with 1.0 mg/kg zanamivir.

2.6. Temperatures

Rectal temperatures were taken twice a day beginning with the afternoon following infection. All temperatures were analyzed for significant fever by calculating the number of standard deviations from a normal average temperature of 101.5 °F (obtained by averaging 72 normal ferret temperatures). A fever of 102.8 was 3 standard deviations (S.D.) from the normal average temperature and was considered fever. Previous publications have used 2 S.D. as an indication of fever [38].

2.7. Nasal washes

Nasal washes, uning to kat catheters, were performed daily at 2:00 PM for 9 days on unanesthetized ferrets. PBS (3 ml) was introduced intranasally and sneezed wash was collected in sterile urine collection cups.

2.8. Viral titration

Nasal wash from each ferret each day was analyzed using an ELISA for the detection of Influenza A antigen in ferret nasal wash. Positive nasal wash samples were titrated on MDCK cells to determine viral titer and on MDCK cells in the presence of 1 μM zanamivir to detect resistant clones of influenza. Resistant plaques were picked, amplified in MDCK cells, and further characterized. Plaques were also picked and amplified if they arose in zanamivir-treated ferret nasal washes after control ferrets cleared the virus.

2.9. Characterization of viral clones

RNA from amplified clones was extracted using a guanidine–phenol extraction method and then reverse transcribed with avian myeloblastosis virus reverse transcriptase (30 U). The product was used in the polymerase chain reaction (PCR) to amplify the cDNA as previously described [39]. The neuraminidase gene was amplified in two fragments using primers NA8—5′GCA GGA GTG AAA ATG AAT CC3′ with NA704R—5′CCG ACT CCT GGG TCC TGA GG3′ and NA605—5′GGG GAT GAT AGA AAT GCA AC3′ with NA1463R—5′GAA ACA AGG AGT TTT TTT C3′. PCR products were purified in agarose and the amplified DNA was extracted from the gel using Promega PCR columns. Amplified NA fragments were sequenced using an ABI-377 automatic sequencer. The NA sequence of each clone isolated was compared to that of the A/Los Angeles/1/89 infecting virus using the GCG analysis package.

3. Results

3.1. Amantadine treatment of ferrets infected with A/LA/1/87

Ferrets treated with 50 mg/kg i.p. daily (Table 1) shed influenza clones resistant to amantadine in their nasal wash following one ferret passage. Results of the Amantadine Experiment are presented in Table 2. Only one ferret shed resistant virus on day 5, but four ferrets out of nine shed resistant virus by day 6 and one continued to shed resistant virus through day 7. It did not seem to matter whether or not they were pretreated or whether they were treated for 9 or 5 days; all groups shed amantadine resistant virus from nasal wash. In resistant influenza clones, mutations were seen in the membrane spanning

Table 1
Amantadine ferret experiment

# Ferrets	Amantadine dose	Virus Used to Infect[a]
3	Not treated	5×10^5 PFU/ml A/LA/1/87 (H3N2) CK1 SE1 39 °C SE3 35 °C
3	50 mg/kg pretreated and treated 9 days	5×10^5 PFU/ml A/LA/1/87 (H3N2) CK1 SE1 39 °C SE3 35 °C
3	50 mg/kg pretreated and treated 5 days	
3	50 mg/kg not pretreated and treated 9 days	

[a] CK1 SE1 39 °C SE3 35 °C refers to isolation in Spafas chick kidney cells, plaque purification in SPAFAS eggs at 39 °C followed by three passages in SPAFAS eggs at 35 °C.

Table 2

M2 influenza mutations arising in ferrets treated with amantadine during one passage

Ferret	Treatment	Day	Resistant	Nucleotide #	Nucleotide	Aa #	Aa
5469	9 days pretreat	5	Cl 2 Neg				
5469		6	Cl 3 Pos	793	C	27	Ala
5469		6	Cl 7 Pos	801	A	30	Thr
5469		6	Cl 14 Pos	805	T	31	Ile
5471	5 days pretreat	5	Cl 1 Neg				
5475	5 days pretreat	6	Cl 3 Pos	802	T	30	Val
5475		6	Cl 5 Neg				
5475		6	Cl 7 Pos	805	A	31	Asn
5475		6	Cl 8 Pos	805	A	31	Asn
5477 very ill	9 days no pretreat	6	Cl 4 Pos	789	T	26	Phe
5477		6	Cl 7 Pos	801	A	30	Thr
5477		6	Cl 9 Pos	805	A/G	31	Asn/Ser
5477		7	Cl 15-A Pos	802	T	30	Val
5477		7	Cl 20 Pos	802	T	30	Val
5477		7	Cl 22-A Pos	802	T	30	Val
5479	9 days no pretreat	6	Cl 3 Neg				
5479		5	Cl 11 Neg				
5479		5	Cl 12 Neg				
5481	9 days no pretreat	6	Cl 1 Pos	805	A	31	Asn
5481		6	Cl 4 Pos	805	A	31	Asn
5481		5	Cl 13 Pos	801	A	30	Thr

M2 amino acids conferring amantadine resistance.

26 (789) Leu (C) → Phe (T).

27 (793) Val (T) → Ala (C).

30 (801) Ala (G) → Thr (A).

30 (802) Ala (C) → Val (T).

31 (805) Ser (G) → Asn (A).

channel of M2 at amino acid positions 26, 27, 30 and 31. Mutations in amino acids 27, 30 and 31 in influenza viruses resistant to amantadine have been isolated in tissue culture [40]; mutations in amino acids 30 and 31 in influenza viruses resistant to amantadine have been isolated clinically from humans [41]; and mutations in amino acids 26, 30 and 31 in influenza viruses resistant to amantadine have been isolated from immunocompromised

Table 3

A/LA/1/87 (H3N2) in the presence of zanamivir. Number of plaques/ml in MDCK cells. Average of two experiments

Zanamivir concentration (μM)	Number of plaques
0	19.0
0.01	30.0
0.1	26.0
1.0	2.5
10.0	5.0
100.0	0

1.0 μM zanamivir is inhibitory to A/LA/1/87 in vitro.

Table 4
Zanamivir ferret experiments—Group I

	# Ferrets	zanamivir Dose	Viruses used to infect
Experiment I	4/Group	0.3 or 0.1 or 0.05 mg/kg	5×10^5 PFU/ml
	Total 20	all pretreated	A/LA/1/87 (H3N2)
Experiment III	4/Group	1.0 mg/kg	5×10^5 A/LA/1/87
	Total 16	pretreated or 1.0 mg/kg	
		not pre-treated or 0.3 mg/kg pretreated	
Experiment IV	3/Group	0.3 mg/kg pretreated	Nasal wash from Exp. III
	Total 12		control ferrets or Nasal wash
			from Exp. III D2, 3, 4 ferrets
			treated with zanamivir

humans [42]. Mutations seen in influenza clones resistant to amantadine and isolated in ferrets are consistent with those mutations seen in human isolates of influenza resistant to amantadine.

Experiments I and III Percent Ferrets with Nasal Wash Titer

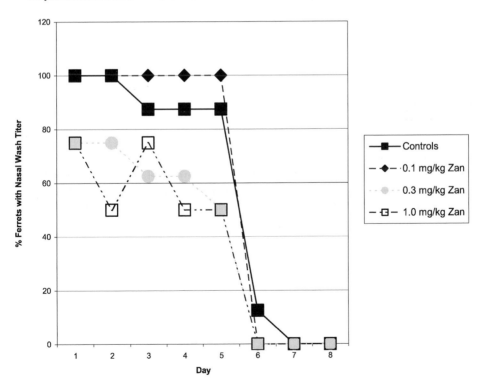

Fig. 1. Ferrets were infected with 5×10^5 PFU/ml A/LA/1/87 (H3N2) and treated with 0.1, 0.3 or 1.0 mg/kg zanamivir. Data from Experiments I and III are combined.

3.2. A/LA/1/87 (H3N2) in the presence of zanamivir in vitro

In MDCK cells, A/LA was sensitive to zanamivir at a concentration of 1 μM (Table 3).

3.3. Ferrets-treated with zanamivir

Four separate ferret experiments in which the only treatment used was zanamivir were performed with the goal of isolating influenza clones of an H3N2 virus resistant to zanamivir. Results from Experiments I, III, and IV are presented here (Table 4).

Although the ferrets treated with zanamivir dose levels of 0.3 and 1 mg/kg and infected with 5×10^5 PFU/ml A/LA/1/87 (H3N2) showed average titers similar to those of the controls throughout the course of the experiments (data not shown), fewer ferrets were infected when pretreated and treated with 0.3 and 1.0 mg/kg zanamivir than were control ferrets and those treated but infected cleared the infection 1–2 days earlier than did the controls (Fig. 1). Seventy-five percent of the control ferrets had fevers of 103 °F or higher on day 1 whereas only 12.5% of ferrets pretreated with zanamivir (even at a dose level of 0.1 mg/kg) had fevers on day 1 (Fig. 2). Zanamivir protected the ferrets throughout the course of the experiment from fever although

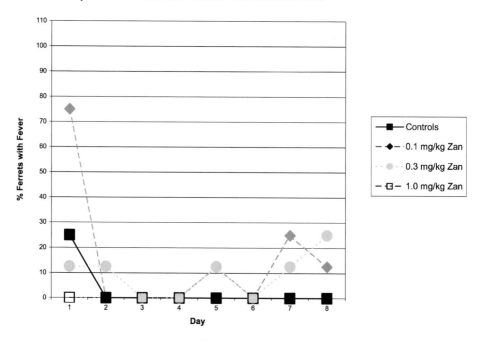

Fig. 2. Data from Experiments I and III are combined. Temperatures of 102.8 °F or over (3 S.D. over the average of 72 normal ferret temperatures) are considered fever.

some of those ferrets with no fever did shed virus. There were no resistant clones generated from Experiment I or III.

In Experiment IV, ferrets were infected with nasal wash from either control ferrets or zanamivir treated ferrets from Experiment III. Ferrets treated with 0.3 mg/kg show no decrease in number of animals infected; nor do they clear the virus faster than the controls (Fig. 3). Data suggests that treated animals that received treated inoculum had fewer animals with nasal wash titers. However, 100% of untreated animals who were infected with control nasal wash exhibited fevers of 102.8 °F or greater (3 S.D.) (Fig. 4) whereas 33% of animals treated with 0.3 mg/kg zanamivir exhibited fevers. Of the animals that were untreated but infected with treated nasal wash, 66% exhibited fevers on day 8; those treated with 0.3 mg/kg zanamivir and infected with treated nasal wash were protected from fever throughout the course of the experiment.

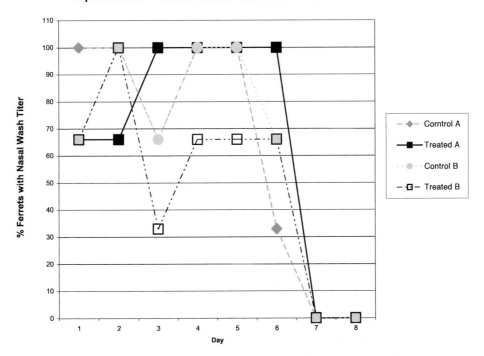

Fig. 3. Control A ferrets were not treated and were infected with nasal wash from untreated but infected ferrets. Treated A ferrets were treated with 0.3 mg/kg zanamivir and were infected with nasal wash from untreated but infected ferrets. Control B ferrets were not treated and were infected with nasal wash from treated and infected ferrets. Treated B ferrets were treated with 0.3 mg/kg zanamivir and were infected with nasal wash from treated and infected ferrets.

Experiment IV Percent Ferrets with Fever

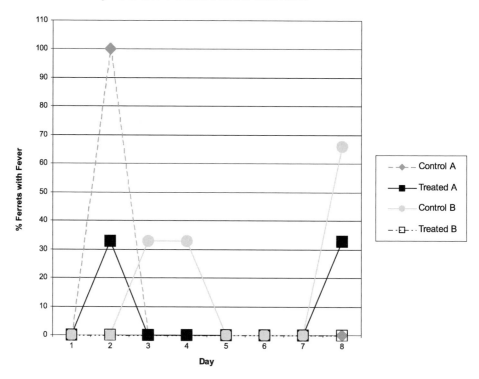

Fig. 4. Control A ferrets were not treated and were infected with nasal wash from untreated but infected ferrets. Treated A ferrets were treated with 0.3 mg/kg zanamivir and were infected with nasal wash from untreated but infected ferrets. Control B ferrets were not treated and were infected with nasal wash from treated and infected ferrets. Treated B ferrets were treated with 0.3 mg/kg zanamivir and were infected with nasal wash from treated and infected ferrets. Temperatures of 102.8 °F or higher (3 S.D. above the average of 72 normal ferrets) are considered fever.

3.4. Clones from Experiment IV growing in the presence of 1 μM zanamivir

A total of 20 pinpoint-sized clones were picked and amplified from 0.3 mg/kg zanamivir-treated ferrets' nasal wash which had been plaqued on MDCK cells in the presence of 1 μM zanamivir. This was the second passage in ferrets for this virus. The neuraminidase gene of all of the clones was sequenced and compared to that of the parent A/LA virus. None of the clones had the amino acids previously shown to confer resistance in the neuraminidase gene. Both amino acids 119 and 292 were glutamic acid and arginine, respectively, as in the A/LA parent virus. However, four out of nine clones from the ferrets treated with zanamivir and infected with nasal wash from treated ferrets had adenine at position 685 instead of cytosine. One out of eleven ferrets treated with zanamivir and infected with nasal wash from control ferrets had adenine at position 685 instead of cytosine. And in 14 out of 14 clones isolated from ferret nasal washes untreated with

Table 5
Neuraminidase gene sequence comparison of pinpoint A/LA/1/87 clones picked from MDCK plates with 1 μM zanamivir. From nasal wash of Experiment IV zanamivir-treated ferrets. With infecting virus A/LA/1/87 (H3N2)

Ferret #	Infection treatment	Day	Clone	NA nucleotide 685	NA AA 119	NA AA 292
A/LA/1/87				**C**	**GAA glu**	AGA arg
5512	Treated inoculum **0.3 mg/kg**	2	cl-1	**A**	GAA glu	AGA arg
5512		2	cl-2	C	GAA glu	AGA arg
5512		3	cl-1	C	GAA glu	AGA arg
5512		3	cl-2	**A**	GAA glu	AGA arg
5512		6	cl-1	C	GAA glu	AGA arg
5512		6	cl-2	C	GAA glu	AGA arg
5522		6	cl-1	C	GAA glu	AGA arg
5522		6	cl-2	**A**	GAA glu	AGA arg
5522		6	cl-4	**A**		AGA arg
5509	Control inoculum **0.3 mg/kg**	2	cl-1	C	GAA glu	AGA arg
5509		2	cl-2	C	GAA glu	AGA arg
5509		2	cl-3	C	GAA glu	AGA arg
5514		2	cl-1	C	GAA glu	AGA arg
5514		2	cl-3	C	GAA glu	AGA arg
5514		2	cl-4	C	GAA glu	AGA arg
5514		2	cl-5	C	GAA glu	AGA arg
5514		2	cl-6	C	GAA glu	AGA arg
5527		2	cl-1	**A**	GAA glu	AGA arg
5527		2	cl-2	C	GAA glu	AGA arg
5527		2	cl-3	C	GAA glu	AGA arg

In 14 plaques picked from animal nasal washes untreated with zanamivir (controls), position 685 was C as in the A/LA NA sequence.

zanamivir, position 685 was cytosine as in the parent A/LA sequence. Position 685 does not code for an amino acid change (Table 5).

4. Discussion

Influenza resistance to zanamivir has not been observed in a clinical setting [38]. Influenza resistance to oseltamivir has been observed in a clinical setting [28–30]; moreover, resistance in H3N2 viruses has been observed [28,29]. We, therefore, tried to raise resistance to zanamivir in an H3N2 virus in vivo. Although A/LA/1/87 (H3N2) influenza became resistant to amantadine treatment in ferrets during 6 days of exposure, A/LA/1/87 (H3N2) resistance to zanamivir in ferrets (as measured by mutations in the neuraminidase gene) was not observed even after two successive ferret passages.

Using the plaque reduction assay, small-sized plaques were rescued in the presence of 1 μM zanamavir on MDCK plates. Although this would seem to be indicative of resistance, plaquing in MDCK cells has not been reliable [11,38]. This was highlighted in the study which identified influenza B resistance in an immunocompromised child [27]. This influenza B virus had mutations in the NA and the HA genes, had a high IC_{50} in the NA assay, but was sensitive to zanamivir in MDCK cells. In our work and in others [38], the reverse is true; clones appear resistant in MDCK cells but are not resistant using any other assay system. NA assays are not currently completed.

It should be pointed out that characterization of the clones isolated in the presence of 1 µM zanamivir are not complete. However, it may be NA mutations alone that are critical [38]. We can say that the two mutations observed in the neuraminidase gene which lead to resistance in vitro are not present in any of our clones. The glutamic acid mutation to glycine at position 119, considered to be a framework mutation, was not present. Nor was the arginine mutation to lysine at position 292, located in the active catalytic site, present in any of our clones. The 119 mutation produces a 30- to 40-fold shift in susceptibility to zanamivir and reduces enzyme stability [24,43].

We did see a silent mutation at nucleotide 685 in four out of nine ferrets treated with zanamivir and infected with treated inoculum. These mutations were isolated from virus present on days 2, 3, and 6 nasal washes. In ferrets treated with zanamivir but infected with control inoculum, we saw the mutation in 1 out of 10 ferrets. In ferrets not treated with zanamivir, all 14 had the cytosine at position 685 seen in the parent A/LA virus. This may be a precursor of resistance; it would be interesting if this mutation was observed in early tissue culture passages which led to in vitro resistance.

The sequence of the HA1 and the HA2 of all isolated clones is currently being investigated. Several mutations in the HA have been identified which appear to contribute to in vitro resistance. They are K68R and G75E in the HA2 peptide [21,23]. In the HA1 polypeptide they are G135D, N 145 S, N 150 S, T 155 A, S 165 N, S 186 F, K 222 T, V 223 I, and R 229I/S [17,19,22,23,25,26]. We cannot say whether there are mutations in either the HA1 or the HA2 of our clones, either of which could contribute to resistance in vivo. However, studies in clinical isolates have shown that HA mutations which lead to resistance in vitro have significantly less effect in vivo [38]. This finding contributed to our decision to sequence the NA gene first. There is one study in which an H2N2 virus resistant to zanamivir in vitro had no mutation in the NA gene but had a gly 135 asp mutation in the HA gene [25] and one study in which an H1N9 virus resistant to zanamivir in vitro had no mutation in the NA gene but mutations in HA1 either in the binding site or on the left edge of the receptor binding pocket [26]. There has also been a report of an H3N2 virus which first became resistant to oseltamivir in tissue culture with only mutations in the HA1 and HA2 and none in the NA gene. Two passages later the 292 NA mutation appeared [30]. These studies argue for the importance of sequencing the hemagglutinin gene in addition to the neuraminidase gene.

Since influenza resistance to zanamivir requires prolonged exposure of the virus to the drug, it would be worth investigating whether resistance could be raised following infection with the nasal wash from a ferret containing the 685 mutation, especially if it is accompanied by mutations in the HA gene, followed by treatment with no more than 0.3 mg/kg zanamivir. Just as full-blown resistance in vitro requires several adaptation steps in tissue culture, resistance may emerge in steps after continued passage in ferrets.

These studies do not mean resistance to zanamivir cannot be raised in vivo; however, it will not occur with either the frequency or the speed observed when treating with amantadine.

Acknowledgements

The authors wish to thank GlaxoWellcome (Stevenage, UK) for sponsoring this study. They also acknowledge the excellent technical assistance of Rachel Truscon, Sean Harrison, Melissa Poschel, and Derek Dimcheff. GCG computer comparisons were supported by General Clinical Research Center grant number MO1 RR00042.

References

[1] B.G. Murphy, R.G. Webster, Orthomyxoviruses, in: B.M. Fields, D.M. Knipe, P.M. Howley (Eds.), Fields Virology, 3rd edn., Lippincott-Raven, New York, 1996, pp. 1397–1445.

[2] S.D. Sears, M.L. Clements, Protective efficacy of low-dose amantadine in adults challenged with wild type influenza A virus, Antimicrob. Agents Chemother. 31 (1987) 1470–1473.

[3] R. Dolin, R.C. Reichman, P.H. Madore, et al., A controlled trial of amantadine and rimantadine in the prophylazis of influenza A infection, N. Engl. J. Med. 307 (1983) 580–584.

[4] A.S. Monto, S.E. Ohmit, K. Hornbuckle, et al., Safety and efficacy of long-term use of rimantadine for prophylaxis of type A influenza in nursing homes, Antimicrob. Agents Chemother. 39 (1995) 2224–2228.

[5] R.G. Douglas, Prophylaxis and treatment of influenza, N. Engl. J. Med. 322 (1990) 443–450.

[6] F.G. Hayden, A.J. Hay, Emergence and transmission of influenza A viruses resistant to amantadine and rimantadine, Curr. Top. Microbiol. Immunol. 176 (1992) 119–130.

[7] A.J. Hay, The action of adamantanamines against influenza A viruses: inhibition of the M2 ion channel protein, Semin. Virol. 3 (1992) 21–30.

[8] P.M. Colman, C.W. Ward, Curr. Top. Microbiol. Immnunol. 114 (1985) 117–255.

[9] H.D. Klenk, R. Rott, Adv. Virus Res. 34 (1988) 247–280.

[10] M. Von Itzstein, W.Y. Wu, G.B. Kok, M.S. Pegg, J.C. Dyason, B. Jin, T.V. Phan, M.L. Smythe, H.F. White, S.W. Oliver, P.M. Colman, J.N. Varghese, D.M. Ryan, J.M. Woods, R.C. Behtell, V.J. Hotham, J.M. Cameron, C.R. Penn, Rational design of potent sialidase-based inhibitors of influenza virus replication, Nature 363 (1993) 418–423.

[11] J.M. Woods, R.C. Bethell, J.A. Coates, N. Healy, S.A. Hiscox, B.A. Pearson, D.M. Ryan, J. Ticehurst, J. Tilling, S.M. Walcott, C.R. Penn, 4-guanidino-2,4-dideoxy-2,3-dehydro-N-acetylneuraminic acid is a highly effective inhibitor both of the sidalidase (neuraminidase) and of growth of a wide range of influenza A and B viruses in vitro, Antimicrob. Agents Chemother. 37 (7) (1993) 1473–1479.

[12] L.V. Gubareva, C.R. Penn, R.G. Webster, Inhibition of replication of avian influenza viruses by the neuraminidase inhibitor 4-guanidino-2,4-dideoxy-2,3-dehydro-N-acetylneuraminic acid, Virology 212 (1995) 323–330.

[13] L.V. Gubareva, J.A. McCullers, R.C. Bethell, R.G. Webster, Characterization of influenza A/HongKong/156/97 (H5N1) virus in a mouse model and protective effect of zanamivir on H5N1 infection in mice, J. Infect. Dis. 178 (1998) 1592–1596.

[14] D.M. Ryan, J. Ticehurst, M.H. Dempsey, C.R. Penn, Inhibition of influenza virus replication in mice by GG167 (4-guanidino-2,4-dideoxy-2,3-dehydro-N-acetylneuraminic acid) is consistent with extracellular activity of viral neuraminidase (sialidase), Antimicrob. Agents Chemother. 38 (10) (1994) 2270–2275.

[15] F.G. Hayden, J.T. Treanor, R.F. Betts, et al., Safety and efficacy of the neuraminidase inhibitor GG167 in experimental influenza, JAMA, J. Am. Med. Assoc. 3 (1992) 21–30.

[16] A.S. Monto, D.P. Robinson, M.L. Herlocher, J.M. Hinson, M.F. Elliott, A. Crisp, Zanamivir in the prevention of influenza among healthy adults — a randomized controlled trial, JAMA, J. Am. Med. Assoc. 282 (1) (1999) 31–35.

[17] J.L. McKimm-Breschkin, M. McDonald, T.J. Blick, P.M. Colman, Mutation in the influenza virus neuraminidase gene resulting in decreased sensitivity to the neuraminidase inhibitor 4-guanidino-Neu5Ac2en leads to instability of the enzyme, Virology 225 (1996) 240–242.

[18] J.L. McKimm-Breschkin, A. Sahasrabudhe, T.J. Blick, M. McDonald, P.M. Colman, G.J. Hart, R.C. Bethell, J.N. Varghese, Mutations in a conserved residue in the influenza virus neuraminidase active site decreases sensitivity to Neu5Ac2en-derived inhibitors, J. Virol. 72 (1998) 2456–2472.

[19] K.A. Staschke, J.M. Colacino, A.J. Baxter, G.M. Air, A. Bansal, W.J. Hornback, J.E. Munroe, W.G. Laver, Molecular basis for the resistance of influenza viruses to 4-guanidino-Neu5Ac2en, Virology 214 (1995) 642–646.

[20] L.V. Gubareva, M.F. Robinson, R.C. Bethell, R.G. Webster, Catalytic and framework mutations in the neuraminidase active site of influenza viruses that are resistant to 4-guanidino-Neu5Ac2en, J. Virol. 71 (5) (1997) 3385–3390.

[21] L.V. Gubareva, R. Bethell, G.J. Hart, K.G. Murti, C.R. Penn, R.G. Webster, Characterization of mutants of influenza a virus selected with the neuraminidase inhibitor 4-guanidino-Neu5Ac2en, J. Virol. 70 (1996) 1818–1827.

[22] T.J. Blick, T. Tiong, A. Sahasrabudhe, J.N. Varghese, P.M. Colman, G.J. Hart, C. Bethell, J.L. McKimm-Breschkin, Generation and characterization of an influenza virus neuraminidase variant with decreased sensitivity to the neuraminidase-specific inhibitor 4-guanidino-Neu5Ac2en, Virology 214 (1995) 475–484.

[23] T.J. Blick, A. Sahasrabudhe, M. McDonald, I.J. Owens, P.J. Morley, F.J. Fenton, J.L. McKimm-Breschkin, The interaction of neuraminidase and hemagglutinin mutations in influenza virus in resistance to 4-guanidino-Neu5Ac2en, Virology 246 (1998) 95–103.

[24] J.M. Colacino, N.Y. Chirgadze, E. Garman, K.G. Murti, R.J. Loncharich, A. Baxter, K.A. Staschke, W.G. Laver, A Single sequence change destabilizes the influenza virus neuraminidase tetramer, Virology 236 (1997) 66–75.

[25] C.R. Penn, J.M. Barnett, R.C. Bethell, R. Fenton, K.L. Gearing, N. Healy, A.J. Jowett, Selection of influenza virus with reduced sensitivity in vitro to the neuraminidase inhibitor GG167 (4-guanidino-Neu5Ac2en): changes in haemagglutinin may compensate for loss of neuraminidase activity, in: L.E. Hampson, A.W. Hampson, R.G. Webster (Eds.), Options for the Control of Influenza III, Elsevier, Amsterdam, 1996, pp. 735–740.

[26] J.L. McKimm-Breschkin, T.J. Blick, A. Sahasrabudhe, T. Tong, D. Marshall, G.J. Hart, R.C. Bethell, C.R. Penn, Generation and characterization of variants of NWS/G70C influenza virus after in vitro passage in 4-amino-Neu5Ac2en and 4-guanidino-Neu5Ac2en, Antimicrob. Agents Chemother. 40 (1996) 40–46.

[27] L.V. Gubareva, M.N. Matrosovich, M.K. Brenner, R.C. Bethell, R.W. Webster, Evidence for zanamivir resistance in an immunocompromised child infected with influenza B virus, J. Infect. Dis. 178 (1998) 1257–1262.

[28] J. Carr, J. Ives, N. Roberts, C.Y. Tai, M. Wang, D.B. Mendel, L. Kelly, R. Lambkin, J. Oxford, An oseltamivir treatment-selected A/Wuhan/359/95 Virus with an E119V mutation in the neuraminidase gene has reduced infectivity in vivo, International Symposium on Influenza and Other Respiratory Viruses, 1999.

[29] J. Ives, J.A. Carr, N.A. Roberts, C. Tai, D.B. Mendel, L. Kelly, R. Lambkin, J.S. Oxford, An oseltamivir treatment-selected influenza A/N2 virus with an R292K mutation in the neuraminidase gene has reduced infectivity in vivo, International Symposium on Influenza and Other Respiratory Viruses, 1999.

[30] J. Carr, J. Ives, N. Roberts, L. Kelly, R. Lambkin, R. Oxford, C.Y. Tai, D. Mendel, F. Hayden, Virological assessment in vitro and in vivo of an influenza H1N1 virus with a H274Y mutation in the neuraminidase gene, Antiviral Res. 46 (1) (2000) A7913th ICAR Conference.

[31] C. Tai, P.A. Escarpe, R.W. Sidwell, M.A. Williams, W. Lew, H. Wu, C.U. Kim, D.B. Mendel, Characterization of human influenza virus variants selected in vitro in the presence of the nuraminidase inhibitor GS 4071, Antimicrob. Agents Chem. 42 (12) (1998) 3234–3241.

[32] J.N. Varghese, P.M. Colman, Three-dimensional structure of the neuraminidase of influenza virus A/Tokyo/3/67 at 2.2 A resolution, J. Mol. Biol. 221 (1991) 473–486.

[33] P.M. Colman, P.A. Hoyne, M.C. Lawence, Sequence and structure alignment of paramyxovirus hemagglutinin-neuraminidase with influenza virus neuraminidase, J. Virol. 67 (8) (1993) 2972–2980.

[34] R.J. Connor, Y. Kawaoka, R.G. Webster, J.C. Paulson, Receptor specificity in human, avian, and equine H2 and H3 influenza virus isolates, Virology 205 (1994) 17–23.

[35] J.L. Schulman, The use of an animal model to study transmission of influenza virus infection, AJPH 58 (11) (1968) 2092–2096.

[36] J.L. Schulman, E.D. Kilbourne, Airborne transmission of influenza virus infection in mice, Nature (1962) 1129–1130.

[37] J.S. Oxford, I.S. Logan, C.W. Potter, In vivo selection of an influenza A2 strain resistant to amantadine, Nature 226 (1970) 82–83.

[38] J.M. Barnett, A. Cadman, D. Gor, M. Dempsey, M. Walters, A. Candlin, M. Tisdale, P.F. Morley, I.J. Owens, R.J. Fenton, A.P. Lewis, E.C.J. Claas, G.F. Rimmelzwaan, R. De Groot, A.D.M.E. Osterhaus, Zanamivir susceptibility monitoring and characterization of influenza virus clinical isolates obtained during phase II clinical efficacy studies, Antimicrob. Agents Chemother. 44 (1) (2000) 78–87.

[39] A. Bressoud, J. Whitcomb, C. Pourzand, O. Haller, P. Cerutti, Rapid detection of influenza virus H1 by the polymerase chain reaction, Biochem. Biophys. Res. Commun. 167 (1990) 42430.

[40] A.J. Hay, A.J. Wolstenholme, J.J. Skehel, M.H. Smith, The molecular Basis of the specific anti-influenza action of amantadine, EMBO J. 4 (11) (1985) 3021–3024.

[41] R.B. Belshe, M.H. Smith, C.B. Hall, R. Betts, A.J. Hay, Genetic basis of resistance to rimantadine emerging during treatment of influenza virus infection, J. Virol. 62 (5) (1988) 1508–1512.

[42] A.I. Klimov, E. Rocha, F.G. Hayden, P.A. Shult, L.F. Roumillat, N.J. Cox, Prolonged shedding of amantadine-resistant influenza a viruses by immunodeficient patients: detection by polymerase chain reaction-restriction analysis, J. Infect. Dis. 172 (1995) 1352–1355.

[43] A. Sahasrabudhe, L. Lawrence, V.C. Epa, J.N. Varghese, P.M. Colman, J.L. McKimm-Breschkin, Substrate, inhibitor, or antibody stabilizes the Glu 119 Gly mutant influenza neuraminidase, Virology 247 (1998) 14–21.

International Congress Series 1219 (2001) 879–886

Methods for determining resistance to neuraminidase inhibitors

Margaret Tisdale*, Janet Daly, Dee Gor

*Clinical Virology and Surrogates Unit, GlaxoWellcome Research and Development,
Gunnels Wood Road, Stevenage, Hertfordshire, SG1 2NY, UK*

Abstract

Various phenotypic methods have been used to monitor viral susceptibility to anti-viral agents in the management of virus diseases. Confirmation of resistance generally requires genotyping of the inhibitor target gene(s) and identification of mutations that confer the phenotypic resistance. While plaque reduction assays are valuable for accurate measurements of susceptibility, they are not ideal for large-scale monitoring. For the influenza inhibitors amantadine/rimantadine, susceptibility of clinical isolates has been monitored predominantly by yield-reduction using EIA-based assays, because plaque formation by influenza clinical isolates is very variable. With the development of the influenza neuraminidase (NA) inhibitors (NIs), it became apparent that current cell-based assays were unsuitable for monitoring susceptibility to this new class of drugs. The reasons for this relate to the close functional interactions between the NA and the HA at virus release and entry, and that weak HA receptor binding may by-pass the NA function in cell assays. Mutations selected in the HA, while not apparently contributing to phenotypic resistance in vivo, may result in cell culture-based resistance, and conversely may mask NA resistance in cell culture by modifying receptor-binding specificity. One important distinction between NIs and other antiviral enzyme inhibitors is that both target enzyme and inhibitor work extracellularly. Therefore, direct NA enzyme susceptibility assays using whole virus are most representative of the in vivo situation for monitoring phenotypic susceptibility. Sequencing of the NA to confirm phenotypic resistance is important. Since no suitable phenotypic assay is available to measure changes in receptor binding, sequencing of the HA, in particular the receptor binding region is an important adjunct to help understand resistance mechanisms. As the clinical use of NIs escalates, a major change will be required in approaches used to monitor susceptibility of influenza isolates in virology laboratories worldwide. © 2001 Elsevier Science B.V. All rights reserved.

Keywords: Neuraminidase inhibitors; Susceptibility monitoring

---

* Corresponding author. Tel.: +44-1438-76-4196; fax: +44-1438-76-4263.
E-mail address: smt40145@glaxowellcome.co.uk (M. Tisdale).

0531-5131/01/$ – see front matter © 2001 Elsevier Science B.V. All rights reserved.
PII: S 0 5 3 1 - 5 1 3 1 (0 1) 0 0 6 5 6 - 2

1. Introduction

Viral resistance may be defined as a reduction or loss of susceptibility of a virus to inhibition by a drug. This results from random genotypic changes which occur during replication and which are selected during inhibitory drug pressure. The resulting phenotypic changes are generally measured by determining the concentration of inhibitor that causes 50% inhibition of virus replication (IC_{50}), and this may be compared with pretreatment isolates, where available, to determine a shift in susceptibility. While virus resistance may be characterised in detail using in vitro techniques, it is important though more difficult to relate this to clinical outcome and to understand the relevance of different shift in susceptibility to clinical efficacy. Detection of drug resistance generally, but not always, relates to failure of therapy. Therapy failure will be dependent on the relative shift in susceptibility compared to the inhibitory concentrations achieved in vivo for each individual drug. Similarly, the consequences of resistance may be less where viral fitness and consequently viral transmission may have been compromised. This may be even more significant with a self-limiting disease such as influenza, where the immune system will play an important part in removing virus present later in infection.

A variety of phenotypic assays have been used to detect changes in susceptibility to anti-viral drugs. These are typically cell-based assays to measure virus replication. All phenotypic assays require amplification of the clinical isolate in cell culture, though virus passage is kept to a minimum to minimise selection of cell-adapted virus. Plaque reduction assays are the gold standard for in vitro studies of resistance but these are not easily automated and not ideal for large-scale clinical monitoring of isolates. Alternative methods for automation include dye-uptake assays that measure the cytopathic effects of the virus and yield reduction assays that measure directly virus infectivity, viral nucleic acid levels or production of a specific viral antigen. Unlike the plaque reduction assays, the alternative methods do not measure absolute IC_{50} values since these will be related to virus inoculum. Careful quantitation of each virus isolate is essential to allow accurate quantitative comparisons between isolates, with inclusion of known virus standards in each assay. For rimantadine/amantadine where > 100-fold shifts in susceptibility are observed, a modified EIA assay is used to detect resistance at one relatively high concentration of inhibitor compared with untreated controls [1].

Genotyping of target genes is used in conjunction with phenotypic assays to determine which mutations are associated with loss of susceptibility. Ideally, in the clinical setting, matched isolates from before and after commencement of treatment should be compared to identify mutations associated with changes in susceptibility. However, this is not always possible, particularly outside of the clinical trial setting, such as during clinical practice or during surveillance of susceptibility within a population. It is especially important to have a comparator sequence where the genes have high natural variability such as the HA and NA genes of influenza. It is essential to compare sequences with the consensus sequence for the different circulating influenza A and B sub-types during the current influenza season. In situations where key resistance mutations are known, as is the case with rimantadine/amantadine, assays to detect point mutations may be used to screen for resistance. However, where relatively new drugs are being evaluated for the potential to develop resistance, such as the NIs, this approach may be too restricted, and sequence analysis of target genes is essential. Direct sequencing of target genes after amplification by PCR from clinical samples has also been used to identify resistance in conjunction with culture [2]. This approach has the advantage that variability due to culture amplification will be avoided. However, interpretation of sequence data in the absence of phenotypic data may be complex and labour intensive. With the development of reverse genetics using relevant clinical isolates, this approach may become more practical. Mutations identified may be re-introduced into viable virus for determination of susceptibility, similar to monitoring undertaken currently with HIV [3].

2. Current status of neuraminidase inhibitors in the clinic

Three NIs in clinical development have been designed based on the structure of the neuraminidase active site. All mimic the natural substrate for the enzyme and are potent and selective inhibitors of influenza A and B [4–6]. The structures of the three NIs are shown in Fig. 1, and compared with the transition state substrate DANA. RWJ-270201 is still in early clinical development, while zanamivir and oseltamivir have been approved for clinical use in many countries. In the US 1999/2000-winter season, both zanamivir and oseltamivir were used extensively in clinical practice for the treatment of influenza A and B infections. NIs were prescribed for more than 1.25 million patients and interestingly, use of both amantadine and rimantadine also increased and exceeded 1 million prescriptions [7]. Although extensive susceptibility monitoring of influenza isolates has been performed during clinical evaluation of these two NIs [8–10] substantially larger numbers of subjects

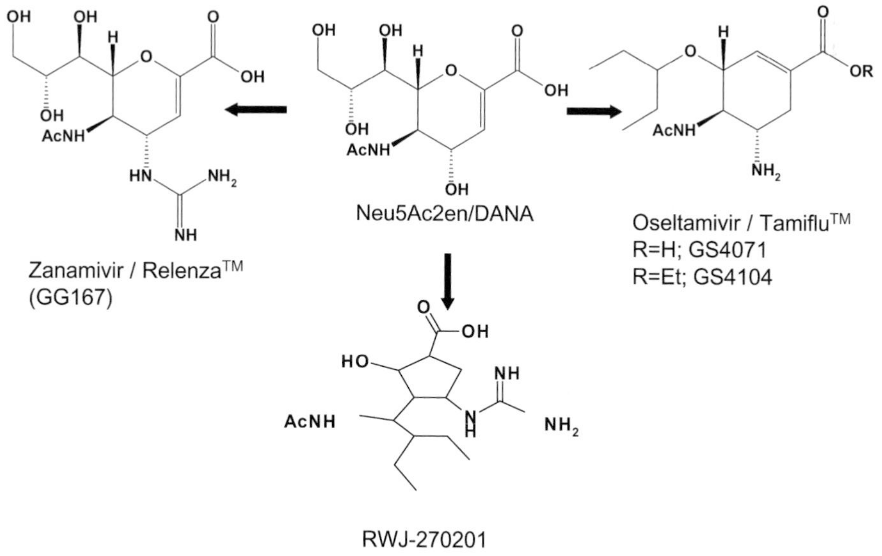

Fig. 1. Structures of NIs, zanamivir (Relenza®), oseltamivir (Tamiflu®), and RWJ-270201 compared to the natural transition state substrate/inhibitor DANA.

will be treated with this new class of inhibitor in clinical practice. Therefore, a global NI Susceptibility Network (NISN) of influenza experts has been set up to continue monitoring for development of resistant variants, for transmission of any such variants and the potential clinical outcome. This group is also evaluating the methodology used for susceptibility monitoring with the aim of encouraging accurate reporting of susceptibility to aid the appropriate management of influenza disease.

3. Susceptibility monitoring for NIs

The strategy currently used for monitoring susceptibility of clinical isolates to NIs has been based on in vitro studies conducted during drug development. With zanamivir and with oseltamivir (GS4071), mutations in the NA were observed following in vitro drug selection, and it was noted that HA and NA either alone or together contributed to phenotypic resistance [11–21]. These studies demonstrated the importance of the balance between the function of the HA and the NA on receptor binding during virus entry and receptor destruction during virus release. It was therefore apparent that clinical monitoring of influenza isolates should include examination of both the HA and NA sequence. Interestingly, in the clinic to date only one HA mutation has been selected during treatment, whereas four NA mutations have been identified (see Table 1; [1,10,22,23]). Monitoring the susceptibility of clinical isolates has been problematic, since there is no suitable cell-based assay to accurately determine IC_{50} values and relative shifts in susceptibility for NIs. NI resistance results in reductions in plaque size rather than plaque number making the plaque assay more variable and interpretation more subjective. As observed with rimantadine/amantadine, plaque assays are not ideal for clinical monitoring due to poor plaque formation by many recent clinical isolates. However, application of the EIA yield reduction assay to NIs also proved too variable for determining shifts in susceptibility. These problems with cell-based assays arise from differences in HA receptor-binding specificity in cell culture compared to the in vivo setting which may allow release of virus, by-passing the NA function, and possibly by direct cell to cell transfer of virus in cell culture. Not only have false positive resistance been observed but also one false negative resistance with the only HA/NA double mutant observed in the

Table 1
NA mutations observed in pre-clinical and clinical studies and their effects on enzyme function

Inhibitor	NA mutations	Selected		Enzyme function	Reference
		In vitro	In clinic		
Zanamivir	E119G/A/D	Yes	No	Reduced stability	[14]
	R292K	Yes	No	Reduced function	[17]
	R152K	No	Yes[a]	Reduced function/infectivity	[2]
Oseltamivir	R292K	Yes	Yes	Reduced function/ infectivity	[10,19]
	E119V	No	Yes	Reduced infectivity	[22]
	H274Y	Yes	Yes	Reduced function	[21,23]
RWJ-270201	R292K	Yes	No data	Reduced infectivity	[27,28]

[a] HA mutation was also observed at Day 8 of therapy, before the NA mutation at Day 12.

clinic [2]. Here, it was postulated that the HA mutation (T198I), which changed receptor binding specificity from Siaα2-6Gal to Siaα2-3Gal, may have masked the NA phenotype observed in the NA enzyme assay. Thus, at present cell-based assays are not recommended for monitoring susceptibility to NIs. Instead, direct NA enzyme inhibition assays are used since they have proved the best predictor of in vivo susceptibility [24]. The in vitro enzyme assays mimic most closely the in vivo environment because NA acts extracell-ularly in the respiratory interstitial fluid facilitating release and spread of virus. None of the NIs enters cells, and therefore NA inhibition occurs independent of cell type. At present, there is no suitable assay for monitoring changes in HA binding affinity and therefore sequencing regions of the HA and NA which include the active sites is recommended. However, care must be taken in interpreting any changes observed due to the natural variability of the antigenic sites surrounding the substrate binding sites.

There are two NA assays that may be used for monitoring susceptibility, both of which use small defined substrates. Undefined substrates such as fetuin are not considered sufficiently specific or sensitive for susceptibility assays. The most widely used is a fluorescent substrate $2'$-(4-methylumbelliferyl)-α-D-N-acetylneuraminic acid (MUN or MUNANA). Assays used are based on the methodology first described by Potier et al. [25], but more recently modifications have been made to this assay to increase sensitivity for clinical monitoring [10]. The second assay uses a chemiluminescent substrate, abbreviated as $2'$-(4-NA-Star)-α-D-N-acetylneuraminic acid (NA-Star), which has also been developed recently to increase sensitivity of detection for clinical isolates with low NA activity or low viral titres [26]. This assay is approximately 60 times more sensitive than the standard fluorescent assay and may detect NA activity for virus titres down to approximately 5×10^2 pfu/ml. Both assays are relatively simple to perform for determin-ing IC_{50} values, provided a fluorimeter or luminometer is accessible. However, because all the NIs are competitive inhibitors, the IC_{50} values determined will vary depending on the substrate concentration used for the assay. It is therefore important to standardise substrate concentration to optimise detection of shifts in susceptibility below substrate saturating concentrations. Similarly, the affinity of different virus isolates for the natural substrate (Km) will vary. This is most marked for influenza A compared to influenza B strains which generally have 10-fold lower Km values than A strains in both NA assays, and this may influence IC_{50} values determined. It is therefore important that the appropriate internal controls are used including both a sensitive and resistant virus. Similarly, affinity for the natural substrate generally changes for resistant variants, which again will influence the IC_{50} values determined. Shifts in susceptibility typically observed for the different NA resistant variants to the selection NI, range from ~ 10 to 10,000 fold, and cross-resistance is generally lower to the other NIs (see Table 2). It is important to look at the shape of the inhibition curve in addition to the IC_{50} value since mixtures of mutant and wild-type may be present. Such mixtures may produce a tail of partial inhibition at higher concentrations compared to wild-type. Any isolate suspected of showing reduced susceptibility in the NA inhibition assay should be further characterised by sequencing the NA before resistance may be confirmed. Ideally, further characterisation of resistant variants should include determination of Ki values, the affinity of the inhibitor for the enzyme-binding site. This would allow more accurate quantification of shifts in susceptibility that could be related to clinical outcome.

Table 2
Comparison of shift in susceptibility with the fluorescent and chemiluminescent NA assays with three NIs

Virus	Zanamivir		Oseltamivir (GS4071)		RWJ-270201	
	MUN assay	NA-Star assay	MUN assay	NA-Star assay	MUN assay	NA-Star assay
B/Memphis[a,b] R152K	94	20	67	338	1380	653
A/NWS/G70C[a] (H1N9)R292K	275	57	11,707[c]	36,795[c]	589	2832
A/NWS/G70C[a] (H1N9) E119G	249	984	2	1	56	40
B/Beijing/1/87[a] E116G	4218[c]	7830[c]	36	119	6619[c]	14,505[c]

[a] 100% mutant, with mixtures shifts in susceptibility would be less, and may show a tail of inhibition at higher concentrations compared with 100% wild-type.

[b] Designated B/Beijing/184/93 like virus.

[c] Extrapolated IC_{50}, above the highest concentration used in the assay.

In the clinical setting, ideally, matched isolates should be obtained from before commencing treatment and following exposure to the drug. In controlled clinical trials, this is generally feasible for therapy but not for prophylaxis studies where circulating strains obtained during surveillance may be used for comparison. However, during clinical practice, generally, only post-exposure isolates would be obtained for analysis. Similarly for global monitoring of susceptibility, diverse groups of isolates circulating worldwide would be analysed. In this setting, it is important to analyse baseline isolates from before the drugs were clinically available, for reference with isolates obtained during clinical use.

Based on data obtained from clinical trials with NIs to date, resistant variants obtained all have reduced viral fitness [2,10,22,23], in contrast to resistant isolates obtained after rimantadine/amantadine therapy [27]. This suggests that NI resistant variants will not be easily transmissible and resistance will be less of a problem with the NI class of inhibitor than with the M2-ion channel inhibitors, amantadine/rimantadine.

References

[1] R.B. Belshe, M.H. Smith, C.B. Hall, R. Betts, A.J. Hay, Genetic basis of resistance to rimantadine emerging during treatment of influenza virus infection, J. Virol. 62 (1988) 1508–1512.

[2] L.V. Gubareva, M.N. Mastrosovich, M.K. Brenner, R.C. Bethell, R.G. Webster, Evidence for zanamivir resistance in an immunocompromised child infected with influenza B virus, J. Infect. Dis. 178 (1998) 1257–1262.

[3] P. Kellam, B.A. Larder, Recombinant virus assay: a rapid, phenotypic assay for assessment of drug susceptibility of human immunodeficiency virus type 1 isolates, Antimicrob. Agents Chemother. 38 (1994) 23–30.

[4] M. von Itzstein, W.Y. Wu, G.B. Kok, J.C. Dyason, B. Jin, T.V. Phan, M.L. Smythe, H.F. White, S.W. Oliver, P.M. Colman, J.N. Varghese, D.M. Ryan, J.M. Woods, R.C. Bethell, V.J. Hotham, J.M. Cameron, C.R. Penn, Rational design of potent sialidase based inhibitors of influenza virus replication, Nature 363 (1993) 418–423.

[5] C.U. Kim, W. Lew, M.A. Williams, et al., Influenza NA inhibitors possessing a novel hydrophobic interaction in the enzyme active site: design, synthesis and structural analysis of carbocyclic sialic acid analogues with potent anti-influenza activity, J. Am. Chem. Soc. 119 (1997) 681–690.

[6] Y. Sudhaker Babu, C. Pooran, S. Bantia, P. Kotian, A. Dehghani, Y. El-Kattan, T.-H. Lin, L. Hutchinson,

A.J. Elliott, C.D. Parker, S.L. Ananth, L.L. Horn, G. Laver, J.A. Montgomery, BCX-1812 (RWJ-270201): discovery of a novel, highly potent, orally active, and selective influenza neuraminidase inhibitor through structure based drug design, J. Med. Chem. 43 (2000) 3482–3486.

[7] Scott-Levin (SPA): TRx Factored MTH/Feb2000.

[8] J.M. Barnett, A. Cadman, D. Gor, M. Dempsey, M. Walters, A. Candlin, M. Tisdale, P.J. Morley, I.J. Owens, R.J. Fenton, A.P. Lewis, E.C.J. Claas, G.F. Rimmelzwaan, R. DeGroot, A.D.M.E. Osterhaus, Zanamivir susceptibility monitoring and characterisation of influenza virus clinical isolates obtained during phase II clinical efficacy studies, Antimicrob. Agents Chemother. 44 (1) (2000) 78–87.

[9] D. Gor, A. Cadman, M. Dempsey, M. Walters, A. Candlin, J. Barnett, M. Tisdale, Antiviral efficacy and sequence analysis of HA and NA genes of influenza isolates from zanamivir phase II/III clinical efficacy trials, 39th ICAAC (San Francisco, September, 1999) Abstract 284.

[10] E. Covington, D.B. Mendel, P. Escarpe, C.Y. Tai, K. Soderbarg, N.A. Roberts, Phenotypic and genotypic assay of influenza neuraminidase indicates a low incidence of viral drug resistance during treatment with oseltamivir, Second International Symposium on Influenza and other Respiratory Viruses, Grand Cayman, Cayman Islands, December 10–12.

[11] T.J. Blick, T. Tiong, A. Sahasrabudhe, J.N. Varghese, P.M. Colman, G.J. Hart, R.C. Bethell, J.L. McKimm-Breschkin, Generation and characterisation of an influenza virus neuraminidase variant with decreased sensitivity to the neuraminidase-specific inhibitor 4-guanidino-Neu5Ac2en, Virology 214 (1995) 475–484.

[12] K.A. Staschke, J.M. Colacino, A.J. Baxter, G.M. Air, A. Bansal, W.J. Hornback, J.E. Munroe, G. Laver, Molecular basis for the resistanec of influenza viruses to 4-Guanidino-Neu5Ac2en, Virology 214 (1995) 642–646.

[13] J.L. McKimm-Breschkin, T.J. Blick, A. Sahasrabudhe, T. Tiong, D. Marshall, G.J. Hart, R.C. Bethell, C.R. Penn, Generation and characterization of variants of NWS/G7OC influenza virus after in vitro passage of 4-amino-Neu5Ac2en and 4-Guanidino-Neu5Ac2en, Antimicrob. Agents Chemother. 40 (1996) 40–46.

[14] J.L. McKimm-Breschkin, M. McDonald, T.J. Blick, P.M. Colman, Mutation in the influenza virus neura-minidase gene resulting in decreased susceptibility to the neuramindiase inhibitor 4-guanidino-Neu5Ac2en leads to instability of the enzyme, Virology 225 (1996) 240–242.

[15] C.R. Penn, J.M. Barnett, R.C. Bethell, et al., Selection of influenza virus with reduced sensitivity in vitro to the NA inhibitor GG167 (4-guanidino-Neu5Ac2en): changes in the HA may compensate for loss of NA activity, in: L.E. Brown, W.A. Hampson, R.G. Webster (Eds.), Options for the Control of Influenza, Elsevier, Amsterdam, Netherlands, 1996.

[16] L.V. Gubareva, R. Bethell, G.J. Hart, K.G. Murti, C.R. Penn, R.G. Webster, Characterisation of mutants of influenza A virus selected with the neuraminidase inhibitor 4-guanidino-Neu5Ac2en, J. Virol. 70 (1996) 1818–1827.

[17] L.V. Gubareva, M.J. Robinson, R. Bethell, R.G. Webster, Catalytic and framework mutations in the neu-raminidase active site of influenza viruses that are resistant to 4-guanidino-Neu5Ac2en, J. Virol. 71 (1997) 3385–3390.

[18] T.J. Blick, A. Sahasrabudhe, M. McDonald, I.J. Owens, P.J. Morley, R.J. Fenton, J.L. McKimm-Breschkin, The interaction of neuraminidase and haemagglutinin mutations in influenza virus in resistance to 4-gua-nidino-Neu5Ac2en, Virology 246 (1998) 95–103.

[19] C.Y. Tai, P.A. Escarpe, R.W. Sidwell, et al., Characterization of human influenza virus variants selected in vitro in the presence of the NA inhibitor GS 4071, Antimicrob. Agents Chemother. 42 (1998) 3234–3241.

[20] J.M. Barnett, A. Cadman, F.M. Burrell, S.H. Madar, A.P. Lewis, M. Tisdale, R. Bethell, In vitro selection and characterisation of influenza B/Beijing/1/87 isolates with altered susceptibility to zanamivir, Virology 265 (1999) 286–295.

[21] Z.M. Wang, C.Y. Tai, D.B. Mendel, Characterization of an influenza virus variant selected in vitro in the presence of the neuraminidase inhibitor GS4071, The 13th International Congress on Antiviral Resesarch, Baltimore, MD, USA, April 16th–21st 2000, Antiviral Research 46 (2000) A60.

[22] J. Carr, J. Ives, N.A Roberts, C.Y. Tai, D.B. Mendel, L. Kelly, R. Lambkin, J. Oxford, An oseltamivir treatment-selected influenza A/Wuhan/359/95 virus with an E119V mutation in the neuraminidasegene has reduced infectivity in vivo, Second International Symposium on Influenza and Other Respiratory Viruses, Grand Cayman, Cayman Islands, December 10–12.

[23] L. Gubareva, C.Y. Tai, D.B. Mendel, J. Ives, N.A. Roberts, F.G. Hayden, Oseltamivir treatment of experimental influenza A/Texas/36/91 (H1N1)virus infections in humans: selection of a novel neuraminidase variant, The 13th International Congress on Antiviral Research, Baltimore MD, USA, April 16th–21st 2000, Antiviral Research 46 (2000) A59.

[24] M. Tisdale, Monitoring of viral susceptibility: new challenges with the development of influenza NA inhibitors, Rev. Med. Virol. 10 (2000) 45–55.

[25] M. Potier, L. Mameli, L. Belisle, L. Dallaire, S.B. Melancon, Fluorometric assay of neuraminidase with a sodium (4-methylumbelliferyl-α-D-N-acetylneuraminate) substrate, Anal. Biochem. 94 (1979) 287–296.

[26] R.C. Buxton, B. Edwards, R.R. Juo, J.C. Voyta, M. Tisdale, R.C. Bethell, Development of a sensitive chemiluminescent neuraminidase assay for the determination of influenza virus susceptibility to zanamivir, Anal. Biochem. 280 (2000) 291–300.

[27] F.G. Hayden, R.B. Belshe, R.D. Clover, A.J. Hay, M.G. Oakes, W. Soo, Emergence and apparent transmission of rimantadine-resistant influenza A virus in families, N. Engl. J. Med. 321 (1989) 1696–1702.

[28] D.F. Smee, R.W. Sidwell, A.C. Morrison, K.W Bailey, L. Ly, E.Z. Baum, P.C. Wagaman, S. Bantia, Influenza A viruses resistant to the neuraminidase inhibitor RWJ-270201, 40th Interscience Conference on Antimicrobial Agents and Chemotherapy. Abstract 1158 (2000) 271.

International Congress Series 1219 (2001) 887–894

Screening of susceptibility to Zanamivir of influenza viruses

M. Aymard*, L. Gérentes, J. Jolly, O. Ferraris, N. Kessler

*Laboratory of Virology, Grp Regional d'Observ de la Gripp and Eur Influenza Surveillance Scheme,
National Influenza Reference Center, 8 Avenue Rockefeller, 69373 Lyon Cedex 08, France*

Keywords: Zanamivir; Susceptibility; Influenza virus

1. Introduction

Influenza produces a significant seasonal morbidity in general population, increases the hospitalisation rate mainly due to respiratory complications and results in excess mortality, particularly in aged and high-risk groups. In spite of efficacy of vaccine prevention, there is a need for antiviral chemotherapy and, it is expected, an increasing use of antiviral drugs for prophylactic and therapeutic treatments.

Several neuraminidase (NA) inhibitors have been designed to interact with conserved residues in the active site of the NA enzyme. Zanamivir is effective against all nine NA subtypes of influenza A and B virus [8,13]. It has been shown to be effective in human experimental influenza and field studies [9,11]. Zanamivir (Relenza®) has been put on the market in most countries (including France) in 1998–1999 and the emergence of resistance could be expected. De novo resistance has not yet been recognised. We isolated in Madin Darby Canine Kidney (MDCK) cells in 1993–1995 [1] A/H3N2 (A/Beij/32/92 related) viruses with poor if any NA enzymatic activity, and currently most of the A/H1N1 strains isolated in MDCK have a very poor NA activity; therefore we could ask the question : "Are those isolates susceptible to NA inhibitors?" They might be checked with a test different from the NI test.

Sequential passages of *influenza viruses* in cells cultures in the presence of Zanamivir lead to resistance [7] and resistant variants have also been identified clinically [3].

It is therefore important to organise a continuous survey of the potential emergence of resistant strains. This is a requirement of the Health Authorities.

---

* Corresponding author. Tel.: +33-4-78-77-70-29; fax: +33-4-78-01-48-87.

As influenza A/H3N2 viruses are responsible for the most frequent and most severe outbreaks and their antigenic variation is also more important than for A/H1N1 and B, we selected A/H3N2 (A/Beij/32/92) to set the susceptibility tests. Then we tested several H3N2 prototypes and a panel of field isolates 1993–2000.

We used the NA enzyme titration and Neuraminidase inhibition [2] test with Zanamivir to determine the IC_{50} NI.

For testing the reduction of virus growth we used a neutralisation test in MDCK. The amount of NP antigen was tested with a capture ELISA test [5].

2. Materials and methods

Cell culture. Madin Darby Canine Kidney (MDCK) cells were purchased from ATCC and routinely passaged in serum-free UltraMDCK medium (BioWhittaker™) supplemented with L-glutamine, 2 mM final concentration.

Virus. Prototypes: influenza A/H3N2 strains came from A.J. Hay (WHO International Collaborating Influenza Center, NIMR, Mill Hill, London, UK)

- A/Beijing/32/92, A/Johannesburg/33/94, A/Nanchang/933/95 egg grown at NIMR were passaged nine times in MDCK cells in infection medium (EMEM BioWhittaker + 1 μg/ml trypsin).
- A/Sydney/5/97, A/Moscow/10/99 have been passaged in the allantoic cavity of 11-day embryonated hen's eggs.

Field strains of human influenza viruses were isolated in MDCK cells from nasal swabs. No one patient has been treated with any anti-viral drug.

The neuraminidase activity (NA) and its inhibition by Zanamivir (GlaxoWellcome) was measured in the NI test using fetuin as substrate and overnight incubation at 37 °C. Zanamivir dilutions ranged from 0.01 to 1000 ng/ml. Each dilution was tested in quadruplicate.

The virus was titrated in MDCK cells grown in 96-well microplates (Nunc), under 10^{-1} to 10^{-7} dilutions in infection medium.

Each dilution was incubated in eight wells containing 100 μl/well of infection medium and microplates were centrifuged at $260 \times g$ for 30 min at 30 °C.

After 24-h incubation at 34 °C, infection medium was replaced and plates incubated for 24 h more. Microplates were read for CPE, hemagglutination (chicken or guinea pig erythrocytes) and NPA/NPB antigen in supernatant medium by ELISA.

In virus growth reduction test, 100 TCID50 of virus giving an $0.530 < OD < 1.136$ at 48 h in NPA ELISA test, were incubated for 1 h at 37 °C with serial concentrations of Zanamivir (0.001–1000 ng/ml). One hundred microliters of each virus/Zanamivir concentration mixture were inoculated to MDCK cells under eight wells and incubated at 34 °C. The infection medium was replaced after 24 h and plates were incubated for 24 h more. The amount of NPA was titrated as previously mentioned. The mean value of OD was calculated for each dilution and the percentage of OD value reduction was deduced by comparison with virus control without Zanamivir. No background was observed ($OD < 0.05$)

3. Results

3.1. Reduction of NA enzyme activity by Zanamivir (NI test)

A/Beijing/32/92 (p9–p10 MDCK) showed a mean neuraminidase enzymatic activity of 1.60 μmol NANA/ml. Virus was diluted in order to give an OD value between 0.425 and 0.700 and tested in six different assays in presence of various concentration of Zanamivir.

The IC_{50} NI determined on the curve is $10^{-3.4}$ μg/ml ($=0.4$ ng/ml) of Zanamivir (Fig. 1). NA activity was completely inhibited by 100 ng/ml Zanamivir.

The reproducibility of the NI test is satisfactory with an IC_{50} regularly found between 0.3 and 0.4 ng/ml. The NA activity and the IC_{50} value of Zanamivir remained stable for 1 year at -20 °C.

3.2. Reduction of virus growth by Zanamivir (NT test)

Results obtained from 11 successive tests with A/Beij/32/92 showed IC_{50} Nt values ranging from 1 to 100 ng/ml Zanamivir and a mean value of 15 ng/ml Zanamivir (Fig. 2).

Moreover, the IC_{50} Nt value greatly varies with the amount of infectious virus used in the test. When we used more than 100 $TCID_{50}$ giving an NPA antigen OD, 48 h post infection, comprised between 0.760 and 1.124, the IC_{50} Nt Zanamivir increased by 600 times (8 μg/ml, mean value of three successive assays).

3.3. Variation in the susceptibility of influenza viruses to Zanamivir

(1) Various prototypes of H3N2 influenza viruses from 1992–1999 have been tested both by NI and Nt tests versus various concentrations of Zanamivir.

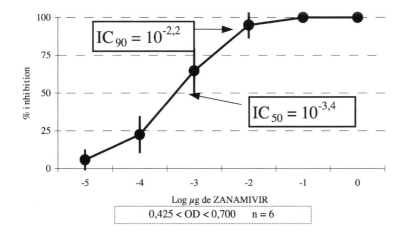

Fig. 1. NI test A/Beijing/32/92 H3N2.

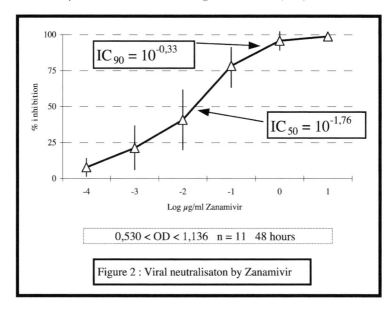

Fig. 2. Viral neutralisation by Zanamivir.

The IC_{50} NI Zanamivir varied from 0.5 to 5 ng/ml, whereas the IC_{50} Nt varies from 3 to 50 ng/ml. But A/Moscow/10/99 showed a reduced susceptibility to Zanamivir with an IC_{50} Nt of 10 μg/ml (Table 1)

(2) A total of 25 H3N2 field strains isolated in MDCK cells from 1993 to 2000, with or without detectable NA enzymatic activity, have been examined.

(2.1) In NI test, strains with a detectable NA enzymatic activity were shown susceptible to Zanamivir, IC_{50} NI varying from 0.08 to 3.5 ng/ml, in the same range as the corresponding prototype strains (Fig. 3).

Table 1
Susceptibility of Influenza virus to Zanamivir

Strains	Plaque inhibition		Neutralisation	NA inhibition	
	(1-2)		(3)	(1-2)	(3)
A/H3N2	0.7 to 565 ng/ml			2.8 ng/ml	
A/Beij/32/92			1 to 100 ng/ml		0.4 ng/ml
Prototypes 1993–97			1 to 50 ng/ml		0.5 to 5 ng/ml
A/Moscow/10/99			1 to 10 μg/ml		
A/H1N1	18 ng/ml to 5.3 μg/ml			0.35 to 0.7 ng/ml	
Prototypes 1991–99			0.5 to 500 ng/ml		1 to 10 ng/ml
B	3.6 to 431 ng/ml			1 ng to 2.8 ng/ml	
Prototypes 1988–94			5 to 50 ng/ml		1 to 10 ng/ml

(1) Woods et al. [14].
(2) Gubarova et al. [8].
(3) Aymard et al. [1].

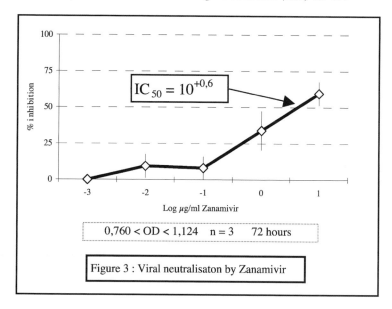

Fig. 3. Viral neutralisation by Zanamivir.

(2.2) In Nt test, we observed a reduced susceptibility to Zanamivir (IC_{50} Nt>1 μg/ml) for both previous and recent isolates, having or not an NA enzymatic activity. A few isolates appeared to be resistant to Zanamivir at concentration over 100 μg/ml. Interestingly, two of these strains, A/Lyon/2063/93 and A/Lyon/7/94, were isolated (1993–1994), before the clinical trials and the marketing of Zanamivir. Both strains had no NA enzymatic activity and exhibited an IC_{50} Nt>100 μg/ml Zanamivir. The sequencing of NA gene [1] did not show any mutation. The sequencing of HA gene showed the existence of five mutations, 47, 121, 124, 133 and 135, the latter one previously identified as associated with Zanamivir resistance [12]. Table 2 summarised results regarding NA activity, Zanamivir susceptibility and NA and HA mutation of five H3N2 strains: A/Beij/32/92, susceptible strain and three different Zanamivir resistant field strains, one of them after either 6 passages in MDCK cells or 6 passages in MDCK cells + 1 passage in embryonated eggs.

Table 2
Comparison of NA activity, Zanamivir susceptibility, and HA/NA mutations of different H3N2 strains

Virus	NA activity	IC50 NI	IC50 Nt	Mutation NA (E119 residue)	Mutation HA (G135 residue)
A/Beij/32/92	+	0.4 ng/ml	17 ng/ml	consensus	consensus
A/Lyon/2036/93	−	NA	>100 μg/ml	0	G 135 K
A/Lyon/493/95	+	0.1 to 1 ng/ml	100 μg/ml	0	G 135 K
A/Lyon/7/94 MDCK	−	NA	>100 μg/ml	0	0
A/Lyon/7/94 MDCK + Egg	+	4 ng/ml	6 μg/ml	0	0

NA: not applicable.

4. Discussion

As the neuraminidase inhibitors have been designed to inhibit the enzymatic activity and consequently to reduce influenza virus multiplication and spread in the respiratory tract, the neuraminidase inhibition test might be the optimal technique for investigating either susceptibility or resistance of influenza viruses to drugs. And this investigation has to be done since influenza viruses may vary (through genetic mutations) in their antiviral susceptibility as they vary in antigenic characteristics and other functions. Increasing use of anti-neuraminidase inhibitors, which may result in an increasing selection pressure, is expected.

The classical neuraminidase inhibition test designed for the titration of anti neuraminidase antibodies could be applied to anti-neuraminidase inhibitors. Nevertheless, 8–10% of A/H3N2 influenza virus isolated in 1993–1995 showing poor if any NA enzymatic activity and most of the A/H1N1 influenza viruses isolates (1993–2000) showing no or very poor enzymatic activity in MDCK cells, it was interesting to develop a substitution test for measuring virus growth inhibition that would be easier to perform than the plaque reduction test.

A neutralisation test in 96-well microplates was performed associated with a quantification of virus growth based on NP-ELISA titration; such a test was shown to be sensitive and reproducible, with a reading adaptable to automation.

With the exception of the A/Moscow/10/99 strain, all A/H3N2, A/H1N1 and B prototype strains exhibited a rather constant susceptibility to Zanamivir when tested in both NI (IC_{50} NI < 10 ng/ml) and Nt (IC_{50} Nt < 500 ng/ml) tests. We wish to propose a preliminary definition of in vitro antiviral susceptibility in Nt test: (i) < 1 μg/ml Zanamivir = susceptible, (ii) between 1 and 100 μg/ml Zanamivir = reduced, (iii) >100 μg/ml Zanamivir = resistant.

It is interesting to note that in vivo, at the maximal single orally dose of 500-mg Zanamivir, only 3 μg/ml was found in throat gargles 1 h after administration [4]. Among the 25 field strains analysed, all strains exhibiting NA activity were susceptible, seven strains showed a reduced susceptibility and six strains were shown to be Zanamivir-resistant.

Several natural variants were compared in terms of NA activity, Zanamivir (NI test–Nt test) and mutations in HA gene (G135 residue) and NA gene (E119 residue). Two strains showed a mutation in HA gene 135 residue (G to K) while change previously mentioned by Penn et al. [12] in variants selected with Zanamivir was a substitution G135D. When examining the NA gene, no substitution was detected in our natural variants and the E119 residue previously described by Gubarva et al. [6] and Mckimm-Breschkin et al. [10] as participating in the specific interaction between the enzyme and the inhibitor, remained unchanged.

The profile of the A/Lyon/493/95 strain appeared highly similar to that of the AS4+ variant selected by Penn et al. [12] after several passages in the presence of Zanamivir. In such viruses a change in HA gene (135 residue) might confer an apparent resistance to Zanamivir in terms of growth inhibition in vitro but not in vivo [3]. Regarding the A/Lyon/2063/93 strain whose profile is similar to A/Lyon/493/95 with the exception of an absence of NA activity, the resistance observed in vitro in the Nt test could be related to the 135 mutation in HA gene; nevertheless due to the absence of a target for the drug, the question of a potential in vivo resistance could be asked. Arguments for an in vivo resistance to Zanamivir of strains devoided of NA activity are brought by the comparative analysis of the A/Lyon/7/94 strain grown in either MDCK or in MDCK with an additional passage in eggs. The A/Lyon/7/94 (MDCK) strain did not show any mutation in HA (135) or NA (119) genes but it appeared as resistant to Zanamivir in Nt test. Such a resistance can be directly associated with the absence of NA activity. Interestingly, after one passage in eggs, this strain recovered simultaneously NA activity and Zanamivir susceptibility.

It is difficult at present to evaluate the impact of NA-deficient natural strains on the clinical use of Zanamivir. Indeed, several points might be considered: (i) the frequency of NA deficient natural strain, (ii) the spontaneous emergence of NA-deficient strains during human infection, (iii) the efficacy of the NA-deficient strains to generate clinical infection.

References

[1] M. Aymard, L. Gerentes, M. Valette, J. Millon-Jolly, B. Lina, N. Kessler, Variation in neuraminidase activity of wild strains of influenza A H3N2 grown in MDCK, Proceeding of Options for the Control of Influenza III, Cairns, Australia, 1996, Elsevier, Amsterdam, pp. 485–490.

[2] M. Aymard-Henry, M.T. Coleman, W.R. Dowdle, V.G. Laver, G.C. Schild, R.G. Webster, Influenza virus neuraminidase and neuraminidase inhibition test procedures, Bull. WHO 48 (1973) 199–202.

[3] J.M. Barnett, A. Cadman, D. Gor, M. Dempsey, M. Walters, A. Candlin, M. Tisdale, P.J. Morley, I.J. Owens, R.J. Fenton, A.P. Lewis, E.C. Claas, G.F. Rimmelzwaan, R. De Groot, A.D. Osterhaus, Zanamivir susceptibility monitoring and characterization of influenza virus clinical isolates obtained during phase II clinical efficacy studies, Antimicrob. Agents Chemother. 44 (1) (2000 Jan) 78–87.

[4] L.M.R. Cass, C. Efthymiopoulos, A. Bye, Pharmacokinetics of Zanamivir after intravenous, oral inhaled or intranasal administration to healthy volunters, Clin. Pharmacokinet. 36 (1999) S1.

[5] J.J. Chomel, D. Thouvenot, M. Onno, C. Kaiser, J.M. Gourreau, M. Aymard, Rapid diagnosis of influenza infection of NP antigen using an immunocapture ELISA test, J. Virol. Methods 25 (1) (1989 Jul) 81–91.

[6] L.V. Gubareva, R.C. Bethell, C.R. Penn, G.R. Webster, In vitro characterization of 4-guanidino-Neu 5-Ac2en-resistant mutants of influenza virus, Options for the Control of Influenza III, Cairns, Australia, 1996, Elsevier, Amsterdam, pp. 753–760.

[7] L.V. Gubareva, L. Kaiser, F.G. Hayden, Influenza virus neuraminidase inhibitors, Lancet 355 (9206) (2000 Mar. 4) 827–835.

[8] L.V. Gubareva, C.R. Penn, R.G. Webster, Inhibition of replication of avian influenza viruses by the neuraminidase inhibitor 4-guanidino-2,4-dideoxy-2,3-dehydro-N-acetylneuraminic acid, Virology 212 (2) (1995 Oct. 1) 323–330.

[9] F.G. Hayden, J.J. Treanor, R.F. Betts, M. Lobo, J.D. Esinhart, E.K. Hussey, Safety and efficacy of the neuraminidase inhibitor GG167 in experimental human influenza, JAMA 275 (4) (1996 Jan. 24–31) 295–299.

[10] J.L. Mckimm-Breschkin, T.J. Blick, A.A. Sahasrabudhe, J.N. Varghese, R.C. Bethell, G.J. Hart, C.R. Penn, P.M. Colman, Influenza virus variants with decrease sensitivity to 4-amino 4-guanidino-2,4-dideoxy-N-acetylneuraminic acid, Options for the Control of Influenza III, Cairns, Australia, 1996, Elsevier, Amsterdam, pp. 726–734.

[11] A.S. Monto, A. Webster, O. Keene, Randomized, placebo-controlled studies of inhaled zanamivir in the treatment of influenza A and B: pooled efficacy analysis, J. Antimicrob. Chemother. 44 (suppl. B) (1999 Nov) 23–29.

[12] C.R. Penn, J.M. Barnett, R.C. Bethell, R. Fenton, K.L. Gearing, N. Healy, A.J. Jowett, Selection of

Influenza virus with reduced sensitivity in votro to the neuraminidase inhibitor GG167 (4-guanidino-2,4-dideoxy-*N*-acetylneuraminic acid) changes in heamagglutinin may compensate for loss of neuraminidase activity, Options for the Control of Influenza III, Cairns, Australia, 1996, Elsevier, Amsterdam, pp. 735–740.

[13] G.P. Thomas, M. Forsyth, C.R. Penn, J.W. Mccauley, Inhibition of the growth of influenza viruses in vitro by 4-guanidino-2,4-dideoxy-*N*-acetylneuraminic acid, Antiviral Res. 24 (4) (1994 Aug) 351–356.

[14] J.M. Woods, R.C. Bethell, J.A. Coates, N. Healy, S.A. Hiscox, B.A. Pearson, D.M. Ryan, et al., 4-Guanidino-2,4-dideoxy-2,3-dehydro-*N*-acetylneuraminic acid is a highly effective inhibitor both of the sialidase (neuraminidase) and of growth of a wide range of influenza A and B viruses in vitro, Antimicrob. Agents Chemother. 37 (7) (1993 Jul) 1473–1479.

Future prospects for improved control

International Congress Series 1219 (2001) 897–903

DNA vaccination with HA or NP encoding plasmids results in rapid viral clearance after viral challenge

Rebecca J. Cox*, Eva Mykkeltvedt, Lars R. Haaheim

Department of Molecular Biology, University of Bergen, N-5020 Bergen, Norway

Abstract

Background: A relevant model for studying the efficacy of DNA vaccines is to examine viral replication in the nasal cavity after non-lethal viral challenge. In this study, we have investigated the humoral cell response after viral challenge of mice vaccinated with plasmids encoding the HA or NP genes. *Methods*: Seven-week-old BALB/c mice were immunised intramuscularly with three doses (100 μg) of HA, NP or backbone plasmid at 3-week intervals and challenged intranasally with homologous virus 13 weeks later. Mice were sacrificed and the antibody secreting cell response was examined systemically and in the respiratory tract. Serum antibody was analysed by haemagglutination inhibition and virus neutralisation assays. *Results*: DNA vaccination with HA and NP encoding plasmids significantly reduced viral replication in the nasal cavity. Antibody secreting cells were maintained in the systemic compartment after vaccination but upon viral challenge were located in the nasal associated lymphoid tissue. *Conclusion*: Intramuscular DNA vaccination resulted in immunological memory in the systemic compartment, which was rapidly reactivated upon viral challenge. © 2001 Elsevier Science B.V. All rights reserved.

Keywords: DNA vaccination; HA or NP encoding plasmids; Rapid viral clearance; Viral challenge

1. Introduction

The protective efficacy of current influenza vaccines depends on the antigenic match between the vaccine strains and those circulating in the community. Thus, annual vaccination is required to combat antigenic drift and there is therefore a need for improved influenza vaccines to provide a broader and longer-lasting immunity.

---

* Corresponding author. Tel.: +47-55584385; fax: +47-55589683.
E-mail address: Rebecca.Cox@mbi.uib.no (R.J. Cox).

0531-5131/01/$ – see front matter © 2001 Elsevier Science B.V. All rights reserved.
PII: S 0 5 3 1 - 5 1 3 1 (0 1) 0 0 3 6 6 - 1

DNA vaccines are a promising new approach to vaccination, eliciting a full spectrum of immune responses including antibody, cytotoxic and helper T cell responses. In 1992, protective immunity was first demonstrated in mice immunised with a DNA vaccine encoding the NP of influenza virus [1]. Subsequently, extensive development has occurred in the field of DNA vaccines with protection demonstrated to many different pathogens in animal models (reviewed in Ref. [2]) and DNA vaccines have now moved into human clinical trials. Influenza DNA vaccines have been extensively studied and constructs encoding NP, HA, NA, M1, and NS1 have all been tested for their ability to induce immune responses [1,3–7].

In this study, we have examined the immune response in the systemic and local compartments after viral challenge with a non-lethal influenza strain in mice vaccinated intramuscularly (i.m.) with HA or NP DNA vaccines. Immunisation with HA plasmids is thought to provide protection by humoral immunity involving neutralising antibodies, although recently a role for Th1 cells has been suggested in protective immunity [3], whereas both cytotoxic CD8+ and cytokine producing CD4+ cells provide protective immunity after i.m. NP DNA vaccination [4].

2. Materials and methods

2.1. Plasmids

Plasmids p1.17 HA, p1.18 NP and p1.18 backbone plasmid were kindly supplied by Dr. J. Robertson (NIBSC, UK).

2.2. Study

Twenty BALB/c mice (7 weeks old) per group were immunised intramuscularly into the quadricep muscles (50 µl per hindleg) with three doses of 100 µg HA or NP expressing plasmid or control backbone plasmid at 3-week intervals. Immunised mice were challenged intranasally with mouse adapted A/Sichuan/2/87 (H3N2) (25 µl 33 MID_{50}) virus 13 weeks after receiving the third dose of vaccine. The mice were awake when intranasally inoculated with a small volume of virus (25 µl), which results in an almost exclusively upper respiratory tract infection. Serum samples were collected pre-vaccination, after each dose of vaccine and at sacrifice (0, 7, 14, 21 and 28 days after challenge) to examine the antibody response using haemagglutination inhibition (HI) and virus neutralisation (VN) assays. The kinetics of the antibody secreting cell (ASC) response were examined in the spleen, bone marrow, lungs and nasal associated lymphoid tissue (NALT) using the ELISPOT assay. Nasal wash samples were analysed for the presence of infectious virus at days 2, 4 and 6 post-infection (p.i.) in MDCK cells.

2.3. Statistics

Student's *t*-test was performed using SPSS for Windows (version 10).

3. Results

3.1. Viral challenge of DNA vaccinated mice

In this study we have immunised mice with 100 μg HA, NP or control plasmid three times at 3-week intervals and challenged by intranasal infection with a non-lethal mouse adapted virus 13 weeks after the third dose of vaccine. We found that the antibody response increased after each dose of vaccine and significantly increased after infection (results not shown).

3.2. Presence of replicative virus in the nasal wash

Nasal wash virus was detected in all of the control mice at all time points (except five mice at 2 days p.i.), whereas only very low nasal wash titres were detected in the HA and NP immunised mice. The control mice had significantly higher ($p < 0.05$ Student's t-test) nasal wash virus titres at 4 days p.i. than the HA or NP immunised groups. Three mice in the HA immunised group and one mouse in the NP group were completely protected from infection with no viral shedding.

3.3. The ASC response after viral challenge

The ELISPOT assay was used to investigate the ASC response after viral challenge to two different antigenic formulations, whole influenza virus and purified NP. The ASC response was investigated in the systemic compartment (spleen and bone marrow) and the local compartment (NALT and lungs, representing the upper respiratory tract [8] and lower respiratory tract, respectively).

3.3.1. Systemic ASC response

Prior to challenge influenza specific ASC were found in the spleen and bone marrow of the HA and NP immunised mice, whereas no ASC were detected in the control group (Table 1). In the HA and NP immunised groups, the numbers of ASC increased in the spleen and bone marrow and peaked at 14 days after viral challenge. In contrast, the lowest number of influenza and NP specific ASC were found in the control group after viral challenge (range 0–11 specific ASC per 500,000 lymphocytes).

3.3.2. Respiratory tract ASC response

No or very low numbers of ASC (1–3 specific ASC per 500,000 lymphocytes) were detected in the lungs or NALT prior to challenge in all mice (Table 1). In all groups, only low numbers of ASC were detected in the lung, except influenza specific ASC in the NP group on days 14 and 21 p.i. Due to the low numbers of cells harvested from the NALT, we only investigated the IgA ASC response. The highest numbers of ASC were found in the NALT and the number of IgA ASC peaked at 7 days p.i. in all groups, the number of ASC were similar in all groups except one mouse in the HA group which had a very high number of ASC (575 specific ASC per 500,000 lymphocytes). Generally, a similar time course of appearance of ASC in the NALT and lungs was observed in the three groups.

Table 1
The presence of influenza and NP specific ASC after viral challenge in mice immunised with HA or NP DNA

Vaccine	Tissue	Antigen	Days post-infection				
			0	7	14	21	28
NP	Spleen	Influenza	+	++	++	++	++
HA			+	++	+++	+	++
Control			−	+	+	+	+
NP		NP	+	++	++	++	++
HA			−	*	+	*	+
Control			−	+	+	*	*
NP	Bone marrow	Influenza	−	+	+	+	++
HA			+	+	+	+	+
Control			−	*	−	*	−
NP		NP	+	+	+++	+	+
HA			*	*	+	*	+
Control			−	*	*	*	*
NP	Lung	Influenza	*	+	++	++	+
HA			*	+	+	*	*
Control			−	+	+	*	*
NP		NP	−	+	*	+	+
HA			−	+	+	−	*
Control			−	+	−	−	*
NP	NALT	Influenza	−	+++	++	−	+
HA			−	+++	++	+++	−
Control			−	+++	++	+	−

The table refers to the number of total (IgG, IgA and IgM) influenza specific ASC per 500,000 lymphocytes, where − no detected ASC, * >1–5 influenza specific ASC, + >5–20 influenza specific ASC, ++ >20–50 influenza specific ASC and +++ >50 influenza specific ASC. Only influenza specific IgA ASC were measured in the NALT. There were 3–4 mice in each group at each time point.

3.3.3. Class and subclass of ASC response

IgG and IgA predominated in the HA and NP immunised groups, whereas IgM was more common in the control group (results not shown). IgG2a ASC were found in the highest number in the HA and NP groups; however, similar numbers of IgG2a and IgG1 ASC were often detected in the control mice. In the NP group, the highest number of ASC were detected towards the NP antigen, whereas much higher numbers of influenza specific ASC were detected in the HA immunised group.

3.4. The serum HI and VN antibody response

Serum samples were collected at sacrifice and analysed by the HI and VN tests. The HI and VN antibody responses were higher in the HA immunised group than in the NP and control groups (Fig. 1). In the HA immunised group, HI and VN antibodies were detected 7 days p.i. and continued to increase up to days 28 p.i., although one mouse had an HI titre of 64 pre-challenge. In contrast, only low concentrations of HI and VN antibodies were

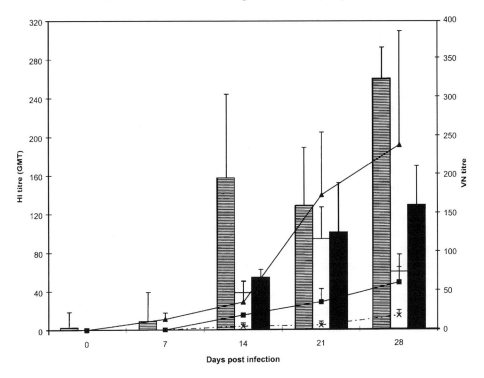

Fig. 1. The HI and VN antibody titres after viral challenge of HA and NP DNA immunised mice. The bars represent the HI antibody titre in the mice immunised with HA (grey striped bar), NP (clear bar) and control (shaded bar) plasmids. The lines represent the VN titres in the mice immunised with HA (solid line, triangle), NP (dashed line, cross) and control (solid line, square) plasmids. The bars represent the standard error of the mean. There were 3–4 mice in each group at each time point.

detected in the NP and control groups from 14 days p.i. Interestingly, the HI and VN titres were lower in the NP immunised group than the control group, probably reflecting more limited viral replication in the NP group.

4. Discussion

The use of influenza DNA vaccines has shown promising results in animal models. The majority of influenza DNA vaccine studies have investigated protection by examining the survival of mice after a lethal viral challenge. Therefore, in our study we examined the humoral response after viral challenge using a non-lethal virus that produces a limited upper respiratory tract infection.

Influenza and NP specific ASC were maintained systemically in the bone marrow and spleen after i.m. immunisation with HA or NP DNA and were reactivated, particularly in the spleen, upon viral challenge. Similarly, gene gun immunisation with HA DNA results in both initial and long-term maintenance of influenza specific ASC in these tissues

[9,10]. The appearance of IgA ASC in the NALT results in the production of sIgA and viral clearance [8]. We found that upon viral challenge, the highest numbers of ASC were found at the site of viral challenge (in the NALT) and appearance of ASC followed a similar time course in all three groups. Generally, only low numbers of ASC were found in the lungs after viral challenge, which is probably due to the viral infection being limited to the upper respiratory tract. The control mice had a primary immune response producing mainly IgM ASC, whereas IgG and IgA were commonly found in the HA and NP vaccinated mice. The presence of ASC and the class has been found previously to require CD4+ cells [9].

In our study, DNA immunisation induced a Th1 type response (dominant IgG2a antibody response and the production of IL-2 and IFN-γ, results not shown). This has been commonly observed after i.m. vaccination with DNA vaccines [3,4] and natural viral infection [3] and contrasts with the typical Th2 type response produced after immunisation with protein vaccines (reviewed in Ref. [11]). The IgG2a/IgG1 ratio and Th1 cytokine concentrations were higher in the HA and NP vaccinated groups after viral challenge than after vaccination, suggesting an increased polarisation of the response to Th1 after challenge.

We found that priming with HA or NP DNA resulted in virtually no viral replication in the upper respiratory tract. Despite no HI antibody titres (except 1 mouse) being found before viral challenge in the HA immunised group, much higher HI and VN titres were observed in this group than in the other groups showing priming of memory B cells by HA DNA vaccination. Repeated immunisation with HA DNA has been found necessary to generate a persistent Th1 response [3] and is probably also necessary to generate a memory B cell response.

In conclusion, immunisation with HA or NP DNA vaccines resulted in priming, which upon viral challenge resulted in significant reduction in viral replication. Our results, in combination with other studies, show the possible role DNA vaccines can have as a priming vehicle in control of influenza virus.

Acknowledgements

We wish to thank Dr. Jim Robertson and Carolyn Nicolson (NIBSC, UK) for kindly supplying the plasmids. This work was supported by the EU Biotechnology programme (EU Bio4-CT96-0637).

References

[1] J.B. Ulmer, J.J. Donnelly, S.E. Parker, G.H. Rhodes, P.L. Felgner, V.J. Dwarki, S.H. Gromkowski, R.R. Deck, C.M. DeWitt, A. Friedman, et al., Heterologous protection against influenza by injection of DNA encoding a viral protein, Science 259 (5102) (1993) 1745–1749.

[2] D.W. Kowalczyk, H.C. Ertl, Immune responses to DNA vaccines, Cell Mol. Life Sci. 55 (5) (1999) 751–770.

[3] P.A. Johnson, M.A. Conway, J. Daly, C. Nicolson, J. Robertson, K.H. Mills, Plasmid DNA encoding influenza virus haemagglutinin induces Th1 cells and protection against respiratory infection despite its limited ability to generate antibody responses, J. Gen. Virol. 81 (Pt. 7) (July 2000) 1737.

[4] J.B. Ulmer, T.M. Fu, R.R. Deck, A. Friedman, L. Guan, C. DeWitt, X. Liu, S. Wang, M.A. Liu, J.J. Donnelly, M.J. Caulfield, Protective CD4+ and CD8+ T cells against influenza virus induced by vaccination with nucleoprotein DNA, J. Virol. 72 (7) (1998) 5648–5653.

[5] Z. Chen, Y. Sahashi, K. Matsuo, H. Asanuma, H. Takahashi, T. Iwasaki, Y. Suzuki, C. Aizawa, T. Kurata, S. Tamura, Comparison of the ability of viral protein-expressing plasmid DNAs to protect against influenza, Vaccine 16 (16) (1998) 1544–1549.

[6] J.J. Donnelly, A. Friedman, J.B. Ulmer, M.A. Liu, Further protection against antigenic drift of influenza virus in a ferret model by DNA vaccination, Vaccine 15 (8) (June 1997) 865–868.

[7] H.L. Robinson, C.A. Boyle, D.M. Feltquate, M.J. Morin, J.C. Santoro, R.G. Webster, DNA immunization for influenza virus: studies using hemagglutinin- and nucleoprotein-expressing DNAs, J. Infect. Dis. 176 (Suppl. 1) (August 1997) S50.

[8] S. Tamura, T. Iwasaki, A.H. Thompson, H. Asanuma, Z. Chen, Y. Suzuki, C. Aizawa, T. Kurata, Antibody-forming cells in the nasal-associated lymphoid tissue during primary influenza virus infection, J. Gen. Virol. 79 (1998) 291–299.

[9] D.M. Justewicz, M.J. Morin, H.L. Robinson, R.G. Webster, Antibody-forming cell response to virus challenge in mice immunized with DNA encoding the influenza virus hemagglutinin, J. Virol. 69 (12) (1995) 7712–7717.

[10] D.M. Justewicz, R.G. Webster, Long-term maintenance of B cell immunity to influenza virus hemagglutinin in mice following DNA-based immunization, Virology 224 (1) (1996) 10–17.

[11] B.P. Mahon, A. Moore, P.A. Johnson, K.H. Mills, Approaches to new vaccines, Crit. Rev. Biotechnol. 18 (4) (1998) 257–282.

International Congress Series 1219 (2001) 905–910

Vaccination with DNA encoding conserved influenza viral proteins

Suzanne L. Epstein[a,*], Abigail Stack[a], Julia A. Misplon[a],
Chia-Yun Lo[a], Howard Mostowski[a], Jack Bennink[b],
Kimberly A. Benton[a], Lynn Cooper[c], Athene Hodges[a],
Kanta Subbarao[c]

[a]*Laboratory of Immunology and Developmental Biology, Division of Cellular and Gene Therapies,
Center for Biologics Evaluation and Research, Food and Drug Administration, Bethesda, MD, USA*
[b]*Laboratory of Viral Diseases, Viral Immunology Section, National Institute of Allergy and Infectious Diseases,
National Institutes of Health, Bethesda, MD, USA*
[c]*Influenza Branch, Centers for Disease Control and Prevention, Atlanta, GA, USA*

Abstract

Background: DNA vaccines encoding conserved antigens of influenza A virus can induce broad cross-protection against multiple influenza A subtypes. Better understanding of the mechanisms of this protection can help guide vaccine development. *Methods*: Mice were vaccinated with plasmids expressing nucleoprotein (NP) and matrix (M) given i.m., followed by lethal i.n. challenge with influenza virus. CTL were analyzed by ^{51}Cr-release using fresh lung lymphocytes. *Results*: A/NP + A/ M vaccination promoted viral clearance and led to recovery, at challenge virus doses that were lethal to controls. CD8+ CTL were induced and were highly specific for influenza A antigens, but were not required for protection. Depletion of both CD4+ and CD8+ T cells during the challenge period abrogated protection. A plasmid expressing influenza B/NP was used to demonstrate specificity of antibodies produced and of protection against influenza B vs. A challenge. *Discussion*: DNA vaccination gave protection corresponding to the influenza A vs. B inserted genes, confirming immunological specificity. For A/NP + A/M DNA, T cells are required, but either CD4+ or CD8+ T cells protected in the absence of the other subset. These findings about DNA vaccines encoding antigens conserved among viral subtypes can be applied to human vaccine development for protection against new pandemic viruses. © 2001 Elsevier Science B.V. All rights reserved.

Keywords: DNA vaccines; Viral immunity; T lymphocytes; Mice; Protective immunity

---

* Corresponding author. FDA, CBER, OTRR, DCGT, 1401 Rockville Pike HFM-521, Rockville, MD 20852-1448, USA. Tel.: +1-301-827-0450; fax: +1-301-827-0449.
E-mail address: epsteins@cber.fda.gov (S.L. Epstein).

1. Introduction

Current influenza vaccines provide considerable public health benefit but are imperfect, both in the nature of the immunity they confer and the practical problems of their production. For instance, in the year 2000, there were difficulties in growing adequate amounts of vaccine strains in eggs, leading to a delay in the planned fall vaccination campaign (http://www.cdc.gov/od/oc/media/pressrel/r2k0622a.htm). If a more broadly protective vaccine could be developed, production would not be tied so tightly to seasonal strain surveillance and predictions about epidemic strains. DNA vaccination using constructs expressing conserved influenza virus proteins is one way to elicit such cross-protection. Such constructs avoid the practical difficulties of vaccine production in eggs and so could be available consistently.

In early studies, DNA vaccination with NP was shown to induce both antibody and CTL responses and to provide protection against lethal challenge [1,2]. Later, combination DNA vaccines encoding NP, M, and hemagglutinin (HA) were studied [3]. A better understanding of the mechanisms of protection by such vaccinations is valuable in guiding vaccine design, optimization of immunization protocols, and the choice of endpoints to monitor in preclinical and clinical trials. We have analyzed the mechanisms of protective immunity induced by plasmids expressing A/NP and A/M proteins, and have tested the specificity of DNA vaccination to influenza using A/NP and B/NP DNA. Results suggest that DNA vaccines expressing conserved components may be a useful part of vaccination strategies.

2. Materials and methods (for further details, see Ref. [4])

2.1. Viruses

Influenza virus strains used were A/PR/8/34 (PR/8, H1N1), B/Ann Arbor/1/86 (B/AA) and A/Philippines/2/82/X-79 (A/Phil; H3N2), which is a reassortant virus with the HA and neuraminidase (NA) genes of A/Philippines/2/82 origin, and the NP and M genes of A/PR/8/34.

2.2. Plasmids

The plasmid VR1012 was obtained from Vical. As described previously [4], influenza NP and M genes from PR/8 were inserted. The plasmid B/NP expresses the full-length NP gene from B/AA subcloned into VR1012 from a baculovirus vector generated by Rota et al. [5].

2.3. Mice

BALB/cAnNCr mice were purchased from the Division of Cancer Treatment, NCI and immunized starting at 6–7 weeks of age.

2.4. Virus quantitation

Influenza virus was quantitated by titration on Madin–Darby canine kidney cells using cytopathic effect as the indicator of presence of virus [6], with results given in tissue culture infectious dose$_{50}$ (TCID$_{50}$) units.

2.5. Immunizations

DNA was injected i.m. in the quadriceps of mice with three doses (100 µg of each plasmid) given i.m. 2 weeks apart. Challenges were done i.n. under anesthesia. In vivo depletions were done by i.p. injection of ascites containing monoclonal antibodies [4].

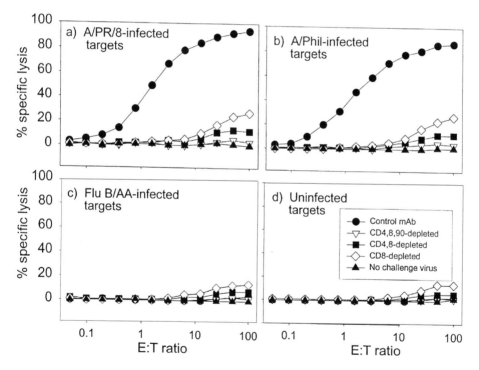

Fig. 1. Cytolytic activity in the lungs of vaccinated mice following challenge. Mice were immunized i.m. three times at intervals of 2 weeks with 100 µg each of A/NP and A/M DNA. They were challenged 2 weeks after the third immunization with A/H3N2 i.n. under anesthesia. T cell depletions on days − 3, − 1, + 2, + 5, + 7, and + 11 relative to challenge used ascites fluids of SFR3-DR5 (control), GK1.5 (anti-CD4), 2.43 (anti-CD8), and 30-H12 (anti-CD90). Solid circles, SFR3-3D5; open diamonds, 2.43; solid squares, GK1.5 + 2.43; open triangles, GK1.5 + 2.43 + 30-H12; solid triangles, no challenge virus. Lungs for CTL analyses were taken 7 days after challenge. Lymphocytes were pooled from six mice per group, and assayed for CTL activity on P815 target cells, uninfected or infected with indicated viruses. Panels a and b were published previously [4], and we acknowledge Oxford University Press for permission to reproduce them.

2.6. CTL assay

Cytotoxic activity was measured in fresh lung lymphocytes after virus challenge without in vitro restimulation, as described [7,8]. P815 cells (H-2^d, MHC class I positive, class II negative) infected with indicated viruses were used as targets. Effectors were incubated with targets for 6 h before harvest.

3. Results

Like previous authors [1,2], we observed that vaccination with DNA encoding conserved antigens NP and M of influenza A, but not empty vector, protected against lethal influenza A challenge, when challenge virus matched the virus strain from which the genes were derived and also with heterosubtypic challenge virus. NP + M vaccination did not completely prevent infection, but prevented mortality.

CTL have long been considered critical components of the protective response to influenza induced by virus [9] or by DNA vaccination [2]. We tested their role in protection by DNA encoding NP and M antigens. In vivo depletion at the time of challenge was used to analyze the need for CD4+ or CD8+ T cells during the effector phase, with completeness of depletion monitored by flow cytometry [4]. Note that a role of CD4+ cells in providing initial help for antibody responses would occur during priming and is unaffected by the later depletion. Unexpectedly, depletion of CD8+ T cells had no significant effect on protection, nor did depletion of CD4+ cells. CTL of course may play a

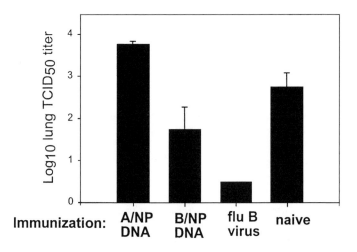

Fig. 2. BALB/c mice were immunized three times with 100 μg of DNA i.m. at 2-week intervals, or once with 10^3 TCID$_{50}$ of influenza B/AA virus i.n., at the time of the first DNA dose. Mice were challenged 2 weeks after the last DNA dose with 5×10^4 TCID$_{50}$ units of influenza B/AA i.n. Lungs were removed on day 6, homogenized, frozen, and titer of virus assayed by TCID$_{50}$.

role, but under these conditions they were not required. Depletion of both subsets abrogated protection [4]. These results show that either CD4+ or CD8+ T cells acting without the other subset can mediate protection, perhaps along with other effectors, such as antibodies, that are not themselves sufficient without some T cells.

The CTL responses were examined in more detail, to confirm complete depletion by anti-CD8. The physiologically relevant CTL populations were studied, namely those present in the lungs of DNA-vaccinated mice during the response to challenge infection. As shown in Fig. 1, very strong cytolytic activity was seen with lung lymphocytes from DNA-vaccinated mice not depleted of any T cells ("control mAb" in panels a and b). The cytolysis was specific, showing only very low levels of lysis on uninfected or influenza B-infected targets (panels c and d), but was reactive with both A/H1N1 and A/H3N2-infected targets. Depletion of CD8+ cells in vivo reduced lytic activity by about 128-fold, and the slight residual activity was partially non-specific.

In the studies described above, a plasmid vector with no inserted gene was used to control for nonspecific effects. As an additional control, we made a construct expressing the NP protein of influenza B virus. This plasmid did not protect against influenza A challenge (data not shown), as would be predicted by the degree of divergence between influenza B and A. But is the influenza B/NP construct active at all? The B/NP construct induced antibodies detectable by ELISA on plates coated with lysates of influenza B-infected cells (data not shown). In addition, as shown in Fig. 2, the B/NP construct protected against influenza B challenge, while A/NP DNA did not.

4. Discussion

Vaccination with NP + M DNA against influenza challenge offers the potential for broad cross-protection without the risks and problems of live virus. A/NP and B/NP constructs showed reciprocal specificity in challenge experiments. Thus, non-specific effects such as those mediated by CpG motifs do not play a significant role in protection. A vector expressing an irrelevant foreign protein, like influenza B NP, provides a better control than an "empty vector" because it triggers cytokine production and various immune responses, though they are not specific for challenge virus. The specificity of protection thus demonstrates true specificity based on antibody or T cell receptor binding sites. T cell depletion showed that T cells were necessary during the challenge period, but either CD4+ or CD8+ T cells were sufficient for protection without the other subset.

While there are other possibilities [4], CD8+ T cells most likely operate as CTL. What could CD4+ T cells be doing? One reasonable possibility is that primed helper cells accelerate and augment the antibody response to the new antigens presented by challenge virus upon infection. The protective response could also include a contribution from antibodies to the portion of M2 accessible on the virion surface, a known epitope for antibodies inhibiting viral replication [10]. Antibodies existing at the time of challenge are not sufficient on their own, though, since T cell depletion abrogates protection. Future studies will further explore the possible roles of these various effectors.

Whether DNA vaccines will be as effective in humans as in animals and whether they will have practical advantages remains to be seen. The limitations of existing vaccines make it important that we study this alternative approach. In mice, NP + M protected against viruses as divergent in their HA and NA proteins (H1N1 and H3N2) as any circulating human strains and more divergent than is avian H5N1 from H1N1 [11]. If these vaccines induce responses in humans reactive with all influenza A strains, they could contribute to a universal vaccine strategy and to pandemic preparedness.

Acknowledgements

This work was supported in part by a grant from the National Vaccine Program to S.E. We thank Anthony Ferrine and other CBER animal care staff for expert animal care, and Drs. Steven Bauer and Lisa Rider for critical review.

References

[1] G.H. Rhodes, V.J. Dwarki, A.M. Abai, J. Felgner, P.L. Felgner, S.H. Gromkowski, S.E. Parker, Injection of expression vectors containing viral genes induces cellular, humoral, and protective immunity, in: R.M. Chanock, F. Brown, H.S. Ginsberg, E. Norrby (Eds.), Vaccines 93, Cold Spring Harbor Laboratory Press, Cold Spring Harbor, NY, 1993, pp. 137–141.

[2] J.B. Ulmer, J.J. Donnelly, S.E. Parker, G.H. Rhodes, P.L. Felgner, V.J. Dwarki, S.H. Gromkowski, R.R. Deck, C.M. DeWitt, A. Friedman, L.A. Hawe, K.R. Leander, D. Martinez, H.C. Perry, J.W. Shiver, D.L. Montgomery, M.A. Liu, Heterologous protection against influenza by injection of DNA encoding a viral protein, Science 259 (1993) 1745–1749.

[3] J.J. Donnelly, A. Friedman, D. Martinez, D.L. Montgomery, J.W. Shiver, S.L. Motzel, J.B. Ulmer, M.A. Liu, Preclinical efficacy of a prototype DNA vaccine: enhanced protection against antigenic drift in influenza virus, Nat. Med. 1 (1995) 583–587.

[4] S.L. Epstein, A. Stack, J.A. Misplon, C.-Y. Lo, J. Bennink, K. Subbarao, Vaccination with DNA encoding internal proteins of influenza virus does not require CD8 + CTL: either CD4+ or CD8+ T cells can promote survival and recovery after challenge, Int. Immunol. 12 (2000) 91–101.

[5] P.A. Rota, R.A. Black, B.K. De, M.W. Harmon, A.P. Kendal, Expression of influenza A and B virus nucleoprotein antigens in baculovirus, J. Gen. Virol. 71 (1990) 1545–1554.

[6] M.H. Snyder, R.F. Betts, D. DeBorde, E.L. Tierney, M.L. Clements, D. Herrington, S.D. Sears, R. Dolin, H.F. Maassab, B.R. Murphy, Four viral genes independently contribute to attenuation of live influenza A/ Ann Arbor/6/60 (H2N2) cold-adapted reassortant virus vaccines, J. Virol. 62 (1988) 488–495.

[7] C.M. Lawson, J.R. Bennink, N.P. Restifo, J.W. Yewdell, B.R. Murphy, Primary pulmonary cytotoxic T lymphocytes induced by immunization with a vaccinia virus recombinant expressing influenza A virus nucleoprotein peptide do not protect mice against challenge, J. Virol. 68 (1994) 3505–3511.

[8] S.L. Epstein, C.-Y. Lo, J.A. Misplon, J.R. Bennink, Mechanism of protective immunity against influenza virus infection in mice without antibodies, J. Immunol. 160 (1998) 322–327.

[9] P.M. Taylor, B.A. Askonas, Influenza nucleoprotein-specific cytotoxic T-cell clones are protective in vivo, Immunology 58 (1986) 417–420.

[10] J.J. Treanor, E.L. Tierney, S.L. Zebedee, R.A. Lamb, B.R. Murphy, Passively transferred monoclonal antibody to the M2 protein inhibits influenza A virus replication in mice, J. Virol. 64 (1990) 1375–1377.

[11] G.M. Air, R.M. Hall, Conservation and variation in influenza gene sequences, in: D.P. Nayak (Ed.), Genetic Variation Among Influenza Viruses, Academic Press, New York, 1981, pp. 29–44.

International Congress Series 1219 (2001) 911–915

Influenza HA DNA induces Th1 cells and protection despite limited antibody responses

Patricia A. Johnson[a], Margaret Conway[a], Janet Daly[b],
Carolyn Nicolson[b], James S. Robertson[b], Kingston H.G. Mills[a,*]

[a]*Infection and Immunity Group, Department of Biology, National University of Ireland,
Maynooth, Co Kildare, Ireland*
[b]*Department of Virology, National Institute for Biological Standards and Control, Blanche Lane,
South Mimms, Potters Bar, Hertfordshire, EN6 3QG, UK*

Abstract

The relative ability of influenza HA DNA vaccines to induce cellular and humoral immunity after one or more doses and the persistence of this response have not been fully elucidated. HA DNA induces a potent Th1 response. Although this response wanes 12 weeks after a single immunisation, Th1 cells persist in the spleen for at least 6 months after two booster immunisations. In contrast, influenza specific ELISA IgG titres reached significant levels only after booster immunisations and HI antibodies were generally weak or undetectable. Nevertheless, two doses of HA DNA confer almost complete protection against respiratory challenge with live virus. © 2001 Elsevier Science B.V. All rights reserved.

Keywords: DNA vaccine; Influenza virus; Haemagglutinin; Th1 cells

1. Introduction

Antigenic variation in the haemagglutinin (HA) surface glycoprotein of influenza virus allows the virus to escape protective immune responses and poses a considerable obstacle to the development of an effective vaccine. Since current influenza vaccines provide limited protection against viruses that have undergone antigenic variation, new versions of the vaccine need to be prepared each year and this presents serious problems for

* Corresponding author. Present Address: Department of Biochemistry, Trinity College, Dublin 2, Ireland.
Tel.: +353-1-608 3573; fax: +353-1-677 2400.
E-mail address: kingston.mills@tcd.ie (K.H.G. Mills).

manufacturers, licensing authorities and health care workers. An alternative approach to conventional whole virus or protein subunit vaccines, which may overcome many of the difficulties associated with current vaccine approaches, involves the direct injection of naked plasmid DNA encoding protective viral proteins [1,4].

Recent studies have demonstrated that immunization of naked plasmid DNA with foreign antigens can generate antibody and immune responses against the encoded antigen. However, there is still some controversy regarding the relative ability of DNA vaccines to generate cell mediated and humoral immunity, the persistence of these responses, and the optimum dose and schedule to selectively prime distinct arms of the immune response. In this study, we have examined the effect of immunising dose and schedule on the induction of cellular and humoral immune response and the persistence of this response using DNA encoding the HA gene from an A(H3N2) influenza virus, A/Sichuan/87.

2. Results

To determine the type and persistence of the local and systemic immune response generated by an HA DNA vaccine, the immune response generated following single (Fig. 1a) or multiple (Fig. 1b) immunisations, BALB/c mice were immunized i.m. with 100 μg HA DNA and T cell responses were assessed in the spleen at 2, 12 and 24 weeks. Two weeks after immunization with a single dose of HA DNA spleen cells from immunised mice secreted significant amounts of IFN-γ (Fig. 1a) but undetectable IL-5 (not shown) following in vitro stimulation with a range of concentrations of influenza virus. These results suggest that DNA vaccination mimics a natural infection which also induces a polarised Th1 response in the spleen (data not shown). In order to examine the effect of

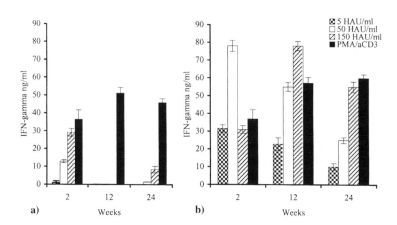

Fig. 1. T cell responses of mice inoculated with HA DNA. Balb/c mice were inoculated i.m. with 100 μg HA DNA and the level of IFN-γ released from spleen cells stimulated in vitro with different amounts of virus determined at 2, 12 and 24 weeks after the final inoculation. (a) single dose of DNA, (b) three doses of DNA at 4-week intervals. Results are mean levels of IFN-γ in supernatants of spleen cells from four to five mice per group.

DNA dose on the T cell response, BALB/c mice were immunized with HA DNA in the dose range 0.01–100 μg. Reduced levels of IFN-γ production were observed from spleen cells isolated from mice which had received lower doses of DNA; however, an antigen-specific response remained detectable at doses as low as 0.1 and 0.01 μg/mouse (data not shown). In contrast, IL-5 production was undetectable in antigen-stimulated spleen cells, regardless of the immunising dose (data not shown).

Fig. 1a indicates that even at high doses, a single immunization with HA DNA did not induce a persistent T cell response. In contrast, spleen cells from mice immunised with 3 doses of 100μg of HA DNA secreted significant amounts of IFN-γ (Fig. 1b) and little or no IL-5 (not shown) at 2, 12 and 24 weeks after immunisation. This suggests that multiple immunisations are required for a persistent T cell response, which remains polarized to the Th1 subtype. However, the response was not as persistent following multiple immuniza- tion with lower doses of DNA (1.0 or 10 μg), with only weak specific responses detected at 12 and 24 weeks (data not shown).

Serum samples taken from mice following natural infection or single or multiple immunizations with HA DNA were examined for influenza virus-specific IgG by ELISA (Fig. 2). DNA immunisation generated weak influenza virus-specific serum IgG titres. A single immunisation of HA DNA at the highest dose of 100 μg induced an antibody titre one log_{10} less than the titre of 4.0 observed following natural infection. Booster immunisations with HA DNA enhanced antibody production, but with titres remaining slightly below that induced by natural infection. After multiple immunisation or natural infection, responses had waned significantly after 6 months.

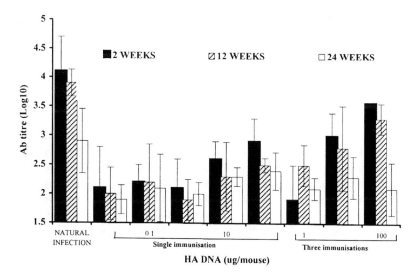

Fig. 2. Anti-influenza virus specific IgG in mice infected with virus or inoculated with HA DNA. Mice were infected intranasally with influenza virus or inoculated i.m. once with 0.01, 0.1, 1.0, 10 or 100 μg HA DNA or three times with 1.0, 10 or 100 μg HA DNA, as indicated. Serum antibody titres were determined by ELISA 2, 12 and 24 weeks after inoculation or infection. Data are the means of titres ($\pm$SD) for four to five mice per group. Reproduced from Johnson et al. [5] with permission.

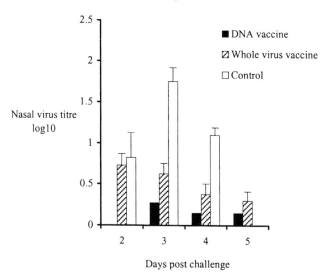

Fig. 3. Protection of mice inoculated with HA DNA versus whole virus vaccine. Mice were inoculated twice with 100 μg HA DNA, one dose of whole virus vaccine or PBS as control and challenged with live homologous virus 2 weeks after the last inoculation. Results are mean viral titres ($\pm$SD) in nasal washes for 5–10 mice per group at each time point. Reproduced from Johnson et al. [5] with permission.

Immunisation with two doses of 100μg HA DNA conferred almost complete protection against influenza virus with little or no virus detectable in the lungs at any time post challenge (Fig. 3). In contrast, mice immunized with the whole virus vaccine, albeit with a single dose, had significantly higher viral shedding at days 2, 3 and 4 post challenge but which was considerably less than control, unvaccinated, mice.

3. Discussion

An approach to vaccine design is to achieve a response that mimics natural infection, without the risk associated with a live virus. We therefore investigated the type and persistence of immune response generated with an HA DNA vaccine and compared these with the responses induced by natural infection. Our results suggest that, similar to intranasal infection with influenza virus, immunisation with HA DNA also selectively primed systemic Th1 cells. In addition, T helper clones generated from the spleens of immunized mice secreted significant amounts of IFN-γ and no IL-5 in response to influenza virus (data not shown), providing direct evidence for the generation of CD4$^+$ Th1 cells following immunization with HA DNA.

In contrast to the potent systemic cellular immune responses, we failed to detect significant circulating anti-influenza virus antibodies following a single immunization of HA DNA over a wide dose range. Booster immunization with high doses of DNA induced modest serum antibody titres, but the levels remained below that observed following infection with influenza virus. Despite the limited ability to induce humoral immunity, the

DNA vaccine provided excellent protection against challenge with live virus. However, the rapid clearance of virus from the lungs is unlikely to reflect an anamnestic antibody response after challenge. Alternatively, the protection observed with the HA DNA vaccine may be mediated solely through the induction of cell mediated immunity. This conclusion is consistent with a report which has demonstrated that mice who lack mature B cells and do not secrete immunoglobulin, are still capable of clearing influenza virus infection from the respiratory tract [2,3].

The present investigation has demonstrated that the humoral immunity induced with a DNA vaccine based on the HA molecule of influenza virus does not approach that observed either by influenza virus respiratory infection or immunization with a whole influenza virus vaccine. Nevertheless the DNA vaccine was capable of conferring protective immunity which surpassed that achieved with a whole virus vaccine, albeit with an additional immunization. Our demonstration that HA DNA was capable of selectively inducing Th1 cells, which mimics that generated following viral infection, point to a role for cellular immunity in protection induced with this and other DNA vaccines.

Acknowledgements

This work was supported by the EU Biotechnology Programme under contract number BIO4 CT96-0637, DG12 SSMI.

References

[1] M.A. Liu, Overview of DNA vaccines, Ann. N. Y. Acad. Sci. 772 (1995) 15–20.
[2] A. Bot, Immunoglobulin deficient mice generated by gene targeting as models for studying the immune response, Int. Rev. Immunol. 13 (1996) 327–340.
[3] D.J. Topham, R.A. Tripp, A.M. Hamilton-Easton, S.R. Sara, P.C. Doherty, Quantitative analysis of the influenza virus-specific CD4+ T cell memory in the absence of B cells and Ig, J. Immunol. 157 (1996) 2947–2952.
[4] J.J. Donnelly, DNA vaccines, Annu. Rev. Immunol. 15 (1997) 617–648.
[5] P.A. Johnson, M.A. Conway, J. Daly, C. Nicolson, J. Robertson, K.H.G. Mills, Plasmid DNA encoding influenza virus haemagglutinin induces Th1 cells and protection against respiratory infection despite its limited ability to generate antibody responses, J. Gen. Virol. 81 (2000) 1737–1745.

International Congress Series 1219 (2001) 917–921

DNA immunization elicits high HI antibody and protects chicken from AIV challenge

H. Chen[1], K. Yu[*], Y. Jiang, X. Tang

Animal Influenza Research Center, Harbin Veterinary Research Institute, Chinese Academy of Agricultural Sciences, 427 Muduan Street, Harbin 150001, PR China

Abstract

Background: A highly pathogenic avian influenza virus of goose origin A/Goose/Guangdong/1/ 96 (H5N1) (GD/96) shared nucleotide homology of 98% in the HA with A/HK/156/97(H5N1). The nucleotide sequences at the cleavage site, all potential glycosylation sites and the receptor binding sites in the HA were conserved. The purpose of this study was to evaluate the immunogenicity and efficacy of a DNA vaccine to against this virus. *Methods*: The HA cDNA from GD/96 was cloned under a CMV promoter to generate vaccine plasmid pCIHA, which was administered to 3-week-old SPF chickens in two doses of 100 µg ($n=9$) or 50 µg ($n=14$) by the intramuscular route, 2 weeks apart. Chickens were challenged with 10 LD50 GD/96 at 2 weeks post-boost. *Results*: Hemagglutinin inhibition (HI) antibody titers were $2^{5.8\pm2.0}$ and $2^{4.7\pm2.5}$, 2 weeks after priming, $2^{8.4\pm2.7}$ and $2^{7.6\pm3.9}$, 2 weeks after boost, and $2^{9.6\pm2.2}$ and $2^{9.0\pm2.4}$, 1 week after challenge in chicken immunized with 100- or 50-µg pCIHA, respectively. All immunized chickens were fully protected from the lethal challenge, with no clinical signs of disease, no virus shedding and 100% survival at 10 days postchallenge. *Conclusion*: The plasmid pCIHA is highly immunogenic and protects SPF chickens from lethal challenge with the homologous avian influenza virus GD/96. © 2001 Elsevier Science B.V. All rights reserved.

Keywords: Avian influenza virus; DNA immunization; H5N1 subtype

[*] Corresponding author. Tel.: +86-451-2730445; fax: +86-451-2733132.
[1] Present address: Influenza Branch, Centers for Disease Control and Prevention, 1600 Clifton Road, MS G-16, Atlanta, GA 30333, USA.

0531-5131/01/$ – see front matter © 2001 Elsevier Science B.V. All rights reserved.
PII: S 0 5 3 1 - 5 1 3 1 (0 1) 0 0 3 6 8 - 5

1. Introduction

In 1996, a highly pathogenic avian influenza virus (HPAIV), A/Goose/Guangdong/1/ 96(H5N1)(GD/96), was isolated in southern China [1]. Molecular analysis revealed that this goose origin AIV shared nucleotide homology of 98% in the hemagglutinin (HA) and 71.9– 93.2% in the other seven gene segments with A/HK/156/97(H5N1), which was directly transmitted from infected poultry to human beings in 18 cases and caused six deaths in Hong Kong in 1997 [2–4]. The nucleotide sequences at the cleavage site, all potential glyco- sylation sites and the receptor binding sites in the HA were conserved. These results indicated that H5N1 AIV was not only a disastrous pathogen for avian species, but was also potentially dangerous for human beings. It is urgent to develop an appropriate strategy for control and eradication in case of an emergency outbreak caused by this dangerous AIV.

Vaccination of chickens with DNA would offer a number of advantages over immunization with other vaccine strategy for AIV control and prevention. Several investigators have demonstrated that HA gene DNA vaccines provide solid immune protection against influenza viruses [5–10], but the immune response to DNA vaccine in chickens was variable and prechallenge HI antibody usually could not be detected when vaccine was delivered by direct intramuscular injection [11–13]. Here, we report that DNA immunization elicited highly HI antibody response and induced complete protection from lethal virus GD/96 challenge in chickens by direct intramuscular injection.

2. Material and methods

2.1. Virus

The AIV GD/96 was isolated from a goose in Guangdong province in China in 1996. Intravenous pathogenicity index test in SPF chickens and plaque-forming assay in MDCK cells showed this strain is an HPAIV [1,2]. The virus was propagated in the allantoic cavities of SPF embryonated eggs.

2.2. Inactivated vaccine preparation

The GD/96 virus was purified by equilibrium density sucrose gradient ultracentrifu- gation [14]. The purified virus was set to 40,000 HA units (HAU)/ml and inactivated by adding 0.025% formalin. The protein concentration was estimated by Bio-Rad protein assay. The HA concentration in the purified virus was determined by polyacrylamide gel electrophoresis. The vaccine was made and homogenized with an equal volume of adjuvant made of mineral oil and Span-Tween.

2.3. Ha gene and expression vector

The HA cDNA of the open reading frame of the HA gene had been cloned and sequenced previously [2]. It was inserted into the Sal I and Sma I sites of the pCI vector (Promega) under the control of the CMV immediate-early promoter. The plasmid, named pCIHA, was grown in *E. coli* JM83 bacteria, purified by polyethylene glycol precipitation, and dissolved in PBS (pH 7.2) for immunization.

2.4. Immunization and challenge infection

Three-week old SPF chickens (SPF Experimental Animal Center of Harbin Veterinary Research Institute) were divided into three groups and inoculated by direct intramuscular injection. Chickens in group I ($n=9$) were inoculated with 100-µg plasmid pCIHA in two shots, 50-µg DNA in 100-µl PBS per shot. Chickens in group II ($n=14$) were inoculated with 50-µg plasmid pCIHA, 25 µg in 100-µl PBS per shot. Chickens in group III ($n=14$) were inoculated with 100-µg plasmid pCI as a control. Two weeks later, chickens were boosted with the same dose by the same route. Chickens in Group IV ($n=12$) were vaccinated with a single dose of the inactivated vaccine containing 10-µg HA in 0.5-ml volume by intramuscular injection. All chickens were challenged with 10 LD_{50} of GD/96 by intramuscular injection. Cloacal swabs were collected at day 7 after challenge from surviving chickens, and the samples were propagated in the allantoic cavities of 10-day-old embryonated eggs for HA tests. Sera were collected preboost (group I, II, III only), prechallenge and 1 week postchallenge for serum HI antibody analyses.

2.5. Serology

HI assays were performed with 0.5% chicken RBCs. Sera from chickens were tested individually and HI titers were determined as the reciprocal of the highest serum dilution that gave complete inhibition of hemagglutination.

3. Results

3.1. Antibody response of chickens immunized with pCIHA

To evaluate the H5 HA DNA vaccine plasmid pCIHA, 3-week-old SPF chickens were immunized with 100- and 50-µg doses, respectively, by intramuscular injection, and boosted 2 weeks later. High HI antibodies titers (2^8) were observed in both the 50- and 100-µg immunization groups with the average being $2^{5.8\pm2.0}$ and $2^{4.7\pm2.5}$, respectively, after priming vaccination. At 2 weeks post-boost, the average HI antibody titers reached $2^{8.4\pm2.7}$ (100-µg group) and $2^{7.6\pm3.9}$ (50-µg group) and the highest HI antibody response reached 2^{12} in both groups. The prechallenge HI antibody of the chickens in the inactivated vaccine group reached 2^6 with an average of $2^{4.3\pm1.0}$. In group III (control), prechallenge HI antibody was zero and postchallenge HI antibody was not detected as all the chickens died before day 7 postchallenge.

3.2. Protection induced by immunization with pCIHA

At 2 weeks post-boost, all chickens were challenged with HPAIV GD/96 to investigate the protective efficacy of the HA DNA vaccine. Besides clinical observation for 10 days

Table 1
Protection against lethal virus GD/96 challenge in SPF chickens

Group	Virus shedding on day 7 postchallenge (no. shedding/total)[a]	Protection on day 10 postchallenge (no. sick/no.dead/total)	Survival (%)
I (pCIHA, 100 μg)	0/9	0/0/9	100
II (pCIHA, 50 μg)	0/14	0/0/14	100
III (pCI, 100 μg)	ND[b]	14/14/14	0
IV (F.I., 10 μg HA)	0/12	0/0/12	100

[a] Cloacal samples were collected at day 7 postchallenge, and were propagated in 9–10-day-old embryonated chicken eggs for checking HA.

[b] All chickens in group III died before day 7 postchallenge.

postchallenge, virus shedding was evaluated in all surviving birds at day 7 postchallenge. All immunized chickens that survived up to day 10 postchallenge were completely protected from the lethal challenge of the GD/96 without any clinical signs and virus shedding (Table 1). One chicken in the 50-μg group, however, did not have detectable HI antibody before challenge. In sharp contrast to the immunized chickens, all chickens in the control group (group III) started to show disease signs of pathogenic AI on day 4 postchallenge and died before day 7 postchallenge (Table 1).

4. Discussion

Although the protective immunity induced by DNA immunization is at least as good as inactivated whole virus vaccines, previous studies in chickens reported that the HA gene DNA vaccine failed to induce detectable prechallenge HI antibody [6,9,10,15]. Direct intramuscular injection, at least in chickens, produced variable immune responses [8,9]. However, in our study, direct intramuscular injection of H5 HA expressing plasmid pCIHA not only induced complete protection from lethal virus challenge, but also elicited higher levels of HI antibody than inactivated vaccine. The prechallenge HI antibody levels in both the 50 μg and 100 μg groups were as high as the HI antibody levels in the inactivated vaccine group.

Protective immunity induced by influenza HA DNA vaccine is antibody-mediated. Antibody production is the critical or major mechanism for protection against influenza infection in chickens, with neutralization of the virus occurring by specific IgG and IgA molecules at the surface of the respiratory or digestive tract mucosa. Antibodies to the HA are necessary to prevent AIV infection and a higher HI antibody response usually means more reliable and durable protection against AIV infection. Compared to inactivated vaccine, DNA immunization has been demonstrated to be more effective in cross protection against different strains within the same subtype [14,16]. In addition, direct intramuscular injection is a very practical and convenient method of vaccine administration to use in the field. Therefore, pCIHA is a promising potential candidate for GD/96- and Hong Kong H5N1-related AIV control in the future.

Acknowledgements

We thank Dr. Gloria Kelly and Dr. Kanta Subbarao for their critical review of the manuscript.

References

[1] X. Tang, G. Tian, C. Zhao, J. Zhou, K. Yu, Isolation and characterization of prevalent strains of avian influenza viruses in China, Chin. J. Anim. Poult. Infect. Dis. 20 (1) (1998) 1–5.
[2] H. Chen, K. Yu, Z. Bu, Molecular analysis of hemagglutinin gene of a goose origin highly pathogenic avian influenza virus, Chin. Agric. Sci. 32 (2) (1999) 87–92.
[3] K. Subbarao, A. Klimov, J.M. Katz, H. Regnery, W. Lim, H. Hall, M. Perdue, D. Swayne, C. Bender, J. Huang, M. Hemphill, T. Rowe, M. Shaw, X. Xu, K. Fukuda, N.J. Cox, Characterization of an avian influenza A (H5N1) virus isolate from a child with a fatal respiratory illness, Science 297 (1998) 393–396.
[4] J. Zhang, K. Yu, H. Chen, G. Deng, X. Tang, G. Tian, Molecular analyses of the entire genes of an avian influenza virus isolate A/Goose/Guangdong/1/96 (H5N1), Chin. J. Prev. Vet. Med. 22 (3) (2000) 232–235.
[5] Z. Chen, K. Matsuo, H. Asanuma, H. Takahashi, T. Iwasaki, Y. Suzuki, C. Aizawa, T. Kurata, S. Tamura, Enhanced protection against a lethal influenza virus challenge by immunization with both hemagglutinin- and neuraminidase-expressing DNAs, Vaccine 17 (7–8) (1999) 653–659.
[6] S. Kodihalli, H. Goto, D.L. Kobasa, S. Krauss, Y. Kawaoka, R.G. Webster, DNA vaccine encoding hemag-glutinin provides protective immunity against H5N1 influenza virus infection in mice, J. Virol. 73 (3) (1999) 2094–2098.
[7] Z. Chen, Y. Sahashi, K. Matsuo, H. Asanuma, H. Takahashi, T. Iwasaki, Y. Suzuki, C. Aizawa, T. Kurata, S. Tamura, Comparison of the ability of viral protein-expressing plasmid DNAs to protect against influenza, Vaccine 16 (16) (1998) 1544–1549.
[8] J.J. Donnelly, A. Friedman, J.B. Ulmer, M.A. Liu, Further protection against antigenic drift of influenza virus in a ferret model by DNA vaccination, Vaccine 15 (8) (1997) 865–868, June.
[9] M.A. Liu, W. McClements, J.B. Ulmer, J. Shiver, J. Donnelly, Immunization of non-human primates with DNA vaccines, Vaccine 15 (8) (1997) 909–912, June.
[10] R.G. Webster, E.F. Fynan, J.C. Santoro, H. Robinson, Protection of ferrets against influenza challenge with a DNA vaccine to the haemagglutinin, Vaccine 12 (16) (1994) 1495–1498.
[11] H.L. Robinson, L.A. Hunt, R.G. Webster, Protection against a lethal influenza virus challenge by immuni-zation with a haemagglutinin-expressing plasmid DNA, Vaccine 11 (9) (1993) 957–960.
[12] H. Chen, K. Yu, G. Tian, X. Tang, J. Lu, Protective immune response to avian influenza virus in chicken induced by DNA inoculation, Chin. Agric. Sci. 31 (5) (1998) 63–68.
[13] S. Kodihalli, J.R. Haynes, H.L. Robinson, R.G. Webster, Cross-protection among lethal H5N2 influenza viruses induced by DNA vaccine to the hemagglutinin, J. Virol. 71 (5) (1997) 3391–3396.
[14] A. Garcia, H. Johnson, D. Srivastava, D.A. Jayawardene, D.R. Wehr, R.G. Webster, Efficacy of inacti-vated H5N2 Influenza vaccines against lethal A/Chicken/Queretaro/19/95 infection, Avian Dis. 42 (1998) 248–256.
[15] M.D. Macklin, D. McCabe, M.W. McGregor, V. Neumann, T. Meyer, R. Callan, V.S. Hinshaw, W.F. Swain, Immunization of pigs with a particle-mediated DNA vaccine to influenza A virus protects against challenge with homologous virus, J. Virol. 72 (2) (1998) 1491–1496.
[16] S. Kodihalli, D.L. Kobasa, R.G. Webster, Strategies for inducing protection against avian influenza A virus subtypes with DNA vaccines, Vaccine 18 (23) (2000) 2592–2599.

International Congress Series 1219 (2001) 923–929

Replicons from positive strand RNA viruses for naked RNA immunization against influenza

Marco Vignuzzi, Sylvie Gerbaud, Sylvie van der Werf*, Nicolas Escriou

Unité de Génétique Moléculaire des Virus Respiratoires, URA 1966 CNRS, Institut Pasteur, 25, rue du Dr Roux, F-75724 Paris Cedex 15, France

Abstract

Background: Genetic immunization is a powerful tool for vaccine development, but faces the potential drawback of persistence of the injected DNA sequences in the host. *Methods*: Replicons derived from poliovirus (PV), attenuated Mengo virus (MV) and Semliki Forest virus (SFV) genomes for which the influenza nucleoprotein (NP) or hemagglutinin (HA) sequences replace structural protein sequences were constructed. Their immunogenicity was evaluated in C57BL/6 mice following intramuscular injection in the form of naked RNA. *Results*: Replicons derived from the SFV, PV or MV genomes were shown to replicate upon transfection of cells and permit NP expression. Expression of the HA in a correctly glycosylated form could be achieved from the SFV-derived genome or from a dicistronic PV-derived genome for which synthesis of the heterologous antigen was uncoupled from that of the truncated poliovirus polyprotein that was placed under the control of the EMCV-IRES. Injection of the NP expressing replicons in the form of naked RNA into mice resulted in the induction of an anti-NP cytotoxic and/or humoral immune response. For the SFV-derived replicon, the response was found to be protective to a level comparable to that achieved by DNA immunization. *Conclusions*: Recombinant replicons derived from positive strand RNA virus genomes could provide a useful alternative to DNA vaccines. © 2001 Elsevier Science B.V. All rights reserved.

Keywords: Cytotoxic T lymphocytes; Humoral response; Vaccine vector; Picornavirus; Semliki Forest virus; Recombinant; Nucleoprotein; Hemagglutinin

---

* Corresponding author. Tel.: +33-1-45-68-87-25; fax: +33-1-40-61-32-41.
E-mail address: svdwerf@pasteur.fr (S. van der Werf).

0531-5131/01/$ – see front matter © 2001 Elsevier Science B.V. All rights reserved.
PII: S 0 5 3 1 - 5 1 3 1 (0 1) 0 0 4 0 9 - 5

1. Introduction

Genetic immunization, an attractive alternative to conventional vaccination based on the injection of DNA expression vectors, has been shown to induce long-lasting humoral and cellular immune responses, as in the case of influenza [1–4]. However, questions remain as to the potential risk of integration of DNA sequences into the host genome.

To avoid such potential hazards, the use of RNA has been proposed for genetic immunization. Development of this approach is, however, limited by the intrinsic instability of RNA that results in short-lived expression of the antigen and overall weak immunogenicity. To overcome these difficulties, RNA vectors derived from the genomes of positive strand RNA viruses may be used to vehicle heterologous sequences into the cell. In such RNA vectors, sequences encoding structural proteins are replaced by heterologous sequences of interest, whereas the non-structural genes required for replication and gene expression are retained. These self-replicating RNAs or replicons are therefore likely to persist longer after injection.

In this study, we investigated the simple injection of naked recombinant RNAs derived from the Semliki Forest virus (SFV), poliovirus (PV) or Mengo virus (MV) genomes, that expressed the influenza virus hemagglutinin (HA) or nucleoprotein (NP) as a means to induce a humoral and cytotoxic T cell (CTL) response against influenza.

2. Material and methods

2.1. Construction of plasmids for the transcription of recombinant replicons

Plasmid pΔP1-E, hereafter named p_PV derived from pT7-PV1-52 [5], contains a subgenomic poliovirus cDNA downstream of the phage T7 promoter, in which a *Sac*I/*Xho*I/*Sal*I polylinker replaces all of the sequences encoding P1 except those coding for the nine C-terminal residues. Plasmid pΔPV-NP was constructed by the in-frame insertion of sequences encoding the nucleoprotein (NP) from the mouse-adapted influenza virus A/PR/8/34(ma) into the Klenow filled *Xho*I site of plasmid pΔPV. Plasmid p_P1-IR contains the IRES sequences (nt 306–845) from the encephalomyocarditis virus (EMCV) cDNA inserted upstream of the first codon of 2A in pΔPV. Plasmid pΔP1-IR-HA was constructed by insertion of the HA sequences of A/PR/8/34(ma) between the *Sac*I and *Sal*I sites of pΔP1-IR. Plasmid pΔMV-NP was constructed by the in-frame insertion of the NP sequences between the *Xho*I and *Sac*I sites of plasmid pΔMV-BB, which contains a subgenomic Mengo virus cDNA downstream of the phage T7 promoter [7]. The pSFV-NP plasmid was constructed by insertion of the NP sequences into the *Sma*I site of pSFV1 that contains a subgenomic cDNA of the SFV, placed downstream of the SP6 RNA polymerase promoter.

2.2. In vitro transcription

The pΔPV, pΔMV and pSFV plasmids were linearized with *Eco*RI, *Bam*HI and *Spe*I, respectively, transcribed by the Promega RiboMax Large-Scale RNA Production kit with

T7 polymerase, or with SP6 polymerase in the presence of 3 mM of cap analogue for the SFV-derived plasmids, and then treated by RQ1 DNase (Promega).

2.3. Immunizations

Groups of five to six C57BL/6 male mice were injected monthly via the intramuscular route with 100 µl of PBS (50 µl in each tibialis anterior muscle) containing either plasmid DNA or replicon RNA.

2.4. Antibody titres

Serum samples prepared 3 weeks after each injection were used to determine NP-specific antibody titers in a standard ELISA using 0.5 µg of detergent-disrupted A/PR/8/34(ma) virus as antigen.

2.5. Cytotoxicity assay

Spleen cells were collected 3 weeks after the last immunization and restimulated for 7 days with syngeneic splenocytes, which had been pulsed for 3 h with 10 µM of NP366 peptide and irradiated (2500 rads). Cytotoxic activity of the restimulated effector cells was measured using a standard ^{51}Cr release cytotoxicity assay towards EL4 target cells that were labelled with $Na_2{}^{51}CrO_4$ and pulsed (or not) with NP366 peptide.

3. Results

3.1. Construction of recombinant replicons derived from the Semliki Forest virus and picornavirus genomes

For the construction of SFV genome-derived replicons, the sequences encoding the structural proteins downstream of the 26S subgenomic promoter were substituted by the influenza A/PR/8/34(ma) virus NP sequences (Fig. 1). Capped in-vitro transcribed rSFV-NP RNA was found to initiate a replication cycle upon transfection of HeLa cells and to permit the expression of the influenza NP as previously described by others [8]. Likewise, recombinant replicons derived from the poliovirus genome were constructed by substitution of the capsid protein-coding sequences. The influenza NP sequences were placed upstream of an optimal 2A cleavage site, consisting of the 9 C-terminal amino acids of VP1 and the first amino acid of 2A, in-frame with the rest of the sequences encoding the poliovirus polyprotein (Fig. 1). In transfected cells, the synthetic rΔPV-NP RNA produced by in vitro transcription with T7 RNA polymerase was competent for replication and the NP-VP1* fusion protein was found to be correctly cleaved from the polyprotein and expressed to high levels (not shown). When the influenza HA sequences were inserted in a similar fashion, the resulting monocistronic RNA was unable to replicate. We therefore constructed a dicistronic replicon in which the IRES of EMCV was inserted to direct the translation of the poliovirus non-structural proteins, while the influenza HA sequences

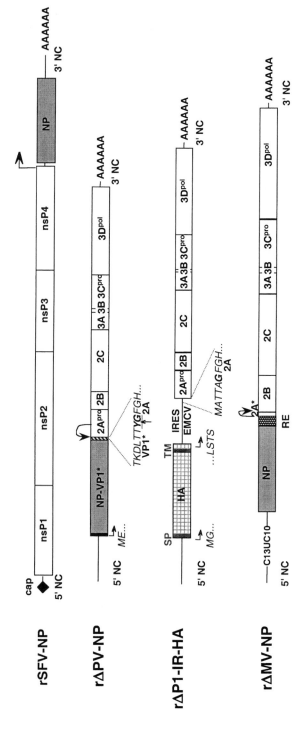

Fig. 1. Schematic representation of recombinant replicons. Subgenomic replicons were derived from the genomes of Semliki Forest virus (SFV), poliovirus (PV) or Mengo virus (MV) by substitution of the structural protein sequences by sequences encoding the influenza virus NP (gray box) or HA (squared box) including the signal peptide (SP) and transmembrane (TM) sequences, while the sequences of the non-structural proteins required for replication of the RNAs were retained (open boxes). Sequences encoding the first amino acids from the poliovirus polyprotein (black boxes) or the nine C-terminal residues of VP1 comprising the optimal context for in *cis* cleavage by the 2A protease (hatched boxes) are indicated with the corresponding amino acid sequences in italics below. The EMCV IRES sequences (nt 306–845) and MV replication element (RE; nt 1137–1267) are indicated.

were under the control of the poliovirus IRES (Fig. 1). Upon transfection of Hela cells, this dicistronic replicon rΔP1-IR-HA was shown to replicate and permitted the expression of the HA in a native and correctly glycosylated form (not shown).

Replicons derived from the MV genome were constructed by a similar approach. It was shown previously that the L-P1-2A regions of the genome may be deleted, with the exception of a replication element present in the VP2 coding region, to give a subgenomic replicon rΔMV-BB that is replication competent [6]. Insertion of the influenza NP sequences resulted in replicon rΔMV-NP (Fig. 1) which was found to replicate efficiently and to permit expression of an NP-2A* fusion protein upon transfection of Hela cells (not shown).

3.2. Immunogenicity of the recombinant replicons administered in the form of naked RNA

C57BL/6 mice were injected via the intramuscular route with naked RNA from poliovirus- or SFV-derived replicons or with pCI-derived plasmid DNA. The induction of a specific anti-NP antibody response was examined by ELISA (Table 1). For rΔPV-NP, three injections of naked RNA permitted the induction of an antibody response against the NP, as strong as that induced by DNA immunization. Two injections of rSFV-NP were sufficient to induce an even stronger response. No specific anti-HA antibody response could be detected with the dicistronic rΔP1-IR-HA replicon even after three injections. This may be due to competition between the poliovirus and EMCV IRES sequences in

Table 1
Induction of NP-specific antibody and CTL responses by naked RNA immunization

Plasmid/replicon	Number of injections[a]	Anti-NP response		
		Antibodies[b]	CTL[c]	
			EL4	EL4 + NP366
pCI 50 μg	1	<50	4	−3
	2	<50	NT[d]	NT
pCI-NP 50 μg	1	1984	2	35
	2	10,593	NT	NT
rSFV 10 μg	1	<50	0	7
	2	<50	−2	5
rSFV-NP 10 μg	1	830	4	27
	2	8400	−1	54
rPV 25 μg	1	<50	NT	NT
	2	<50	NT	NT
	3	<50	−1	9
rPV-NP 25 μg	1	<50	NT	NT
	2	<50	NT	NT
	3	2051	−1	8

[a] C57BL/6 mice were immunized via the intramuscular route at monthly intervals.

[b] Serum antibody titers as determined by ELISA, 3 weeks after each injection.

[c] % Specific lysis in a standard ^{51}Cr release assay of EL4 cells loaded or not with peptide NP366; effector splenocytes were collected 3 weeks after last injection, stimulated in vitro for 1 week with peptide NP366 and used at an effector to target ratio of 20:1.

[d] NT: not tested.

murine cells in vivo, in which the EMCV IRES could dominate and preclude high expression of the HA from the poliovirus IRES.

Using the NP-encoding replicons, we evaluated the induction of a CTL response directed against the immunodominant CTL epitope of the influenza NP (NP366) in a classical cytolysis assay (Table 1). A single injection of plasmid DNA pCI-NP elicited a specific CTL response towards the immunodominant epitope. An even stronger response was observed after two injections of rSFV-NP in the form of naked RNA. This response conferred the same degree of protection against a challenge infection with 0.1 LD_{50} (100 PFU) of A/PR/8/34(ma), as determined by measuring the lung virus titers at 7 days post-challenge (not shown). However, three injections of rΔPV-NP did not result in the induction of a detectable anti-NP CTL response. A general explanation could be that the poliovirus genome replicates poorly in murine cells in vivo. It will therefore be of interest to analyze the immunogenicity of the Mengo virus-derived replicons.

4. Discussion

The injection of recombinant replicons in the form of naked RNA was shown to constitute a new approach to gene immunization. Induction of antibodies specific of an influenza protein by SFV-derived replicons administered as naked RNA has already been described [8,9]. Here, we showed that in addition to antibodies, a CTL response targeting the NP366 epitope at least as strong as that induced by plasmid DNA could be elicited and was able to bring about protection towards a homologous virus challenge. It will be of interest to evaluate the role of anti-NP CTL induced by naked RNA immunization against a heterologous virus (of different sub-type) as well as the potency of combined or sequential immunization with different replicons that express different antigens.

Acknowledgements

The technical assistance of Ida Rijks, for the production of A/PR/8/34(ma) is gratefully acknowledged.

This work was supported in part by the Ministère de l'Education Nationale, de la Recherche et de la Technologie (EA 302).

References

[1] J.B. Ulmer, J.J. Donnelly, S.E. Parker, G.H. Rhodes, P.L. Felgner, V.J. Dwarki, et al., Heterologous protection against influenza by injection of DNA encoding a viral protein, Science 259 (5102) (1993) 1745–1749.

[2] J.J. Donnelly, J.B. Ulmer, M.A. Liu, Immunization with DNA, J. Immunol. Methods 176 (2) (1994) 145–152.

[3] J.J. Donnelly, A. Friedman, D. Martinez, D.L. Montgomery, J.W. Shiver, S.L. Motzel, et al., Preclinical efficacy of a prototype DNA vaccine: enhanced protection against antigenic drift in influenza virus, Nat. Med. 1 (6) (1995) 583–587.

[4] B.S. Bender, J.B. Ulmer, C.M. DeWitt, R. Cottey, S.F. Taylor, A.M. Ward, et al., Immunogenicity and efficacy of DNA vaccines encoding influenza A proteins in aged mice, Vaccine 16 (18) (1998) 1748–1755.

[5] D. Marc, G. Drugeon, A.L. Haenni, M. Girard, S. van der Werf, Role of myristoylation of poliovirus capsid protein VP4 as determined by site-directed mutagenesis of its N-terminal sequence, EMBO J. 8 (9) (1989) 2661–2668.

[6] P.E. Lobert, N. Escriou, J. Ruelle, T. Michiels, A coding RNA sequence acts as a replication signal in cardioviruses, Proc. Natl. Acad. Sci. U. S. A. 96 (20) (1999) 11560–11565.

[7] P. Liljestrom, H. Garoff, A new generation of animal cell expression vectors based on the Semliki Forest virus replicon, Bio/Technology 9 (12) (1991) 1356–1361.

[8] X. Zhou, P. Berglund, G. Rhodes, S.E. Parker, M. Jondal, P. Liljeström, Self-replicating Semliki Forest virus RNA as recombinant vaccine, Vaccine 12 (1994) 1510–1514.

[9] W. Dalemans, A. Delers, C. Delmelle, F. Denamur, R. Meykens, C. Thiriart, et al., Protection against homologous influenza challenge by genetic immunization with SFV-RNA encoding Flu-HA, Ann. N. Y. Acad. Sci. 772 (1995) 255–256.

International Congress Series 1219 (2001) 931–937

Efficacy and effectiveness of attenuated, cold-adapted, trivalent intranasal influenza vaccine

Robert B. Belshe*

Department of Medicine, Division of Infectious Diseases, Health Sciences Center, Saint Louis University, 3635 Vista Avenue (FDT-8N), St. Louis, MO 63110, USA

Abstract

Cold-adapted, live, attenuated, trivalent, intranasal influenza vaccine (CAIV-T) is well accepted, well-tolerated, highly protective against culture-confirmed influenza, and provides significant health benefits to children and adults. A 2-year, multicenter, double-blind, placebo-controlled efficacy field trial of CAIV-T in children aged 15–71 months with annual re-immunization revealed the vaccine to be highly protective against culture-confirmed influenza. Overall, during 2 years of study, vaccine was 92% protective against culture-confirmed influenza. During the second year of study, the vaccine was 86% protective against A/Sydney, a significantly drifted strain not well-matched to the vaccine. Antibody studies on children given CAIV-T revealed that high titers of cross-reacting antibodies to influenza A/Sydney were induced with vaccination by live attenuated influenza A/Wuhan. Effectiveness measures revealed significant reductions in febrile illness (21% reduction in year 1, 19% reduction in year 2), febrile otitis media (33% reduction in year 1, 16% reduction in year 2) and associated antibiotic use among vaccinated children compared with placebo recipients. In adults, vaccination with CAIV-T resulted in protection during experimental challenge with virulent wild-type viruses. An effectiveness trial in adults demonstrated significant benefits of CAIV-T vaccine (28% reduction in days of missed work for febrile illness days with associated 45% reduction in days taking antibiotics). General use of CAIV-T has the potential to significantly reduce the impact of influenza in children and adults. © 2001 Elsevier Science B.V. All rights reserved.

Keywords: Intranasal influenza vaccine; Influenza vaccine efficacy; Influenza vaccine in children

1. Introduction

Despite the availability of inactivated vaccine, influenza A and B remain significant causes of serious respiratory diseases. In children, significant secondary diseases including

* Tel.: +1-314-577-8648; fax: +1-314-771-3816.
  E-mail address: belsherb@slu.edu (R.B. Belshe).

0531-5131/01/$ – see front matter © 2001 Elsevier Science B.V. All rights reserved.
PII: S 0 5 3 1 - 5 1 3 1 (0 1) 0 0 3 9 3 - 4

otitis media (OM) often accompany these common viral infections, and viruses may be isolated from middle ear fluid in some cases [1–3]. In adults, significant loss of work productivity is due to influenza. The recent demonstration that trivalent, cold-adapted, live, attenuated, intranasally administered vaccine (CAIV-T) is safe and effective in children and adults represents a new opportunity to reduce the impact of influenza and to prevent its complications [4–6]. This communication summarizes the results of recent clinical trials designed to measure efficacy and effectiveness in children and adults.

1.1. Vaccine

Trivalent cold-adapted influenza vaccine was supplied by Aviron (Mountain View, CA) and was frozen in single-dose intranasal applicators described below. The vaccine contained approximately $10^{7.0}$ TCID$_{50}$/dose of each of the three attenuated strains that matched the antigens as recommended for the trivalent inactivated influenza vaccine by the Food and Drug Administration for the 1996–1997 and 1997–1998 influenza seasons, respectively, for field trials [4–6], and as described for adult challenge studies [7]. The vaccine was stored frozen at -20 °C or below. The spray applicator consisted of a syringe-like device, which was calibrated and divided for delivery of two 0.25-ml aliquots (one per nostril) as a large particle aerosol for a total delivered volume of 0.5 ml of study vaccine or placebo.

1.2. Studies in adults

To assess vaccine efficacy in adults, challenge studies were conducted after vaccination of volunteers with either CAIV-T, trivalent inactivated vaccine (TIV) or placebo. Virulent virus was given intranasally approximately 1 month after vaccination to evaluate the efficacy of vaccines [7].

To assess vaccine effectiveness in adults, 4561 participants were randomized 2:1 to receive CAIV-T ($n = 3041$) or placebo ($n = 1520$) [6]. Data on side effects during the 7 days following vaccination and on clinical outcomes for each month, November 1997 through March 1998, were collected from diaries completed by the participants. Vaccine effectiveness was assessed for several illness syndromes during the peak and total outbreak periods [6].

1.3. Studies in children

An efficacy field trial was conducted with CAIV-T in 1602 healthy children who were aged 15–71 months at the time of initial vaccination. Informed consent was obtained from a parent or guardian. Two doses of CAIV-T or placebo were given to the majority of children in year 1. In September of 1997, 1358 of the original study group of 1602 children (85%) were revaccinated with a single dose of live attenuated influenza vaccine or placebo by nasal spray.

The study was prospective, randomized, double-blind, placebo-controlled, and multi-center in design. The primary efficacy endpoint was the first episode of culture-confirmed influenza illness in each year. Details of the study design have been published [4,5].

H1N1 did not circulate during either of the 2 years of the pivotal efficacy field trial. Therefore, to develop surrogate data on vaccine efficacy against viral shedding, children were challenged with monovalent H1N1 vaccine strain 6 months after vaccination in the second year [8].

In a parallel study conducted at Vanderbilt University, 31 seronegative children aged 6–18 months were given the recommended two doses of inactivated trivalent influenza vaccine (Fluzone, split®, Connaught Laboratories, Swiftwater, PA) [9]. Pre- and post-vaccination sera from these children were used for the assessment of antibody responses to inactivated vaccine. For this comparison, we tested sera from 25 children from the CAIV-T field trial who were initially seronegative for H3N2 and compared antibody responses stimulated by two doses of live, attenuated, intranasal influenza vaccine to the antibody responses in the cohort of children described above who received two doses of trivalent inactivated vaccine [9,10].

2. Results

2.1. Studies in adults

A summary of the results of challenge studies in adults is shown in Table 1. Placebo subjects had significantly more infections and illnesses than either vaccine group. CAIV-T had 85% efficacy and TIV had 71% efficacy against infection and illness after experimental challenge with H1, H3 or B viruses [7].

A summary of key effectiveness results in healthy working adults is shown in Table 2. CAIV-T was safe and well-tolerated. Vaccine significantly reduced days of severe febrile illnesses and days of febrile upper respiratory tract illnesses among healthy, working adults (Table 2). Vaccine also led to lower rates of work absenteeism, health care provider visits, and the use of prescription antibiotics and non-prescription medications. These benefits were observed during a season in which the predominant circulating influenza virus strain, A/Sydney/05/97 (H3N2), was not well-matched to strains contained in the vaccine [6].

2.2. Studies in children

No serious adverse events were associated with vaccination [4,5,8]. Transient, minor symptoms of respiratory illness were present after dose 1 of year 1 when more vaccinated children, relative to placebo children, exhibited mild upper respiratory symptoms (rhinor-

Table 1
Summary of virulent influenza challenge studies in adults after live attenuated (CAIV-T) or inactivated vaccine (TIV). Results of challenge with virulent H1N1, H3N2 and B viruses are combined (data from Ref. [7])

Vaccine	Number vaccinated and challenged	Number with infection and illness (%)	Efficacy (%)
CAIV-T	29	2 (7)	85
TIV	32	4 (13)	71
Placebo	31	14 (45)	–

Table 2
Effectiveness of CAIV-T in adults during influenza A/Sydney outbreak of 1997–1998 (data from Ref. [6])

Outcome	Reduction (95% CI)
Number of severe febrile illnesses	19 (7–29)
Number of days with febrile URI (FURI)	24 (13–33)
Days of missed work for FURI	28 (16–39)
Days of antibiotic use for FURI	45 (35–54)

rhea or nasal congestion (on days 2, 3, 8, 9 post vaccine), low grade fever (on day 2 post vaccine) or decreased activity (on day 2 post vaccine) [4,5]. After revaccination, no significant differences in rhinorrhea, fever or decreased activity were present [5]. Live vaccine induced significantly more frequent HAI responses and higher titered responses to a range of H3N2 viruses including A/Sydney/5/97 (H3N2), Thessalonika/1/95 (H3N2), Russia/13919/95 (H3N2), and Johannesburg/33/94 (H3N2) in young children compared to the inactivated vaccine (Fig. 1) [9,10]. Although significant differences in age between children in the live vaccine and inactivated vaccine groups may account for this more broad immune response, live vaccine will induce antibodies in children as young as 2 months of age [11,12].

Live attenuated vaccine was highly efficacious at preventing culture-confirmed influenza (Table 3); in year 1, vaccine had 95% efficacy vs. H3N2 (Wuhan or Nanchang-like viruses) and 91% efficacy vs. B. In year 2, the epidemic consisted largely of a variant not contained in the vaccine, influenza A/Sydney. In year 2, the epidemic of A/Sydney/5/97-like viruses caused 66 of 71 cases with the remaining cases associated with

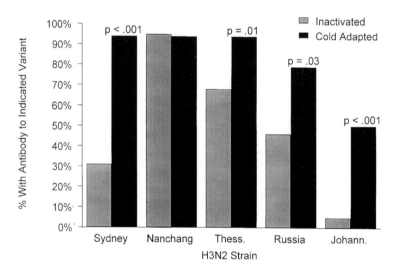

Fig. 1. Percentage of children given two doses of live attenuated influenza vaccine (dark bars) or two doses of inactivated influenza vaccine (light bars) with HAI antibody post vaccine to the indicated variant of H3N2. *P*-values indicate significant differences. Vaccines contained Nanchang antigen (inactivated vaccine) or Nanchang-like antigen (live vaccine contained A/Wuhan). Reproduced with permission from Pediatric Infectious Diseases Journal, Lippincott William and Wilkins, Philadelphia, PA.

Table 3

Occurrence of culture-positive influenza among study children in 1996–1997 (year 1) and 1997–1998 (year 2)

	Year 1		Year 2	
	Vaccine[a]	Placebo	Vaccine	Placebo
Number of children	1070	532	917	441
Influenza A	7	63	15	55
Influenza B	7	37	0	1
Either	14	94[b]	15	56

Children in the vaccine group received live attenuated intranasal vaccine in each year of this study (data from Refs. [4] and [5]).

[a] Overall vaccine efficacy was 92% (95% CI 88–94) during the 2 years of study. In year 1, vaccine efficacy was 95% (95% CI, 88, 97) vs. influenza A and 91% (95% CI 79–96) vs. influenza B. In year 2, vaccine was 86% effective vs. influenza A/Sydney (95% CI 75–92).

[b] Six children had two illnesses, one A and one B.

A/Wuhan/359/95-like viruses (four cases) or influenza B (one case). Vaccine was 100% efficacious in year 2 against strains included in the vaccine and 86% efficacious against the variant, A/Sydney/5/97. Overall, during the 2 years of study, vaccine was 92% efficacious at preventing culture-confirmed influenza [5]. Challenge studies with H1N1 vaccine strain confirmed high efficacy against this virus [8].

Influenza-associated otitis media was significantly reduced in each year of the study. In year 1, there was only one case of influenza-associated otitis media in the vaccine group, but there were 20 cases of otitis media among the placebo recipients associated with culture-positive influenza (vaccine efficacy = 98%). In year 2, only two cases of otitis media were associated with influenza in the vaccine group, but 17 occurred in the placebo recipients (vaccine efficacy = 94%). Cases of lower respiratory disease associated with culture-positive influenza were also significantly reduced in the vaccine group; only one case occurred in the 2 years in the vaccine group, but there were 11 cases in the 2 years in the placebo recipients (vaccine efficacy = 95% against influenza culture-positive lower respiratory disease).

Table 4

Effectiveness of live attenuated influenza vaccine in children in 1996–1997 (year 1) and 1997–1998 (year 2) (data from Ref. [10])

Effectiveness measure	Reduction in vaccine group (%)	
	Year 1	Year 2
Febrile illness	21*	19*
OM	9	8
Febrile OM	33*	16
Febrile illness with Abx	29*	13
Febrile OM with Abx	33*	18
Days of missed day care	11	18*
Days of present missing work	18	6
Visits to doctor	13*	8

* $p < 0.05$.

Several measures of vaccine effectiveness were assessed as indicators of benefit from annual vaccination (Table 4). Significant reduction in all febrile illness (regardless of result of viral cultures), reduction in febrile otitis media and reduction in associated antibiotic use was apparent in the vaccine groups [10]. Similarly, reduction in lost day care or lost school days, and reduction in lost work days by parents were present in the vaccinated children. Vaccinated children also visited health care workers significantly less often.

3. Discussion

Live attenuated influenza vaccine provided high efficacy and effectiveness against influenza and influenza-associated illnesses in children and adults. These studies included a year (1997–1998) in which the influenza strains selected for inclusion in the vaccine did not closely match the circulating predominant strain, influenza A/Sydney/5/97. The high efficacy against a variant influenza strain suggests that the live attenuated vaccine may provide superior immunity compared to inactivated vaccine in years when there is a poor match between vaccine and circulating viruses. The 2 years of study allowed us to estimate the efficacy of natural infection in year 1 against repeat infection in year 2. Of 53 placebo children with culture-positive H3N2 in year 1, only one (1.9%) had H3N2 in year 2, but of 393 placebo children without culture-positive H3N2 in year 1, 54 (14%) had H3N2 in year 2. When these data are used to estimate the protective efficacy of natural infection with A/Wuhan (year 1) against A/Sydney (year 2), the result is 85% (95% CI = 27–98). Point estimate of vaccine efficacy for the live attenuated vaccine (86%) was nearly identical to the point estimate of protection afforded by previous natural infection with A/Wuhan/369/95-like virus (85% efficacy) [5].

By what mechanism does the vaccine work? The induction of secretory IgA antibodies in the upper respiratory tract or the development of serum antibodies has been correlated with protection [8]. Seropositive children infrequently develop serum antibodies in response to the live vaccine, and yet, these children were also highly protected with the live attenuated vaccine [4]. Therefore, the fact that serum antibody is not boosted in seropositive individuals or in adults should not discourage the use of the vaccine to prevent influenza. The development of secretory IgA is an important addition to immunity against influenza. Other mediators of protection, including cell-mediated immunity, may also be induced by live attenuated vaccine. The safety, ease of administration of the vaccine, high efficacy, and high effectiveness make CAIV-T suitable for use in adults and children annually to prevent influenza and its complications.

References

[1] F.W. Henderson, A.M. Collier, M.A. Sanyal, A longitudinal study of respiratory viruses and bacteria in the etiology of acute otitis media with effusion, NEJM 306 (1982) 1377.
[2] T. Heikkinen, M. Thint, T. Chonmaitree, Prevalence of various respiratory viruses in the middle ear during acute otitis media, NEJM 340 (1999) 260–264.
[3] T. Chonmaitree, M.J. Owen, J.A. Patel, D. Hedgpeth, D. Horlick, V.M. Howie, Effect of viral respiratory tract infection on outcome of acute otitis media, J. Pediatr. 120 (1992) 856–862.

[4] R.B. Belshe, P.M. Mendelman, J. Treanor, J. King, W.C. Gruber, P. Piedra, D.I. Bernstein, F.G. Hayden, K. Kotloff, K. Zangwill, D. Iacuzio, M. Wolff, The efficacy of live attenuated, cold-adapted, trivalent, intranasal influenza virus vaccine in children, NEJM 338 (1998) 11405–11412.

[5] R.B. Belshe, W.B. Gruber, P.M. Mendelman, I. Cho, K. Reisinger, S.L. Block, J. Wittes, D. Iacuzio, P. Piedra, J. Treanor, J. King, K. Kotloff, D.I. Bernstein, F.G. Hayden, K. Zangwill, L. Yan, M. Wolff, Efficacy of vaccination with live attenuated, cold-adapted, trivalent, intranasal influenza virus vaccine against a variant (A/Sydney) not contained in the vaccine, J. Pediatr. 136 (2000) 168–175.

[6] K.L. Nichol, P.M. Mendelman, K.P. Mallon, L.A. Jackson, G.J. Gorse, R.B. Belshe, W.P. Glezen, J. Wittes, for the Live Attenuated Influenza Virus Vaccine in Healthy Adults Trial Group, Effectiveness of live, attenuated intranasal influenza virus vaccine in healthy, working adults: A randomized controlled trial, JAMA 282 (1999) 137–144.

[7] J.J. Treanor, K. Kotloff, R.F. Betts, R. Belshe, F. Newman, D. Iacuzio, J. Wittes, M. Bryant, Evaluation of trivalent, live, cold-adapted (CAIV-T) and inactivated (TIV) influenza vaccines in prevention of virus infection and illness following challenge of adults with wild-type influenza A (H1N1), A (H3N2), and B viruses, Vaccine 18 (1999) 899–906.

[8] R.B. Belshe, W.B. Gruber, P.M. Mendelman, B. Harshvardhan, H.B. Mehta, I. Cho, K. Reisinger, J. Treanor, K. Zangwill, F.G. Hayden, D.I. Bernstein, K. Kotloff, J. King, P.A. Piedra, S.L. Block, L. Yan, M. Wolff, Correlates of immune protection induced by live attenuated, cold-adapted, trivalent, intranasal influenza virus vaccine, J. Infect. Dis. 181 (2000) 1133–1137.

[9] W.C. Gruber, R. Belshe, P. Mendelman, L. Yan, M. Wolff, for the NIAID Vaccine and Treatment Evaluation Units and Aviron. Immunologic Response to Heterotypic H3N2 Strains After Live Intranasal or Inactivated Influenza Vaccine in Children, Presented at the 36th Annual IDSA Meeting, Denver, CO, November 1998.

[10] R.B. Belshe, W.C. Gruber, Prevention of otitis media in children with live attenuated influenza vaccine given intranasally, Pediatr. Infect. Dis. J. 19 (2000) S66–S71.

[11] R.B. Belshe, E.M. Swierkosz, E.L. Anderson, F.K. Newman, S.L. Nugent, J. Maassab, Immunization of infants and young children with live attenuated trivalent cold recombinant influenza A H1N1, H3N2, and B vaccine, JID 165 (1992) 727–732.

[12] E. Swierkosz, F. Newman, E. Anderson, S. Nugent, G. Mills, R. Belshe, Multidose live attenuated, cold-recombinant, trivalent influenza vaccine in infants and young children, JID 169 (1994) 1121–1124.

International Congress Series 1219 (2001) 939–943

Safety and effectiveness of the trivalent, cold-adapted influenza vaccine (CAIV-T) in children

Pedro A. Piedra[a,b,*], Manjusha Gaglani[c], Gayla Herschler[d],
Mark Riggs[e], Melissa Griffith[d], Claudia Kozinetz[b],
W. Paul Glezen[a,b]

[a]Department of Molecular Virology and Microbiology, Baylor College of Medicine, Houston, TX, USA
[b]Department of Pediatrics, Baylor College of Medicine, Houston, TX, USA
[c]Department of Pediatrics, Scott & White Clinic, Temple, TX, USA
[d]Office of Research, Scott & White Clinic, Temple, TX, USA
[e]Department of Biostatistics, Scott & White Clinic, Temple, TX, USA

Abstract

Background: We report on the safety and effectiveness of trivalent, cold-adapted influenza vaccine (CAIV-T) in children in the largest community trial to date. *Methods*: Enrolled children 18 months through 18 years of age received CAIV-T in years 1 (1998) and 2 (1999). All were surveyed for serious adverse events (SAEs). The relative risk (RR) of medically attended acute respiratory illness (MAARI) was estimated in the first 14 days after CAIV-T and compared to the reference interval pre-vaccine and > 14 days after CAIV-T. Vaccine effectiveness against MAARI during the influenza outbreak was determined for vaccinees compared to age-eligible non-participants. *Results*: 4298 and 5250 children received CAIV-T in years 1 and 2. Twenty-two SAEs were identified; none were vaccine associated. No excess MAARI attributed to CAIV-T was observed: the RRs 0–14 days after CAIV-T were 1.0 (95% CI 0.8–1.3) and 1.1 (95% CI 0.8–1.4) for years 1 and 2, respectively. Similar safety was seen in a subgroup of children with mild wheezing illness. In year 1, vaccine effectiveness was detected during the intense period of the influenza season: RR 0.9 (95% CI: 0.81–0.99); year 2 is pending. *Conclusions*: CAIV-T was safe in children including those with mild wheezing illness. Effectiveness of CAIV-T was detected against MAARI. © 2001 Elsevier Science B.V. All rights reserved.

Keywords: Community trial; Serious adverse event (SAE); Medically attended acute respiratory illness (MAARI); Mild wheezing illness

---

* Corresponding author. Department of Molecular Virology and Microbiology, Baylor College of Medicine, Rm. 248E, One Baylor Plaza, Houston, TX 77030, USA. Tel.: +1-713-798-5240; fax: +1-713-798-6802.
E-mail address: ppiedra@bcm.tmc.edu (P.A. Piedra).

0531-5131/01/$ – see front matter © 2001 Elsevier Science B.V. All rights reserved.
PII: S0531-5131(01)00019-X

1. Introduction

Influenza is a vaccine preventable disease that causes widespread infection and morbidity in all age groups. The attack rate is greatest among individuals with minimal prior exposure to influenza, particularly children. The licensed influenza vaccine administered by an injection is recommended for people at risk for complications of influenza. The main strategy has been the annual vaccination of high-risk individuals to reduce excess mortality. Vaccination of healthy children is being considered because they have high rates of infection, and are important in the spread of influenza. It is postulated that immunization of children would be effective for epidemic influenza control [1,2]. In a pre-licensure phase III efficacy trial in children 15 to 71 months of age, the trivalent, cold-adapted influenza vaccine (CAIV-T) was well tolerated, safe and efficacious [3]. CAIV-T was 93% efficacious against culture confirmed influenza, and during the second year of the trial, CAIV-T was 86% efficacious against a variant strain (A/Sydney/05/97).

We report on the safety and effectiveness of the CAIV-T in children in the largest study to date. A primary objective is to demonstrate that immunization of children ages 18 months through 18 years with CAIV-T will reduce medically attended acute respiratory illnesses (MAARI) in the vaccinated children. A secondary objective is to assess the general safety of the CAIV-T. The goal is to determine if immunization of children with CAIV-T will provide herd immunity that will be effective for the control of epidemic influenza and may serve as a model for control of pandemic influenza.

2. Materials and methods

2.1. Study design

The study was approved by the local Institutional Review Boards and signed informed consent was obtained. This is an ongoing open label, community trial enrolling children 18 months through 18 years of age. The trial is focused in Temple-Belton, located in Central Texas. The principal vaccination sites are the Scott & White clinics, which provide health care to approximately 80% of the population. The study aims to enroll 80% of the approximately 20,000 children in Temple-Belton.

Prior to vaccination, a brief medical history and physical assessment was performed. All children received by nasal spray a 0.5-ml dose of CAIV-T (approximately 10^7 $TCID_{50}$ of each of the three vaccine components) manufactured by Aviron. The vaccine strains were comparable to those chosen by the FDA. The parent of enrolled children received a laminated card and refrigerator magnet that instructed the parents to call if their child was hospitalized or developed any serious condition within 6 weeks of vaccination. Approximately 6 weeks after the date of vaccination, an automated phone call was made to remind parents to report any serious adverse events (SAEs) and pregnancies. In addition, study participants who were not members of the managed care program of Scott & White (SWHP) were contacted by study personnel approximately 6 weeks after vaccination to ascertain the occurrence of SAEs and pregnancies.

Children 18 months through 18 years were enrolled after satisfying the inclusion criteria and none of the exclusion criteria. The latter were children who had a chronic disease for which the licensed inactivated flu vaccine is recommended, who lived with a household member who had an immunosuppressive disease or therapy, who had a history of significant hypersensitivity to eggs, or who were pregnant or planned to become pregnant within 42 days after vaccination. Postponement of vaccination occurred with an acute febrile illness within 2 days of vaccination, with significant nasal discharge or congestion, or with use of a live vaccine or inactivated vaccine within 4 or 2 weeks, respectively. Children were not excluded if they used daily nasal steroids, had mild, intermittent wheezing or exercise induced asthma with use of bronchodilator prior to exercise. Subjects not eligible to receive CAIV-T were offered inactivated influenza vaccine.

2.2. Virologic surveillance

Surveillance for influenza viruses was performed in children and adults with a history of a febrile respiratory illness who presented to a Scott & White medical care facility. Throat cultures were processed for isolation and identification of influenza viruses by standard methods.

2.3. Data analysis

Administrative files extracted from the fully integrated online computerized database at Scott & White were used to determine the safety and effectiveness of CAIV-T. Monthly searches for SAEs were performed by screening the administrative files for all hospital and emergency room encounters. Pregnancies were sought by screening for ICD-9 pregnancy codes (hospital, emergency room and clinic visits). A final SAE search was conducted at least 6 weeks from the date the last child was vaccinated. For additional safety assessment, the relative risk (RR) of MAARI (ICD-9 codes for acute otitis media and sinusitis, acute upper respiratory illness, and acute lower respiratory illness) 0–14 days after vaccination was compared to that occurring in the interval pre- and >14 days post-vaccine. Each study subject was assumed to have contributed the same number of days of observation regardless of the date of vaccination. Poisson regression analysis, a multivariate analysis for log-linear modeling of incidence rates, was used to estimate the relative risk of an event while controlling for age category and season [4,5]. The logarithm of a rate was modeled as a weighted sum of the independent variables. The models were fit by maximum likelihood. The estimated coefficients were transformed to incidence rate ratios, i.e., e^b rather than b. The 95% confidence intervals (95% CIs) were similarly transformed. The goodness-of-fit test was used to test the appropriateness of the models. The SWHP administrative files were used to ascertain the direct effectiveness of CAIV-T in SWHP members by comparing MAARI rates in CAIV-T vaccinees to age-eligible unvaccinated children in Temple-Belton during the intense period of the influenza season. To assess direct effectiveness, point estimates and 95% confidence intervals for the incidence rate ratio were calculated for the vaccinated and age-eligible, unvaccinated.

3. Results

In years 1 (1998–99) and 2 (1999–2000), 4298 children and 5250 children, respectively, received CAIV-T. For both years, a total of 7448 children received 9548 doses of CAIV-T of which 2101 children were enrolled in both years. The vaccine virus strains (A/Beijing/262/95-like (H1N1), A/Sydney/05/97-like (H3N2) and B/Beijing/184/93-like) in CAIV-T were the same for both years and were antigenically similar to the virus strains in the licensed inactivated influenza vaccines.

Six-week follow up for SAEs was successful for 4145 (96.43%) of 4298 children immunized in year 1 and 5146 (95.8%) of 5250 children immunized in year 2. In total, 20 SAEs (year 1: 8 SAEs and year 2: 14 SAEs) were identified, and none were attributed to the vaccine. Five pregnancies were identified and there were no congenital anomalies detected. The administrative files were searched for rare serious illnesses that may be associated with natural influenza virus infections within 6 weeks of vaccination. These illnesses included myocarditis, encephalitis, Guillain–Barre' syndrome, myositis, febrile seizures, etc. No such instances were discovered in year 1 (year 2 pending). Furthermore, in years 1 and 2, SWHP vaccinees were studied for excess occurrence of MAARI during the first 14 days after vaccination (Table 1). An excess in the rate of MAARI was not observed in the first 14 days after vaccination compared to the comparison period. A similar evaluation was performed in SWHP vaccinees with a history of a wheezing illness (Table 1). These children were eligible to receive CAIV-T if they were not on chronic treatment for asthma and had not had an acute wheezing attack requiring emergency room care or hospitalization in the past year (or past 6 months for children 18 months to 2 years of age). No excess in the rate of MAARI was detected.

In year 1, influenza A/Sydney (H3N2) and influenza B/Yamanashi accounted for 60% and 40% of the influenza viruses identified in Temple-Belton. The influenza outbreak occurred from January 17, 1999 to April 3, 1999 with no overlap in the vaccination-safety phase. The intense period of the outbreak was from January 31 to March 13. In year 2, influenza A/Sydney (H3N2) accounted for 99% of the strains isolated in Temple-Belton. The influenza outbreak occurred from December 5, 1999 to January 29, 2000, which was encompassed by the vaccination-safety phase. Vaccine effectiveness was detected during

Table 1
Relative risk (RR) of medically attended acute respiratory illness for acute otitis media/sinusitis, acute upper respiratory illness, and acute lower respiratory illness in the first 14 days after vaccine

Study year	Period	Population	Child-days	Number	RR	95% CI
1	Pre-vaccine, 0–14 days post-vaccine	SWHP ($n=2031$)	251,844, 30,465	980, 115	1, 1.0	Reference, 0.9–1.4
1	Pre-vaccine, 0–14 days post-vaccine	Hx of wheeze ($n=302$)	37,448, 4530	247, 30	1, 1.06	Reference, 0.72–1.55
2	Pre-vaccine, 0–14 days post-vaccine	SWHP ($n=2304$)	248,832, 34,560	1257, 171	1, 1.0	Reference, 0.8–1.2
2	Pre-vaccine, 0–14 days post-vaccine	Hx of wheeze ($n=463$)	50,004, 6945	368, 52	1, 0.99	Reference, 0.74–1.33

Table 2
CAIV-T effectiveness against medically attended acute respiratory illnesses (MAARI) during the intense period of the influenza season in year 1

Age group	Number of SWHP children in Temple-Belton		MAARI rate/10,000 child-day		RR 95% CI
	CAIV-T	Non-CAIV-T	CAIV-T	Non-CAIV-T	
1.5–4 years	454	1962	89.2	107.8	0.8 0.7 –0.98
5–9 years	799	3030	57.5	65.9	0.9 0.74–1.02
10–18 years	749	5986	38.5	49.3	0.8 0.64–0.94
All	2002	10,978	57.6	64.3	0.9 0.81–0.99

the intense period of the influenza season: RR 0.9 (95% CI: 0.81–0.99) (Table 2). Year 2 is pending.

4. Discussion

In the largest community trial to date with CAIV-T, 7448 children received 9548 doses of CAIV-T during the first 2 years of this ongoing trial. The vaccine was shown to be well tolerated and safe and well accepted by the parents. CAIV-T was not associated with an increase in health care utilization for acute respiratory illnesses, and no serious adverse events were attributed to CAIV-T.

A significant reduction in MAARI was observed in vaccinated children in year 1 (year 2 analysis is pending). This reduction was still detectable in the face of higher than usual community immunity to A/Sydney because A/Wuhan (H3N2) and A/Sydney have been the major circulating viruses since the 1996–1997 influenza season. A significant reduction in MAARI should impact on the wellness of the vaccinees and reduce the utilization of medical services during one of the busiest times of the year for health care providers.

The indirect effect or herd immunity was not detected in year 1 (data not shown). The year 2 data for an indirect effect has not yet been examined. With approximately 40% of children in Temple-Belton vaccinated with CAIV-T, we will begin to develop an estimate of the percent of vaccinated children required for the detection of an indirect effect in the community against influenza-related morbidity.

References

[1] W.P. Glezen, Emerging infections: pandemic influenza, Epidemiol. Rev. 18 (1996) 1–13.
[2] I.M. Longini, M.E. Halloran, A. Nizam, M. Wolff, P.M. Mendelman, P.E. Fast, R.B. Belshe, Estimation of the live, attenuated influenza vaccine from a two-year, multi-center trial: implication for influenza epidemic control, Vaccine 18 (2000) 1902–1909.
[3] R.B. Belshe, W.C. Gruber, P.M. Mendelman, I. Cho, K. Reisinger, S.L. Block, J. Wittes, D. Iacuzio, P. Piedra, J. Treanor, J. King, K. Kotloff, D.I. Bernstein, F.G. Hayden, K. Zangwill, L. Yan, M. Wolff, Efficacy of vaccination with live attenuated, cold-adapted, trivalent, intranasal influenza virus vaccine against a variant (A/Sydney) not contained in the vaccine, J. Pediatr. 136 (2000) 168–175.
[4] M.R. Griffin, J.A. Taylor, J.R. Daugherty, W.A. Ray, No increased risk for invasive bacterial infection found following diphtheria–tetanus–pertussis immunization, Pediatrics 89 (1992) 640–642.
[5] N. Breslow, Multivariate cohort analysis, Natl. Cancer Inst. Monogr. 67 (1985) 149–156.

International Congress Series 1219 (2001) 945–950

Current strategies for the prevention of influenza by the Russian cold-adapted live influenza vaccine among different populations

L.G. Rudenko*, G.I. Alexandrova

*Department of Virology, Institute for Experimental Medicine RAMS, Acad. Pavlov Str. 12,
197376 St. Petersburg, Russia*

Abstract

Trivalent live attenuated influenza vaccine (LIV) prepared from the donor strains A/Len/134/17/57 (H2N2) and B/USSR/60/69 demonstrated safety, immunogenicity, genetic stability for a single dose in children from 3 years old. The vaccine efficacy against serologically and virologically confirmed influenza virus infection was 94.4% for children 7–14 years old and 92.9% for children 3–6 years old. An improved strategy for immunizing the elderly with a combination of LIV and inactivated vaccine has been developed. This strategy has been estimated to be 68% effective against influenza. The proposed strategy uses LIV based on the donor strains A/Len/134/17/57 (H2N2) and B/USSR/60/69 for different population groups. The LIV may also have a potential use in the event of an influenza pandemic. © 2001 Elsevier Science B.V. All rights reserved.

Keywords: Cold-adapted live vaccine; Influenza; Donor strains; Immunogenicity; Safety; Efficacy

Russia is the only country in the world where live influenza vaccine (LIV) has been licensed and used. Special attention has been paid to the vaccines following the first preparation of cold-adapted (ca) variants of influenza viruses A and B used to prevent influenza in adults and children from 1 year old. The safety and efficacy of the vaccines have been amply demonstrated following widespread public health use across different geographical areas and varied ethnic groups.

---

* Corresponding author. Tel.: +7-812-234-9214; fax: +7-812-234-9489.
E-mail address: iem@iem.spb.ru (L.G. Rudenko).

0531-5131/01/$ – see front matter © 2001 Elsevier Science B.V. All rights reserved.
PII: S0531-5131(01)00661-6

The results from 126 efficacy trials involving > 500,000 adults (500–45,000/trial) can be summarized as follows:

- statistical analysis of each trial confirmed vaccine efficacy;
- index of efficacy (as measured clinically against all acute respiratory diseases) was 2.4 (58%);
- the minimum index of efficacy was 1.37 (29%), which occurred when vaccine trials were conducted between epidemics;
- the mean efficacy was 1.80 (45%);
- single-dose vaccination was shown to be as effective as two or three doses [1].

Clinical and laboratory examination of children vaccinated with additionally attenuated 'ca' live influenza vaccine demonstrated a reactogenicity and safety of the tested vaccine for children 1–7 years. Even utilising clinically assessed non-specific acute respiratory disease (ARD) as the key parameter of vaccine efficacy, the LIV was 23–40% effective, whereas serologically confirmed influenza morbidity (not virus isolation confirmed) demonstrated the vaccine was 69–80% effective. In addition, vaccinated children had a 53% lower incidence of pneumonia and bronchitis and 47% lower incidence of otitis media than unvaccinated children.

Subsequently, cold-adapted strain A/Leningrad/134/17/57 (H2N2), further attenuated variant A/Leningrad/134/47/57 (H2N2) and B/USSR/60/69 have proven to be reliable donors of attenuation for preparation of live reassortant influenza vaccine for use in adults and children [2]. Live cold-adapted reassortant mono-, di- and trivalent influenza type A and B vaccines have been studied in a series of controlled clinical and epidemiological investigations involving nearly 150,000 children 3–14 years old. These investigations confirmed safety and efficacy LIV [3].

However, the need to produce two vaccines, one for adults and one for children, the two-dose regimen for vaccinating children and the absence of a suitable strategy to protect high-risk individuals, necessitated a further series of studies which have provided the basis for the current strategy for LIV use.

From 1993 to 1997, we conducted a randomized, placebo-controlled, double-blind study to compare the Russian 17 passage LIV, administered alone and in combination with US inactivated split-virus influenza vaccine (IIV), among the elderly with chronic diseases such as cardiovascular, diabetes or pulmonary diseases of mild to moderate severity. The results of the safety evaluations have been reported previously [4]. The study was complex and involved monitoring humoral, secretory and cellular immunity, the age dependence of cytokine production (IL-2, IL-4, gamma-IFN), the method of antigen administration and antigen type. LIV had advantages over the inactivated influenza vaccine (IIV) in providing a greater intensity of secretory immunity among young and elderly recipients, plus gamma-IFN and IL-2 production and T-cell factors in the elderly people. IIV induced a higher level of humoral antibodies compared with LIV; however, the qualitative characteristics (functional activity) of the immunoglobulins were lower than those stimulated by LIV. Following separate LIV and IIV administration, the qualitative parameters of local, humoral and cellular immunity induction were lower among elderly than the young. Simultaneous LIV and IIV administration promoted the stimulation of these immunity factors among elderly people to

Table 1
Systemic, local, cellular and cytokine immune response in elderly and young patients vaccinated with a combination of live and inactivated influenza trivalent vaccines

| Preparation | Age group | Number in group | Geometric mean values (GMT) and arithmethic mean values (AMV) to the A(H1N1) antigen after immunization | | | | | |
| | | | Serum antibody GMT | Local IgA-antibody GMT | Lymphocytes in vitro stimulation index | Levels (pg/ml) in supernatants lymphocyte cultures | | |
						γ-IFN	IL-2	IL-4
Live (i.n.)+ inactivated (i.m.)	Elderly	19	8.7	3.6	2.0	1.6	2.0	1.2
	Young	20	6.5	1.8	2.2	1.8	2.0	1.1

the level observed in young people. In elderly people, an important chain of immunity—prolonged T- and B-cell memory (Table 1)—was actively induced in response to the combined immunization. Among the elderly, vaccination with either LIV or IIV resulted in a vaccine efficacy of 51–53%. The combination vaccine strategy resulted in a vaccination efficacy of 65–73% and was significantly different from the placebo group (Table 2).

The next stage of investigation involved combined clinical trials, which commenced in Vologda [5] utilising LIV based on A/Leningrad/134/17/57 (H2N2) and B/USSR/60/69 among preschool and school children aged 3–14 years.

The first clinical trial involved schoolchildren 7–14 years old to compare a live trivalent influenza vaccine based on the master strain A/Leningrad/134/17/57 with one based on the master strain A/Leningrad/134/47/57, during the epidemic period 1999–2000 in St. Petersburg region. Schoolchildren were 94% and 83% protected against serologically and virologically confirmed influenza infection, with LIV based on either A/Len/134/17/57 or A/Len/134/47/57, respectively (Table 3). Against all clinically diagnosed acute respiratory diseases, the above vaccines were 43.3% and 48.8% effective, respectively, during the peak of influenza epidemic period and were 28.1–30.9% effective when calculated over the entire epidemic period of 35 days. LIV for adults reduced bronchitis in children 7–14 years old by 4.2-fold during the epidemic. Less than 1% school children (7–9 years) developed acute respiratory disease (ARD) within 1 week of receiving LIV based on master strain A/Len/134/17/57 and approximately 1.6% children developed ARD

Table 2
Estimated vaccine efficacy for live and inactivated influenza vaccines administered in combination or separately to nursing home residents (St. Petersburg, 1996–1997)

Study group	Vaccine preparation	Number	Number (%) of ill with lab-confirmed influenza	Vaccine efficacy (%) (95% CI)
I	IMV and LV + LV	109	5 (4.6)	67.4 (6.0–88.7)
II	IMV and LV + lp	103	5 (4.6)	65.4 (0.1–88.0)
III	Imp and LV + LV	111	7 (6.3)	54.3 (18.0–82.3)
IV	IMV and lp + lp	93	6 (6.5)	53.2 (−27.2–82.8)
V	Imp and lp + lp	109	14 (12.8)	−
VI	IMV and lp + LV	77	3 (3.9)	72.5 (−0.7–92.4)
I, II, VI		289	13 (4.5)	68.0 (29.6–85.5)

Table 3
Efficacy of LIV in school children determined by serological and virological diagnosis (winter 2000)

Number of children tested with ARD	Serological/virological confirmation of influenza		Group	Number (%) with confirmation of influenza		Efficacy
	Total	Percentage		Number	Percentage	
58	22	37.9	LIV for adults	1	4.6	94.4
			LIV for children	3	13.6	83.3
			Placebo	18	81.8	

within 1 week of receiving LIV based on master strain A/Len/134/47/57. The highest percentage of seroconversions, protective HI titers and geometric mean titer rises was achieved among those children who received a single dose of LIV based on master strain A/Len/134/17/57 (Table 4).

The second clinical trial of trivalent LIV based on the master strain A/Len/134/17/57 was made among children 3–6 years old during the 1999–2000 flu season. Reactogenicity and immunogenicity studies were undertaken among 256 kindergarten children aged 3–6 years old. The vaccine was well tolerated. Vaccines exhibited very low reactogenicity with 0% temperature reactions > 37.5 °C and with 0.5% showing headache/catarrhal symptoms. Following a single vaccination, 59% seronegative children seroconverted to the influenza A strain and 36% seroconverted to the influenza B strain. It is notable that a single dose of vaccine induced similar geometric mean titer rises as a two-dose vaccine regimen.

In the event of an influenza pandemic, most countries in the world have prepared vaccination programs to protect the population. LIV use in pre-epidemic and pre-pandemic periods is recommended for the reasons discussed below.

(1) LIV is a potent interferon inducer; its use, independent of the strains included in its composition, reduces all ARD morbidity by 40% for 10 days post-administration.

Table 4
HI antibody response in seronegative children (7–9 years old) to vaccination with trivalent LIV for adults and for children

Preparation	Number of doses	Antigen	Number in group	Sero-conversions (%)	Percentage with protective titer $\geq$ 1:40	Pre-GMT	Post-GMT	GMT rise
LIV for adults	1	A(H1N1)	50	64.0	52.0	7.6	32.0	4.0
		A(H3N2)	40	67.5	62.5	8.9	42.1	4.8
		B	39	48.7	43.6	9.7	29.0	3.0
LIV for children	2	A(H1N1)	32	56.2	25.0	6.0	16.5	2.8
		A(H3N2)	30	66.7	46.7	6.9	26.4	3.8
		B	25	36.0	34.6	8.7	20.6	2.4
LIV for children	1	A(H1N1)	13	23.1	21.3	6.9	11.1	1.6
		A(H3N2)	12	41.7	38.2	6.3	14.1	2.1
		B	11	36.4	36.4	8.3	24.2	2.9
Placebo	1	A(H1N1)	42	2.4	0	6.6	6.7	1.0
		A(H3N2)	45	2.9	2.9	6.4	6.8	1.1
		B	45	8.0	4.0	10.9	12.8	1.2

(2) LIV confers significant levels of "herd immunity" as shown by the Novgorod school study, in which it was observed that influenza morbidity was significantly lower among non-vaccinated pupils and staff where more than 50% pupils were vaccinated, compared with those schools where pupils received IIV. [6].

(3) Using cold-adapted viruses as a basis for IIV in the event that especially virulent strains appear. A similar approach was undertaken with gene modification of avian H5 virus.

Conclusion

Live influenza vaccine preparations based on the attenuated donor A/Len/134/17/57 is safe, genetically stable, stimulates a high level of all components of the immune system, and ensures reliable protection against influenza infection. The recommended vaccination strategy could be a single vaccine dose for all age groups (from 3 years).

Live influenza vaccine should be included in the immunization calendar, especially for schoolchildren who are the source of spread of the infection during epidemics.

For influenza prophylaxis among elderly people with chronic diseases of the cardio-vascular system, lungs and metabolic disorders, the most effective immunization regimen is combined administration of live and inactivated vaccine.

Live influenza vaccine could be recommended in the case of an influenza pandemic since:

(a) it has an interferon inducing effect;
(b) it has indirect effect on unimmunized people (herd immunity);
(c) cold-adapted viruses could be used for obtaining vaccine strains for IIV in case of especially dangerous influenza viruses.

Acknowledgements

We thank the Influenza Branch of CDC, and personally N. Cox, A. Klimov, A. Kendal, J. Katz, N. Arden and Professor A. Monto for their long-time cooperation and support in research with live influenza vaccine.

References

[1] Y.G. Ivannikov, I.G. Marinich, V.A. Kondrat'ev, et al., The statistical analysis of long-term experience of efficacy study live influenza vaccines, in: G.I. Jophe, G.I. Alexandrova (Eds.), Immunology and Specific Influenza Prophylaxis in Children, 1971, pp. 75–92, Leningrad.
[2] G.I. Alexandrova, Live influenza vaccine in Russia, in: L.E. Brown, A.W. Hampson, R.G. Webster (Eds.), Options for the Control of Influenza III, Elsevier, Amsterdam, 1996, pp. 123–128.
[3] L.G. Rudenko, N.I. Lonskaya, A.I. Klimov, et al., Clinical and epidemiological evaluation of live, cold-adapted influenza vaccine for 3–14-years-olds, Bull. WHO 74 (1987) 77–84.
[4] L.G. Rudenko, N. Arden, E.P. Grigorieva, et al., Safety and immunogenicity of Russian live-attenuated and US inactivated trivalent influenza vaccines in the elderly, in: L.E. Brown, A.W. Hampson, R.G. Webster (Eds.), Options for the Control of Influenza III, Elsevier, Amsterdam, 1996, pp. 572–578.

[5] A.S. Khan, F.I. Polezhaev, R.I. Vasiljeva, et al., Comparison of US inactivated and Russian live attenuated, cold-adapted trivalent influenza vaccines in Russian schoolchildren, J. Infect. Dis. 173 (1996) 453–456.
[6] L.G. Rudenko, A.N. Slepuskin, A.S. Monto, et al., Efficacy of live attenuated and inactivated influenza vaccines in schoolchildren and their unvaccinated contacts in Novgorod, Russia, J. Infect. Dis. 168 (1993) 881–887.

International Congress Series 1219 (2001) 951–954

Live attenuated reassortant influenza vaccine prepared using A/Leningrad/134/17/57 (H2N2) donor strain is genetically stable after replication in children 3-6 years of age

A.I. Klimov[a,*], I.V. Kiseleva[b], J.A. Desheva[b], G.I. Alexandrova[b], N.J. Cox[a], L.G. Rudenko[b]

[a]*Influenza Branch, G-16, Centers for Disease Control and Prevention, 1600 Clifton Rd., NE, Atlanta, GA, USA*
[b]*Department of Virology, Institute of Experimental Medicine, RAMS, St. Petersburg, Russia*

Abstract

Background: Live influenza A vaccines (LIVs) for adults and children are prepared in Russia by reassorting current epidemic strains with cold-adapted (ca) attenuated donor viruses A/Leningrad/134/17/57 (H2N2) (Len/17) and A/Leningrad/134/47/57 (H2N2) (Len/47), respectively. Len/17 and Len/47 were derived from the A/Leningrad/134/57 (H2N2) wild-type virus after 17 and 47 passages in eggs at 25 °C. Two doses of Len/47-based vaccine have been used for vaccinating children. In a recent study, children were vaccinated with the Len/17-based LIV in order to determine if this vaccine is safe and immunogenic after a single dose vaccination. As part of this study, type A isolates obtained from children 3–6 years of age on the third day after vaccination were analyzed for genetic stability. *Methods*: PCR-restriction (RFLP) analysis was used to detect mutations in genomes of isolates. *Results*: Internal genes of Len/17 contain eight coding mutations in the PB2 (1), PB1 (2), PA (2), M1 (1), M2 (1) and NS (1) genes. All of these mutations, except one, were conserved in the genomes of all 28 strains studied. Similar to other studies with Len/17, the A-86-T change in the M2 protein, which was shown to be heterogeneous in the parent donor strain, was absent in 13 isolates. Since it was shown that mutations in polymerase genes play a leading role in the attenuation of Len/17, it is important to emphasize their conservation in all of the isolates. Moreover, an additional mutation in the PB2 protein (S-478-R), previously known only for the more attenuated Len/47 ca donor strain, was detected in 9 of 28 isolates, indicating that this mutation may also be heterogeneous in the donor virus. *Conclusion*: The Len/17-based LIV is genetically stable in children. © 2001 Elsevier Science B.V. All rights reserved.

Keywords: Live influenza vaccine; Genetic stability

* Corresponding author. Tel.: +1-404-639-3591; fax: +1-404-639-2334.
E-mail address: axk0@cdc.gov (A.I. Klimov).

0531-5131/01/$ – see front matter © 2001 Elsevier Science B.V. All rights reserved.
PII: S 0 5 3 1 - 5 1 3 1 (0 1) 0 0 0 2 0 - 6

1. Introduction

Live influenza A vaccines (LIVs) for adults and children are prepared in Russia by reassorting current epidemic strains with cold-adapted (ca) attenuated donor viruses A/Leningrad/134/17/57 (H2N2) (Len/17) and A/Leningrad/134/47/57 (H2N2) (Len/47), respectively. Len/17 and Len/47 were derived from the A/Leningrad/134/57 (H2N2) wild-type virus (Len/wt) after 17 and 47 passages in eggs at 25 °C [1, 2]. For many years, Len/17 has been used for preparing reassortant attenuated LIVs for adults and Len/47 for preparing LIVs for children. Vaccine reassortants that inherited the hemagglutinin (HA) and neuraminidase genes from epidemic viruses and all internal genes from Len/17 or Len/47 ca donors (6:2 reassortants) were shown to be safe, immunogenic and genetically stable after replication in adults and children [1–6]. To obtain the necessary level of immunity, however, two doses of Len/47-based vaccine have been used for vaccinating children. Several years ago, the possibility of using one dose of Len/17-based vaccine for immunizing children was evaluated and the vaccine was shown to be safe and immunogenic for seronegative school children [7]. Isolates from these children revealed preservation of Len/17-specific mutations in all internal genes except the M2 gene. Approximately 50% of the isolates lacked the Ala-96-Thr mutation in the M2 protein. It was shown, however, that heterogeneity at nucleotide 969 of the M2 gene of the Len/17 donor was responsible for the lack of this mutation in some isolates [6]. The Len/17-based vaccine was further studied recently in preschool children. In October 1999, 150 children (3–6 years of age) were vaccinated with the Len/17-based LIV in order to determine if this vaccine is safe and immunogenic after a single-dose vaccination. The trivalent LIV included reassortants prepared using epidemic strains recommended by WHO for the 1999–2000 epidemic season: A/Sydney/5/97 (H3N2), A/Beijing/262/95 (H1N1) and B/St. Petersburg/92/95 (B/Beijing/184/93-like; the B vaccine reassortant was prepared using B/USSR/60/69 ca donor strain). As part of this study, type A isolates obtained from vaccinated children were analyzed for genetic stability.

2. Methods

Virus isolation. Viruses were isolated from nasal swabs collected from children on the third day after vaccination and passed 1–2 times in embryonated hens' eggs.

Virus typing. Primers specific for HAs of influenza A(H3N2), A(H1N1) and B viruses were used for PCR amplification of virus RNAs to type/subtype the isolates.

PCR-restriction (RFLP) analysis [8] was modified to detect preservation in type A isolates of all mutations known for internal genes of Len/17 and Len/47 donor strains.

3. Results

Internal genes of Len/17 contain eight coding mutations in the PB2 (G-1459-A), PB1 (G-819-T, G-1795-A), PA (T-107-C, G-1045-T), M (A-68-G, G-969-A), and NS (G-798-A) genes. All of these mutations were detected in genomes of both A(H1N1) and

Table 1
PCR-restriction analysis of mutations in genomes of isolates from children 3–6 years of age vaccinated with Len/17-based attenuated LIV

Strain	Internal genes								
	PB2		PB1		PA		M		NS
	1459	1497	819	1795	107	1045	68	969	798
Len/wt	G	C	G	G	T	G	A	G	G
Len/17	T	C	T	A	C	T	G	A	A
H3N2 vaccine	T	C	T	A	C	T	G	A	A
H1N1 vaccine	T	C	T	A	C	T	G	A	A
12 isolates	T	C	T	A	C	T	G	A	A
3 isolates	T	A[a]	T	A	C	T	G	A	A
7 isolates	T	C	T	A	C	T	G	G	A
6 isolates	T	A[a]	T	A	C	T	G	G	A

[a] The C-1497-A mutation coding for Ser-490-Arg amino acid change was known for the PB2 gene of the more attenuated Len/47 ca donor strain.

A(H3N2) components of the trivalent LIV used in the study (Table 1). All of the mutations, except one in the M gene, were also conserved in the genomes of all 28 strains studied (Table 1). Similar to other studies with Len/17 [6], the A-86-T, G-969-A (Ala-86-Thr) change in the M2 protein gene, which was shown to be heterogeneous in the parent donor strain, was absent in 13 of 28 isolates.

An additional coding mutation in the PB2 protein (C-1497-A coding for the Ser-478-Arg change), previously known only for the more attenuated Len/47 ca donor virus, was detected in genomes of 9 out of 28 isolates.

4. Discussion

The results of this study provide additional evidence of the high degree of genetic stability of ca attenuated reassortant LIVs. All of the mutations known for internal genes of Len/17, except one in the M gene, were conserved in genomes of all 28 strains studied. Although about 50% of the isolates from children lacked one of coding mutations known for the Len/17 donor, it was shown that heterogeneity at nucleotide 969 of the M2 gene of the Len/17 donor was responsible for the lack of this mutation in these isolates [6]. It is important to point out that the absence of this mutation in the M2 protein did not affect attenuation of the reassortant LIV for pre-school children.

Since it was shown that mutations in polymerase genes play a leading role in the attenuation of Len/17 [9], it is important to emphasize their conservation in all of the isolates. Moreover, an additional coding mutation in the PB2 protein was detected in genomes of 9 out of 28 isolates. Previously this mutation (Ser-478-Arg) was known only for the more attenuated Len/47 ca donor virus that was obtained after 30 additional passages of Len/17 in eggs at 25 °C. Selection of such a mutation during replication of the Len/17-based LIV in some children can provide additional attenuation and genetic stability to the vaccine.

References

[1] A.P. Kendal, H.F. Maassab, G.I. Alexandrova, et al., Development of cold-adapted recombinant live, attenuated influenza vaccines in USA and USSR, Antiviral Res. 1 (1981) 339–365.

[2] G.I. Alexandrova, Live influenza vaccine in Russia, in: L.E. Brown, A.W. Hampson, R.G. Webster (Eds.), Options for the Control of Influenza III, Elsevier, Amsterdam, 1996, pp. 123–128.

[3] Y.Z. Ghendon, A.I. Klimov, G.I. Alexandrova, et al., Analysis of genome composition and reactogenicity of recombinants of cold-adapted and virulent influenza virus strains, J. Gen. Virol. 53 (1981) 215–224.

[4] L.G. Rudenko, N.I. Lonskaya, A.I. Klimov, et al., Clinical and epidemiological evaluation of a live, cold-adapted influenza vaccine for 3–14-year-olds, Bull. WHO 74 (1966) 77–84.

[5] A.I. Klimov, A.Y. Egorov, M.I. Gushchina, et al., Genetic stability of cold-adapted A/Leningrad/134/47/57 (H2N2) influenza virus: sequence analysis of live cold-adapted reassortant vaccine strains before and after replication in children, J. Gen. Virol. 76 (1995) 1521–1525.

[6] A.I. Klimov, L.G. Rudenko, A.Y. Egorov, et al., Genetic stability of Russian cold-adapted live attenuated reassortant influenza vaccines, in: L.E. Brown, A.W. Hampson, R.G. Webster (Eds.), Options for the Control of Influenza III, Elsevier, Amsterdam, 1996, pp. 129–136.

[7] A.S. Khan, F.I. Polezhaev, R. Vasiljeva, et al., Comparison of US inactivated split-virus and Russian live attenuated, cold-adapted trivalent influenza vaccines in Russian schoolchildren, J. Infect. Dis. 173 (1996) 453–456.

[8] A.I. Klimov, N.J. Cox, PCR restriction analysis of genome composition and stability of cold-adapted reassortant live influenza vaccines, J. Virol. Methods 52 (1995) 41–49.

[9] A.I. Klimov, I.V. Kiseleva, G.I. Alexandrova, et al., Genes coding for polymerase proteins are essential for attenuation of the cold-adapted A/Leningrad/134/17/57 (H2N2) influenza virus, Options for the Control of Influenza IV, Elsevier, Amsterdam, 2001, pp. 917–921.

International Congress Series 1219 (2001) 955–959

Genes coding for polymerase proteins are essential for attenuation of the cold-adapted A/Leningrad/134/17/57 (H2N2) influenza virus

A.I. Klimov[a,*], I.V. Kiseleva[b], G.I. Alexandrova[b], N.J. Cox[a]

[a]*Influenza Branch, G-16, Centers for Disease Control and Prevention, 1600 Clifton Rd., NE Atlanta, GA 30333, USA*
[b]*Department of Virology, Institute of Experimental Medicine, RAMS, St. Petersburg, Russia*

Abstract

Background: The A/Leningrad/134/17/57 (H2N2) (Len/17) cold-adapted (ca) master strain used as a donor of attenuation for preparing live attenuated influenza vaccine was derived from the A/Leningrad/134/57 wild-type virus (Len/wt) after 17 passages in eggs at 25 °C. In contrast to Len/wt, the Len/17 virus is sensitive to high (40 °C) temperature (*ts*), is able to grow at low (25 °C) temperature (*ca*), and is attenuated (*att*) for humans. Len/17 is different from Len/wt by eight coding mutations in internal genes PB2 (V-478-L), PB1 (K-265-N, V-591-I), PA (L-28-P, V-341-L), M1 (I-15-V), M2 (A-86-T) and NS2 (M-100-I). However, the role of individual mutant genes in the manifestation of the *ts*, *ca*, and *att* phenotypes was not established. To evaluate this, single gene reassortants (SGRs) with one mutated gene in the background of the Len/wt genome were studied. *Methods*: Since heterogeneity (A- or T-86 in the M2 gene) was noted in Len/17, the *ts* and *ca* clone 28 of this donor (Len/17-cl28) that has A-86 in M2 was used to prepare the SGRs. Preservation of mutations in SGRs was monitored by PCR-restriction (RFLP) analysis. Virus replication in ferret lungs was observed to evaluate the *att* phenotype of SGRs. *Results*: PB2- and PB1-SGRs each manifested the *ts* phenotype, and PB2-SGR demonstrated the *ca* phenotype as well. PA-SGR was *ca*, but not *ts*. Mutations in the M1 and NS2 genes did not affect the *ts* or *ca* phenotypes of corresponding SGRs. Ferrets infected with Len/17-cl28, Len/wt and PB2-, PB1- or PA-SGRs demonstrated comparable titers in nasal turbinates on the third day, while infectious virus was found only in the lungs of ferrets infected with Len/wt and PA-SGR. *Conclusion*: These data suggest that mutations in the PB2 (V-478-L) and PB1 (K-265-N, V-591-I) genes play a critical role in the attenuation of the ca Len/17 vaccine donor strain. © 2001 Elsevier Science B.V. All rights reserved.

Keywords: Live influenza vaccine; Attenuation; Polymerase genes

* Corresponding author. Tel.: +1-404-639-3591; fax: +1-404-639-2334.
E-mail address: axk0@cdc.gov (A.I. Klimov).

0531-5131/01/$ – see front matter © 2001 Elsevier Science B.V. All rights reserved.
PII: S 0 5 3 1 - 5 1 3 1 (0 1) 0 0 3 6 9 - 7

1. Introduction

The A/Leningrad/134/17/57 (H2N2) (Len/17) cold-adapted (ca) master strain has been used in Russia for many years to prepare attenuated reassortant live influenza vaccines (LIVs). This master strain was derived from A/Leningrad/134/57 (H2N2) wild-type virus (Len/wt) after 17 passages in eggs at 25 °C [1,2]. In contrast to Len/wt, Len/17 is sensitive to high (40 °C) temperature (*ts* phenotype), is able to grow at low (25 °C) temperature (*ca* phenotype), and is attenuated for humans (*att* phenotype) [1,2]. Len/17 is different from Len/wt by eight coding mutations in internal genes PB2 (V-478-L), PB1 (K-265-N, V-591-I), PA (L-28-P, V-341-L), M1 (I-15-V), M2 (A-86-T) and NS2 (M-100-I) [3] and three coding mutations in the hemagglutinin (HA) gene (not published). It was shown that Len/17 itself as well as ca reassortant LIVs prepared using Len/17 were safe for adults and children [2,4,5]. Since ca reassortant LIVs inherited their HA and neuraminidase genes from non-attenuated epidemic viruses, it is clear that mutations in internal genes of Len/17 are responsible for the attenuation. However, the role of individual internal mutant genes in the manifestation of the *ts*, *ca*, and *att* phenotypes of Len/17 was not established. To evaluate this, single gene reassortants (SGRs) with one mutated gene in the background of the Len/wt genome were obtained and studied.

2. Methods

2.1. Obtaining SGRs

Since heterogeneity (A- or T-86) in the M2 gene of Len/17 was noted previously [6], the *ts* and *ca* clone 28 of this donor (Len/17-cl28) that has A-86 in M2 was selected and used to prepare the SGRs. Reassortants were obtained after mixed infection of eggs with Len/17-cl28 and Len/wt followed by cloning at limit dilution at different temperatures (25, 34 and 40 °C). Preservation of mutations in reassortants was monitored by PCR-restriction (RFLP) analysis [7]. Reassortants that inherited more than one gene from Len/17 were crossed again with Len/wt virus. For some internal genes, up to three rounds of crossing with Len/wt were needed to obtain the corresponding SGRs. As a result of the cloning, 3 PB2-, 3 PB1-, 5PA-, 6 M-, and 1 NS-SGRs were selected (as indicated above, Len/17 does not have mutations in the NP gene). Also we obtained a number of reassortants that inherited two (29 clones), three (15 clones) or four (11 clones) internal genes from Len/17-cl28.

2.2. Determining ts and ca phenotypes

ts and *ca* phenotypes were determined by titration in eggs and expressed as reproduction capacity at elevated (*ts*) or low (*ca*) temperature: RCT40 (log EID_{50})=log EID_{50}/0.2 ml at 34 °C−log EID_{50}/0.2 ml at 40 °C, and RCT25 (log EID_{50})=log EID_{50}/0.2 ml at 34 °C−log EID_{50}/0.2 ml at 25 °C.

2.3. Study of att phenotype

Virus replication in ferret lungs was observed to evaluate the *att* phenotype of SGRs. Ferrets (two per virus) were infected intranasally with 7.0 log $EID_{50}/0.2$ ml of tested viruses. Nasal turbinates and lungs were collected on the third day after infection. Virus titers in the homogenized organs were determined by titration in eggs at 34 °C, normalized by the organs weight (in grams) and expressed in log $EID_{50}/ml/g$.

3. Results

3.1. ts phenotype of SGRs

RCT40 for Len/wt was shown to be 2.0 ± 0.2 log EID_{50} (non-*ts* phenotype), while for both Len/17 and Len/17-cl28, it was 7.0 ± 0.2 log EID_{50} (*ts* phenotype). SGRs that inherited PA, M, or NS genes from Len/17-cl28 all demonstrated non-*ts* phenotype (RCT40=2.1 ± 0.3 log EID_{50} for PA-SGRs, 2.2 ± 0.3 log EID_{50} for M-SGRs, and 2.2 ± 0.4 log EID_{50} for the NS-SGR). Transferring the PB2 or PB1 gene from Len/17-cl28 into the Len/wt genome led to a dramatic decrease of infectivity of corresponding SGRs at 40 °C (*ts* phenotype): RCT40=5.8 ± 0.3 log EID_{50} for PB2-SGRs and $5.85+0.3$ log EID_{50} for PB1-SGRs. Table 1 summarizes data on the *ts* phenotype of SGRs.

3.2. ca phenotype of SGRs

For Len/wt, the RCT25 was 6.5 ± 0.2 log EID_{50} (non-*ca* phenotype), while for Len/17-cl28 and Len/17, the RCT25 was 2.0 ± 0.2 log EID_{50} and 2.2 ± 0.2 log EID_{50}, respectively (*ca* phenotype). SGRs that inherited PB1, M, or NS genes from Len/17-cl28 all demonstrated non-*ca* phenotype (RCT25=6.0 ± 0.3 log EID_{50} for PB1-SGRs, 6.2 ± 0.3 log EID_{50} for M-SGRs, and 6.1 ± 0.4 log EID_{50} for the NS-SGR). Transferring the PB2 or PA gene from Len/17-cl28 into the Len/wt background significantly increased the ability of

Table 1

ts, ca and *att* phenotypes of SGRs between Len/17-cl28 and Len/wt

Virus/SGR	Amino acid changes	*ts* phenotype	*ca* phenotype	*att* phenotype
Len/wt	–	non-*ts*	non-*ca*	non-*att*
Len/17-cl28	eight	*ts*	*ca*	*att*
PB2	Val-478-Leu	*ts*	*ca*	*att*
PB1	Lys-265-Asn, Val-591-Ile	*ts*	non-*ca*	*att*
PA	Leu-28-Pro, Val-341-Leu	non-*ts*	*ca*	non-*att*
M	Ile-15-Val	non-*ts*	non-*ca*	n.d.[a]
NS	Met-100-Ile	non-*ts*	non-*ca*	n.d.[a]

[a] Not done.

corresponding SGRs to grow at 25 °C (*ca* phenotype): RCT25=2.8±0.3 log EID_{50} for PB2-SGRs and 2.7±0.3 log EID_{50} for PA-SGRs (Table 1).

3.3. ts and ca phenotypes of reassortants that inherited more than one gene from Len/17

Reproduction at 40 °C of multi-gene reassortants that inherited both PB2 and PB1 genes from Len/17 was repeatedly ~1 log lower than reproduction of reassortants that received only one of these genes, thus indicating that combination of the PB2 and PB1 mutations reinforced manifestation of the *ts* phenotype. A combination of mutations in the PB2 and PA genes seemed to reinforce the manifestation of the *ca* phenotype since growth at 25 °C of reassortants that inherited both these genes was 0.5–1.0 log lower than reproduction of any reassortant that inherited only one of the genes.

3.4. att phenotype of SGRs

Only PB2-, PB1- and PA-SGRs (one of each) that demonstrated *ts* and/or *ca* phenotypes were tested for attenuation in ferrets. Virus replication in nasal turbinates of ferrets infected with these SGRs as well as with Len/17-cl28, and Len/wt was within the range of 4–5 log $EID_{50}/ml/g$. Only Len/wt and PA-SGR were able to replicate in lungs. Corresponding titers were 3.8–4.1 log $EID_{50}/ml/g$ for Len/wt and 3.2–3.7 for the PA-SGR. Virus titers in lungs were <0.5 log $EID_{50}/ml/g$ for Len/17-cl28 as well as for PB2-SGR and PB1-SGR, thus demonstrating their *att* phenotype for ferrets (Table 1).

4. Discussion

Results of this study demonstrate that mutations in polymerase genes are essential for attenuation of the Len/17 master strain. The Val-478-Leu substitution in the PB2 gene as well as Lys-265-Asn and Val-591-Ile amino acid changes in the PB1 gene independently contribute to attenuation of the Len/17 master strain. Importantly, mutations in both these genes are responsible for the manifestation of the *ts* phenotype (Table 1). Although two mutations in the PA gene (Leu-28-Pro and Val-341-Leu) were responsible for the *ca* phenotype, they did not lead to the attenuation of the corresponding SGR. These data demonstrated a close relationship between attenuation and the *ts* rather than *ca* phenotype of cold-adapted viruses. Data suggesting that a combination of polymerase genes seems to reinforce the manifestation of *ts* (PB2+PB1) or *ca* (PB2+PA) phenotypes can explain the genetic stability of ca reassortant LIVs during their replication in humans [6,8].

Acknowledgements

We thank Anne Tomasi and Lois Zitzow for their assistance in experiments with ferrets and Dr. Larisa Rudenko for helpful discussion.

References

[1] A.P. Kendal, H.F. Maassab, G.I. Alexandrova, et al., Development of cold-adapted recombinant live, atte-nuated influenza vaccines in USA and USSR, Antiviral Res. 1 (1981) 339–365.

[2] G.I. Alexandrova, Live influenza vaccine in Russia, in: L.E. Brown, A.W. Hampson, R.G. Webster (Eds.), Options for the Control of Influenza III, Elsevier, Amsterdam, 1996, pp. 123–128.

[3] A.I. Klimov, N.J. Cox, W.V. Yotov, et al., Sequence changes in the live attenuated, cold-adapted variants of influenza A/Leningrad/134/57 (H2N2) virus, Virology 86 (1992) 795–797.

[4] Y.Z. Ghendon, A.I. Klimov, G.I. Alexandrova, et al., Analysis of genome composition and reactogenicity of recombinants of cold-adapted and virulent influenza virus strains, J. Gen. Virol. 53 (1981) 215–224.

[5] A.S. Khan, F.I. Polezhaev, R. Vasiljeva, et al., Comparison of US inactivated split-virus and Russian live attenuated, cold-adapted trivalent influenza vaccines in Russian schoolchildren, J. Infect. Dis. 173 (1996) 453–456.

[6] A.I. Klimov, L.G. Rudenko, A.Y. Egorov, et al., Genetic stability of Russian cold-adapted live attenuated reassortant influenza vaccines, in: L.E. Brown, A.W. Hampson, R.G. Webster (Eds.), Options for the Control of Influenza III, Elsevier, Amsterdam, 1996, pp. 129–136.

[7] A.I. Klimov, N.J. Cox, PCR restriction analysis of genome composition and stability of cold-adapted re-assortant live influenza vaccines, J. Virol. Methods 52 (1995) 41–49.

[8] A.I. Klimov, A.Y. Egorov, M.I. Gushchina, et al., Genetic stability of cold-adapted A/Leningrad/134/47/57 (H2N2) influenza virus: sequence analysis of live cold-adapted reassortant vaccine strains before and after replication in children, J. Gen. Virol. 76 (1995) 1521–1525.

International Congress Series 1219 (2001) 961–964

A new intranasal, modified-live virus vaccine for equine H3N8 influenza

P. Whitaker-Dowling[b], J.S. Youngner[b], T.M. Chambers[c,*],
Heska Corporation Collaborative Group[a]

[a]*Heska Corporation, Fort Collins, CO, USA*
[b]*Department of Molecular Genetics and Biochemistry, University of Pittsburgh School of Medicine,
Pittsburgh, PA, USA*
[c]*Department of Veterinary Science, 108 Gluck Equine Research Center, University of Kentucky,
Lexington, KY 40546-0099, USA*

Abstract

Background: Equine-2 (H3N8) influenza is the most frequent cause of infectious upper respiratory disease in horses in the USA. Conventional inactivated-virus vaccines have been largely ineffective for prevention of this disease, even following repeated doses. We developed a modified-live virus vaccine derived by cold-adaptation from a wild-type strain of equine-2 influenza virus, and demonstrated its safety and efficacy in equines. *Methods*: The wild-type influenza A/equine/2/Kentucky/91 virus was serially passed in embryonated eggs at temperatures reduced stepwise from 34 to 26 °C. Temperature sensitivity and stability was tested in MDCK cells. Safety and efficacy tests, including experimental challenges with wild-type viruses, were conducted in seropositive and seronegative equines. *Results*: Randomly selected clones from the 49th passage were temperature sensitivity (ts) with 34/39.5° infectivity ratios $>10^4$. The ts phenotype was retained through five serial passages in MDCK cells. The clone selected as vaccine candidate (P821) was further tested in equines and had the desired degree of attenuation: it successfully infected seropositive animals based on detectable virus shedding, yet induced no significant disease symptoms in seronegative animals. The candidate vaccine was tested for stability of ts phenotype through five serial horse-to-horse passages; for safety and efficacy in exercised–stressed animals; for efficacy against challenge with heterologous strains of equine-2 influenza virus; and for safety in large-scale field studies. Each of these tests was passed successfully. Efficacy following single doses was established on the basis of protection from clinical disease, as the vaccine induced little serum antibody in single-dosed animals.

* Corresponding author. Tel.: +1-859-257-3407; fax: +1-859-257-8542.
E-mail address: tmcham1@pop.uky.edu (T.M. Chambers).

0531-5131/01/$ – see front matter © 2001 Elsevier Science B.V. All rights reserved.
PII: S 0 5 3 1 - 5 1 3 1 (0 1) 0 0 3 7 0 - 3

Conclusion: A modified-live virus vaccine for equine-2 influenza has been developed which is safe and effective in horses following a single dose administered intranasally. © 2001 Elsevier Science B.V. All rights reserved.

Keywords: Horse; Cold-adaptation; Temperature-sensitive; Challenge

---

1. Introduction

Equine influenza remains in circulation in most parts of the world despite the existence and widespread use of vaccines. Among the causes of this, antigenic drift is clearly contributory. We previously identified a bifurcation of the circulating strains into two lineages, called the 'American' and 'Eurasian' lineages although the viruses have sometimes crossed those geographic bounds [1]. Antigenic differences between these are great enough that the Office International des Epizooties recommends vaccines should be formulated to protect against both lineages. However, another major cause is believed to have been the use of vaccines of limited potency. In our experience in the USA, horses of 2–3 years of age, which had not encountered natural influenza but had been vaccinated multiple times, frequently failed to exhibit an antibody response of clinically significant titer or duration.

Equine influenza vaccines commercially available in the USA have been adjuvanted inactivated virus vaccines administered by intramuscular injection. We have developed and tested a new equine influenza vaccine, which is a modified live virus vaccine, unadjuvanted, and administered intranasally. The vaccine, called Flu Avert™ I.N. vaccine, is produced by Heska and was licensed in 1999 for sale and use in the USA. This article is an overview of the vaccine's development and testing, which will be described in detail elsewhere.

2. Materials and methods

The vaccine virus was derived from a wild-type equine-2 (H3N8) influenza virus, strain A/equine/KY/91, isolated during an outbreak of influenza from a horse exhibiting typical clinical signs of fever, cough, and nasal discharge. Attenuation was done by cold adaptation through serial passage at gradually reduced temperatures down to 26°, in embryonated eggs. Virus clones from selected passages were phenotypically characterized on MDCK cells for temperature sensitivity (ts), based on cytopathic effect and virus protein synthesis at 34° versus 39.5°. A candidate vaccine strain and method of administration were evaluated by various tests for safety and efficacy in seronegative horses/ponies, including challenge infections with wild-type viruses administered by inhalation of virus aerosols produced by a nebulizer. Challenge-infected vaccinates and controls were evaluated by expert veterinarians based on clinical signs, virus shedding, and seroconversion, with most trials single- or double-blinded.

3. Results

Several protocols for cold adaptation of the wild-type virus were pursued, with the ts phenotype of the resulting viruses assessed at each passage. The ts phenotype was achieved by passage 34. Clones from the 49th passage were entirely ts, with plaquing efficiency $(34/39.5°) > 10^4$. Ten clones were tested by $5 \times$-repeated serial passage at $34°$ in both eggs and MDCK cells, and the ts phenotype remained stable throughout. One such clone, P821, became the basis for the Flu Avert™ I.N. vaccine strain. This clone grew to equivalent titers at both $26°$ and $34°$, but not at all at $39.5°$. P821 viral protein synthesis in MDCK cells, based on SDS-PAGE, was similar to the parental virus at $34°$, but nearly absent at $39.5°$. Inhibition of host protein synthesis was reduced at $34°$ and absent at $39.5°$.

P821 virus, along with numerous similar clones, was tested for attenuation in vivo in experimentally infected horses or ponies based on appearance of clinical signs. Virus shedding of $4-5$ days duration, yet without clinical signs, was produced by the P821 clone in both seropositive and seronegative animals, and this clone was chosen for further in vivo studies using preparations or production runs from a master seed stock, and a custom-designed intranasal applicator device. These tests included the following.

(a) Egg- versus MDCK-grown vaccine: MDCK-grown virus was similarly attenuated and immunogenic and replicated longer in vivo than did egg-grown virus.

(b) Safety/efficacy studies in exercise–stressed ponies: vaccination was safe and a single dose protected the animals from challenge 3 months later [2].

(c) Stability of ts phenotype in vivo through five serial horse-to-horse passages: viruses isolated from horses in the last group of serial passages had completely retained its original ts phenotype [3]. Studies [b and c] were performed by Lunn et al. (University of Wisconsin).

(d) Duration of immunity following a single dose of vaccine in 9- to 12-month-old seronegative ponies. Challenge was with wild-type KY/91 virus. At 5 weeks and 3 months post-vaccination, vaccinates showed highly significant protection from clinical disease, whereas most controls showed typical clinical signs. At 6 months post-vaccination, the clinical differences were still significant but less marked [4]. At 12 months post-vaccination, there was no clear protection but still a trend of reduced clinical signs compared to age-matched controls, and anamnestic serological responses.

(e) Heterologous protection: challenges were done using wild-type equine-2 virus strains including a recent 'American'-lineage isolate, KY/98, and a 'Eurasian'-lineage equine-2 virus, Saskatoon/90. The vaccine protected against these challenge viruses at 1 month following a single dose [3]. The vaccine also provided protection against KY/99 virus challenge.

(f) When administered simultaneously with another equine intranasal vaccine (against *Streptococcus equi*), the vaccine retained its safety and effectiveness. Many of studies [d–f] were done by Townsend et al. (University of Saskatchewan).

(g) Large-scale field trials of safety were done, involving 482 horses in six states across the USA. Adverse effects were noted in only 2% and were uniformly minor.

(h) The vaccine proved safe for use in pregnant mares.

(i) Shed-spread: vaccine virus spread from 39 vaccinates to only 1/13 sentinel animals maintained together with them, indicating such spread is rare.

4. Discussion

The Flu Avert® I.N. modified live virus vaccine exhibits many characteristics of an ideal equine influenza virus vaccine. Its attenuation phenotype was stable in both in vitro and in vivo backpassage studies. It has demonstrated safety and efficacy in equines under the conditions in which it is used in the field, and also demonstrated protection against heterologous equine-2 influenza viruses of both the 'American' and 'Eurasian' lineages. Work of Lunn et al. [2] indicates that Flu Avert® I.N. vaccine induces an antibody response in horses more similar to that from natural infection, than does conventional killed-virus vaccination. Interestingly, a single dose of vaccine in a naive animal protects for up to 6 months yet may not induce detectable serum antibodies. Thus, this intranasal vaccine induces other immune mechanisms, likely including respiratory mucosal immunity.

The concept of attenuation by cold adaptation has also led to development of a human modified live virus vaccine (FluMist®, Aviron). In principle, attenuation results in part from ts mutations restricting virus growth at normal body temperature; and in part from mutations arising from adaptation to a heterologous host. The genotype of the Flu Avert® I.N. vaccine virus is presently being determined. A concern with modified live influenza virus vaccines is the possibility of reassortment with wild-type strains. Accumulating field experience with Flu Avert® I.N. vaccine will provide further information on the likelihood of this occurrence. There is evidence that cold-adapted influenza A viruses such as Flu Avert® I.N. vaccine exhibit dominance over wild-type viruses and impair their growth [5].

References

[1] J.M. Daly, A.C.K. Lai, M.M. Binns, T.M. Chambers, M. Barrandeguy, J.A. Mumford, Recent worldwide antigenic and genetic evolution of equine H3N8 influenza A viruses, J. Gen. Virol. 77 (1996) 661–671.

[2] D. Lunn, D. Horohov, S. Hussey, P. Whitaker-Dowling, J. Youngner, T. Chambers, R. Holland, K. Rushlow, R. Sebring, A potent modified-live equine influenza virus vaccine: safe even after exercise-induced immunosuppression, AAEP Proc. 45 (1999) 43–44.

[3] R. Holland, T. Chambers, H. Townsend, A. Cook, J. Bogdan, D. Lunn, S. Hussey, P. Whitaker-Dowling, J. Youngner, R. Sebring, S. Penner, G. Stiegler, New modified-live equine influenza virus vaccine: safety and efficacy studies in young equids, AAEP Proc. 45 (1999) 38–40.

[4] H. Townsend, A. Cook, T. Watts, J. Bogdan, D. Haines, S. Griffin, T. Chambers, R. Holland, P. Whitaker-Dowling, J. Youngner, S. Penner, R. Sebring, Efficacy of a cold-adapted, modified-live virus influenza vaccine: a double-blind challenge trial, AAEP Proc. 45 (1999) 41–42.

[5] P. Whitaker-Dowling, W. Lucas, J.S. Youngner, Cold-adapted vaccine strains of influenza A act as dominant-negative mutants in mixed infections with wild-type influenza A virus, Virology 175 (1990) 358–364.

International Congress Series 1219 (2001) 965–967

Intranasal influenza vaccine: protective efficacy in children and adults

Pietro Crovari[a,*], Elio Garbarino[a], Bianca Bruzzone[a], Christian Herzog[b], Reinhard Glück[b]

[a]*Health Sciences Department, University of Genoa, Genoa, Italy*
[b]*Swiss Serum and Vaccine Institute, Berne, Switzerland*

Keywords: Intranasal influenza vaccine; Mucosal immunity; Influenza

1. Introduction

During the last few years, increased knowledge of the mechanisms of mucosal immunity [1] has enabled the identification of better mucosal adjuvants for increased adherence and penetration capacity by inactivated antigens [2]. Starting from these premises, we have turned our attention to influenza and the possibility of utilizing an intranasal influenza vaccine, firstly, because influenza is a disease with a high social and health-care burden [3] and is caused by viruses whose natural access to an organism is the mucosa of the upper respiratory tract; secondly, because present parenteral vaccines have shown sub-optimal protective efficacy (70–80% in adults; 50–60% in the elderly) [4–6]. Moreover, parenteral vaccines usually produce a general immunity with little effect on the interpersonal dissemination of the virus while intranasal vaccines could offer the advantage of creating a specifically immune defense barrier right at the access level of the virus, thus blocking its replication/diffusion and further passage to the lower respiratory tract.

Throughout the winter of 1996-1997 we tested, with satisfactory results, a trivalent inactivated vaccine, with HLT as adjuvant, administered intra-nasally to adult subjects [7].

---

* Corresponding author. Dept. di Scienze della Salute, Facolta di Medicina e Chirurgia, dell'Univ degli Studi di Genova, Genoa, Italy. Tel.: +39-10-353-8520; fax: +39-10-353-8407.
E-mail address: crovari@csita.unique.it (P. Crovari).

0531-5131/01/$ – see front matter © 2001 Elsevier Science B.V. All rights reserved.
PII: S 0 5 3 1 - 5 1 3 1 (0 1) 0 0 3 7 1 - 5

2. Materials and methods

During the month of October 1998, we recruited for this prospective and randomized study a group of subjects to be vaccinated and a control group. In November, the subjects of the study were vaccinated by nasal spray with two doses of inactivated trivalent vaccine administered 8 days apart. The follow-up program was from December 1998 to April 1999. In collaboration with general practitioners and family pediatricians, we recruited 250 adults and 250 children. After randomization, the vaccine was administered to 100 adults and 100 children while 150 adults and 150 children were included in the control group.

The composition of the antigen for the vaccine, prepared by the Swiss Serum and Vaccine Institute, Berne, was in accordance with the WHO recommendations for that season:

A/Beijing/262/95-like-H1N1: 11.3 μg
A/Sydney/5/97-like-H3N2: 12.1 μg
B/Beijing/184/93-like: 12.5 μg

These antigens were inserted into liposomes (virosomes) composed of lecithin vesicles (112.5 μg) using as adjuvant a small quantity of heat-labile *E. coli* toxin (2 μg) in PBS solution (200 μl).

The vaccine was administered with a disposable dispenser especially designed to ensure the homogeneous distribution of the atomized solution in the turbinates and the nasal cavity; one insufflation in both nostrils was regarded as corresponding to one dose.

For the evaluation of tolerability, we recorded both local and systemic reactions during 4 days after each vaccination, i.e. at day 1 and at day 8±1. We asked each adult and each parent to record on a special clinical diary the temperature and the occurrence of specific symptoms such as stuffy nose, sneezing, runny nose, pain, discomfort, headache, shivers, nausea and diarrhea.

To evaluate immunogenicity, we used the HAI test on blood samples taken before day 1 and after vaccination (day 29±2) while we calculated the extent of seroprotection using the geometric mean titre (GMT) as parameter.

The production of IGA. antibodies was assessed with the Elispot method and the immunoenzymatic assay of different classes of antibodies against the hemagglutinin antigen.

The protective efficacy was assessed among vaccinated and control subjects during the follow-up period from December 1998 to April 1999. Adults and parents were told to contact immediately a toll-free number in case of onset of influenza-like illness (ILI). Nasopharyngeal and oropharyngeal swabs were immediately taken from these subjects and the presence of influenza virus was detected by PCR and MDCK cell culture. Each case of ILI associated with a positive result in at least one of these tests was diagnosed as influenza.

3. Results

The vaccine was well tolerated by both adults and children and we observed no serious adverse reactions. As for the occurrence of adverse reactions in similar studies, where a vaccine without or with the addition of different concentrations of heat-labile toxin was administered, the results did not show any significant differences.

In vaccinated adults, the GMT parameter increased from 2.5 to as much as 4 times depending on the type of virus tested (A/H1N1 from 7.9 to 31.6; A/H3N2 from 14.7 to 47.2; B from 13.9 to 35.5). Vaccinated subjects with a protective titre ($\geq$1:40) had a range from 57% to 70%. Similarly, in vaccinated children, the GMT parameter increased from 2.6 to as much as 6.5 times depending on the type of virus tested (A/H1N1 from 10.7 to 69.6; A/H3N2 from 23 to 59; B from 20.3 to 62.2) while seroprotection was found to be in the range of 75% to 85%.

As shown by other studies [8], the Elispot test showed an increase in post-vaccine plasma cells secreting Ig A.

During the 1998/1999 season, the epidemic in the city of Genoa lasted 11 weeks, with a considerable peak in morbidity, and was characterized by the co-circulation of both A and B virus types. There was only one virologically confirmed case of influenza in the group of vaccinated adults compared with 10 cases in the non-vaccinated control group, representing a protective efficacy of 85% by the vaccine. In the group of vaccinated children, there were two cases of influenza that occurred compared with 26 cases in the non-vaccinated group, thus confirming a protective efficacy of 90%.

4. Conclusions

This study demonstrates the safety, immunogenicity and effectiveness of the trivalent virosomal adjuvant vaccine, administered by nasal spray in both adults and children, against influenza virus A and B infections. These results open up important prospects for vaccines in the prevention of influenza. The administration of vaccines by nasal spray is much more acceptable and could, therefore, be more convenient and effective in preventing the disease, especially in children where the use of parenteral vaccines is rare.

References

[1] K.A. Brokstad, R.J. Cox, J.C. Eriksen, J. Oiofsson, R. Jonsson, A. Davidsson, The basal levels of influenza specific antibody secreting B-cells and antibodies in blood, lymphoid tissue and nasal mucosa of healthy subjects,Options Control Influenza IV, Crete-Greece, (2000) 44 abstract W52-3.

[2] E.T.S. Ben-Ahmeida, G. Gregoriadis, C.W. Potter, R. Jennings, Immunopotentiation of local and systemic humoral immune responses by ISCOMs, liposomes and FCA: role in protection against influenza A in mice,Vaccine 11 (1993) 1302–1308.

[3] S.C. Schoenbaum, Economic impact of influenza: the individual's perspective, Am. J. Med. 82 (1987) 26–30.

[4] F. Davenport, Control of influenza, Med. J. Aust. 1 (special suppl.) (1973) 33–38.

[5] K.L. Nichol, A. Lind, K.L. Margiolis, et al., The effectiveness of vaccination against influenza in healthy, working adults, N. Engl. J. Med. 333 (1995) 889–893.

[6] P.A. Gross, A.W. Hermogenes, H.S. Sacks, J. Lau, R.A. Levandowski, The efficacy of influenza vaccine in elderly persons, Ann. Intern. Med. 123 (1995) 518–527.

[7] P. Crovari, F. Ansaldi, B.M. Bruzzone, E. Garbarino, C. Di Pietroantonj, C. Herzog, R. Glück, Safety and immunogenicity of mucosal, inactivated virosome-formulated influenza vaccine with Escherichia Coli heat labile toxin as an adjuvant, J Prev Med Hyg 40 (3) (1999) 83–88.

[8] R. Gluck, J.O. Gebbers, R. Gluck, Phase 1 evaluation of intranasal virosomal influenza vaccine with and without Escherichia coli heat-labile toxin in adult volunteers, J. Virol. 73 (1999) 7780–7786.

International Congress Series 1219 (2001) 969–978

Preclinical and clinical evaluation of a new virosomal intranasal influenza vaccine

Reinhard Glück*

Swiss Serum and Vaccine Institute Berne, P.O. Box CH3001, Berne, Switzerland

Abstract

Virosome-formulated and Escherigen-adjuvanted inactivated intranasal influenza vaccine (Nasalflu Berna®), when given as two intranasal spray doses on both days 1 and 8 ± 1, achieved a high level of influenza-specific hemagglutination inhibition IgG antibody titers measured in serum, to the strains incorporated in the administered vaccine. This nasal vaccine fulfills the European Agency for Evaluation of Medicinal Products (EMEA) immunogenicity requirements for parenteral vaccines. Likewise, influenza-specific IgA antibodies were elicited in the nasal mucosa (lavage fluid) and in saliva. This additional mucosal IgA antibody response may provide additional local protection by the inhibition of viral replication and further spread in the respiratory tract as documented in a ferret challenge model. Furthermore, preliminary data from an epidemiological protection study conducted in 1998/1999 in Genoa showed a protective efficacy against laboratory-confirmed influenza infection of 85.0% in adults and 89.7% in 6–12-year-old children. © 2001 Elsevier Science B.V. All rights reserved.

Keywords: Virosomal; Intranasal; Influenza vaccine

1. Introduction

1.1. Current influenza vaccines

There are three types of vaccines commercially available for protection from influenza. The first contains intact virions inactivated by treatment with formaldehyde. Such vaccines are considered to be the most reactogenic and are in many countries recommended only for use in adults [1]. The split and subunit vaccines are composed of purified influenza antigens, of which hemagglutinin predominates. These vaccines are less reactogenic and

---

* Tel.: +41-31-980-6111; fax: +41-31-980-6775.

0531-5131/01/$ – see front matter © 2001 Elsevier Science B.V. All rights reserved.
PII: S0531-5131(01)00654-9

usually recommended for individuals of all ages. The currently used vaccines suffer from several limitations, including the need for the application of two doses of vaccine at an interval of 1–2 months for the immunization of infants and young children [1]. The lack of a high and long-lasting protective immune response, particularly in this age group [2], is another disadvantage. Newer vaccines with improved immunogenicity are clearly needed [3,4]. Attempts to increase immunogenicity by increasing the antigen content per dose have not always resulted in an improvement of the antibody response [4,5]. The use of reformulated whole virus or subunit vaccines with new adjuvants or antigen-free delivery systems has been shown to greatly potentiate the immune response in animals and humans.

1.2. Mucosal immunization

The presently used injectable influenza vaccines stimulate hemagglutinin (HA)-specific serum immunoglobulin G (IgG) in the majority of healthy individuals, but they give a significant rise in HA-specific nasal IgA antibodies in only a minority of subjects. This reduced ability of injectable vaccines to elicit an immunological response at the mucosa, the site of virus entry and propagation, confirmed by animal experiments, could be an important determinant of the non-ideal overall protective capacity of these vaccines. It may also be particularly relevant, when considering that mucosal immunity represents the first line of defense for the host and is a major component of the immunological cell-mediated response in the upper and lower respiratory tract passages.

The route of immunization appears to play a significant role in the achievement of an effective immune response. This hypothesis is supported by the findings in the prophylaxis against, for example, cholera, a disease with the gastrointestinal tract as the primary site of infection and in which oral immunization appears to elicit a more effective immune response than immunization by the parenteral route. Furthermore, the triggering of mucosal immune responses involving both the humoral and cellular arms of the immune system after oral or intranasal vaccination [6,7] are in agreement with recently established concepts of vaccination, which postulate that interference with the establishment and colonization of the pathogen at the earliest possible stage of infectivity is the most efficient way of preventing the development of the infection. The activation of mucosal immunity after intranasal vaccination, through the production of HA-specific secretory immunoglobulin type A (sIgA) should therefore greatly increase the resistance to influenzal infection by this route.

1.3. Virosome-formulated influenza vaccine for nasal administration

The new approach employed at the Swiss Serum and Vaccine Institute is to develop an easy-to-administer intranasal influenza vaccine based on the biodegradable virosome carrier system. Intranasal administration delivers the vaccine directly at the mucosal surface, where viral invasion and replication takes place. The objective is to improve immunogenicity without causing increased toxicity.

Virosomes, produced by inserting glycoproteins obtained from inactivated influenza virus purified hemagglutinin and neuraminidase into a bilayer of phospholipid vesicles, have been shown to posses significant adjuvant properties and increased immunoprotective activity, when administered parenterally as a trivalent influenza vaccine formulation to elderly subjects [8]. This clinical investigation demonstrated a higher seroconversion rate (a ≥ four-fold rise in anti-HA titer) and a significantly greater protection rate (antibody titers ≥ 1:40) in subjects vaccinated with the virosome formulation, when compared with the existing commercial formula (whole virion and subunit vaccines). The excellent immunogenicity and safety of the virosomal influenza vaccine was also confirmed in a subsequent study conducted in geriatric patients [9]. Nevertheless, for the use by the intranasal route, a virosomal vaccine adjuvanted with Escherigen (HLT Berna) has proven to be superior. Escherigen Berna (HLT Berna) is an *Escherichia coli* heat labile toxin (HLT) preparation.

Animal experiments employing pro-cholera genoid (PCG) and Escherigen have demonstrated the potent adjuvant properties of these antigens in eliciting a mucosal immune response, when added to other antigens [6,7]. HLT seems to be less toxic than PCG, and in contrast with the latter, also requires proteolytic activation, which makes it safer for use as an adjuvant [10]. The toxin is required for the adjuvant function, while the antigen-presenting capacity of macrophages and the differentiation and growth of both B and T lymphocytes are profoundly modulated [7,10]. In animal experiments, the adjuvant activity was achieved with doses 100-fold below the dose needed for fluid accumulation in the gut.

In non-human primates, the adjuvant effects of holotoxin and HLT have been observed without any adverse effects [11]. The use of HLT (100 μg) containing trace amounts of holotoxin as adjuvant to an intranasal influenza vaccine administered as two doses, 4 weeks apart, has been reported to elicit in humans a significant greater increase in serum antibody titers and salivary IgA antibody titers than in the control group, vaccinated by the same route with an influenza vaccine without toxin as adjuvant [12]. Although the volunteers receiving the HLT-containing vaccine reported twice as many adverse events as the control group, these were mainly non-severe and self-limiting local effects. None of the volunteers developed diarrhea.

2. Pre-clinical development of Nasalflu Berna®

Two key animal trials, carried out in mice [13] and ferrets [14], demonstrated the mucosal immunogenicity of an Escherigen-adjuvanted virosomal influenza vaccine when administered intranasally. The intramuscular and the intranasal route, respectively, were compared with virosomal test vaccines with or without Escherigen. In the ferrets, protection was tested by the challenge of the animals 21 days post vaccination with a homologous virus, i.e. A/Sydney/5/97 (H_3N_2). The results from these animal trials lead to the following conclusions.

2.1. Mice model

In a murine model, Escherigen was an effective adjuvant in eliciting a mucosal anti-influenza immune response following intranasal vaccination. Mice vaccinated with two intranasal doses of Escherigen-adjuvanted vaccine administered 7 days apart were found to respond 1 month after vaccination with significantly higher influenza-specific IgA anti-body titers (ELISA) in nasal washes (2.1–5.6 times) and with higher IgG antibody titers (hemagglutination inhibition [HI] test) in serum (up to 5.4 times) compared to animals receiving non-adjuvanted vaccine intranasally. After intramuscular administration of Escherigen-free vaccine, the HI antibody response in the serum was comparable to the response to intranasal, Escherigen-adjuvanted vaccine, but no influenza-specific IgA antibodies could be detected in nasal washes.

The difference between Escherigen-containing vaccine and vaccine without Escherigen were, regarding influenza-specific IgA antibodies (ELISA), found to be even more pronounced regarding broncho-alveolar lavages: IgA antibodies were found only from mice vaccinated intranasally with vaccine containing Escherigen and not in mice vaccinated intranasally or intramuscularly with the Escherigen-free virosomal influenza vaccine.

2.2. Ferret challenge model

The results from this animal model demonstrated the value of vaccination with the intranasal formulation in providing greater protection against a homologous virus challenge, when compared to the intramuscular vaccine. This is based on the four parameters studied: body temperature, body weight change, inflammatory cell counts and the amount of challenge virus recovered in nasal washes.

• The intranasal vaccine was found to effectively control the post challenge (+3 days) pyrexia observed particularly in the control animals, and less significantly, in animals vaccinated intramuscularly.

• Ferrets vaccinated intranasally showed no loss of body weight when measured 3 days post-infection and the animals continued to gain weight throughout the length of the experiment. These results compared very favorably with the significant decrease of body mass observed in the control group. Ferrets receiving the intramuscular vaccine showed only a minimal weight loss.

• Vaccination with the intramuscular and intranasal vaccines was associated with a 10-fold reduction in mean inflammatory cell counts measured in the nasal washes, when compared with the unvaccinated control group. This reduction was maintained throughout the length of the experiment and was more marked in the intranasal than in the intramuscular group.

• Proof of the protection against viral infection afforded by the intranasal vaccination, most likely through the production of a strain-specific anti-hemagglutinin and virus neutralizing immune response, was obtained from the quantitative evaluation of virus shedding measured in the nasal washes for a period of 6 days after challenge with virus. In the intranasally vaccinated animals, only a marginal production of virus was found, peaking below 1 log, 2 days post challenge, decreasing gradually to 0.1 log by the sixth day. In comparison, the intramuscularly vaccinated animals exhibited a rapid increase in virus shedding, peaking at 4.69 logs, 3 days post challenge, followed by a rapid decrease by over 3 logs over 2 days. In the control group, the maximum shedding of virus (5 logs) was also recorded 3 days post challenge, decreasing slowly over 2 logs over the next 2 days.

3. Animal safety testing of Nasalflu Berna®

The test program of toxicological studies performed to evaluate the safety of the Nasalflu Berna® vaccine and also of the Escherigen adjuvant alone has been carried out in five relevant animal species. The toxicological results are summarized in Tables 1 and 2.

Nasalflu Berna® (Escherigen-adjuvanted), tested in mice, shows no overt signs of toxicity at the highest dose administered (20 ml/kg) equivalent to $> \times 1000$ (p.o.) and $\times 630$ (i.v.), the daily highest dose (DHD) to be administered to a young child weighing 10 kg. The results from the intranasal repeated dose study (RDS) in the baboon at equivalents of human doses, have also demonstrated the good local tolerability of the vaccine and the absence of mucosal inflammatory markers, when administered using a commercial intranasal spray. Further assurance about the good local tolerability was also obtained from the acute eye irritation study in the rabbit. The vaccine does not enter the central nervous system through the blood–brain barrier (mice and baboon).

The adjuvant Escherigen was well tolerated after acute dosing to mice and rats by the oral and intravenous routes, at doses equivalent to $\times 1000$, the DHD administered to a child of 10-kg weight.

In the mini-pig (a species known to be susceptible to diarrhea following oral HLT), no overt signs of toxicity were detected following intranasal dosing of up to $500 \times$ the DHD and no diarrhea was detected after oral administration of more than $500 \times$ the DHD with previous neutralization of the stomach, which added an even greater safety margin. Intranasal dosing to the baboon at equivalents of human doses also failed to demonstrate any signs of local or systemic toxicity.

Intranasal distribution studies in the baboon using radiolabelled Nasalflu Berna® failed to demonstrate the passage of radioactivity into adjacent neural structures, brain or the cerebrospinal fluid. An autoradiographic intranasal study in mice also using Nasalflu Berna® showed that radioactivity was restricted primarily to the stomach and, to a low degree, in the heart, lungs and blood, 1 h after dosing. Radioactivity was excreted in urine 6 h after nasal application. In a ^{125}I-labeled HLT and Nasalflu® Berna tolerability study in baboons, the absence of radioactivity in the feces of Nasalflu® Berna-dosed animals, 24 and 72 h after application, and only minimal radioactivity in Escherigen-dosed animals at

Table 1

Nasalflu Berna	
Main tox program—summary of findings	
Acute tox, mice	No significant toxicity at $1000 \times HD$ (oral); $LD_{50} = 630 \times HD$ (i.v.)
Repeat tox, mice	No significant toxicity at $50 \times HD$ (i.v.)
Eye irritation, rabbit	No general or local clinical signs
Nasal safety, baboons	Chemical and blood parameters normal; T and B lymphocyte population normal; No inflammation of nerve and brain structure
^{125}I-PK, baboons	No radioactivity in CNS (nasal)
^{125}I-PK, mice	No radioactivity in CNS (i.v., nasal)
Challenge, ferrets	Prevention of fever and weight loss

Table 2

Escherigen Berna	
Main tox program — summary of findings	
Acute tox, mice	No significant toxicity at $1000 \times HD$ (oral, i.v.)
Acute tox, rats	No significant toxicity at $1000 \times HD$ (oral, i.v.)
Gene mutation	No significant findings in mouse lymphoma cells (L5178Y), ± microsomal enzymes
Nasal MTD, mini-pigs	No significant toxicity at $500 \times HD$
Oral MTD, mini-pigs	No significant toxicity at $500 \times HD$

24 h, were observed. No radioactivity was found in the stomach or ileum of both animal groups 24 h after dosing.

4. Clinical testing

4.1. Systemic tolerability

Nasalflu Berna® was well tolerated locally following intranasal vaccination in the 1218 subjects vaccinated, with 26.8% of vaccinees reporting upon solicited questioning ≥ 1 systemic adverse event, mainly mild or moderate and lasting for 1–3 days only. Headache (15%), malaise (9%) and arthralgias (6%) were the most frequently reported symptoms after the first dose. These rates did not increase after the second dose. In addition to the adverse events (AE) reported based on solicited questioning, 71 other AEs were reported. However, only pharyngitis (2.2%) was seen with a frequency of more than 1.0% after the first dose. The incidence of pharyngitis decreased to 0.4% after the second dose.

In young adults ($n = 909$, including 46 asthma patients), headache after the first vaccination had an incidence of 18% and was the most frequently reported symptom. This was followed in decreasing order by malaise (11%), arthralgias (7%), coughing (6%), shivering (5%), nausea (3%), fatigue and diarrhea (2%). The corresponding figures reported after the second vaccination basically did not change the tolerability profile. Overall, 29.9% and 24.7% of the vaccinees reported AEs after the first and second vaccination, respectively.

The overall rate of systemic AEs reported after the first and second vaccinations by subjects immunized intranasally with the vaccine without Escherigen ($n = 633$) was with 30.6% and 23.0% similar to those reported by subjects receiving Nasalflu Berna®. The fact that a higher rate of nausea (4%) was reported in this group indicates that this event, when reported, cannot necessarily be ascribed to Escherigen. The addition of Escherigen to the vaccine did not really increase the overall incidence of systemic symptoms with 33.9% of vaccinees reporting ≥ 1 systemic AE compared to 30.6% with the HLT-free vaccine.

In adult subjects aged >60 years ($n = 209$, including five asthma patients), the overall reported incidence of systemic symptoms was 24.9% and 21.8% after the first and second vaccinations, respectively. This was lower than those observed by the group of young adults. A similar spectrum and intensity of symptoms was observed, i.e. mainly mild events lasting 1–2 days only.

Concerning the subjects with bronchial asthma vaccinated with Nasalflu Berna® (*n* = 51), the incidences of vaccination-related systemic events, were lower than in the adults aged over 18 years after the first and second vaccination with 9% and 10%, respectively.

The systemic tolerability of Nasalflu Berna® in children aged ≥ 6 to ≤ 12 years (*n* = 100) and adolescents (*n* = 3) was good with only 2% and 3% of vaccinees reporting ≥ 1 systemic symptoms after the first and the second dose, respectively.

The rate of systemic symptoms after the administration of the PCG-adjuvanted vaccine (*n* = 52) was higher than that reported for the group of young adults vaccinated with Nasalflu Berna®. PCG adjuvant appears to be less well tolerated than Escherigen, particularly concerning gastrointestinal events.

4.2. Nasal tolerability

Nasalflu Berna® was well tolerated locally following intranasal vaccination in the 1218 subjects vaccinated, with 39.7% of vaccinees reporting upon solicited questioning ≥ 1 nasal adverse event, mainly mild or moderate and lasting for 1–3 days only. "Runny" nose (rhinitis) (24%), stuffy nose (20%) and sneezing (18%) were the most frequently reported symptoms after the first dose. These rates increased slightly for the second dose.

In young adults (*n* = 909, including 46 asthma patients), 43.1% of subjects vaccinated reported ≥ 1, mainly mild to moderate nasal symptoms. Runny nose was, with 26%, the most frequently reported symptom, followed by 'stuffy' nose (23%), sneezing (21%), and local discomfort (14%). The corresponding figures reported after the second vaccination were very similar in terms of overall incidence (40.8%), intensity, duration and regarding the individual symptoms recorded. Runny nose (27%) 'stuffy nose' (27%), and sneezing (24%) were slightly higher compared to the first vaccination, whereas localized discomfort (12%) was slightly lower.

In adult subjects aged >60 years (*n* = 209, including five asthma patients), the overall reported incidences of nasal symptoms were 37.3% and 27.7% after the first and second vaccination, respectively. This was lower than those observed by the group of young adults. A similar spectrum and intensity of symptoms was observed, i.e. mainly mild events lasting 1–2 days only.

The local tolerability reported by the adult subjects immunized with the vaccine without Escherigen (*n* = 633) was superior to that observed after vaccination with Nasalflu Berna®. Differences for nasal discomfort, sneezing, stuffy nose and runny nose/rhinitis were already significant after the first vaccination in favour of the Escherigen-free vaccine and increased further after the second dose. The addition of Escherigen to the vaccine did increase the overall incidence of nasal symptoms from 41.7–51.1% when compared to the HLT-free vaccine.

The nasal tolerability of Nasalflu Berna® in adults with bronchial asthma (*n* = 51) was good, considering the overall nasal AE rates of 7.8% and 10.0% reported after the first and second vaccination, respectively.

The nasal tolerability of Nasalflu Berna® in children aged ≥ 6 to ≤ 12 years ($n = 100$) and adolescents ($n = 3$) was good, with 13% of vaccinees only reporting ≥ 1 nasal symptoms after the first and the second dose, respectively.

The nasal tolerability following vaccination with PCG-adjuvanted vaccine ($n = 52$) was inferior to Nasalflu Berna® with a higher overall AE incidence of 61.5% and, e.g. discomfort in 17.3% and runny nose in 44.2% of vaccinees.

4.3. Laboratory results

The hematological and biochemical parameters investigated in two studies showed a high percentage of subjects with results slightly outside the reference limits before vaccination. They became normalized after vaccination. Clinically not relevant variations within or slightly outside the reference limits were observed 7–28 days after vaccination.

5. Immunogenicity

5.1. Humoral immune response

The immunogenicity of the virosome formulated and Escherigen-adjuvanted intranasal, trivalent subunit influenza vaccine (Nasalflu Berna®) has been evaluated in 1218 volunteer subjects (including 863) subjects aged ≥ 18 to <60 years, 204 subjects aged >60 years, 46 young and 5 elderly adult patients with mild/moderate bronchial asthma and 103 children/adolescents). These subjects were enrolled into nine clinical trials conducted in Italy and Switzerland. Three additional groups comprising young and elderly adult subjects, were also evaluated, for comparative purposes, after the administration of an intranasal vaccine containing an alternative adjuvant (PCG) ($n = 52$), an intranasal vaccine devoid of the standard HLT adjuvant ($n = 633$), or the commercial vaccines Inflexal Berna V ($n = 164$) and Fluarix ($n = 74$) for intramuscular use, respectively.

The standard dosage of Nasalflu Berna® used was 100 μl sprayed into each nostril on day 1 and day 8 ± 1 by the use of a nasal spray. The full immunization schedule thus consisted of 400 μl of the vaccine containing the influenza hemagglutinin, according the requirements of the European Agency for Evaluation of Medicinal Products (EMEA), and a total dose of 4 μg HLT.

The clinical experience demonstrated a good humoral immune response following intranasal administration of Nasalflu Berna® according to the EMEA immunogenicity criteria of seroconversion, GMT-fold increase and seroprotection. These criteria set by the EMEA for yearly relicensing were fulfilled for all age groups regarding all strains in all four seasons (1996/1997, 1997/1998, 1998/1999, 1999/2000, 2000/2001) the nasal vaccine had been tested.

In a clinical trial, the HLT-adjuvanted vaccine elicited a strong strain-specific IgA antibody response at the nasal mucosa (nasal lavage fluid). This effect was observed between 10 and 28 days after vaccination and was clearly superior to the weak response observed after IM Inflexal V Berna or to the moderate response observed after intranasal use of the vaccine devoid of the Escherigen adjuvant. This Escherigen-mediated enhancement of the post vaccination nasal immune response was not dependent on the immune response against Escherigen. The serological results were confirmed in a study assessing cellular immunity, where the increase in specific antibody secreting cells could be shown as well. Furthermore, it could be shown that the vaccination via the nasal route was able to sensitize T-helper cells, promoting the cytotoxic defense mechanisms.

During the influenza season 1998/1999, an epidemiological trial was conducted in Genoa, Italy. During a 2-month follow-up, there were significantly fewer episodes of virologically confirmed influenza infections in the vaccinated compared to the non-vaccinated groups, showing a protective efficacy of the intranasal vaccine, of 89.7% in children (95% CI, 57.6–97.5%) and 85.0% in adults (95% CI, −15.4–98.1%).

6. Conclusion

Nasalflu Berna[R], developed by the Swiss Serum and Vaccine Institute, is a novel, highly immunogenic, and safe influenza subunit vaccine, which can be easily administered as a nasal spray. This new route of administration is likely to increase compliance to vaccination, and could become an important tool to promote vaccination in population groups that show high resistance to vaccination.

References

[1] CDC Atlanta, Prevention and control of influenza: Part I, vaccines. Recommendations of the Advisory Committee on Immunization Practices (ACIP), MMWR 48 (No. RR-4) (1999) 1–28.

[2] P.F. Wright, J.D. Cherry, H.M. Foy, Antigenicity and reactogenicity of influenza A/USSR/77 virus vaccine in children—a multicentered evaluation of dosage and safety, Rev. Infect. Dis. 5 (1983) 758–764.

[3] W.B. Ershler, Influenza vaccination in the elderly: can efficacy be enhanced? Geriatrics 43 (1988) 79–83.

[4] R.B. Couch, W.A. Keitel, T.R. Cate, Improvement of inactivated influenza vaccines, J. Infect. Dis. 176 (Suppl. 1) (1997) 38–44.

[5] T. Zei, M. Neri, A.M. Ioro, Immunogenicity of trivalent subunit and split influenza vaccines (1989–1990) winter season in volunteers of different age groups, Vaccine 9 (1991) 613–617.

[6] J.R. McGhee, H. Kiyono, New perspectives in vaccine development: mucosal immunity to infections, Infect. Agents Dis. 2 (1993) 55–73.

[7] J. Holmgren, Mucosal immunity and vaccination, FEMS Microbiol. Immunol. 89 (1991) 1–10.

[8] R. Glück, R. Mischler, B. Finkel, J.U. Que, B. Scarpa, S.J. Cryz Jr., Immunogenicity of new virosome influenza vaccine in elderly people, Lancet 344 (1994) 160–163.

[9] P. Conne, L. Gauthey, P. Vernet, B. Althaus, J. Que, B. Finkel, R. Glück, S.J. Cryz Jr., Immunogenicity of trivalent subunit versus virosome-formulated influenza vaccines in geriatric patients, Vaccine 15 (1997) 1675–1679.

[10] R.I. Walker, New strategies for using mucosal vaccination to achieve more effective immunization, Vaccine 12 (1994) 387–400.

[11] S. Baqar, A.L. Burgeois, P.J. Schultheiss, R.I. Walker, D.M. Rollins, R.L. Haberberger, O.R. Pavloskis, Safety and immunogenicity of a prototype oral whole-cell killed *Campylobacter* vaccine administered with a mucosal adjuvant in non-human primates, Vaccine 13 (1995) 22–28.

[12] K. Hashigucci, H. Ogawa, T. Ishidate, R. Yamashita, H. Kamiya, K. Watanabe, N. Hattori, T. Sato, Y. Suzuki, T. Nagamine, C. Aizawa, S. Tamura, T. Kurata, A. Oya, Antibody responses in volunteers induced by nasal influenza vaccine combined with *Escherichia coli* heat-labile enterotoxin B subunit containing a trace amount of the holotoxin, Vaccine 14 (1996) 113–119.

[13] M.G. Cusi, P.E. Lomagistro, M. Valassino, P.E. Valensin, R. Glück, Immunopotentiating of mucosal and systemic antibody responses in mice by intranasal immunization with HLT-combinated influenza virosomal vaccine, Vaccine 18 (2000) 2838–2842.

[14] F. Swaby, L. Kelly, R. Lambkin, J. Oxford, The efficacy of a test vaccine in the ferret influenza model when challenged with homologous virus. Internal SSVI Final Report dated May 7, 1999.

International Congress Series 1219 (2001) 979–984

Nasal proteosome subunit flu vaccine elicits enhanced mucosal IgA, serum HAI and protection comparable to conventional injectable flu vaccine

M. Plante[*], D. Jones, F. Allard, K. Torossian, J. Gauthier, G. White, G. Lowell, D. Burt

Intellivax International Inc., 7150 Frederick Banting, Suite 200, Ville St-Laurent, Québec, Canada H4S 2A1

Abstract

Background: Protective immunity against infection by influenza virus may be enhanced by vaccines that induce immune responses at mucosal surfaces of the respiratory tract. Since proteosomes are safe and induce antigen-specific systemic and mucosal immune responses in animals and humans, the efficacy of a nasal proteosome subunit flu vaccine was investigated. *Methods*: BALB/c mice were immunized twice intranasally (i.n.) or intramuscularly (i.m.) with detergent Split flu virus (SFV; strain A/Taiwan/1/86 (H1N1)) formulated with proteosomes (Pr) at different Pr:hemagglutinin (HA) ratios or with SFV alone. Mice were then challenged intranasally with 4 LD_{50} of the mouse-adapted homologous influenza virus. *Results*: Intranasal immunization with Pr-SFV induced levels of serum IgG, hemagglutination inhibition activity and viral neutralizing activity comparable to those elicited by i.m. administered SFV. Serum IgG_1/IgG_{2a} ratios suggested that the proteosome influenza vaccine converts the Type 2 immune response induced by SFV alone to a balanced Type 1/Type 2 response. Nasal and lung IgA levels were increased 14- and 19-fold, respectively, in mice immunized nasally with Pr-SFV compared to SFV alone. Mice that received nasal Pr-SFV vaccines were protected against morbidity to the same extent as animals immunized i.m. with the split influenza vaccine alone. *Conclusions*: Proteosomes are a potent mucosal adjuvant delivery system for influenza vaccines. © 2001 Elsevier Science B.V. All rights reserved.

Keywords: Proteosomes; Influenza vaccine; Intranasal

[*] Corresponding author. Tel.: +1-514-338-3883; fax: +1-514-334-0606.
E-mail address: mplante@intellivax.com (M. Plante).

0531-5131/01/$ – see front matter © 2001 Elsevier Science B.V. All rights reserved.
PII: S 0 5 3 1 - 5 1 3 1 (0 1) 0 0 0 2 4 - 3

1. Introduction

Conventional influenza vaccines are administered as split virus preparations or as subunit components. In children and healthy young adults, immunization with inactivated influenza vaccines is 70–90% effective in inducing immunity, thereby reducing the severity and incidence of illness [1]. The immune response to influenza vaccines is strain-specific and short-lived [2]. The efficacy of influenza vaccines is lower in the elderly suggesting that current injectable vaccines are less immunogenic in this high-risk population group. It has been postulated that a mucosally delivered influenza vaccine which stimulates both secretory and systemic antibody responses would provide protection against both initial infection and disease progression. Inactivated virus vaccines [3–5] and subunit vaccines [6] are weakly immunogenic when applied via mucosal surfaces and require co-administration of mucosal adjuvants. Intranasal immunization with antigens non-covalently formulated with proteosomes (Pr) formed from outer membrane proteins of *Neisseria meningitidis* has been shown to induce antigen-specific systemic and mucosal immune responses. Examples include, staphylococcal enterotoxin B [7], O-polysaccharide antigen of *Shigella sonnei* and *S. flexneri* 2a [8–10], and rgp160 from the human immunodeficiency virus [11,12]. Nasal administration of *S. flexneri* lipopolysaccharides formulated with proteosomes was also shown to be safe and immunogenic in human phase 1 and 2 clinical trials (manuscripts in preparation). Since proteosome vaccines are safe and induce antigen-specific systemic and mucosal immune responses in animals and humans, the potential of a nasal proteosome flu vaccine was investigated.

2. Materials and methods

2.1. Vaccine formulation, immunization, challenge and sample collection

SFV was formulated with empigen-solubilized proteosome proteins at a weight ratio of proteosome protein to HA of 8:1. Thirteen female BALB/C mice (6–8 weeks old) were immunized intranasally (i.n.) or intramuscularly (i.m.) at day 0 and day 21 with 3 μg (based on HA content determined by SRID) of Pr-SFV formulation or SFV alone. For i.n. immunizations, mice were lightly anesthetized by methophane inhalation and 12.5 μl of vaccine was applied to each nostril. Intramuscular immunizations were achieved by injection of 25 μl into mouse hind limbs. Animals (eight per group) were challenged on day 38 with 4 LD_{50} of homologous, mouse adapted influenza virus. Body weights were monitored for 14 days post-challenge and weight loss was used as a surrogate for morbidity.

2.2. Sampling, antibody and functional assays

Five unchallenged mice per group were euthanized and exsanguinated by cardiac puncture. Nasal and lung wash samples were also collected from these mice. Influenza-specific antibody levels (serum IgG's and mucosal IgA) were measured by ELISA using whole virus as the solid phase. Hemagglutination inhibition (HAI) assays were performed by standard methods using chicken red blood cells. Viral neutralization assays were performed using 100 $TCID_{50}$ of the homologous virus strain.

3. Results

As shown in Table 1, intranasal immunization with Pr-SFV induced levels of serum IgG1, IgG2a, IgG2b and IgG3 against whole virus that was substantially higher than those induced by SFV alone administered by the same route. Levels of total influenza-specific IgG (Table 3) induced by Pr-SFV administered intranasally or intramuscularly were comparable to, or higher than, respectively, SFV vaccine at the same dose of HA administered intramuscularly. In addition, the serum IgG1/IgG2a ratios following nasal immunization with Pr-SFV were 3.5–10-fold less than that for the split product given intramuscularly (Table 1). This strongly suggests that administration of proteosome-formulated SFV induces a switch from a Type 2 phenotype towards a balanced Type1/ Type 2 response. Importantly, only Pr-SFV vaccine administered intranasally elicited significant virus-reactive lung and nasal IgA as shown in Table 2. Lung and nasal IgA titers were 19 and 14 times higher, respectively, compared to SFV alone administered by the same route. The serum hemagglutination inhibition (HAI) and viral neutralizing (VN) antibody titers elicited by intranasal immunization with Pr-SFV were 8 and 19 times greater, respectively, compared to nasal SFV alone (Table 3). Although the HAI titers induced following intramuscular injection were comparable for Pr-SFV and SFV alone,

Table 1

Influenza-specific systemic antibody response in mice immunized intranasally or intramuscularly with proteosome-subunit influenza formulations

Vaccine formulation[a]	Immunization route[b]	Influenza-specific IgG subclass antibody titer (ng/ml)[c]				IgG1/IgG2a ratio
		IgG1	IgG2a	IgG2b	IgG3	
Pr-SFV (HA)	i.n.	615,561	303,911	1,724,235	35,625	2.0
SFV (HA)	i.n.	98,916	4554	31,322	3171	21.0
Pr-SFV (HA)	i.m.	1,474,974	405,675	2,825,934	323,822	3.6
SFV (HA)	i.m.	1,673,652	134,178	249,914	7945	12.5
Live influenza virus[d]	i.n.	47,814	190,592	670,376	19,424	0.25
Pr-Ctrl Ag[e]	i.n.	<49	<24	500	<49	n.d.

[a] Mice were immunized on days 0 and 21 with 3 μg of influenza vaccine formulation based on HA content as determined by SRID.

[b] Mice were anesthetized by methophane inhalation prior to intranasal immunization.

[c] Titers of IgG1, IgG2a, IgG2b and IgG3 subclasses were measured by ELISA on pooled sera using formalin-inactivated whole influenza virus as solid-phase antigen.

[d] Mice were given an intranasal instillation of approximately 0.04 LD_{50} of mouse passaged live influenza virus strain A/Taiwan/1/86 (H1N1).

[e] A hepatitis surface antigen (HBsAg) was used as control antigen.

Table 2
Mucosal IgA antibody response elicited following immunization with Pr-SFV formulations

Vaccine formulation	Immunization route	Mucosal antibody titer[a,b]	
		Lung IgA (ng/ml)	Nasal IgA (ng/ml)
Pr-SFV (HA) 8:1	i.n.	1133 ± 364	135 ± 41
SFV (HA)	i.n.	59 ± 24	10 ± 4
Pr-SFV (HA) 8:1	i.m.	4 ± 2	2 ± 0
SFV (HA)	i.m.	2 ± 0	2 ± 0
Live influenza virus	i.n.	176 ± 94	7 ± 2
Pr-Ctrl Ag	i.n.	2 ± 0	3 ± 0

[a] Nasal IgA, lung IgA and functional antibody titers were determined on samples collected from a subset of the original groups that were not challenged with the influenza virus.

[b] Influenza-specific nasal and lung IgA concentrations were determined by ELISA on individual nasal and lung lavage fluids. Results are expressed as the mean IgA concentration ± SEM for each group.

viral neutralization titers were approximately four times higher in sera from mice immunized with Pr-SFV compared with SFV alone. Mice immunized nasally with Pr-SFV vaccine were completely protected against weight loss and mortality following challenge with live homologous influenza virus. The degree of protection was identical to that observed for mice immunized by the i.m. route with SFV alone. In contrast, a proteosome formulation containing an irrelevant protein antigen (Pr-CtrlAg) failed to protect the mice as shown by the 24% weight loss and 50% mortality. Mice immunized intranasally with SFV alone lost 10% of their starting weight by 6 days after challenge.

Table 3
Immunogenicity and efficacy of Pr-SFV (HA) vaccines in BALB/c mice

Vaccine formulation	Immunization route	Total influenza-specific serum IgG (ng/ml)	HAI titer[a]	VNA titer[b]	Weight change on day 6 (%)[c]	Survival on day 14 (%)[d]
Pr-SFV (HA) 8:1	i.n.	2,679,332	1280	3428	1.15 ± 0.5	100
SFV (HA)	i.n.	134,863	160	182	− 9.91 ± 2.7	88
Pr-SFV (HA) 8:1	i.m.	5,030,405	1280	5382	1.15 ± 0.7	100
SFV (HA)	i.m.	2,065,689	1280	1467	2.80 ± 0.6	100
Live influenza virus	i.n.	928,206	160	363	0.63 ± 1.6	100
Pr-Ctrl Ag	i.n.	<622	10	77	− 24.14 ± 1.4	50

[a] HAI assays were performed using chicken red blood cells and 8 HAU of the homologous influenza virus strain. Results are expressed as the reciprocal of the last dilution producing complete agglutination inhibition.

[b] Viral neutralization titers were calculated using the Kärber formula and are expressed as the reciprocal of the dilution at which the cytopathic effect on MDCK cells was inhibited by 50%.

[c] Mice were challenged by intranasal instillation of 4 LD_{50} of mouse-passaged live influenza virus, strain A/Taiwan/1/86 and body weight was monitored over a period of 14 days. Body weight changes were compared at day 6 post-challenge (time at which body weight loss was maximal for control animals). Results are presented as mean body weight change (percentage) ± SEM for each group.

[d] Mice reaching 30% body weight loss were euthanized by CO_2 inhalation.

4. Discussion

Intranasal or intramuscular immunization with a proteosome-split flu vaccine formulation was shown to induce serum IgG levels, viral neutralizing and HAI titers comparable to injected subunit vaccine. The ability to induce serum hemagglutination inhibition activity remains a key criterion for the registration of influenza vaccines for humans. Our results demonstrate that intranasal administration of a subunit influenza vaccine formulated with proteosomes increases its systemic immunogenicity to match that of injectable subunit influenza vaccines. Serum antibody isotypes generated following immunization with Pr-SFV formulations suggest a switch from a Type 2 phenotype towards a balanced Type 1/Type 2 response. Studies of the pattern of cytokines produced by T cells from Pr-SFV immunized mice are ongoing to confirm these results. A shift in the immune response towards a Type 1 phenotype is a desirable property for a vaccine since virus clearance depends on the generation of cytotoxic lymphocytes and the release of IFN-γ and TNF-α [13] In contrast to SFV administered intranasally or intramuscularly, only intranasal immunization with Pr-SFV induced high levels of lung and nasal IgA that may provide protection at the site of entry of the influenza virus. Importantly, mice immunized intranasally or intramuscularly with Pr-SFV formulations were protected against homologous challenge, to the same degree as mice immunized intramuscularly with a conventional subunit influenza vaccine, confirming the functional relevance of the immune responses elicited by the proteosome influenza vaccine.

Intranasal administration of a Pr-SFV formulation was shown to be an effective and non-invasive means of delivering a protective subunit influenza vaccine in an animal model. Ongoing clinical trials will determine whether these vaccines are immunogenic in human volunteers.

References

[1] N.J. Cox, K. Subbarao, Influenza, Lancet 354 (1999) 1277–1282.

[2] K.M. Edwards, W.D. Dupont, M.K. Westrich, W.D. Plummer Jr., P.S. Palmer, P.F. Wright, A randomized controlled trial of cold-adapted and inactivated vaccines for the prevention of influenza A disease, J. Infect. Dis. 169 (1994) 68–76.

[3] Z. Moldoveanu, M.L. Clements, S.J. Prince, B.R. Murphy, J. Mestecky, Human immune responses to influenza virus vaccines administered by systemic or mucosal routes, Vaccine 13 (1995) 1006–1012.

[4] R.V. Fulk, D.S. Fedson, M.A. Huber, J.R. Fitzpatrick, B.F. Howar, J.A. Kasel, Antibody responses in children and elderly persons following local or parenteral administration of an inactivated influenza virus vaccine, A2/Hong Kong/68 variant, J. Immunol. 102 (1969) 1102–1105.

[5] P.F. Wright, B.R. Murphy, M. Kervina, E.M. Lawrence, M.A. Phelan, D.T. Karzon, Secretory immunological response after intranasal inactivated influenza virus vaccinations: evidence for immunoglobulin A memory, Infect. Immun. 40 (1983) 1092–1095.

[6] T.G. Boyce, H.H. Hsu, E.C. Sannella, S.D. Coleman-Dockery, E. Baylis, Y. Zhu, G. Barchfeld, A. Di-Francesco, M. Paranandi, B. Culley, K.M. Neuzil, P.F. Wright, Safety and immunogenicity of adjuvanted and unadjuvanted subunit influenza vaccines administered to healthy adults, Vaccine 19 (2000) 217–226.

[7] G.H. Lowell, R.W. Kaminski, S. Grate, R.E. Hunt, C. Charney, S. Zimmer, C. Colleton, Intranasal and intramuscular proteosome-staphylococcal enterotoxin B (SEB) toxoid vaccine: immunogenicity and efficacy against lethal SEB intoxication in mice, Infect. Immun. 64 (1996) 1706–1713.

[8] N. Orr, G. Rubin, D. Cohen, R. Arnon, G.H. Lowell, Immunogenicity and efficacy of oral or intranasal

Shigelle flexneri 2a and *Shigella sonnei* proteosome-lipopolysaccharide vaccines in animal models, Infect. Immun. 61 (1993) 2390–2395.

 [9] N. Orr, R. Arnon, G. Rubin, D. Cohen, H. Bercovier, G.H. Lowell, Enhancement of anti-*Shigella* lipopolysaccharide (LPS) response by addition of the cholera toxin B subunit to oral and intranasal proteosome-*Shigella flexneri* 2a LPS vaccine, Infect. Immun. 62 (1994) 5198–5200.

[10] C.P. Mallett, T.L. Hale, R.W. Kaminski, T. Larsen, N. Orr, D. Cohen, G.H. Lowell, Intranasal or intragastric immunization with proteosome-*Shigella* lipopolysaccharide vaccines protects against lethal pneumonia in a murine model of *Shigella* infection, Infect. Immun. 63 (1995) 2382–2386.

[11] G.H. Lowell, R.W. Kaminski, T.C. VanCott, B. Slike, K. Kersey, E. Zawoznik, L. Loomis-Price, G. Smith, R.R. Redfield, S. Amselem, D.L. Birx, Proteosomes, emulsomes, and cholera toxin B improve nasal immunogenicity of human immunodeficiency virus gp160 in mice: induction of serum, intestinal, vaginal, and lung IgA and IgG, J. Infect. Dis. 175 (1997) 292–301.

[12] T.C. VanCott, R.W. Kaminski, J.R. Mascola, V.S. Kalyanaraman, N.M. Wassef, C.R. Alving, J.T. Ulrich, G.H. Lowell, D.L. Birx, HIV-1 neutralizing antibodies in the genital and respiratory tracts of mice intranasally immunized with oligomeric gp160, J. Immunol. 160 (1998) 2000–2001.

[13] F.V. Chisari, C. Ferrari, Hepatitis B virus immunopathogenesis, Ann. Rev. Immunol. 13 (1995) 29–60.

International Congress Series 1219 (2001) 985–992

Mucosal vaccination protects mice against influenza A heterosubtypic challenge

T.M. Tumpey[a], J.D. Clements[b,1], J.M. Katz[a,*]

[a]*Influenza Branch, Division of Viral and Rickettsial Diseases (DVRD), National Center for Infectious Diseases (NCID), Centers for Disease Control and Prevention, Mailstop G-16, 1600 Clifton Road, N.E., Atlanta, GA 30333, USA*
[b]*Department of Microbiology and Immunology, Tulane University Medical Center, New Orleans, LA 70112, USA*

Abstract

Background: The introduction of an influenza A virus possessing a novel hemagglutinin (HA) into an immunologically naive human population has the potential to cause the next influenza pandemic. The recent emergence of avian H5 and H9 influenza subtypes into the human population has renewed the search for a vaccine strategy that induces broadly cross-reactive or heterosubtypic immunity (Het-I), with the potential to protect individuals against multiple subtypes of influenza A virus. *Methods*: Mice vaccinated mucosally with a formalin-inactivated X-31 (H3N2) virus vaccine coadministrated with a mutant form of heat-labile enterotoxin (mLT) from *Escherichia coli* as an adjuvant were challenged with the highly pathogenic human H5N1 influenza A (A/HK/483/97) subtype. As the indicator of Het-I, survival and reduction in virus shedding from the respiratory tract were determined. Serum and mucosal antibody responses were compared between immune and non-immune control mice. *Results*: Mice that received three intranasal immunizations of H3N2 vaccine coadministered with $1-5$ µg of mLT had increased levels of antiviral IgG and IgA antibodies, and lower levels of infectious virus observed in lung tissues when compared with mice which received vaccine alone. Mice administered H3N2/mLT vaccine were completely protected against lethal H5N1 challenge and had viral titers that were at least 1000-fold lower than control mice receiving mLT alone. *Conclusions*: These results suggest a strategy of mucosal vaccination that stimulates cross-protection against an influenza subtype with pandemic potential. Published by Elsevier Science B.V.

Keywords: Vaccines; Influenza H5N1; Mouse model

* Corresponding author. Tel.: +1-404-639-3591; fax: +1-404-639-2334.
E-mail address: jmk9@cdc.gov (J.M. Katz).
1 Present address: Southeast Poultry Research Laboratory, Agricultural Research Service, US Department of Agriculture, 934 College Station Road, Athens, GA 30605, USA.

0531-5131/01/$ – see front matter. Published by Elsevier Science B.V.
PII: S 0 5 3 1 - 5 1 3 1 (0 1) 0 0 6 5 3 - 7

1. Introduction

Influenza is still a serious threat to public health throughout the world. The current licenced influenza vaccine has limitations in its protective ability because the virus alters its surface glycoproteins, hemagglutinin (HA) and neuraminidase (NA), thus escaping the presence of preexisting immunity. To control influenza, the vaccine needs to be updated annually in order to provide sufficient protection against new circulating human strains. However, the late emergence of variant strains of influenza, which are not antigenically closely matched with those in the vaccine, can result in increased morbidity and mortality. Such antigenic drift occurred most recently in 1997 with the emergence of A/Sydney/5/97 which resulted in increased morbidity. Additionally, antigenic shift involving the introduction of an influenza A virus possessing a novel HA into an immunologically naive human population can also result in severe disease. Antigenic shifts have contributed to the pandemics of 1918, 1957 and 1968 [1]. In 1997, an avian influenza A (H5N1) virus emerged in humans in Hong Kong and caused 18 cases of human respiratory disease, six of them fatal [2–4]. This outbreak and the recently reported transmission of avian H9N2 influenza virus to humans has renewed interest in developing vaccines that are capable of inducing more broadly cross-reactive immunity against novel influenza variants.

In animals models, live virus infection with an influenza A virus of one subtype can provide protection against subsequent infection of another subtype, and this is termed heterosubtypic immunity (Het-I) [5–7]. Therefore, the design of inactivated influenza vaccines which mimic the efficacy of live vaccines by inducing cross-protection would benefit in years when there is a poor antigenic match between vaccine and circulating viruses and perhaps offer protection against the emergence of novel influenza subtypes with pandemic potential. We demonstrate here that a human influenza H3N2 inactivated-virus vaccine administrated mucosally together with adjuvant induced Het-I and protected mice against lethal H5N1 virus challenge. Data from this study suggest that a non-invasive mucosal vaccine would improve the efficacy of the current influenza vaccine by providing greater cross-reactive immunity to influenza.

2. Materials and methods

2.1. Viruses and mice

Female BALB/c mice 6–10 weeks of age were obtained from Jackson Laboratories (Bar Harbor, ME). The influenza viruses used in this study were: A/Hong Kong/483/97 (HK/483) H5N1, the reassortant human influenza A virus, X-31 (which possesses the surface glycoprotein genes of A/Aichi/2/68 [H3N2] and the internal protein genes of A/Puerto Rico/8/34), and A/Taiwan/1/86 (A/TW) H1N1, originally derived by Dr. P Wyde (Baylor College of Medicine Houston, TX) and was kindly provided by Dr. J. Matthews, (Aventis Pasteur, Swiftwater, PA). Virus stocks were propagated in the allantoic cavity of 10-day-old embryonated hens' eggs at 35 °C. The allantoic fluids were harvested 24–48 h post-inoculation and stored at −70 °C until use. Fifty percent mouse infectious dose

(MID_{50}) titers were determined as previously described [8]. MID_{50} titers were calculated by the method of Reed and Muench [9] and are expressed as mean $log_{10}EID_{50}/ml \pm$ standard error (SE).

2.2. Vaccine preparation and immunization

Viruses used as vaccines or purified proteins on ELISA plates were concentrated from allantoic fluid and purified by equilibrium density centrifugation through a 30–60% linear sucrose gradient as previously described [10]. The X-31 (H3N2) inactivated whole virus vaccine was prepared by treating purified virus at a concentration of 1 mg/ml with 0.025% formalin at 4 °C for 3 days. The vaccine doses given throughout are expressed as amounts of total protein measured by Bradford assay (Bio-Rad Laboratories, Hercules, CA). For immunization, groups of mice were lightly anesthetized with CO_2 and vaccinated intranasally (i.n.) three times at weekly intervals with 50 µl containing 20 µg of purified X-31 (H3N2) virus suspended in PBS in the presence or absence of the indicated dose of

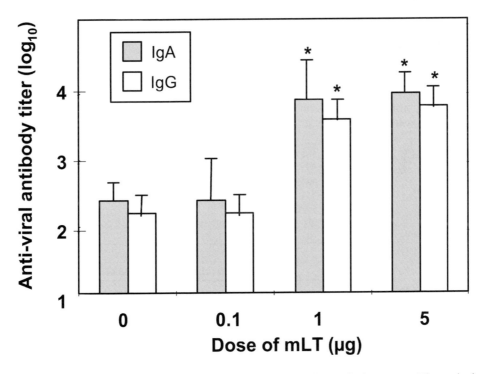

Fig. 1. Dose dependence of mLT activity on the induction of IgG and IgA lung antibody responses. Mice received three intranasal inoculations at weekly intervals of 20 µg of formalin-inactivated H3N2 (X-31) virus in the presence or absence of indicated concentrations of mLT adjuvant. Two weeks after the final vaccine boost, five mice from each vaccine and mLT control group were euthanized for lung wash collection. Titers are expressed as the highest dilution of lung wash having a mean $(OD)_{405}$ greater than the mean plus two standard deviations of similarly diluted mLT-control sera. (*) Indicates the H3N2/mLT-vaccinated group was significantly ($p < 0.05$) different from the vaccine-only group by ANOVA.

mutant LT (R192G). The LT mutant (mLT) used in these studies was genetically engineered and purified as described [11]. Two weeks after final vaccination, mice were challenged i.n. with 100 MID_{50} of A/TW(H1N1), X-31 (H3N2) or HK/483 (H5N1) in a volume of 50 μl. Following infection, mice were monitored daily for disease signs for 14 days post-infection (p.i.). For determination of infectious virus, nose and lung tissue samples of four to five mice per group were removed on day 5 p.i. Individual tissues were homogenized in 1 ml of PBS and titrated for virus infectivity in eggs and endpoint titers are expressed as mean $\log_{10}EID_{50}$/ml. Initial dilutions of 1:10 gave a limit of virus detection of $10^{1.2}$ EID_{50}/ml.

2.3. Antibody sampling and assay

Two weeks after the final vaccine boost, four to five mice from each group were anesthetized by intraperitoneal administration of Avertin; 2,2,2-tribromoethanol (Sigma, St. Louis, MO) at 0.15 ml/10 g of body weight. Blood samples collected from the orbital plexus provided immune sera. Bronchoaveolar (lung) wash samples were obtained from euthanized animals as previously described [12]. Serum and lung washes were tested by ELISA for the presence of antiviral IgG and IgA. All sera were initially diluted 1:10 in receptor-destroying enzyme from V. cholera, (Denka Seiken, Tokyo) and incubated at 37 °C overnight to destroy nonspecific serum inhibitor activity. Immunolon II plates (Dynatech Laboratories, Chantilly, VA) were coated with 50 hemagglutinating units of purified homologous H3N2 (X-31) virus in PBS. Bound antibody was detected by the addition of goat anti-mouse IgG or IgA conjugated to horseradish peroxidase and absorbance was measured at 405 nm 30 min following the addition of ABTS (Kirkegaard and Perry, Gaithersburg, MD). Titers are expressed as the highest dilution that yielded an optical density greater than the mean plus two standard deviations of similarly diluted mLT-control sera.

Table 1

Heterosubtypic immunity following intranasal vaccination with H3N2 in the presence or absence of increasing doses of mutant LT (mLT) adjuvant

Group	Treatment[a]	Mean lung virus titer ± SE, $\log_{10}$ EID_{50}/ml	
		Homologous virus challenge	Heterologous virus challenge
1	mLT (5.0 μg)	7.3 ± 0.3	8.2 ± 0.3
2	H3N2 only	4.0 ± 0.8	7.6 ± 0.3
3	H3N2 + 0.1 μg mLT	5.1 ± 0.8	7.0 ± 0.3
4	H3N2 + 1.0 μg mLT	2.3 ± 0.3*	3.5 ± 0.4*
5	H3N2 + 5.0 μg mLT	1.9 ± 0.4*	3.0 ± 0.3*

[a] Eight-week-old mice (four/group) received three intranasal inoculations at weekly intervals of 5 μg of formalin-inactivated H3N2 virus in the presence or absence of indicated concentrations of mLT adjuvant. Two weeks after the final vaccine boost, mice were challenged intranasally with 100 MID_{50} of mouse-adapted homologous H3N2 (X-31) or heterologous (H1N1) A/Taiwan/86 virus and euthanized 5 days later. Lung tissues were homogenized in 1 ml of PBS and titrated for virus infectivity in eggs. Virus end-point titers are expressed as mean $\log_{10}$ EID_{50}/ml ± SE.

* Indicates the H3N2/mLT-vaccinated group was significantly ($p < 0.05$) different from the H3N2 vaccine-only group by ANOVA.

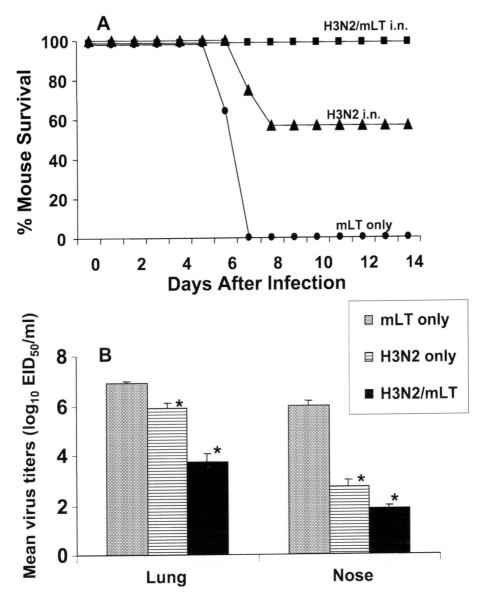

Fig. 2. Mucosal delivery of H3N2 influenza vaccine induces heterosubtypic protection against lethal influenza A H5N1 virus infection. Groups of BALB/c mice received three intranasal (i.n.) inoculations at weekly intervals of 20 μg of formalin-fixed H3N2 virus in the presence or absence of 2 μg of mLT adjuvant. Control mice received mLT adjuvant only. Two weeks after the final vaccine boost, mice were challenged i.n. with lethal H5N1 (HK/483) virus and monitored for survival (A) or euthanized 5 days later for collection of lung and nose tissue (B). (*) Indicates the H3N2/mLT-vaccinated group was significantly ($p < 0.05$) different from the adjuvant-only control group by ANOVA.

3. Results

Initial mouse experiments were performed to determine the optimum dose of mLT adjuvant given mucosally. Formalin-inactivated purified whole X-31 (H3N2) vaccine (20 µg) was coadministrated i.n. with or without the indicated doses of mLT three times at weekly intervals. In comparison to mice which received inactivated H3N2 vaccine alone, without adjuvant, significant increases of antiviral IgG and IgA antibodies were observed in the lungs of mice which were immunized with $1-5$ µg of mLT (Fig. 1). S subgroups of mice were challenged i.n. with 100 MID_{50} of homologous (H3N2) or heterosubtypic (H1N1) virus and euthanized 5 days later for determination of virus titers in tissues. As shown in Table 1, accelerated virus clearance was observed in the lungs of mice that were immunized with $1-5$ µg of mLT.

To further assess the effectiveness of H3N2/mLT mucosal vaccine, mice were challenged with 100 MID_{50} of A/HK483/97 (H5N1) virus isolated from a fatal human case in Hong Kong. The extent of Het-I was measured as (i) survival over a 14-day post-challenge period and (ii) virus titers in the upper respiratory tract (nose) and lower respiratory tract (lung) tissue of individual mice 5 days post-challenge (p.c.). Hetero-subtypic immune mice were completely protected from death, whereas 57% of mice administered vaccine alone i.n., without mLT, survived the lethal H5N1 heterosubtypic challenge (Fig. 2A). Mean lung virus titers detected in mice administered H3N2/mLT vaccine were at least 1500-fold lower than that of control mice receiving mLT alone and were 150-fold lower than that of mice administered H3N2 vaccine alone (Fig. 2B). Virus recovered from nose tissue of H3N2/mLT vaccinated mice was 15,000-fold lower than that of control mice. These results suggest that mucosal influenza immunization can provide Het-I against multiple subtypes of influenza A, including novel influenza variants with pandemic potential.

4. Discussion

Influenza A viruses continue to cause widespread disease in humans, with significant morbidity and mortality each year. This is because the current influenza vaccine licenced for parenteral administration vaccines has been optimally effective in controlling influenza if the epidemic virus strains are antigenically closely matched with those in the vaccine. Thus, influenza vaccines that induce greater cross-reactive immunity may overcome limitations in vaccine efficacy imposed by the antigenic variability of influenza A viruses. The recent avian H5N1 outbreak in Hong Kong has further highlighted the need for development of vaccines that are universally protective against multiple subtypes of influenza A. We investigated the use of a formalin-inactivated whole H3N2 virus vaccine coadministrated with mLT adjuvant for the ability to induce Het-I to an H5N1 virus. The Hong Kong H5N1 (HK/483) challenge virus selected for these studies was isolated from a fatal human case in 1997 and was among a group of H5N1 viruses previously characterized to be of high pathogenicity in mice [8,13,14]. The results clearly demonstrate that an intranasal vaccination induced Het-I and that a mutant derivative of heat-labile enterotoxin from *Escherichia coli* (mLT) delivered with vaccine serves as a potent mucosal adjuvant resulting in increased protection. The genetically altered mLT (R192G) protein possesses negligible toxicity, retains adjuvant properties similar to the native LT molecule and, as a result, has been given consideration as a useful mucosal adjuvant in humans [11,15]. The H3N2-immune mice were protected against mortality, and had accelerated virus clearance from respiratory tissues following a lethal H5N1 virus challenge. Characterization of the post-vaccination antibody responses identified an increase in antibody responses induced by mLT adjuvant, which correlates with increased Het-I. Administration of vaccine induced a substantial local IgA and IgG antibody response (Fig. 1) but also induced high antibody responses detected in the sera (data not shown). In a comparison study, the H3N2/mLT vaccine administrated subcutaneously was unable to induce Het-I and these animals succumbed to H5N1 virus challenge (data not shown), suggesting that mucosal vaccination was superior to parenteral vaccination for induction of Het-I. Taken together, these results demonstrate cross-reactive immunity to influenza subtypes and were such immunity inducible in humans, would provide a strategy for pandemic preparedness. Such a vaccine formulation could be rapidly prepared as an important first line of prevention, allowing time for a pandemic strain-specific vaccine to be developed.

References

[1] R.G. Webster, W.J. Bean, O.T. Gorman, T.M. Chambers, Y. Kawaoka, Evolution and ecology of influenza A viruses, Microbiol. Rev. 56 (1992) 152.

[2] E.C. Claas, A.D. Osterhaus, R. van Beek, J.C. de Jong, G.F. Rimmelzwaan, D.A. Senne, S. Krauss, K.F. Shortridge, R.G. Webster, Human influenza A H5N1 virus related to a highly pathogenic avian influenza virus, Lancet 351 (1998) 472–477.

[3] K. Subbarao, A. Klimov, J.M. Katz, H. Regnery, W. Lim, H. Hall, M. Perdue, D. Swayne, C. Bender, J. Huang, M. Hemphill, T. Rowe, M. Shaw, X. Xu, K. Fukuda, N. Cox, Characterization of an avian influenza A (H5N1) virus isolated from a child with a fatal respiratory illness, Science 279 (1998) 393–396.

[4] K.Y. Yuen, P.K. Chan, M. Peiris, D.N. Tsang, D.L. Que, K.F. Shortridge, P.T. Cheung, W.K. To, E.T. Ho, R. Sung, A.F. Cheng, Members of the H5N1 study group, Clinical features and rapid viral diagnosis of human disease associated with avian influenza A H5N1 virus, Lancet 351 (1999) 467–471.

[5] S.L. Epstein, C.Y. Lo, J. Misplon, C.M. Lawson, B.A. Hendrickson, E.E. Max, K. Subbarao, Mechanisms of heterosubtypic immunity to lethal influenza A virus infection in fully immunocompetent, T cell-depleted, β_2-microglobulin-deficient, and J chain-deficient mice, J. Immunol. 158 (1997) 1222–1230.

[6] S. Liang, K. Mozdzanowska, G. Pallandino, W. Gerhard, Heterosubtypic immunity to influenza type A virus in mice, J. Immunol. 152 (1994) 1653–1661.

[7] H.H. Nguyen, Z. Moldoveanu, M.J. Novak, F.W. van Ginkel, E. Ban, H. Kiyono, J.R. McGhee, J. Mestecky, Heterosubtypic immunity to lethal influenza A virus infection is associated with virus-specific CD8(+) cytotoxic T lymphocyte responses induced in mucosa-associated tissues, Virology 254 (1999) 50–60.

[8] X.T. Lu, T.M. Tumpey, T. Morken, S. Zaki, N.J. Cox, J.M. Katz, A mouse model for the evaluation of pathogenesis and immunity to influenza A (H5N1) virus isolated from humans, J. Virol. 73 (1999) 5903–5911.

[9] L.J. Reed, H. Muench, A simple method of estimating fifty percent endpoints, Am. J. Hyg. 27 (1938) 493–497.

[10] N.J. Cox, A.P. Kendal, Genetic stability of A/Ann Arbor/6/60 cold-mutant (temperature-sensitive) live influenza virus genes: analysis by oligonucleotide mapping of recombinant vaccine strains before and after replication in volunteers, J. Infect. Dis. 149 (1984) 194–200.

[11] B.L. Dickinson, J.D. Clements, Dissociation of *Escherichia coli* heat-labile enterotoxin adjuvanticity form ADP-ribosyltransferase activity, Infect. Immun. 63 (1995) 1617–1623.

[12] J.M. Katz, X. Lu, S.A. Young, J.C. Galphin, Adjuvant activity of the heat-labile enterotoxin from enterotoxigenic *Escherichia coli* for oral administration of inactivated influenza virus vaccine, J. Infect. Dis. 175 (1997) 352–363.

[13] P.S. Gao, S. Watanabe, T. Ito, H. Goto, K. Wells, M. McGregor, A.J. Cooley, Y. Kawaoka, Biological heterogeneity, including systemic replication in mice, of H5N1 influenza A virus isolates from humans in Hong Kong, J. Virol. 73 (1999) 3184–3189.

[14] T.M. Tumpey, X. Lu, T. Morken, S.R. Zaki, J.M. Katz, Depletion of lymphocytes and diminished cytokine production in mice infected with a highly virulent influenza A (H5N1) virus isolated from humans, J. Virol. 74 (2000) 6105–6116.

[15] M.L. Oplinger, S. Baqar, A.F. Trofa, J.D. Clements, P. Gibbs, G. Pazzaglia, A.L. Bourgeois, D.A. Scott, Safety and immunogenicity in volunteers of a new candidate oral mucosal adjuvant, LT(R192G), abstr. G-10, Program and Abstracts of the 37th Interscience Conference on Antimirobial Agents and Chemotherapy, 1997, p. 193.

International Congress Series 1219 (2001) 993–998

Lipopeptide vaccines: a strategy for improving protective immunity against influenza

Georgia Deliyannis[a,*], David C. Jackson[a], Leanne Harling-McNabb[a],
Weiguang Zeng[a], Nicholas J. Ede[a], Irene Hourdakis[a], Michael Rudd[b],
Anne Kelso[b], Lorena E. Brown[a]

[a]*Cooperative Research Centre for Vaccine Technology, Department of Microbiology and Immunology,
University of Melbourne, Parkville, Victoria 3052, Australia*
[b]*Cooperative Research Centre for Vaccine Technology, Queensland Institute of Medical Research,
Bancroft Centre, Post Office Royal Brisbane Hospital, Queensland, 4029, Australia*

Abstract

Background: Lipopeptide vaccines containing minimal CTL determinants have been shown to induce CTL responses against a variety of viruses, however, few have been reported to induce viral clearance. This study examines the ability of a lipopeptide vaccine incorporating palmitic acid, a CTL and a helper T cell (TH) determinant from influenza virus, to induce CTL-mediated viral clearing responses. The efficacy of the immunogen was examined after one or two doses, delivered either in the absence of an adjuvant or formulated with either CFA or Montanide ISA-720. *Methods*: The lipopeptide was administered subcutaneously (s.c.) to mice and at different times post-priming, mice were challenged with nonlethal doses of influenza virus and the titres in the lungs determined 5 days later. *Results*: High levels of anti-viral protection of the lung were achieved when the lipopeptide was administered with or without an adjuvant and only a single dose of vaccine was necessary to elicit long-lived immunity. The best reduction in lung virus titres was obtained when the construct was administered in Montanide ISA-720. *Conclusions*: These findings demonstrate the ability of T cell-based lipopeptide vaccines to induce effective influenza viral clearing responses, highlighting their potential as an adjunct to vaccines eliciting antibody responses. © 2001 Elsevier Science B.V. All rights reserved.

Keywords: Cytotoxic T lymphocytes; Helper T cells; Adjuvant

* Corresponding author. Tel.: +61-3-9344-3867; fax: +61-3-9347-1540.
E-mail address: g.deliyannis@microbiology.unimelb.edu.au (G. Deliyannis).

0531-5131/01/$ – see front matter © 2001 Elsevier Science B.V. All rights reserved.
PII: S 0 5 3 1 - 5 1 3 1 (0 1) 0 0 4 0 5 - 8

1. Introduction

Cross-reactive CTL immunity would be expected to aid in the clearance of newly emerging pandemic viruses as well as providing benefit against strains arising by antigenic drift in situations where strain prediction for inclusion in the current vaccine provides a less than adequate match. Therefore, an improved vaccine for induction of comprehensive protection against influenza might aim to incorporate a component that elicits cross-reactive CTL responses in addition to the viral glycoproteins, which elicit neutralising antibody.

Peptide vaccines containing CTL epitopes formulated with different adjuvants have been shown to induce CTL against a variety of viruses. In addition, anti-viral CTL induction can be achieved with peptides to which lipid has been covalently attached, even in the absence of an exogenous adjuvant [1–4]. Despite these numerous reports, however, very few of the vaccines have proven capable of inducing viral clearing responses [5–8].

This study focuses on the ability of a T cell-based lipopeptide vaccine incorporating a minimal CTL and a TH determinant from influenza virus, to induce CTL-mediated viral clearing responses and on determining any benefits derived from eliciting such responses in the face of challenge with heterologous virus. The efficacy of this synthetic immunogen was examined when delivered in the absence of an adjuvant or formulated with either complete Freund's adjuvant (CFA) or Montanide ISA-720 which, unlike CFA, has potential for use in humans.

2. Materials and methods

2.1. Mice and viruses

BALB/c mice were bred at the Department of Microbiology and Immunology, University of Melbourne. The influenza viruses used were PR8 = A/Puerto Rico/8/34 (H1N1), and the recombinant viruses Mem 71 (H3N1), a reassortant of A/Memphis/1/71 (H3N2) × A/Bellamy/42 (H1N1), and X-31 (H3N2), a reassortant of A/Aichi/2/68 (H3N2) × A/Puerto Rico/8/34 (H1N1).

2.2. Preparation of lipopeptide

The lipopeptide construct (pal2-CTL-TH) incorporates the dominant $H-2^d$-restricted CTL determinant NP (147–155) TYQRTRALV, derived from the nucleoprotein of PR8 virus together with the TH determinant, HA2 (166–180) ALNNRFQIKGVELKS, identified within the HA2 of Mem 71 [9]. The CTL determinant is common to type A influenza strains while the TH determinant is present on viruses of the H3 subtype. The peptide construct was assembled by conventional solid phase methodology using Fmoc chemistry. The CTL determinant was synthesised first to provide a free carboxyl group at the C-terminus. Two lysine residues were then added in tandem at the N-terminus and a palmitic acid introduced onto each of the two amino groups of the N-terminal lysine.

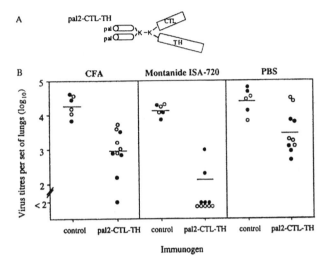

Fig. 1. (A) Schematic representation of the pal2-CTL-TH synthetic lipopeptide vaccine. (B) Viral clearing responses in BALB/c mice after immunisation s.c. either in the scruff of the neck (closed circles) or the base of the tail (open circles) with 9 nmol of the pal2-CTL-TH emulsified in CFA, Montanide ISA-720, or PBS. Seven days later the mice were challenged with $10^{4.5}$ pfu of Mem 71 virus and the lung viral titres determined 5 days post-challenge. Individual titres calculated from duplicate samples are shown with the mean values represented by a bar.

Finally, the TH determinant was synthesised from the ε amino group of the remaining lysine residue as shown in Fig. 1A.

2.3. Intranasal challenge of mice and preparation of mouse lung extracts

Vaccinated mice were challenged intranasally (i.n.) under penthrane anaesthesia with $10^{4.5}$ plaque forming units (pfu) of either Mem 71 or X-31 virus, or with 50 pfu of PR8 virus in 50 μl PBS. On day 5 post-challenge, mice were killed, lungs removed and homogenates prepared. The titre of infectious virus in each lung extract was subsequently determined by plaque assay on confluent monolayers of Madin–Darby canine kidney (MDCK) cells.

3. Results

3.1. The lipopeptide vaccine induces potent viral clearing responses when delivered in different formulations

Groups of 5 BALB/c mice were immunized in either the scruff of the neck or the base of the tail with 9 nmol of the pal2-CTL-TH construct emulsified in CFA (Sigma, USA), Seppic Montanide ISA-720 (kindly donated by CSL, Australia) or phosphate buffered saline (PBS). The mice were challenged 7 days later in order to evaluate the primary effector population induced by vaccination. Challenge was with Mem 71 virus, which bears both the CTL and TH determinants present in the lipopeptide immunogen.

Delivering pal2-CTL-TH in Montanide ISA-720 produced the highest levels of viral clearance with the virus load in the lungs on day 5 post-challenge being reduced by 99% (Fig. 1B). Delivering this construct in CFA was slightly less effective ($p = 0.0017$, Mann–Whittney test) with an average reduction of 93%. Pal2-CTL-TH was also effective in the absence of an adjuvant; the virus load in the lungs was reduced by 88% when the construct was administered in PBS. No significant differences ($p = 0.694$) were observed between the two s.c. routes.

3.2. Ability of lipopeptide to elicit immunity that aids in the clearance of different influenza viruses

Mice were immunized with pal2-CTL-TH emulsified in Montanide ISA-720, and subsequently challenged i.n. with either Mem 71, X-31 or PR8 viruses. Lipopeptide primed mice produced a high percentage of viral clearance against challenge with Mem 71 and X-31 viruses (both H3 subtype), which possess the CTL and TH determinants used in the lipopeptide. A lower percentage but a greater absolute reduction in viral titre was observed after challenge with PR8 virus (H1 subtype), which has only the CTL determinant in common with the immunogen (Fig. 2). The inability of the lipopeptide to reduce titres of PR8 to the very low levels (400–2000 pfu/lung) seen with the H3

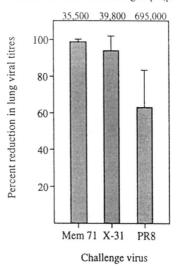

Fig. 2. Percent reduction in lung viral titres of mice (8 per group) immunized in the base of the tail with 9 nmol of pal2-CTL-TH emulsified in Montanide ISA-720 and challenged 7 days later with either Mem 71, X-31 or PR8 viruses. Five days post challenge, the lungs were collected and the titre of infectious virus determined. Data are expressed as percentages relative to the mean lung viral titres of the corresponding control groups that received adjuvant only.

Table 1
Levels of protection following s.c. administration of one or two doses of 9 nmol pal2-CTL-TH and i.n. challenge with Mem 71 virus

	Mean control[a]	Mean pal2-CTL-TH[b]	Virus reduction (%)
(A) Prime day 0, challenge day 28			
CFA	4.72 ± 0.10^c	3.40 ± 0.36^c	95.0
Montanide ISA-720	4.74 ± 0.08	3.28 ± 0.27	96.5
PBS	4.65 ± 0.11	3.83 ± 0.50	85
(B) Prime day 0, challenge day 56			
CFA	4.63 ± 0.09	3.64 ± 0.09	90
Montanide ISA-720	4.75 ± 0.04	3.39 ± 0.38	95.6
PBS	4.66 ± 0.11	3.65 ± 0.12	90
(C) Prime day 0, boost day 28, challenge day 56			
CFA	4.60 ± 0.17	3.73 ± 0.27	87
Montanide ISA-720	4.62 ± 0.08	3.45 ± 0.17	93
PBS	4.74 ± 0.04	3.77 ± 0.04	89

[a] Mice received adjuvant or PBS only prior to challenge.
[b] Mice were vaccinated with the lipopeptide pal2-CTL-TH prior to challenge with $10^{4.5}$ pfu of Mem 71 virus.
[c] Geometric mean titre and standard deviation of virus in the lung homogenates as determined by plaque assay on MDCK cells. The data for group A is derived from two different experiments.

viruses, may be due to PR8 not being able to restimulate the lipopeptide-primed T helper cell population or due to the greater virulence of PR8, which grows to at least tenfold higher titre in the lungs of mice than the H3 viruses.

3.3. Longevity of lipopeptide-induced viral clearing responses after one or two doses of vaccine

Mice were immunized with pal2-CTL-TH emulsified in either CFA, Montanide ISA-720 or PBS. One group of mice was challenged 28 days later with Mem 71 virus. A second group was boosted with the above formulations 4 weeks after priming and challenged on day 56 post-vaccination. The remaining mice did not receive a booster dose but were challenged on day 56 after the initial vaccination. On day 5 post-challenge, the lungs of the mice were assessed for the presence of infectious virus. As shown in Table 1, when combining the different formulations together, no significant differences ($p = 0.51$) were observed in the percentage of virus reduction in the lungs of the mice immunized with one (group A) or two doses (group C) of pal2-CTL-TH. Again, the Montanide ISA-720 formulation appeared to give slightly greater efficacy than CFA or PBS in each challenge group. High levels of clearance were achieved even after 2 months.

4. Discussion

This study represents one of the few reported examples of determinant-based immu-nogens that impact on the rate of clearance of a viral infection. High levels of anti-viral protection of the lung were achieved when the synthetic peptide construct was administered with or without the use of an adjuvant. Only a single dose of the lipopeptide was necessary to elicit long-lived immunity. The lipopeptide vaccine was capable of providing greatest protection against moderately virulent H3 influenza viruses bearing both $CD4^+$ and $CD8^+$ T cell determinants in common with the immunogen but also showed significant reduction of viral load with the highly virulent PR8 virus. The ability of T cell-based synthetic lipopeptide vaccines to induce immunity resulting in effective viral clearing responses in the influenza system highlights their potential as candidates for inclusion in an improved vaccine against this disease. For combination with the current split virus vaccine, for example, the practicalities of inclusion of sufficient numbers of epitopes to cover the MHC molecules of the target population would need to be addressed. Nevertheless, this strategy would be of particular significance in the face of a new pandemic where strong cross-reactive T cell responses may prove to be an important line of defence in the absence of specific antibody.

Acknowledgements

This work was supported by grants from the CRC for Vaccine Technology and the National Health and Medical Research Council of Australia. We thank Joanne Pagnon for laboratory assistance.

References

[1] B. Deprez, J.P. Sauzet, C. Boutillon, F. Martinon, A. Tartar, C. Sergheraert, J.G. Guillet, E. Gomard, H. Gras-Masse, Comparative efficiency of simple lipopeptide constructs for in vivo induction of virus-specific CTL, Vaccine 14 (1996) 375–382.

[2] K. Deres, H. Schild, K.H. Wiesmuller, G. Jung, G. Rammensee, In vivo priming of virus-specific cytotoxic T lymphocytes with synthetic lipopeptide vaccine, Nature 342 (1989) 561–564.

[3] F. Martinon, H. Gras-Masse, C. Boutillon, F. Chirat, B. Deprez, J.G. Guillet, E. Gomard, A. Tartar, J.P. Levy, Immunization of mice with lipopeptides bypasses the prerequisite for adjuvant. Immune response of BALB/c mice to human immunodeficiency virus envelope glycoprotein, J. Immunol. 149 (1992) 3416–3422.

[4] C. Oseroff, A. Sette, P. Wentworth, E. Celis, A. Maewal, C. Dahlberg, J. Fikes, R.T. Kubo, R.W. Chesnut, H.M. Grey, J. Alexander, Pools of lipidated HTL-CTL constructs prime for multiple HBV and HCV CTL epitope responses, Vaccine 16 (1998) 823–833.

[5] W.M. Kast, L. Roux, J. Curren, H.J. Blom, A.C. Voordouw, R.H. Meloen, D. Kolakofsky, C.J. Melief, Protection against lethal Sendai virus infection by in vivo priming of virus-specific cytotoxic T lymphocytes with a free synthetic peptide, Proc. Natl. Acad. Sci. U. S. A. 88 (1991) 2283–2287.

[6] M. Schulz, R.M. Zinkernagel, H. Hengartner, Peptide-induced antiviral protection by cytotoxic T cells, Proc. Natl. Acad. Sci. U. S. A. 88 (1991) 991–993.

[7] A.A. Scalzo, S.L. Elliott, J. Cox, J. Gardner, D.J. Moss, A. Suhrbier, Induction of protective cytotoxic T cells to murine cytomegalovirus by using a nonapeptide and a human-compatible adjuvant (Montanide ISA 720), J. Virol. 69 (1995) 1306–1309.

[8] R.G. van-der-Most, A. Sette, C. Oseroff, J. Alexander, K. Murali-Krishna, L.L. Lau, S. Southwood, J. Sidney, R.W. Chesnut, M. Matloubian, R. Ahmed, Analysis of cytotoxic T cell responses to dominant and subdominant epitopes during acute and chronic lymphocytic choriomeningitis virus infection, J. Immunol. 157 (1996) 5543–5554.

[9] D.C. Jackson, H.E. Drummer, L.E. Brown, Conserved determinants for CD4+T cells within the light chain of the H3 hemagglutinin molecule of influenza virus, Virology 198 (1994) 613–623.

International Congress Series 1219 (2001) 999–1005

Immunogenicity and protection in mice given inactivated influenza vaccine, MPL, QS-21 or QS-7

Philip R. Wyde*, Efrain Guzman, Brian E. Gilbert, Robert B. Couch

Department of Molecular Virology and Microbiology, Baylor College of Medicine, One Baylor Plaza, Houston, TX 77030, USA

Abstract

Background: Monophosphoryl lipid A (MPL), QS-21 and QS-7 were evaluated in mice for their ability to increase the immunogenicity and protective efficacy of formalin-inactivated (FI) influenza A/Texas/91 virus vaccine. Freund's incomplete adjuvant (FIA) was used as a positive control. *Methods*: Mice were inoculated twice, 28 days apart, either intramuscularly (I.M.) with vaccine mixed with phosphate buffered saline, FIA, MPL or QS21, or intranasally (I.N.) with vaccine containing QS-21 or QS-7. The mice were bled on days 0, 28 and 49 and challenged I.N. on this last day with live virus. Four days later, the lungs from each animal were assessed for influenza virus. All sera were tested for virus-specific neutralizing (Nt), hemagglutination inhibiting (HI) and ELISA antibodies. Studies to account for the mechanism(s) of adjuvant activity have been initiated. *Results*: FIA, MPL and QS-21 all enhanced the production of virus-specific antibodies and increased protection from pulmonary virus infection following I.M. administration. Maximal adjuvanticity occurred in groups inoculated with "low" doses of vaccine and in groups administered vaccine mixed with QS-21. Both QS adjuvants exhibited significant adjuvant activity following I.N. inoculation. Protection correlated best with levels of virus-specific serum Nt and HI antibodies. *Conclusions*: The present studies support continued development of adjuvants for inactivated influenza virus vaccines. © 2001 Elsevier Science B.V. All rights reserved.

Keywords: Adjuvants; Influenza vaccines; Antibodies; QS-21; MPL

1. Introduction

Influenza viruses annually cause significant morbidity and mortality worldwide. Although new and innovative vaccines are being developed, inactivated vaccines remain

---

* Corresponding author. Tel.: +1-713-798-5255; fax: +1-713-798-6802.
E-mail address: pwyde@bcm.tmc.edu (P.R. Wyde).

0531-5131/01/$ – see front matter © 2001 Elsevier Science B.V. All rights reserved.
PII: S0531-5131(01)00411-3

the only major modality for prevention of serious disease in the USA and other countries. Unfortunately, these vaccines generally are less effective in the elderly [1–3] than in younger individuals, and may not provide full protection from infection in the latter [4]. New adjuvants are being evaluated as one means to improve the immune responses induced by inactivated vaccines [5,6].

In the present studies, monophosphoryl lipid A (MPL; Ribi Adjuvants), QS-21 (Aquila Biopharmaceuticals), QS-7 (Aquila Biopharmaceuticals) and traditional Freund's incomplete adjuvant (FIA) were compared in mice for their ability to enhance the immunogenicity and protective efficacy of a commercially produced inactivated mono-valent influenza A/Texas/91 (H1N1) virus vaccine. MPL and the two QS compounds have been shown to enhance the immunogenicity of different antigens in clinical trials [7,8]. Freund's incomplete adjuvant (FIA) was included to provide comparisons to an adjuvant that was extensively utilized in the 1950s and 1960s in humans and that has been shown to significantly enhance antibody responses to inactivated influenza virus vaccines [9–11].

2. Materials and methods

2.1. Viruses

The concentrated inactivated monovalent influenza A/Texas/91 (H1N1) virus vaccine (IVV; Aventis Pasteur Laboratories, Swiftwater, PA), live A/Mississippi/86 (H3N2) influenza virus (used to prime mice) and live A/Texas/91 virus (used to challenge mice) utilized in these experiments were all obtained from the Respiratory Pathogens Research Unit, Baylor College of Medicine (BCM).

2.2. Experimental design

Groups of five or seven outbred ICR mice were injected intramuscularly (I.M.) or intranasally (I.N.) with IVV mixed with phosphate buffered saline (PBS), FIA, MPL, QS-21 or QS-7. Four weeks later, the animals were revaccinated using the same route, adjuvant and dose they had received initially.

The mice were bled from the retro-orbital sinus plexus on Day 0, Day 28 and again on Day 49 just before they were challenged I.N. with approximately 100 median infectious doses of live influenza virus. Four days later, each animal was sacrificed and its lungs were removed, processed and assessed for influenza virus as described previously [12]. All sera were tested for virus-specific neutralizing (Nt), hemagglutinin-inhibiting (HI) and ELISA antibodies using previously described methods [13,14].

2.3. Statistics

Titers were transformed to logs and then tested for normal distribution using Bartlett's test of homogeneity [15]. A parametric analysis of variances (ANOVA) was used for normally distributed data and a nonparametric ANOVA for non-Guassian data.

3. Results

3.1. Serum antibody responses in mice vaccinated I.M.

In initial studies, IVV was tested in unprimed mice using doses of vaccine ranging from 1 to 10 μg virus hemagglutinin (HA)/dose. In addition, an experiment was performed using doses ranging from 1 to 100 μg HA/dose and mice primed with influenza A/Mississippi/86 (H3N2) virus 8 weeks prior to administering influenza A/Texas vaccine. Data from these experiments are not shown. However, the findings from them closely mirrored those presented in Figs. 1 (virus-specific serum HI response) and 2 (virus-specific serum ELISA antibody response) obtained from an experiment in which unprimed mice and vaccine doses ranging from 1 to 100 μg/dose were used.

As Fig. 1 reveals, the serum antibody responses in these experiments followed a dose–response curve, regardless of whether the vaccine was given with or without an adjuvant. However, antibody levels were consistently greater in groups of mice inoculated with vaccine mixed with an adjuvant than in groups inoculated with vaccine without an adjuvant. Maximal fold enhancement of antibody with adjuvant was consistently observed in mice given lower doses of vaccine and in the groups administered vaccine mixed with QS-21. Nevertheless, MPL and FIA given with 1 or 10-μg doses of IVV also induced significantly increased levels of virus-specific antibodies compared to the vaccine–PBS control group. Serum Nt antibody responses in all experiments were similar to the serum HI antibody responses. However, adjuvant effects were less apparent for the virus-specific serum ELISA antibody titers (data not shown).

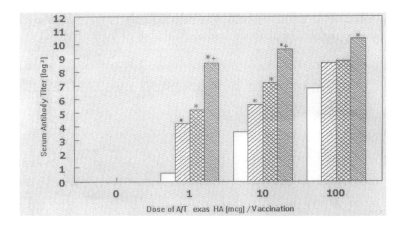

Fig. 1. Serum hemagglutination-inhibiting (HI) antibody levels on day 49 (21 days post boost) in mice vaccinated twice, 28 days apart, with formalin-inactivated influenza virus vaccine mixed with phosphate buffered saline (PBS; open bars), Freund's incomplete adjuvant (FIA; diagonal pattern), monophosphoryl lipid A (MPL; hatched pattern) or QS-21 (thin diagonal pattern). Asterisks indicate the mean titer is significantly greater than the titer obtained for animals given the same dose of vaccine and PBS. A + symbol indicates the mean titer is significantly greater than the titer obtained for sera from the mice given vaccine mixed with FIA or MPL.

3.2. Pulmonary virus titers after virus challenge

Pulmonary virus levels in the same mice shown in Fig. 1, 4 days after virus challenge, are displayed in Fig. 2. Lower virus levels were seen in all of the groups of animals given two 1-μg doses of vaccine HA, but only the group inoculated with vaccine and QS-21 had a significantly lower mean virus titer than was seen in the unvaccinated control groups ($p \leq 0.001$). The mean virus titer of this group was also significantly less than the groups given two injections containing 1 μg vaccine HA mixed with either FIA or MPL ($p \leq 0.05$).

In contrast to these results, all of the groups of mice injected with 10-μg doses of vaccine HA mixed with an adjuvant had significantly reduced pulmonary virus titers compared to the titers seen in the unvaccinated control animals. These reductions were also significantly lower than the mean titer of mice given two 10-μg doses of IVV in PBS. However, they were not significantly different from each other. All of the groups vaccinated twice with 100-μg doses of IVV had similar, marked reductions in virus titers that were significantly lower than the mean titers seen in the unvaccinated control mice. Correlation curves indicated that the protection from pulmonary infection was strongly inversely related to the virus-specific Nt and HI antibody titers in sera ($R^2 \geq 0.9$), and less related to levels of virus-specific ELISA antibodies ($R^2 = 0.6$, data not shown).

3.3. Responses in mice vaccinated I.N. With QS compounds

The mean virus-specific HI antibody titers measured on day 49 in sera of mice inoculated I.N. with two 1-μg doses of virus HA mixed with PBS, QS-21 (10 μg/dose) or QS-7 (50 μg/dose) 28 days apart are shown in the top portion of Fig. 3. As indicated, virus-specific serum antibody was detected only in the groups given vaccine mixed with an adjuvant. The antibody responses in both of the responding groups were

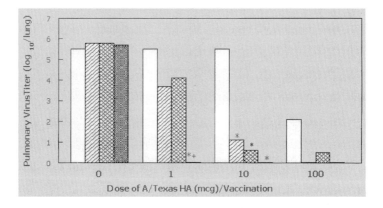

Fig. 2. Pulmonary virus titers determined on day 53, 4 days after virus challenge of the same mice shown in Fig. 1 and this figure. Symbols for statistically significant differences are as in Fig. 1.

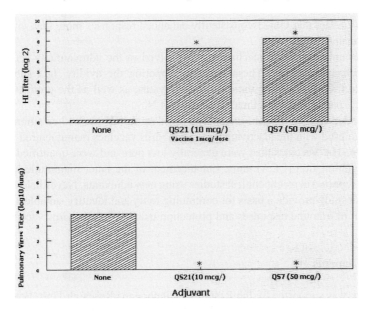

Fig. 3. (Top panel)Virus-specific serum HI antibody levels on day 49 (21 days post boost) in mice intranasally inoculated twice, 28 days apart, with formalin-inactivated influenza virus vaccine mixed with phosphate buffered saline (left bar), QS-21 (10 μg/vaccination; middle bar) or QS-7 (50 μg/vaccination; right-most bar). Asterisks indicate the mean antibody titer is significantly higher than the mean titer obtained for animals given the same dose of vaccine and PBS. (Bottom panel) Pulmonary virus titers determined on day 53, 4 days after virus challenge, in the same mice shown in the top portion of this figure. Asterisks indicate the mean virus titer is significantly lower than the mean titer obtained for animals given the same dose of vaccine and PBS.

equivalent although five-fold more QS-7 than QS-21 was administered with each vaccination.

The mean pulmonary virus titers seen in these animals 4 days after virus challenge are shown in the bottom portion of Fig. 3. As indicated, protection of mice from pulmonary virus infection correlated inversely with their serum HI antibody levels and was only seen in the animals given adjuvant.

4. Discussion

The data obtained in these studies clearly show that addition of MPL, QS-21 or QS-7 to influenza vaccine led to increased levels of virus-specific antibodies in the sera of test mice (Fig. 1), and increased protection of these animals from pulmonary infection (Fig. 2) when compared to mice given non adjuvanted vaccine. Serum Nt and HI antibody responses exhibited the well-described pattern of an increase with increasing doses of antigen and after a booster inoculation. Of interest was the finding that each of the adjuvants consistently increased serum antibody responses at all doses including the 100-μg HA dose although the adjuvant effect was less pronounced with increasing dose. Of further interest was the fact that QS-21 consistently enhanced responses more than either the FIA or MPL adjuvants.

To further understand the mechanism(s) involved in the adjuvanticity seen, we have initiated mechanism studies. These include comparing the avidity, IgG subclasses and virus-specific CTL induced by the different adjuvants, as well as the production of local IgA antibody, particularly in animals inoculated I.N.

FIA provided a 4- to 20-fold enhancement of serum HI antibodies among mice and humans when used with the inactivated influenza virus vaccines manufactured in the 1950s and 1960s [9–11]. Vaccines then were generally less pure and were quantified with HA or chick cell agglutination (CCA) units. Enhancement of the latter magnitude has not been consistently reported in recent clinical studies using new adjuvants. Nevertheless, the results of the present study provide a basis for continuing to try and identify suitable adjuvants for enhancement of immune responses and protection using influenza virus vaccines.

Acknowledgements

This work was supported by the Respiratory Pathogens Research Unit, Baylor College of Medicine and National Institutes of Health contract AI 65298.

References

[1] E.J. Remarque, Influenza vaccination in elderly people, Exp. Gerontol. 34 (1999) 445–452.

[2] A.M. Palache, W.E. Beyer, M.J. Sprenger, N. Masurel, S. de Jonge, A. Vardy, et al., Antibody response after influenza immunization with various vaccine doses: a double-blind, placebo-controlled, multi-centre, dose–response study in elderly nursing-home residents and young volunteers, Vaccine 11 (1993) 3–9.

[3] D.C. Powers, R.B. Belshe, Effect of age on cytotoxic T lymphocyte memory as well as serum and local antibody responses elicited by inactivated influenza virus vaccine, J. Infect. Dis. 167 (1993) 584–592.

[4] R.B. Couch, W.A. Keitel, T.R. Cate, J.A. Quarles, L.A. Taber, W.P. Glezen, Prevention of influenza virus infections by current inactivated influenza virus vaccines, in: L.E. Brown, A.W. Hampson, R.G. Webster (Eds.), Options for the Control of Influenza III, 1996, pp. 97–106. Elsevier, Amsterdam.

[5] R.K. Gupta, G.R. Siber, Adjuvants for human vaccines—current status, problems and future prospects, Vaccine 13 (1995) 1263–1276.

[6] D.T. O'Hagan, Recent advances in vaccine adjuvants for systemic and mucosal administration, J. Pharm. Pharmacol. 49 (1997) 1–10.

[7] J.R. Baldridge, R.T. Crane, Monophosphoryl lipid A (MPL) formulations for the next generation of vaccines, Methods 19 (1999) 103–107.

[8] C.R. Kensil, J.Y. Wu, C.A. Anderson, D.A. Wheeler, J. Amsden, QS-21 and QS-7: purified saponin adjuvants, Dev. Biol. Stand. 92 (1998) 41–47.

[9] A.C. Allison, N.E. Byars, Immunological adjuvants and their mode of action, in: R.W. Ellis (Ed.), Vaccines: New Approaches to Immunologic Problems, Butterworth-Heinemann, Stoneham, MA, 1992, pp. 431–449.

[10] A.V. Hennessy, F.M. Davenport, Relative merits of aqueous and adjuvant influenza vaccines when used in a two-dose schedule, Public Health Rep. 76 (1961) 411–419.

[11] J.E. Salk, M.L. Bailey, A.M. Laurent, The use of adjuvants in studies on influenza immunization: II. Increased antibody formation in human subjects inoculated with influenza virus vaccine in a water-in-oil emulsion, Am. J. Hyg. 55 (1952) 439–456.

[12] P.R. Wyde, B.E. Gilbert, B.M. Levy, Evidence that T-lymphocytes are part of the blood–brain barrier to virus dissemination, J. Neuroimmunol. 5 (1983) 47–58.

[13] R.Q. Robinson, W.R. Dowdle, Influenza viruses, in: E.H. Schmidt, N.J. Lennette (Eds.), Diagnostic Procedures for Viral and Rickettsial Infections, American Public Health Association, New York, NY, 1969, pp. 414–433.

[14] S.-I. Tamura, Y. Samegai, H. Kurate, T. Nagamine, C. Aizawa, T. Kurata, Protection against influenza virus infection by vaccine inoculated intranasally with cholera toxin B subunit, Vaccine 6 (1988) 409–413.

[15] R.R. Sokal, F.J. Rohlf, Biometry, Freeman, San Francisco, 1969, p. 370.

International Congress Series 1219 (2001) 1007–1013

Eight-plasmid rescue system for influenza A virus

Erich Hoffmann*, Nannan Zhou, Robert G. Webster

*Department of Virology and Molecular Biology, St. Jude Children's Research Hospital,
332 North Lauderdale Memphis, TN 38105-2794, USA*

Abstract

Plasmid-driven synthesis of viral RNA and protein allows the recovery of infectious influenza virus without the need for helper virus infection. Because no selection system is required for this approach, genetic manipulation of all eight viral gene segments without technical limitations is possible. We have developed a system which requires the construction and transfection of only eight plasmids for the recovery of influenza A viruses. In this DNA transfection system, viral cDNA is inserted between the human RNA polymerase I (pol I) promoter and murine terminator sequences. The entire pol I transcription unit is flanked by an RNA polymerase II (pol II) promoter and a poly(A) site. As a first step to evaluate the utility of this plasmid-based system for the production of vaccines, we generated the master strain A/PR/8/34 (H1N1) currently used for the production of inactivated vaccines entirely from cloned cDNAs. The virus yield as determined by HA-assay after passage of the recombinant virus in eggs was as high as the virus yield of the parental wild-type virus. These results prove that the generated recombinant virus has the same growth properties as the parental egg grown virus and indicate that the eight-plasmid transfection method has the potential to improve currently used methods for the production of vaccine viruses. © 2001 Elsevier Science B.V. All rights reserved.

Keywords: Reverse genetics; RNA polymerase I; RNA polymerase II; Transcription; Vaccine

1. Introduction

The licensed influenza vaccines currently used are inactivated influenza vaccines. The viruses representing epidemiologically important influenza A and influenza B strains are grown in embryonated hens' eggs and the virus particles are subsequently purified and inactivated by chemical means. Each year the World Health Organisation (WHO) selects

---

* Corresponding author. Tel.: +1-901-495-3400; fax: +1-901-523-2622.
E-mail address: robert.webster@stjude.org (E. Hoffmann).

0531-5131/01/$ – see front matter © 2001 Elsevier Science B.V. All rights reserved.
PII: S 0 5 3 1 - 5 1 3 1 (0 1) 0 0 3 7 5 - 2

subtypes that most likely will circulate. For the production of a safe and effective vaccine, it is important that the selected vaccine strains are closely related to the circulating strains thereby ensuring that the antibodies in the vaccinated population are able to neutralize the antigenetically similar virus. However, not all viruses that are found to be closely related are suitable for vaccine production because some grow poorly in eggs. Therefore, it is now a practice to generate a high growth reassortant by combining the high virus yield of a laboratory strain A/PR/8/34 (H1N1) with the glycoproteins of currently circulating strains. However, the coinfection with two influenza viruses containing eight segments results in the generation of theoretically $2^8=256$ different progeny viruses. To obtain a virus with the required glycoproteins, a selection method is needed to eliminate the gene segments from the parental laboratory strain. The selection procedure to obtain the reassortant virus with the appropriate glycoproteins and the verification of the gene constellation is a cumbersome and time-consuming task. Although the reverse genetics method based on the transfection of in vitro generated ribonucleoproteins (RNP) into cells reduces the possible number of progeny viruses, an efficient selection method is still required [1–3].

The establishment of the RNA polymerase I (pol I)-driven synthesis of vRNA molecules in vivo allowed the intracellular production of RNP complexes [4]. In this system, virus-like cDNA was inserted between the pol I promoter and terminator sequences [4]. Unlike the mRNA transcripts synthesized by RNA polymerase II (pol II), pol I-generated RNAs lack both a $5'$ cap and a $3'$ poly (A) tail. Functional vRNP molecules could be generated by infection with helper virus. The establishment of plasmid-based systems eliminates the need for a selection system [5–7]. In principle, these systems should allow the construction of designer viruses. Thus, the manipulation of all eight segments should permit changing the antigenic properties and optimizing the virus yield of generated viruses used for the production of vaccines. As a first step in achieving this goal, we report here the generation of A/PR/8/34 (H1N1) from cloned cDNA by using the eight-plasmid transfection system that we have recently developed [7].

2. Materials and methods

2.1. Viruses and transfection

The influenza virus A/PR/8/34 (H1N1) was obtained from the repository of St. Jude Childrens's Research Hospital and propagated in 10-day-old embryonated chicken eggs. Madin-Darby canine kidney (MDCK) cells were maintained in MEM containing 10% FBS. 293T human embryonic kidney cells and Vero cells were cultured in Opti-MEM I (Life Technologies, Gaithersburg, MD) containing 5% fetal bovine serum (FBS). For the transfection experiments, six-well tissue culture plates were used. The cocultured MDCK and 293T cells ($0.2–1\times10^6$ each of cells per well) were used for the transfection experiments. TransIT LT-1 (Panvera, Madison, WI) was used according to the manufacturer's instructions to transfect the cells. Briefly, 2 µl of TransIT LT-1 per 1 µg of DNA was mixed, incubated at room temperature for 45 min, and added to the cells. Six hours later, the DNA-transfection mixture was replaced by Opti-MEM I. Twenty-four hours after transfection, 1 ml of Opti-MEM I containing TPCK-trypsin was added to the cells; this addition resulted in a final concentration of TPCK-trypsin of 0.5 μg/ml in the cell supernatant. The virus titer was determined by passage of the cell supernatant on MDCK cells by plaque assay.

2.2. RT-PCR and construction of plasmids

Viral RNA was extracted from 200 μl of virus containing allantoic fluid of embryonated eggs using Qiagen RNeasy Kit. Two-step RT-PCR was employed to amplify each of the viral gene segments. Briefly, the RNA was transcribed into cDNA using AMV reverse transcriptase (Roche Diagnostics, Germany) according to the protocol provided and then the cDNA was amplified using Expand High Fidelity PCR system (Roche Diagnostics, Germany). The amplification program started with 1 cycle at 94 °C for 2 min; followed by 30 cycles at 94° for 20 s, 54 °C for 30 s, 72 °C for 3 min; the program ended with one cycle at 72° for 5 min. The primers used contained either sequences for *Bsa*I or *Bsm*BI to allow the precise insertion of the digested PCR-fragments into the cloning vector pHW2000 [7].

For cloning of the HA, NP, NA, M, NS genes, the PCR-fragments were digested with *Bsm*BI or *Bsa*I and ligated into the cloning vector pHW2000. For cloning of the P-genes, two (PB2, PA) or three (PB1) fragments were isolated, digested and ligated into pHW2000-*Bsm*BI. To ensure that the genes were free of unwanted mutations, the PCR-derived fragments were sequenced. The eight plasmids containing the full-length cDNA of A/PR/8/34 (H1N1) were designated pHW191-PB2, pHW192-PB1, pHW193-PA, pHW194-HA, pHW195-NP, pHW196-NA, pHW197-M, and pHW198-NS. The Center for Biotechnology at St. Jude Children's Research Hospital determined the sequence of template DNA by using rhodamine or dRhodamine dye-terminator cycle sequencing ready reaction kits with AmpliTaq® DNA polymerase FS (Perkin-Elmer, Applied Biosystems. [PE/ABI], Foster City, CA) and synthetic oligonucleotides. Samples were subjected to electrophoresis, detection, and analysis on PE/ABI model 373, model 373 Stretch, or model 377 DNA sequencers.

3. Results

To allow intracellular synthesis of virus-like vRNAs and mRNAs, we have established the RNA polI–polII expression system. In this system, viral cDNA is inserted between the human RNA polymerase I (pol I) promoter and a terminator sequences. This entire pol I transcription unit is flanked by an RNA polymerase II (pol II) promoter and a poly(A) site. The orientation of the two transcription units allows the synthesis of negative-sense viral RNA and positive-sense mRNA from one viral cDNA template. This pol I–pol II system starts with the initiation of transcription of the two cellular RNA polymerase enzymes from their own promoters, presumably in different compartments of the nucleus (Fig. 1). Transfection of eight plasmids into 293T cells results in the interaction of all molecules derived from the cellular and viral transcription and translation machinery, ultimately generating infectious influenza A virus. This system proved to be very efficient

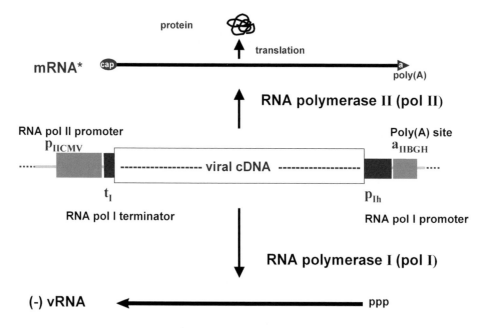

Fig. 1. Schematic representation of the RNA pol I–pol II transcription system. The cDNA of each of the eight influenza virus segments is inserted between the pol I promoter (p_{Ih}) and the pol I terminator (t_I). This pol I transcription unit is flanked by the pol II promoter (p_{II}CMV) of the human cytomegalovirus and the polyadenylation signal (a_{II}BGH) of the gene encoding bovine growth hormone. After transfection of the eight expression plasmids, two types of molecules are synthesized. From the human pol I promoter, negative-sense vRNA is synthesized by cellular pol I. Transcription by pol II yields mRNAs with $5'$ cap structures and $3'$ poly(A) tails; these mRNAs are translated into viral proteins.

for the formation of the influenza viruses A/WSN/33 (H1N1) and A/Teal/HK/W312/97 (H6N1) [7].

Since the current master strain for production of inactivated influenza vaccine is A/PR/8/34 (H1N1), we attempted to generate this virus entirely from cloned cDNA. The cDNAs representing the eight RNA-segments were inserted into the vector pHW2000. The resultant plasmids (pHW191-PB2, pHW192-PB1, pHW193-PA, pHW194-HA, pHW195-NP, pHW196-NA, pHW197-M, and pHW198-NS) were transfected into cocultured 293T-MDCK or Vero-MDCK cells (Fig. 2). Seventy-two hours after transfection, the virus titer was determined by titration in MDCK cells. The supernatant of cocultured Vero-MDCK cells contained 1×10^4 pfu and the supernatant of cocultured 293T-MDCK cells contained 2×10^6 pfu per ml. The higher yield in 293T-MDCK cells is most likely caused by the higher transfection efficiency of 293T cells compared to Vero cells. These results show that the eight-plasmid system allows the generation of A/PR/8/34 (H1N1) from cloned cDNA.

To compare the growth between the wild-type virus and the generated recombinant virus, embryonated hen's eggs were inoculated with wild-type virus or recombinant virus. The allantoic fluid was harvested 48 h after infection. The virus yield was determined by HA-assay. Although the HA-titers differed between individual eggs, we found that both

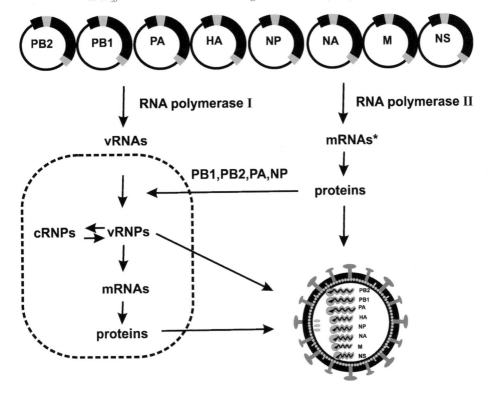

Fig. 2. Generation of infectious influenza A virus A/PR/8/34 (H1N1) by cotransfecting eight plasmids. The eight plasmids containing transcription units were transfected into 293T or Vero cells. Cellular RNA pol I and pol II synthesized virus-like vRNAs and mRNAs, presumably in different compartments of the nucleus. PB1, PB2, PA, and NP translated from transcripts synthesized by RNA pol II bound to the eight naked vRNAs to form vRNPs. The vRNPs constituted replication-competent transcription units that are required for the replication–transcription cycle (shown inside the dashed rectangle). Ultimately, the vRNPs and structural proteins are assembled into new virus particles. The mRNAs synthesized by pol II (mRNAs*) are different from those synthesized by the viral polymerase proteins, because the pol II–synthesized mRNAs possess pol I promoter and terminator sequences in their noncoding regions (Fig. 1).

viruses had HA-titers between 5120 and 10,240 hemagglutination units indicating that both viruses are high-yielding isolates. Thus, the recombinant virus that was generated by DNA transfection has the same phenotypic characteristics as the parental isolate.

4. Discussion

The first reverse genetics system developed for influenza virus, the RNP transfection system, allowed the creation of reassortant viruses suitable for vaccine production [3]. It was shown that eight RNP segments could be transfected into cells resulting in the generation of virus without the need for helper virus infection [8]. However, the disadvantage of this method is the purification of viral proteins and the purification/

reconstitution of viral RNPs in vitro. Plasmid-based systems that produce virus-like molecules intracellularly eliminate the burden of purification of viral proteins [5–7,9]. The plasmid systems developed by Neumann et al. [5] and Fodor et al. [6] require the construction and cotransfection of 12 or more plasmids. Eight plasmids encoding the vRNA-segments and at least four plasmids encoding proteins that are needed for replication and transcription (PB1, PB2, PA, and NP) are required by this approach. It was shown that the protein expression of the structural proteins increases the virus yield [5]. With the eight-plasmid system, the use of separate plasmids for protein expression is not required, thus simplifying the method of generation of influenza A virus entirely from cloned cDNA.

The production of vaccines involves the generation of a virus that is used as virus seed for the production of a vaccine virus either in eggs or in cell culture. For the efficiency of a vaccination program, it is important that the selected subtype matches the circulating pathogenic strains closely to stimulate a high antibody titer in the vaccinated population resulting in efficient protection. The six master plasmids (pHW191-PB2, pHW192-PB1, pHW193-PA, pHW195-NP, pHW197-M, and pHW198-NS) encoding the internal genes can now be used in cotransfection with plasmids encoding the glycoproteins HA and NA of a currently circulating strain. It is expected that the ability to manipulate each gene segment will allow us to evaluate what gene segment(s) are important for high-yield growth of the reassortant viruses in eggs as well as in cell culture.

The fact that we were able to generate two laboratory influenza virus strains (A/WSN/33 (H1N1) and A/PR/8/34 (H1N1) and one field isolate (A/Teal/HK/W312/97 (H6N1)) by cotransfecting only eight plasmids suggests that this system should also be applicable for the development of live attenuated influenza vaccines. Live attenuated influenza virus vaccines administered intranasally induce local, mucosal, cell-mediated and humoral immunity. Cold-adapted (ca) reassortant (CR) viruses containing the six internal genes of live, attenuated influenza A/Ann Arbor/6/60 (H2N2) and the haemagglutinin (HA) and neuraminidase (NA) of contemporary wild-type influenza viruses appear to be reliably attenuated. This vaccine has been shown to be efficacious in children and young adults [10]. However, it may be too attenuated to stimulate an ideal immune response in elderly people, the major group of the 20,000–40,000 individuals in the USA dying each year as a result of influenza infection. The contribution of each segment to the attenuated phenotype is still not well defined [10]. This lack of information can be acquired only by the sequential introduction of specific, defined attenuating mutations into a virus. Since a detailed analysis requires the testing of a large number of manipulated viruses, the construction and transfection of only eight plasmids simplifies this task and reduces the time and cost to achieve this goal.

Acknowledgements

These studies were supported by Public Health Research Grants AI95357 and AI29680 from the National Institute of Allergy and Infectious Diseases, by Cancer Center Support CORE Grant CA-21765, and by the American Lebanese Syrian Associated Charities. The excellent technical support of Scott Krauss and David Walker is gratefully acknowledged.

References

[1] W. Luytjes, M. Krystal, M. Enami, J.D. Parvin, P. Palese, Amplification, expression, and packaging of a foreign gene by influenza virus, Cell 59 (1989) 1107–1113.

[2] M. Enami, W. Luytjes, M. Krystal, P. Palese, Introduction of site-specific mutations into the genome of influenza virus, Proc. Natl. Acad. Sci. U. S. A. 87 (1990) 3802–3805.

[3] S. Li, C. Liu, A. Klimov, K. Subbarao, M.L. Perdue, D. Mo, Y. Ji, L. Woods, S. Hietala, M. Bryant, Recombinant influenza A virus vaccines for the pathogenic human A/Hong Kong/97 (H5N1) viruses, J. Infect. Dis. 179 (1999) 1132–1138.

[4] G. Neumann, A. Zobel, G. Hobom, RNA polymerase I-mediated expression of influenza viral RNA molecules, Virology 202 (1994) 477–479.

[5] G. Neumann, T. Watanabe, H. Ito, S. Watanabe, H. Goto, P. Gao, M. Hughes, D.R. Perez, R. Donis, E. Hoffmann, G. Hobom, Y. Kawaoka, Generation of influenza A viruses entirely from cloned cDNAs, Proc. Natl. Acad. Sci. U. S. A. 96 (1999) 9345–9350.

[6] E. Fodor, L. Devenish, O.G. Engelhardt, P. Palese, G.G. Brownlee, A. García-Sastre, Rescue of influenza A virus from recombinant DNA, J. Virol. 73 (1999) 9679–9682.

[7] E. Hoffmann, G. Neumann, Y. Kawaoka, G. Hobom, R.G. Webster, A DNA transfection system for generation of influenza A virus from eight plasmids, Proc. Natl. Acad. Sci. U. S. A. 97 (2000) 6108–6113.

[8] M. Enami, K. Enami, Characterization of influenza virus NS1 protein by using a novel helper-virus-free reverse genetic system, J. Virol. 74 (2000) 5556–5561.

[9] S. Pleschka, R. Jaskunas, O.G. Engelhardt, T. Zürcher, P. Palese, A. García-Sastre, A plasmid-based reverse genetics system for influenza A virus, J. Virol. 70 (1996) 4188–4192.

[10] W.A. Keitel, P.A. Piedra, Live cold-adapted, reassortant influenza vaccines (USA), in: K.G. Nicholson, R.G. Webster, A.J. Hay (Eds.), Textbook of Influenza, 1998, pp. 373–390.

International Congress Series 1219 (2001) 1015–1017

An efficient plasmid-driven system for the generation of influenza virus-like particles for vaccine

Tokiko Watanabe[a,b], Shinji Watanabe[a], Gabriele Neumann[a], Hiroshi Kida[b], Yoshihiro Kawaoka[a,c,*]

[a]*Department of Pathobiological Sciences, School of Veterinary Medicine, University of Wisconsin-Madison, 2015 Linden Drive West, Madison, WI 53706, USA*
[b]*Department of Disease Control, Graduate School of Veterinary Medicine, Hokkaido University, Sapporo 060-0818, Japan*
[c]*Institute of Medical Science, University of Tokyo, 4-6-1, Shirokanedai, Minato-ku, Tokyo 108-8639, Japan*

Abstract

We established an efficient plasmid-driven system for the generation of infectious influenza VLPs containing a virus-like RNA segment entirely from cDNAs. To generate influenza VLPs, we used the RNA polymerase I system for the intracellular synthesis of influenza virus RNAs. Human embryonic kidney cells (293T) were transfected with plasmids encoding the influenza A virus structural proteins and with a plasmid encoding an influenza virus-like viral RNA (vRNA), which contained an antisense copy of the cDNA for green fluorescence protein (GFP) flanked by an RNA polymerase I promoter and terminator (pPolI-GFP). Influenza virus-like particles containing GFP vRNA that were infectious and expressed GFP in infected cells were generated. We also generated VLPs lacking the NS gene by eliminating the plasmid for the NS RNA segment from the set of plasmids required for infectious influenza virus production. Because of its efficiency, this system would be useful in studies of influenza virus replication and particle formation as well as for production of vaccines. © 2001 Elsevier Science B.V. All rights reserved.

Keywords: Reverse genetics; NS; Vaccine vector

* Corresponding author. Tel.: +1-608-265-4925; fax: +1-608-265-5622.
E-mail address: kawaokay@svm.vetmed.wisc.edu (Y. Kawaoka).

1. Introduction

Influenza A viruses possess a genome of eight single-stranded negative-sense viral RNAs (vRNAs) that encode a total of 10 proteins. Mena et al. [1] established a vaccinia virus-based system for generation of influenza virus-like particles (VLPs). In this system, an influenza virus-like vRNA carrying a reporter gene is transcribed in vitro and transfected into eukaryotic cells. All 10 influenza virus proteins are expressed from plasmids under the control of a T7 RNA polymerase promoter. When the transfected cells are infected with recombinant vaccinia virus that expresses T7 RNA polymerase, they produce influenza VLPs containing the vRNA of an artificial reporter gene [1]. However, vaccinia virus expresses more than 80 proteins, any of which could affect the influenza virus life cycle. We therefore generated infectious influenza VLPs containing a virus-like RNA segment without using vaccinia virus. In addition, we explored the possibility of using the reverse genetics system we recently established [2,3] for vaccine purposes.

2. Materials and methods

To generate influenza VLPs, nine plasmids for nine structural proteins and an RNA polymerase I reporter gene construct (pPolI-GFP) were mixed with transfection reagent (Trans IT LT-1; Panvera, Madison, WI), incubated at room temperature for 15 min, and added to 1×10^6 293T cells. Six hours later, the DNA-transfection reagent mixture was replaced with Opti-MEM (GIBCO/BRL) containing 0.3% BSA and 0.01% FCS. Forty-eight hours later, MDCK cells were infected with the VLPs in the culture supernatant, along with A/WSN/33 virus. At 10-h post-infection, we observed the level of GFP expression. To generate influenza VLPs lacking one of the influenza gene segments, we followed the procedure for the generation of infectious influenza virus as described, but eliminated the plasmid for the NS RNA segment.

3. Results and discussion

To generate influenza VLPs, we used the RNA polymerase I system for the intracellular synthesis of influenza virus RNAs [4]. In this system, a cDNA carrying a reporter gene in antisense orientation is flanked by the 5′ and 3′ noncoding regions of an influenza virus RNA. This cassette is inserted between an RNA polymerase I promoter and terminator. Transfection of such constructs into eukaryotic cells leads to transcription of the reporter gene by cellular RNA polymerase I, thereby generating influenza virus-like RNAs [4]. Upon influenza virus infection, artificial vRNAs are replicated and transcribed by the viral polymerase complex, resulting in the expression of the reporter gene [4].

To generate VLPs, we transfected 293T cells with pPolI-GFP and plasmids for expression of nine influenza viral proteins: PB2, PB1, PA, HA, NP, NA, M1, M2, and NS2. Culture supernatants were harvested 48 h after transfection and mixed with A/WSN/ 33 virus to provide the virus polymerase proteins and NP protein required for replication and transcription of GFP vRNA. The mixture was then inoculated into MDCK cells. At

10-h post-infection, we detected GFP-positive MDCK cells, corresponding to $\sim 10^4$ particles per ml of supernatant. Thus, plasmid-driven expression of all influenza virus structural proteins resulted in the efficient formation of infectious influenza VLPs containing GFP vRNA that could be delivered into subsequent cells.

We next attempted to generate influenza VLPs lacking the NS gene. To this end, we followed the procedure for influenza virus production, but eliminated the plasmid for the NS gene segment. When the supernatant of 293T cells transfected with the plasmids were incubated with MDCK cells, NP was immunologically detected 16-h post-inoculation. The number of NP-positive cells corresponded to 10^4 infectious VLPs/ml. The plasmid-based system for producing influenza VLPs we established is highly efficient and would be useful in studies of influenza virus replication and particle formation. In addition, one can now generate VLPs that contain vRNAs encoding the proteins required for transcription and replication (i.e., the NP and the polymerase), as well as a vRNA encoding the protein of interest. Although these particles are infectious and some viral proteins are expressed in these infected cells, they cannot produce infectious progeny virus since they do not contain a full complement of viral genes. Therefore, we suggest that these VLPs may be effective vaccines for influenza and useful as virus vectors expressing foreign proteins.

Acknowledgements

We thank members of our laboratory for the production of data presented in this manuscript. Support for this work was provided by NIAID Public Health Service research grants and from the Japan Health Science Foundation and the Ministry of Education and Culture of Japan. T.W. is the recipient of a Research Fellowship for Young Scientists from the Japan Society for the Promotion of Science. S.W. is the recipient of the Japan Society for Promotion of Science Postdoctoral Fellowship for Research Abroad.

References

[1] I. Mena, A. Vivo, E. Perez, A. Portela, Rescue of a synthetic chloramphenicol acetyltransferase RNA into influenza virus-like particles obtained from recombinant plasmids, J. Virol. 70 (1996) 5016–5024.

[2] G. Neumann, T. Watanabe, H. Ito, S. Watanabe, H. Goto, P. Gao, H. Hughes, D.R. Perez, R. Donis, E. Hoffmann, G. Hobom, Y. Kawaoka, Generation of influenza A viruses entirely from cloned cDNAs, PNAS 96 (1999) 9345–9350.

[3] E. Fodor, L. Devenish, O.G. Engelhardt, P. Palese, G.G. Brownlee, A. Garcia-Sastre, Rescue of influenza A virus from recombinant DNA, J. Virol. 73 (1999) 9679–9682.

[4] G. Neumann, A. Zobel, G. Hobom, RNA polymerase I-mediated expression of influenza viral RNA molecules, Virology 202 (1994) 477–479.

International Congress Series 1219 (2001) 1019–1021

Genetic incompatibility among influenza A viruses

Masato Hatta[a], Peter Halfmann[a], Krisna Wells[a],
Yoshihiro Kawaoka[a,b,*]

[a]*Department of Pathobiological Sciences, School of Veterinary Medicine, University of Wisconsin-Madison, Madison, WI 53706, USA*
[b]*Institute of Medical Science, University of Tokyo, 4-6-1, Shirokanedai, Minato, Tokyo 108-8639, Japan*

Abstract

Although influenza A viruses occasionally transmit from one species to another, host range restriction exists among these viruses. Current human influenza A viruses are thought to originate from avian viruses. However, human influenza A viruses do not replicate in duck intestine, a major replication site of avian viruses. Although previous studies identified that the HA and NA genes restrict human virus replication in ducks, the contribution of the other genes remains unknown. To determine the genetic basis for host range restriction in ducks, we first established a reverse genetics system for generating A/Memphis/8/88 (H3N2) and A/Mallard/NY/6750/78 (H2N2) viruses from cloned cDNA. Using this system, we attempted to generate reassortant viruses with various combinations of genes. However, reassortant viruses with some of the gene combinations were not generated, suggesting that there may be incompatibility between the genes of avian and human strains. © 2001 Elsevier Science B.V. All rights reserved.

Keywords: Host range; Reassortant; Reverse genetics

1. Introduction

Influenza A viruses infect swine, horses, seals, and a large variety of birds as well as humans. Phylogenetic studies have revealed species-specific lineages of viral genes and have demonstrated that the prevalence of interspecies transmission depends on the host animal species. Aquatic birds are thought to be the source of all influenza A viruses in

---
* Corresponding author. Department of Microbiology and Immunology, Institute of Medical Science, University of Tokyo, 4-6-1, Shirokanedai, Minato, Tokyo 108-8639, Japan. Tel.: +81-3-5449-5310; fax: +81-3-5449-5408.
E-mail address: kawaoka@ims.u-tokyo.ac.jp (Y. Kawaoka).

0531-5131/01/$ – see front matter © 2001 Elsevier Science B.V. All rights reserved.
PII: S 0 5 3 1 - 5 1 3 1 (0 1) 0 0 4 0 0 - 9

other animal species. There have been three human influenza pandemics in this century. Avian influenza A viruses are thought to contribute to all of these pandemic strains [1,2]. However, avian influenza viruses replicate poorly in humans, and similarly, human viruses do not replicate efficiently in birds, demonstrating host range restriction among these viruses [3–6]. The HA and NA genes restrict human virus replication in duck intestinal tracts. However, the contribution of the other genes remains unknown. As an initial step in determining the genetic basis for host range restriction in ducks, we attempted to generate reassortant viruses with various combinations of genes using a reverse genetics system [7,8].

2. Generation of reassortant viruses using reverse genetics

We attempted to generate the human influenza A/Memphis/8/88 (H3N2) and avian influenza A/Mallard/NY/6750/78 (H2N2) viruses entirely from cloned cDNA using plasmid-driven reverse genetics [8]. To this end, the cDNAs encoding all eight segments of these viruses were cloned between the human RNA polymerase I promoter and mouse RNA polymerase I terminator. Transfectant viruses were generated as reported earlier [8].

To determine which of the genes are important for host range restriction in ducks, we next generated single- or multiple-gene reassortant viruses possessing only one or some of the genes from A/Memphis/8/88 and the rest from A/Mallard/NY/6750/78 virus. Single-gene reassortant viruses possessing the PB2 or NP gene of A/Memphis/8/88 virus and the rest from A/Mallard/NY/6750/78 virus were obtained. Other single-gene reassortant viruses were not generated. Also, multiple-gene reassortant viruses possessing the HA and NA; PB1, PB2, and PA; or PB1, PB2, PA and NP of A/Memphis/8/88 virus and the rest from A/Mallard/NY/6750/78 virus were obtained. These results indicate that there may be incompatibility between the genes of avian and human strains.

3. Discussion

High-frequency reassortment is characteristic of influenza A viruses. However, genetic variation of the HA/NA subtype combinations is limited. In this study, we demonstrate that there may be some restriction on generating reassortant viruses between avian and human species because multiple-gene reassortant viruses were generated easier than single-gene reassortants. Our findings provide a molecular basis for the mechanisms of generating reassortant viruses among influenza A viruses.

Acknowledgements

We thank Martha McGregor, Nicole Poznik, and Ryo Kawaoka for excellent technical assistance. Automated sequencing was performed at the University of Wisconsin-Madison, Biotechnology Center.

References

[1] W.G. Laver, R.G. Webster, Studies on the origin of pandemic influenza: III. Evidence implicating duck and equine influenza viruses as possible progenitors of the Hong Kong strain of human influenza, Virology 51 (1973) 383–391.

[2] O.T. Gorman, W.J. Bean, Y. Kawaoka, I. Donatelli, Y.J. Guo, R.G. Webster, Evolution of influenza A virus nucleoprotein genes: implications for the origins of H1N1 human and classical swine viruses, J. Virol. 65 (1991) 3704–3714.

[3] R.G. Webster, M. Yakhno, V.S. Hinshaw, W.J. Bean, K.G. Murti, Intestinal influenza: replication and characterization of influenza viruses in ducks, Virology 84 (1978) 268–278.

[4] V.S. Hinshaw, R.G. Webster, C.W. Naeve, B.R. Murphy, Altered tissue tropism of human–avian reassortant influenza viruses, Virology 128 (1983) 260–263.

[5] A.S. Beare, R.G. Webster, Replication of avian influenza viruses in humans, Arch. Virol. 119 (1991) 37–42.

[6] B.R. Murphy, A.J. Buckler-White, W.T. London, J. Harper, E.L. Tierney, N.T. Miller, L.J. Reck, R.M. Chanock, V.S. Hinshaw, Avian–human reassortant influenza A viruses derived by mating avian and human influenza A viruses, J. Infect. Dis. 150 (1984) 841–850.

[7] E. Fodor, L. Devenish, O.G. Engelhardt, P. Palese, G.G. Brownlee, A. Garcia-Sastre, Rescue of influenza A virus from recombinant DNA, J. Virol. 73 (1999) 9679–9682.

[8] G. Neumann, T. Watanabe, H. Ito, S. Watanabe, H. Goto, P. Gao, M. Hughes, D.R. Perez, R. Donis, E. Hoffmann, G. Hobom, Y. Kawaoka, Generation of influenza A viruses entirely from cloned cDNAs, Proc. Natl. Acad. Sci. U. S. A. 96 (1999) 9345–9350.

International Congress Series 1219 (2001) 1023–1027

Compatibility of various avian HA subtypes with the genome of human influenza A viruses

Christoph Scholtissek*, Jurgen Stech, Scott Krauss,
Robert G. Webster

Department of Virology and Molecular Biology, St. Jude Children's Research Hospital, Memphis, TN, USA

Abstract

So far, with human influenza A viruses, only hemagglutinin (HA) subtypes 1, 2, or 3 were found. For pandemic planning, the question, whether other HA subtypes are compatible to create new human pandemic strains by reassortment, arises. Therefore, we crossed an amantadine-resistant variant of the human A/Singapore/57 (Sing) strain (H2N2) with various avian strains of different HA subtypes in the presence of amantadine and of anti-H2-antibodies. With A/Duck/Ukraine/63 (H3N8) and some other avian strains isolated recently in Hong Kong, large plaque-forming reassortants with the Sing-M-gene and the avian HA could be obtained in high yields, while with A/Chicken/Germany N/49 (Virus N) (H10N7) and some other avian strains, the yields were extremely low, and the remaining plaques were very small, and partly turbid and fuzzy. These observations may indicate that certain avian HA subtypes are not compatible to replace the HA-gene of the present human influenza A viruses to create a viable pandemic strain. © 2001 Elsevier Science B.V. All rights reserved.

Keywords: Reassortment between avian HA and human M genes; Pandemic planning

1. Introduction

Pandemic human influenza A viruses may be created by replacement of the hemagglutinin (HA) gene of the prevailing human strain by at least the HA gene of an avian influenza A virus by reassortment, as it had happened in 1957 and 1968 [1,2]. Now the question arises — important for pandemic planning — whether all of the 15 HA subtypes are compatible for the formation of such a new pandemic human influenza A virus. From influenza "archeology", we know that in human influenza A viruses, only HA subtypes 1,

* Corresponding author. Waldstr. 53, D-35440 Linden, Germany. Tel.: +49-6403-61246; fax: +49-6403-68824.

2, and 3 were found [3]. The question is, whether we can expect any other HA subtype in the next pandemic strain as well, and do we need to be prepared for that.

In our previous studies on the rescue of the temperature-sensitive mutants of fowl plague virus (FPV, H7N1) with human isolates, we never observed segregation of the FPV HA- and M-genes [4]. Only under strong selection pressure, using specific antisera, reassortants carrying the human HA- and FPV M-genes could be obtained. However, these reassortants multiplied only to very low titers, and they formed turbid and fuzzy plaques. It is not expected that such badly growing reassortants become dominant pandemic human influenza A strains. Segregation of HA- and M-genes by rescue with avian strains was normal [5]. In this sense, the combination of human HA and FPV M-gene products, and vice versa, seem not to be compatible.

2. Materials and methods

With these observations in mind, we have developed a test system to show how far human virus M-gene products can cooperate well with the various avian HA subtypes to create a corresponding well-growing reassortant carrying the avian HA- and the human M-genes. For this purpose, we have isolated an amantadine-resistant variant of A/Singapore/ 57 (H2N2) (mutation in the ion channel of the M2 protein [6]), and we have crossed this human strain by double-infection of MDCK cells with amantadine-sensitive avian strains of various subtypes (see Table 1) in the presence of amantadine and anti-H2-antibodies. In this way, we select reassortants which carry the avian HA and the human M-gene.

3. Results

In Table 1, the results of 12 different viruses are shown. After double infection with Duck/Ukraine H3N8 virus, under the selection pressure of anti-H2-antibodies and amantadine, we were able to obtain high yields of large plaque formers, which could be easily passaged. Those plaque isolates, which were further analyzed, carried the H3 HA of the avian virus, and — as shown by sequencing — the M-gene of the amantadine-resistant human Singapore strain.

Similar results were obtained with two recent avian isolates from Hong Kong. In crosses with an H4 and an H11 avian virus, large plaque formers could be obtained in relatively high yields. By sequencing, it was shown that these large plaques contain the M-gene of the A/Singapore/57 strain.

After crossing with the H5N3 Duck/Singapore/3/97 virus, only a low yield of virus was left using selection by anti-H2 serum and amantadine. Most of the remaining plaques were small. The H6N1 Teal/Hong Kong virus behaved intermediately in that the virus yield after the selection procedure was still relatively high and a few plaques which were left had a diameter of about 3 mm. However, when the M-gene of these large plaque formers was sequenced, it turned out that they carried the M-gene of the teal virus with a mutation in the ion channel of the M2-protein, which rendered it amantadine resistant. Thus, during the course of the experiment, an amantadine resistant variant M-gene of the teal virus was

Table 1
Plaque yield and maximum plaque size after single- or double-infection of MDCK cells overnight and plaque test
with selection by anti-H2 antiserum (1:200 dilution into PBS) and amantadine (4 mg/ml in agar overlay) (right) or
without selection (left)

Virus strain	PFU (max. plaque size, mm)	
	None	Amantadine + anti-H2
Singapore/57 (H2N2) (Amantadine-resist.)	2×10^8 (2)	$< 10^2$
Duck/Ukraine/63 (H3N8)	2×10^8 (6)	$< 10^5$
Duck/Ukraine × Singapore	2×10^8 (6)	1.3×10^8 (6)
Chick/Germany N/49 (H10N7)	5×10^7 (2)	$< 10^5$
Chick/Germany N × Singapore	8×10^7 (2)	1.5×10^5 (0.2)
Mallard/Astrachan/82 (H14N5)	2×10^7 (4)	$< 10^4$
Mallard/Astrachan × Singapore	3×10^7 (4)	5×10^4 (0.4)
Wedge-tailed Sh./Austr./79 (H15N9)	8×10^8 (6)	tiny
Wedge-tailed Sh./Austr. × Singapore	8×10^7 (4)	5×10^5 (0.4)
Red knot/DE/254/94 (H8N4)	2×10^7 (4)	$< 10^4$
Red knot/DE × Singapore	3×10^7 (3)	2×10^5 (0.2)
Pintail/Alberta/121/79 (H7N8)	2×10^7 (5)	$< 10^4$
Pintail/Alberta × Singapore	6×10^7 (5)	4×10^4 (0.4)
Duck/Alberta/35/76 (H1N1)	4×10^7 (2)	$< 10^3$
Duck/Alberta × Singapore	1×10^8 (2)	2×10^4 (0.2)
Oystercatcher/Germany/87 (H1N1)	4×10^6 (1.5)	$< 10^3$
Oystercatcher/Germany × Singapore	1×10^6 (2)	2×10^2 (0.1)
Duck/Hong Kong/Y 264/97 (H4N8)	3×10^7 (4)	$< 10^3$
Duck/Hong Kong × Singapore	1×10^7 (4)	1×10^6 (5)
Duck Singapore/3/97 (H5N3)	2×10^8 (3)	tiny
Duck/Singapore × Singapore	2×10^8 (3)	2×10^5 (0.5)
Teal/Hong Kong/W312/97(H6N1)	5×10^8 (4)	tiny
Teal/Hong Kong × Singapore	8×10^7 (5)	8×10^6 (3)
Duck/Hong Kong/P50/97 (H11N9)	3×10^8 (3)	$< 10^3$
Duck/Hong Kong × Singapore	2×10^8 (4)	2×10^7 (4)

accidentally picked up. When this experiment was repeated twice, no large plaque formers
showed up after the selection procedure. This emphasizes the importance of sequencing
the M-gene of the large plaque formers obtained after selection.

After crossing all the other avian viruses only low yields of virus, forming exclusively
small plaques, were left after selection with anti-H2 serum and amantadine. Although in
two cases we are dealing with avian H1 viruses, their HA seems not to be well adapted to
cooperate with the M-gene products of the human virus.

4. Discussion and conclusion

Pandemic influenza A viruses are created from time to time by replacement of at least
the HA gene of the prevailing human virus by the allelic gene of an avian virus as it
happened in 1957 and in 1968 [1,2]. In order to become a dominant, fast growing and
easily spreading virus with a different surface antigen, the new HA glycoprotein has to
cooperate optimally with the remaining virus gene products in close contact to the HA,

like the neuraminidase (NA) and the M-gene products, the M1- and M2-proteins. Here, we have developed a test system for the functional cooperation of the M-gene products of a human virus with the HA of various avian isolates. In this respect, the H3 hemagglutinin of the Duck/Ukraine/63 virus cooperated very well with the M-gene products of the human H2 virus (Table 1), mimicking the situation of 1968, when the pandemic Hong Kong virus was created. During crosses with several other avian viruses involving HA's belonging to other subtypes, such well growing reassortants could not be obtained. Exceptions were recent isolates from Hong Kong (subtypes H4 and H11). This is an interesting observation in so far as in recent years in this area avian viruses were transmitted directly to humans causing diseases and even fatalities [7–9], without, however, spreading further among humans.

From our results, we cannot yet conclude whether the cooperation or lack of cooperation respectively, between the M-gene products of the human viruses and the HAs of the avian strains relates to a certain HA-subtype, or only to the individual HAs tested. In order to answer this question, more individual isolates of the same subtype need to be tested. Furthermore, we do not know whether better growing reassortants can be created if both the HA and M-genes of the avian virus are reassorted into the prevailing human viruses. However, such pandemic strains have not yet been discovered. There might be other restrictions to avoid this.

In conclusion, the test system presented here should be able to give us an idea how potentially dangerous an avian influenza virus might be for the creation of a pandemic human virus. This holds true especially for the region of Southeast Asia, where we might have the greatest chance for such an event of reassortment to occur [10,11].

If we can correlate the creation of such a dominant, well growing and well spreading reassortant to certain HA subtypes, also excluding other subtypes, then pandemic planning will be easier. Such a test might be included in the influenza surveillance programs.

Acknowledgements

We would like to thank ALSAC for their support. We also thank Patrick Seiler for excellent technical assistance and Sydney Gray and Margot Seitz for typing the manuscript.

References

[1] C. Scholtissek, W. Rohde, V. von Hoyningen, R. Rott, On the origin of the human influenza subtypes H2N2 and H3N2, Virology 87 (1978) 13–20.

[2] Y. Kawaoka, S. Krauss, R.G. Webster, Avian-to-human transmission of the PB1 gene of influenza A viruses in the 1957 and 1968 pandemics, J. Virol. 63 (1989) 4603–4608.

[3] S.W. Potter, Chronicle of influenza pandemics, in: K.G. Nicholson, R.G. Webster, A. Hay (Eds.), Textbook of Influenza, Blackwell Science, Oxford, 1998, pp. 3–18.

[4] C. Scholtissek, R. Rott, M. Orlich, E. Harms, W. Rohde, Correlation of pathogenicity and gene constellation of an influenza A virus (fowl plague): I. Exchange of a single gene, Virology 81 (1977) 74–80.

[5] R. Rott, M. Orlich, C. Scholtissek, Correlation of pathogenicity and gene constellation of influenza A

viruses: III. Non-pathogenic recombinants derived from highly pathogenic parent strains, J. Gen. Virol. 44 (1979) 471–477.

[6] A.J. Hay, A.J. Wolstenholm, J.J. Skehel, M.H. Smith, The molecular basis of the specific anti-influenza action of amantadine, EMBO J. 4 (1985) 3021–3024.

[7] E.J.C. Class, A.D.M.E. Osterhaus, R. van Beek, J.C. de Jong, G.F. Rimmelzwaan, D.A. Senne, S. Krauss, K.F. Shortridge, R.G. Webster, Human influenza A H5N1 virus related to a highly pathogenic avian influenza virus, Lancet 351 (1998) 472–477.

[8] K. Subbarao, A. Klimov, J. Katz, H. Regnery, W. Lim, H. Hall, M. Perdue, D. Swayne, C. Bender, J. Huang, M. Hemphill, T. Rowe, M. Shaw, X. Xu, K. Fukuda, N. Cox, Characterization of an avian influenza A (H5N1) virus isolated from a child with a fatal respiratory illness, Science 279 (1998) 393–396.

[9] M. Peiris, K.Y. Yean, C.W. Leung, K.H. Chan, P.L.S. Ip, R.W.M. Lai, W.K. Orr, K.F. Shortridge, Human infection with influenza H9N2, Lancet 354 (1999) 916–917.

[10] K.F. Shortridge, C.H. Stuart-Harris, An influenza epicentre? Lancet ii (1982) 812–813.

[11] C. Scholtissek, E. Naylor, Fish farming and influenza pandemics, Nature 331 (1988) 215.

International Congress Series 1219 (2001) 1029–1035

Potential applications of influenza A virus vectors as tumor vaccines

Hongyong Zheng, Adolfo García-Sastre*

Department of Microbiology, Mount Sinai School of Medicine, One Gustave Levy Place, Box 1124, New York, NY 10029 USA

Abstract

Reverse genetics techniques have been established for the introduction of specific mutations into the influenza A virus genes. These techniques allowed the generation of influenza virus vectors expressing foreign antigens. Expression of tumor-associated antigens (TAAs) by influenza virus vectors might represent a promising way to induce potent cellular immune responses against cancer cells, leading to tumor regression. © 2001 Elsevier Science B.V. All rights reserved.

Keywords: Influenza virus; Tumor-associated antigens; Reverse genetics; Cancer therapy

1. Introduction

Despite the accumulated evidence demonstrating expression of specific tumor-associated antigens (TAAs) by cancer cells, the host immune response is usually ineffective in eliminating cancer cells [1]. One of the factors that contributes to the evasion of the immune system by tumors is the poor immunogenicity of the tumor cells. Therefore, a major focus in the development of novel therapeutic strategies against cancer relates to the development of methods to elicit a strong cellular immune response against tumor cells capable of clearing these cells. This might be achieved by expressing TAAs in a highly immunogenic context. For example, the administration of immuno-potentiating cytokines might result in higher immunogenicity of tumor cells. In another approach, TAAs are cloned and administered to tumor patients using delivery strategies which are known to induce efficient cellular immune responses.

* Corresponding author. Tel.: +1-212-241-7769; fax: +1-212-534-1684.
 E-mail address: adolfo.garcia-sastre@mssm.edu (A. García-Sastre).

0531-5131/01/$ – see front matter © 2001 Elsevier Science B.V. All rights reserved.
PII: S 0 5 3 1 - 5 1 3 1 (0 1) 0 0 6 6 2 - 8

Highly immunogenic viruses are attractive delivery vehicles for expression of TAAs. It is now possible to genetically engineer several groups of viruses to achieve expression of foreign antigens. Some of these viruses are being considered as promising vectors for the induction of immune responses against foreign antigens. Thus, viral vectors expressing TAAs are being explored as potential anti-tumor agents. Poxviruses [2–4], herpesviruses [5], adenoviruses [6–8], adeno-associated viruses [9], picornaviruses [10] and alphaviruses [11] are among the viral vectors which are being investigated in cancer therapies. Non-viral vectors, such as bacterial vectors [12,13], recombinant DNA or RNA molecules [14–16], and the use of potent adjuvants, such as dendritic cells [17–21], are also under consideration. This review article will describe our recent research on the potential use of influenza viruses expressing TAAs as therapeutic tumor vaccines.

2. Generation of transfectant influenza A viruses

The first requirement before considering a particular virus as a delivery vaccine agent is the availability of techniques to manipulate the genome of this virus. The generation of recombinant DNA and positive strand RNA viruses can usually be achieved by transfecting a plasmid which express the viral genome. However, this is not the case for influenza viruses. The genome of negative strand RNA viruses, such as influenza A virus, cannot initiate infection without the viral transcriptase/replicase. Techniques for the genetic manipulation of influenza A viruses became available in 1990 [22]. First, one of the eight viral RNAs of influenza A virus is synthesized in vitro from recombinant DNA. This RNA is assembled into functional ribonucleoprotein (RNP) complexes by incubation with purified nucleoprotein and RNA polymerase from influenza virus particles. These RNP complexes are then transfected into cells previously infected with a helper influenza A virus, which replicates and transcribes the transfected RNPs and provides the remaining seven RNPs required for the generation of infectious influenza viruses. This technique further requires the use of a selection method to eliminate viruses still containing all eight RNA segments of the helper virus. Using this technique, it was possible to replace one of the RNA segments of a helper influenza virus by the corresponding DNA-derived RNA segment [23].

It was possible to eliminate the in vitro RNP reconstitution step for the generation of transfectant influenza A viruses by cotransfecting cells with five plasmids, one encoding the viral RNA segment, and the other four encoding the viral NP and polymerase proteins (PB2, PB1 and PA) [24]. In order to generate the precise 5' (uncapped) and 3' ends of the viral RNA segment, the RNA was expressed from a truncated polymerase I promoter and was engineered to be cleaved by a ribozyme sequence. When these transfected cells were infected with a helper influenza A virus, the plasmid-derived RNPs were rescued into infectious virus particles. Again, selective pressure was used in order to eliminate viruses containing all eight RNPs derived from the helper virus.

Recently, the requirement for a helper virus was eliminated by cotransfecting 12 different plasmids, eight encoding the eight viral RNA segments from a polymerase I promoter, and four expressing the NP and viral polymerase proteins [25,26]. These techniques allow the generation of transfectant influenza A virus entirely from recombinant DNA. The number of required plasmids for the generation of infectious particles can be reduced from twelve to eight by using strategies that allow expression of positive sense mRNA (encoding the viral proteins) and negative sense viral RNA (encoding the viral genome) from the same plasmid [27].

3. Influenza A virus expression vectors

Using reverse genetics techniques to manipulate the genome of influenza A virus, it was possible to construct influenza virus vectors expressing foreign antigens. This was first achieved by inserting (grafting) foreign sequences into the amino acid sequence of the hemagglutinin (HA) protein of the virus [28]. Interestingly, the insertion of short amino acid sequences into antigenic site B of the HA molecule did not prevent virus viability [29]. Moreover, these chimeric influenza A viruses elicited a vigorous and long-lasting antibody response against their inserted epitopes at the systemic and mucosal levels when they were intranasally administered into mice [30–32]. The insertion of epitopes recognized by MHC class I molecules into recombinant influenza viruses expressing chimeric proteins resulted in virus vectors inducing high levels of CTL responses against their expressed epitopes in mice [29,33,34]. Strikingly, prime-boosting strategies based on the sequential administration of a recombinant influenza virus followed a few weeks later by a recombinant vaccinia virus expressing the same MHC class I-restricted epitope increased even further the number of CD8$^+$ T cells elicited against the shared epitope [33,35–37]. These results suggest that influenza A virus expressing TAAs might induce high levels of CTLs against tumor cells specially when used in combined prime-boosting strategies with heterologous vectors.

Expression of foreign antigens by influenza virus vectors is not only restricted to the generation of recombinant viruses expressing chimeric proteins. It was possible to engineer recombinant influenza viruses expressing bicistronic genes encoding foreign polypeptides by inserting an internal ribosomal entry site into an influenza virus RNA segment [38]. It was also possible to construct influenza virus vectors encoding polyproteins which contained a proteolytic signal responsible for the generation of an extra (foreign) polypeptide in cells infected with these vectors [39]. Finally, recombinant influenza viruses with an additional RNA segment encoding a novel polypeptide have also been constructed [40]. If desired, the foreign polypeptide can be incorporated into the virus envelope by including a transmembrane and cytoplasmic domain derived from the HA protein of influenza virus [38,40].

4. Influenza A virus vectors as tumor vaccines

We are investigating the potential use of influenza virus vectors expressing selected TAAs as therapeutic agents in anti-cancer strategies. For this purpose, we have first characterized the anti-tumor properties in mice of recombinant influenza viruses expressing a model TAA. The tumor model we have used is based on the malignant properties of the CT26.CL25 cell line [3]. This cell line is a derivative of the highly invasive murine tumor cell line CT26, in which the β-galactosidase (β-gal) gene has been transfected and expressed. β-Gal can then be used as a model TAA for this cell line. The growth rate and lethality of the tumor cell line is not affected by the expression of the model TAA β-gal.

We have generated three transfectant influenza viruses expressing a CD8$^+$ T-cell, H-2L^d-restricted epitope (TPHPARIGL) which is present in the amino acid sequence of β-gal [41]. The first transfectant influenza virus, MINIGAL, has been designed to express the β-gal epitope as a minicistron from a bicistronic viral neuraminidase (NA) gene. The epitope has been directed to the endoplasmic reticulum (ER) by using a leader peptide derived from the adenovirus E3/19K protein. Targeting peptides to the ER has been shown to greatly enhance the CD8$^+$ T-cell response in some cases [42]. The second transfectant influenza virus, NAGAL, encodes an NA protein which contains the β-gal epitope inserted into the stalk region of this protein. The third transfectant influenza virus (BHAGAL) has the β-gal epitope inserted into the antigenic site B of the viral hemagglutinin (HA) protein. All three recombinant influenza A viruses elicited a β-gal-specific CTL response in mice when administered i.p. or i.v. [41]. Moreover, this response mediated the regression of established CT26.CL25 metastases in mice.

Mice inoculated with CT26.CL25 cells were followed for survival rates after treatment with the recombinant β-gal influenza viruses [43]. Animals with a high tumor burden showed extended survival times when treated with a recombinant β-gal influenza virus, but they finally succumbed to death. Death was associated with the presence of a small number of large tumors in lungs. Interestingly, these tumors were found to express undetectable levels of the TAA due to a down-regulation in the TAA-specific mRNA levels. On the other hand, mice with five times lower tumor burden showed complete tumor regression and survival for more than 6 months when treated with the recombinant virus. These animals were still protected against a tumor challenge 6 months after treatment. Our results suggest that recombinant influenza viruses might be good therapeutic agents for the prevention and treatment of cancers with known TAAs.

5. Discussion

The search for viral vector candidates to be used in cancer therapy is still ongoing. One reason for this is that there is no good evidence that would allow us to predict which vector would be the best for inducing a strong cellular immune response in humans against the tumor cells, while being a safe delivery agent. In addition, the presence of pre-existing immunity in tumor patients against some of the considered vectors could prevent the efficient induction of the desired antitumor response. Furthermore, the availability of different vectors makes it possible to design novel boosting protocols that could result in more potent immune responses.

Influenza A viruses are very strong inducers of cellular immune responses. In addition, influenza A viruses are non-integrating, non-oncogenic viruses. There are also non-transmissible attenuated strains of influenza viruses available that could be used in humans [44]. Moreover, the insertion of attenuating mutations into transfectant influenza viruses by reverse genetics techniques is also possible [45–47]. Finally, since influenza viruses change their antigenic determinants very quickly, one could also choose among different viral strains to avoid the presence of pre-existing immunity against the virus in patients. In this respect, we found that recombinant influenza A viruses expressing a model TAA were still efficacious in mediating tumor regression in mice with pre-existing immunity against a different subtype of influenza [41]. Nevertheless, further experimentation is required to assess the efficacy of attenuated recombinant influenza viruses expressing human TAAs in the treatment of human cancer.

Acknowledgements

This work has been funded in part by National Institutes of Health Grant CA77432 to A.G.-S.

References

[1] N.P. Restifo, The new vaccines: building viruses that elicit antitumor immunity, Curr. Opin. Immunol. 8 (1996) 658–663.

[2] J.W. Hodge, J. Schlom, S.J. Donohue, J.E. Tomaszewski, C.W. Wheeler, B.S. Levine, L. Gritz, D. Panicali, J.A. Kantor, A recombinant vaccinia virus expressing human prostate-specific antigen (PSA): safety and immunogenicity in a non-human primate, Int. J. Cancer. 63 (1995) 231–237.

[3] M. Wang, V. Bronte, P.W. Chen, L. Gritz, D. Panicali, S.A. Rosenberg, N.P. Restifo, Active immunotherapy of cancer with a nonreplicating recombinant fowlpox virus encoding a model tumor-associated antigen, J. Immunol. 154 (1995) 4685–4692.

[4] M.Z. Zhu, J. Marshall, D. Cole, J. Schlom, K.Y. Tsang, Specific cytolytic T-cell responses to human CEA from patients immunized with recombinant avipox-CEA vaccine, Clin. Cancer. Res. 6 (2000) 24–33.

[5] H.M. Karpoff, D. Kooby, M. D'Angelica, J. Mack, D.H. Presky, M.D. Brownlee, H. Federoff, Y. Fong, Efficient cotransduction of tumors by multiple herpes simplex vectors: implications for tumor vaccine production, Cancer Gene. Ther. 7 (2000) 581–588.

[6] P.W. Chen, M. Wang, V. Bronte, Y. Zhai, S.A. Rosenberg, N.P. Restifo, Therapeutic antitumor response after immunization with a recombinant adenovirus encoding a model tumor-associated antigen, J. Immunol. 156 (1996) 224–231.

[7] R.E. Toes, R.C. Hoeben, E.I. van der Voort, M.E. Ressing, A.J. van der Eb, C.J. Melief, R. Offringa, Protective anti-tumor immunity induced by vaccination with recombinant adenoviruses encoding multiple tumor-associated cytotoxic T lymphocyte epitopes in a string-of-beads fashion, Proc. Natl. Acad. Sci. U. S. A. 94 (1997) 14660–14665.

[8] S.A. Rosenberg, Y. Zhai, J.C. Yang, D.J. Schwartzentruber, P. Hwu, F.M. Marincola, S.L. Topalian, N.P. Restifo, C.A. Seipp, J.H. Einhorn, B. Roberts, D.E. White, Immunizing patients with metastatic melanoma using recombinant adenoviruses encoding MART-1 or gp100 melanoma antigens, J. Natl. Cancer. Inst. 90 (1998) 1894–1900.

[9] D.W. Liu, Y.P. Tsao, J.T. Kung, Y.A. Ding, H.K. Sytwu, X. Xiao, S.L. Chen, Recombinant adeno-associated virus expressing human papillomavirus type 16 E7 peptide DNA fused with heat shock protein DNA as a potential vaccine for cervical cancer, J. Virol. 74 (2000) 2888–2894.

[10] D.C. Ansardi, Z. Moldoveanu, D.C. Porter, D.E. Walker, R.M. Conry, A.F. LoBuglio, S. McPherson, C.D. Morrow, Characterization of poliovirus replicons encoding carcinoembryonic antigen, Cancer Res. 54 (1994) 6359–6364.

[11] P. Colmenero, P. Liljestrom, M. Jondal, Induction of P815 tumor immunity by recombinant Semliki Forest virus expressing the P1A gene, Gene. Ther. 6 (1999) 1728–1733.

[12] E. Medina, C.A. Guzman, L.H. Staendner, M.P. Colombo, P. Paglia, Salmonella vaccine carrier strains: effective delivery system to trigger anti-tumor immunity by oral route, Eur. J. Immunol. 29 (1999) 693–699.

[13] R. Xiang, H.N. Lode, T.H. Chao, J.M. Ruehlmann, C.S. Dolman, F. Rodriguez, J.L. Whitton, W.W. Overwijk, N.P. Restifo, R.A. Reisfeld, An autologous oral DNA vaccine protects against murine melanoma, Proc. Natl. Acad. Sci. U. S. A. 97 (2000) 5492–5497.

[14] R.M. Conry, A.F. LoBuglio, D.T. Curiel, Polynucleotide-mediated immunization therapy of cancer, Semin. Oncol. 23 (1996) 135–147.

[15] H. Ying, T.Z. Zaks, R.F. Wang, K.R. Irvine, U.S. Kammula, F.M. Marincola, W.W. Leitner, N.P. Restifo, Cancer therapy using a self-replicating RNA vaccine, Nat. Med. 5 (1999) 823–827.

[16] W.W. Leitner, H. Ying, D.A. Driver, T.W. Dubensky, N.P. Restifo, Enhancement of tumor-specific immune response with plasmid DNA replicon vectors, Cancer. Res. 60 (2000) 51–55.

[17] S.K. Nair, D. Boczkowski, M. Morse, R.I. Cumming, H.K. Lyerly, E. Gilboa, Induction of primary carcinoembryonic antigen (CEA)-specific cytotoxic T lymphocytes in vitro using human dendritic cells transfected with RNA, Nat. Biotechnol. 16 (1998) 364–369.

[18] M.L. De Bruijn, D.H. Schuurhuis, M.P. Vierboom, H. Vermeulen, K.A. de Cock, M.E. Ooms, M.E. Ressing, M. Toebes, K.L. Franken, J.W. Drijfhout, T.H. Ottenhoff, R. Offringa, C.J. Melief, Immunization with human papillomavirus type 16 (HPV16) oncoprotein-loaded dendritic cells as well as protein in adjuvant induces MHC class I-restricted protection to HPV16-induced tumor cells, Cancer. Res. 58 (1998) 724–731.

[19] R.C. Fields, K. Shimizu, J.J. Mule, Murine dendritic cells pulsed with whole tumor lysates mediate potent antitumor immune responses in vitro and in vivo, Proc. Natl. Acad. Sci. U. S. A. 95 (1998) 9482–9487.

[20] P.A. Lodge, L.A. Jones, R.A. Bader, G.P. Murphy, M.L. Salgaller, Dendritic cell-based immunotherapy of prostate cancer: immune monitoring of a phase II clinical trial, Cancer. Res. 60 (2000) 829–833.

[21] S.K. Nair, A. Heiser, D. Boczkowski, A. Majumdar, M. Naoe, J.S. Lebkowski, J. Vieweg, E. Gilboa, Induction of cytotoxic T cell responses and tumor immunity against unrelated tumors using telomerase reverse transcriptase RNA transfected dendritic cells, Nat. Med. 6 (2000) 1011–1017.

[22] M. Enami, W. Luytjes, M. Krystal, P. Palese, Introduction of site-specific mutations into the genome of influenza virus, Proc. Natl. Acad. Sci. U. S. A. 87 (1990) 3802–3805.

[23] A. García-Sastre, Negative-strand RNA viruses: applications to biotechnology, TIBTECH 16 (1998) 230–235.

[24] S. Pleschka, R. Jaskunas, O.G. Engelhardt, T. Zürcher, P. Palese, A. García-Sastre, A plasmid-based reverse genetics system for influenza A virus, J. Virol. 70 (1996) 4188–4192.

[25] G. Neumann, T. Watanabe, H. Ito, S. Watanabe, H. Goto, P. Gao, M. Hughes, D.R. Perez, R. Donis, E. Hoffmann, G. Hobom, Y. Kawaoka, Generation of influenza A viruses entirely from cloned cDNAs, Proc. Natl. Acad. Sci. U. S. A. 96 (1999) 9345–9350.

[26] E. Fodor, L. Devenish, O.G. Engelhardt, P. Palese, G.G. Brownlee, A. García-Sastre, Rescue of influenza A virus from recombinant DNA, J. Virol. 73 (1999) 9679–9682.

[27] E. Hoffmann, G. Neumann, Y. Kawaoka, G. Hobom, R.G. Webster, A DNA transfection system for generation of influenza A virus from eight plasmids, Proc. Natl. Acad. Sci. U. S. A. 97 (2000) 6108–6113.

[28] S.Q. Li, J.L. Schulman, T. Moran, C. Bona, P. Palese, Influenza A virus transfectants with chimeric hemagglutinins containing epitopes from different subtypes, J. Virol. 66 (1992) 399–404.

[29] S. Li, V. Polonis, H. Isobe, H. Zaghouani, R. Guinea, T. Moran, C. Bona, P. Palese, Chimeric influenza virus induces neutralizing antibodies and cytotoxic T cells against human immunodeficiency virus type 1, J. Virol. 67 (1994) 6659–6666.

[30] T. Muster, R. Guinea, A. Trkola, M. Purtscher, A. Klima, F. Steindl, P. Palese, H. Katinger, Cross-neutralizing activity against divergent human immunodeficiency virus type 1 isolates induced by the gp41 sequence ELDKWAS, J. Virol. 68 (1994) 4031–4034.

[31] T. Muster, B. Ferko, A. Klima, M. Purtscher, A. Trkola, P. Schulz, A. Grassauer, O.G. Engelhardt, A. García-Sastre, P. Palese, H. Katinger, Mucosal model of immunization against human immunodeficiency virus type 1 with a chimeric influenza virus, J. Virol. 69 (1995) 6678–6686.

[32] J. Staczek, H.E. Gilleland Jr., L.B. Gilleland, R.N. Harty, A. García-Sastre, O.G. Engelhardt, P. Palese, A chimeric influenza virus expressing an epitope of outer membrane protein F of *Pseudomonas aeruginosa* affords protection against challenge with *P. aeruginosa* in a murine model of chronic pulmonary infection, Infect. Immun. 66 (1998) 3990–3994.

[33] S. Li, M. Rodrigues, D. Rodriguez, J.R. Rodriguez, M. Esteban, P. Palese, R.S. Nussenzweig, F. Zavala, Priming with recombinant influenza virus followed by administration of recombinant vaccinia virus induces

CD8$^+$ T-cell-mediated protective immunity against malaria, Proc. Natl. Acad. Sci. U. S. A. 90 (1993) 5214–5218.

[34] M.R. Castrucci, S. Hou, P.C. Doherty, Y. Kawaoka, Protection against lethal lymphocytic choriomeningitis virus (LCMV) infection by immunization of mice with an influenza virus containing an LCMV epitope recognized by cytotoxic T lymphocytes, J. Virol. 68 (1994) 3486–3490.

[35] K. Murata, A. García-Sastre, M. Tsuji, M. Rodrigues, D. Rodriguez, J.R. Rodriguez, R.S. Nussenzweig, P. Palese, M. Esteban, F. Zavala, Characterization of in vivo primary and secondary CD8$^+$ T cell responses induced by recombinant influenza and vaccinia viruses, Cell. Immunol. 173 (1996) 96–107.

[36] Y. Miyahira, A. García-Sastre, D. Rodriguez, J.R. Rodriguez, K. Murata, M. Tsuji, P. Palese, M. Esteban, F. Zavala, R.S. Nussenzweig, Recombinant viruses expressing a human malaria antigen can elicit potentially protective immune CD8$^+$ responses in mice, Proc. Natl. Acad. Sci. U. S. A. 31 (1998) 3954–3959.

[37] R.M. Gonzalo, D. Rodriguez, A. García-Sastre, J.R. Rodriguez, P. Palese, M. Esteban, Enhanced CD8$^+$ T cell response to HIV-1 env by combined immunization with influenza and vaccinia virus recombinants, Vaccine 17 (1999) 887–892.

[38] A. García-Sastre, T. Muster, W.S. Barclay, N. Percy, P. Palese, Use of a mammalian internal ribosomal entry site element for expression of a foreign protein by a transfectant influenza virus, J. Virol. 68 (1994) 6254–6261.

[39] N. Percy, W.S. Barclay, A. García-Sastre, P. Palese, Expression of a foreign protein by influenza A virus, J. Virol. 68 (1994) 4486–4492.

[40] Y. Zhou, M. Konig, G. Hobom, E. Neumeier, Membrane-anchored incorporation of a foreign protein in recombinant influenza virions, Virology 246 (1998) 83–94.

[41] N.P. Restifo, D.R. Surman, H. Zheng, P. Palese, S.A. Rosenberg, A. García-Sastre, Transfectant influenza A viruses are effective recombinant immunogens in the treatment of experimental cancer, Virology 249 (1998) 89–97.

[42] N.P. Restifo, I. Bacik, K.R. Irvine, J.W. Yewdell, B.J. McCabe, R.W. Anderson, L.C. Eisenlohr, S.A. Rosenberg, J.R. Bennink, Antigen processing in vivo and the elicitation of primary CTL responses, J. Immunol. 154 (1995) 4414–4422.

[43] H. Zheng, P. Palese, A. García-Sastre, Antitumor properties of influenza virus vectors. Cancer Res. (in press).

[44] H.F. Maassab, J.R. LaMontagne, D.C. DeBorde, Live influenza virus vaccines, in: S.A. Plotkin, E.A. Mortimer (Eds.), Vaccines, Saunders, Philadelphia, 1998, pp. 435–457.

[45] T. Muster, E.K. Subbarao, M. Enami, B.R. Murphy, P. Palese, An influenza A virus containing influenza B virus 5′ and 3′ noncoding regions on the neuraminidase gene is attenuated in mice, Proc. Natl. Acad. Sci. U. S. A. 88 (1991) 5177–5181.

[46] A. Solorzano, H. Zheng, E. Fodor, G.G. Brownlee, P. Palese, A. García-Sastre, Reduced levels of neuraminidase of influenza A viruses correlate with attenuated phenotypes in mice, J. Gen. Virol. 81 (2000) 737–742.

[47] J. Talon, M. Salvatore, R.E. O'Neill, Y. Nakaya, H. Zheng, T. Muster, A. García-Sastre, P. Palese, Influenza A and B viruses expressing altered NS1 proteins: a vaccine approach, Proc. Natl. Acad. Sci. U. S. A. 97 (2000) 4309–4314.

Index of authors

Keyword index